M000047956

LE	lupus erythematos		
LH	luteinizing hormo		
LLQ	left lower quadrar		
LMP	last menstrual per		
LOC	level of conscious		
LR	lactated Ringer's		
LUQ	left upper quadrar		

Abbr.	Definition	Abbr.	Definition
M	meter	q12h	every 12 hours
m	minim	r	right
m²	square meter	RAIU	radioactive iodine uptake
MAOI	monoamine oxidase inhibitor	RBC(s)	red blood count or cell(s)
mEq	milliequivalent	RLQ	right lower quadrant
mg	milligram	ROM	range of motion
μg	microgram	RUQ	right upper quadrant
MI	myocardial infarction	SC	subcutaneous
min	minute	SIMV	synchronous intermittent mandatory ventilation
ml	milliliter	SL	sublingual
mm	millimeter	SLE	systemic lupus erythematosus
mo	month	SOB	short of breath
Na	sodium	sol	solution
neg	negative	ss	one half
NPO	nothing by mouth (Lat. *nulla per os*)	supp	suppository
NS	normal saline	Sus rel	sustained release
O₂	oxygen	syr	syrup
OBS	organic brain syndrome	T&A	tonsillectomy and adenoidectomy
OD	right eye	tab	tablet
OR	operating room	tbsp	tablespoon
OS	left eye	temp	temperature
os	mouth	tid	three times daily
OTC	over the counter	tinc	tincture
OU	each eye	TPN	total parenteral nutrition
oz	ounce	top	topical
p̄	after	TRANS	transdermal
P56	plasma-lyte 56	TSH	thyroid-stimulating hormone
Paco₂	arterial carbon dioxide tension (pressure)	tsp	teaspoon
Pao₂	arterial oxygen tension (pressure)	TT	thrombin time
PBI	protein-bound iodine	U	unit
PAT	paroxysmal atrial tachycardia	UA	urinalysis
PCWP	pulmonary capillary wedge pressure	UTI	urinary tract infection
PEEP	positive end expiratory pressure	UV	ultraviolet
PERRLA	pupils equal, round, react to light and accommodation	vag	vaginal
pH	hydrogen ion concentration	VMA	vanillylmandelic acid
PO	by mouth	vol	volume
postop	postoperatively	VS	vital signs
PP	postprandial	WBC	white blood count
preop	preoperatively	wk	week
prn	as needed	wt	weight
pro-time, PT	prothrombin time	yr	year
PTT	partial thromboplastin time	>	greater than
PVC	premature ventricular contraction	<	less than
q	every	=	equal
qAM	every morning	°	degree
qd	every day	%	percent
qh	every hour	γ	gamma
qid	four times a day	β	beta

Relevant subscripts rendered: O_2, $Paco_2$, Pao_2, m^2.

Rebecca
Cordeiro

Mosby's

1995

Nursing
Drug
Reference

Linda Skidmore-Roth, R.N., M.S.N., N.P.

Formerly, New Mexico State University,
Nursing Faculty, Las Cruces, New Mexico;
El Paso Community College, El Paso, Texas

 Mosby

St. Louis Baltimore Berlin Boston Carlsbad Chicago London Madrid

Naples New York Philadelphia Sydney Tokyo Toronto

Mosby

Dedicated to Publishing Excellence

Publisher: Alison Miller
Editor-in-Chief: Nancy Coon
Editor: Robin Carter
Developmental editor: Gina Gay Wright
Project manager: Carol Sullivan Wiseman
Designer: Betty Schulz
Manufacturing supervisor: Betty Richmond
Cover design: Rokusek Design

A NOTE TO THE READER

The authors and publisher have made every attempt to check dosages and nursing content for accuracy. Because the science of pharmacology is continually advancing, our knowledge base continues to expand. Therefore we recommend that the reader always check product information for changes in dosage or administration before administering any medication. This is particularly important with new or rarely used drugs.

Copyright © 1995 by Mosby–Year Book, Inc.

All rights reserved. No part of this publication may be reproduced, stored in a retrieval system, or transmitted, in any form or by any means, electronic, mechanical, photocopying, recording, or otherwise, without prior written permission from the publisher.

Permission to photocopy or reproduce solely for internal or personal use is permitted for libraries or other users registered with the Copyright Clearance Center, provided that the base fee of $4.00 per chapter plus $.10 per page is paid directly to the Copyright Clearance Center, 27 Congress Street, Salem, MA 01970. This consent does not extend to other kinds of copying, such as copying for general distribution, for advertising or promotional purposes, for creating new collected works, or for resale.

Printed in the United States of America.
Composition by Graphic World, Inc.
Printing/binding by R.R. Donnelley

Mosby–Year Book, Inc.
11830 Westline Industrial Drive
St. Louis, Missouri 63146

ISSN 1044-8470
ISBN 0-8016-6742-9

95 96 97 98 99 / 9 8 7 6 5 4 3 2 1

Clinical nursing consultants

Marie B. Andrews, R.N., Ph.D.
Lecturer, Texas Woman's
University, Houston, Texas

Phyllis Baker, R.N., M.S.N.
Assistant Professor, Saint Xavier
University, Chicago, Illinois

Janet T. Barrett, R.N., Ph.D.
Director, BSN Program, Deaconess
College of Nursing, St. Louis,
Missouri

Jean Krajicek Bartek, Ph.D., R.N.,
C.A.R.N.
Assistant Professor, University of
Nebraska Medical Center, Colleges
of Nursing and Medicine, Omaha,
Nebraska

Alice Bledig, R.N., Ph.D.
Professor, Southeastern Illinois
Community College, Harrisburg,
Illinois

Donnie F. Booth, R.N., Ph.D.
Director, School of Nursing,
Southeastern Louisiana University,
Hammond, Louisiana

Ruth Bowen, R.N., M.S.
Lecturer, Texas Woman's
University, Denton, Texas

Sheri L. Bremer, R.N., M.S.N.
Professor of Nursing, Community
College of Denver, Denver,
Colorado

Barbara A. Brunow, R.N., M.S.N.
Instructor, Providence Hospital
School of Nursing, Sandusky, Ohio

Margaret A. Burns, R.N., D.N.Sc.
Associate Professor, Loma Linda
University School of Nursing,
Loma Linda, California

Connie L. Bush, R.N., M.S.
Associate Professor, Nursing,
Niagara County Community
College, Sanborn, New York

Judith Chapin Buzby, R.N., M.S.N.
Associate Professor, Niagara
County Community College,
Sanborn, New York

June Chandler, R.N., Ed.D.
Instructor, Florida Community
College, Jacksonville, Florida

Rosemary Chappell, R.N., M.S.
Coordinator, Undergraduate
Curriculum, South Dakota State
University, College of Nursing,
Brookings, South Dakota

Mary Lou Cheatham, R.N., M.S.N.
Associate Professor, Ball State
University, Muncie, Indiana

Leah M. Cleveland, R.N., Ed.D.
Professor, Saddleback College,
Mission Viejo, California

Julia Korontjis Dattolo, B.S.N.,
R.N., M.S.N.
Clinical Nurse Specialist, Surgery
and Burns, University of California
San Diego Medical Center, San
Diego, California

Judy E. Davidson, R.N., M.S., C.C.R.N.
Clinical Nurse Specialist, University
of California San Diego Medical
Center, San Diego, California

Susan Donckers, R.N., Ed.D.
Consultant, Formerly Associate
Professor, Radford University,
Radford, Virginia

Jane G. Doyle, R.N., M.S., M.B.A.
Instructor, Nursing, Mount
Wachusett Community College,
Gardner, Massachusetts

Sister M. Ellene Egan, R.N., Ed.D.
Assistant Professor, University of
San Francisco, San Francisco,
California

Laurel A. Eisenhauer, R.N., Ph.D.
Professor of Nursing, Boston
College, Chestnut Hill,
Massachusetts

Anne Marie Frey, R.N., B.S.N., C.R.N.I.
I.V. Nurse Clinician, St. Christopher's
Hospital for Children, Philadelphia,
Pennsylvania

Mary B. Gardner, R.N., M.S.
Nursing Faculty, Assumption
College, Worcester, Massachusetts

Barbara H. Goodkin, R.N., M.S.
Instructor, Washtenaw Community
College, Ann Arbor, Michigan

Brenda Goodner, R.N., M.S.N., C.S.
Assistant Professor, Abilene
Intercollegiate School of Nursing,
Abilene, Texas

Patricia Graham, R.N., M.S., C.C.R.N.
Clinical Nurse Specialist SICU,
University of California San Diego
Medical Center, San Diego,
California

Jyneal Linton Greer, R.N., M.S.N.
Instructor, Nursing, Normandale
Community College, Bloomington,
Minnesota

Kathy Gutierrez, R.N., M.S.N.
Assistant Professor, Regis
University, Denver, Colorado

Milly Gutkoski, R.N.C., M.N.
Assistant Professor, Montana State
University, Bozeman, Montana

Mark Hamelink, R.N., M.S.N., C.R.N.A.
Lakeshore Anesthesia, P.C., South
Haven, Michigan

Jane Hartsock, R.N., M.A.
Instructor, Nursing, Minneapolis
Community College, Minneapolis,
Minnesota

Marcia Jo Hill, R.N., M.S.N.
Manager, Nursing, The Methodist
Hospital; Assistant Clinical
Professor, Dermatology, Baylor
College of Medicine, Houston,
Texas

Judith Ann Holton, R.N., M.S.N., C.C.R.N.
Professor of Science in Nursing,
Los Angeles Valley College, Van
Nuys, California

Patricia Hong, R.N., M.A.
Instructor, Anchorage Community
College, Anchorage, Alaska

Barbara D. Horton, R.N., M.S.
Nurse Educator, Arnot-Ogden
Medical Center, School of Nursing,
Elmira, New York

Linda A. Howe, R.N., M.S., M.A.E.
Director, Roper Hospital School of
Nursing, Charleston, South Carolina

Ann Hoye, R.N., M.S.N., O.C.N.
Oncology Clinical Nurse Specialist,
University of California San Diego
Medical Center, San Diego,
California

Joan M. Jenks, R.N., M.S.N.
Assistant Professor, Thomas
Jefferson University,
Philadelphia, Pennsylvania

Barbara Johnston, R.N., M.S.
Assistant Professor, Molloy
College, Rockville Centre, New
York

Mary F. Johnston, R.N., M.S.N.
Coordinator of Nursing, Front
Range Community College,
Westminster, Colorado

Sandra Jones, R.N., M.A.
Assistant Professor, John Tyler
Community College, Chester,
Virginia

Natalie G. Ledbetter, R.N., M.S.N.,
C.C.R.N.
Nursing Instructor, Galveston
College, Galveston, Texas

Linda L. Lilley, R.N., M.S.
Assistant Professor, Old Dominion
University, Norfolk, Virginia

Adrianne Dill Linton, R.N., C., Ph.D.
Assistant Professor, The University
of Texas Health Science Center at
San Antonio School of Nursing,
San Antonio, Texas

Sandra N. Long, B.S.N., R.N.
Associate Instructor, Harding
University, School of Nursing,
Searcy, Arkansas

Carolyn W. Lyon, R.N., M.S.N.
Director, Roanoke Memorial
Hospitals School of Practical
Nursing, Roanoke, Virginia

Edwina McConnell, R.N., Ph.D.
Independent Nurse Consultant,
Madison, Wisconsin; Professor,
Texas Tech University Health
Sciences Center School of Nursing,
Lubbock, Texas

Bernadette Maucher McKay,
R.N.C., M.S.
Nurse Practitioner and Assistant
Professor, School of Nursing, The
University of Texas, Galveston,
Texas

Cheryl Macejkovik, R.N., M.S.
Adult Health Instructor, University
of North Dakota, Grand Forks,
North Dakota

Suzanne E. Malloy, R.N., M.S.N.
Assistant Professor, San Jose State
University, San Jose, California

Marylou Medlin, R.N., B.S.N., M.N.
Instructor, Charity Hospital School
of Nursing, New Orleans, Louisiana

Mary Mirch, R.N., M.S.
Associate Professor, Glendale
Community College, Glendale,
California

Michaelene P. Mirr, R.N., Ph.D.,
C.C.R.N.
Assistant Professor, School of
Nursing, University of Wisconsin-
Eau Claire, Eau Claire, Wisconsin

Shirley Moore, R.N., M.S.N., M.S.
Faculty, Barnes College, St. Louis,
Missouri

M. Joan Owen, R.N., M.A.
Instructor, Mesa College,
Mesa, Arizona

Judy A. Peterson, R.N., M.S.N., C.S.
Associate Professor, University of
Alaska, Anchorage, Alaska

Elaine E. Phifer, R.N., M.N.
Professor of Nursing, Los Angeles
Pierce College, Woodland,
California

Celeste Phillips, R.N., Ed.D.
Principal, Phillips & Fenwick,
Scotts Valley, California

Rosemary A. Pine, R.N., M.S.N.
Assistant Professor of Nursing,
Department Chair ADN Program,
Houston Baptist University,
Houston, Texas

Michele Poradzisz, R.N., M.S.
Instructor, De Paul University,
Chicago, Illinois

Carolyn Smith Powell, A.D.N.,
B.S.N., M.S.N.
Assistant Professor of Nursing,
Abraham Baldwin College, Tifton,
Georgia

Joyce Powers, R.N., M.S.N., C.S.
Clinical Nurse Specialist,
Cardiology Consultants,
Albuquerque, New Mexico

Camille Rabitoy, R.N., M.A.Ed.
Nursing Educator, Bay de Noc
Community College,
Escanaba, Michigan

Tracy Riley, R.N., B.S.N.
Instructor, Aultman Hospital School
of Nursing, Canton, Ohio

Janet S. Rose, R.N., B.S.N.
Project Manager, Vitas Healthcare
Corporation, Miami, Florida

Carol Ruscin, R.N., B.S.
Level I Faculty, Baptist Medical
System School of Nursing, Little
Rock, Arkansas

Robert E. St. John, R.N., R.R.T.,
B.S.N., B.A.
Cardiopulmonary Nurse Clinician,
Jewish Hospital, St. Louis,
Missouri

Joanne Santangelo, R.N., M.S.N.,
C.F.N.P.
Clinical Nurse Practitioner,
University of California San Diego
Student Health Services, La Jolla,
California

Jean Schneewind, R.N., M.S.N.
Assistant Professor, Imperial Valley
College, Imperial, California

Brenda K. Shelton, R.N., B.S.,
C.C.R.N., O.C.N.
Critical Care Instructor, The Johns
Hopkins Oncology Center,
Baltimore, Maryland

Debora Signoracci, B.S.N., R.N.C.
Practical Nursing Instructor,
Northland Career Center, Platte
City, Missouri

Janet D. Smith, R.N., M.S.N.
Professor, Quinsigamond
Community College, Worcester,
Massachusetts

Cynthia Mills Spiro, R.N., M.S.N.
Faculty, Barnes College, St. Louis,
Missouri

Carol A. Stephenson, R.N., Ed.D.
Associate Professor, Texas Christian
University, Fort Worth, Texas

Ruth Stieglitz-Hooley, R.N., Ph.D.
Associate Professor, University of
Wyoming, Laramie, Wyoming

Regina Stroud, R.N., M.S.
Instructor, Rancho Santiago
College, Santa Ana, California

Janice A. Traylor, R.N., M.Ed., M.S.
Nurse Educator, Casper College,
Casper, Wyoming

Carole Jean Petrosky Vozel,
R.N., C., Ph.D.
Instructor, Western Pennsylvania
Hospital, School of Nursing,
Pittsburgh, Pennsylvania

Richard E. Watters, R.N., M.Ed.
Nursing Consultant, Wembley,
Western Australia

Pamela Becker Weilitz, R.N., M.S.N. (R)
Clinical Nurse Specialist, Barnes Hospital at Washington University Medical Center, St. Louis, Missouri

Kathleen Whalen, R.N., M.S.N.
Instructor, Community College of Denver, Arvada, Colorado

Judith M. Wilkinson, R.N.C., M.A., M.S.N.
Instructor, Johnson County Community College, Overland Park, Kansas

Anita Lee Wynne, R.N., Ph.D.
Associate Professor of Nursing, University of Portland, Portland Oregon

Rita Yaeger, R.N., M.S.N., M.A.
Associate Professor of Nursing, West Virginia Northern Community College, Wheeling, West Virginia

Clinical pharmacology consultants

Carmen Aceves-Blumenthal, M.S., R.Ph.
Assistant Professor, Southeastern College of Pharmaceutical Sciences, North Miami Beach, Florida

Richard H. Alper, Ph.D.
Assistant Professor, The University of Kansas Medical Center, Kansas City, Kansas

Danial E. Baker, Pharm.D., F.A.S.C.P., F.A.S.H.P.
Director, Drug Information Center, College of Pharmacy, Washington State University at Spokane, Spokane, Washington

Lance K. Campbell, Pharm.D.
Clinical Pharmacy Resident, Group Health Cooperative of Puget Sound, Seattle, Washington

R. Keith Campbell, F.A.S.H.P., R.Ph.
Associate Dean and Professor of Pharmacy, Certified Diabetes Educator, Washington State University College of Pharmacy, Pullman, Washington

Catherine Celestin, Pharm.D.
Assistant Professor, Southeastern College of Pharmaceutical Sciences, North Miami Beach, Florida

Bruce D. Clayton, Pharm.D.
Professor, University of Arkansas, Little Rock, Arkansas

Edward H. Clouse, Ph.D.
Associate Professor, Southeastern College of Pharmaceutical Sciences, North Miami Beach, Florida

Jackson Como, Pharm.D.
Director, Drug Information, University of Alabama Hospital, Birmingham, Alabama

David E. Domann, M.S., F.A.S.C.P.
Professional Services Manager,
E.R. Squibb and Sons,
Princeton, New Jersey

Mark W. Garrison, Pharm.D.
Assistant Professor of Pharmacy,
Washington State University at
Spokane, College of Pharmacy,
Spokane, Washington

William Gerthoffer, Ph.D.
Associate Professor, University of
Nevada School of Medicine,
Reno, Nevada

Kevin Patrick Haley, Ph.D.
Associate Professor of Biology,
College of St. Mary, Omaha,
Nebraska

Patricia A. Howard, B.S., R.Ph.
Clinical Instructor, University of
Kansas Medical Center,
Kansas City, Kansas

Norman L. Keltner, R.N., Ed.D.
Associate Professor, Graduate
Program, University of Alabama
School of Nursing, University of
Alabama at Birmingham,
Birmingham, Alabama

James Lipp, Ph.D.
Associate Professor, Grand Valley
State University,
Allendale, Michigan

Lori A. Mangels, B.S.
Pharmacologist, The University of
Michigan Medical School,
Ann Arbor, Michigan

Judith K. Marquis, Ph.D.
Assistant Professor, Boston
University School of Medicine,
Boston, Massachusetts

Lori A. Martell, Ph.D.
Research Investigator, The
University of Michigan; Lecturer,
Eastern Michigan University, Ann
Arbor, Michigan

Bozena B. Michniak, Ph.D., M.P.S.
Assistant Professor, University of
South Carolina,
Columbia, South Carolina

Keith M. Olsen, Pharm.D.
Assistant Professor, University of
Arkansas, Little Rock, Arkansas

Rosemarie Pincus, Ph.D.
Faculty, Department of Biology,
Adelphi University, Garden City,
New York

Claire H. Raymond, Pharm.D.
Clinical Pharmacist, Critical Care
Medicine, Jewish Hospital of St.
Louis, Clinical Assistant Professor,
St. Louis College of Pharmacy, St.
Louis, Missouri

Robert T. Reilly, Pharm.D.
Assistant Director of Pharmacy,
Clinical Services, Thomason
Hospital, El Paso, Texas

Roberta J. Secrest, Ph.D., Pharm.D.,
R.Ph.
Associate Scientist, Marion Merrell
Dow Research Institute, Cincinnati,
Ohio

Kay See-Lasley, M.S.
Pharmacology Consultant,
Lawrence, Kansas

Donald J. Sefcik, D.O., R.Ph.
Adjunct Assistant Professor, Butler
University, Indianapolis, Indiana

Katherine Stefos, Ph.D., R.Ph.
Staff Development Coordinator,
Division of Pharmacy, The
University of Texas M.D. Anderson
Cancer Center, Houston, Texas

Carol Walsh, Ph.D.
Associate Professor, Boston
University School of Medicine,
Boston, Massachusetts

John R. White, Jr., Pharm.D.
Assistant Professor, Washington
State University,
Spokane, Washington

Lynn Roger Willis, Ph.D.
Professor, Indianapolis University
School of Medicine,
Indianapolis, Indiana

Canadian consultants

Linda Albert, R.N., B.N.
Instructor, Prince Edward Island
School of Nursing, Charlottetown,
Prince Edward Island

Susanne Guy Alcolado, R.N.,
B.N., M.Ed.
Assistant Director, Halifax
Infirmary Hospital School of
Nursing, Halifax, Nova Scotia

Linda M. Cameron, R.N., B.N.
Instructor, Foothills Hospital School
of Nursing, Calgary, Alberta

Margaret Chad, B.S.N.
Instructor, Diploma Nursing
Program, Saskatchewan Institute of
Applied Science and Technology,
Saskatoon, Saskatchewan

Tim Engelhardt, B.Sc., Pharm.D.
Manager, Pharmacy Services,
Calgary District Hospital Group,
Calgary, Alberta

Edythe Ann Fleming, B.Sc.N.
Professor, Fanshawe College,
London, Ontario

Jacqueline Murphy, R.N., M.Sc.
Instructor and Staff Nurse, Foothills
Hospital School of Nursing,
Calgary, Alberta

Maureen J. Osis, R.N., M.N.
Clinical Nurse Specialist,
Calgary, Alberta

Kenneth W. Renton, Ph.D.
Professor and Head, Dalhousie
University Department of
Pharmacology, Halifax, Nova Scotia

Roberta Ronayne, R.N., B.Sc.N., M.Sc.
Assistant Professor, University of
Ottawa, School of Nursing, Ottawa,
Ontario

Shiela M. Stanton, R.N., M.S.N.
Associate Professor Emerita
Nursing, University of British
Columbia, Vancouver, British
Columbia

Linda Strand, Ph.D.
Executive Director, Saskatchewan
Health, Regina, Saskatchewan

Sheila Rankin Zerr, R.N., M.Ed.
Assistant Professor, University of
Victoria, Victoria, British Columbia

Preface

Mosby's 1995 Nursing Drug Reference has been completely revised and updated with the addition of over 2500 new drug facts—including 21 new drugs recently approved by the FDA. Nursing considerations have been extensively revised to include over 800 new nursing guidelines. In addition, hundreds of newly researched side effects, adverse reactions, precautions, interactions, contraindications, and IV therapy facts have been added. To keep our readers as up-to-date as possible, Appendix J, Selected New Drugs, contains monographs for the most recently FDA-approved drugs at press time. New drugs throughout the book include beta-interferon (Betaseron), used to treat ambulatory patients with relapsing-remitting multiple sclerosis; cisapride (Propulsid), for treatment of nocturnal heartburn due to gastroesophageal reflux disease; cladribine (Leustatin), for treatment of hairy cell leukemia; and enoxaparin sodium (Lovenox), used for prevention of deep vein thrombosis. Other important new drugs include venlafaxine HCl (Effexor), a second-generation antidepressant; levomethydyle acetate HCl (Orlamm), used for management of opiate dependence; and tacrine HCl (Cognex), for treatment of mild-to-moderate dementia in Alzheimer's disease.

Although drug references abound, few are available that are truly portable and geared specifically for clinical use by the practicing nurse or student. The guiding principle of this reference remains to provide the user with a book that allows easy access to drug information and nursing considerations that specifically tell the nurse what to do in terms consistent with the nursing process. Every detail—down to the choice of paper, typeface, cover, binding, use of color, and appendixes—has been carefully chosen with the user in mind.

Over 1300 generic and 4500 trade medications, alphabetized by generic name, are included. Trade names are given for all medications commonly used in the United States and Canada. Drugs available only in Canada are identified by an asterisk. The following information is provided, whenever possible, for safe and effective administration of each drug:

Pronunciations: Pronunciations are provided to help the nursing student master the more complex generic names.

Functional and chemical classifications: All known broad functional and chemical classifications are given. These classifications allow the nurse to see similarities and dissimilarities among drugs in the same functional but different chemical classes.

Controlled-substance schedule: Schedules are included for the United States (I, II, III, IV, V) and Canada (F, G).

Action: Pharmacologic properties are described in concise terms. Action is discussed to the cellular level when known.

Uses: Provides drug application.

Dosages and routes: All available and approved dosages and routes are given for adult, pediatric, and geriatric patients.

Available forms: All available forms—including tablets, capsules, extended-release, injectables (IV, IM, SC), solutions, creams, ointments, lotions, gels, shampoos, elixirs, suspensions, suppositories, sprays, aerosols, and lozenges—are provided.

Side effects/adverse reactions: Grouped by body system, common side effects are *italicized,* and life-threatening reactions are in ***bold italic type,*** allowing the nurse to quickly identify common and life-threatening reactions.

Contraindications: Contraindications are instances in which a medication should absolutely not be given. When the FDA has assigned pregnancy safety category D or X, it appears here.

Precautions: Special precautionary steps are given here, including FDA pregnancy safety categories A, B, and C.

Pharmacokinetics: Metabolism, distribution, and elimination are provided for all dosage forms, if known.

Interactions/incompatibilities: This section includes confirmed drug, food, and smoking interactions. The reaction is listed first, followed by the drug or nutrient causing that interaction, when applicable.

Lab test interferences: When known, lab test interferences are provided.

Nursing considerations: Highlighted nursing considerations are organized to foster use of the nursing process: Assess, Administer, Perform/provide, Evaluate, and Teach patient/family. Nursing considerations are consistently grouped under these headings to help the nurse group interventions that can be used for planning nursing care.

Treatment of overdose: Drugs and treatment for overdoses are provided for appropriate drugs.

Two new appendixes, Appendix E (Home Care Medication Record) and Appendix J (Selected New Drugs), keep our readers abreast of late-breaking developments. The following appendixes are also included to further enhance the usability of this reference: weights and equivalents, formulas for drug calculations, commonly used antibiotics in adults and children, nomogram, controlled substances, FDA pregnancy categories, bibliography, and combination products. Commonly used abbreviations have been printed on the inside front cover, and drug-to-drug and drug-to-solution IV compatibility charts have been printed immediately inside the back cover for quick access.

I am indebted to the nursing and pharmacology consultants who reviewed the manuscript and galley pages and thank them for their criticism and encouragement. I would also like to thank Robin Carter and Gina Gay Wright, my editors, whose active encouragement and enthusiasm have made this book better than it might otherwise have been. I am likewise grateful to Carol Sullivan Wiseman and Graphic World, Inc. for the coordination of the production process, and Betty Schulz for her creativity and cooperative spirit. In addition, I want to extend a special note of gratitude to Don Ladig, who has supported and encouraged my efforts since the inception of this project.

Linda Skidmore-Roth

Contents

Individual drugs, 69

Appendixes

Generic and trade index, 1135

ALPHA-ADRENERGIC BLOCKERS

Action: Acts by binding to α-adrenergic receptors, causing dilation of peripheral blood vessels. Lowers peripheral resistance, resulting in decreased blood pressure.

Uses: Used for pheochromocytoma, prevention of tissue necrosis and sloughing associated with extravasation of IV vasopressors.

Side effects/adverse reactions: The most common side effects are: hypotension, tachycardia, nasal stuffiness, nausea, vomiting, and diarrhea.

Contraindications: Hypersensitive reactions may occur, and allergies should be identified before these products are given. Patients with myocardial infarction, coronary insufficiency, angina, or other evidence of coronary artery disease should not use these products.

Pharmacokinetics: Onset, peak, and duration vary among products.

Interactions/incompatibilities: Vasoconstrictive and hypertensive effects of epinephrine are antagonized by α-adrenergic blockers.

Possible nursing diagnoses:
• Altered tissue perfusion *[uses]*
• High risk for injury *[adverse reactions]*
• Sleep pattern disturbance *[adverse reactions]*

NURSING CONSIDERATIONS

Assess:
• Electrolytes: K, Na, Cl, CO_2
• Weight daily, I&O
• B/P lying, standing before starting treatment, q4h thereafter

Administer:
• Starting with low dose, gradually increasing to prevent side effects
• With food or milk for GI symptoms

Evaluate:
• Therapeutic response: decreased B/P, increased peripheral pulses
• Nausea, vomiting, diarrhea
• Skin turgor, dryness of mucous membranes for hydration status

Teach patient/family:
• To avoid alcoholic beverages
• To report dizziness, palpitations, fainting
• To change position slowly or fainting may occur
• To take drug exactly as prescribed
• To avoid all OTC products (cough, cold, allergy) unless directed by physician

Generic names:

phenoxybenzamine (p. 850)   phentolamine (p. 853)

ANESTHETICS—GENERAL/LOCAL

Action: Anesthetics (general) act on the CNS to produce tranquilization and sleep before invasive procedures. Anesthetics (local) inhibit conduction of nerve impulses from sensory nerves.

Uses: General anesthetics are used to premedicate for surgery, induction and maintenance in general anesthesia. For local anesthetics, refer to individual product listing for indications.

Side effects/adverse reactions: The most common side effects are dystonia, akathisia, flexion of arms, fine tremors, drowsiness, restlessness, and hypotension. Also common are chills, respiratory depression, and laryngospasm.

Contraindications: Persons with CVA, increased intracranial pressure, severe hypertension, cardiac decompensation should not use these products since severe adverse reactions can occur.

Precautions: Anesthetics (general) should be used with caution in the elderly, cardiovascular disease (hypotension, bradydysrhythmias), renal disease, liver disease, Parkinson's disease, children <2 yr. The precaution for anesthetics (local) is pregnancy.

Pharmacokinetics: Onset, peak, and duration vary widely among products. Most products are metabolized in the liver and excreted in urine.

Interactions/incompatibilities: MAOIs, tricyclics, phenothiazines may cause severe hypotension or hypertension when used with local anesthetics. CNS depressants will potentiate general and local anesthetics.

Possible nursing diagnoses:

General:

• High risk for injury *[adverse reactions]*
• Knowledge deficit *[teaching]*

Local:

• Pain *[uses]*
• Knowledge deficit *[teaching]*

NURSING CONSIDERATIONS

Assess:

• VS q10min during IV administration, q30min after IM dose

Administer:

• Anticholinergic preoperatively to decrease secretions
• Only with crash cart, resuscitative equipment nearby

Perform/provide:

• Quiet environment for recovery to decrease psychotic symptoms

Evaluate:

• Therapeutic response: maintenance of anesthesia, decreased pain

- Hallucinations, delusions, separation from environment
- Extrapyramidal reactions: dystonia, akathisia
- Increasing heart rate or decreasing B/P, notify physician at once

Generic names (Injectables only):

General anesthetics
droperidol (p. 415)
etomidate (p. 462)
fentanyl citrate (p. 473)
fentanyl citrate/droperidol
(p. 474)
ketamine HCl (p. 610)
methohexital sodium (p. 695)
procaine HCl (p. 899)
tetracaine HCl (p. 1006)

Local anesthetics
bupivacaine HCl (p. 193)
chloroprocaine HCl (p. 267)
etidocaine HCl (p. 459)
lidocaine HCl (p. 625)
mepivacaine HCl (p. 677)
midazolam (p. 727)
propofol (p. 911)
thiopental sodium (p. 1018)

ANTACIDS

Action: Antacids are basic compounds that neutralize gastric acidity and decrease the rate of gastric emptying. Products are divided into those containing aluminum, magnesium, calcium, or a combination of these.
Uses: Hyperacidity is decreased by antacids in conditions such as peptic ulcer disease, reflux esophagitis, gastritis, or hiatal hernia.
Side effects/adverse reactions: The most common side effect caused by aluminum-containing antacids is constipation, which may lead to fecal impaction and bowel obstruction. Diarrhea occurs often when magnesium products are given. Alkalosis may occur when systemic products are used. Constipation occurs more frequently than laxation with calcium carbonate. The release of CO_2 from carbonate-containing antacids causes belching, abdominal distention, and flatulence. Sodium bicarbonate may act as a systemic antacid and produce systemic electrolyte disturbances and alkalosis. Calcium carbonate and sodium bicarbonate may cause rebound hyperacidity and milk-alkali syndrome. Alkaluria may occur when products are used on a long-term basis, particularly in persons with abnormal renal function.
Contraindications: Sensitivity to aluminum or magnesium products may cause hypersensitive reactions. Aluminum products should not be used by persons sensitive to aluminum; magnesium products should not be used by persons sensitive to magnesium. Check for sensitivity before administering.
Precautions: Magnesium products should be given cautiously to patients

with renal insufficiency and during pregnancy and lactation. Sodium content of antacids may be significant; use with caution for patients with hypertension, CHF, or those on a low-sodium diet.

Pharmacokinetics: Duration is 20-40 min. If ingested 1 hr after meals, acidity is reduced for at least 3 hr.

Interactions/incompatibilities: Drugs whose effects may be increased by some antacids: quinidine, amphetamines, pseudoephedrine, levodopa, valproic acid, dicumarol. Drugs whose effects may be decreased by some antacids: cimetidine, corticosteroids, ranitidine, iron salts, phenothiazines, phenytoin, digoxin, tetracyclines, ketoconazole, salicylates, isoniazid.

Possible nursing diagnoses:

• Pain *[uses]*
• Constipation *[adverse reactions]*
• Diarrhea *[adverse reactions]*

NURSING CONSIDERATIONS

Assess:

• Aggravating and alleviating factors of epigastric pain or hyperacidity; identify the location, duration, and characteristics of epigastric pain
• GI symptoms, including constipation, diarrhea, abdominal pain; if severe abdominal pain with fever occurs, these drugs should not be given
• Renal symptoms, including increasing urinary pH, electrolytes

Administer:

• All products with an 8-oz glass of water to ensure absorption in the stomach
• Another antacid if constipation occurs with aluminum products

Evaluate:

• The therapeutic effectiveness of the drug; absence of epigastric pain and decreased acidity should occur

Teach patient/family:

• Not to take other drugs within 1-2 hr of antacid administration, since antacids may impair absorption of other drugs

Generic names:

aluminum carbonate gel (p. 96)
aluminum hydroxide (p. 97)
aluminum phosphate (p. 98)
bismuth subsalicylate (p. 182)
calcium carbonate (p. 206)

dihydroxyaluminum (p. 390)
magaldrate (p. 647)
magnesium carbonate (p. 648)
magnesium oxide (p. 648)
magnesium trisilicate (p. 653)
sodium bicarbonate (p. 961)

ANTIANGINALS

Action: The antianginals are divided into the nitrates, calcium channel blockers, and β-adrenergic blockers. The nitrates dilate coronary arteries causing decreased preload and dilate systemic arteries causing decreased afterload. Calcium channel blockers dilate coronary arteries, decrease SA/AV node conduction. Beta-adrenergic blockers decrease heart rate so that myocardial O_2 use is decreased. Dipyridamole selectively dilates coronary arteries to increase coronary blood flow.

Uses: Antianginals are used in chronic stable angina pectoris, unstable angina, vasospastic angina. Some (i.e., calcium channel blockers and β-blockers) may be used as dysrhythmias and in hypertension.

Side effects/adverse reactions: The most common side effects are postural hypotension, headache, flushing, dizziness, nausea, edema, and drowsiness. Also common are rash, dysrhythmias, and fatigue.

Contraindications: Persons with known hypersensitivity, increased intracranial pressure, or cerebral hemorrhage should not use some of these products.

Precautions: Antianginals should be used with caution in postural hypotension, pregnancy, lactation, children, renal disease, and hepatic injury.

Pharmacokinetics: Onset, peak, and duration vary widely among coronary products. Most products are metabolized in the liver and excreted in urine.

Interactions/incompatibilities: Please check individual monographs since interactions vary widely among products.

Possible nursing diagnoses:
• Altered tissue perfusion: cardiopulmonary [uses]
• Pain [uses]
• High risk for injury [uses]
• Knowledge deficit [teaching]
• Decreased cardiac output [adverse reactions]

NURSING CONSIDERATIONS

Assess:
• Orthostatic B/P, pulse

Perform/provide:
• Storage protected from light, moisture; placed in cool environment

Evaluate:
• Therapeutic response: decrease, prevention of anginal pain
• Pain: duration, time started, activity being performed, character
• Tolerance if taken over long period of time

• Headache, light-headedness, decreased B/P; may indicate a need for decreased dosage

Teach patient/family:

• To keep tabs in original container
• Not to use OTC products unless directed by physician
• To report bradycardia, dizziness, confusion, depression, fever
• To take pulse at home, advise when to notify physician
• To avoid alcohol, smoking, sodium intake
• To comply with weight control, dietary adjustments, modified exercise program
• To carry Medic Alert ID to identify drug that you are taking, allergies
• To make position changes slowly to prevent fainting

Generic names:

Nitrates
amyl nitrite (p. 132)
erythrityl tetranitrate (p. 433)
isosorbide dinitrate (p. 601)
isosorbide mononitrate (p. 603)
nitroglycerin (p. 774)
pentaerythritol tetranitrate
(p. 832)

Beta-adrenergic blockers
atenolol (p. 144)
dipyridamole (p. 399)
metoprolol (p. 717)

Calcium channel blockers
amlodipine (p. 114)
bepridil HCl (p. 173)
diltiazem HCl (p. 390)
nicardipine (p. 767)
nifedipine (p. 771)
verapamil HCl (p. 1087)

nadolol (p. 746)
propranolol HCl (p. 914)

ANTICHOLINERGICS

Action: Anticholinergics inhibit the muscarinic actions of acetylcholine at receptor sites in the autonomic nervous system; anticholinergics are also known as antimuscarinic drugs.

Uses: Anticholinergics are used for a variety of conditions: gastrointestinal anticholinergics are used to decrease motility (smooth muscle tone) in the GI, biliary, and urinary tracts and for their ability to decrease gastric secretions (propantheline, glycopyrrolate); decreasing involuntary movements in parkinsonism (benztropine, trihexyphenidyl); bradydysrhythmias (atropine); nausea and vomiting (scopolamine); and as cycloplegic mydriatics (atropine, hematropine, scopalamine, cyclopentolate, tropicamide).

Side effects/adverse reactions: The most common side effects are dry mouth, constipation, urinary retention, urinary hesitancy, headache, and dizziness. Also, common is paralytic ileus.

Contraindications: Persons with narrow-angle glaucoma, myasthenia gravis, or GI/GU obstruction should not use some of these products.

Precautions: Anticholinergics should be used with caution in patients who are elderly, pregnant, or lactating or in those with prostatic hypertrophy, CHF, or hypertension; use with caution in presence of high environmental temperature.

Pharmacokinetics: Onset, peak, and duration vary widely among products. Most products are metabolized in the liver and excreted in urine.

Interactions/incompatibilities: Increased anticholinergic effects may occur when used with MAOIs and tricyclic antidepressants and amantadine. Anticholinergics may cause a decreased effect of phenothiazines and levodopa.

Possible nursing diagnoses:
• Decreased cardiac output [uses]
• Constipation [adverse reactions]
• Knowledge deficit [teaching]

NURSING CONSIDERATIONS

Assess:
• I&O ratio; retention commonly causes decreased urinary output

Administer:
• Parenteral dose with patient recumbent to prevent postural hypotension
• With or after meals to prevent GI upset; may give with fluids other than water
• Parenteral dose slowly; keep in bed for at least 1 hr after dose, monitor vital signs
• After checking dose carefully, even slight overdose could lead to toxicity

Perform/provide:
• Storage at room temperature
• Hard candy, frequent drinks, sugarless gum to relieve dry mouth

Evaluate:
• Therapeutic response: decreased secretions, absence of nausea and vomiting
• Urinary hesitancy, retention; palpate bladder if retention occurs
• Constipation; increase fluids, bulk, exercise if this occurs
• For tolerance over long-term therapy, dose may need to be increased or changed
• Mental status: affect, mood, CNS depression, worsening of mental symptoms during early therapy

Teach patient/family:
• To avoid driving or other hazardous activities; drowsiness may occur
• To avoid OTC medication: cough, cold preparations with alcohol, antihistamines unless directed by physician

Generic names:

atropine sulfate (p. 147)
belladonna alkaloids (p. 165)
benztropine (p. 172)
biperiden (p. 180)
clidinium bromide (p. 297)
cyclopentolate (p. 331)
dicyclomine HCl (p. 374)
glycopyrrolate (p. 523)
hexocyclium methylsulfate (p. 544)
homatropine (p. 545)
hyoscyamine (p. 563)

hyoscyamine sulfate (p. 563)
mepenzolate bromide (p. 672)
methantheline bromide (p. 688)
methscopolamine bromide (p. 701)
procyclidine (p. 903)
propantheline bromide (p. 910)
scopolamine (transdermal) (p. 949)
scopolamine hydrobromide (p. 950)
trihexyphenidyl (p. 1061)
tropicamide (p. 1075)

ANTICOAGULANTS

Action: Anticoagulants interfere with blood clotting by preventing clot formation.

Uses: Anticoagulants are used for deep vein thrombosis, pulmonary emboli, myocardial infarction, open heart surgery, disseminated intravascular clotting syndrome, atrial fibrillation with embolization and in transfusion and dialysis

Side effects/adverse reactions: The most serious adverse reactions are hemorrhage, agranulocytosis, leukopenia, eosinophilia, and thrombocytopenia, depending on the specific product. The most common side effects are diarrhea, rash, and fever.

Contraindications: Persons with hemophilia, leukemia with bleeding, peptic ulcer disease, thrombocytopenic purpura, blood dyscrasias, acute nephritis, and subacute bacterial endocarditis should not use these products.

Precautions: Anticoagulants should be used with caution in alcoholism, elderly, and pregnancy.

Pharmacokinetics: Onset, peak, and duration vary widely among products. Most products are metabolized in the liver and excreted in urine.

Interactions/incompatibilities: Salicylates, steroids, and nonsteroidal antiinflammatories will potentiate the action of anticoagulants. Anticoagulants may cause serious effects; please check individual monographs.

Possible nursing diagnoses:
• Altered tissue perfusion *[uses]*
• High risk for injury *[side effects]*
• Knowledge deficit *[teaching]*

NURSING CONSIDERATIONS

Assess:
• Blood studies (Hct, platelets, occult blood in stools) q3mo
• Partial prothrombin time, which should be 1½-2 × control, PPT; often qd, APTT, ACT
• B/P, watch for increasing signs of hypertension

Administer:
• At same time each day to maintain steady blood levels
• Do not massage area or aspirate when giving SC injection, give in abdomen between pelvic bone, rotate sites; do not pull back on plunger, leave in for 10 sec; apply gentle pressure for 1 min
• Without changing needles
• Avoiding all IM injections that may cause bleeding

Perform/provide:
• Storage in tight container

Evaluate:
• Therapeutic response: decrease of deep vein thrombosis
• Bleeding gums, petechiae, ecchymosis, black tarry stools, hematuria
• Fever, skin rash, urticaria
• Needed dosage change q1-2wk

Teach patient/family:
• To avoid OTC preparations that may cause serious drug interactions unless directed by physician
• That drug may be held during active bleeding (menstruation), depending on condition
• To use soft-bristle toothbrush to avoid bleeding gums, avoid contact sports, use electric razor
• To carry a Medic-Alert ID identifying drug taken
• To report any signs of bleeding: gums, under skin, urine, stools

---

Generic names:

heparin calcium (p. 539)   warfarin sodium (p. 1097)
heparin sodium (p. 539)

ANTICONVULSANTS

Action: Anticonvulsants are divided into the barbiturates (p. 36), benzodiazepines (p. 37), hydantoins, succinimides, and miscellaneous products. Barbiturates and benzodiazepines are discussed in separate sections. Hydantoins act by inhibiting the spread of seizure activity in the motor cortex. Succinimides act by inhibiting spike and wave formation; they also decrease amplitude, frequency, duration, and spread of discharge in seizures.

Uses: Hydantoins are used in generalized tonic-clonic seizures, status epilepticus, and psychomotor seizures. Succinimides are used for absence (petit mal) seizures. Barbiturates are used in generalized tonic-clonic and cortical focal seizures.

Side effects/adverse reactions: Bone marrow depression is the most life-threatening adverse reaction associated with hydantoins or succinimides. The most common side effects are GI symptoms. Other common side effects for hydantoins are gingival hyperplasia and CNS effects such as nystagmus, ataxia, slurred speech, and mental confusion.

Contraindications: Hypersensitive reactions may occur, and allergies should be identified before these products are given.

Precautions: Persons with renal or hepatic disease should be watched closely.

Pharmacokinetics: Onset, peak, and duration vary widely among products. Most products are metabolized in the liver and excreted in urine, bile, and feces.

Interactions/incompatibilities: Decreased effects of estrogens, oral contraceptives (hydantoins).

Possible nursing diagnoses:
- High risk for injury *[uses]*
- Noncompliance *[teaching]*
- Sleep pattern disturbance *[adverse reactions]*

NURSING CONSIDERATIONS
Assess:
- Renal function studies, including BUN, creatinine, serum uric acid, urine creatinine clearance before and during therapy
- Blood studies: RBC, Hct, Hgb, reticulocyte counts qwk for 4 wk then qmo
- Hepatic studies: AST, ALT, bilirubin, creatinine

Administer:
- With food, milk to decrease GI symptoms

Perform/provide:
- Good oral hygiene is important for hydantoins

Evaluate:

• Therapeutic response, including decreased seizure activity; document on patient's chart
• Mental status, including mood, sensorium, affect, behavorial changes; if mental status changes, notify physician
• Eye problems, including need for ophthalmic examinations before, during, and after treatment (slit lamp, funduscopy, tonometry)
• Allergic reaction, including red raised rash; if this occurs, drug should be discontinued
• Blood dyscrasia, including fever, sore throat, bruising, rash, jaundice
• Toxicity, including bone marrow depression, nausea, vomiting, ataxia, diplopia, cardiovascular collapse, Stevens-Johnson syndrome

Teach patient/family:

• To carry ID card or Medic-Alert bracelet stating drugs taken, condition, physician's name, phone number
• To avoid driving, other activities that require alertness

Generic names:

Hydantoins: ethotoin (p. 456)
mephenytoin (p. 675)
phensuximide (p. 851)
phenytoin (p. 858)

Succinimides: ethosuximide (p. 454)
methsuximide (p. 702)
phensuximide (p. 851)

Miscellaneous: acetazolamide (p. 73)

carbamazepine (p. 212)
clonazepam (p. 306)
diazepam (p. 368)
febamate (p. 468)
gabapentin (p. 509)
magnesium sulfate (p. 651)
paraldehyde (p. 815)
paramethadione (p. 817)
phenacemide (p. 843)
primidone (p. 895)
trimethadione (p. 1065)
valproate sodium (p. 1083)

ANTIDEPRESSANTS

Action: Antidepressants are divided into the tricyclics, MAOIs, and miscellaneous antidepressants. The tricyclics work by blocking reuptake of norepinephrine and serotonin into nerve endings and increasing action of norepinephrine and serotonin in nerve cells. MAOIs act by increasing concentrations of endogenous epinephrine, norepinephrine, serotonin, dopamine in storage sites in CNS by inhibition of MAO; increased concentration reduces depression.

Uses: Antidepressants are used for depression and in some cases enuresis in children.

Side effects/adverse reactions: The most serious adverse reactions are paralytic ileus, acute renal failure, hypertension, and hypertensive crisis depending on the specific product. Common side effects are dizziness, drowsiness, diarrhea, dry mouth, retention, and orthostatic hypotension.

Contraindications: The contraindications for antidepressants are convulsive disorders, prostatic hypertrophy, severe renal, hepatic, cardiac disease depending on the type of medication.

Precautions: Antidepressants should be used cautiously in suicidal patients, severe depression, schizophrenia, hyperactivity, diabetes mellitus, pregnancy, and the elderly.

Pharmacokinetics: Onset, peak, and duration vary widely among products. Most products are metabolized in the liver and excreted in urine.

Interactions/incompatibilities: Please check individual monographs since interactions vary widely among products.

Possible nursing diagnoses:
• Ineffective individual coping *[uses]*
• High risk for injury *(uses/adverse reactions)*
• Knowledge deficit *[teaching]*

NURSING CONSIDERATIONS
Assess:
• B/P (lying, standing), pulse q4h; if systolic B/P drops 20 mm Hg hold drug, notify physician; take vital signs q4h in patients with cardiovascular disease
• Blood studies: CBC, leukocytes, differential, cardiac enzymes if patient is receiving long-term therapy
• Hepatic studies: AST, ALT, bilirubin, creatinine
• Weight qwk, appetite may increase with drug
Administer:
• Increased fluids, bulk in diet if constipation, urinary retention occur
• With food or milk for GI symptoms
• Gum, hard candy, or frequent sips of water for dry mouth
Perform/provide:
• Storage in tight container at room temperature, do not refreeze
• Assistance with ambulation during beginning therapy since drowsiness/dizziness occurs
• Safety measures including siderails primarily in elderly
• Checking to see PO medication swallowed
Evaluate:
• Therapeutic response: decreased depression

• EPS primarily in elderly: rigidity, dystonia, akathisia
• Mental status: mood, sensorium, affect, suicidal tendencies, increase in psychiatric symptoms: depression, panic
• Urinary retention, constipation; constipation is more likely to occur in children, elderly
• Withdrawal symptoms: headache, nausea, vomiting, muscle pain, weakness; do not usually occur unless drug was discontinued abruptly
• Alcohol consumption; if alcohol is consumed, hold dose until morning

Teach patient/family:
• That therapeutic effects may take 2-3 wk
• To use caution in driving or other activities requiring alertness because of drowsiness, dizziness, blurred vision
• To avoid alcohol ingestion, other CNS depressants
• Not to discontinue medication quickly after long-term use, may cause nausea, headache, malaise
• To wear sunscreen or large hat since photosensitivity may occur

Generic names:

Tricyclics
amitriptyline HCl (p. 112)
amoxapine (p. 119)
clomipramine HCl (p. 304)
desipramine HCl (p. 350)
doxepin HCl (p. 409)
imipramine HCl (p. 571)
nortriptyline HCl (p. 781)
protriptyline HCl (p. 918)
trimipramine maleate (p. 1070)

Miscellaneous
bupropion HCl (p. 195)
fluoxetine HCl (p. 495)
maprotiline HCl (p. 655)
paroxetine (p. 821)
trazodone HCl (p. 1048)
venlafaxine HCl (p. 1133)
MAOI
isocarboxazid (p. 595)
phenelzine sulfate (p. 846)
sertraline (p. 957)
tranylcypromine sulfate (p. 1046)

ANTIDIABETICS

Action: Antidiabetics are divided into the insulins that decrease blood sugar, phosphate, and potassium and increase blood pyruvate and lactate; and oral antidiabetics that cause functioning beta cells in the pancreas to release insulin, improves the effect of endogenous and exogenous insulin.
Uses: Insulins are used for ketoacidosis and diabetes mellitus types I (IDDM) and II (NIDDM); oral antidiabetics are used for stable adult-onset diabetes mellitus type II (NIDDM).
Side effects/adverse reactions: The most common side effect of insulin

and oral antidiabetics is hypoglycemia. Other adverse reactions for oral antidiabetics include blood dyscrasias, hepatotoxicity, and, rarely, cholestatic jaundice. Adverse reactions for insulin products include allergic responses and, more rarely, anaphylaxis.

Contraindications: Hypersensitive reactions may occur, and allergies should be identified before these products are given. Oral antidiabetics should not be used in juvenile or brittle diabetes, diabetic ketoacidosis, severe renal disease, or severe hepatic disease.

Precautions: Oral antidiabetics should be used with caution in the elderly, in cardiac disease, pregnancy, lactation, and in the presence of alcohol.

Pharmacokinetics: Onset, peak, and duration vary widely among products. Oral antidiabetics are metabolized in the liver, with metabolites excreted in urine, bile, and feces.

Interactions/incompatibilities: Interactions vary widely among products. Check individual monograph for specific information.

Possible nursing diagnosis:

• Altered nutrition: more than body requirements *[uses]*

NURSING CONSIDERATIONS

Assess:

• Blood, urine glucose levels during treatment to determine diabetes control (oral products)
• Fasting blood glucose, 2 hr PP (60-100 mg/dl normal fasting level) (70-130 mg/dl—normal 2-hr level)

Administer:

• Insulin, after warming to room temperature by rotating in palms to prevent lipodystrophy from injecting cold insulin
• Human insulin to those allergic to beef or pork
• Oral antidiabetic 30 min before meals

Perform/provide:

• Rotation of injection sites when giving insulin; use abdomen, upper back, thighs, upper arm, buttocks; rotate sites within one of these regions; keep a record of sites

Evaluate:

• Therapeutic response, including decrease in polyuria, polydipsia, polyphagia, clear sensorium, absence of dizziness, stable gait
• Hypoglycemic reaction that can occur during peak time

Teach patient/family:

• To avoid alcohol and salicylates except on advice of physician
• Symptoms of ketoacidosis: nausea, thirst, polyuria, dry mouth, decreased B/P, dry, flushed skin, acetone breath, drowsiness, Kussmaul respiration

• Symptoms of hypoglycemia: headache, tremors, fatigue, weakness; and that candy or sugar should be carried to treat hypoglycemia
• To test urine for glucose/ketones tid if this drug is replacing insulin
• To continue weight control, dietary restrictions, exercise, hygiene

Generic names:

Oral antidiabetics: acetohexamide (p. 75)
chlorpropamide (p. 278)
insulin, regular (p. 580)
insulin, regular concentrated (p. 582)

insulin, zinc suspension (extended) (p. 584)
insulin, zinc suspension (Lente) (p. 583)
insulin, zinc suspension (prompt) (p. 586)

ANTIDIARRHEALS

Action: Antidiarrheals work by various actions including direct action on intestinal muscles to decrease GI peristalsis; or by inhibiting prostaglandin synthesis responsible for GI hypermotility; acting on mucosal receptors responsible for peristalsis; or decreasing water content of stools.

Uses: Antidiarrheals are used for diarrhea of undetermined causes.

Side effects/adverse reactions: The most serious adverse reactions of some products are paralytic ileus, toxic megacolon, and angioneurotic edema. The most common side effects are constipation, nausea, dry mouth, and abdominal pain.

Contraindications: Persons with severe ulcerative colitis, pseudomembranous colitis with some products.

Precautions: Antidiarrheal should be used with caution in the elderly, pregnancy, lactation, children, dehydration.

Pharmacokinetics: Onset, peak, and duration vary widely among products. Most products are metabolized in the liver and excreted in urine.

Interactions/incompatibilities: Please check individual monographs since interactions vary widely among products.

Possible nursing diagnoses:
• Diarrhea *[uses]*
• Constipation *[adverse reactions]*
• Fluid volume deficit *[adverse reactions]*
• Knowledge deficit *[teaching]*

NURSING CONSIDERATIONS

Assess:
• Electrolytes (K, Na, Cl) if on long-term therapy

Administer:
• For 48 hr only
Evaluate:
• Therapeutic response: decreased diarrhea
• Bowel pattern before; for rebound constipation after termination of medication
• Response after 48 hr; if no response, drug should be discontinued
• Dehydration in children
Teach patient/family:
• To avoid OTC products
• Not to exceed recommended dose

Generic names:

bismuth subsalicylate (p. 182)   kaolin/pectin (p. 609)
difenoxin HCl (p. 381)   loperamide HCl (p. 639)
diphenoxylate HCl (p. 397)   opium tincture (p. 789)

ANTIDYSRHYTHMICS

Action: Antidysrhythmics are divided into four classes and miscellaneous antidysrhythmics:
• Class I increases the action potential duration and the effective refractory period and reduces disparity in the refractory period between a normal and infarcted myocardium; further subclasses include Ia, Ib, Ic
• Class II decreases the rate of SA node discharge, increases recovery time, slows conduction through the AV node, and decreases heart rate, which decreases O_2 consumption in the myocardium
• Class III increases the action potential duration and the effective refractory period
• Class IV inhibits calcium ion influx across the cell membrane during cardiac depolarization; decreases SA node discharge, decreases conduction velocity through the AV node
• Miscellaneous antidysrhythmics include those such as adenosine, which slows conduction through the AV node, and digoxin, which decreases conduction velocity and prolongs the effective refractory period in the AV node
Uses: These products are used for PVCs, tachycardia, hypertension, atrial fibrillation, angina pectoris.

Side effects/adverse reactions: Side effects and adverse reactions vary widely among products.

Contraindications: Contraindications vary widely among products.

Precautions: Precautions vary widely among products.

Pharmacokinetics: Onset, peak, and duration vary widely among products.

Interactions/incompatibilities: Interactions vary widely among products; check individual monograph for specific information.

Possible nursing diagnoses:

• Altered tissue perfusion: cardiopulmonary *[uses]*

• Decreased cardiac output *[uses]*

• Diarrhea *[adverse reactions]*

• Impaired gas exchange *[adverse reactions]*

NURSING CONSIDERATIONS

Assess:

• ECG continuously to determine drug effectiveness, PVCs or other dysrhythmias

• IV infusion rate to avoid causing nausea, vomiting

• For dehydration or hypovolemia

• B/P continuously for hypotension, hypertension

• I&O ratio

• Serum potassium

Evaluate:

• Therapeutic response, including decrease in B/P in hypertension, decreased B/P, edema moist rales in CHF

• Edema in feet and legs daily

Teach patient/family:

• To comply with dosage schedule, even if patient is feeling better

• To report bradycardia, dizziness, confusion, depression, fever

Generic names:

Class I: moricizine (p. 739)

Class Ia: disopyramide (p. 400)
procainamide (p. 898)
quinidine (p. 932)

Class Ib: lidocaine (p. 625)
mexiletine (p. 722)
phenytoin (p. 858)
tocainide (p. 1038)

Class Ic: flecainide (p. 481)
indecainide (p. 574)
propafenone (p. 909)

Class II: acebutolol (p. 69)
esmolol (p. 438)
propranolol (p. 914)

Class III: amiodarone HCl (p. 111)
bretylium (p. 187)

Class IV: verapamil HCl
(p. 1087)

Miscellaneous: adenosine
(p. 82)
digoxin (p. 385)

ANTIFUNGALS (SYSTEMIC)

Action: Antifungals act by increasing cell membrane permeability in susceptible organisms by binding sterols and decreasing potassium, sodium, and nutrients in the cell.

Uses: Antifungals are used for infections of histoplasmosis, blastomycosis, coccidiomycosis, cryptococcosis, aspergillosis, phycomycosis, candidiasis, sporotrichosis causing severe meningitis, septicemia, and skin infections.

Side effects/adverse reactions: The most serious adverse reactions include renal tubular acidosis, permanent renal impairment, anuria, oliguria, hemorrhagic gastroenteritis, and acute liver failure, blood dyscrasias. Some common side effects include hypokalemia, nausea, vomiting, anorexia, headache, fever, and chills.

Contraindications: Persons with severe bone depression or hypersensitivity should not use these products.

Precautions: Antifungals should be used with caution in renal disease, pregnancy, and hepatic disease.

Pharmacokinetics: Onset, peak, and duration vary widely among products. Most products are metabolized in the liver and excreted in urine.

Interactions/incompatibilities: Please check individual monographs since interactions vary widely among products.

Possible nursing diagnoses:

• High risk for infection *[uses]*

- High risk for injury *[adverse reactions]*
- Knowledge deficit *[teaching]*

NURSING CONSIDERATIONS

Assess:
- VS q15-30min during first infusion; note changes in pulse, B/P
- I&O ratio; watch for decreasing urinary output, change is sp gr; discontinue drug to prevent permanent damage to renal tubules
- Blood studies: CBC, K, Na, Ca, Mg q2wk
- Weight weekly; if weight increases over 2 lb/wk, edema is present, renal damage should be considered

Administer:
- IV using in-line filter (mean pore diameter >1 μm) using distal veins, check for extravasation, necrosis q8h
- Drug only after C&S confirms organism, drug needed to treat condition; make sure drug is used in life-threatening infections

Perform/provide:
- Protection from light during infusion, cover with foil
- Symptomatic treatment as ordered for adverse reactions: aspirin, antihistamines, antiemetics, antispasmodics
- Storage, protected from moisture and light; diluted solution is stable for 24 hr

Evaluate:
- Therapeutic response: decreased fever, malaise, rash, negative C&S for infecting organism
- For renal toxicity: increasing BUN, is >40 mg/dl or if serum creatinine >3 mg/dl; drug may be discontinued or dosage reduced
- For hepatotoxicity: increasing AST, ALT, alk phosphatase, bilirubin
- For allergic reaction: dermatitis, rash; drug should be discontinued, antihistamines (mild reaction) or epinephrine (severe reaction) administered
- For hypokalemia: anorexia, drowsiness, weakness, decreased reflexes, dizziness, increased urinary output, increased thirst, paresthesias
- For ototoxicity: tinnitus (ringing, roaring in ears), vertigo, loss of hearing (rare)

Teach patient/family:
- That long-term therapy may be needed to clear infection (2 wk-3 mo depending on type of infection)

Generic names:

amphotericin B (p. 125)
fluconazole (p. 483)
flucytosine (p. 484)
griseofulvin microsize (p. 526)
griseofulvin ultramicrosize
(p. 526)

itraconazole (p. 606)
ketoconazole (p. 611)
miconazole (p. 726)
nystatin (p. 784)

ANTIHISTAMINES

Action: Antihistamines compete with histamines for H₁ receptor sites. They antagonize in varying degrees most of the pharmacologic effects of histamines.

Uses: Products are used to control the symptoms of allergies, rhinitis, and pruritus.

Side effects/adverse reactions: Most products cause drowsiness; however, two of the newer products, astemizole and terfenadine, produce little, if any, drowsiness. Other common side effects are headache and thickening of bronchial secretions. Serious blood dyscrasias may occur, but are rare. Urinary retention, GI effects occur with many of these products.

Contraindications: Hypersensitivity to H₁-receptor antagonists occurs rarely. Patients with acute asthma and lower respiratory tract disease should not use these products, since thick secretions may result. Other contraindications include narrow-angle glaucoma, bladder neck obstruction, stenosing peptic ulcer, symptomatic prostatic hypertrophy, newborn, lactation.

Precautions: These products must be used cautiously in conjunction with intraocular pressure, since they increase intraocular pressure. Caution should also be used in patients with renal and cardiac disease, hypertension, and seizure disorders, pregnancy, lactation and in the elderly.

Pharmacokinetics: Onset varies from 20-60 min, with duration lasting 4-12 hr. In general, pharmacokinetics vary widely among products.

Drug interactions/incompatibilities: Barbiturates, narcotics, hypnotics, tricyclic antidepressants, or alcohol can increase CNS depression when taken with antihistamines.

Possible nursing diagnoses:
• Ineffective airway clearance *[uses]*

NURSING CONSIDERATIONS

Assess:
• I&O ratio; be alert for urinary retention, frequency, dysuria; drug should be discontinued if these occur

• CBC during long-term therapy, since hemolytic anemia, although rare, may occur

Administer:
• With food or milk to decrease GI symptoms; absorption may be decreased slightly
• Whole (sustained release tabs)

Perform/provide:
• Hard candy, gum, frequent rinsing of mouth for dryness

Evaluate:
• Therapeutic response, including absence of allergy symptoms, itching
• Blood dyscrasias: thrombocytopenia, agranulocytosis (rare)
• Respiratory status, including rate rhythm, increase in bronchial secretions, wheezing, chest tightness
• Cardiac status, including palpitations, increased pulse, hypotension

Teach patient/family:
• To notify physician if confusion, sedation, hypotension occur
• To avoid driving or other hazardous activity if drowsiness occurs
• To avoid concurrent use of alcohol or other CNS depressants
• To discontinue a few days before skin testing

Generic names:

astemizole (p. 143)
azatadine maleate (p. 153)
brompheniramine maleate
(p. 190)
chlorpheniramine maleate
(p. 274)
clemastine fumarate (p. 296)
cyproheptadine HCl
(p. 326)
dexchlorpheniramine maleate
(p. 359)

diphenhydramine HCl
(p. 395)
loratadine (p. 641)
promethazine HCl
(p. 908)
terfenadine (p. 1000)
trimeprazine tartrate (p. 1064)
tripelennamine HCl (p. 1072)
triprolidine HCl
(p. 1073)

ANTIHYPERTENSIVES

Action: Antihypertensives are divided into angiotensin-converting enzyme (ACE) inhibitors, β-adrenergic blockers, calcium channel blockers, centrally acting adrenergics, diuretics, peripherally acting antiadrenergics, and vasodilators. Beta blockers, calcium channel blockers, and diuretics are discussed in separate sections. Angiotensin-converting enzyme inhibitors act by selectively suppressing renin-angiotensin I to angiotensin II; dilation of arterial and venous vessels occurs. Centrally acting adrenergics act by inhibiting the sympathetic vasomotor center in the CNS that reduces impulses in the sympathetic nervous system; blood pressure, pulse rate, and cardiac output decrease. Peripherally acting antiadrenergics inhibit sympathetic vasoconstriction by inhibiting release of norepinephrine and/or depleting norepinephrine stores in adrenergic nerve endings. Vasodilators act on arteriolar smooth muscle by producing direct relaxation or vasodilation; a reduction in blood pressure, with concomitant increases in heart rate and cardiac output, occurs.

Uses: Used for hypertension and for heart failure not responsive to conventional therapy. Some products are used in hypertensive crisis, angina, and for some cardiac dysrhythmias.

Side effects/adverse reactions: The most common side effects are marked hypotension, bradycardia, tachycardia, headache, nausea, and vomiting. Side effects and adverse reactions may vary widely between classes and specific products.

Contraindications: Hypersensitive reactions may occur, and allergies should be identified before these products are given. Antihypertensives should not be used in patients with heart block or children.

Precautions: Antihypertensives should be used with caution in the elderly, in dialysis patients, and in the presence of hypovolemia, leukemia, and electrolyte imbalances.

Pharmacokinetics: Onset, peak, and duration vary widely among products. Most products are metabolized in the liver, with metabolites excreted in urine, bile, and feces.

Interactions/incompatibilities: Interactions vary widely among products; check individual monograph for specific information.

Possible nursing diagnoses:
- Altered tissue perfusion *[uses]*
- Decreased cardiac output *[uses]*
- Diarrhea *[adverse reactions]*
- Impaired gas exchange *[adverse reactions]*

NURSING CONSIDERATIONS
Assess:
- Blood studies: neutrophil; decreased platelets occur with many of the products
- Renal studies: protein, BUN, creatinine; watch for increased levels that may indicate nephrotic syndrome; obtain baselines in renal and liver function studies before beginning treatment

Perform/provide:
• Supine or Trendelenburg position for severe hypotension
Evaluate:
• Therapeutic response, including decrease in B/P in hypotension; decreased B/P, edema, moist rales in CHF
• Edema in feet and legs daily
• Allergic reaction, including rash, fever, pruritus, urticaria: drug should be discontinued if antihistamines fail to help
• Symptoms of CHF: edema, dyspnea, wet rales, B/P
• Renal symptoms: polyuria, oliguria, frequency
Teach patient/family:
• To comply with dosage schedule, even if feeling better
• To rise slowly to sitting or standing position to minimize orthostatic hypotension

---

Generic names:

Angiotensin-converting enzyme inhibitors: benazepril HCl (p. 166)
enalapril (p. 422)
fosinopril sodium (p. 506)
perindopril (p. 1129)
quinapril HCl (p. 930)
ramipril (p. 937)

Centrally acting adrenergics:
clonidine HCl (p. 307)
guanabenz (p. 528)
guanfacine (p. 531)
methyldopa (p. 704)

Peripherally acting antiadrenergics: guanadrel (p. 529)

guanethidine (p. 530)
prazosin (p. 889)
reserpine (p. 939)
terazosin (p. 997)

Vasodilators: diazoxide (p. 369)
hydralazine (p. 546)
minoxidil (p. 731)
nitroprusside (p. 775)

Antiadrenergic: combined alpha/beta blocker—labetalol (p. 614)

ANTIINFECTIVES

Action: Antiinfectives are divided into several groups, which include but are not limited to penicillins, cephalosporins, aminoglycosides, sulfonamides, tetracyclines, monobactam, erythromycins, and quinolones. These drugs act by inhibiting the growth and replication of susceptible bacterial organisms.
Uses: Used for infections of susceptible organisms. These products are effective against bacterial, rickettsial, and spirochete infections.

Side effects/adverse reactions: The most common side effects are nausea, vomiting, and diarrhea. Adverse reactions include bone marrow depression and anaphylaxis.

Contraindications: Hypersensitive reactions may occur, and allergies should be identified before these products are given. Cross-sensitivity can occur between products of different classes (penicillins or cephalosporins). Often persons allergic to penicillins will also be allergic to cephalosporins.

Precautions: Antiinfectives should be used with caution in persons with renal and liver disease.

Pharmacokinetics: Onset, peak, and duration vary widely among products. Most products are metabolized in the liver, and metabolites are excreted in urine, bile, and feces.

Interactions/incompatibilities: Interactions vary widely among products; check individual monograph for specific information.

Possible nursing diagnoses:
• High risk for infection [uses]
• Diarrhea [adverse reactions]

NURSING CONSIDERATIONS
Assess:
• Nephrotoxicity, including increased BUN, creatinine
• Blood studies: AST, ALT, CBC, Hct, bilirubin; test monthly if patient is on long-term therapy
• Bowel pattern qd; if severe diarrhea occurs, drug should be discontinued
Administer:
• For 10-14 days to ensure organism death, prevention of superimposed infection
• After C&S completed, drug may be taken as soon as culture is taken
Evaluate:
• Therapeutic response, including absence of fever, fatigue, malaise, draining wounds
• Urine output; if decreasing, notify physician; may indicate nephrotoxicity
• Allergic reaction, including rash, fever, pruritus, urticaria; drug should be discontinued
• Bleeding: ecchymosis, bleeding gums, hematuria, stool guaiac daily
• Overgrowth of infection: perineal itching, fever, malaise, redness, pain, swelling, drainage, rash, diarrhea, change in cough, sputum
Teach patient/family:
• To comply with dosage schedule, even if feeling better

• To report sore throat, bruising, bleeding, joint pain; may indicate blood dyscrasias (rare)

Generic names:

Aminoglycosides: amikacin sulfate (p. 101)
azithromycin (p. 155)
clarithromycin (p. 294)
gentamicin (p. 514)
kanamycin (p. 607)
neomycin (p. 760)
netilmicin (p. 764)
streptomycin (p. 974)
tobramycin (p. 1036)

Cephalosporins: cefaclor (p. 224)
cefadroxil (p. 225)
cefamandole (p. 227)
cefazolin (p. 228)
cefixime (p. 230)
cefmetazole (p. 231)
cefonicid (p. 232)
cefoperazone (p. 234)
ceforanide (p. 235)
cefotaxime (p. 237)
cefprozil monohydrate (p. 243)
cefuroxime axetil (p. 248)
cefuroxime sodium (p. 250)
cephalexin (p. 252)
cephalothin (p. 253)
cephapirin (p. 255)
cephradine (p. 257)
moxalactam disodium (p. 742)

Penicillins: amoxicillin/
clavulanate (p. 121)
ampicillin/sulbactam (p. 129)
azlocillin (p. 156)
bacampicillin (p. 159)

cloxacillin (p. 311)
dicloxacillin (p. 373)
imipenem/cilastatin (p. 569)
methicillin (p. 691)
mezlocillin (p. 723)
nafcillin (p. 748)
oxacillin (p. 793)
penicillin G benzathine (p. 824)
penicillin G potassium (p. 825)
penicillin G procaine (p. 827)
penicillin G sodium (p. 829)
penicillin V (p. 830)
piperacillin (p. 868)
ticarcillin (p. 1029)
ticarcillin/clavulanate (p. 1030)

Sulfonamides: sulfasalazine (p. 985)
sulfisoxazole (p. 987)

Tetracyclines: demeclocycline HCl (p. 349)
doxycycline (p. 413)
minocycline (p. 730)
oxytetracycline (p. 807)
tetracycline (p. 1008)

ANTINEOPLASTICS

Action: Antineoplastics are divided into alkylating agents, antimetabolites, antibiotic agents, hormonal agents, and miscellaneous agents. Alkylating agents act by cross-linking strands of DNA. Antimetabolites act by inhibiting DNA synthesis. Antibiotic agents act by inhibiting RNA synthesis and by delaying or inhibiting mitosis. Hormones alter the effect of androgens, luteinizing hormone, follicle-stimulating hormone, or estrogen by changing the hormonal environment.

Uses: Uses vary widely among products and classes of drugs. They are used to treat leukemia, Hodgkin's disease, lymphomas, and other tumors throughout the body.

Side effects/adverse reactions: Most products cause thrombocytopenia, leukopenia, and anemia, and, if these reactions occur, the drug may need to be stopped until the problem is corrected. Other side effects include nausea, vomiting, glossitis, and hair loss. Some products also cause hepatotoxicity, nephrotoxicity, and cardiotoxicity.

Contraindications: Hypersensitive reactions may occur, and allergies should be identified before these products are given. Also, persons with severe liver and kidney disease should not use these products unless the benefits outweigh the risks.

Precautions: Persons with bleeding, severe bone marrow depression, or renal or hepatic disease should be watched closely.

Pharmacokinetics: Onset, peak, and duration vary widely among products. Most products cross the placenta and are excreted in breast milk and in urine.

Interactions/incompatibilities: Toxicity may occur when used with other antineoplastics or radiation.

Possible nursing diagnoses:
• High risk for infection [adverse reactions]
• Altered nutrition: less than body requirements [adverse reactions]
• Altered oral mucous membrane [adverse reactions]

NURSING CONSIDERATIONS

Assess:
• CBC, differential, platelet count weekly; withhold drug if WBC is <4000 or platelet count is <75,000; notify physician of results
• Renal function studies, including BUN, creatinine, serum uric acid, and urine creatinine clearance before and during therapy
• I&O ratio; report fall in urine output of 30 ml/hr
• Monitor temperature q4h (may indicate beginning infection)
• Liver function tests before and during therapy (bilirubin, AST, ALT, LDH) as needed or monthly

Administer:
• Checking IV site for irritation; phlebitis
• Epinephrine for hypersensitivity reaction
• Antibiotics for prophylaxis of infection

Perform/provide:
- Strict medical asepsis, protective isolation if WBC levels are low
- Comprehensive oral hygiene, using careful technique and soft-bristle brush

Evaluate:
- Therapeutic response, including decreased tumor size
- Bleeding, including hematuria, guaiac, bruising or petechiae, mucosa, or orifices q8h; obtain prescription for viscous xylocaine
- Yellowing of skin, sclera, dark urine, clay-colored stools, itchy skin, abdominal pain, fever, diarrhea
- Edema in feet, joint pain, stomach pain, shaking
- Inflammation of mucosa, breaks in skin

Teach patient/family:
- To report signs of infection, including increased temperature, sore throat, malaise
- To report signs of anemia, including fatigue, headache, faintness, shortness of breath, irritability
- To report bleeding and avoid use of razors or commercial mouthwash

---

Generic names:

Alkylating agents: busulfan (p. 197)
carboplatin (p. 216)
carmustine (p. 219)
chlorambucil (p. 260)
cisplatin (p. 291)
cyclophosphamide (p. 332)
dacarbazine (p. 339)
lomustine (p. 637)
mechlorethamine (p. 661)
melphalan (p. 669)
streptozocin (p. 976)
thiotepa (p. 1021)
uracil mustard (p. 1077)

Antimetabolites: cytarabine (p. 337)
doxorubicin (p. 411)
fludarabine phosphate (p. 485)
fluorouracil (p. 493)
mercaptopurine (p. 679)

methotrexate (p. 696)
mitomycin (p. 733)
mitoxantrone (p. 735)
plicamycin (p. 875)

Hormonal agents:
aminoglutethimide (p. 108)
estramustine (p. 445)
flutamide (p. 503)
goserelin acetate (p. 525)
leuprolide (p. 617)
megestrol (p. 668)
mitotane (p. 734)
tamoxifen (p. 993)
testolactone (p. 1002)
trilostane (p. 1063)

Miscellaneous agents:
altretamine (p. 94)
asparaginase (p. 139)
cladribine (p. 293)

etoposide (p. 462)
thioguanine (6-TG) (p. 1017)

Antibiotic agents: bleomycin
(p. 186)
dactinomycin (p. 340)
daunorubicin HCl (p. 346)

interferon alfa-2A (p. 587)
interferon alfa-2B (p. 587)
pentostatin (p. 837)
procarbazine (p. 900)
vinblastine (p. 1090)
vincristine (p. 1092)

ANTIPARKINSON AGENTS

Action: Antiparkinson agents are divided into cholinergics and dopamine
agonists. Cholinergics work by the blocking or competing at central
acetylcholine receptors; dopamine agonists work by decarboxylation to
dopamine or by activation of dopamine receptors; monoamine oxidase
type B inhibitors work by increase dopamine activity by inhibiting MAO
type B activity.

Uses: Antiparkinson agents are used alone or in combination for patients
with Parkinson's disease.

Side effects/adverse reactions: Side effects and adverse reactions vary
widely among products. The most common side effects include involuntary movements, headache, numbness, insomnia, nightmares, nausea,
vomiting, dry mouth, and orthostatic hypotension.

Contraindications: Persons with hypersensitivity, narrow-angle glaucoma, and undiagnosed skin lesions should not use these products.

Precautions: Antiparkinson agents should be used with caution in pregnancy, lactation, children, renal, cardiac, hepatic disease, and affective
disorder.

Pharmacokinetics: Onset, peak, and duration vary widely among products. Most products are metabolized in the liver and excreted in urine.

Interactions/incompatibilities: Please check individual monographs
since interactions vary widely among products.

Possible nursing diagnoses:
• High risk for injury *[uses]*
• High risk for impaired mobility *[uses]*
• Knowledge deficit *[teaching]*

NURSING CONSIDERATIONS
Assess:
• B/P, respiration
Administer:
• Drug up until NPO before surgery

- Adjust dosage depending on patient response
- With meals; limit protein taken with drug
- Only after MAOIs have been discontinued for 2 wk

Perform/provide:
- Assistance with ambulation, during beginning therapy
- Testing for diabetes mellitus, acromegaly if on long-term therapy

Evaluate:
- Therapeutic response: decrease in akathisia, increased mood
- Mental status: affect, mood, behavioral changes, depression, complete suicide assessment

Teach patient/family:
- To change positions slowly to prevent orthostatic hypotension
- To report side effects: twitching, eye spasm; indicate overdose
- To use drug exactly as prescribed; if drug is discontinued abruptly, parkinsonian crisis may occur

---

Generic names:

amantadine (p. 98)
benztropine mesylate (p. 172)
biperiden HCl (p. 180)
biperiden lactate (p. 180)
bromocriptine mesylate (p. 189)

levodopa (p. 619)
carbidopa/levodopa (p. 215)
procyclidine HCl (p. 903)
selegiline HCl (p. 955)
trihexyphenidyl HCl (p. 1061)

ANTIPSYCHOTICS

Action: Antipsychotics/neuroleptics are divided into several subgroups: phenothiazines, thioxanthenes, butyrophenones, dibenzoxazepines, dibenzodiazepines, and indolones and other heterocyclic compounds. Although chemically different, these subgroups share many pharmacologic and clinical properties. All antipsychotics work to block postsynaptic dopamine receptors in the brain that are responsible for psychotic behavior, including hallucinations, delusions, and paranoia.

Uses: Antipsychotic behavior is decreased in conditions such as schizophrenia, paranoia, and mania. These agents are also effective for severe anxiety, intractable hiccups, nausea, vomiting, behavioral problems in children, and before surgery for relaxation.

Side effects/adverse reactions: The most common side effects include extrapyramidal symptoms such as pseudoparkinsonism, akathisia, dystonia, and tardive dyskinesia, which may be controlled by use of antiparkinsonian agents. Serious adverse reactions such as hypotension, agranulocytosis, cardiac arrest, and laryngospasm have occurred. Other common side effects include dry mouth and photosensitivity.

Contraindications: Persons with liver damage, severe hypertension or coronary disease, cerebral arteriosclerosis, blood dyscrasias, bone marrow depression, parkinsonism, severely depressed persons, narrow-angle glaucoma, children <12 yr, or persons withdrawing from alcohol or barbiturates should not use antipsychotics until these conditions are corrected.

Precautions: Caution must be used when antipsychotics are given to the elderly, since metabolism is slowed and adverse reactions can occur rapidly. Hepatic and renal disease may cause poor metabolism and excretion of the drug. Seizure threshold is decreased with these products; increases in the dose of anticonvulsants may be required. Persons with diabetes mellitus, prostatic hypertrophy, chronic respiratory disease, and peptic ulcer disease should be monitored closely.

Pharmacokinetics: Onset, peak, and duration vary widely with different products and routes. Products are metabolized by the liver, are excreted in urine as metabolites, are highly bound to plasma proteins, cross the placenta, and enter breast milk. Half-life can be extended over 3 days.

Interactions/incompatibilities: Because other CNS depressants can cause oversedation, these combinations should be used carefully. Anticholinergics may decrease the therapeutic actions of phenothiazines and also cause increased anticholinergic effects.

Possible nursing diagnoses:
• Altered thought processes *[uses]*
• Sensory-perceptual alterations *[uses]*

NURSING CONSIDERATIONS
Assess:
• Bilirubin, CBC, liver function studies monthly, since these drugs are metabolized in the liver and excreted in urine
• I&O ratio: palpate bladder if low urinary output occurs, since urinary retention occurs with many of these products
• Affect, orientation, LOC, reflexes, gait, coordination, sleep pattern disturbances
• Dizziness, faintness, palpitations, tachycardia on rising

Administer:
• Antiparkinsonian agent if extrapyramidal symptoms occur
• Liquid concentrates mixed in glass of juice or cola, since taste is unpleasant; avoid contact with skin when preparing liquid concentrate or parental medications

Perform/provide:

• Supervised ambulation until stabilized on medication; do not involve in strenuous exercise program because fainting is possible; patient should not stand still for long periods of time

• Increased fluids to prevent constipation

• Sips of water, candy, gum for dry mouth

Evaluate:

• Therapeutic response: decrease in excitement, hallucinations, delusions, paranoia, reorganization of thought patterns, speech

• B/P lying and standing; wide fluctuations between lying and standing B/P may require dosage or product change since orthostatic hypotension is occurring

• Extrapyramidal symptoms, including akathisia, tardive dyskinesia, pseudoparkinsonism

Teach patient/family:

• To rise from sitting or lying position gradually, since fainting may occur

• To remain lying down for at least 30 min after IM injections

• To avoid hot tubs, hot showers, or tub baths, since hypotension may occur

• To wear a sunscreen or protective clothing to prevent burns

• To take extra precautions during hot weather to stay cool; heat stroke can occur

• To avoid driving or other activities requiring alertness until response to medication is known

• That drowsiness or impaired mental/motor activity is evident the first 2 wk, but tends to decrease over time

---

Generic names:

Phenothiazines: chlorpromazine HCl (p. 275)
fluphenazine (p. 498)
mesoridazine (p. 682)
perphenazine (p. 841)
prochlorperazine (p. 902)
promazine (p. 905)
thioridazine (p. 1019)
thiothixene (p. 1023)

trifluoperazine (p. 1056)

Butyrophenone: haloperidol (p. 536)

Miscellaneous: loxapine (p. 644)
molindone (p. 738)
risperidone (p. 1130)

ANTITUBERCULARS

Action: Antituberculars act by inhibiting RNA or DNA, or interfering with lipid and protein synthesis, thereby decreasing tubercle bacilli replication.

Uses: Antituberculars are used for pulmonary tuberculosis.

Side effects/adverse reactions: They vary widely among products. Most products can cause nausea, vomiting, anorexia, and rash. Serious adverse reactions include renal failure, nephrotoxicity, ototoxicity, and hepatic necrosis.

Contraindications: Persons with severe renal disease or hypersensitivity should not use these products.

Precautions: Antituberculars should be used with caution with pregnancy, lactation, and hepatic disease.

Pharmacokinetics: Onset, peak, and duration vary widely among products. Most products are metabolized in the liver and excreted in urine.

Interactions/incompatibilities: Please check individual monographs since interactions vary widely among products.

Possible nursing diagnoses:
• High risk for infection *[uses]*
• High risk for injury *[adverse reactions]*
• Knowledge deficit *[teaching]*
• Noncompliance *[teaching]*

NURSING CONSIDERATIONS

Assess:
• Signs of anemia: Hct, Hgb, fatigue
• Liver studies qwk: ALT, AST, bilirubin
• Renal status before, qmo: BUN, creatinine, output, sp. gr., urinalysis

Administer:
• For some of these agents on empty stomach, 1 hr ac (only for isoniazid and rifampin) or 2 hr pc
• Antiemetic if vomiting occurs
• After C&S is completed; qmo to detect resistance

Evaluate:
• Therapeutic response: decreased symptoms of TB, culture negative
• Hepatic status: decreased appetite, jaundice, dark urine, fatigue

Teach patient/family:
• That compliance with dosage schedule, duration is necessary
• That scheduled appointments must be kept; relapse may occur
• To avoid alcohol while taking drug
• To report flu-like symptoms: excessive fatigue, anorexia, vomiting, sore throat; unusual bleeding, yellowish discoloration of skin/eyes

Generic names:

capremycin sulfate (p. 205)   kanamycin (p. 607)
cycloserine (p. 334)   pyrazinamide (p. 922)
ethambutol HCl (p. 450)   rifabutin (p. 942)
ethionamide (p. 454)   rifampin (p. 943)
isoniazid (p. 599)   streptomycin (p. 974)

ANTITUSSIVES/EXPECTORANTS

Action: Antitussives act by suppressing the cough reflex by direct action on the cough center in the medulla. Expectorants act by liquefying and reducing the viscosity of thick, tenacious secretions.

Uses: Antitussives/expectorants are used to treat cough occurring in pneumonia, bronchitis, TB, cystic fibrosis, and emphysema; as an adjunct in atelectasis (expectorants); and nonproductive cough (antitussives).

Side effects/adverse reactions: The most common side effects are drowsiness, dizziness, and nausea.

Contraindications: Some products are contraindicated in hypothyroidism, iodine sensitivity, pregnancy, and lactation.

Precautions: Some products should be used cautiously in asthma, elderly, and debilitated patients.

Pharmacokinetics: Onset, peak, and duration vary widely among products. Some products are metabolized in the liver and excreted in urine.

Interactions/incompatibilities: Please check individual monographs since interactions vary widely among products.

Possible nursing diagnoses:
• Ineffective breathing pattern *[uses]*
• Ineffective airway clearance *[uses]*
• Knowledge deficit *[teaching]*

NURSING CONSIDERATIONS

Administer:
• Decreased dose to elderly patients; their metabolism may be slowed

Perform/provide:
• Increased fluids to liquefy secretions
• Humidification of patient's room

Evaluate:
• Therapeutic response: absence of cough
• Cough: type, frequency, character including sputum

Teach patient/family:
• To avoid driving or other hazardous activities until patient is stabilized on this medication

• To avoid smoking, smoke-filled rooms, perfumes, dust, environmental pollutants, cleaners that increase cough

---

Generic names:

ANTIVIRALS

Action: Antivirals act by interfering with DNA synthesis that is needed for viral replication.

Uses: Antivirals are used for mucocutaneous herpes simplex virus, herpes genitalis (HSV_1, HSV_2), advanced HIV infections, herpes simplex virus encephalitis, varicella-zoster encephalomyelitis.

Side effects/adverse reactions: Serious adverse reactions are fatal metabolic encephalopathy, blood dyscrasias, and acute renal failure. Common side effects are nausea, vomiting, anorexia, diarrhea, headache, vaginitis, and moniliasis.

Contraindications: Persons with hypersensitivity, herpes zoster in immunosuppressed individuals should not use these products.

Precautions: Antivirals should be used with caution in renal disease, liver disease, lactation, pregnancy, and dehydration.

Pharmacokinetics: Onset, peak, and duration vary widely among products. Most products are metabolized in the liver and excreted in urine.

Interactions/incompatibilities: Please check individual monographs since interactions vary widely among products.

Possible nursing diagnoses:
• High risk for infection *[uses]*
• High risk for injury *[adverse reactions]*
• Knowledge deficit *[teaching]*

NURSING CONSIDERATIONS
Assess:
• Signs of infection, anemia
• I&O ratio; report hematuria, oliguria, fatigue, weakness; may indicate nephrotoxicity; check for protein in urine during treatment

• Any patient with compromised renal system, since drug is excreted slowly in poor renal system function; toxicity may occur rapidly
• Liver studies: AST, ALT
• Blood studies: WBC, RBC, Hct, Hgb, bleeding time; blood dyscrasias may occur; drug should be discontinued
• Renal studies: urinalysis, protein, BUN, creatinine, CrCl
• C&S before drug therapy; drug may be taken as soon as culture is taken; repeat C&S after treatment

Administer:
• Increased fluids to 3 L/day to decrease crystalluria when given IV

Perform/provide:
• Storage at room temperature for up to 12 hr after reconstitution
• Adequate intake of fluids (2000 ml) to prevent deposit in kidneys

Evaluate:
• Therapeutic response: absence of control of infection
• Bowel pattern before, during treatment; if severe abdominal pain with bleeding occurs, drug should be discontinued
• Skin eruptions: rash, urticaria, itching
• Allergies before treatment, reaction of each medication; place allergies on chart, Kardex in bright red letters

Teach patient/family:
• That drug does not cure infection, just controls symptoms
• To report sore throat, fever, fatigue; could indicate superimposed infection
• That drug must be taken in equal intervals around the clock to maintain blood levels for duration of therapy
• To notify physician of side effects of bruising, bleeding, fatigue, malaise; may indicate blood dyscrasias

---

Generic names:

acyclovir sodium (p. 81)
amantadine HCl (p. 98)
didanosine (p. 376)
foscarnet sodium (p. 504)
ganciclovir (p. 512)
rimantadine (p. 944)
vidarabine (p. 1089)
zalcitabine (p. 1099)
zidovudine (p. 1100)

BARBITURATES

Action: Barbiturates act by decreasing impulse transmission to the cerebral cortex.

Uses: All forms of epilepsy can be controlled, since the seizure threshold is increased. Uses also include febrile seizures in children, sedation, insomnia, hyperbilirubinemia, chronic cholestasis with some of these products. Ultra-short acting barbiturates are used as anesthetics.

Side effects/adverse reactions: The most common side effects are drowsiness and nausea. Serious adverse reactions such as Stevens-Johnson syndrome and blood dyscrasias may occur with high doses and long-term treatment.

Contraindications: Hypersensitivity may occur, and allergies should be identified before administering. Barbiturates are identified as pregnancy category (D) and should not be used in pregnancy. Other contraindications include porphyria and marked impairment of liver function.

Precautions: Caution must be used when these products are given to the elderly or debilitated; usually smaller doses are needed, since metabolism is slowed. Persons with renal and hepatic disease may show delayed excretion. Barbiturates may produce excitability in children.

Pharmacokinetics: Onset of action can be slow, up to 1 hr, with a peak of 8 hr and a duration of 3-10 hr. These drugs are metabolized by the liver, excreted by the kidneys, cross the placenta, and enter breast milk.

Drug interactions/incompatibilities: Increased CNS depressant effect may occur with alcohol, MAOIs, sedatives, or narcotics. These products should be used together cautiously. Oral anticoagulants, corticosteroids, griseofulvin, quinidine, oral contraceptives, and theophylline may show a decreased effect when used with barbiturates.

Possible nursing diagnoses:
• Sleep pattern disturbance *[uses]*
• High risk for injury *[adverse reactions]*

NURSING CONSIDERATIONS

Assess:
• Hepatic and renal studies: AST, ALT, bilirubin, creatinine, LDH, alkaline phosphatase, BUN if patient is on long-term therapy, since these products are metabolized and excreted by the liver and kidney
• Blood studies: CBC, hematocrit, hemoglobin, and prothrombin time if patient is on long-term therapy, since these products increase the possibility of bleeding and blood dyscrasias

Evaluate:
• Therapeutic response, including appropriate sedation or seizure control

• Barbiturate toxicity: hypotension, pulmonary constriction; cold, clammy skin; cyanosis of lips; insomnia; nausea; vomiting, hallucinations, delirium, weakness

Teach patient/family:

• That physical dependency may result when used for extended periods of time (45-90 days, depending on dose)

• To avoid driving and activities that require alertness, since drowsiness and dizziness may occur

• To abstain from alcohol or other psychotropic medications unless prescribed by physician

• Not to discontinue medication abruptly after long-term use; withdrawal symptoms will occur

---

Generic names:

amobarbital (p. 117)   secobarbital (p. 952)
mephobarbital (p. 676)   talbutal (p. 992)
pentobarbital (p. 835)   thiopental (p. 1018)
phenobarbital (p. 848)

BENZODIAZEPINES

Action: Benzodiazepines potentiate the effects of γ-aminobutyrate (GABA), including any other inhibitory transmitters in the CNS, resulting in decreased anxiety.

Uses: Anxiety is relieved in conditions such as phobic disorders. Benzodiazepines are also used for acute alcohol withdrawal to relieve the possibility of delirium tremens, and some products are used before surgery for relaxation.

Side effects/adverse reactions: The most common side effects are dizziness, drowsiness, blurred vision, and orthostatic hypotension. Most adverse effects are mediated through the CNS. There is a risk for physicial dependence and abuse.

Contraindications: Hypersensitivity, acute narrow-angle glaucoma, children <6 months, liver disease (clonazepam), lactation (diazepam).

Precautions: Caution must be used when these products are given to the elderly or debilitated; usually smaller doses are needed, since metabolism is slowed. Persons with renal and hepatic disease may show delayed excretion. Clonazepam may increase incidence of seizures.

Pharmacokinetics: Onset of action is ½-1 hr, with a peak of 1-2 hr and a duration of 4-6 hr. These drugs are metabolized by the liver, excreted by the kidneys, cross the placenta, and enter breast milk.

Drug interactions/incompatibilities: Increased CNS depressant effect may occur with other CNS depressants. These products should be used together cautiously. Alcohol should not be used; fatal reactions can occur. The serum concentration and toxicity of digoxin may be increased.

Possible nursing diagnoses:
• Anxiety *[uses]*
• High risk for injury *[adverse reactions]*

NURSING CONSIDERATIONS
Assess:
• B/P (lying, standing), pulse; if systolic B/P drops 20 mm Hg, hold drug, notify physician; orthostatic hypotension is severe
• Hepatic and renal studies: AST, ALT, bilirubin, creatinine, LDH, alkaline phosphatase

Administer:
• With food or milk for GI symptoms; may give crushed if patient is unable to swallow medication whole

Evaluate:
• Therapeutic response, including relaxation or decreased anxiety
• Physical dependency, withdrawal symptoms, including headache, nausea, vomiting, muscle pain, weakness after long-term use

Teach patient/family:
• That drug should not be used for everyday stress or long-term; not to take more than prescribed amount, since drug is habit forming
• To avoid driving and activities that require alertness, since drowsiness and dizziness occur
• To abstain from alcohol or other psychotropic medications unless prescribed by physician
• Not to discontinue medication abruptly after long-term use; withdrawal symptoms will occur

---

Generic names:

alprazolam (p. 91)
chlordiazepoxide HCl (p. 265)
clonazepam (p. 306)
diazepam (p. 368)
flurazepam (p. 501)
halazepam (p. 533)
lorazepam (p. 642)

midazolam (p. 727)
oxazepam (p. 798)
prazepam (p. 887)
quazepam (p. 927)
temazepam (p. 995)
triazolam (p. 1054)

BETA-ADRENERGIC BLOCKERS

Action: Beta blockers are divided into selective and nonselective blockers. Nonselective blockers produce a fall in blood pressure without reflex tachycardia or reduction in heart rate through a mixture of beta blocking effects; elevated plasma renins are reduced. Selective beta blockers competitively block stimulation of β-1 receptors in cardiac smooth muscle; these drugs produce chronotropic and inotropic effects.

Uses: Beta blockers are used for hypertension, ventricular dysrhythmias, and prophylaxis of angina pectoris.

Side effects/adverse reactions: The most common side effects are orthostatic hypotension, bradycardia, diarrhea, nausea, vomiting. Serious adverse reactions include blood dyscrasias, bronchospasm, and CHF.

Contraindications: Hypersensitive reactions may occur, and allergies should be identified before these products are given. β-adrenergic blockers should not be used in heart block, CHF, or cardiogenic shock.

Precautions: Beta blockers should be used with caution in the elderly or in renal and thyroid disease, COPD, CAD, diabetes mellitus, pregnancy, or asthma.

Pharmacokinetics: Onset, peak, and duration vary widely among products. Most products are metabolized in the liver, with metabolites excreted in urine, bile, and feces.

Interactions/incompatibilities: Interactions vary widely among products; check individual monograph for specific information.

Possible nursing diagnoses:
- Altered tissue perfusion *[uses]*
- Decreased cardiac output *[uses]*
- Diarrhea *[adverse reactions]*
- Impaired gas exchange *[adverse reactions]*

NURSING CONSIDERATIONS

Assess:
- Renal studies, including protein, BUN, creatinine; watch for increased levels that may indicate nephrotic syndrome; obtain baselines in renal and liver function studies before beginning treatment
- I&O, weight daily
- B/P during beginning treatment and periodically thereafter, pulse q4h, note rate, rhythm, quality
- Apical/radial pulse before administration; notify physician of significant changes

Administer:
- PO ac, hs, tablets may be crushed or swallowed whole
- Reduced dosage in renal dysfunction

Evaluate:
• Therapeutic response, including decrease in B/P in hypertension, decreased B/P, edema, moist rales in CHF
• Edema in feet and legs daily

Teach patient/family:
• To comply with dosage schedule, even if feeling better
• To rise slowly to sitting or standing position to minimize orthostatic hypotension
• To report bradycardia, dizziness, confusion, depression, fever
• To take pulse at home; advise when to notify physician
• To comply with weight control, dietary adjustment, modified exercise program
• To wear support hose to minimize effects of orthostatic hypotension
• Not to discontinue drug abruptly; taper over 2 wk; may precipitate angina

---

Generic names:

Selective β-1 receptor blockers:
acebutolol (p. 69)
atenolol (p. 144)
esmolol (p. 438)
metoprolol (p. 717)

nadolol (p. 746)
pindolol (p. 865)
propranolol (p. 914)
timolol maleate (p. 1032)

Nonselective β-1 and β-2 blockers: carteolol (p. 221)

Combined α-1, β-1, and β-2 receptor blocker: labetalol (p. 614)

BRONCHODILATORS

Action: Bronchodilators are divided into anticholinergics, α/β-adrenergics agonists, β-adrenergic agonist, and phosphodiesterase inhibitors. Anticholinergics act by inhibiting interaction of acetylcholine at receptor sites on bronchial smooth muscle; α/β-adrenergic agonist by relaxing bronchial smooth muscle and increasing diameter of nasal passages; β-adrenergic agonists by action on β-2 receptors, which relaxes bronchial smooth muscle; phosphodiesterase inhibitors by blocking phosphodiesterase increase cAMP, which mediates smooth muscle relaxation in the respiratory system.

Uses: Bronchodilators are used for bronchial asthma, bronchospasm associated with bronchitis, emphysema, or other obstructive pulmonary diseases, Cheyne-Stokes respirations, prevention of exercise-induced asthma.

Side effects/adverse reactions: The most common side effects are tremors, anxiety, nausea, vomiting, and irritation in throat. The most serious adverse reactions include bronchospasm and dyspnea.

Contraindications: Persons with hypersensitivity, narrow-angle glaucoma, tachydysrhythmias, and severe cardiac disease should not use some of these products.

Precautions: Bronchodilators should be used with caution in lactation, pregnancy, hyperthyroidism, hypertension, prostatic hypertrophy, and seizure disorders.

Pharmacokinetics: Onset, peak, and duration vary widely among products. Most products are metabolized in the liver and excreted in urine.

Interactions/incompatibilities: Please check individual monographs since interactions vary widely among products.

Possible nursing diagnoses:
• Ineffective airway clearance *[uses]*
• Activity intolerance *[uses]*
• High risk for injury *[adverse reactions]*
• Knowledge deficit *[teaching]*

NURSING CONSIDERATIONS

Assess:
• Respiratory function: vital capacity, forced expiratory volume, ABGs, lung sounds, heart rate and rhythm

Administer:
• After shaking, exhale, place mouthpiece in mouth, inhale slowly, hold breath, remove, exhale slowly
• Gum, sips of water for dry mouth
• PO with meals to decrease gastric irritation

Perform/provide:
• Storage in light-resistant container, do not expose to temperatures over 86° F

Evaluate:
• Therapeutic response: absence of dyspnea, wheezing

Teach patient/family:
• Not to use OTC medications, extra stimulation may occur
• Use of inhaler, review package insert with patient
• To avoid getting aerosol in eyes
• To wash inhaler in warm water qd and dry
• To avoid smoking, smoke-filled rooms, persons with respiratory infections

Generic names:

albuterol (p. 84)
aminophylline (p. 109)
atropine sulfate (p. 147)
bitolterol mesylate (p. 185)
dyphylline (p. 416)
ephedrine sulfate (p. 426)
epinephrine (p. 428)
epinephrine bitartrate (p. 428)
epinephrine HCl (p. 429)
ethylnorepinephrine HCl (p. 458)
ipratropium bromide (p. 593)

isoetharine HCl (p. 597)
isoetharine mesylate (p. 597)
isoproterenol (p. 600)
metaproterenol (p. 684)
oxtriphylline (p. 799)
pirbuterol acetate (p. 872)
terbutaline sulfate (p. 999)
theophylline (p. 1013)
theophylline sodium glycinate
(p. 1013)

CALCIUM-CHANNEL BLOCKERS

Action: These products act by inhibiting calcium ion influx across the cell membrane in cardiac and vascular smooth muscle. This action produces relaxation of coronary vascular smooth muscle, dilates coronary arteries, slows SA/AV node conduction, and dilates peripheral arteries.

Uses: These products are used for chronic stable angina pectoris, vasospastic angina, dysrhythmias, hypertension, and unstable angina.

Side effects/adverse reactions: The most common side effects are dysrhythmias and edema. Also common are headache, fatigue, drowsiness, and flushing.

Contraindications: Persons with 2nd or 3rd degree heart block, sick sinus syndrome, hypotension of <90 mm Hg systolic, Wolff-Parkinson-White syndrome or cardiogenic shock should not use these products, since worsening of those conditions may occur.

Precautions: CHF may worsen, since edema may be increased. Hypotension may worsen, since B/P is decreased. Patients with renal and liver disease should use these products cautiously, since they are metabolized in the liver and excreted by the kidneys.

Pharmacokinetics: Onset, peak, and duration vary widely with route of administration. Drugs are metabolized by the liver and excreted in the urine primarily as metabolites.

Interactions/incompatibilities: Increased levels of digoxin and theophylline may occur when used with these products. Increased effects of beta blockers and antihypertensives may occur with calcium channel blockers.

Possible nursing diagnoses:
• Altered tissue perfusion: cardiopulmonary [uses]
• Decreased cardiac output [adverse reactions]

NURSING CONSIDERATIONS

Assess:
• Cardiac system, including B/P, pulse, respirations, ECG intervals (PR, QRS, QT)

Administer:
• PO before meals and hs

Evaluate:
• Therapeutic response, including decreased anginal pain, decreased B/P, dysrhythmias

Teach patient/family:
• How to take pulse before taking drug; patient should record or graph pulses to identify changes
• To avoid hazardous activities until stabilized on this drug, since dizziness occurs frequently
• Need for compliance to all areas of medical regimen, including diet, exercise, stress reduction, drug therapy

---

Generic names:

diltiazem (p. 390)
felodipine (p. 470)
nicardipine (p. 767)

nifedipine (p. 771)
verapamil HCl (p. 1087)

CARDIAC GLYCOSIDES

Action: Products act by inhibiting sodium and potassium ATPase and then making more calcium available to activate contracted proteins. Cardiac contractility and cardiac output are increased.

Uses: These products are used for CHF, atrial fibrillation, atrial flutter, atrial tachycardia, and rapid digitalization in these disorders.

Side effects/adverse reactions: The most common side effects are cardiac disturbances, headache, hypotension, GI symptoms. Also common are blurred vision and yellow-green halos.

Contraindications: Hypersensitive reactions may occur, and allergies should be identified before these products are given. Also, persons with ventricular tachycardia, ventricular fibrillation, and carotid sinus syndrome should not use these products.

Precautions: Persons with acute MI and those who have or may develop serum potassium, calcium, or magnesium imbalances should use these products cautiously. Also, persons with AV block, severe respiratory disease, hypothyroidism, renal and liver disease, and the elderly should exercise caution when these drugs are prescribed.

Pharmacokinetics: Onset, peak, and duration vary widely with the route of administration. Digitoxin is inactivated by the liver, and inactive metabolites are excreted in urine. Digoxin is excreted in urine mainly as the parent drug and metabolites.

Interactions/incompatibilities: Toxicity may occur when used with diuretics, succinylcholine, quinidine, and thioamines. Increased blood levels may occur with propantheline bromide, spironolactone, quinidine, verapamil, aminoglycosides (PO), amiodarone, anticholinergics, and quinine. Diuretics may increase toxicity.

Possible nursing diagnoses:
• Altered tissue perfusion: cardiopulmonary *[uses]*
• Decreased cardiac output *[adverse reactions]*

NURSING CONSIDERATIONS
Assess:
• Cardiac system, including B/P, pulse, respirations, and increased urine output
• Apical pulse for 1 min before giving drug; if pulse <60, take again in 1 hr; if <60 notify physician
• Electrolytes, including potassium, sodium, chloride, calcium, magnesium; renal function studies, including BUN and creatinine; and blood studies, including AST, ALT, bilirubin
• I&O ratio, daily weights
• Monitor therapeutic drug levels
Administer:
• Potassium supplements if ordered for potassium levels <3.0
Evaluate:
• Therapeutic response, including decreased weight, edema, pulse, respiration, and increased urine output
Teach patient/family:
• How to take pulse before taking drug; patient should record or graph pulse to identify changes
• To avoid hazardous activities until stabilized on this drug, since dizziness occurs frequently
• Need for compliance to all areas of medical regimen, including diet, exercise, stress reduction, drug therapy

---

Generic names:

digitoxin (p. 384)   digoxin (p. 385)

CHOLINERGICS

Action: Cholinergics act by preventing destruction of acetylcholine, which increases concentration at sites where acetylcholine is released; this exaggerates the effects of acetylcholine and facilitates transmission of impulses across myoneural junction. Cholinergics may also act by stimulating receptors for acetylcholine.

Uses: Cholinergics are used for myasthenia gravis, as antagonists of nondepolarizing neuromuscular blockade, postoperative bladder distention and urinary distention, postoperative ileus.

Side effects/adverse reactions: The most serious adverse reactions are respiratory depression, bronchospasm, constriction, laryngospasm, respiratory arrest, convulsions, and paralysis. The most common side effects are nausea, diarrhea, and vomiting.

Contraindications: Persons with obstruction of the intestine or renal system should not use these products.

Precautions: Caution should be used in patients with bradycardia, hypotension, seizure disorders, bronchial asthma, coronary occlusion, hyperthyroidism, lactation, and children.

Pharmacokinetics: Onset, peak, and duration vary widely among products. Most products are metabolized in the liver and excreted in urine.

Interactions/incompatibilities: Please check individual monographs since interactions vary widely among products.

Possible nursing diagnoses:

• Altered urinary elimination *[uses]*
• Ineffective breathing pattern *[uses]*
• Knowledge deficit *[teaching]*
• Noncompliance *[teaching]*

NURSING CONSIDERATIONS

Assess:

• VS, respiration q8h
• I&O ratio; check for urinary retention of incontinence

Administer:

• Only with atropine sulfate available for cholinergic crisis
• Only after all other cholinergics have been discontinued
• Increased doses if tolerance occurs
• Larger doses after exercise or fatigue
• On empty stomach for better absorption

Perform/provide:

• Storage at room temperature

Evaluate:

• Therapeutic response: increased muscle strength, hand grasp, improved muscle gait, absence of labored breathing (if severe)
• Bradycardia, hypotension, bronchospasm, headache, dizziness, convulsions, respiratory depression; drug should be discontinued if toxicity occurs

Teach patient/family:

• That drug is not a cure; it only relieves symptoms (myasthenia gravis)
• To wear Medic Alert ID specifying myasthenia gravis, drugs taken

---

Generic names:

ambenonium chloride (p. 100)
bethanechol chloride (p. 179)
edrophonium chloride (p. 421)
neostigmine bromide (p. 762)

neostigmine methylsulfate (p. 762)
physostigmine salicylate (p. 861)
pyridostigmine bromide (p. 924)

CHOLINERGIC BLOCKERS

Action: Cholinergic blockers inhibit or block acetylcholine at receptor sites in the autonomic nervous system.

Uses: Many products are used to decrease secretions before surgery, to reverse neuromuscular blockade, and to decrease motility of GI, biliary, urinary tracts. Other products are used for parkinsonian symptoms, including dystonia associated with neuroleptic drugs.

Side effects/adverse reactions: The most common side effects are dryness of the mouth and constipation, which can be prevented by frequent rinsing of the mouth and increasing water and bulk in the diet.

Contraindications: Hypersensitivity can occur, and allergies should be identified before administering these products. Persons with GI and GU obstruction should not use these products, since constipation and urinary retention may occur. They are also contraindicated in angle-closure glaucoma and myasthenia gravis.

Precautions: Caution must be used when these products are given to the elderly, since metabolism is slowed. Also, persons with tachycardia or prostatic hypertrophy should use these products with caution.

Pharmacokinetics: Onset, peak, and duration vary with route.

Drug interactions/incompatibilities: Increase in anticholinergic effect occurs when used with narcotics, barbiturates, antihistamines, MAOIs, phenothiazines, amantadine.

Possible nursing diagnoses:

• Impaired physical mobility [uses]
• Pain [uses]

NURSING CONSIDERATIONS
Assess:
• I&O ratio; be alert for urinary retention, frequency, dysuria; drug should be discontinued if these occur
Administer:
• With food or milk to decrease GI symptoms
• Parenteral dose with patient recumbent to prevent postural hypotension; give parenteral dose slowly, monitoring vital signs
Perform/provide:
• Hard candy, gum, frequent rinsing of mouth for dryness
Evaluate:
• Therapeutic response, including absence of cramps, absence of extra-pyramidal symptoms
• Urinary hesitancy, retention; palpate bladder if retention occurs
• Constipation; increase fluids, bulk, exercise
• For tolerance over long-term therapy, dose may need to be increased or changed
• Mental status: affect, mood, CNS depression, worsening of mental symptoms during early therapy
Teach patient/family:
• To avoid driving or other hazardous activity if drowsiness occurs
• To avoid concurrent use of cough, cold preparations with alcohol, antihistamines unless directed by physician
• To use with caution in hot weather, since medication may increase susceptibility to heat stroke

---

Generic names:
atropine sulfate (p. 147)
benztropine mesylate (p. 172)
biperiden HCl (p. 180)
biperiden lactate (p. 180)
glycopyrrolate (p. 523)

procyclidine HCl (p. 903)
scopolamine hydrobromide (p. 950)
trihexyphenidyl HCl (p. 1061)

CORTICOSTEROIDS

Action: Corticosteroids are divided into glucocorticoids and mineralocorticoids. Glucocorticoids decrease inflammation by the suppression of migration of polymorphonuclear leukocytes, fibroblasts, increased capillary permeability, and lysosomal stabilization. They also have varied metabolic effects and modify the body's immune responses to many

different stimuli. Mineralocorticoids act by increasing resorption of sodium by increasing hydrogen and potassium excretion in the distal tubule.
Uses: Glucocorticoids are used to decrease inflammation and for immunosuppression. In addition, some products may be given for allergy, adrenal insufficiency, or cerebral edema. Mineralocorticoids are given for adrenal insufficiency or adrenogenital syndrome.

Side effects/adverse reactions: The most common side effects include change in behavior, including insomnia and euphoria; GI irritation, including peptic ulcer; metabolic reactions, including hypokalemia, hyperglycemia, and carbohydrate intolerance; and sodium and fluid retention. Most adverse reactions are dose dependent.

Contraindications: Hypersensitivity may occur and should be identified before administering. Since these products mask infection, they should not be used in systemic fungal infections or amebiasis. Mothers taking pharmacologic doses of corticosteroids should not nurse.

Precautions: Caution must be used when these products are prescribed for diabetic patients, since hyperglycemia may occur. Also, patients with glaucoma, seizure disorders, peptic ulcer, impaired renal function, CHF, hypertension, ulcerative colitis, or myasthenia gravis should be monitored closely if corticosteroids are given. Use with caution in children and the elderly and during pregnancy.

Pharmacokinetics: For oral preparations the onset of action occurs between 1-2 hr, and duration can be up to 2 days, with a half-life of 2-4 days. Pharmacokinetics vary widely among products. These products cross the placenta and appear in breast milk.

Drug interactions/incompatibilities: Decreased corticosteroid effect may occur with barbiturates, rifampin, phenytoin; corticosteroid dose may need to be increased. There is a possibility of GI bleeding when used with salicylates, indomethacin. Steroids may reduce salicylate levels. When using with digitalis glycosides, potassium-depleting diuretics, and amphotericin, serum potassium levels should be monitored.

Possible nursing diagnoses:
- High risk for infection [adverse reactions]
- Body-image disturbance [adverse reactions]
- High risk for violence: self-directed (suicide) [adverse reactions]

NURSING CONSIDERATIONS
Assess:
- Potassium, blood sugar, urine glucose while on long-term therapy; hypokalemia and hyperglycemia are common
- Weight daily; notify physician if weekly gain of >5 lb, since these products alter fluid and electrolyte balance

- I&O ratio; be alert for decreasing urinary output and increasing edema
- Plasma cortisol levels during long-term therapy (normal level is 138-635 nmol/L SI U when drawn at 8 AM
- Infection, including increased temperature, WBC, even after withdrawal of medication; drug masks symptoms of infection
- Adrenal insufficiency: nausea, anorexia, fatigue, dizziness, dyspnea, weakness, joint pain

Administer:
- With food or milk to decrease GI symptoms

Evaluate:
- Therapeutic response, including decreased inflammation
- Potassium depletion, including paresthesias, fatigue, nausea, vomiting, depression, polyuria, dysrhythmias, weakness
- Mental status, including affect, mood, behavioral changes, aggression; if severe personality changes occur, including depression, drug may need to be tapered and then discontinued

Teach patient/family:
- That ID as steroid user should be carried
- Not to discontinue this medication abruptly or adrenal crisis can result
- Teach patient all aspects of drug use, including cushingoid symptoms
- That single daily or alternate-day doses should be taken in the morning before 9 AM (for replacement therapy)
- To take with meals or a snack

Generic names:

Glucocorticoids: beclomethasone
dipropionate (p. 164)
betamethasone (p. 176)
betamethasone benzoate (p. 178)
betamethasone disodium
phosphate (p. 176)
betamethasone sodium phosphate
(p. 176)
cortisone acetate (p. 320)
dexamethasone (p. 355)
dexamethasone acetate (p. 355)
dexamethasone sodium phosphate
(p. 355)
flunisolide (p. 489)
hydrocortisone (p. 550)
hydrocortisone acetate (p. 550)
hydrocortisone sodium phosphate
(p. 552)
hydrocortisone sodium succinate
(p. 552)
methylprednisolone (p. 708)
methylprednisolone acetate
(p. 708)
methylprednisolone sodium
succinate (p. 708)
paramethasone acetate (p. 818)
prednisolone (p. 890)
prednisolone acetate (p. 890)
prednisolone phosphate (p. 890)
prednisolone sodium phosphate
(p. 892)
prednisolone tebutate (p. 890)
prednisone (p. 893)
triamcinolone (p. 1050)
triamcinolone acetonide (p. 1050)

triamcinolone diacetate (p. 1050)
triamcinolone hexacetonide
(p. 1050)

Mineralocorticoid: fludrocortisone
acetate (p. 487)

DIURETICS

Action: Diuretics are divided into subgroups: thiazides and thiazide-like diuretics, loop diuretics, carbonic anhydrase inhibitors, osmotic diuretics, and potassium-sparing diuretics. Each one of these subgroups differs in its mechanism of action. Thiazides and thiazide-like diuretics increase excretion of water and sodium by inhibiting resorption in the early distal tubule. Loop diuretics inhibit resorption of sodium and chloride in the thick ascending limb of the loop of Henle. Carbonic anhydrase inhibitors increase sodium excretion by decreasing sodium–hydrogen ion exchange throughout the renal tubule. Carbonic anhydrase inhibitors also decrease secretion of aqueous humor in the eye and thus decrease intraocular pressure. Osmotic diuretics increase the osmotic pressure of glomerular filtrate, thus decreasing net absorption of sodium. The potassium-sparing diuretics interfere with sodium resorption at the distal tubule, thus decreasing potassium excretion.

Uses: Blood pressure is reduced in hypertension; edema is reduced in CHF; intraocular pressure is decreased in glaucoma.

Side effects/adverse reactions: Hypokalemia, hyperuricemia, and hyperglycemia occur most frequently with thiazide diuretics. Aplastic anemia, blood dyscrasias, volume depletion, and dehydration may occur when thiazide-like diuretics, loop diuretics, or carbonic anhydrase inhibitors are given. Side effects and adverse reactions vary widely for the miscellaneous products.

Contraindications: Persons with electrolyte imbalances (sodium, chloride, potassium), dehydration, or anuria should not be given these products until the problem is corrected.

Precautions: Caution must be used when diuretics are given to the elderly, since electrolyte disturbances and dehydration can occur rapidly. Hepatic and renal disease may cause poor metabolism and excretion of the drug.

Pharmacokinetics: Onset, peak, and duration vary widely among the different subgroups of these drugs.

Interactions/incompatibilities: Cholestyramine and colestipol will decrease the absorption of thiazide diuretics. Concurrent use of thiazides with diazoxide may increase hyperuricemia, hyperglycemia, and antihypertensive effects of thiazides. Ototoxicity may occur when loop diuretics are used with aminoglycosides. Thiazide and loop diuretics may increase therapeutic and toxic effects of lithium.

Possible nursing diagnoses:
• Fluid volume excess *[uses]*
• Decreased cardiac output *[adverse reactions]*

NURSING CONSIDERATIONS

Assess:
• Weight, I&O daily to determine fluid loss; check skin turgor for dehydration
• Electrolytes: potassium, sodium, chloride: include BUN, blood sugar, CBC, serum creatinine, blood pH, ABGs, uric acid, calcium; electrolyte imbalances may occur quickly
• B/P lying, standing; postural hypotension may occur, since fluid loss occurs from intravascular spaces first

Administer:
• In AM to avoid interference with sleep if using drug as a diuretic
• Potassium replacement if potassium is less than 3.0

Evaluate:
• Therapeutic response: improvement in edema of feet, legs, sacral area daily if medication is being used in CHF; improvement in B/P if medication is being used as a diuretic; improvement in intraocular pressure if medication is being used to decrease aqueous humor in the eye
• Signs of metabolic alkalosis, including drowsiness and restlessness
• Signs of hypokalemia with some products, including postural hypotension, malaise, fatigue, tachycardia, leg cramps, weakness

Teach patient/family:
• To take drug early in the day (diuretic) to prevent nocturia

Generic names:

Thiazides: chlorothiazide (p. 269)
hydrochlorothiazide (p. 547)

Thiazide-like: chlorthalidone (p. 280)
indapamide (p. 573)
metolazone (p. 716)

Loop: bumetanide (p. 192)
ethacrynate acid (p. 449)
ethacrynate sodium (p. 449)
furosemide (p. 508)
torsemide (p. 1044)

Carbonic anhydrase inhibitors:
acetazolamide (p. 73)
acetazolamide sodium (p. 73)
methazolamide (p. 689)

Potassium-sparing: amiloride HCl (p. 103)
spironolactone (p. 970)
triamterene (p. 1053)

Osmotic: mannitol (p. 653)
urea (p. 1079)

HISTAMINE H₂ ANTAGONISTS

Action: Histamine (H_2) antagonists act by inhibiting histamine at H_2 receptor site in parietal cells, which inhibits gastric-acid secretion.

Uses: Histamine H_2 antagonists are used for short-term treatment of duodenal and gastric ulcers and maintenance therapy for duodenal ulcer; gastroesophageal reflux disease.

Side effects/adverse reactions: The most serious adverse reactions are agranulocytosis, thrombocytopenia, neutropenia, aplastic anemia, exfoliative dermatitis. The most common side effects are confusion (not with rantidine), headache and diarrhea.

Contraindications: Persons with hypersensitivity should not use these products.

Precautions: Caution should be used in pregnancy, lactation, child <16 yr, organic brain syndrome, hepatic disease, renal disease.

Pharmacokinetics: Onset, peak, and duration vary widely among products. Most products are metabolized in the liver and excreted in urine.

Interactions/incompatibilities: Antacids interfere with absorption of histamine (H_2) antagonists. Check individual monographs for other interactions.

Possible nursing diagnoses:
- Pain *[uses]*
- High risk for injury *[bleeding]*
- Knowledge deficit *[teaching]*

NURSING CONSIDERATIONS
Assess:
- Gastric pH (>5 should be maintained)
- I&O ratio, BUN, creatinine

Administer:
- With meals for prolonged drug effect
- Antacids 1 hr before or 1 hr after cimetidine
- IV slowly, bradycardia may occur, give over 30 min

Perform/provide:
- Storage of diluted solution at room temperature for up to 48 hr

Evaluate:
- Therapeutic response: decreased pain in abdomen

Teach patient/family:
- That gynecomastia, impotence may occur, but is reversible
- To avoid driving or other hazardous activities until patient is stabilized on this medication
- To avoid black pepper, caffeine, alcohol, harsh spices, extremes in temperature of food

- To avoid OTC preparations: aspirin, cough, cold preparations
- That drug must be continued for prescribed time to be effective
- To report bruising, fatigue, malaise; blood dyscrasias may occur

---

Generic names:

cimetidine (p. 287)   ranitidine (p. 938)
famotidine (p. 466)

IMMUNOSUPPRESSANTS

Action: Immunosuppressants act by producing immunosuppression by inhibiting lymphocytes (T).

Uses: Most products are used for organ transplants to prevent rejection.

Side effects/adverse reactions: The most serious adverse reactions are albuminuria, hematuria, proteinuria, renal failure, and hepatotoxicity. The most common side effects are oral *Candida*, gum hyperplasia, tremors, and headache. The most serious adverse reactions for azatheoprine are hematologic (leukopenia and thrombocytopenia) and GI (nausea and vomiting). There is a risk of secondary infection.

Contraindications: Products are contraindicated in hypersensitivity.

Precautions: Caution should be used in severe renal disease, severe hepatic disease, and pregnancy.

Pharmacokinetics: Onset, peak, and duration vary widely among products. Most products are metabolized in the liver and excreted in urine.

Interactions/incompatibilities: Please check individual monographs since interactions vary widely among products.

Possible nursing diagnoses:
- High risk for infection *[adverse reactions]*
- High risk for injury *[uses]*
- Knowledge deficit *[teaching]*

NURSING CONSIDERATIONS

Assess:
- Renal studies: BUN, creatinine at least monthly during treatment, 3 mo after treatment
- Liver function studies: alk phosphatase, AST, ALT, bilirubin
- Drug blood levels during treatment

Administer:
- For several days before transplant surgery
- With meals for GI upset or drug placed in chocolate milk
- With oral antifungal for *Candida* infections

Evaluate:
• Therapeutic response: absence of rejection
• Hepatotoxicity: dark urine, jaundice, itching, light-colored stools; drug should be discontinued

Teach patient/family:
• To report fever, chills, sore throat, fatigue since serious infections may occur
• To use contraceptive measures during treatment, for 12 wk after ending therapy

Generic names:

azathioprine (p. 154)   muromonab-CD3 (p. 744)
cyclosporine (p. 335)

LAXATIVES

Action: Laxatives are divided into bulk products, lubricants, osmotics, saline laxative stimulants, and stool softeners. Bulks work by absorbing water and expanding to increase moisture content and bulk in the stool. Lubricants increase water retention in the stool, causing reabsorption of water in the bowel. Stimulants act by increasing peristalsis by direct effect on the intestine. Saline draws water into the intestinal lumen. Osmotics results increase distention and promote peristalsis. Stool softeners reduce surface tension of liquids of the bowel.

Uses: Laxatives are used as a preparation for bowel, rectal examination, constipation, or stool softener.

Side effects/adverse reactions: The most common side effects are nausea, abdominal cramps, and diarrhea.

Contraindications: Persons with GI obstruction, perforation, gastric retention, toxic colitis, megacolon, abdominal pain, nausea, vomiting, and fecal impaction should not use these products.

Precautions: Caution should be used in rectal bleeding, large hemorrhoids, and anal excoriation.

Pharmacokinetics: Onset, peak, and duration vary among products.

Interactions/incompatibilities: Please check individual monographs since interactions vary widely among products.

Possible nursing diagnoses:
• Constipation [uses]
• Diarrhea [adverse reactions]
• Knowledge deficit [teaching]

NURSING CONSIDERATIONS

Assess:

• Blood, urine electrolytes if drug is used often by patient
• I&O ratio: to identify fluid loss

Administer:

• Alone only with water for better absorption; do not take within 1 hr of antacids, milk, or cimetidine

Evaluate:

• Therapeutic response: decrease in constipation
• Cause of constipation; identify whether fluids, bulk, or exercise is missing from lifestyle
• Cramping, rectal bleeding, nausea, vomiting; if these symptoms occur, drug should be discontinued

Teach patient/family:

• To swallow tabs whole; do not chew
• Not to use laxatives for long-term therapy; bowel tone will be lost
• That normal bowel movements do not always occur daily
• Not to use in presence of abdominal pain, nausea, vomiting
• To notify physician of abdominal pain, nausea, vomiting
• To notify physician if constipation is unrelieved or if symptoms of electrolyte imbalance occur: muscle cramps, pain, weakness, dizziness

---

Generic names:

Bulk laxative
   calcium polycarbophil (p. 208)
   methylcellulose (p. 703)
   psyllium (p. 920)

Lubricants
   mineral oil (p. 729)

Osmotic agents
   glycerin (p. 522)
   lactulose (p. 615)

Saline
   magnesium salts (p. 651)
   sodium phosphate (p. 963)
   sodium phosphate/biphosphate (p. 963)

Stimulants
   bisacodyl (p. 181)
   cascara (p. 222)
   castor oil (p. 223)
   phenolphthalein (p. 849)
   senna (p. 956)

Stool softeners
   docusate (p. 404)

NARCOTICS

Action: Narcotics act by depressing pain impulse transmission at the spinal cord level by interacting with opioid receptors. Products are divided into opiates and nonopiates.

Uses: Most products are used to control moderate-to-severe pain and are used before and after surgery.

Side effects/adverse reactions: GI symptoms, including nausea, vomiting, anorexia, constipation, and cramps are the most common side effects. Other common side effects include lightheadedness, dizziness, sedation. Serious adverse reactions such as respiratory depression, respiratory arrest, circulatory depression, and increased intracranial pressure may result, but are less common and usually dose dependent.

Contraindications: Hypersensitive reactions occur frequently. Check for sensitivity before administering. These drugs should not be used if narcotic addiction is suspected, and they are also contraindicated in acute bronchial asthma and upper airway obstruction.

Precautions: Caution must be used when these products are given to persons with an addictive personality, since the possibility of addiction is so great. Also, persons with increased intracranial pressure may experience an even greater increase in intracranial pressure. Persons with severe heart disease, hepatic or renal disease, respiratory conditions, and seizure disorders should be monitored closely for worsening condition.

Pharmacokinetics: Onset of action is immediate by IV route and rapid by IM and PO routes. Peak occurs from 1-2 hr, depending on route, with a duration of 2-8 hr. These agents cross the placenta and appear in breast milk.

Drug interactions/incompatibilities: Barbiturates, other narcotics, hypnotics, antipsychotics, or alcohol can increase CNS depression when taken with narcotics.

Possible nursing diagnoses:
• Pain *[uses]*
• Impaired gas exchange *[adverse reactions]*

NURSING CONSIDERATIONS
Assess:
• I&O ratio; be alert for urinary retention, frequency, dysuria; drug should be discontinued if these occur

Administer:
• With antiemetic if nausea or vomiting occurs
• When pain is beginning to return; determine dosage interval by patient response

Perform/provide:
• Assistance with ambulation; patient should not be ambulating during drug peak

Evaluate:
• Therapeutic response, including decrease in pain
• Respiratory dysfunction, including respiratory depression, rate, rhythm, character; notify physician if respirations are <12/min
• CNS changes: dizziness, drowsiness, hallucinations, euphoria, LOC, pupil reaction
• Allergic reactions: rash, urticaria
• Need for pain medication, physical dependence

Teach patient/family:
• To report any symptoms of CNS changes, allergic reactions, or shortness of breath
• That physical dependency may result when used for extended periods of time
• That withdrawal symptoms may occur, including nausea, vomiting, cramps, fever, faintness, anorexia
• To avoid alcohol and other CNS depressants

Generic names:

alfentanil HCl (p. 88)
buprenorphine HCl (p. 194)
butorphanol tartrate (p. 199)
codeine phosphate (p. 315)
codeine sulfate (p. 315)
dezocine (p. 366)
fentanyl citrate (p. 473)
fentanyl transdermal (p. 475)
hydromorphone HCl (p. 554)
levorphanol tartrate (p. 622)

meperidine HCl (p. 673)
methadone HCl (p. 685)
morphine sulfate (p. 740)
nalbuphine HCl (p. 750)
oxycodone HCl (p. 801)
oxymorphone HCl (p. 805)
pentazocine HCl (p. 834)
pentazocine lactate (p. 834)
propoxyphene HCl (p. 913)
propoxyphene napsylate (p. 913)

NEUROMUSCULAR BLOCKING AGENTS

Action: Neuromuscular blocking agents are divided into depolarizing and nondepolarizing blockers. They act by inhibiting transmission of nerve impulses by binding with cholinergic receptor sites.

Uses: Neuromuscular blocking agents are used to facilitate endotracheal intubation and skeletal muscle relaxation during mechanical ventilation, surgery, or general anesthesia.

Side effects/adverse reactions: The most serious adverse reactions are prolonged apnea, bronchospasm, cyanosis, respiratory depression, and malignant hyperthermia. The most common side effects are bradycardia and decreased motility.

Contraindications: Persons that are hypersensitive should not be given this product.

Precautions: Caution should be used in pregnancy, thyroid disease, collagen disease, cardiac disease, lactation, children <2 yr, electrolyte imbalances, dehydration, neuromuscular disease (myasthenia gravis), and respiratory disease.

Pharmacokinetics: Onset, peak, and duration vary widely among products. Most products are metabolized in the liver and excreted in urine.

Interactions/incompatibilities: Aminoglycosides potentiate neuromuscular blockade. See individual monographs.

Possible nursing diagnoses:
- Ineffective breathing pattern *[uses]*
- High risk for injury *[adverse reactions]*
- Knowledge deficit *[teaching]*

NURSING CONSIDERATIONS
Assess:
- For electrolyte imbalances (K, Mg); may lead to increased action of this drug
- Vital signs (B/P, pulse, respirations, airway) q15min until fully recovered; rate, depth, pattern of respirations, strength of hand grip
- I&O ratio; check for urinary retention, frequency, hesitancy

Administer:
- Using nerve stimulator by anesthesiologist to determine neuromuscular blockade
- Anticholinesterase to reverse neuromuscular blockade
- IV undiluted over 1-2 min (only by qualified person, usually an anesthesiologist)

Perform/provide:
- Storage in light-resistant, cool area
- Reassurance if communication is difficult during recovery from neuromuscular blockade

Evaluate:
- Therapeutic response: paralysis of jaw, eyelid, head, neck, rest of body
- Recovery: decreased paralysis of face, diaphragm, leg, arm, rest of body
- Allergic reactions: rash, fever, respiratory distress, pruritus; drug should be discontinued

Generic names:

atracurium besylate (p. 146)

doxacurium chloride (p. 406)

gallamine triethiodide (p. 510)

metocurine iodide (p. 715)

mivacurium chloride (p. 737)

pancuronium bromide (p. 813)

pipecuronium bromide (p. 867)

succinylcholine chloride (p. 978)

tubocurarine chloride (p. 1076)

vecuronium bromide (p. 1086)

NONSTEROIDAL ANTIINFLAMMATORIES

Action: Nonsteroidals decrease prostaglandin synthesis by inhibiting an enzyme needed for biosynthesis.

Uses: Nonsteroidal antiinflammatories are used to treat mild to moderate pain, osteoarthritis, rheumatoid arthritis, and dysmenorrhea.

Side effects/adverse reactions: The most serious adverse reactions are nephrotoxicity (dysuria, hematuria, oliguria, azotemia), blood dyscrasias, and cholestatic hepatitis. The most common side effects are nausea, abdominal pain, anorexia, dizziness, and drowsiness.

Contraindications: Persons with hypersensitivity, asthma, severe renal disease, and severe hepatic disease should not use these products.

Precautions: Caution should be used in pregnancy, lactation, children, bleeding disorders, GI disorders, cardiac disorders, hypersensitivity to other antiinflammatory agents, and the elderly.

Pharmacokinetics: Onset, peak, and duration vary widely among products. Most products are metabolized in the liver and excreted in urine.

Interactions/incompatibilities: Please check individual monographs since interactions vary widely among products.

Possible nursing diagnoses:

• Chronic pain *[uses]*

• Impaired physical mobility *[uses]*

• Knowledge deficit *[teaching]*

• Noncompliance *[teaching]*

NURSING CONSIDERATIONS

Assess:

• Renal, liver, blood studies: BUN, creatinine, AST, ALT, Hgb, before treatment, periodically thereafter

• Audiometric, ophthalmic examination before, during, and after treatment

Administer:

• With food to decrease GI symptoms; however, best to take on empty stomach to facilitate absorption

Perform/provide:
- Storage at room temperature

Evaluate:
- Therapeutic response: decreased pain, stiffness in joints, decreased swelling in joints, ability to move more easily
- For eye, ear problems: blurred vision, tinnitus; may indicate toxicity

Teach patient/family:
- To report blurred vision, ringing, roaring in ears; may indicate toxicity
- To avoid driving, other hazardous activities if dizziness, drowsiness occurs, especially elderly
- To report change in urine pattern, increased weight, edema, increased pain in joints, fever, blood in urine; indicate nephrotoxicity
- That therapeutic effects may take up to 1 mo

Generic names:

diclofenac (p. 372)
etodolic acid (p. 461)
fenoprofen calcium (p. 472)
flurbiprofen sodium (p. 502)
ibuprofen (p. 565)
indomethacin (p. 575)
indomethacin sodium trihydrate (p. 575)
ketoprofen (p. 612)
ketorolac (p. 613)
meclofenamate (p. 663)

mefenamic acid (p. 666)
nabumetone (p. 745)
naproxen (p. 757)
naproxen sodium (p. 757)
oxyphenbutazone (p. 806)
phenylbutazone (p. 854)
piroxicam (p. 873)
sulindac (p. 989)
tolmetin sodium (p. 1043)

SALICYLATES

Action: Salicylates have analgesic, antipyretic, and antiinflammatory effects. The antiinflammatory and analgesic activities may be mediated through the inhibition of prostaglandin synthesis. Antipyretic action results from inhibition of the hypothalamic heat-regulating center.

Uses: The primary uses of salicylates are relief of mild-to-moderate pain and fever and in inflammatory conditions such as arthritis, thromboembolic disorders, and rheumatic fever.

Side effects/adverse reactions: The most common side effects are GI symptoms and rash. Serious blood dyscrasias and hepatotoxicity may result when used for long periods of time at high doses. Tinnitus or impaired hearing may indicate that blood salicylate levels are reaching or exceeding the upper limit of the therapeutic range.

Contraindications: Hypersensitivity to salicylates is common. Check for sensitivity before administering. Persons with bleeding disorders, GI bleeding, and vitamin K deficiency should not use these products, since salicylates increase prothrombin time. Children should not use these products, since salicylates have been associated with Reye's syndrome.

Precautions: Caution is needed when salicylates are given to patients with anemia, hepatic or renal disease, or Hodgkin's disease. Caution should also be exercised in pregnancy and lactation.

Pharmacokinetics: Onset of action occurs in 15-30 min, with a peak of 1-2 hr and a duration up to 6 hr. These drugs are metabolized by the liver and excreted by the kidneys.

Drug interactions/imcompatibilities: Increased effects of anticoagulants, insulin, methotrexate, heparin, valproic acid, and oral sulfonylureas may occur when used with salicylates. Aspirin may decrease serum concentrations of nonsteroidal antiinflammatory agents.

Possible nursing diagnoses:
- Pain [uses]
- Impaired physical mobility [uses]
- Activity intolerance [uses]
- Sensory/perceptual alteration: auditory [adverse reactions]
- Thermoregulation [uses]

NURSING CONSIDERATIONS

Assess:
- Hepatic and renal studies: AST, ALT, bilirubin, creatinine, LDH, alkaline phosphatase, BUN if patient is on long-term therapy, since these products are metabolized and excreted by the liver and kidney
- Blood studies: CBC, hematocrit, hemoglobin, and prothrombin time if patient is on long-term therapy, since these products increase the possibility of bleeding and blood dyscrasias

Administer:
- With food or milk to decrease gastric irritation; give 30 min before or 1 hr after meals with a full glass of water

Evaluate:
- Therapeutic response/including decreased pain, fever
- Hepatotoxicity: dark urine, clay-colored stools, yellowing of skin, sclera, itching, abdominal pain, fever, diarrhea, which may occur with long-term use
- Ototoxicity: tinnitus, ringing, roaring in ears; audiometric testing is needed before and after long-term therapy

Teach patient/family:
- That blood sugar levels should be monitored closely, if patient is diabetic

- Not to exceed recommended dosage; acute poisoning may result
- That therapeutic response takes 2 wk in arthritis
- To avoid use of alcohol, since GI bleeding may result
- To notify physician if ringing in the ears or persistent GI pain occurs
- To take with full glass of H_2O to reduce risk of lodging in esophagus

Generic names:

aspirin (p. 141)
choline salicylate (p. 283)

magnesium salicylate (p. 649)
salsalate (p. 947)
sodium thiosalicylate (p. 965)

THROMBOLYTICS

Action: Thrombolytics act by activating conversion of plasminogen to plasmin (fibrinolysin): plasmin is able to break down clots (fibrin).

Uses: Thrombolytics are used to treat deep vein thrombosis, pulmonary embolism, arterial thrombosis, arterial embolism arteriovenous cannula occlusion, lysis of coronary artery thrombi after MI, acute evolving transmural MI.

Side effects/adverse reactions: Serious adverse reactions include GI, GU, intracranial retroperitoneal bleeding, and anaphylaxis. The most common side effects are decreased Hct, urticaria, headache, and nausea.

Contraindications: Persons with hypersensitivity, active bleeding, intraspinal surgery, neoplasms of the CNS, ulcerative colitis/enteritis, severe hypertension, renal disease, hepatic disease, hypocoagulation, COPD, subacute bacterial endocarditis, rheumatic valvular disease, cerebral embolism/thrombosis/hemorrhage, intraarterial diagnostic procedure or surgery (10 days), and recent major surgery should not use these products.

Precautions: Caution should be used in arterial emboli from left side of heart and pregnancy.

Pharmacokinetics: Onset, peak, and duration vary widely among products. Most products are metabolized in the liver and excreted in urine.

Interactions/incompatibilities: Please check individual monographs since interactions vary widely among products.

Possible nursing diagnoses:

- High risk for injury [uses]

NURSING CONSIDERATIONS

Assess:

- VS, B/P, pulse, resp, neuro signs, temp at least q4h, temp <104° F are indicators of internal bleeding, cardiac rhythm following intracoronary administration; systolic pressure increase of >25 mm Hg should be reported to physician

• For neurologic changes that may indicate intracranial bleeding
• Retroperitoneal bleeding: back pain, leg weakness, diminished pulses

Administer:
• As soon as thrombi identified; not useful for thrombi over 1 wk old
• Cryoprecipitate or fresh, frozen plasma if bleeding occurs
• Loading dose at beginning of therapy may require increased loading doses
• Heparin after fibrinogen level is over 100 mg/dl. Heparin infusion to increase PTT to 1.5–2 × baseline for 3-7 days
• About 10% patients have high streptococcal antibody titers requiring increased loading doses
• IV therapy using 0.8 μm filter

Perform/provide:
• Storage of reconstituted in refrigerator; discard after 24 hr
• Bed rest during entire course of treatment
• Avoidance of venous or arterial puncture, inj, rectal temp
• Treatment of fever with acetaminophen or aspirin
• Pressure for 30 sec to minor bleeding sites; inform physician if this does not attain hemostasis; apply pressure dressing

Evaluate:
• Therapeutic response: resolution of thrombosis, embolism
• Allergy: fever, rash, itching, chill; mild reaction may be treated with antihistamines
• For bleeding during 1st hr of treatment: hematuria, hematemesis, bleeding from mucous membranes, epistaxis, ecchymosis
• Blood studies (Hct, platelets, PTT, PT, TT, APTT) before starting therapy; PT or APTT must be less than ×2 control before starting therapy TT or PT q3-4h during treatment

Generic names:
alteplase (p. 93)
anistreplase (p. 133)
streptokinase (p. 972)
urokinase (p. 1081)

THYROID HORMONES

Action: Acts by increasing metabolic rates, resulting in increased cardiac output, O_2 consumption, body temperature, blood volume, growth, development at cellular level, respiratory rate, enzyme system activity.

Uses: Products are used for thyroid replacement.

Side effects/adverse reactions: The most common side effects include insomnia, tremors, tachycardia, palpitations, angina, dysrhythmias, weight loss, and changes in appetite. Serious adverse reactions include thyroid storm.

Contraindications: Persons with adrenal insufficiency, myocardial infarction, or thyrotoxicosis should not use these products.

Precautions: The elderly and patients with angina pectoris, hypertension, ischemia, cardiac disease, or diabetes mellitus or insipidus should be watched closely when using these products. Caution should be used in pregnancy (A) and lactation.

Pharmacokinetics: Pharmacokinetics vary widely among products; check specific monographs.

Interactions/incompatibilities:
• Impaired absorption of thyroid products may occur when administered with cholestyramine (separate by 4-5 hr)
• Increased effects of anticoagulants, sympathomimetics, tricyclic antidepressants, catecholamines may occur
• Decreased effects of digitalis, glycosides, insulin, hypoglycemics may occur
• Decreased effects of thyroid products may occur with estrogens

Possible nursing diagnoses:
• Knowledge deficit
• Noncompliance
• Body image disturbance [adverse reactions]

NURSING CONSIDERATIONS
Assess:
• B/P, pulse before each dose
• I&O ratio
• Weight qd in same clothing, using same scale, at same time of day
• Height, growth rate if given to a child
• T3, T4, which are decreased; radioimmunoassay of TSH, which is increased; ratio uptake, which is decreased if patient is on too low a dosage of medication

Administer:
• At same time each day to maintain drug level

• Only for hormone imbalances, not to be used for obesity, male infertility, menstrual conditions, lethargy

Perform/provide:
• Removal of medication 4 wk before RAIU test

Evaluate:
• Therapeutic response: absence of depression; increased weight loss; diuresis; pulse; appetite; absence of constipation; peripheral edema; cold intolerance; pale, cool, dry skin; brittle nails; alopecia; coarse hair; menorrhagia; night blindness; paresthesias; syncope; stupor; coma; rosy cheeks
• Increased nervousness, excitability, irritability; may indicate too high doses of medication usually after 1-3 wk of treatment
• Cardiac status: angina, palpitation, chest pain, change in VS

Teach patient/family:
• That hair loss will occur in child and is temporary
• To report excitability, irritability, anxiety; indicates overdose
• Not to switch brands unless directed by physician
• That hypothyroid child will show almost immediate behavior/personality change
• That treatment drug is not to be taken to reduce weight
• To avoid OTC preparations with iodine; read labels
• To avoid iodine food, salt-iodinized, soy beans, tofu, turnips, some seafood, some bread

---

Generic names:

levothyroxine sodium (T_4) (p. 623)
liothyronine sodium (T_3) (p. 631)
liotrix (p. 632)

thyroglobulin (p. 1025)
thyroid USP (p. 1027)
thyrotropin (TSH) (p. 1028)

VASODILATORS

Action: Vasodilators act by various actions. Please check individual monograph for specific action.

Uses: Vasodilators are used to treat intermittent claudication, arteriosclerosis obliterans, vasospasm and muscular ischemia, ischemic cerebral vascular disease, hypertension, and angina.

Side effects/adverse reactions: The most common side effects are headache, nausea, hypotension or hypertension, and ECG changes.

Contraindications: Some drugs are contraindicated in acute MI, paroxysmal tachycardia, and thyrotoxicosis.

Precautions: Caution should be used in uncompensated heart disease or peptic ulcer disease.

Pharmacokinetics: Onset, peak, and duration vary widely among products. Most products are metabolized in the liver and excreted in urine.

Interactions/incompatibilities: Please check individual monographs since interactions vary widely among products.

Possible nursing diagnoses:
- Decreased cardiac output *[uses]*
- Altered tissue perfusion: cardiovascular/pulmonary *[uses]*
- Knowledge deficit *[teaching]*

NURSING CONSIDERATIONS

Assess:
- Bleeding time in individuals with bleeding disorders

Administer:
- With meals to reduce GI symptoms

Perform/provide:
- Storage in tight container at room temperature

Evaluate:
- Therapeutic response: ability to walk without pain, increased temperature in extremities, increased pulse volume
- Cardiac status: B/P, pulse, rate, rhythm, character; watch for increasing pulse

Teach patient/family:
- That medication is not cure, may need to be taken continuously
- That it is necessary to quit smoking to prevent excessive vasoconstriction
- That improvement may be sudden, but usually occurs gradually over several weeks
- To report headache, weakness, increased pulse, as drug may need to be decreased or discontinued
- To avoid hazardous activities until stabilized on medication; dizziness may occur

---

Generic names:

amyl nitrite (p. 132)
cyclandelate (p. 328)
dipyridamole (p. 399)
hydralazine HCl (p. 546)

isoxsuprine HCl (p. 604)
minoxidil (p. 731)
nylidrin HCl (p. 783)
papaverine HCl (p. 814)
tolazoline HCl (p. 1040)

VITAMINS

Action: Action varies widely among products and classes; check specific monographs.

Uses: Vitamins are used to correct and prevent vitamin deficiencies.

Side effects/adverse reactions: There is an absence of side effects or adverse reactions with the water-soluble vitamins (C, B). However, fat-soluble vitamins (A, D, E, K) may accumulate in the body and cause adverse reactions (refer to specific monographs).

Contraindications: Hypersensitive reactions may occur, and allergies should be identified before these products are given.

Pharmacokinetics: Onset, peak, and duration vary widely among products; check individual monograph for specific information.

Possible nursing diagnosis:
• Nutrition, less than body requirements *[uses]*

NURSING CONSIDERATIONS

Administer:
• PO with food for better absorption

Perform/provide:
• Storage in tight, light-resistant container

Evaluate:
• Therapeutic response

Teach patient/family:
• Not to take more than prescribed amount

Generic names:

Fat-soluble: phytonadione (p. 862)
vitamin A (p. 1093)
vitamin D (p. 1095)
vitamin E (p. 1096)
menadione/menadiol sodium diphosphate (vitamin K₃) (p. 670)

Water-soluble: ascorbic acid (C) (p. 138)

cyanocobalamin hydroxocobalimin (B₁₂) (p. 327)
pyridoxine (B₆) (p. 925)
riboflavin (B₂) (p. 941)
thiamine (B₁) (p. 1015)

Miscellaneous: multivitamins (p. 743)

absorbable gelatin
Gelfoam, Gelfilm, Gelfilm
Ophthalmic
Func. class.: Hemostatic
Chem. class.: Purified gelatin
solution

Action: Absorbs blood, provides
area for clot formation, healthy tissue growth

Uses: Hemostasis during surgery,
decubitus ulcers

Dosage and routes:
• *Adult:* TOP hold in place for 15
sec after saturating with isotonic
NaCl injection
Decubitus ulcer
• *Adult:* TOP place into ulcer, may
add more as needed, not to be re-
moved
Available forms: Sponge, pack,
cone, powder

Side effects/adverse reactions:
SYST: Sponge may form media for
infection and abscess

Contraindications: Hypersensitivity, frank infection, abnormal
bleeding, postpartum bleeding,
closure of skin incisions

Precautions: Blood dyscrasias

Pharmacokinetics:
IMPLANT: Absorbed in 4-6 wk

NURSING CONSIDERATIONS
Assess:
• Infection: fever, redness, inflam-
mation

Administer:
• By lightly packing; do not over-
pack foam
• Dry, hold for 10-15 sec, remove
• Moist, place in sterile saline or
thrombin solution, squeeze after removing, blot before applying
• After debridement of decubiti unless dressing change qd; do not remove sponge; may add more
sponges over top of old ones

Perform/provide:
• Discard unused portion; do not
resterilize

Evaluate:
• Therapeutic response: Control of
bleeding during surgery or healing
of decubitus ulcer

Teach patient/family:
• That foam is absorbed in 4-6 wk,
does not need to be removed

acebutolol
(ase-bute'-oh-lole)
Monitan,* Sectral
Func. class.: Antihypertensive
Chem. class.: Nonselective β-
blocker

Action: Competitively blocks stimulation of β-adrenergic receptor
within vascular smooth muscle;
produces chronotropic, inotropic
activity (decreases rate of SA node
discharge, increases recovery
time), slows conduction of AV
node, decreases heart rate, which
decreases O_2 consumption in myocardium; also decreases renin-aldosterone-angiotensin system at
high doses, inhibits β-2 receptors
in bronchial system (high doses)

Uses: Mild to moderate hypertension, sinus tachycardia, persistent
atrial extrasystoles, tachydysrhythmias, prophylaxis of angina pectoris

Dosage and routes:
Hypertension
• *Adult:* PO 400 mg qd or in 2 di-
vided doses, may be increased to
desired response
Ventricular dysrhythmia
• *Adult:* PO 200 mg bid, may in-
crease gradually, usual range 600-
1200 mg daily
Available forms: Caps 200, 400

mg, tabs 100, 200, 400 mg (Canada only)

Side effects/adverse reactions:
*CV: **Profound hypotension, bradycardia, CHF,** cold extremities, postural hypotension, **2nd or 3rd degree heart block***
CNS: Insomnia, fatigue, dizziness, mental changes, memory loss, hallucinations, depression, lethargy, drowsiness, strange dreams, catatonia
GI: Nausea, diarrhea, vomiting, ***mesenteric arterial thrombosis, ischemic colitis***
INTEG: Rash, fever, alopecia
*HEMA: **Agranulocytosis, thrombocytopenia, purpura***
EENT: Sore throat, dry burning eyes
GU: Impotence
ENDO: Increased hypoglycemic response to insulin
*RESP: **Bronchospasm,** dyspnea, wheezing*

Contraindications: Hypersensitivity to β-blockers, cardiogenic shock, heart block (2nd, 3rd degree), sinus bradycardia, CHF, cardiac failure

Precautions: Major surgery, pregnancy (B), lactation, diabetes mellitus, renal disease, thyroid disease, COPD, asthma, well-compensated heart failure, aortic, mitral valve disease

Pharmacokinetics:
PO: Onset 1-1½ hr. Peak 2-4 hr; duration 10-12 hr; half-life 6-7 hr, excreted unchanged in urine, protein binding 5%-15%

Interactions/incompatibilities:
• Increased hypotension, bradycardia: reserpine, hydralazine, methyldopa, prazosin, anticholinergics
• Decreased antihypertensive effects: indomethacin

• Increased hypoglycemic effect: insulin
• Decreased bronchodilation: theophyllines β₂ agonist

Lab test interferences:
Interference: Glucose/insulin tolerance tests
Increase: Uric acid, potassium, triglyceride, lipoproteins

NURSING CONSIDERATIONS
Assess:
• B/P during beginning treatment, periodically thereafter; pulse q4h; note rate, rhythm, quality
• Apical/radial pulse before administration; notify physician of any significant changes (pulse <50 bpm)
• Baselines in renal, liver function tests before therapy begins
• Edema in feet, legs daily: monitor I & O, daily weight
• Skin turgor, dryness of mucous membranes for hydration status, especially elderly

Administer:
• PO ac, hs, tablet may be crushed or swallowed whole; give with food to prevent GI upset
• Reduced dosage in renal dysfunction

Perform/provide:
• Storage protected from light, moisture; placed in cool environment

Evaluate:
• Therapeutic response: decreased B/P after 1-2 wk; decreased dysrhythmias

Teach patient/family:
• Not to discontinue drug abruptly, taper over 2 wk; may cause precipitate angina if stopped abruptly
• Not to use OTC products containing α-adrenergic stimulants (such as nasal decongestants, OTC cold preparations) unless directed by physician

- To report bradycardia, dizziness, confusion, depression, fever
- To take pulse at home, advise when to notify physician
- To avoid alcohol, smoking, sodium intake
- To comply with weight control, dietary adjustments, modified exercise program
- To carry Medic Alert ID to identify drug that you are taking, allergies
- To avoid hazardous activities if dizziness is present
- To report symptoms of CHF: difficult breathing, especially on exertion or when lying down, night cough, swelling of extremities

Treatment of overdose: Lavage, IV atropine for bradycardia, IV theophylline for bronchospasm, digitalis, O_2, diuretic for cardiac failure, hemodialysis, IV glucose for hyperglycemia, IV diazepam (or phenytoin) for seizures

acetaminophen

(a-seat-a-mee'noe-fen)
Acetaminophen Uniserts, Anacin-3 Infant's Drops, Anacin-3 Maximum Strength, Apacet, Aspirin Free Pain Relief, Atasol*, Banesin, Campain*, Children's Feverall, Dapa Extra Strength, Datril Extra Strength, Dolane, Dorcol Children's Fever and Pain Reducer, Genapap Extra Strength, Genapap Infant's Drops, Geners Extra Strength, Halenol Children's, Junior Strength Feverall, Liquiprin Elixir, Liquiprin Infant Drops, Meda Cap, Myapap Drops, Oraphen-PD, Panadol, Panadol Infant's Drops, Panex 500, Parten, Pedric, Phenaphen Caplets, Redutemp, Robigesic*, Rounax*, St. Joseph Aspirin-free Infant Drops, Tapanol Extra Strength, Tempra, Tempra Drops, Tylenol, Tylenol Caplets, Tylenol Extra Strength, Tylenol Infant's Drops

Func. class.: Nonnarcotic analgesic

Chem. class.: Nonsalicylate, paraaminophenol derivative

Action: May block pain impulses peripherally that occur in response to inhibition of prostaglandin synthesis; does not possess antiinflammatory properties; antipyretic action results from inhibition of prostaglandins in the CNS (hypothalamic heat-regulating center).

Uses: Mild to moderate pain or fever

Dosage and routes:
- *Adult and child >10 yr:* PO 325-650 mg q4h prn, not to exceed 4 g/day; REC: 325-650 mg q4h prn, not to exceed 4 g/day

---

italics = common side effects   ***bold italic*** = life threatening reactions

- *Child 0-3 mo:* 40 mg/dose
- *Child 4-11 mo:* 80 mg/dose
- *Child <1 yr:* PO/REC 15-60 mg/dose q4-6h, not to exceed 65 mg/kg/day
- *Child 1-2 yr:* PO/REC 60 mg/dose
- *Child 2-3 yr:* PO/REC 120 mg/dose
- *Child 3-4 yr:* PO/REC 180 mg/dose
- *Child 4-5 yr:* PO/REC 240 mg/dose
- *Child 5-10 yr:* PO/REC 325 mg/dose

Available forms: Rectal supp 120, 125, 325, 600, 650 mg; chewable tab 80 mg; caps 325, 500, 650 mg; elix 120, 160, 325 mg/5 ml; liq 160 mg/5 ml, 500mg/15ml; sol 100 mg/1 ml, 120 mg/2.5 ml

Side effects/adverse reactions:

SYST: Anaphylaxis

HEMA: Leukopenia, neutropenia, hemolytic anemia (long-term use), thrombocytopenia, pancytopenia

CNS: Stimulation, drowsiness

GI: Nausea, vomiting, abdominal pain, *hepatotoxicity*

INTEG: Rash, urticaria, *angioedema*

TOXICITY: Cyanosis, anemia, neutropenia, jaundice, pancytopenia, CNS stimulation, delirium followed by vascular collapse, convulsions, coma, death

Contraindications: Hypersensitivity, intolerance to tartrazine (yellow dye #4), alcohol, table sugar, saccharin

Precautions: Anemia, hepatic disease, renal disease, chronic alcoholism, pregnancy (B), elderly, lactation

Pharmacokinetics: Well-absorbed PO, rectal absorption varies

PO: Onset 10-30 min, peak ½-2 hr, duration 3-4 hr

REC: Onset slow, peak 1-2 hrs., duration 3-4 hr 85%-90% metabolized by liver, excreted by kidneys; metabolites may be toxic if overdose occurs; widely distributed, crosses placenta, excreted in breast milk, half-life 3-4 hr)

Interactions/incompatibilities:

- Increased effects of chloramphenicol
- Decreased effects of acetaminophen: cholestyramine, oral contraceptives, anticholinergics, colestipol
- Increased effect of acetaminophen: diflunisal, caffeine
- Severe hypothermia: phenothiazines
- Increased chance of hepatotoxicity: alcohol

NURSING CONSIDERATIONS
Assess:

- Liver function studies: AST, ALT, bilirubin, creatinine prior to therapy if long-term therapy is anticipated
- Renal function studies: BUN, urine creatinine, occult blood, albumin, if patient is on long-term therapy; presence of blood or albumin indicates nephritis
- Blood studies: CBC, pro-time if patient is on long-term therapy
- I&O ratio; decreasing output may indicate renal failure (long-term therapy)
- For fever and pain: type of pain, location, intensity, duration
- Mucosa, fingernail beds for cyanosis; inquire about dyspnea, vertigo, headache, weakness; symptoms indicate methemoglobinemia; notify physician immediately
- For chronic poisoning: rapid, weak pulse; dyspnea; cold, clammy extremities; report immediately to physician
- Hepatotoxicity: dark urine; clay-

colored stools; yellowing of skin, sclera; itching, abdominal pain; fever; diarrhea if patient is on long-term therapy

• Allergic reactions: rash, urticaria; if these occur, drug may have to be discontinued

Administer:

• To patient crushed or whole; chewable tablets may be chewed; give with full glass of water

• With food or milk to decrease gastric symptoms if needed

Perform/provide:

• Storage of suppositories <80° F (27° C)

Evaluate:

• Therapeutic response: absence of pain, fever

Teach patient/family:

• Not to exceed recommended dosage; acute poisoning with liver damage may result. Acute toxicity includes symptoms of nausea, vomiting, and abdominal pain; physician should be notified immediately.

• To read label on other OTC drugs; many contain acetaminophen and may cause toxicity if taken concurrently

• To recognize signs of chronic overdose: bleeding, bruising, malaise, fever, sore throat

• That urine may become dark brown as a result of phenacitin (metabolite of acetaminophen)

• To notify physician for pain or fever lasting over 3 days

Treatment of overdose: Drug level q4h, gastric lavage, activated charcoal; administer oral acetylcysteine to prevent hepatic damage (see acetylcystine monograph)

acetazolamide/ acetazolamide sodium

(a-set-a-zole'a-mide)

Acetazolamide, AK-Zol, Cetazol, Dazamide, Diamox, Diamox Sequels, Hydrazol/Diamox Parenteral

Func. class.: Diuretic; carbonic anhydrase inhibitor

Chem. class.: Sulfonamide derivative

Action: Inhibits carbonic anhydrase activity in proximal renal tubules to decrease reabsorption of water, sodium, potassium, bicarbonate; decreases carbonic anhydrase in CNS, increasing seizure threshold; able to decrease aqueous humor in eye, which lowers intraocular pressure

Uses: Open-angle glaucoma, narrow-angle glaucoma (preoperatively, if surgery delayed), epilepsy (petit mal, grand mal, mixed), edema in CHF, drug-induced edema, acute mountain sickness

Dosage and routes:

Narrow-angle glaucoma

• *Adult:* PO/IM/IV 250 mg q4h or 250 mg bid, to be used for short-term therapy

Open-angle glaucoma

• *Adult:* PO/IM/IV 250 mg-1g/day in divided doses for amounts over 250 mg

Edema

• *Adult:* IM/IV 250-375 mg/day in AM

• *Child:* IM/IV 5 mg/kg/day in AM

Seizures

• *Adult:* PO/IM/IV 8-30 mg/kg/day, usual range 375-1000 mg/day

• *Child:* PO/IM/IV 8-30 mg/kg/day in divided doses tid or qid, or

300-900 mg/m²/day, not to exceed 1.5 g/day

Mountain sickness
• *Adult:* PO 250 mg q8-12h

Available forms: Tabs 125, 250 mg; caps sust rel 500 mg; inj IM/IV 500 mg

Side effects/adverse reactions:

GU: Frequency, hypokalemia, polyuria, **uremia,** glucosuria, hematuria, dysuria, crystalluria, renal calculi

CNS: Drowsiness, paresthesia, anxiety, depression, headache, dizziness, confusion, stimulation, fatigue, **convulsions,** sedation, nervousness

GI: Nausea, vomiting, anorexia, constipation, diarrhea, melena, weight loss, **hepatic insufficiency,** taste alterations

EENT: Myopia, tinnitus

INTEG: Rash, pruritus, urticaria, fever, **Stevens-Johnson syndrome,** photosensitivity

ENDO: Hyperglycemia

*HEMA: **Aplastic anemia, hemolytic anemia, leukopenia, agranulocytosis, thrombocytopenia, purpura, pancytopenia***

Contraindications: Hypersensitivity to sulfonamides, severe renal disease, severe hepatic disease, electrolyte imbalances (hyponatremia, hypokalemia), hyperchloremic acidosis, Addison's disease, long-term use in narrow-angle glaucoma, COPD

Precautions: Hypercalciuria, pregnancy (C)

Pharmacokinetics:

PO: Onset 1-1½ hr, peak 2-4 hr, duration 6-12 hr

PO—SUS REL: Onset 2 hr, peak 8-12 hr, duration 18-24 hr

IV: Onset 2 min, peak 15 min, duration 4-5 hr

65% absorbed if fasting (oral), 75% absorbed if given with food; half-life 2½-5½ hr; excreted unchanged by kidneys (80% within 24 hr), crosses placenta

Interactions/incompatibilities:

• Increased action of amphetamines, procainamide, quinidine, tricyclics, flecainide, ephedrine, pseudoephedrine

• Increased excretion of barbiturates, ASA, lithium

• Toxicity: salicylates

• Hypokalemia: with other diuretics, corticosteroids, amphotericin B

• IV compatibility: cimetidine, D_5W, $D_{10}W$, NaCl, LR, Ringer's Sol

• Improvement in CVP q8h

• Signs of metabolic acidosis: drowsiness, restlessness

• Signs of hypokalemia: postural hypotension, malaise, fatigue, tachycardia, leg cramps, weakness

• Rashes, temperature elevation qd

• Confusion, especially in elderly; take safety precautions if needed

Lab test interferences:

False positive: Urinary protein, 17 hydroxysteroid

Increase: Blood glucose levels, bilirubin, blood ammonia, calcium, chloride

Decrease: Urine citrate, potassium

NURSING CONSIDERATIONS

Assess:

• Weight daily, I&O daily to determine fluid loss; effect of drug may be decreased if used qd

• Rate, depth, rhythm of respiration, effect of exertion

• B/P lying, standing; postural hypotension may occur

• Electrolytes: potassium, sodium, chloride; include BUN, blood sugar, CBC, serum creatinine, blood pH, ABGs, liver function tests

---

* Available in Canada only

Administer:

• After diluting 500 mg in >5 ml sterile H$_2$O for injection; direct IV—give at 100-500 mg/min; may be diluted further in LR, D$_5$W, D$_{10}$W 0.45% NaCl, 0.9% NaCl, or Ringer's Sol and infused over 4-8 hr; use within 24 hr of dilution.

• PO or IV if possible; IM administration is painful

• In AM to avoid interference with sleep if using drug as diuretic

• Potassium replacement if potassium level is less than 3.0

• With food if nausea occurs; absorption may be decreased slightly

Perform/provide:

• Storage in dark, cool area; use reconstituted solution within 24 hr

Evaluate:

• Therapeutic response: improvement in edema of feet, legs, sacral area daily if medication is being used in CHF; or decrease in aqueous humor if medication is being used in glaucoma

Teach patient/family:

• To increase fluid intake by 2-3 L/day unless contraindicated; to rise slowly from lying or sitting position

• To notify physician if sore throat, unusual bleeding, bruising, paresthesias, tremors, flank pain, or skin rash occurs

• To use sunscreen to prevent photosensitivity

• To avoid hazardous activities if drowsiness occurs

Treatment of overdose: Lavage if taken orally; monitor electrolytes; administer dextrose in saline; monitor hydration, CV, renal status

acetohexamide
(a-seat-oh-hex'a-mide)
Acetohexamide, Dimelor,* Dymelor
Func. class.: Antidiabetic
Chem. class.: Sulfonylurea (1st generation)

Action: Causes functioning β-cells in pancreas to release insulin, leading to drop in blood glucose levels; may improve binding between insulin and insulin receptors or increase number of insulin receptors with prolonged administration. May also reduce basal hepatic glucose secretion. Not effective if patient lacks functioning β-cells

Uses: Stable adult-onset diabetes mellitus (type II), NIDDM

Dosage and routes:

• *Adult:* PO 250 mg-1.5 g/day; usually given before breakfast, unless large dose is required; then dose is divided in two

Available forms: Tabs 250, 500 mg scored

Side effects/adverse reactions:

CNS: Headache, weakness, tinnitus, fatigue, dizziness, vertigo

GI: Nausea, vomiting, diarrhea, **hepatotoxicity, jaundice,** heartburn

HEMA: **Leukopenia, thrombocytopenia, agranulocytosis, aplastic anemia, hemolytic anemia,** increased AST, ALT, alk phosphatase

INTEG: Rash, allergic reactions, pruritus, urticaria, eczema, photosensitivity, erythema

ENDO: **Hypoglycemia,** hyponatremia

Contraindications: Hypersensitivity to sulfonylureas, juvenile or brittle diabetes, renal failure

Precautions: Pregnancy (C), el-

---

italics = common side effects   ***bold italic*** = life threatening reactions

derly, cardiac disease, renal disease, hepatic disease, thyroid disease, severe hypoglycemic reactions

Pharmacokinetics:
PO: Completely absorbed by GI route, onset 1 hr, peak 2-4 hr, duration 12-24 hr, half-life 6-8 hr, metabolized in liver, excreted in urine (active metabolites, unchanged drug)

Interactions/incompatibilities:
• Increased hypoglycemic effects: oral anticoagulants, salicylates, sulfonamides, nonsteroidal antiinflammatories, guanethidine, methyldopa, MAOIs, chloramphenicol, insulin, cimetidine
• Decreased action of acetohexamide: calcium channel blockers, corticosteroids, oral contraceptives, thiazide diuretics, thyroid preparations, estrogens, phenobarbital, phenothiazines, phenytoin, rifampin, sympathomimetics
• Decreased effect of both drugs: diazoxide

NURSING CONSIDERATIONS
Assess:
• Hypoglycemic/hyperglycemic reaction that can occur soon after meals

Administer:
• Drug 30 min before meals

Perform/provide:
• Storage in tight container in cool environment

Evaluate:
• Therapeutic response: decrease in polyuria, polydipsia, polyphagia, clear sensorium, absence of dizziness, stable gait

Teach patient/family:
• To check for symptoms of cholestatic jaundice: dark urine, pruritus, yellow sclera; if these occur, physician should be notified

• To use capillary blood glucose test or Chemstrip 3 ×/day
• Symptoms of hypo/hyperglycemia, what to do about each
• That drug must be continued on daily basis; explain consequence of discontinuing drug abruptly
• To take drug in morning to prevent hypoglycemic reactions at night
• To avoid OTC medications unless prescribed by physician
• That diabetes is lifelong illness; that this drug is not a cure
• That all food included in diet plan must be eaten to prevent hypoglycemia
• To carry Medic-Alert ID for emergency purposes, carry a glucagon emergency kit

Treatment of overdose: Glucose 25g IV, via dextrose 50% sol, 50 cc or 1 mg glucagon

---

acetohydroxamic acid
(a-set-oh-hye-drox-am'ic)
Lithostat

Func. class.: Ammonia detoxicant, reversible urease inhibitor
Chem. class.: Hydroxylamine, ethyl acetate compound

Action: Inhibits bacterial enzyme urease, which decreases conversion of urea to ammonia; the reduced ammonia levels and decreased pH increase the effectiveness of antimicrobial agents

Uses: Adjunctive treatment in chronic urea-splitting urinary infection

Dosage and routes:
• *Adult:* PO 250 mg tid-qid q6-8h when stomach is empty, not to exceed 1.5 g/day
• *Child:* PO 10 mg/kg/day in 2-3 divided doses
Available forms: Tabs 250 mg

Side effects/adverse reactions:
*HEMA: **Hemolytic anemia, reticulocytosis***
CNS: Headache, depression, restlessness, anxiety, nervousness, malaise
GI: Nausea, vomiting, anorexia
INTEG: Rash on face, arms, alopecia
CV: Phlebitis, ***deep vein thrombosis, pulmonary embolism,*** palpitations
Contraindications: Hypersensitivity, severe renal disease, non-urease-producing organisms, pregnancy (X)
Precautions: Deep vein thrombosis, hepatic disease, renal disease, lactation
Pharmacokinetics:
PO: Peak 15-60 min, half-life 3½-10 hr, metabolized, excreted in urine as unchanged drug (15%-60%)
Interactions/incompatibilities:
• Decreased absorption of both drugs: iron preparations
• Rash: alcohol
NURSING CONSIDERATIONS
Assess:
• I&O ratio; observe for decrease in urinary output
• CBC, platelets, reticulocytes before, during therapy (q3 mo)
Administer:
• On empty stomach only, to facilitate absorption
Perform/provide:
• Storage in tight container at room temperature
Evaluate:
• Therapeutic response: decrease in stone formation on x-ray, decreased pain in kidney region, absence of hematuria, signs of anemia
Teach patient/family:
• To avoid alcohol, OTC preparations that contain alcohol, rashes have occurred
• To report any pain, redness, or hard area, usually in legs; may indicate phlebitis
• The importance of patient compliance with medical regimen; bone marrow depression may occur
• To increase fluids to 3-4 L/day
• To use contraception during treatment

acetylcholine chloride
(a-se-teel-koe'leen)
Miochol direct-acting
Func. class.: Miotic, cholinergic
Chem. class.: Quaternary ammonium compound

Action: Intense, immediate miosis (pupil constriction) by causing contraction of sphincter muscle of iris
Uses: Miosis during anterior segment surgery; cataract removal keratoplasty, peripheral iridectomy or cyclodialysis
Dosage and routes:
• *Adult and child:* INSTILL 0.5-2 ml of a 1% sol in anterior chamber of eye (instillation by physician)
Available forms: Sol 1:100
Side effects/adverse reactions:
CV: Hypotension, bradycardia
EENT: Blurred vision, lens opacities
Contraindications: Hypersensitivity; when miosis is undesirable
Precautions: Acute cardiac failure, bronchial asthma
Pharmacokinetics:
INSTILL: Miosis occurs immediately, duration 10 min
NURSING CONSIDERATIONS
Administer:
• Check vial for percentage of solution
• Check label for expiration date

italics = common side effects   ***bold italic*** = life threatening reactions

o mix drug to
stopper to mix
er; do not use if
forced down
g stopper with al-
cohol or other germicidal
• IV atropine 0.6-0.8 mg for systemic reactions

Perform/provide:
• Use reconstituted solution immediately; discard unused portion

Evaluate:
• Therapeutic response: miosis
during surgery

Teach patient/family:
• To report change in vision, blurring or loss of sight, trouble breathing, sweating, flushing

---

acetylcysteine
(a-se-til-sis'tay-een)
Airbron,* Mucomyst, Mucosil
Func. class.: Mucolytic
Chem. class.: Amino acid
L-cysteine

Action: Decreases viscosity of secretions by breaking disulfide links
of mucoproteins; increases hepatic
glutathione, which is necessary to
inactivate toxic metabolites in
acetaminophen overdose

Uses: Acetaminophen toxicity;
bronchitis; pneumonia; cystic fibrosis; emphysema; atelectasis; tuberculosis; complications of thoracic,
cardiovascular surgery; diagnosis
in bronchial lab tests

Dosage and routes:
• *Adult and child:* INSTILL 1-2 ml
(10%-20% sol) q1-4h prn or 3-5 ml
(20% sol) or 6-10 ml (10% sol) tid
or qid

Acetaminophen toxicity
• *Adult and child:* PO 140 mg/kg,
then 70 mg/kg q4h × 17 doses to
total of 1330 mg/kg

Available forms: Sol 10%, 20%

Side effects/adverse reactions:
CNS: Dizziness, drowsiness, head-
ache, fever, chills
GI: Nausea, stomatitis, constipa-
tion, vomiting, anorexia, ***hepato-
toxicity***
EENT: Rhinorrhea, tooth damage
CV: Hypotension
INTEG: Urticaria, rash, fever, clam-
miness
RESP: **Bronchospasm,** burning,
hemoptysis, chest tightness

Contraindications: Hypersensitivity, increased intracranial pressure,
status asthmaticus

Precautions: Hypothyroidism,
Addison's disease, CNS depression, brain tumor, asthma, hepatic
disease, renal disease, COPD, psychosis, alcoholism, convulsive disorders, lactation, pregnancy (B)

Pharmacokinetics:
INH/INSTILL: Onset 1 min, duration
5-10 min, metabolized by liver, excreted in urine

Interactions/incompatibilities:
• Do not use with iron, copper, rubber
• Do not mix with antibiotics: tetracycline, chlortetracycline, oxytetracycline, erythromycin, lactobionate, amphotericin-B, sodium
ampicillin; iodized oil, chymotryp-
sin, trypsin, hydrogen peroxide

NURSING CONSIDERATIONS
Assess:
• Cough: type, frequency, character, including sputum
• Rate, rhythm of respirations, increased dyspnea; discontinue if
bronchospasm occurs
• Antidotal use: decrease in hepatic
encephalopathy
• VS, cardiac status including
checking for dysrhythmias, increased rate, palpitations
• ABGs for increased CO_2 retention in asthma patients

• Antidotal use: liver function tests, acetaminophen levels; inform physician if dose is vomited or vomiting is persistent

Administer:

• Store in refrigerator: use within 96 hr of opening

• Before meals ½-1 hr for better absorption, to decrease nausea

• 20% solutions diluted with NS or water for injection; may give 10% solution undiluted

• Only after patient clears airway by deep breathing, coughing

• Antidotal use: give within 24 hr; give with cola or soft drink to disguise taste; can be given with H_2O through tubes; use within 1 hr

• By syringe 2-3 doses of 1-2 ml of 20% or 2-4 ml of 10% solution

• Decreased dose to elderly patients; their metabolism may be slowed

• Gum, hard candy, frequent rinsing of mouth for dryness of oral cavity

• Only if suction machine is available

Perform/provide:

• Storage in refrigerator after opening

• Assistance with inhaled dose: bronchodilator if bronchospasm occurs

• Mechanical suction if cough insufficient to remove excess bronchial secretions

Evaluate:

• Therapeutic response: absence of purulent secretions when coughing; absence of hepatic damage in acetaminophen toxicity

Teach patient/family:

• To avoid driving or other hazardous activities until patient is stabilized on this medication

• To avoid alcohol, other CNS depressants; will enhance sedating properties of this drug

• That unpleasant odor will decrease after repeated use

• That discoloration of solution after bottle is opened does not impair its effectiveness

• To avoid smoking, smoke-filled rooms, perfume, dust, environmental pollutants, cleaners

---

activated charcoal

Arm-a-char, Actidose-Aqua, Liqu-Char, Superchar, Charcoaide, Charcocaps, Charcodote, Charcotabs, Digestalin

Func. class.: Antiflatulent/antidote

Action: Binds poisons, toxins, irritants; increases adsorption in GI tract; inactivates toxins and binds until excreted

Uses: Flatulence, poisoning, dyspepsia, distention, deodorant in wounds, diarrhea

Dosage and routes:

Poisoning

• *Adult and child:* PO 5-10 × weight of substance ingested, minimum dose 30 g/250 ml of water, may give 20-40g q6h for 1-2 days in severe poisoning

Flatulence/dyspepsia

• *Adult:* PO 520-975 mg p.c. up to 4.16 g/day

Available forms: Powder; liq 12.5, 25, 30,50 g; caps 260 mg; tabs 325 mg

Side effects/adverse reactions:

GI: Nausea, black stools, vomiting, constipation, diarrhea

Contraindications: Hypersensitivity to this drug, unconsciousness, semiconsciousness, poisoning of cyanide, mineral acids, alkalies

---

Pharmacokinetics:
PO: Excreted in feces
Interactions/incompatibilities:
• Decreased effectiveness of both drugs: ipecac, laxatives
• Do not mix with dairy products

NURSING CONSIDERATIONS
Assess:
• Respiration, pulse, B/P to determine charcoal effectiveness if taken for barbiturate/narcotic poisoning
Administer:
• After inducing vomiting unless vomiting contraindicated (i.e., cyanide or alkalies)
• After mixing with water or fruit juice to form thick syrup; do not use dairy products to mix charcoal
• Repeat dose if vomiting occurs soon after dose
• After spacing at least 1 hr before or after other drugs, or absorption will be decreased
• With a laxative to promote elimination
• Alone; do not administer with ipecac
• Through a nasogastric tube if patient unable to swallow
• Keeping container tightly closed to prevent absorption of gases
Evaluate:
• Therapeutic response: LOC-alert (poisoning)
Teach patient/family:
• That stools will be black

---

acyclovir (topical)
(ay-sye'kloe-ver)
Zovirax
Func. class.: Local antiinfective
Chem. class.: Antiviral

Action: Interferes with viral DNA replication
Uses: Simple mucocutaneous herpes simplex, in immunocompromised clients with initial herpes genitalis
Dosage and routes:
• *Adult and child:* TOP apply to all lesions q3h while awake, 6 times/day × 1 wk
Available forms: TOP oint 5% (50 mg/g)
Side effects/adverse reactions:
INTEG: Rash, urticaria, stinging, burning, pruritus, vulvitis
Contraindications: Hypersensitivity
Precautions: Pregnancy (C), lactation

NURSING CONSIDERATIONS
Assess:
• Allergic reaction: burning, stinging, swelling, redness, rash, vulvitis, pruritus
Administer:
• Using finger cot or rubber glove to prevent further infection
• Enough medication to cover lesions completely
• After cleansing with soap, water before each application, dry well
Perform/provide:
• Storage at room temperature in dry place
Evaluate:
• Therapeutic response: decrease in size, number of lesions
Teach patient/family:
• Not to use in eyes or use when there is no evidence of infection
• To apply with glove to prevent further infection
• To avoid use of OTC creams, ointments, lotions unless directed by physician
• To use medical asepsis (hand washing) before, after each application and avoid contact with eyes
• To adhere strictly to prescribed regimen to maximize successful treatment outcome

• To begin taking drug when symptoms arise

---

acyclovir sodium
(ay-sye-kloe-ver)
Zovirax
Func. class.: Antiviral
Chem. class.: Acylic purine nucleoside analog

Action: Interferes with DNA synthesis by conversion to acyclovir triphosphate, causing decreased viral replication, time of lesional healing
Uses: Mucocutaneous herpes simplex virus, herpes genitalis (HSV-1, HSV-2), herpes zoster
Dosage and routes:
Herpes simplex
• *Adult and child >12 yr:* IV INF 5 mg/kg over 1 hr q8h × 5 days
• *Child <12 yr:* IV INF 250 mg/m² over 1 hr q8h × 5 days
Genital herpes
• *Adult:* PO 200 mg q4h 5 × /day while awake for 5 days to 6 mo depending on whether initial, recurrent, or chronic
Herpes simplex encephalitis
• *Child >6 mo:* IV 500 mg/m² q8h × 10 days
Herpes zoster
• *Adult:* PO 800 mg × 5 days IV 5 mg/kg q8h
Children with immunosuppression:
• *Child >2 yr:* 20 mg/kg qid × 5 days
Available forms: Caps 200 mg; inj IV 500 mg
Side effects/adverse reactions:
CNS: Tremors, confusion, lethargy, hallucinations, **convulsions,** *dizziness, headache,* encephalopathic changes
GI: Nausea, vomiting, diarrhea, in-creased ALT, AST, abdominal pain, glossitis, colitis
GU: **Oliguria, proteinuria, hematuria,** vaginitis, moniliasis, **glomerulonephritis, acute renal failure,** changes in menses, polydypsia
EENT: gingival hyperplasia
INTEG: Rash, urticaria, pruritus, pain or phlebitis at IV site, unusual sweating, alopecia
MS: Joint pain, leg pain, muscle cramps
Contraindications: Hypersensitivity
Precautions: Lactation, hepatic disease, renal disease, electrolyte imbalance, dehydration, pregnancy (C)
Pharmacokinetics:
IV: Peak 1 hr, half-life 20 min-3 hr (terminal); metabolized by liver, excreted by kidneys as unchanged drug (95%); crosses placenta; absorbed minimally (PO), distributed widely-crosses placenta, CSF concentrations are 50% plasma
PO: onset unknown, peak 1½-2 hours, terminal half-life 3½ hours
Interactions/incompatibilities:
• Increased neurotoxicity, nephrotoxicity: aminoglycosides, amphotericin, interferon, probenecid, methotrexate
• IV incompatibility: dobutamine, dopamine, all protein products, blood products, ondansetron, verapamil
• IV-compatible solutions: D_5W, LR, or NaCl (D_5 0.9% NaCl, 0.9% NaCl) solutions
NURSING CONSIDERATIONS
Assess:
• Signs of infection, anemia
• I&O ratio; report hematuria, oliguria, fatigue, weakness; may indicate nephrotoxicity; check for protein in urine during treatment

---

italics = common side effects   ***bold italic*** = life threatening reactions

• Any patient with compromised renal system, since drug is excreted slowly in poor renal system function; toxicity may occur rapidly

• Liver studies: AST, ALT

• Blood studies: WBC, RBC, Hct, Hgb, bleeding time; blood dyscrasias may occur; drug should be discontinued

• Renal studies: urinalysis, protein, BUN, creatinine, CrCl

• C&S before drug therapy; drug may be taken as soon as culture is taken; repeat C&S after treatment Determine the presence of other sexually transmitted diseases.

• Bowel pattern before, during treatment; if severe abdominal pain with bleeding occurs, drug should be discontinued

• Skin eruptions: rash, urticaria, itching

• Allergies before treatment, reaction of each medication; place allergies on chart in bright red letters

Administer:

• Increased fluids to 3 L/day to decrease crystalluria when given IV

• After reconstituting with 10 ml compatible solution/500 mg of drug, concentration of 50 mg/ml, shake, use within 12 hr (<7 mg/ml); give over at least 1 hr (constant rate) by infusion pump to prevent nephrotoxicity; do not reconstitute with sol containing benzyl alcohol in neonates

• Lower dose in acute or chronic renal failure

Perform/provide:

• Storage at room temperature for up to 12 hr after reconstitution; if refrigerated, sol may show a precipitate that clears at room temperature

• Adequate intake of fluids (2000 ml) to prevent deposit in kidneys

Evaluate:

• Therapeutic response: absence of itching, painful lesions; crusting and healed lesions

Teach patient/family:

• That drug may be taken orally before infection occurs; drug should be taken when itching or pain occurs, usually before eruptions

• That partners need to be told that patient has herpes; they can become infected, condoms must be worn to prevent reinfections

• That drug does not cure infection, just controls symptoms and does not prevent infection to others

• To report sore throat, fever, fatigue; may indicate superimposed infection

• That drug must be taken in equal intervals around the clock to maintain blood levels for duration of therapy

• To notify physician of side effects of bruising, bleeding, fatigue, malaise; may indicate blood dyscrasias

Treatment of overdose: Discontinue drug, hemodialysis, resuscitate if needed

• To seek dental care during treatment to prevent gingival hyperplasia

---

adenosine

(ah-den'oh-seen)

Adenocard

Func. class.: Antidysrhythmic
Chem. class.: Endogenous nucleoside

Action: Slows conduction through AV node, can interrupt reentry pathways through AV node, and can restore normal sinus rhythm in patients with paroxysmal supraventricular tachycardia (PSVT)

Uses: PSVT

Dosage and routes:
• *Adult:* IV BOL 6 mg; if conversion to normal sinus rhythm does not occur within 1-2 min, give 12 mg by rapid IV BOL; may repeat 12 mg dose again in 1-2 min
Available forms: Inj 3 mg/ml
Side effects/adverse reactions:
GI: Nausea, metallic taste, throat tightness, groin pressure
RESP: Dyspnea, chest pressure, hyperventilation
CNS: Lightheadedness, dizziness, arm tingling, numbness, apprehension, blurred vision, headache
CV: Chest pain, **atrial tachydysrhythmias,** sweating, palpitations, hypotension, *facial flushing*
Contraindications: Hypersensitivity, 2nd or 3rd degree heart block, AV block, sick sinus syndrome, atrial flutter, atrial fibrillation, ventricular tachycardia
Precautions: Pregnancy (C), lactation, children, asthma, elderly
Pharmacokinetics: Cleared from plasma in <30 sec, half-life 10 sec
Interactions/incompatibilities:
• Increased effects of adenosine: dipyridamole
• Decreased activity of adenosine; theophylline or other methylxanthines (caffeine)
• Higher degree of heart block: carbamazepine
• Incompatible with any other drug in solution or syringe
Lab test interferences:
Increase: Liver function tests
NURSING CONSIDERATIONS
Assess:
• Cardiac status continually
• B/P continuously for fluctuations
• I&O ratio, electrolytes (K, Na, Cl)
• Cardiac status: B/P, pulse, respiration, ECG intervals (PR, QRS, QT)

• Respiratory status: rate, rhythm, lung fields for rales, watch for respiratory depression
• CNS effects: dizziness, confusion, psychosis, paresthesias, convulsions; drug should be discontinued
• Lung fields, bilateral rales may occur in CHF patient
• Increased respiration, increased pulse; drug should be discontinued
Administer:
• IV bolus undiluted; give 6 mg or less over 1 min; if using an IV line, use port near insertion site, flush with normal saline (50 cc)
Perform/provide
• Storage at room temperature; sol should be clear
Evaluate:
• Therapeutic response: decreased anginal pain, decreased B/P, dysrhythmias, decreased heart rate
Treatment of overdose: Defibrillation, vasopressor for hypotension

---

albumin, normal serum 5%/25%
(al-byoo'min)
Albuminar 5%, Albutein 5%, Buminate 5%, Plasbumin 5%, Albuminar 25%, Albutein 25%, Buminate 25%, Plasbumin-25%
Func. class.: Blood derivative
Chem. class.: Placental human plasma

Action: Exerts oncotic pressure, which expands volume of circulating blood and maintains cardiac output
Uses: Restores plasma volume in burns, hyperbilirubinemia, shock, hypoproteinemia, prevention of cerebral edema, cardiopulmonary bypass procedures, ARDS

---

italics = common side effects   ***bold italic*** = life threatening reactions

Dosage and routes:
Burns
• *Adult:* IV dose to maintain plasma albumin at 30-50 g/L, use 5% sol initially, then 25% sol after 24 hr
Shock
• *Adult:* IV 500 ml of 5% sol q30 min, as needed
• *Child:* ¼-½ adult dose in non-emergencies
Hypoproteinemia
• *Adult:* IV 1000-2000 ml of 5% sol qd, not to exceed 5-10 ml/min or 25-100 g of 25% sol qd, not to exceed 3 ml/min, titrated to patient response
Hyperbilirubinemia / erythroblastosis fetalis
• *Infant:* IV 1 g of 25% sol/kg before transfusion
Available forms: Inj IV 50, 250 mg/ml; (5%, 25%)
Side effects/adverse reactions:
GI: Nausea, vomiting, increased salivation
INTEG: Rash, urticaria
CNS: Fever, chills, flushing, headache
RESP: Altered respirations, *pulmonary edema*
CV: Fluid overload, hypotension, erratic pulse, tachycardia
Contraindications: Hypersensitivity, CHF, severe anemia, renal insufficiency
Precautions: Decreased salt intake, decreased cardiac reserve, lack of albumin deficiency, hepatic disease, renal disease, pregnancy (C)
Pharmacokinetics: In hyponutrition states, metabolized as protein/energy source.
Lab test interferences:
False increase: Alk phosphatase
NURSING CONSIDERATIONS
Assess:
• Blood studies Hct, Hgb; if serum protein declines, dyspnea, hypoxemia can result
• Decreased B/P, erratic pulse, respiration
• I&O ratio: urinary output may decrease
• CVP, pulmonary wedge pressure will increase if overload occurs
• Allergy: fever, rash, itching, chills, flushing, urticaria, nausea, vomiting, hypotension, requires discontinuation of infusion, use of new lot if therapy reinstituted
• CVP reading: distended neck veins indicate circulatory overload; shortness of breath, anxiety, insomnia, expiratory rales, frothy blood-tinged cough, cyanosis indicate pulmonary overload
Administer:
• IV slowly, to prevent fluid overload; dilute with NS for injection or D₅W; 5% may be given undiluted; 25% may be given diluted or undiluted, give over 4 hr, use infusion pump
Perform/provide:
• Adequate hydration before, during administration
• Check type of albumin, some stored at room temperature, some need to be refrigerated
Evaluate:
• Therapeutic response: increased B/P, decreased edema, increased serum albumin

---

albuterol
(al-byoo'ter-ole)
Albuterol, Proventil, Proventil Repetabs, Salbutamol,* Ventolin, Ventolin Rotacaps, Volmax

Func. class.: Adrenergic β₂ agonist

Action: Causes bronchodilation by

action on β_2 (pulmonary) receptors by increasing levels of cAMP, which relaxes smooth muscle; produces bronchodilation, CNS, cardiac stimulation, as well as increased diuresis and gastric acid secretion; longer acting than isoproterenol

Uses: Prevention of exercise-induced asthma, bronchospasm, production of premature labor

Dosage and routes:
To prevent exercise-induced asthma
• *Adult:* INH 2 puffs 15 min before exercising, NEB/LPPB 5 mg tid-qid
Bronchospasm
• *Adult:* INH 1-2 puffs q4-6h PO 2-4 mg tid-qid, not to exceed 8 mg
Prevention of premature labor
Available forms: Aerosol 90 μg/actuation; tabs 2, 4 mg; syr 2 mg/5 ml, cont rel 4, 8 mg

Side effects/adverse reactions:
CNS: Tremors, anxiety, insomnia, headache, dizziness, stimulation, *restlessness,* hallucinations, flushing, irritability
EENT: Dry nose, irritation of nose and throat
CV: Palpitations, tachycardia, hypertension, angina, hypotension, dysrhythmias
GI: Heartburn, nausea, vomiting
MS: Muscle cramps

Contraindications: Hypersensitivity to sympathomimetics, tachydysrhythmias, severe cardiac disease

Precautions: Lactation, pregnancy (C), cardiac disorders, hyperthyroidism, diabetes mellitus, hypertension, prostatic hypertrophy, narrow-angle glaucoma, seizures, exercise-induced bronchospasm (aerosol) in children <12 years

Pharmacokinetics: Well absorbed

PO, extensively metabolized in the liver, excreted in urine, crosses placenta, breast milk, blood-brain barrier
PO: Onset ½ hr, peak 2½ hr, duration 4-6 hr, half-life 2½ hr
PO-ER: Onset ½ hour; peak 2-3 hr; duration 12 hr
INH: Onset 5-15 min, peak 1-1½ hr, duration 4-6 hr, half-life 4 hr

Interactions/incompatibilities:
• Increased action of aerosol bronchodilators
• Increased action of albuterol: tricyclic antidepressants, MAOIs, other adrenergics
• May inhibit action of albuterol: other β-blockers

NURSING CONSIDERATIONS
Assess:
• Respiratory function: vital capacity, forced expiratory volume, ABGs, lung sounds, heart rate and rhythm (baseline)
• That patient has not received theophylline therapy before giving dose
• Client's ability to self-medicate
• For evidence of allergic reactions

Administer:
• After shaking, exhale, place mouthpiece in mouth, inhale slowly, hold breath, remove, exhale slowly
• Gum, sips of water for dry mouth
• PO with meals to decrease gastric irritation
• Syrup to children (no alcohol, sugar)

Perform/provide:
• Storage in light-resistant container, do not expose to temperatures over 86° F (30° C)

Evaluate:
• Therapeutic response: absence of dyspnea, wheezing after 1 hr, improved airway exchange, improved ABGs

---

italics = common side effects   ***bold italic*** = life threatening reactions

Teach patient/family:
• Not to use OTC medications; extra stimulation may occur
• Use of inhaler; review package insert with patient
• To avoid getting aerosol in eyes; blurring may result
• To wash inhaler in warm water qd and dry
• To avoid smoking, smoke-filled rooms, persons with respiratory infections
• That paradoxical bronchospasm may occur and to stop drug immediately
• To limit caffeine products such as chocolate, coffee, tea, and colas
Treatment of overdose: Administer a β_2-adrenergic blocker

---

aldesleukin (interleukin-2, IL-2)

(al-dess'-loo-kin)
Proleukin
Func. class.: Miscellaneous antineoplastics
Chem. class.: Interleukin-2, human recombinant

Action: Enhancement of lymphocyte mitogenesis and stimulation of IL-2–dependent cell lines; enhancement of lymphocyte cytotoxicity; induction of killer cell activity; induction of interferon γ-production; results in activation of cellular immunity, cytokines and inhibition of tumor growth
Uses: Metastatic renal cell carcinoma in adults
Dosage and routes:
• *Adult:* IV INF 600,000 IU/kg (0.037 mg/kg) q8h over 15 min × 14 doses; off 9 days, repeat schedule for another 14 doses, for a max of 28 doses/course

Available forms: Powder for inj, lyophilized
Side effects/adverse reactions:
CV: Hypotension, sinus tachycardia, dysrhythmias, bradycardia, PVCs, PACs, myocardial ischemia, *myocardial infarction, cardiac arrest*
RESP: Pulmonary congestion, dyspnea, *pulmonary edema, respiratory failure,* tachypnea, pleural effusion, wheezing
GI: Nausea, vomiting, diarrhea, stomatitis, anorexia, GI bleeding, dyspepsia, constipation, *intestinal perforation*/ileus, jaundice, ascites
HEMA: Anemia, *thrombocytopenia, leukopenia, coagulation disorders, leukocytosis, eosinophilia*
CNS: Mental status changes, dizziness, sensory dysfunction, syncope, motor dysfunction, fever, chills, headache
GU: Oliguria/anuria, proteinuria, hematuria, dysuria, *renal failure*
INTEG: Pruritus, erythema, rash, dry skin, *exfoliative dermatitis,* purpura, petechiae, urticaria
MS: Arthralgia, myalgia
SYST: Infection
Contraindications: Hypersensitivity, abnormal thallium stress test or pulmonary function tests, organ allografts
Precautions: CNS metastases, bacterial infections, renal/hepatic disease, pregnancy (C), lactation, children, anemia, thrombocytopenia
Pharmacokinetics: Renal elimination half-life 85 min
Interactions/incompatibilities:
• Potentiate hypotension: antihypertensives
• Reduced antitumor effectiveness: corticosteroids

• Increased toxicity: aminoglycosides, indomethacin, cytotoxic chemotherapy, methotrexate, asparaginase, doxorubicin

Lab test interferences:

Increase: Bilirubin, BUN, serum creatinine, transaminase, alk phosphatase; hypomagnesemia, acidosis hypocalcemia, hypophosphatemia, hypokalemia, hyperuricemia, hypoalbuminemia, hypoproteinemia, hyponatremia, hyperkalemia, alkalosis

NURSING CONSIDERATIONS

Assess:

• CBC, differential, platelet count weekly; withhold drug if WBC is $<4000/mm^3$ or platelet count is $<75,000/mm^3$; notify physician of these results

• Capillary leak syndrome (CLS) including a drop in mean arterial pressure (2-12 hr after initiating therapy); hypotension and hypoperfusion will occur

• Renal function studies: BUN, serum uric acid, urine CrCl, electrolytes before, during therapy

• I&O ratio; report fall in urine output to <30 ml/hr

• Monitor temperature q4h; fever may indicate beginning infection

• Liver function tests before, during therapy: bilirubin, AST, ALT, alk phosphatase as needed or monthly

• ECG; watch for ST-T wave changes, low QRS and T, possible dysrhythmias (sinus tachycardia, PVCs)

• Baselines in pulmonary function; document FEV >2 L or $\geq75\%$ prior to therapy

• Stress thallium study prior to therapy; document normal ejection fraction, unimpaired wall motion

• Bleeding: hematuria, guaiac, bruising or petechiae, mucosa or orifices q8h

• Food preferences; list likes, dislikes

• Inflammation of mucosa, breaks in skin

• Buccal cavity q8h for dryness, sores, ulceration, white patches, oral pain, bleeding, dysphagia

• Alkalosis if severe vomiting is present

• Local irritation, pain, burning at injection site

• GI symptoms: frequency of stools, cramping

• Acidosis, signs of dehydration: rapid respirations, poor skin turgor, decreased urine output, dry skin, restlessness, weakness

• Cardiac status: B/P, pulse, character, rhythm, rate, ABGs, ECG

Administer:

• Hydrocortisone, dexamethasone or sodium bicarbonate (1 mEq/1 ml) for extravasation, apply ice compresses

• Antiemetic 30-60 min before giving drug to prevent vomiting

• IV after diluting 22 million IU (1.3 mg)/1.2 sterile H_2O for inj at site of vial and swirl, do not shake; dilute dose with 50 ml D_5W and give over 15 min; use plastic bag; do not use an in-line filter, give through Y-tube or 3-way stopcock

• Topical or systemic analgesics for pain

• Transfusion for anemia

• Antispasmodic for GI symptoms

Perform/provide:

• Strict hand-washing technique, gloves, protective clothing

• Liquid diet: carbonated beverage, gelatin (Jell-O) may be added if patient is not nauseated or vomiting

• Rinsing of mouth tid-qid with water, club soda; brushing of teeth bid-tid with soft brush or cotton-

---

italics = common side effects   ***bold italic*** = life threatening reactions

tipped applicators for stomatitis; use unwaxed dental floss
• Storage in refrigerator of diluted drug; do not freeze; administer within 48 hr; bring to room temperature before infusing; discard unused portion

Evaluate:
• Therapeutic response: decreased tumor size, spread of malignancy

Teach patient/family:
• To report any complaints, side effects to nurse or physician
• To avoid foods with citric acid, hot or rough texture
• To report any bleeding, white spots, ulcerations in mouth to physician; tell patient to examine mouth qd
• To avoid crowds and persons with infections when granulocyte count is low

---

alfentanil HCl

(al-fen'ta-nil)
Alfenta
Func. class.: Narcotic analgesic
Chem. class.: Opiate, synthetic

Controlled Substance Schedule II
Action: Inhibits ascending pain pathways in limbic system, thalamus, midbrain, hypothalamus
Uses: In combination with other drugs in general anesthesia, as a primary anesthetic in general surgery

Dosage and routes:
Combination
• *Adult:* IV 8-50 µg/kg, may increase by 3-15 µg/kg
Anesthetic induction
• *Adult:* IV 130-245 µg/kg, then 0.5-1.5 µg/kg/min
Available forms: Inj 500 µg/ml

Side effects/adverse reactions:
CNS: Drowsiness, dizziness, confusion, headache, sedation, euphoria, delirium, agitation, anxiety
GI: Nausea, vomiting, anorexia, constipation, cramps, dry mouth
GU: Urinary retention, dysuria
INTEG: Rash, urticaria, bruising, flushing, diaphoresis, pruritus
EENT: Tinnitus, blurred vision, miosis, diplopia
CV: Palpitation, bradycardia, change in B/P, facial flushing, syncope, asystole
RESP: Respiratory depression, apnea
MS: Rigidity

Contraindications: Child <12 yr, hypersensitivity
Precautions: Pregnancy (C), lactation, increased intracranial pressure, acute MI, severe heart disease, renal disease, hepatic disease, asthma, respiratory conditions, convulsive disorders, elderly
Pharmacokinetics: Half-life 1-2 hr, 90% bound to plasma proteins, duration 30 min
Interactions/incompatibilities:
• Respiratory depression, hypotension, profound sedation: alcohol, sedative, hypnotics, or other CNS depressants, antihistamines, phenothiazines
• Compatible IV solution: LR, 0.9% NaCl, D₅W, D₅/0.9% NaCl
Lab test interferences: *Increase:* Amylase

NURSING CONSIDERATIONS
Assess:
• I&O ratio, check for decreasing output; may indicate urinary retention, especially in elderly
• CNS changes: dizziness, drowsiness, hallucinations, euphoria, LOC, pupil reaction
• Allergic reactions: rash, urticaria
• Respiratory dysfunction: respi-

ratory depression, character, rate, rhythm: notify physician if respirations are <12/min; CV status: bradycardia, syncope
• Use pain scoring to determine pain perception
Administer:
• Direct IV over 1½-3 min; use tuberculin syringe
• Cont. IV by diluting 20 ml of drug in 230 ml of diluent (40 µg/ml); discontinue inf 15 mins before surgery is completed
Perform/provide:
• Storage in light-resistant area at room temperature
Evaluate:
• Therapeutic response: maintenance of anesthesia
Treatment of overdose: Narcan 0.2-0.8 IV, O₂, IV fluids, vasopressors

---

alglucerase
(all-gloo-ser'-ase)
Ceredase
Func. class.: Enzyme

Action: Catalyzes the breakdown of glucocerebroside, which accumulates in macrophages primarily in the liver, spleen, and bone marrow in Gaucher's disease
Uses: Long-term enzyme replacement for a confirmed diagnosis of type I Gaucher's disease
Dosage and routes:
• *Adult and child:* IV 60 U/kg diluted in up to 100 ml of 0.9% NaCl given over 1-2 hr; dose is repeated q2 wk, but may be given QOD or as infrequently as q4wk; dose should be adjusted downward at intervals of 3-6 mo
Available forms: Inj 80 IU/ml
Side effects/adverse reactions:
CNS: Fever, malaise, chills

GI: Nausea, vomiting, diarrh abdominal discomfort
INTEG: Pain on injection, burning and swelling at site of injection
Contraindications: Hypersensitivity
Precautions: Pregnancy (C), lactation
Pharmacokinetics: Steady-state enzymatic activity occurs within 60 min after a single injection; elimination half-life 4-20 min
NURSING CONSIDERATIONS
Assess:
• GI status: transient nausea, vomiting, abdominal discomfort
• Hypersensitive reactions; rashes and local injection site reactions may occur
• For increased fluid retention in cardiac disease
Administer:
• By IV infusion over 1-2 hr
• Dilute 60 U/kg in up to 10 ml of 0.9% NaCl
Perform/provide:
• Storage in refrigerator; do not freeze; do not shake, as this may inactivate the drug
Evaluate:
• Therapeutic response: Reduction of splenomegaly and hepatomegaly; improvement of hematologic deficiencies, reduced cachexia and wasting in children
Teach patient/family:
• To use medication only as directed by physician
• To report unusual side effects and avoid all other medications unless prescribed by physician

allopurinol,*
...purin, Purimol,*
Zyloprim

Func. class.: Antigout drug
Chem. class.: Enzyme inhibitor

Action: Inhibits the enzyme xanthine oxidase, reducing uric acid synthesis

Uses: Chronic gout, hyperuricemia associated with malignancies, recurrent calcium oxalate calculi

Dosage and routes:
Gout/hyperuricemia
• *Adult:* PO 200-600 mg qd depending on severity, not to exceed 800 mg/day
• *Child 6-10 yr:* 300 mg qd
• *Child <6 yr:* 150 mg qd
Impaired renal function
• *Adult:* PO 200 mg qd when CrCl is 20 to 10 ml/min
Recurrent calculi
• *Adult:* PO 200-300 mg qd
Uric acid nephropathy prevention
• *Adult:* PO 600-800 mg qd × 2-3 days

Available forms: Tabs 100, 300 mg
Side effects/adverse reactions:
HEMA: Agranulocytosis, thrombocytopenia, aplastic anemia, pancytopenia, leukopenia, bone marrow depression, eosinophilia
CNS: Headache, drowsiness, neuritis, paresthesia
GI: Nausea, vomiting, anorexia, malaise, metallic taste, cramps, peptic ulcer, diarrhea, stomatitis
MISC: Myopathy, arthralgia, hepatomegaly, *cholestatic jaundice, renal failure*
EENT: Retinopathy, cataracts, epistaxis
INTEG: Fever, chills, dermatitis, pruritus, purpura, erythema, ecchymosis, alopecia

Contraindications: Hypersensitivity

Precautions: Pregnancy (B), lactation, renal disease, hepatic disease, children

Pharmacokinetics:
PO: Peak 2-4 hr; excreted in feces, urine, half-life 2-3 hr, terminal half-life 18-30 hr

Interactions/incompatibilities:
• Increased action of oral anticoagulants, chlorpropamide, cyclophosphamide, hydantoin, theophylline, vidarabine, ACE inhibitors
• Decreased effects of probenecid
• Rash: ampicillin, amoxicillin
• Increased hypersensitivity: thiazide diuretics
• Decreased effects of allopurinol: aluminum salts

Lab test interferences:
Increase: AST/ALT, alk phosphatase
Decrease: Hct/Hgb, leukocytes, serum glucose

NURSING CONSIDERATIONS
Assess:
• Uric acid levels q2 wk; uric acid levels should be 6 mg/dl
• CBC, AST, BUN, creatinine before starting treatment, monthly
• I&O ratio; increase fluids to prevent stone formation
• Nutritional status: discourage organ meat, sardines, salmon, legumes, gravies (high-purine foods)
Administer:
• With meals, to prevent GI symptoms
• A few days before antineoplastic therapy
Evaluate:
• Therapeutic response: decreased pain in joints, decreased stone formation in kidney

*Available in Canada only

Teach patient/family:
• To increase fluid intake to 3-4 L/day
• To report skin rash, stomatitis, malaise, fever, aching; drug should be discontinued
• To avoid hazardous activities if drowsiness or dizziness occurs
• To avoid alcohol, caffeine; will increase uric acid levels
• To avoid large doses of vitamin C; kidney stone formation may occur
• To maintain a diet enhancing urine alkalinity e.g., milk

---

alprazolam
(al-pray'zoe-lam)
Xanax
Func. class.: Antianxiety
Chem. class.: Benzodiazepine

Controlled Substance Schedule IV
Action: Depresses subcortical levels of CNS, including limbic system, reticular formation
Uses: Anxiety, panic disorders, anxiety with depressive symptoms
Dosage and routes:
• *Adult:* PO 0.25-0.5 mg tid, not to exceed 4 mg/day in divided doses
• *Geriatric:* PO 0.25 mg bid-tid
Available forms: Tab 0.25, 0.5, 1 mg
Side effects/adverse reactions:
CNS: Dizziness, drowsiness, confusion, headache, anxiety, tremors, stimulation, fatigue, depression, insomnia, hallucinations
GI: Constipation, dry mouth, nausea, vomiting, anorexia, diarrhea
INTEG: Rash, dermatitis, itching
CV: Orthostatic hypotension, **ECG changes, tachycardia,** hypotension

EENT: Blurred vision, tinnitus, mydriasis
Contraindications: Hypersensitivity to benzodiazepines, narrow-angle glaucoma, psychosis, pregnancy (D), child <18 yr
Precautions: Elderly, debilitated, hepatic disease, renal disease
Pharmacokinetics:
PO: Onset 30 min, peak 1-2 hr, duration 4-6 hr, therapeutic response 2-3 days; metabolized by liver, excreted by kidneys; crosses placenta, breast milk; half-life 12-15 hr
Interactions/incompatibilities:
• Increased CNS depression: anticonvulsants, alcohol, antihistamines, sedative/hypnotics
• Decreased action of alprazolam: disulfiram, cimetidine
• Decreased action of levodopa
Lab test interferences:
Increase: AST/ALT, serum bilirubin
False increase: 17-OHCS
Decrease: RAIU
NURSING CONSIDERATIONS
Assess:
• B/P (lying, standing), pulse; if systolic B/P drops 20 mm Hg, hold drug, notify physician
• Blood studies: CBC during long-term therapy; blood dyscrasias have occurred rarely
• Hepatic studies: AST, ALT, bilirubin, creatinine, LDH, alk phosphatase
• I&O; may indicate renal dysfunction
• For indications of increasing tolerance and abuse
• Mental status: mood, sensorium, affect, sleeping pattern, drowsiness, dizziness, especially elderly
• Physical dependency, withdrawal symptoms: anxiety, panic attacks, agitation, convulsions, headache,

---

italics = common side effects   ***bold italic*** = life threatening reactions

nausea, vomiting, muscle pain, weakness
• Suicidal tendencies
Administer:
• With food or milk for GI symptoms
• Crushed if patient is unable to swallow medication whole
• Sugarless gum, hard candy, frequent sips of water for dry mouth
Perform/provide:
• Assistance with ambulation during beginning therapy; drowsiness/dizziness occurs
• Safety measures, including side rails
• Check that PO medication has been swallowed
Evaluate:
• Therapeutic response: decreased anxiety, restlessness, sleeplessness
Teach patient/family:
• That drug may be taken with food
• Not to use for everyday stress or longer than 3 mo unless directed by physician; not to take more than prescribed amount; may be habit forming
• To avoid OTC preparations unless approved by physician
• To avoid driving, activities that require alertness, since drowsiness may occur
• To avoid alcohol ingestion or other psychotropic medications unless prescribed by physician
• Not to discontinue medication abruptly after long-term use
• To rise slowly or fainting may occur, especially elderly
• That drowsiness may worsen at beginning of treatment
Treatment of overdose: Lavage, VS, supportive care

---

alprostadil
(al-pros'ta-dil)
Prostin VR Pediatric
Func. class.: Hormone
Chem. class.: Prostaglandin E₁

Action: Relaxes smooth muscles of ductus arteriosus; results in increased O_2 content throughout body
Uses: To maintain patent ductus arteriosus (temporary treatment)
Dosage and routes:
• *Infants:* IV INF 0.1 μg/kg/min, until desired response, then reduce to lowest effective amount, 0.4 μg/kg/min not likely to produce greater beneficial effects
Available forms: Inj IV 500 μg/ml
Side effects/adverse reactions:
*MISC: **Sepsis,** hypokalemia, **peritonitis,** hypoglycemia, hyperkalemia*
*RESP: **Apnea, bradypnea, wheezing, respiratory depression***
*HEMA: **DIC** (disseminated intravascular coagulation), **thrombocytopenia,** anemia, **bleeding***
*CNS: Fever, **convulsions,** lethargy, hypothermia, stiffness, hyperirritability, **cerebral bleeding***
GI: Diarrhea, regurgitation, hyperbilirubinemia
*GU: Oliguria, hematuria, **anuria***
*CV: **Bradycardia, tachycardia,** hypotension, **CHF, ventricular fibrillation, shock,** flushing, **cardiac arrest,** edema*
Contraindications: *Hypersensitivity,* respiratory distress syndrome (RDS)
Precautions: Bleeding disorders
Pharmacokinetics: Up to 80% metabolized in lungs, excreted in urine (metabolites)
Interactions/incompatibilities:
• Do not mix in sol or syringe with

other drugs; compatibility not known

NURSING CONSIDERATIONS
Assess:
• ABGs, arterial pH, arterial pressure, continuous ECG; if arterial pressure decreases, reduce or stop drug
• Apnea and bradycardia; if these occur, discontinue drug
• Increased pH, B/P, output, decreased ratio of PA to AP (restricted systemic blood flow)

Administer:
• Only with emergency equipment available by trained clinicians
• After diluting with NS or D₅W injection to a concentration of 500 μg/ml, dilute further with 0.9% NaCl, D₅W; 500 μg of drug/250 ml of dilute = 2 μg/ml; 0.1 μg/kg/min run at 0.05 ml/kg/min, use infusion pump

Perform/provide:
• Arterial pressure measurement during infusion
• Refrigeration for drug; discard all mixed unused portion

Evaluate:
• Therapeutic response: increased PO₂ (cyanotic heart disease)

Teach patient/family:
• About diagnosis, prognosis, treatment

Treatment of overdose:
Discontinue drug, provide supportive measures

---

alteplase
(al-teep′lase)
Activase
Func. class.: Antithrombotic
Chem. class.: Tissue plasminogen activator (TPA)

Action: Produces fibrin conversion of plasminogen to plasmin; able to bind to fibrin, convert plasminogen in thrombus to plasmin, which leads to local fibrinolysis, limited systemic proteolysis

Uses: Lysis of obstructing thrombi associated with acute MI; although not currently approved, alteplase will be used for other conditions requiring thrombolysis, i.e., PE, DUT, unclotting arteriovenous shunts

Dosage and routes:
• *Adult:* IV a total of 100 mg; 6-10 mg given IV BOL over 1-2 min, 60 mg given over first hour, 20 mg given over second hour, 20 mg given over third hour; or 1.25 mg/kg given over 3 hr for smaller patients

Available forms: Powder for inj 20 mg (11.6 million IU)/vial, 50 mg (29 million IU)/vial

Side effects/adverse reactions:
*SYST: **GI, GU, intracranial, retroperitoneal bleeding,** surface bleeding*
*CV: **Sinus bradycardia, ventricular tachycardia, accelerated idioventricular rhythm***
INTEG: Urticaria, rash

Contraindications: Hypersensitivity, active internal bleeding, recent CVA, severe uncontrolled hypertension, intracranial/intraspinal surgery/trauma, aneurysm

Precautions: Pregnancy (C), lactation, children

Pharmacokinetics: Cleared by liver, 80% cleared within 10 min of drug termination

Interactions/incompatibilities:
• Increased bleeding: heparin, acetylsalicylic acid, dipyridamole
• Do not add other drugs to IV solution

Lab test interferences:
Increase: PT, APTT, TT

---

italics = common side effects   ***bold italic*** = life threatening reactions

NURSING CONSIDERATIONS
Assess:

• VS, B/P, pulse, respirations, neurologic signs, temperature at least q4h; temperature >104° F (40° C) indicates internal bleeding; monitor rhythm closely; ventricular dysrhythmias may occur with hyperfusion; monitor heart, breath sounds, neuro status, peripheral pulses

• For bleeding during first hr of treatment: hematuria, hematemesis, bleeding from mucous membranes, epistaxis, ecchymosis; guaiac all body fluids, stools

• Allergy: fever, rash, itching, chills; mild reaction may be treated with antihistamines

• Blood studies (Hct, platelets, PTT, PT, TT, APTT) before starting therapy; PT or APTT must be less than 2 × control before starting therapy TT or PT q3-4h during treatment

Administer:

• After reconstituting with provided diluent, add appropriate amount of sterile water for injection (no preservatives) 20 mg vial/20 ml or 50 mg vial/50 ml to make 1 mg/ml, mix by slow inversion or dilute with NaCl, D₅W to a concentration of 0.5 mg/ml further dilution, 1.5 to <0.5 mg/ml may result in precipitation of drug; use 18G needle; flush line with NaCl after administration

• Heparin therapy after thrombolytic therapy is discontinued, TT, ACT, or APTT less than 2 × control (about 3-4 hr)

• Reconstituted IV solution within 8 hr

• Within 6 hr of coronary occlusion for best results

Perform/provide:

• Avoidance of invasive procedures, injection, rectal temperature

• Pressure for 30 sec to minor bleeding sites; 30 min to sites of atrial puncture, followed by pressure dressing; inform physician if this does not attain hemostasis; apply pressure dressing

• Storage of powder at room temperature or refrigerate; protect from excessive light

Evaluate:

• Therapeutic response: lysis of thrombi

---

altretamine
(al-tray'ta-meen)
Hexalen
Func. class.: Misc. antineoplastic
Chem. class.: s-triazine derivative (formerly known as hexamethylmelamine)

Action: Products of metabolism form covalent adducts with tissue macromolecules including DNA, which may be responsible for cytotoxicity; activity is not cell cycle phase specific

Uses: Palliative treatment of recurrent, persistent ovarian cancer following first-line treatment with cisplatin or alkylating agent–based combination

Dosage and routes:

• *Adult:* PO 260 mg/m² day for 14 or 21 days in a 28-day cycle; give in 4 divided doses after meals and at hs

Available forms: Caps 50 mg

Side effects/adverse reactions:

GI: Nausea, anorexia, vomiting, increased alk phosphatase, *hepatic toxicity*

CNS: Peripheral sensory neuropathy, fatigue, *seizures,* mood dis-

orders, disorders of consciousness, ataxia, dizziness, vertigo
*HEMA: **Leukopenia, thrombocytopenia, anemia***
GU: Increased BUN, serum creatinine
INTEG: Rash, pruritus, alopecia
Contraindications: Hypersensitivity, severe bone marrow depression, severe neurologic toxicity
Precautions: Pregnancy (D), lactation, children
Pharmacokinetics:
PO: Well absorbed orally, rapidly metabolized in liver, metabolites excreted in urine; peak ½-3 hr
Interactions/incompatibilities:
• Possible increased toxicity of altretamine: cimetidine
• Severe orthostatic hypotension: MAOI
NURSING CONSIDERATIONS
Assess:
• CBC, differential, platelet count weekly, withhold drug if WBC is <2000 or platelet count is <75,000 or granulocyte count is <1000/mm³; notify physician of results
• Renal function studies: BUN, serum uric acid, urine CrCl before, during therapy
• I&O ratio; report fall in urine output of 30 ml/hr
• Temperature q4h; may indicate beginning infection
• Liver function tests before, during therapy (bilirubin, AST, ALT, LDH) as needed or monthly
Administer:
• Antacid before oral agent, give drug after meals, at hs
• Antiemetic 30-60 min before giving drug to prevent vomiting
• Antibiotics for prophylaxis of infection
Perform/provide:
• Strict medical asepsis, protective isolation if WBC levels are low

Evaluate:
• Therapeutic response: decreased tumor size, spread of malignancy
Teach patient/family:
• To report signs of infection: increased temperature, sore throat, flu symptoms
• To report signs of anemia: fatigue, headache, faintness, shortness of breath, irritability
• To report bleeding; avoid use of razors or commercial mouthwash
• To avoid use of aspirin products or ibuprofen
• That hair may be lost during therapy; a wig or hairpiece may make patient feel better; new hair may be different in color, texture (rare)

---

aluminum acetate
Bluboro Powder, Boropak Powder, Burow's Solution, Domeboro, Modified Burow's Solution, Pedi-boro Soak Paks
Func. class.: Astringent
Chem. class.: Aluminum product

Action: Maintains skin acidity, which is protective to skin surface
Uses: Skin irritation, inflammation, athlete's foot, insect bites, poison ivy, eczema, acne, rash, bruises, pruritus (anal)
Dosage and routes:
• *Adult and child:* TOP apply for 15-30 min, q4-8h (1:10-40); gargle use 1:10 sol prn
Available forms: Solution, cream (Canada only)
Side effects/adverse reactions:
INTEG: Irritation, increasing inflammation
Contraindications: Tight, occlusive dressing
Interactions/incompatibilities:
• Inhibits action of topical collagenase ointment

• Decreased action of aluminum acetate: soap

NURSING CONSIDERATIONS
Assess:
• Area of body to receive topical application, irritation, rash, breaks, dryness

Administer:
• 1 pk/1 pt water (1:10-40 water)

Perform/provide:
• Wet dressings using only loose-fitting dressing

Evaluate:
• Therapeutic response: decreased skin irritation

Teach patient/family:
• To discontinue use if irritation occurs
• To avoid using near eye area
• To retain otic preparation for 2-3 min

---

aluminum carbonate gel
Basaljel

Func. class.: Antacid
Chem. class.: Aluminum product

Action: Neutralizes gastric acidity, binds phosphates in GI tract; these phosphates are excreted

Uses: Antacid, phosphate stones (prevention), phosphate binder in chronic renal failure

Dosage and routes:
Urinary phosphate stones
• *Adult:* SUSP 5-10 ml as needed; EXTRA STREN SUSP 2.5-5 ml as needed; PO 2-6 1 hr pc, hs

Antacid
• *Adult:* SUSP 15-45 ml in water or juice 1 hr pc, hs; EXTRA STREN SUSP 5-15 ml in water or juice 1 hr pc, hs; PO 1-2 tabs or caps as needed

Available forms: Caps 500, 608 mg; tabs 500, 608 mg; susp 400 mg/5 ml; extra stren susp 1000 mg/ml

Side effects/adverse reactions:
GI: Constipation, anorexia, obstruction, fecal impaction
META: Hypophosphatemia, hypercalciuria

Contraindications: Hypersensitivity to this drug or aluminum products, appendicitis

Precautions: Elderly, fluid restriction, decreased GI motility, GI obstruction, dehydration, renal disease, sodium-restricted diets, pregnancy (C)

Pharmacokinetics:
PO: Excreted in feces

Interactions/incompatibilities:
• Decreased effectiveness of tetracyclines, ketoconazole
• Decreased absorption of anticholinergics, chlordiazepoxide, cimetidine, corticosteroids, iron salts, phenothiazines, phenytoin, digitalis
• Enteric-coated drugs: separate by 1 hr

NURSING CONSIDERATIONS
Assess:
• Hypophosphatemia: anorexia, weakness, fatigue, bone pain, hyporeflexia
• Constipation; if product is being used as an antacid, may need to switch to magnesium antacid
• Phosphate levels, urinary pH, Ca^{++}, electrolytes

Administer:
• Laxatives or stool softeners if constipation occurs, especially elderly
• After shaking

Perform/provide:
• I&O; strain urine if using for urinary calculi

Evaluate:
• Therapeutic response: absence of pain, decreased acidity

---

*Available in Canada only

Teach patient/family:
• Increase fluids to 2000 ml/day unless contraindicated
• Avoid phosphate foods (most dairy products, eggs, fruits, carbonated beverages) during drug therapy
• Add cheese, corn, pasta, plums, prunes, lentils after drug is discontinued
• Limit sodium intake

aluminum hydroxide

AlternaGEL, Alternagel, Alu-Cap, Aluminum Hydroxide, Aluminum Hydroxide Gel, Alu-Tab, Amphojel, Basaljel,* Concentrated Aluminum Hydroxide, Dialume

Func. class.: Antacid
Chem. class.: Aluminum product

Action: Neutralizes gastric acidity, binds phosphates in GI tract; these phosphates are excreted
Uses: Antacid, hyperphosphatemia in chronic renal failure
Dosage and routes:
• *Adult:* SUSP 5-10 ml 1 hr pc, hs; PO 600 mg 1 hr pc, hs, chewed with milk or water
Hyperphosphatemia in renal failure
• *Adult:* SUSP 500 mg-2 g bid-qid
Available forms: Caps 475, 500 mg; tabs 300, 500 mg; chewable tabs 600 mg; susp (4%) 600 mg/5 ml; liq 320 mg/5ml, 600 mg/5 ml
Side effects/adverse reactions:
GI: Constipation, anorexia, **obstruction,** fecal impaction
META: Hypophosphatemia, hypercalciuria
Contraindications: Hypersensitivity to this drug or aluminum products

Precautions: Elderly, fluid restriction, decreased GI motility, GI obstruction, dehydration, renal disease, sodium-restricted diets, pregnancy (C)
Pharmacokinetics:
PO: Onset 20-40 min, excreted in feces
Interactions/incompatibilities:
• Decreased effectiveness of tetracyclines, anticholinergics, phenothiazines, isoniazid, quinidine, phenytoin, digitalis, iron salts, warfarin, ketoconazole; separate by at least 2 hr
NURSING CONSIDERATIONS
Assess:
• Phosphate levels, since drug is bound in GI system
• Hypophosphatemia: anorexia, weakness, fatigue, bone pain, hyporeflexia
• Constipation; increase bulk in diet if needed
• Phosphate levels, urinary pH, Ca^{++}, electrolytes
Administer:
• Laxatives or stool softeners if constipation occurs, especially elderly
• After shaking liquid
• By nasogastric tube if patient unable to swallow
• With small amount of water or milk
Evaluate:
• Therapeutic response: absence of pain, decreased acidity
Teach patient/family:
• To increase fluids to 2000 ml/day unless contraindicated
• To avoid phosphate foods (most dairy products, eggs, fruits, carbonated beverages) during drug therapy
• Not to use for prolonged periods in patients with low serum phosphate or if on a low-sodium diet

---

italics = common side effects   ***bold italic*** = life threatening reactions

• To add cheese, corn, pasta, plums, prunes, lentils after drug is discontinued
• Stools may appear white or speckled
• To check with physician after 2 wk of self-prescribed antacid use

---

aluminum phosphate
Phosphaljel

Func. class.: Antacid
Chem. class.: Aluminum products

Action: Neutralizes gastric acidity, binds phosphates in GI tract; these phosphates are excreted
Uses: Antacid
Dosage and routes:
• *Adult:* SUSP 15-30 ml 1 hr pc, hs
• *Adult:* Intragastric dilute 1:3 or 1:4
Available forms: Susp 233 mg/5 ml
Side effects/adverse reactions:
GI: Constipation, anorexia, *obstruction,* fecal impaction
META: Hyperphosphatemia
Contraindications: Hypersensitivity to this drug or aluminum products
Precautions: Elderly, fluid restriction, decreased GI motility, GI obstruction, dehydration, renal disease, sodium-restricted diets, pregnancy (C)
Pharmacokinetics:
PO: Onset 20-40 min, excreted in feces
Interactions/incompatibilities:
• Decreased effectiveness of tetracyclines, ketoconazole, isoniazid, phenothiazines, iron salts, digitalis
NURSING CONSIDERATIONS
Assess
• Constipation; increase bulk in

diet if needed or alternate with magnesium antacids
• Phosphate levels, urinary pH, Ca^{++}, electrolytes
Administer:
• Laxatives or stool softeners if constipation occurs, especially elderly
• After shaking solution
Evaluate:
• Therapeutic response: absence of pain, decreased acidity
Teach patient/family:
• To increase fluids to 2000 ml unless contraindicated
• Not to switch antacids unless directed by physician
• To use PO meds 1-2 hr after antacid
• That antacid may cause premature dissolution of enteric-coated tablets

---

amantadine HCl
(a-man'ta-deen)
Amantadine HCl, Symadine, Symmetrel

Func. class.: Antiviral, antiparkinsonian agent
Chem. class.: Tricyclic amine

Action: Prevents uncoating of nucleic acid in viral cell, preventing penetration of virus to host; causes release of dopamine from neurons
Uses: Prophylaxis or treatment of influenza type A, extrapyramidal reactions, parkinsonism, respiratory tract infections
Dosage and routes:
Influenza type A
• *Adult and child >12 yr:* PO 200 mg/day in single dose or divided bid
• *Child 9-12 yr:* PO 100 mg bid
• *Child 1-9 yr:* PO 4.4-8.8 mg/kg/

day divided bid-tid, not to exceed
200 mg/day
Extrapyramidal reaction/parkin-
sonism
• *Adult:* PO 100 mg bid, up to 400
mg/day in EPS; give for 1 wk then
100 mg as needed up to 400 mg in
parkinsonism
Available forms: Caps 100 mg; syr
50 mg/5 ml
Side effects/adverse reactions:
CNS: Headache, dizziness, drowsiness, fatigue, anxiety, psychosis,
depression, hallucinations, tremors, *convulsions*
CV: Orthostatic hypotension, ***CHF***
INTEG: Photosensitivity, dermatitis
EENT: Blurred vision
HEMA: ***Leukopenia***
GI: Nausea, vomiting, constipation, dry mouth
GU: Frequency, retention
Contraindications: Hypersensitivity, lactation, child <1 yr,
pregnancy (C), eczematic rash
Precautions: Epilepsy, CHF, orthostatic hypotension, psychiatric
disorders, hepatic disease, renal
disease, peripheral edema
Pharmacokinetics:
PO: Onset 48 hr, half-life 24 hr, not
metabolized, excreted in urine
(90%) unchanged, crosses placenta, excreted in breast milk
Interactions/incompatibilities:
• Increased anticholinergic response: atropine, other anticholinergics
• Increased CNS stimulation: CNS
stimulants

NURSING CONSIDERATIONS
Assess:
• I&O ratio; report frequency, hes-
itancy
• CHF, confusion, mottling of skin
• Bowel pattern before, during
treatment

• Skin eruptions, photosensitivity
after administration of drug
• Respiratory status: rate, character, wheezing, tightness in chest
• Allergies before initiation of
treatment, reaction of each medication; place allergies on chart in
bright red letters
• Signs of infection
Administer:
• Before exposure to influenza;
continue for 10 days after contact
• At least 4 hr before hs to prevent
insomnia
• After meals for better absorption,
to decrease GI symptoms
• In divided doses to prevent CNS
disturbances: headache, dizziness,
fatigue, drowsiness
Perform/provide:
• Storage in tight, dry container
Evaluate:
• Therapeutic response: absence of
temperature, malaise, cough, dyspnea in infection; tremors, shuffling gait in Parkinson's disease
Teach patient/family:
• To change body position slowly
to prevent orthostatic hypotension
• About aspects of drug therapy:
need to report dyspnea, weight
gain, dizziness, poor concentration, dysuria, behavioral changes
• To avoid hazardous activities if
dizziness occurs
• To take drug exactly as prescribed; parkinsonian crisis may
occur if drug is discontinued
abruptly
• To avoid alcohol
Treatment of overdose: Withdraw
drug, maintain airway, administer
epinephrine, aminophylline, O₂, IV
corticosteroids, physostigmine

---

italics = common side effects   ***bold italic*** = life threatening reactions

ambenonium chloride
(am-be-noe'nee-um)
Mytelase caplets
Func. class.: Cholinergics, Anticholinesterase
Chem. class.: Synthetic quaternary ammonium compound

Action: An acetylcholinesterase inhibitor; inhibits destruction of acetylcholine, which increases concentration at sites where acetylcholine is released; this facilitates transmission of impulses across myoneural junction

Uses: Myasthenia gravis when other drugs cannot be used

Dosage and routes:
• *Adult:* PO 5 mg q3-4h, then gradually increased q1-2 days; usually 5-40 mg per dose is sufficient

Available forms: Tabs 10 mg

Side effects/adverse reactions:
INTEG: Rash, urticaria, sweating

CNS: Dizziness, headache, weakness, *convulsions,* incoordination, *paralysis, loss of consciousness,* drowsiness

GI: Nausea, diarrhea, vomiting, cramps, increased salivary, gastric secretions, dysphagia, increased peristalsis

CV: Tachycardia, dysrhythmias, bradycardia, hypotension, AV block, ECG changes, *cardiac arrest,* sycope

GU: Frequency, incontinence, urgency

RESP: Respiratory depression, bronchospasm, constriction, laryngospasm, respiratory arrest, increased secretions, dyspnea

EENT: Miosis, blurred vision, lacrimation, visual changes

Contraindications: Obstruction of intestine, renal system, hypersensitivity

Precautions: Seizure disorders, bronchial asthma, coronary occlusion, hyperthyroidism, dysrhythmias, peptic ulcer, megacolon, poor GI motility, pregnancy (C), bradycardia, hypotension, lactation, children

Pharmacokinetics:
PO: Onset 20-30 min, duration 3-8 hr

Interactions/incompatibilities:
• Decreased action of ambenonium: aminoglycosides, anesthetics, antidysrhythmics, mecamylamine, polymyxin, quinidine, magnesium, corticosteroids
• Increased action of neuromuscular blockers, succinylcholine

NURSING CONSIDERATIONS
Assess:
• VS, respiration q2h
• I&O ratio; check for urinary retention or incontinence
• Bradycardia, hypotension, bronchospasm, headache, dizziness, convulsions, respiratory depression; drug should be discontinued if toxicity occurs
• Muscle strength: hand grasp

Administer:
• Only with atropine sulfate available for cholinergic crisis
• Only after all other cholinergics have been discontinued
• Increased doses if tolerance occurs
• Larger doses after exercise or fatigue
• On empty stomach for better absorption

Perform/provide:
• Storage at room temperature

Evaluate:
• Therapeutic response: increased muscle strength, improved gait, absence of labored breathing (if severe)

*Available in Canada only

Teach patient/family:
• To take drug exactly as prescribed
• That drug is not a cure; it only relieves symptoms
• To wear Medic Alert ID specifying myasthenia gravis, drugs taken
Treatment of overdose: Discontinue medication, respiratory support, atropine 1-4 mg

---

amcinonide
(am-sin'oh-nide)
Cyclocort
Func. class.: Topical corticosteroid
Chem. class.: Synthetic fluorinated agent, group II potency

Action: Antipruritic, antiinflammatory
Uses: Psoriasis, eczema, contact dermatitis, pruritus
Dosage and routes:
• *Adult and child:* Apply to affected area bid-tid; rub completely into skin
Available forms: Cream 0.1%; oint 0.1%
Side effects/adverse reactions:
INTEG: Burning, dryness, itching, irritation, acne, folliculitis, hypertrichosis, perioral dermatitis, hypopigmentation, atrophy, striae, miliaria, allergic contact dermatitis, secondary infection
Contraindications: Hypersensitivity to corticosteroids, fungal infections
Precautions: Pregnancy (C), lactation, viral infections, bacterial infections
NURSING CONSIDERATIONS
Assess:
• Temperature, worsening of rash;

if fever develops drug should be discontinued
• For systemic absorption: increased temperature, inflammation, irritation
Administer:
• Only to affected areas; do not get in eyes
• Medication, then cover with occlusive dressing (only if prescribed), seal to normal skin, change q12h; systemic absorption may occur
• Only to dermatoses; do not use on weeping, denuded, or infected area
Perform/provide:
• Cleansing before application of drug
• Treatment for a few days after area has cleared
• Storage at room temperature
Evaluate:
• Therapeutic response: absence of severe itching, patches on skin, flaking
Teach patient/family:
• To avoid sunlight on affected area; burns may occur
• To discontinue drug, notify physician if local irritation or fever develops

---

amikacin sulfate
(am-i-kay'sin)
Amikacin Sulfate, Amikin
Func. class.: Antibiotic
Chem. class.: Aminoglycoside

Action: Interferes with protein synthesis in bacterial cell by binding to ribosomal subunit, which causes misreading of genetic code; inaccurate peptide sequence forms in protein chain, causing bacterial death
Uses: Severe systemic infections of

---

italics = common side effects   **bold italic** = life threatening reactions

CNS, respiratory, GI, urinary tract, bone, skin, soft tissues caused by *P. aeruginosa, E. coli, Enterobacter, Acinetobacter, Providencia, Citrobacter, Staphylococcus, Serratia, Proteus, Klebsiella* pneumonia

Dosage and routes:

Severe systemic infections

• *Adult and child:* IV INF 15 mg/kg/day in 2-3 divided doses q8-12h in 100-200 ml D₅W over 30-60 min, not to exceed 1.5 g; decreased doses are needed in poor renal function as determined by blood levels, renal function studies; IM 15 mg/kg/day in divided doses q8-12h

• *Neonates:* IV INF 10 mg/kg initially, then 7.5 mg/kg q12h in D₅W over 1-2 hr

Severe urinary tract infections

• *Adults:* IM 250 mg bid

• *Adults with poor renal function:* 7.5 mg/kg initially, then increased as determined by blood levels, renal function studies

Available forms: Inj IM, IV 50, 250 mg/ml

Side effects/adverse reactions:

GU: Oliguria, hematuria, renal damage, azotemia, failure, nephrotoxicity

CNS: Confusion, depression, numbness, tremors, *convulsions,* muscle twitching, *neurotoxicity,* dizziness, vertigo, tinnitus

EENT: Ototoxicity, deafness, visual disturbances

HEMA: Agranulocytosis, thrombocytopenia, leukopenia, eosinophilia, anemia

GI: Nausea, vomiting, anorexia, increased ALT, AST, bilirubin, hepatomegaly, *hepatic necrosis,* splenomegaly

CV: Hypotension or hypertension, palpitations

INTEG: Rash, burning, urticaria, dermatitis, alopecia

Contraindications: Mild to moderate infections, hypersensitivity to aminoglycosides

Precautions: Neonates, mild renal disease, pregnancy (D), myasthenia gravis, lactation, hearing deficits, Parkinson's disease, elderly

Pharmacokinetics:

IM: Onset rapid, peak 1-2 hr

IV: Onset immediate, peak 1-2 hr

Plasma half-life 2-3 hr; not metabolized, excreted unchanged in urine, crosses placental barrier

Interactions/incompatibilities:

• Increased ototoxicity, neurotoxicity, nephrotoxicity: other aminoglycosides, amphotericin B, polymyxin, vancomycin, ethacrynic acid, furosemide, mannitol, methoxyflurane, cisplatin, cephalosporins

• Increased neuromuscular blockade, respiratory depression: anesthetics, nondepolarizing neuromuscular blockers, succinylcholine

• Do not mix in solution or syringe: carbenicillin, ticarcillin, amphotericin B, cephalothin, erythromycin, heparin, ampicillin, cefazolin, chlorothiazide, phenytoin, thiopental, vitamin B complex with C, warfarin, methicillin

NURSING CONSIDERATIONS

Assess:

• Weight before treatment; calculation of dosage is usually based on ideal body weight but may be calculated on actual body weight

• I&O ratio; urinalysis daily for proteinuria, cells, casts; report sudden change in urine output

• VS during infusion; watch for hypotension, change in pulse

• IV site for thrombophlebitis including pain, redness, swelling q30 min; change site if needed; apply

---

*Available in Canada only

warm compresses to discontinued site
• Serum peak, drawn at 30-60 min after IV infusion or 60 min after IM injection, trough level drawn just before next dose; Peak 20-30 min; peak serum level, trough <8 h; adjust dosage per levels
• Urine pH if drug is used for UTI; urine should be kept alkaline
• Renal impairment by securing urine for CrCl testing, BUN, serum creatinine; lower dosage should be given in renal impairment (CrCl <80 ml/min)
• Deafness by audiometric testing, ringing, roaring in ears, vertigo; assess hearing before, during, after treatment
• Dehydration: high sp. gr., decrease in skin turgor, dry mucous membranes, dark urine
• Overgrowth of infection, including increased temperature, malaise, redness, pain, swelling, perineal itching, diarrhea, stomatitis, change in cough, sputum
• C&S before starting treatment to identify organism
• Vestibular dysfunction: nausea, vomiting, dizziness, headache; drug should be discontinued if severe
• Injection sites for redness, swelling, abscesses; use warm compresses at site

Administer:
• IV, dilute 500 mg of drug/100-200 ml of IV D₅W, D₅NaCl or 0.9% NaCl and give over ½-1hr; flush after administration with D₅W or 0.9% NaCl
• IM injection in large muscle mass; rotate injection sites
• In evenly spaced doses to maintain blood level
• Bicarbonate to alkalinize urine if

ordered for UTI, as drug is most active in alkaline environment

Perform/provide:
• Adequate fluids of 2-3 L/day, unless contraindicated, to prevent irritation of tubules
• Flush of IV line with NS or D₅W after infusion
• Supervised ambulation, other safety measures with vestibular dysfunction

Evaluate:
• Therapeutic response: absence of fever, draining wounds, negative C&S after treatment

Teach patient/family:
• To report headache, dizziness, symptoms for overgrowth of infection, renal impairment
• To report loss of hearing, ringing, roaring in ears or feeling of fullness in head

Treatment of overdose: Hemodialysis, exchange transfusion in the newborn, monitor serum levels of drug, may give ticarcillin or carbenicillin

---

amiloride HCl
(a-mill'oh-ride)
Amiloride HCl, Midamor
Func. class.: Potassium-sparing diuretic
Chem. class.: Pyrazine

Action: Acts primarily on distal tubule, secondarily by inhibiting reabsorption of sodium, H₂O, and increasing potassium retention
Uses: Edema in CHF in combination with other diuretics, for hypertension, adjunct with other diuretics to maintain potassium
Dosage and routes:
• *Adult:* PO 5 mg qd, may be increased to 10-20 mg qd if needed
Available forms: Tab 5 mg

italics = common side effects   **bold italic** = life threatening reactions

Side effects/adverse reactions:
GU: Polyuria, dysuria, frequency, impotence
ELECT: Acidosis, hyponatremia, **hyperkalemia,** hypochloremia
CNS: Headache, dizziness, fatigue, weakness, paresthesias, tremor, depression, anxiety
GI: Nausea, diarrhea, dry mouth, *vomiting, anorexia,* cramps, constipation, abdominal pain, jaundice, bleeding
EENT: Loss of hearing, tinnitus, blurred vision, nasal congestion, increased intraocular pressure
INTEG: Rash, pruritus, alopecia, urticaria
MS: Cramps, joint pain
CV: Orthostatic hypotension, dysrhythmias, angina
*HEMA: **Agranulocytopenia, leukopenia, thrombocytopenia** (rare)*
Contraindications: Anuria, hypersensitivity, hyperkalemia, impaired renal function
Precautions: Dehydration, pregnancy (B), diabetes, acidosis, lactation
Pharmacokinetics:
PO: Onset 2 hr, peak 6-10 hr, duration 24 hr; excreted in urine, feces, half-life 6-9 hr
Interactions/incompatibilities:
• Enhanced action of antihypertensives; lithium toxicity may be provoked
• Hyperkalemia: other potassium-sparing diuretics, potassium products, ACE inhibitors, salt substitutes
Lab test interferences:
Interfere: GTT
NURSING CONSIDERATIONS
Assess:
• Weight, I&O daily to determine fluid loss; effect of drug may be decreased if used qd

• Rate, depth, rhythm of respiration, effect of exertion
• B/P lying, standing; postural hypotension may occur
• Electrolytes: potassium, sodium, chloride; glucose (serum), BUN, CBC, serum creatinine, blood pH, ABGs
• Improvement in CVP q8h
• Signs of drowsiness, restlessness
• Rashes, temperature elevation qd
• Confusion, especially in elderly; take safety precautions if needed
Administer:
• In AM to avoid interference with sleep if using drug as a diuretic
• With food, if nausea occurs, absorption may be decreased slightly
Evaluate:
• Therapeutic response: improvement in edema of feet, legs, sacral area daily if medication is being used in CHF
Teach patient/family:
• About adverse reactions: muscle cramps, weakness, nausea, dizziness, blurred vision
• To take with food or milk for GI symptoms
• To take early in day to prevent nocturia
• To avoid potassium-rich foods: oranges, bananas; salt substitutes, dried fruits except dried apricots
Treatment of overdose: Lavage if taken orally, monitor electrolytes, administer sodium bicarbonate for $K^+ > 6.5$ mEq/L, monitor hydration, CV, renal status

amino acid injection
(a-mee'noe)
FreAmine HBC, HepatAmine
Func. class.: Nitrogen product

Action: Needed for anabolism to

maintain structure, decrease catabolism, promote healing

Uses: Hepatic encephalopathy, cirrhosis, hepatitis, nutritional support in cancer

Dosage and routes:
• *Adult:* IV 80-120 g/day; 500 ml of amino acids/500 ml D_{50} given over 24 hr

Available forms: Inj IV many strengths, types

Side effects/adverse reactions:
CNS: Dizziness, headache, confusion, *loss of consciousness*
CV: Hypertension, ***CHF, pulmonary edema***
GI: Nausea, vomiting, liver fat deposits, abdominal pain
GU: Glycosuria, osmotic diuresis
ENDO: Hyperglycemia, rebound hypoglycemia, electrolyte imbalances, hyperosmolar syndrome, hyperosmolar hyperglycemic nonketotic syndrome, alkalosis, acidosis, hypophosphatemia, hyperammonemia, dehydration, hypocalcemia
INTEG: Chills, flushing, warm feeling, rash, urticaria, extravasation necrosis, phlebitis at injection site

Contraindications: Hypersensitivity, severe electrolyte imbalances, anuria, severe liver damage, maple syrup urine disease, PKU

Precautions: Renal disease, pregnancy (C), children, diabetes mellitus, CHF

Interactions/incompatibilities:
• Do not add any drug to sol or syringe

NURSING CONSIDERATIONS
Assess:
• Electrolytes (K, Na, Ca, Cl, Mg), blood glucose, ammonia, phosphate, ketones
• Renal, liver function studies: BUN, creatinine, ALT, AST, bilirubin

• Injection site for extravasation: redness along vein, edema at site, necrosis, pain, hard tender area; site should be changed immediately
• Monitor respiratory function q4h: auscultate lung fields bilaterally for crackles, respirations, quality, rate, rhythm
• Monitor temperature q4h for increased fever, indicating infection; if infection suspected, infusion is discontinued, tubing bottle cultured
• Monitor for impending hepatic coma: asterixis, confusion, fetor, lethargy
• Urine glucose q6h using Chemstrips, which are not affected by infusion substances
• Hyperammonemia: nausea, vomiting, malaise, tremors, anorexia, convulsions

Administer:
• Up to 40% protein and dextrose (up to 12.5%) via peripheral vein; stronger solutions require central IV administration
• TPN only mixed with dextrose to promote protein synthesis
• Immediately after mixing in pharmacy under strict aseptic technique using laminar flowhood, use infusion pump, in-line filter (0.22 μm) unless mixed with fat emulsion and dextrose (3 in 1)
• Using careful monitoring technique; do not speed up infusion; pulmonary edema, glucose overload will result

Perform/provide:
• Storage depends on type of solution; consult manufacturer
• Changing dressing and IV tubing to prevent infection q24-48h or q5-7 days if transparent dressing is used

Evaluate:
• Therapeutic response: weight

---

italics = common side effects   ***bold italic*** = life threatening reactions

gain, decrease in jaundice in liver disorders, increased LOC

Teach patient/family:
• Reason for use of TPN
• If chills, sweating are experienced, report at once

---

amino acid solution
Aminosyn, Aminosyn II, Aminosyn-PF, FreAmine III, Novamine, Travasol, Trophmine
Func. class.: Nitrogen product

Action: Needed for anabolism to maintain structure, decrease catabolism, promote healing

Uses: Nutritional support in cancer, trauma, intestinal obstruction, short bowel syndrome, severe malabsorption

Dosage and routes:
• *Adult:* IV 1-1.5 g/kg/day titrated to patient's needs
• *Child:* IV 2-3 g/kg/day titrated to patient's needs

Available forms: Inj IV many types, strengths

Side effects/adverse reactions:
CNS: Dizziness, headache, confusion, *loss of consciousness*
CV: Hypertension, *CHF, pulmonary edema*
GI: Nausea, vomiting, liver fat deposits, abdominal pain, jaundice
GU: Glycosuria, osmotic diuresis
ENDO: Hyperglycemia, rebound hypoglycemia, electrolyte imbalances, hyperosmolar syndrome, hyperosmolar hyperglycemic nonketotic syndrome, alkalosis, acidosis, hypophosphatemia, hyperammonemia, dehydration, hypocalcemia
INTEG: Chills, flushing, warm feeling, rash, urticaria, extravasation necrosis, phlebitis at injection site

Contraindications: Hypersensitivity, severe electrolyte imbalances, anuria, severe liver damage, maple syrup urine disease, PKU

Precautions: Renal disease, pregnancy (C), children, diabetes mellitus, CHF

Interactions/incompatibilities:
• Do not add any drug to sol or syringe

NURSING CONSIDERATIONS
Assess:
• Electrolytes (K, Na, Ca, Cl, Mg), blood glucose, ammonia, phosphate
• Renal, liver function studies: BUN, creatinine, ALT, AST, bilirubin
• Injection site for extravasation: redness along vein, edema at site, necrosis, pain, hard tender area; site should be changed immediately
• Monitor respiratory function q4h: auscultate lung fields bilaterally for crackles, respirations, quality, rate, rhythm
• Monitor temperature q4h for increased fever, indicating infection; if infection suspected, infusion is discontinued, tubing, bottle cultured
• Urine glucose q6h using Tes-Tape, Clinistix, Keto-Diastix, which are not affected by infusion substances; blood glucose is preferred testing method
• Hyperammonemia: nausea, vomiting, malaise, tremors, anorexia, convulsions

Administer:
• Up to 40% protein and dextrose (up to 12.5%) via peripheral vein; stronger solutions require central IV administration
• TPN only mixed with dextrose to promote protein synthesis
• Immediately after mixing in pharmacy under strict aseptic technique using laminar flowhood, use infu-

sion pump, in-line filter (0.22 μm) unless mixed with fat emulsion and dextrose (3 in 1)
• Using careful monitoring technique; do not speed up infusion; pulmonary edema, glucose overload will result

Perform/provide:
• Storage depends on type of solution; consult manufacturer
• Changing dressing and IV tubing to prevent infection q24-48h

Evaluate:
• Therapeutic response: weight gain, decrease in jaundice in liver disorders, increased serum albumin

Teach patient/family:
• Reason for use of TPN
• If chills, sweating are experienced, they should be reported at once

---

aminocaproic acid
(a-mee-noe-ka-proe'ik)
Amicar, Aminocaproic Acid
Func. class.: Hemostatic
Chem. class.: Synthetic monoaminocarboxylic acid

Action: Inhibits fibrinolysis by inhibiting plasminogen activator substances

Uses: Hemorrhage from hyperfibrinolysis, adjunctive therapy in hemophilia

Dosage and routes:
• *Adult:* PO/IV 5 g loading dose, then 1-1.25 g q1h if needed, not to exceed 30 g/day

Available forms: Inj IV 250 mg/ml; tab 500 mg; syr 250 mg/ml

Side effects/adverse reactions:
*GU: Dysuria, frequency, oliguria, **renal failure**, ejaculatory failure, menstrual irregularities*
GI: Nausea, vomiting, abdominal cramps, diarrhea

INTEG: Rash
*CNS: Headache, dizziness, malaise, fatigue, hallucinations, delirium, psychosis, **convulsions**, weakness*
*HEMA: **Thrombosis***
*CV: **Dysrhythmias**, orthostatic hypotension, bradycardia*
EENT: Tinnitus, nasal congestion, conjunctival suffusion

Contraindications: Hypersensitivity, abnormal bleeding, postpartum bleeding, DIC, upper urinary tract bleeding, new burns

Precautions: Neonates/infants, mild or moderate renal disease, hepatic disease, thrombosis, cardiac disease, pregnancy (C)

Pharmacokinetics:
PO/IV: Peak 2 hr, excreted by kidneys as unmetabolized drug rapidly absorbed

Interactions/incompatibilities:
Increased coagulation: estrogens, oral contraceptives
• Do not mix with sodium lactate in solution

Lab test interferences:
Increased: K^+, CPK

NURSING CONSIDERATIONS
Assess:
• I&O; if urinary output decreases, notify physician and stop drug
• Blood studies: coagulation factors, platelets, protamine coagulation test for extravascular clotting, thrombophlebitis
• B/P, pulse for increase
• Drug level: 0.13 mg/ml is required to decrease fibrinolysis
• Creatine phosphokinase, urinalysis
• Allergy: fever, rash, itching, jaundice
• Myopathy: if weakness, fever, myoglobinemia, or oliguria; discontinue drug
• Bleeding: mucous membrane,

---

italics = common side effects   ***bold italic*** = life threatening reactions

epistaxis, ecchymosis, petechiae, hematuria, hematemesis

Administer:
• Give IV loading dose over 30 min to avoid hypotension
• IV after dilution with 4-5 g/250 ml NS, D₅W, LR, give over 1 hr; may give by continuous infusion after loading dose(s) of 1 g/hr diluted in 50-100 ml of compatible solutions; use infusion pump; do not give by direct IV

Perform/provide:
• Storage in tight container in cool environment; do not freeze

Evaluate:
• Therapeutic response: decreased bleeding

Teach patient/family:
• To report any signs of bleeding (gums, under skin, urine, stools, emesis) or myopathy
• To change position slowly to decrease orthostatic hypotension
• Proper administration for 8-10 days following dental procedure in hemophilia
• To inform physicians that drug is being taken
• To change position slowly

---

aminoglutethimide

(a-meen-noe-gloo-teth′i-mide)
Cytadren
Func. class.: Antineoplastic, adrenal steroid inhibitor
Chem. class.: Hormone

Action: Acts by inhibiting DNA, RNA, protein synthesis; is derived from *Streptomyces verticillus;* replication is decreased by binding to DNA, which causes strand splitting; phase specific in G₂ and M phases; blocks biosynthesis of all steroid hormones (cortisol, androgens, progestins)

Uses: Suppression of adrenal function in Cushing's syndrome, metastatic breast cancer, adrenal cancer

Dosage and routes:
• *Adult:* PO 250 mg qid at 6 hr intervals, may increase by 250 mg/day q1-2 wk, not to exceed 2 g/day

Available forms: Tabs 250 mg

Side effects/adverse reactions:
GI: Nausea, vomiting, anorexia, **hepatotoxicity**
INTEG: Rash, pruritus, hirsutism
CV: **Hypotension,** tachycardia
CNS: Drowsiness, morbilliform skin rash, dizziness, headache, lethargy

Contraindications: Hypersensitivity, hypothyroidism, pregnancy (D)

Precautions: Renal disease, hepatic disease, respiratory disease

Pharmacokinetics: Half-life 13 hr, metabolized in liver, excreted in urine, crosses placenta

Interactions/incompatibilities:
• Accelerated metabolism of dexamethasone

NURSING CONSIDERATIONS
Assess:
• Renal function studies: BUN, serum uric acid, urine CrCl, electrolytes before, during therapy
• I&O ratio; report fall in urine output of 30 ml/hr
• Monitor temperature q4h; may indicate beginning infection
• Liver function tests before, during therapy (bilirubin, AST, ALT, LDH) as needed or monthly
• RBC, Hct, Hgb, since these may be decreased
• Food preferences; list likes, dislikes
• Inflammation of mucosa, breaks in skin
• Yellowing of skin, sclera, dark urine, clay-colored stools, itchy

---

* Available in Canada only

skin, abdominal pain, fever, diarrhea
• Symptoms indicating severe allergic reaction: rash, pruritus, urticaria, purpuric skin lesions, itching, flushing
Administer:
• Antacid before oral agent; give last dose of the day after evening meal before bedtime
• Local or systemic drugs for infection if indicated
Perform/provide:
• Special skin care
• Liquid diet, including cola, Jell-O; dry toast or crackers as ordered may be added if patient is not nauseated or vomiting
• Nutritious diet with iron and vitamin supplements as ordered
Evaluate:
• Therapeutic response: decrease in size of tumor or decrease in Cushing's syndrome
Teach patient/family:
• To report any complaints, side effects to nurse or physician
• That masculinization can occur, is reversible after discontinuing treatment
• To avoid self-administration of adjuvant corticosteroids
• That drowsiness may occur and to avoid driving or operating heavy machinery

---

aminophylline (theophylline ethylenediamine)
(am-in-off'i-lin)
Corophyllin,* Phyllocontin, Truphylline
Func. class.: Spasmolytic
Chem. class.: Xanthine, ethylenediamide

Action: Relaxes smooth muscle of respiratory system by blocking phosphodiesterase, which increases cyclic AMP. Increased cyclic AMP alters intracellular calcium ion movements; produces bronchodilation, increased pulmonary blood flow, relaxation of respiratory tract
Uses: Bronchial asthma, bronchospasm, Cheyne-Stokes respirations
Dosage and routes:
• *Adult:* PO 500 mg, then 250-500 mg q6-8h; CONT IV 0.3-0.9 mg/kg/hr (maintenance); RECT 500 mg q6-8h
• *Child:* PO 7.5 mg/kg, then 3-6 mg/kg q6-8h; IV 7.5 mg/kg, then 3-6 mg/kg q6-8h injected over 5 min; do not exceed 25 mg/min; may give loading dose of 5.6 mg/kg over ½ hr; CONT IV 1 mg/kg/hr (maintenance); for children/infants use drug without preservative of alcohol
• *Neonates:* IV/PO 1 mg/kg initially for plasma increases of each 2 μg/ml, then 1 mg/kg q6h
Available forms: Inj IV, IM, rectal supp 250, 500 mg; rectal sol 300 mg/5 ml; elix 250 mg/5 ml; oral liq 105 mg/5 ml; tabs 100, 200 mg, tabs con-rel 225 mg; tabs sust-rel 300 mg
Side effects/adverse reactions:
CNS: Anxiety, restlessness, insomnia, *dizziness,* **convulsions,** headache, light-headedness, muscle twitching
CV: Palpitations, sinus tachycardia, hypotension, flushing, dysrhythmias, increased respiratory rate
GI: Nausea, vomiting, anorexia, diarrhea, bitter taste, dyspepsia, anal irritation (suppositories), epigastric pain
RESP: Increased rate

---

italics = common side effects   ***bold italic*** = life threatening reactions

INTEG: Flushing, urticaria, *rectal supp (irritation)*

GU: Urinary frequency

Contraindications: Hypersensitivity to xanthines, tachydysrhythmias

Precautions: Elderly, CHF, cor pulmonale, hepatic disease, active peptic ulcer disease, diabetes mellitus, hyperthyroidism, hypertension, children, pregnancy (C), glaucoma, prostatic hypertrophy

Pharmacokinetics: Well absorbed PO, extended rel well absorbed slowly, rectal supp is erratic, rectal sol is absorbed quickly; metabolized by liver (caffeine); excreted in urine; crosses placenta; appears in breast milk

Half-life: 3-12 hr; half-life increased in geriatric patients, hepatic disease or CHF

PO: Onset ¼ hr., peak 1-2 hr., duration 6-8 hr.

PO-ER: Unknown, peak 4-7 hr., duration 8-12 hr.

IV: Onset rapid, duration 6-8 hr.

REC: Onset erratic, peak 1-2 hr., duration 6-8 hr.

Interactions/incompatibilities:

• Incompatible with amikacin, Vit C, bleomycin, cephalothin, cephaprin, chloramphenicol, chlorpromazine, cimetidine, clindamycin, codeine, corticotropin, diphenhydrinate, dobutamine, doxapram, doxorubicin, epinephrine, erythromycin, fructose sol, heparin, hydralazine, hydroxyzine, insulin, invert sugar, isoproterenol, levarterenol, meperidine, methadone, methicillin, methylprednisolone, morphine, nafcillin, papaverine, penicillin G, pentazocine, phenobarbital, phenytoin, procaine, prochlorperazine, promazine, promethazine, succinylcholine, tetracycline, vancomycin, Vit B with C

• Increased action of aminophylline: cimetidine, propranolol, erythromycin, troleandomycin

• Dysrhythmias: halothane

• May increase effects of: anticoagulants

• Cardiotoxicity: β-blockers

• Increased elimination: smoking

• Increased toxicity: erythromycin, influenza vaccine, oral contraceptives, glucocorticoids, disulfiram

• Decreased effects of: lithium

• Decreased effects of this drug: rifampin, barbiturates, adrenergics, ketoconozole

Lab test interferences:

Increased: Plasma free fatty acids

NURSING CONSIDERATIONS

Assess:

• Theophylline blood levels (therapeutic level is 10-20 μg/ml); toxicity may occur with small increase above 20 μg/ml, especially elderly

• Monitor I&O; diuresis occurs; dehydration may result in elderly or children

• Whether theophylline was given recently (24 hrs)

• Respiratory rate, rhythm, depth; auscultate lung fields bilaterally; notify physician of abnormalities

• Allergic reactions: rash, urticaria; if these occur, drug should be discontinued

Administer:

• PO after meals to decrease GI symptoms; absorption may be affected with a full glass of water; do not crush or chew enteric coated or ER tabs.

• IV after diluting in 5% dextrose to decrease burning sensation at injection site; only clear solutions

• May be diluted for IV INF in 100-200 ml in D_5W, $D_{10}W$, $D_{20}W$, 0.9% NaCl, 0.45% NaCl, LR

• Avoid IM injection; pain LR and tissue damage may occur

• Only clear solution; flush IV line before dose
• Rectal dose if patient is unable to take PO; retain rectal dose for ½ hour

Perform/provide:
• Storage of diluted solution for 24 hr if refrigerated

Evaluate:
• Therapeutic response: decreased dyspnea, respiratory stimulation in infancy, clear lung fields bilaterally

Teach patient/family:
• To take doses as prescribed, not to skip dose
• To check OTC medications, current prescription medications for ephedrine; will increase CNS stimulation, not to drink alcohol or caffeine products (tea, coffee, chocolate, colas)
• To avoid hazardous activities; dizziness may occur
• If GI upset occurs, to take drug with 8 oz water; avoid food, since absorption may be decreased
• To remain in bed 15-20 min after rectal suppository is inserted to avoid removal
• To notify physician of toxicity: insomnia, anxiety, nausea, vomiting, rapid pulse, convulsions
• To notify physician of change in smoking habit; a change in dose may be required
• To increase fluids to 2L/day to decrease secretion viscosity.

---

amiodarone HCl
(a-mee'-oh-da-rone)
Cordarone
Func. class.: Antidysrhythmic (Class III)
Chem. class.: Iodinated benzofuran derivative

Action: Prolongs action, potential duration, and effective refractory period, noncompetitive α- and β-adrenergic inhibition

Uses: Severe ventricular tachycardia, supraventricular tachycardia, ventricular fibrillation not controlled by first-line agents

Dosage and routes:
• *Adult:* PO Loading dose 800-1600 mg/day 1-3 wk; then 600-800 mg/day 1 mo; maintenance 200-600 mg/day

Available forms: Tabs 200 mg

Side effects/adverse reactions:
CNS: Headache, dizziness, involuntary movement, tremors, peripheral neuropathy, malaise, fatigue, ataxia, paresthesias, insomnia
GI: Nausea, vomiting, diarrhea, abdominal pain, anorexia, constipation, ***hepatotoxicity***
*CV: Hypotension, bradycardia, **sinus arrest, CHF,** dysrhythmias, **SA node dysfunction***
INTEG: Rash, photosensitivity, blue-gray skin discoloration, alopecia, spontaneous ecchymosis
EENT: Blurred vision, halos, photophobia, ***corneal microdeposits,*** dry eyes
ENDO: Hyperthyroidism or hypothyroidism
MS: Weakness, pain in extremities
*RESP: **Pulmonary fibrosis,*** pulmonary inflammation
MISC: Flushing, abnormal taste or smell, edema, abnormal salivation, coagulation abnormalities

Precautions: Goiter, Hashimoto's thyroiditis, SN dysfunction, 2nd or 3rd degree AV block, electrolyte imbalances, pregnancy (C), bradycardia, lactation

Pharmacokinetics:
PO: Onset 1-3 wk, peak 2-10 hr; half-life 15-100 days; metabolized by liver, excreted by kidneys

---

italics = common side effects   **bold italic** = life threatening reactions

Interactions/incompatibilities:
• Bradycardia: β-blockers, calcium channel blockers
• Increased levels of digitalis, quinidine, procainamide, flecainide, disopyramide, phenytoin
• Increased anticoagulant effects: warfarin
• Bradycardia, arrest: lidocaine

NURSING CONSIDERATIONS
Assess:
• I&O ratio; electrolytes: (K, Na, Cl)
• Liver function studies: AST, ALT, bilirubin, alk phosphatase
• ECG continuously to determine drug effectiveness, measure PR, QRS, QT intervals, check for PVCs, other dysrhythmias
• For dehydration or hypovolemia
• B/P continuously for hypotension, hypertension
• For rebound hypertension after 1-2 hr
• CNS symptoms: confusion, psychosis, numbness, depression, involuntary movements; if these occur, drug should be discontinued
• Hypothyroidism: lethargy, dizziness, constipation, enlarged thyroid gland, edema of extremities, cool, pale skin
• Hyperthyroidism: restlessness, tachycardia, eyelid puffiness, weight loss, frequent urination, menstrual irregularities, dyspnea, warm, moist skin
• Pulmonary toxicity: dyspnea, fatigue, cough, fever, chest pain; drug should be discontinued
• Cardiac rate, respiration: rate, rhythm, character, chest pain
Administer:
• Reduced dosage slowly with ECG monitoring
Evaluate:
• Therapeutic response: decrease in

ventricular tachycardia, supraventricular tachycardia or fibrillation
Teach patient/family:
• To use sunscreen or stay out of sun to prevent burns
• To report side effects immediately
• That skin discoloration is usually reversible
• That dark glasses may be needed for photophobia
Treatment of overdose: O_2, artificial ventilation, ECG, administer dopamine for circulatory depression, administer diazepam or thiopental for convulsions, isoproterenol

---

amitriptyline HCl
(a-mee-trip'ti-leen)
Amitriptylline HCl, Apo-Amitriptyline,* Elavil, Endep, Enovil, Levate,* Meravil,* Novotriptyn,* Rolavil*
Func. class.: Antidepressant—tricyclic
Chem. class.: Tertiary amine

Action: Blocks reuptake of norepinephrine, serotonin into nerve endings, increasing action of norepinephrine, serotonin in nerve cells
Uses: Major depression
Dosage and routes:
• *Adult:* PO 50-100 mg hs, may increase to 200 mg qd, not to exceed 300 mg/day; IM 20-30 mg qid, or 80-120 mg hs
• *Adolescent/geriatric:* PO 30 mg/day in divided doses, may be increased to 150 mg/day
Available forms: Tabs 10, 25, 50, 75, 100, 150 mg; inj IM 10 mg/ml
Side effects/adverse reactions:
HEMA: Agranulocytosis, throm-

bocytopenia, eosinophilia, leukopenia

CNS: Dizziness, drowsiness, confusion, headache, anxiety, tremors, stimulation, weakness, insomnia, nightmares, EPS (elderly), increased psychiatric symptoms

GI: Diarrhea, dry mouth, nausea, vomiting, **paralytic ileus,** increased appetite, cramps, epigastric distress, jaundice, **hepatitis,** stomatitis

GU: Retention

INTEG: Rash, urticaria, sweating, pruritus, photosensitivity

CV: Orthostatic hypotension, **ECG changes, tachycardia, hypertension,** palpitations

EENT: Blurred vision, tinnitus, mydriasis, ophthalmoplegia

Contraindications: Hypersensitivity to tricyclic antidepressants, recovery phase of myocardial infarction

Precautions: Suicidal patients, convulsive disorders, prostatic hypertrophy, schizophrenia, psychosis, severe depression, increased intraocular pressure, narrow-angle glaucoma, urinary retention, cardiac disease, hepatic disease/renal disease, hyperthyroidism, electroshock therapy, elective surgery, child <12 yr, pregnancy (C), elderly

Pharmacokinetics:

PO/IM: Onset 45 min, peak 2-12 hr, therapeutic response 2-3 wk; metabolized by liver, excreted in urine/feces, crosses placenta, excreted in breast milk, half-life 10-50 hr

Interactions/incompatibilities:

• Decreased effects of guanethidine, clonidine, indirect acting sympathomimetics (ephedrine)

• Increased effects of direct acting sympathomimetics (epinephrine), alcohol, barbiturates, benzodiazepines, CNS depressants

• Hyperpyretic crisis, convulsions, hypertensive episode: MAOI (pargyline [Eutonyl])

Lab test interferences:

Increase: Serum bilirubin, blood glucose, alk phosphatase

Decrease: VMA, 5-HIAA

False increase: Urinary catecholamines

NURSING CONSIDERATIONS

Assess:

• B/P (lying, standing), pulse q4h; if systolic B/P drops 20 mm Hg hold drug, notify physician; take vital signs q4h in patients with cardiovascular disease

• Blood studies: CBC, leukocytes, differential, cardiac enzymes if patient is receiving long-term therapy

• Hepatic studies: AST, ALT, bilirubin

• Weight qwk; appetite may increase with drug

• ECG for flattening of T wave, bundle branch block, AV block, dysrhythmias in cardiac patients

• EPS primarily in elderly: rigidity, dystonia, akathisia

• Mental status: mood, sensorium, affect, suicidal tendencies; increase in psychiatric symptoms: depression, panic

• Urinary retention, constipation; constipation is more likely to occur in children or elderly

• Withdrawal symptoms: headache, nausea, vomiting, muscle pain, weakness; do not usually occur unless drug was discontinued abruptly

• Alcohol consumption; if alcohol is consumed, hold dose until morning

Administer:

• Increased fluids, bulk in diet

if constipation, urinary retention occur, especially elderly
• With food or milk for GI symptoms
• Crushed if patient is unable to swallow medication whole
• Dosage hs if oversedation occurs during day; may take entire dose hs; elderly may not tolerate once/day dosing
• Gum, hard sugarless candy, or frequent sips of water for dry mouth
Perform/provide:
• Storage at room temperature; do not freeze
• Assistance with ambulation during beginning therapy, since drowsiness/dizziness occurs
• Safety measures, including side rails primarily in elderly
• Checking to see PO medication swallowed
Evaluate:
• Therapeutic response: decrease in depression, absence of suicidal thoughts
Teach patient/family:
• That therapeutic effects may take 2-3 wk
• To use caution in driving or other activities requiring alertness because of drowsiness, dizziness, blurred vision; to avoid rising quickly from sitting to standing, especially elderly
• To avoid alcohol ingestion, other CNS depressants
• Not to discontinue medication quickly after long-term use: may cause nausea, headache, malaise
• To wear sunscreen or large hat, since photosensitivity occurs
Treatment of overdose: ECG monitoring, induce emesis, lavage, activated charcoal, administer anticonvulsant

amlodipine besylate
(am-loh-dye'-peen)
Norvasc
Func. class.: Calcium channel blocker
Chem. class.: Dihydropyridine

Action: Inhibits calcium ion influx across cell membrane during cardiac depolarization; produces relaxation of coronary vascular smooth muscle, peripheral vascular smooth muscle; dilates coronary vascular arteries; increases myocardial oxygen delivery in patients with vasospastic angina
Uses: Chronic stable angina pectoris, hypertension, vasospastic angina
Dosage and routes:
Angina
• *Adult:* PO 5-10 mg qd
Hypertension
• *Adult:* PO 5 mg qd initially, may increase up to 10 mg/day
Available forms: Tabs 2.5, 5, 10 mg
Side effects/adverse reactions:
CV: Dysrhythmia, edema, bradycardia, hypotension, palpitations, syncope, AV block
GI: Nausea, vomiting, diarrhea, gastric upset, constipation, abdominal cramps, flatulence, anorexia
GU: Nocturia, polyuria, *acute renal failure*
INTEG: Rash, pruritus, urticaria, hair loss
CNS: Headache, fatigue, dizziness, anxiety, depression, insomnia, paresthesia, somnolence, asthenia
OTHER: Flushing, nasal congestion, sweating, shortness of breath, sexual difficulties, muscle cramps, cough, weight gain, tinnitus, epistaxis

Contraindications: Sick sinus syndrome, 2nd or 3rd degree heart block, hypotension less than 90 mm Hg systolic, hypersensitivity
Precautions: CHF, hypotension, hepatic injury, pregnancy (C), lactation, children, renal disease, elderly
Pharmacokinetics:
PO: Onset not determined, peak 6-12 hr, half-life 30-50 hr; metabolized by liver, excreted in urine (90% as metabolites)
Interactions/incompatibilities:
• Increased effects of digitalis, neuromuscular blocking agents, theophylline, prazosin, β blockers, fentanyl
NURSING CONSIDERATIONS
Assess:
• Cardiac status: B/P, pulse, respiration, ECG
Administer:
• Once a day
Evaluate:
• Therapeutic response: decreased anginal pain, decreased B/P
Teach patient/family:
• To avoid hazardous activities until stabilized on drug, dizziness is no longer a problem
• To limit caffeine consumption
• To avoid OTC drugs unless directed by physician
• To comply in all areas of medical regimen: diet, exercise, stress reduction, drug therapy
• To notify physician of irregular heart beat, shortness of breath, swelling of feet and hands, pronounced dizziness, constipation, nausea, hypotension
Treatment of overdose: Defibrillation, β-agonists, IV calcium inotropic agents, diuretics, atropine for AV block, vasopressor for hypotension

ammonia, aromatic spirit
Func. class.: Respiratory stimulants
Chem. class.: Aromatic hydroalcoholic solution of ammonia

Action: Stimulates medulla (respiratory, vasomotor areas) by irritation of sensory receptors in mucosa of nasal passages, esophagus, stomach
Uses: To treat, prevent fainting
Dosage and routes:
• *Adult and child:* INH prn; PO 2-4 ml diluted in water
Available forms: Inh 0.33, 0.4 ml; sol
Side effects/adverse reactions:
None known
NURSING CONSIDERATIONS
Assess:
• Vital signs, B/P after administration of inhalant
• Cause of fainting
Administer:
• By inhalation; do not place packets in pockets, may open, cause caustic burns
• Orally by diluting 2-4 ml in >30 ml of water
Perform/provide:
• Storage protected from light at room temperature
Evaluate:
• Therapeutic response: revival after fainting

ammonium chloride
Func. class.: Acidifier
Chem. class.: Ammonium ion

Action: Lowers urinary pH, liberates hydrogen and chloride ions in blood and extracellular fluid with decreased pH and correction of alkalosis

Uses: Alkalosis (metabolic), systemic and urinary acidifer, expectorant, diuretic

Dosage and routes:
Alkalosis
• *Adult and child:* IV INF 0.9-1.3 ml/min of a 2.14% sol, not to exceed 5 ml/min
Acidifier
• *Adult:* PO 4-12 g/day in divided doses
• *Child:* PO 75 mg/kg/day in divided doses
Expectorant
• *Adult:* PO 250-500 mg q2-4h as needed

Available forms: Tabs 500 mg, 1 g; inj IV 0.4, 5 mEq/ml

Side effects/adverse reactions:
CNS: Drowsiness, headache, confusion, stimulation, tremors, *twitching, hyperreflexia,* **tetany,** *EEG changes*
CV: Bradycardia, dysrhythmias, bounding pulse
GU: Glycosuria, thirst
GI: Gastric irritation, nausea, vomiting, anorexia, diarrhea
INTEG: Rash, pain at infusion site
META: Acidosis, hypokalemia, hyperchloremia, hyperglycemia
RESP: **Apnea,** irregular respirations, hyperventilation

Contraindications: Hypersensitivity, severe hepatic disease, severe renal disease

Precautions: Severe respiratory disease, cardiac edema, respiratory acidosis, infants, pregnancy (C), children, elderly

Pharmacokinetics:
PO: Absorbed in 3-6 hr; metabolized in liver, excreted in urine and feces

Interactions/incompatibilities:
• Increased toxicity: PAS

• Decreased effects of: amphetamines, tricyclic antidepressants, salicylates, sulfonylureas
• Increased risk of systemic acidosis: spironolactone
• Incompatible with chlortetracycline, codeine, dimenhydrinate, levorphanol, methadone, warfarin, alkal. sol or drugs

Lab test interferences:
Increase: Blood ammonia, AST/ALT
Decrease: Serum magnesium, urine urobilinogen

NURSING CONSIDERATIONS
Assess:
• Respiratory rate, rhythm, depth; notify physician of abnormalities that may indicate acidosis
• Electrolytes and CO_2, chloride before and during treatment
• Urine pH, urinary output, urine glucose, specific gravity during beginning treatment
• I&O ratio, report large increases or decreases
• For CNS symptoms: confusion, twitching, hyperreflexia, stimulation, headache that may indicate ammonia toxicity
• For cardiac dysrhythmias
• For respiratory symptoms: hyperventilation

Administer:
• PO with meals if GI symptoms occur
• IV slowly to avoid pain at infusion site and toxicity
• After diluting solutions to 2.14% (IV), each 20-ml vial must be further diluted by adding 1-2 vials/500-1000 ml of compatible solution given at a rate of 5 ml/min or less; KCl 20-40 mEq/L may be added to the infusion; infants dilute 1 ml of drug/5-10 ml of diluent
• With water for expectorant not

compatible with milk or other alkaline solutions

Evaluate:
• Therapeutic response: decreasing metabolic alkalosis or increasing urinary acidity or diuresis

Teach patient/family:
• To increase potassium in diet: bananas, oranges, cantaloupe, honeydew, spinach, potatoes, dry fruit

---

amobarbital/amobarbital sodium

(am-oh-bar'bi-tal)
Amobarbital Sodium, Amytal, Amytal Sodium, Amytal Sodium Pulvules

Func. class.: Sedative/hypnotic-barbiturate (intermediate acting)
Chem. class.: Amylobarbitone

Controlled Substance Schedule II (USA), Schedule G (Canada)

Action: Depresses activity in brain cells primarily in reticular activating system in brain stem; also selectively depresses neurons in posterior hypothalamus, limbic structures; able to decrease seizure activity by inhibition of impulses in CNS; depresses REM sleep

Uses: Sedation, preanesthetic sedation, insomnia, anticonvulsant, adjunct in psychiatry, hypnotic

Dosage and routes:
Preanesthetic sedation
• *Adult and child:* PO/IM 200 mg 1-2 hr preoperatively
Sedation
• *Adult:* PO 30-50 mg bid or tid, may be 15-120 mg bid-qid
• *Child:* PO 2 mg/kg/day in 4 divided doses
Anticonvulsant/psychiatry
• *Adult:* IV 65-500 mg given over several min, not to exceed 100 mg/min; not to exceed 1 g
• *Child <6 yr:* IV/IM 3-5 mg/kg over several min
Insomnia
• *Adult:* PO/IM 65-200 mg hs, not to exceed 5 ml in one site
• *Child:* IM 3-5 mg/kg at hs, not to exceed 5 ml in one site

Available forms: Tabs 30, 50, 100 mg; caps 65, 200 mg; powder for inj IM, IV 250, 500 mg/vial

Side effects/adverse reactions:
CNS: Lethargy, drowsiness, hangover, dizziness, stimulation in the elderly and children, light-headedness, physical dependence, CNS depression, mental depression, slurred speech
GI: Nausea, vomiting, diarrhea, constipation
INTEG: Rash, urticaria, pain, abscesses at injection site, *angioedema,* thrombophlebitis, *Stevens-Johnson syndrome*
CV: Hypotension, bradycardia
RESP: Depression, apnea, laryngospasm, bronchospasm
HEMA: Agranulocytosis, thrombocytopenia, megaloblastic anemia (long-term treatment)

Contraindications: Hypersensitivity to barbiturates, respiratory depression, addiction to barbiturates, severe liver impairment, porphyria

Precautions: Anemia, pregnancy (B), lactation, hepatic disease, renal disease, hypertension, elderly, acute/chronic pain

Pharmacokinetics:
PO: Onset 45-60 min, duration 6-8 hr
IV: Onset 5 min, duration 3-6 hr
Metabolized by liver, excreted by kidneys (inactive metabolites), crosses placenta, highly protein

---

italics = common side effects   ***bold italic*** = life threatening reactions

bound, excreted in breast milk, half-life 16-40 hr

Interactions/incompatibilities:
• Increased CNS depression: alcohol, MAOIs, sedative, narcotics, general anesthetics, antipsychotics
• Decreased effect of oral anticoagulants, corticosteroids, griseofulvin, quinidine, oral contraceptives, estrogens
• Increased half-life of doxycycline
• Incompatible with cefazolin, cephalothin, chlorpromazine, cimetidine, clindamycin, codeine, dimenhydrinate, droperidol, hydrocortisone, hydroxyzine, insulin, levarterenol, levorphanol, meperidine, methadone, morphine, pentazocine, penicillin G, phytonadione, procaine, prochlorperazine, streptomycin, tetracycline, thiamine, trifluoperazine, vancomycin in sol or syringe

Lab test interferences:
False increase: Sulfobromophthalein

NURSING CONSIDERATIONS
Assess:
• VS q30 min after parenteral route for 2 hr
• Blood studies: Hct, Hgb, RBCs, serum folate, vitamin D (if on long-term therapy); pro-time in patients receiving anticoagulants
• Hepatic studies: AST, ALT, bilirubin; if increased, drug is usually discontinued
• Mental status: mood, sensorium, affect, memory (long, short), especially elderly
• Physical dependency: more frequent requests for medication, shakes, anxiety; elderly may be more sensitive due to decreased metabolism
• Barbiturate toxicity: hypotension; pulmonary constriction; cold,

clammy skin; cyanosis of lips; CNS depression; nausea; vomiting; hallucinations; delirium; weakness; coma, pupillary constriction, mild symptoms may occur in 8-12 hr without drug
• Respiratory dysfunction: respiratory depression, character, rate, rhythm; hold drug if respirations are <10/min or if pupils are dilated
• Blood dyscrasias: fever, sore throat, bruising, rash, jaundice, epistaxis

Administer:
• After removal of cigarettes, to prevent fires
• Deep IM injection in large muscle mass to prevent tissue sloughing, abscesses, no more than 5 ml/site
• After trying conservative measures for insomnia
• After diluting each 125 mg/1.25 ml, give by direct IV at a rate of 100 mg or less/1 min (adult), or 60 mg/min child; titrate slowly to desired response with sterile water for injection to a concentration of 100 mg/ml inject within 30 min of preparation; do not shake solution or use cloudy solution; use large vein, may cause thrombosis, extravasation
• IV only with resuscitative equipment available, administer at <100 mg/min (only by qualified personnel)
• ½-1 hr before hs for expected sleeplessness
• On empty stomach for best absorption

Perform/provide:
• Assistance with ambulation after receiving dose
• Safety measures: side rails, nightlight, call bell within easy reach

A

• Checking to see PO medication swallowed

Evaluate:

• Therapeutic response: ability to sleep at night, decreased amount of early morning awakening if taking drug for insomnia, or decrease in number, severity of seizures if taking drug for seizure disorder

Teach patient/family:

• That hangover is common

• That drug is indicated only for short-term treatment of insomnia and is probably ineffective after 2 wk

• That physical dependency may result when used for extended time (45-90 days depending on dose)

• To avoid driving or other activities requiring alertness

• To avoid alcohol ingestion or CNS depressants; serious CNS depression may result

• Not to discontinue medication quickly after long-term use; drug should be tapered over 1 wk

• To tell all prescribers that a barbiturate is being taken

• That withdrawal insomnia may occur after short-term use; do not start using drug again, insomnia will improve in 1-3 nights, may experience increased dreaming

• That effects may take 2 nights for benefits to be noticed

• Alternate measures to improve sleep: reading, exercise several hours before hs, warm bath, warm milk, TV, self-hypnosis, deep breathing

Treatment of overdose: Lavage, activated charcoal, warming blanket, vital signs, hemodialysis, alkalinize urine; give IV volume expanders, IV fluids

amoxapine

(a-mox′a-peen)

Amoxapine, Asendin

Func. class.: Antidepressant—tricyclic

Chem. class.: Dibenzoxazepine derivative—secondary amine

Action: Blocks reuptake of norepinephrine, serotonin into nerve endings, increasing action of norepinephrine, serotonin in nerve cells

Uses: Depression

Dosage and routes:

• *Adult:* PO 50 mg tid, may increase to 100 mg tid on 3rd day of therapy; not to exceed 300 mg/day unless lower doses have been given for at least 2 wk, may be given daily dose hs, not to exceed 600 mg/day in hospitalized patients

Available forms: Tabs 10, 25, 50, 75, 100, 150 mg

Side effects/adverse reactions:

*HEMA: **Agranulocytosis, thrombocytopenia, eosinophilia, leukopenia***

CNS: Dizziness, drowsiness, confusion, headache, anxiety, tremors, stimulation, weakness, insomnia, nightmares, EPS (elderly), increased psychiatric symptoms, paresthesia, impairment of sexual functioning

GI: Diarrhea, dry mouth, constipation, nausea, vomiting, ***paralytic ileus,*** increased appetite, cramps, epigastric distress, jaundice, ***hepatitis,*** stomatitis

GU: Retention, ***acute renal failure***

INTEG: Rash, urticaria, sweating, pruritus, photosensitivity

*CV: Orthostatic hypotension, ECG changes, tachycardia, **hypertension,*** palpitations

---

EENT: Blurred vision, tinnitus, mydriasis, ophthalmoplegia

Contraindications: Hypersensitivity to tricyclic antidepressants, recovery phase of myocardial infarction, convulsive disorders, prostatic hypertrophy

Precautions: Suicidal patients, severe depression, increased intraocular pressure, narrow-angle glaucoma, urinary retention, cardiac disease, hepatic disease, hyperthyroidism, electroshock therapy, elective surgery, elderly, pregnancy (C)

Pharmacokinetics:

PO: Steady state 7 days; metabolized by liver, excreted by kidneys, crosses placenta, half-life 8 hr

Interactions/incompatibilities:

• Decreased effects of guanethidine, clonidine, indirect-acting sympathomimetics (ephedrine)

• Increased effects of direct-acting sympathomimetics (epinephrine), alcohol, barbiturates, benzodiazepines, CNS depressants

• Hyperpyretic crisis, convulsions, hypertensive episode: MAOI (pargyline [Eutonyl])

Lab test interferences:

Increase: Serum bilirubin, blood glucose, alk phosphatase

False increase: Urinary catecholamines

Decrease: VMA, 5-HIAA

NURSING CONSIDERATIONS

Assess:

• B/P (lying, standing), pulse q4h; if systolic B/P drops 20 mm Hg hold drug, notify physician; take vital signs q4h in patients with cardiovascular disease

• Blood studies: CBC, leukocytes, differential, cardiac enzymes if patient is receiving long-term therapy

• Hepatic studies: AST, ALT, bilirubin

• Weight qwk, appetite may increase with drug

• ECG for flattening of T wave, bundle branch block, AV block, dysrhythmias in cardiac patients

• EPS primarily in elderly: rigidity, dystonia, akathisia

• Mental status: mood, sensorium, affect, suicidal tendencies, increase in psychiatric symptoms: depression, panic

• Urinary retention, constipation; constipation is more likely to occur in children, elderly

• Withdrawal symptoms: headache, nausea, vomiting, muscle pain, weakness; do not usually occur unless drug was discontinued abruptly

• Alcohol consumption; if alcohol is consumed, hold dose until morning

Administer:

• Increased fluids, bulk in diet if constipation, urinary retention occur, especially in elderly

• With food or milk for GI symptoms

• Crushed if patient is unable to swallow medication whole

• Dosage hs if oversedation occurs during day; may take entire dose hs; elderly may not tolerate once/day dosing

• Gum, hard candy, or frequent sips of water for dry mouth

Perform/provide:

• Storage at room temperature; do not freeze

• Assistance with ambulation during beginning therapy, since drowsiness/dizziness occurs

• Safety measures including side rails primarily for elderly

• Check to see PO medication swallowed

Evaluate:

• Therapeutic response: decreased

depression, absence of suicidal thoughts

Teach patient/family:

• That therapeutic effects may take 2-3 wk

• To use caution in driving or other activities requiring alertness because of drowsiness, dizziness, blurred vision

• To avoid alcohol ingestion, other CNS depressants

• Not to discontinue medication quickly after long-term use, may cause nausea, headache, malaise

• To wear sunscreen or large hat, since photosensitivity occurs

Treatment of overdose: ECG monitoring, induce emesis, lavage, activated charcoal, administer anticonvulsant

---

amoxicillin/clavulanate potassium

(a-mox-i-sill'in)

Augmentin, Clavulin*

Func. class.: Broad-spectrum antibiotic

Chem. class.: Aminopenicillin-B lactamase inhibitor

Action: Interferes with cell wall replication of susceptible organisms; the cell wall, rendered osmotically unstable, swells and bursts from osmotic pressure; combination increases spectrum of activity, β-lactamase resistance

Uses: Sinus infections, pneumonia, otitis media, skin, UTI; effective for strains of *E. coli, P. mirabilis, H. influenzae, S. faecalis, S. pneumoniae,* and β-lactamase-producing organisms

Dosage and routes:

• *Adult:* PO 250-500 mg q8h depending on severity of infection

• *Child:* PO 20-40 mg/kg/day in divided doses q8h

Available forms: Tabs 250, 500 mg; chew tabs 125, 250 mg; powder for oral susp 125, 250 mg/5 ml

Side effects/adverse reactions:

HEMA: Anemia, **bone marrow depression, granulocytopenia, leukopenia, eosinophilia,** thrombocytopenic purpura

GI: Nausea, diarrhea, vomiting, increased AST, ALT, abdominal pain, glossitis, colitis, black tongue, pseudomembranous colitis

GU: Oliguria, proteinuria, hematuria, *vaginitis, moniliasis,* **glomerulonephritis**

CNS: Headache, fever

META: Hyperkalemia, hypokalemia, alkalosis, hypernatremia

Contraindications: Hypersensitivity to penicillins; neonates

Precautions: Pregnancy (B), hypersensitivity to cephalosporins

Interactions/incompatibilities:

• Decreased antimicrobial effectiveness of amoxicillin: tetracyclines, erythromycins

• Increased amoxicillin concentrations: aspirin, probenecid

Pharmacokinetics:

PO: Peak 2 hr, duration 6-8 hr; half-life 1-1⅓ hr, metabolized in liver, excreted in urine, crosses placenta, enters breast milk

Lab test interferences:

False positive: Urine glucose, urine protein

NURSING CONSIDERATIONS

Assess:

• I&O ratio; report hematuria, oliguria, since penicillin in high doses is nephrotoxic

• Any patient with a compromised renal system, since drug is excreted slowly in poor renal system function; toxicity may occur rapidly

• Liver studies: AST, ALT

---

italics = common side effects   ***bold italic*** = life threatening reactions

- Blood studies: WBC, RBC, H&H, bleeding time
- Renal studies: urinalysis, protein, blood
- Culture, sensitivity before drug therapy; drug may be given as soon as culture is taken
- Bowel pattern before, during treatment
- Skin eruptions after administration of penicillin to 1 wk after discontinuing drug
- Respiratory status: rate, character, wheezing, tightness in chest
- Allergies before initiation of treatment, reaction of each medication; place allergies on chart, Kardex in bright red

Administer:
- After C&S completed
- Only as directed 2 (250 mg tab) are ≠ to 1 (500 mg tab) due to strength of clavulanate

Perform/provide:
- Adrenaline, suction, tracheostomy set, endotracheal intubation equipment on unit
- Adequate intake of fluids (2 L) during diarrhea episodes
- Scratch test to assess allergy after securing order from physician; usually done when penicillin is only drug of choice
- Storage refrigerated for 2 wk or room temperature for 1 wk

Evaluate:
- Therapeutic response: absence of fever, draining wounds

Teach patient/family:
- Aspects of drug therapy: need to complete entire course of medication to ensure organism death (10-14 days); culture may be taken after completed course of medication
- To report sore throat, fever, fatigue (may indicate a superimposed infection or agranulocytosis); vaginal candidiasis

- That drug must be taken in equal intervals around the clock to maintain blood levels; take on empty stomach with full glass of water
- To wear or carry a Medic Alert ID if allergic to penicillins
- To notify nurse of diarrhea

Treatment of overdose: Withdraw drug, maintain airway, administer epinephrine, aminophylline, O_2, IV corticosteroids for anaphylaxis

---

amoxicillin trihydrate
(a-mox-i-sill′in)
Amoxican,* Amoxicillin, Amoxil, Amoxil Pediatric Drops, Apo-Amoxi,* Biomox, Novamoxin,* Polymox, Polymox Drops, Trimox 125, Trimox 250, Trimox 500, Wymox
Func. class.: Broad-spectrum antibiotic
Chem. class.: Aminopenicillin

Action: Interferes with cell wall replication of susceptible organisms; the cell wall, rendered osmotically unstable, swells and bursts from osmotic pressure

Uses: Effective for gram-positive cocci *(S. aureus, S. pyogenes, S. faecalis, S. pneumoniae)*, gram-negative cocci *(N. gonorrhoeae, N. meningitidis, E. coli)*, gram-positive bacilli *(C. diphtheriae, L. monocytogenes)*, gram-negative bacilli *(H. influenzae, P. mirabilis, Salmonella)*

Dosage and routes:
Systemic infections
- *Adult:* PO 750 mg-1.5 g qd in divided doses q8h
- *Child:* PO 20-40 mg/kg/day in divided doses q8h

Gonorrhea/urinary tract infections

• *Adult:* PO 3 g given with 1 g probenecid as a single dose

Available forms: Caps 250, 500 mg; chew tabs 125, 250 mg; powder for oral susp 50, 125, 250 mg/ 5 ml

Side effects/adverse reactions:

HEMA: Anemia, increased bleeding time, *bone marrow depression, granulocytopenia*

GI: Nausea, vomiting, diarrhea, increased AST, ALT, abdominal pain, glossitis, colitis, *pseudomembranous colitis*

CNS: Headache, fever

SYST: Anaphylaxis, respiratory distress

Contraindications: Hypersensitivity to penicillins; neonates

Precautions: Pregnancy (B), hypersensitivity to cephalosporins

Interactions/incompatibilities:

• Decreased antimicrobial effectiveness of amoxicillin: tetracyclines, erythromycins

• Increased amoxicillin concentrations: aspirin, probenecid

Pharmacokinetics:

PO: Peak 2 hr, duration 6-8 hr; half-life 1-1⅓ hr, metabolized in liver, excreted in urine, crosses placenta, enters breast milk

Lab test interferences:

False positive: Urine glucose, urine protein

NURSING CONSIDERATIONS
Assess:

• I&O ratio; report hematuria, oliguria, since penicillin in high doses is nephrotoxic

• Any patient with a compromised renal system, since drug is excreted slowly in poor renal system function; toxicity may occur rapidly

• Liver studies: AST, ALT

• Blood studies: WBC, RBC, H&H, bleeding time

• Renal studies: urinalysis, protein, blood

• Culture, sensitivity before drug therapy; drug may be given as soon as culture is taken

• Bowel pattern before, during treatment

• Skin eruptions after administration of penicillin to 1 wk after discontinuing drug

• Respiratory status: rate, character, wheezing, tightness in the chest

• Allergies before initiation of treatment, reaction of each medication; place allergies on chart, in bright red

Administer:

• After C&S completed

Perform/provide:

• Adrenaline, suction, tracheostomy set, endotracheal intubation equipment on unit

• Adequate intake of fluids (2 L) during diarrhea episodes

• Scratch test to assess allergy after securing order from physician; usually done when penicillin is only drug of choice

• Storage in tight container; after reconstituting, oral suspension refrigerated for 2 wk or stored at room temperature for 1 wk

Evaluate:

• Therapeutic response: absence of temperature, draining wounds

Teach patient/family:

• Aspects of drug therapy: need to complete entire course of medication to ensure organism death (10-14 days); culture may be taken after completed course of medication

• To report sore throat, fever, fatigue, diarrhea (may indicate a superimposed infection or agranulocytopenia)

• That drug must be taken in equal intervals around the clock to maintain blood levels, take on empty

---

italics = common side effects   ***bold italic*** = life threatening reactions

stomach with a full glass of water
• To wear or carry a Medic Alert ID if allergic to penicillins

Treatment of overdose: Withdraw drug, maintain airway, administer epinephrine, aminophylline, O_2, IV corticosteroids for anaphylaxis

---

amphetamine sulfate

(am-fet'a-meen)
Amphetamine Sulfate
Func. class.: Cerebral stimulant
Chem. class.: Amphetamine

Controlled Substance Schedule II

Action: Increases release of norepinephrine, dopamine in cerebral cortex to reticular activating system

Uses: Narcolepsy, exogenous obesity, attention deficit disorder

Dosage and routes:

Narcolepsy
• *Adult:* PO 5-60 mg qd in divided doses
• *Child >12 yr:* PO 10 mg qd increasing by 10 mg/day at weekly intervals
• *Child 6-12 yr:* PO 5 mg qd increasing by 5 mg/wk, max 60 mg/day

Attention deficit disorder
• *Child >6 yr:* PO 5 mg qd-bid increasing by 5 mg/day at weekly intervals
• *Child 3-6 yr:* PO 2.5 mg qd increasing by 2.5 mg/day at weekly intervals

Obesity
• *Adult:* PO 5-30 mg in divided doses 30-60 min before meals

Available forms: Tabs 5, 10 mg; long-acting capsules 5, 10 mg

Side effects/adverse reactions:

CNS: Hyperactivity, insomnia, restlessness, talkativeness, dizziness, headache, chills, stimulation, dysphoria, irritability, aggressiveness, tremor, dependence, addiction
GI: Nausea, vomiting, anorexia, dry mouth, diarrhea, constipation, weight loss, metallic taste, cramps
GU: Impotence, change in libido
CV: Palpitations, tachycardia, hypertension, dysrhythmias, decreased heart rate
INTEG: Urticaria

Contraindications: Hypersensitivity to sympathomimetic amines, hyperthyroidism, hypertension, glaucoma, severe arteriosclerosis, drug abuse, cardiovascular disease, anxiety

Precautions: Gilles de la Tourette's disorder, pregnancy (X), lactation, child <3 yr

Pharmacokinetics:
PO: Onset 30 min, peak 1-3 hr, duration 4-20 hr, metabolized by liver, excreted by kidneys, crosses placenta, breast milk, half-life 10-30 hr

Interactions/incompatibilities:
• Hypertensive crisis: MAOIs or within 14 days of MAOIs or furazolidine
• Increased effect of amphetamine: acetazolamide, antacids, sodium bicarbonate urinary alkalinizers
• Decreased effect of amphetamine: barbiturates, tricyclics, urinary acidifiers (ascorbic acid, ammonium chloride)
• Decreased effect of guanethidine

NURSING CONSIDERATIONS

Assess:
• VS, B/P, since this drug may reverse antihypertensives; check patients with cardiac disease more often
• CBC, urinalysis, in diabetes: blood sugar, urine sugar; insulin changes be required, since eating will decrease

---

• Height, growth rate in children may be decreased

• Mental status: mood, sensorium, affect, stimulation, insomnia; aggressiveness may occur

• Physical dependency; should not be used for extended time; dose should be discontinued gradually

• Withdrawal symptoms: headache, nausea, vomiting, muscle pain, weakness

• Drug tolerance will develop after long-term use

• Dosage should not be increased if tolerance develops

Administer:

• At least 6 hr before hs to avoid sleeplessness

• For obesity only if patient is on weight-reduction program that includes dietary changes, exercise; patient will develop tolerance, and weight loss won't occur without additional methods; give 30-60 min before meals

• Gum, hard candy, frequent sips of water for dry mouth

Evaluate:

• Therapeutic response: decreased activity in attention deficit disorder; absence of sleeping during day in narcolepsy; decrease in weight

Teach patient/family:

• To decrease caffeine consumption (coffee, tea, cola, chocolate), which may increase irritability, stimulation

• To avoid OTC preparations unless approved by physician

• To taper off drug over several weeks, or depression, increased sleeping, lethargy may occur

• To avoid alcohol ingestion

• To avoid hazardous activities until patient is stabilized on medication

• To get needed rest; patients will feel more tired at end of day

Treatment of overdose: Administer fluids, hemodialysis, peritoneal dialysis, antihypertensives for increased B/P; ammonium Cl for increased excretion

amphotericin B

(am-foe-ter'i-sin)
Amphotericin B, Fungizone IV
Func. class.: Antifungal
Chem. class.: Amphoteric polyene

Action: Increases cell membrane permeability in susceptible organisms by binding sterols; decreases K, Na, and nutrients in cell

Uses: Histoplasmosis, blastomycosis, coccidioidomycosis, cryptococcosis, aspergillosis, phycomycosis, candidiasis, sporotrichosis causing severe meningitis, septicemia, skin infections

Dosage and routes:

• *Adult and child:* IV INF 1 mg/250 ml D₅W (0.1 mg/ml) over 2-4 hr or 0.25 mg/kg/day over 6 hr; may be increased gradually up to 1 mg/kg/day, not to exceed 1.5 mg/kg; INTRATHECAL 25 μg/0.1 ml diluted in 10-20 ml CSF given by barbotage 2-3 times a wk, gradually increased to 0.5 mg q48-72 hr

Candida infection of GI tract: Adults: 100 mg PO qid × 2 wks
Candida oral infection: 1 loz qid × 7-14 days; allow loz to dissolve slowly in mouth

Available forms: Powder for inj 50 mg

Side effects/adverse reactions:

EENT: Tinnitus, deafness, diplopia, blurred vision

INTEG: Burning, irritation, pain, necrosis at injection site with ex-

---

italics = common side effects   ***bold italic*** = life threatening reactions

travasation, flushing, dermatitis, skin rash (topical route)

CNS: Headache, fever, chills, peripheral nerve pain, paresthesias, peripheral neuropathy, *convulsions,* dizziness

GU: Hypokalemia, axotemia, hyposthenuria, *renal tubular acidosis,* nephrocalcinosis, *permanent renal impairment, anuria, oliguria*

GI: Nausea, vomiting, anorexia, diarrhea, cramps, *hemorrhagic gastroenteritis, acute liver failure*

MS: Arthralgia, myalgia, generalized pain, weakness, weight loss

HEMA: Normochromic, normocytic anemia, *thrombocytopenia, agranulocytosis, leukopenia, eosinophilia,* hypokalemia, hyponatremia, hypomagnesemia

Contraindications: Hypersensitivity, severe bone marrow depression

Precautions: Renal disease, pregnancy (B)

Pharmacokinetics:

IV: Peak 1-2 hr, initial half-life 24 hr, metabolized in liver, excreted in urine (metabolites), breast milk, highly bound to plasma proteins; penetrates poorly CSF, bronchial secretions, aqueous humor, muscle, bone

Interactions/incompatibilities:

• Increased nephrotoxicity: other nephrotoxic antibiotics (aminoglycosides, cisplatin, vancomycin, cyclosporine, polymyxin B)

• Increased hypokalemia: corticosteroids, digitalis, skeletal muscle relaxants

• Antagonism: miconazole

• Incompatible in amikacin, calcium sol, carbenicillin, chlorpromazine, chlortetracycline, cimetidine, diphenhydramine, dopamine, gentamicin, heparin, kananycin, metaraminol, penicillin G, polymycin B, KCL, prochlorperazine, ranitidine, tetracycline, Vit B with C in sodium solutions or diluent with preservatives

NURSING CONSIDERATIONS

Assess:

• VS q15-30 min during first infusion; note changes in pulse, B/P

• I&O ratio; watch for decreasing urinary output, change in sp gr; discontinue drug to prevent permanent damage to renal tubules

• Blood studies: CBC, K, Na, Ca, Mg q2 wk, BUN, creatinine weekly

• Weight weekly; if weight increases over 2 lb/wk, edema is present; renal damage should be considered

• For renal toxicity: increasing BUN, serum creatinine; if BUN is >40 mg/dl or if serum creatinine >3 mg/dl, drug may be discontinued or dosage reduced

• For hepatotoxicity: increasing AST, ALT, alk phosphatase, bilirubin

• For allergic reaction: dermatitis, rash; drug should be discontinued, antihistamines (mild reaction) or epinephrine (severe reaction) administered

• For hypokalemia: anorexia, drowsiness, weakness, decreased reflexes, dizziness, increased urinary output, increased thirst, paresthesias

• For ototoxicity: tinnitus (ringing, roaring in ears) vertigo, loss of hearing (rare)

Administer:

• After diluting 50 mg/10 ml sterile water (no preservatives) or NS, (5 mg-1 ml) shake, dilute with 500 ml of solution to concentration of 0.1 mg/ml

• Test dose of 1 mg/20 ml D_5W; give over 10-30 min

• IV using in-line filter (mean pore diameter >1 μm) using distal veins; check for extravasation, necrosis q8h; use an infusion pump; administer over 6 hr; rapid infusion may result in circulation collapse

• Drug only after C&S confirms organism, drug needed to treat condition; make sure drug is used in life-threatening infections

Perform/provide:

• Protection from light during infusion, cover with foil

• Symptomatic treatment as ordered for adverse reactions: aspirin, antihistamines, antiemetics, antispasmodics

• Storage, protected from moisture and light; diluted solution is stable for 24 hr at room temperature

Evaluate:

• Therapeutic response: decreased fever, malaise, rash, negative C&S for infecting organism

Teach patient/family:

• That long-term therapy may be needed to clear infection (2 wk-3 mo depending on type of infection)

---

amphotericin B (topical)

(am-foe-ter′i-sin)
Fungizone
Func. class.: Local antiinfective
Chem. class.: Antifungal (polyene)

Action: Increases cell membrane permeability in susceptible organisms by binding sterols

Uses: Cutaneous, mucocutaneous infections caused by *Candida*

Dosage and routes:

• *Adult and child:* TOP bid-qid for 7-21 days or longer if needed

Available forms: Cream, lotion, oint 3%

Side effects/adverse reactions:

INTEG: Urticaria, stinging, burning, dry skin, pruritus, contact dermatitis, erythema, staining of nail lesions

Contraindications: Hypersensitivity

Precautions: Pregnancy (B), lactation

NURSING CONSIDERATIONS

Assess:

• Allergic reaction: burning, stinging, swelling, redness

Administer:

• Enough medication to cover lesions completely; apply liberally and rub thoroughly into affected area

• After cleansing with soap, water before each application, dry well (as ordered)

Perform/provide:

• Storage at room temperature in dry place

Evaluate:

• Therapeutic response: decrease in size, number of lesions

Teach patient/family:

• That skin and clothing may become discolored

• To apply with glove to prevent further infection; not to cover with occlusive dressing

• To avoid use of OTC creams, ointments, lotions unless directed by physician

• To use medical asepsis (hand washing) before, after each application to prevent further infection

• To continue even if condition improves

• To report increased itching, burning, rash, redness; ointment may irritate most hairy areas

---

italics = common side effects   ***bold italic*** = life threatening reactions

ampicillin/ampicillin sodium/ampicillin trihydrate

(am-pi-sill'in)

Amcill, D-Amp, Omnipen, Polycillin, Omnipen-N, Polycillin-N, Totacillin,Totacillin-N

Func. class.: Broad-spectrum antibiotic

Chem. class.: Aminopenicillin

Action: Interferes with cell wall replication of susceptible organisms; the cell wall, rendered osmotically unstable, swells, bursts from osmotic pressure

Uses: Effective for gram-positive cocci *(S. aureus, S. pyogenes, S. faecalis, S. pneumoniae),* gram-negative cocci *(N. gonorrhoeae, N. meningitidis),* gram-negative bacilli *(H. influenzae, P. mirabilis, Salmonella, Shigella, L. monocytogenes),* gram-positive bacilli

Dosage and routes:

Systemic infections

• *Adult:* PO 1-2 g qd in divided doses q6h; IV/IM 2-8 g qd in divided doses q4-6h

• *Child:* PO 50-100 mg/kg/day in divided doses q6h; IV/IM 100-200 mg/kg/day in divided doses q6h

Meningitis

• *Adult:* IV 8-14 g/day in divided doses q3-4h × 3 days

• *Child:* IV 200-300 mg/kg/day in divided doses q3-4h × 3 days

Gonorrhea

• *Adult:* PO 3.5 g given with 1 g probenecid as a single dose

Available forms: Powder for inj IV, IM 125, 250, 500 mg, 1, 2, 10 g; IV inf 500 mg, 1, 2 g; caps 250, 500 mg; powder for oral susp 100/1 ml, 125, 250, 500 mg/5 ml

Side effects/adverse reactions:

INTEG: Rash, urticaria

HEMA: Anemia, increased bleeding time, *bone marrow depression, granulocytopenia*

GI: Nausea, *vomiting, diarrhea*

GU: Oliguria, proteinuria, hematuria, *vaginitis, moniliasis, glomerulonephritis*

CNS: Lethargy, hallucinations, anxiety, depression, twitching, *coma, convulsions*

Contraindications: Hypersensitivity to penicillins

Precautions: Pregnancy (B); hypersensitivity to cephalosporins; neonates

Pharmacokinetics:

PO: Peak 2 hr

IV: Peak 5 min

IM: Peak 1 hr

Half-life 50-110 min; metabolized in liver, excreted in urine, bile, breast milk, crosses placenta

Interactions/incompatibilities:

• Possible increased bleeding: oral anticoagulants

• Decreased antimicrobial effectiveness of ampicillin: tetracyclines, erythromycins

• Increased ampicillin concentrations: aspirin, probenecid

• Decreased effectiveness of: oral contraceptives

• Increased ampicillin-induced skin rash: allopurinol

• Do not add mix with any other drug

Lab test interferences:

False positive: Urine glucose, urine protein

NURSING CONSIDERATIONS

Assess:

• I&O ratio; report hematuria, oliguria since penicillin in high doses is nephrotoxic

• Any patient with compromised renal system, since drug is excreted

slowly in poor renal system function; toxicity may occur rapidly
• Liver studies: AST, ALT
• Blood studies: WBC, RBC, H&H, bleeding time
• Renal studies: urinalysis, protein, blood
• Culture, sensitivity before drug therapy; drug may be taken as soon as culture is taken
• Sodium levels when high doses of injectables are given to cardiac patients
• Bowel pattern before, during treatment
• Skin eruptions after administration of penicillin to 1 wk after discontinuing drug
• Respiratory status: rate, character, wheezing, tightness in chest
• Allergies before initiation of treatment; reaction of each medication; place allergies on chart in bright red

Administer:
• After diluting with sterile H₂O 0.9-1.2 ml/125 mg drug, administer over 3-5 min (up to 500 mg), 10-15 min, (>500 mg) by direct IV; may be diluted in 50 ml or more of D₅W, D₅ ½ NaCl, 10% invert sugar in water, ⅙ sodium lactate solutions to a concentration of 30 mg/ml or less; IV sol is stable for 1 hr; give at prescribed rate
• After C&S completed
• On empty stomach for best absorption (1-2 hr ac or 2-3 hr pc)

Perform/provide:
• Adrenaline, suction, tracheostomy set, endotracheal intubation equipment on unit
• Adequate intake of fluids (2 L) during diarrhea episodes
• Scratch test to assess allergy after securing order from physician; usually done when penicillin is only drug of choice

• Storage in tight container; after reconstituting, oral suspension refrigerated for 2 wk or stored at room temperature for 1 wk

Evaluate:
• Therapeutic response: absence of temperature, draining wounds

Teach patient/family:
• To take oral penicillin on empty stomach with full glass of water
• Aspects of drug therapy: need to complete entire course of medication to ensure organism death (10-14 days); culture may be taken after completed course of medication
• To report sore throat, fever, fatigue, diarrhea (may indicate superimposed infection); report rash or other signs of allergy
• That drug must be taken in equal intervals around the clock to maintain blood levels
• To wear or carry a Medic Alert ID if allergic to penicillins

Treatment of overdose: Withdraw drug, maintain airway, administer epinephrine, aminophylline, O₂, IV corticosteroids for anaphylaxis

---

ampicillin sodium, sulbactam sodium
Unasyn

Func. class.: Broad-spectrum antibiotic
Chem. class.: Aminopenicillin

Action: Interferes with cell wall replication of susceptible organisms; the cell wall, rendered osmotically unstable, swells, bursts from osmotic pressure; combination extends spectrum of activity, β-lactamase inhibition

Uses: Skin infections (*S. aureus, E. coli, Klebsiella, P. mirabilis, B. fragilis, Enterobacter, A. calcoac-*

---

italics = common side effects   ***bold italic*** = life threatening reactions

eticus), intraabdominal infections (*Enterobacter, Klebsiella, Bacteroides, E. coli*) gynecologic infections (*E. coli, Bacteroides.*)

Dosage and routes:
• *Adult:* IV 1 g ampicillin, 0.5 g sulbactam to 2 g ampicillin and 1 g sulbactam q6h, not to exceed 4 g/day sulbactam

Available forms: Powder for inj 1.5 g (1 g ampicillin, 0.5 g sulbactam), 3.0 g (2 g ampicillin, 1 g sulbactam)

Side effects/adverse reactions:
HEMA: Anemia, increased bleeding time, *bone marrow depression, granulocytopenia*
GI: Nausea, vomiting, diarrhea, increased AST, ALT, abdominal pain, glossitis, colitis
GU: Oliguria, proteinuria, hematuria, *vaginitis, moniliasis, glomerulonephritis*
CNS: Lethargy, hallucinations, anxiety, depression, twitching, *coma, convulsions*

Contraindications: Hypersensitivity to penicillins

Precautions: Pregnancy, hypersensitivity to cephalosporins, neonates

Pharmacokinetics:
IV: Peak 5 min; half-life 50-110 min; little metabolized in liver, 75% to 85% of both drugs excreted in urine, diffuses to breast milk, crosses placenta

Interactions/incompatibilities:
• Decreased antimicrobial effectiveness of ampicillin: tetracyclines, erythromycins
• Increased ampicillin concentration: aspirin, probenecid
• Do not admix with any other drug

Lab test interferences:
False positive: Urine glucose, urine protein

NURSING CONSIDERATIONS
Assess:
• Bowel pattern before, during treatment
• Respiratory status: rate, character, wheezing, tightness in chest
• I&O ratio; report hematuria, oliguria, since penicillin in high doses is nephrotoxic
• Any patient with compromised renal system, since drug is excreted slowly in poor renal system function; toxicity may occur rapidly
• Liver studies: AST, ALT
• Blood studies: WBC, RBC, Hct/Hgb, bleeding time
• Renal studies: urinalysis, protein, blood
• C&S before drug therapy; drug may be given as soon as culture is taken
• Skin eruptions after administration of ampicillin 1 wk after discontinuing drug
• Allergies before initiation of treatment; reaction of each medication; report allergies on chart

Administer:
• IV after diluting 1.5 g/4 ml or more sterile H$_2$O for inj (375 mg/ml); allow to stand until foaming stops; dilute further in 50 ml or more of D$_5$W, D$_5$y$_2$ NaCl, 10% invert sugar in water, LR, y$_6$ sodium lactate, isotonic NaCl; administer within 1 hr after reconstitution; give as an intermittent inf over 15-30 min
• After C&S completed; on empty stomach

Perform/provide:
• Adrenaline, suction, tracheostomy set, endotracheal intubation equipment on unit for possible anaphylaxis
• Adequate intake of fluids (2 L) during diarrhea episode
• Scratch test to assess allergy after

securing order from physician; usually done when penicillin is only drug choice
• Storage in tight container, out of light

Evaluate:
• Therapeutic response: absence of fever, draining wounds, negative C&S

Teach patient/family:
• To report sore throat, fever, fatigue (may indicate superimposed infection)
• To wear or carry Medic Alert ID if allergic to penicillin products

Treatment of overdose: Withdraw drug, maintain airway, administer epinephrine, aminophylline, O₂, IV corticosteroids for anaphylaxis

---

amrinone lactate
(am′ri-none)
Inocor
Func. class.: Cardiac inotropic agent
Chem. class.: Bipyrimidine derivative

Action: Positive inotropic agent with vasodilator properties; reduces preload and afterload by direct relaxation of vascular smooth muscle

Uses: Short-term management of CHF that has not responded to other medication; can be used with digitalis

Dosage and routes:
• *Adult:* IV BOL 0.75 mg/kg given over 2-3 min; start infusion of 5-10 µg/kg/min; may give another bolus ½ hr after start of therapy, not to exceed 10 mg/kg total daily dose

Available forms: Inj 5 mg/ml

Side effects/adverse reactions:
HEMA: Thrombocytopenia

CV: Dysrhythmias, hypotension, headache, chest pain
GI: Nausea, vomiting, anorexia, abdominal pain, **hepatotoxicity, ascites,** jaundice, hiccups
INTEG: Allergic reactions, burning at injection site
RESP: Pleuritis, **pulmonary densities, hypoxemia**

Contraindications: Hypersensitivity to this drug or bisulfites, severe aortic disease, severe pulmonic valvular disease, acute MI

Precautions: Lactation, pregnancy (C), children, renal disease, hepatic disease, atrial flutter/fibrillation, elderly

Pharmacokinetics:
IV: Onset 2-5 min, peak 10 min, duration variable; half-life 4-6 hr, metabolized in liver, excreted in urine as drug and metabolites 60%-90%

Interactions/incompatibilities:
• Excessive hypotension: antihypertensives
• Additive effect: cardiac glycosides
• Incompatible in furosemide or dextrose sol other than for direct dilution

NURSING CONSIDERATIONS
Assess:
• B/P and pulse q5 min during infusion; if B/P drops 30 mm Hg, stop infusion and call physician
• Electrolytes: K, S, Cl, Ca; renal function studies: BUN, creatinine; blood studies: platelet count
• ALT, AST, bilirubin daily
• I&O ratio and weight qd; diuresis should increase with continuing therapy
• If platelets are <150,000/mm³, drug is usually discontinued and another drug started
• Extravasation; change site q48h

italics = common side effects   ***bold italic*** = life threatening reactions

Administer:
• Do not mix directly with glucose solutions; chemical reaction occurs over 24 hr; precipitate forms if amrinone and furosemide come in contact
• Into running dextrose infusion through Y-connector or directly into tubing; may give undiluted over 2-3 min or dilute with normal saline to concentration of 1-3 mg/ml, run at prescribed rate
• By infusion pump for doses other than bolus
• Potassium supplements if ordered for potassium levels <3.0

Evaluate:
• Therapeutic response: increased cardiac output, decreased PCWP, adequate CVP, decreased dyspnea, fatigue, edema, ECG

Treatment of overdose: Discontinue drug, support circulation

---

amyl nitrite
(am′il)

Amyl nitrite, Amyl Nitrite Aspirols, Amyl Nitrite Vaporole
Func. class.: Coronary vasodilator
Chem. class.: Nitrite

Action: Relaxes vascular smooth muscle; may dilate coronary blood vessels, resulting in reduced venous return, decreased cardiac output; reduces preload, afterload, which decreases left ventricular end diastolic pressure, systemic vascular resistance; converts hemoglobin to methemoglobin, which is able to bind cyanide

Uses: Acute angina pectoris, cyanide poisoning

Dosage and routes:
Angina
• *Adult:* INH 0.18-0.3 ml as needed, 1-6 inhalations from 1 cap, may repeat in 3-5 min

Cyanide poisoning
• *Adult:* INH 0.3 ml ampule inhaled 15 sec until preparation of sodium nitrite infusion is ready

Available forms: Inh pearls 0.18, 0.3 ml

Side effects/adverse reactions:
*CV: Postural hypotension, **tachycardia, cardiovascular collapse,** palpitations*
CNS: Headache, dizziness, weakness, syncope
GI: Nausea, vomiting, abdominal pain
INTEG: Flushing, pallor, sweating
MISC: Muscle twitching, **hemolytic anemia, methemoglobinemia**

Contraindications: Hypersensitivity to nitrites, severe anemia, increased intracranial pressure, hypertension, pregnancy (X)

Precautions: Lactation, children, drug abuse, head injury, cerebral hemorrhage, hypotension

Pharmacokinetics:
INH: Onset 30 sec, duration 3-5 min; metabolized by liver, ⅓ excreted in urine, half-life 1-4 min

Interactions/incompatibilities:
• Increased hypotension: alcohol, β-blockers, antihypertensive

NURSING CONSIDERATIONS
Assess:
• B/P, supine and sitting, pulse during treatment until stable
• For drug tolerance: the need for more medication for each attack
• For postural hypotension, headache during treatment, which are common side effects because of vasodilation

Administer:
• After wrapping, crushing ampule to avoid cuts
• Ordered analgesic if headache develops

• To patient who is sitting or lying down during treatment; keep head low, use deep breaths, which will decrease dizziness

• Drug, and have patient rest for 15 min

Perform/provide:

• Storage in light-resistant area in cool environment or refrigerate

Evaluate:

• Therapeutic response: relief of chest pain (angina)

Teach patient/family:

• To keep a record of angina attacks and what aggravates condition; prolonged chest pain may indicate MI: seek emergency treatment

• That medication may explode in presence of flame

• To take several deep breaths despite foul odor

• To make position changes slowly to prevent orthostatic hypotension

• To keep drug out of reach of children and in secure place, as there is high abuse potential

---

anistreplase (APSAC)
(an-ih-strep'layz)
Eminase
Func. class.: Thrombolytic enzyme
Chem. class.: Anisolated plasminogen streptokinase activator complex

---

Action: Promotes thrombolysis by promoting conversion of plasminogen to plasmin

Uses: Management of acute MI; although not yet approved, anistreplase will also be used for other conditions requiring thrombolysis, i.e., PE, DUT, unclotting arteriovenous shunts.

Dosage and routes:

• *Adult:* IV 30 U over 4-5 min as soon as possible after onset of symptoms

Available forms: Powder, lyophilized 30 U/vial

Side effects/adverse reactions:

HEMA: Decreased Hct, *GI, GU, intracranial, retroperitoneal,* surface bleeding, *thrombocytopenia*

INTEG: Rash, urticaria, phlebitis at site, itching, flushing

CNS: Headache, fever, sweating, agitation, dizziness, paresthesia, tremor, vertigo

GI: Nausea, vomiting

RESP: Altered respirations, dyspnea, *bronchospasm, lung edema*

MS: Low back pain, arthralgia

CV: Hypotension, dysrhythmias, conduction disorders

SYST: Anaphylaxis

Contraindications: Hypersensitivity, active internal bleeding, intraspinal or intracranial surgery, neoplasms of CNS, severe hypertension, cerebral embolism/thrombosis/hemorrhage

Precautions: Arterial emboli from left side of heart, pregnancy (B), ulcerative colitis/enteritis, renal disease, hepatic disease, hypocoagulation, COPD, subacute bacterial endocarditis, rheumatic valvular disease, intraarterial diagnostic procedure or surgery (10 days), recent major surgery

Pharmacokinetics: Half-life 105 min

Interactions/incompatibilities:

• Increased bleeding potential: aspirin, indomethacin, phenylbutazone, anticoagulants

• Do not mix with any other sol or drug

Lab test interferences:

Increase: PT, APTT, TT

Decrease: Fibrinogen, plasminogen

---

italics = common side effects   ***bold italic*** = life threatening reactions

NURSING CONSIDERATIONS
Assess:

• VS, B/P, pulse, respirations, neurologic signs, temperature at least q4h, temp >104° F (40° C) or indicators of internal bleeding, cardiac rhythm after intracoronary administration

• Allergy: fever, rash, itching, chills; mild reaction may be treated with antihistamines

• Bleeding during 1st hr of treatment (hematuria, hematemesis, bleeding from mucous membranes, epistaxis, ecchymosis)

• Blood studies (Hct, platelets, PTT, PT, TT, APTT) before starting therapy; PT or APTT must be less than 2 × control before starting therapy; TT or PT q3-4h during treatment

Administer:

• Reconstitute single-dose vial/5 ml sterile water for injection (not bacteriostatic water), and roll (not shake) to enhance reconstitution; give over 2-5 mins by direct IV; give within 6 hr of thrombi identification for best results

• Cryoprecipitate or fresh frozen plasma if bleeding occurs

• Heparin therapy after thrombolytic therapy is discontinued, TT or APTT less than 2 × control (about 3-4 hr)

• About 10% of patients have high streptococcal antibody titers, requiring increased loading doses

Perform/provide:

• Bed rest during entire course of treatment; handle patient as little as possible during therapy

• Storage of powder in refrigerator; use within 30 min after reconstitution

• Avoid invasive procedures: inj, rectal temperature

• Treat fever with acetaminophen

• Pressure of 30 sec to minor bleeding sites, 30 min to sites of arterial puncture followed by dressing; inform physician if hemostasis not attained; apply pressure dressing

Evaluate:

• Therapeutic response: absence of thrombi formation in MI, improved ventricular function

antihemophilic Factor (AHF)

(an-tee-hee-moe-fill'ik)
Antihemophilic Factor, Humate-P, Monoclate-P, Profilate HP, Hemofil M, Koate H.P., Koate H.S., Kryobulin VH,* Monoclate

Func. class.: Hemostatic
Chem. class.: Factor VIII

Action: Necessary for clotting, activates factor X in conjunction with activated factor IX; transforms prothrombin to thrombin

Uses: Hemophilia A, patients with acquired circulating factor VIII inhibitors, factor VIII deficiency

Dosage and routes: Depends on severity of deficiency

• *Adult and child:* IV 10-20 U/kg q8-24 h; INF 2 ml/min

Available forms: Inj IV (number of units noted on label)

Side effects/adverse reactions:

GI: Nausea, vomiting, abdominal cramps, jaundice, *viral hepatitis*

INTEG: Rash, flushing, *urticaria,* stinging at injection site

CNS: Headache, *lethargy, chills, fever, flushing*

HEMA: **Thrombosis, hemolysis, AIDS**

CV: Hypotension, tachycardia

RESP: **Bronchospasm**

Contraindications: Hypersensitivity, monoclonal antibody–derived factor VIII

Precautions: Neonates/infants, hepatic disease, blood types A, B, AB, pregnancy (C), factor VIII inhibitor

Pharmacokinetics:

IV: Half-life 4 hr, terminal 15 hr

Interactions/incompatibilities:

• Do not admix with other drugs

NURSING CONSIDERATIONS
Assess:

• Blood studies (coagulation factors assay by % normal: 5% prevents spontaneous hemorrhage, 30%-50% for surgery, 80%-100% for severe hemorrhage)

• I&O, urine color; notify physician if urine becomes orange, red

• Pulse: discontinue infusion if significant increase

• Hct, Coombs' test with blood types A, B, AB

• Test for factor VIII inhibitors before starting treatment, may require concomitant antiinhibitor coagulant complex therapy

• Allergy: fever, rash, itching, jaundice; give diphenhydramine HCl (Benadryl), continue therapy if reaction is mild

• Blood group of patient, donors (if applicable; most factor VIII not from specific blood group donors)

• Bleeding: ankles, knees, elbows, other joints

Administer:

• After rotating gently to mix

• IV slowly, plastic syringe to reconstitute, and administer; adheres to glass; use another needle as a vent when reconstituting

• After dilution with warm NS, D$_5$W, LR, give within 3 hr

• IV INF: give at ≤2 ml/min if concentration exceeds 34 U/ml or over 3 min if concentration is less than 34 U/ml

Perform/provide:

• Storage in refrigerator; do not freeze; after reconstitution, do not refrigerate; give within 3 hrs

Evaluate:

• Therapeutic response: absence of bleeding

Teach patient/family:

• To report any signs of bleeding: gums, under skin, urine, stools, emesis; review methods to prevent bleeding

• To avoid salicylates (increase bleeding tendencies)

• To prepare, administer factor VIII concentrates at first sign of danger

• To advise health professionals of treatment for hemophilia

• Signs of viral hepatitis, AIDS

• That immunization for hepatitis B may be given first

• To report hives, urticaria, chest tightness, hypotension; may be monoclonal antibody-derived factor VIII

• To be checked q2-3 mo for HIV screen

• To carry ID describing disease process

---

antithrombin III, human
ATnativ, Thombate III

Func. class.: Antithrombin
Chem. class.: Pooled human plasma

Action: Inactivates thrombin and the activated forms of factors IX, X, XI, XII, resulting in inhibition of coagulation

Uses: Hereditary antithrombin III deficiency in connection with surgical or obstetric procedures or for thromboembolism

Dosage and routes: Dosage is in-

---

dividualized. After first dose, antithrombin III level should increase to about 120% of normal; thereafter maintain at levels >80%; this is usually achieved by administering maintenance doses q24h

Available forms: Lyophilized powder, 50 ml infusion bottles containing 500 IU antithrombin III with 10 ml sterile water for injection

Side effects/adverse reactions:
SYST: Bleeding, surface bleeding, *anaphylaxis,* vasodilatory effects

Precautions: Pregnancy (C), children

Pharmacokinetics: Unknown

Interactions/Incompatibilities:
• Increased anticoagulant effect: heparin

NURSING CONSIDERATIONS
Assess:
• VS, B/P, pulse, respirations, neurologic signs, temperature at least q4h, temperature 104° F (40° C) or indicators of internal bleeding, cardiac rhythm
• For neurologic changes that may indicate intracranial bleeding
• Retroperitoneal bleeding: back pain, leg weakness, diminished pulses

Administer:
• Heparin after fibrinogen level is over 100 mg/dl; heparin infusion to increase PTT to 1.5-2 × baseline for 3-7 days
• After reconstituting 500 IU/10 ml of NS or D_5W; do not shake; rotate to dissolve; allow to warm to room temperature; use within 3 hr of reconstitution; give 50 IU or less/min; do not exceed 100 IU/min
• IV therapy using 0.22 or 0.45 micro filter

Perform/provide:
• Bed rest during entire course of treatment
• Avoidance of venous or arterial

puncture, inj, rectal temperature
• Treatment of fever with acetaminophen or aspirin

Evaluate:
• Therapeutic response: absence of thrombi formation

---

apomorphine HCl
(a-poe-mor'feen)

Func. class.: Emetic, dopamine agonist
Chem. class.: Morphine, hydrochloric acid

Controlled Substance Schedule II
Action: Acts centrally by stimulating chemoreceptor trigger zone, which in turn acts on vomiting center

Uses: In poisoning/drug overdose to induce vomiting promptly (10-15 min); is almost 100% effective

Dosage and routes:
• *Adult:* IM/SC 2-10 mg, then 7-10 oz evaporated milk or water; do not repeat
• *Child >1 yr:* IM/SC 0.07 mg/kg then 16 oz evaporated milk or water; do not repeat
• *Child <1 yr:* IM/SC 0.07 mg/kg, then 8 oz evaporated milk or water; do not repeat

Available forms: Soluble tabs (parenteral) 6 mg

Side effects/adverse reactions:
CNS: Euphoria, depression, restlessness, tremor, muscle weakness
GI: Nausea, anorexia, dry mouth, diarrhea, constipation, weight loss, metallic taste, cramps, salivation
CV: Circulatory failure, tachycardia, irregular rapid pulse, decreased B/P
RESP: Respiratory depression

Contraindications: Hypersensitivity to narcotics, respiratory depression, corrosive poisoning, coma,

shock, narcosis from CNS depressants

Precautions: Children, cardiac decompensation, elderly, pregnancy (C)

Pharmacokinetics:

PO: Onset 10-15 min

SC: Onset 1-2 min, metabolized by liver, excreted by kidneys

Interactions/incompatibilities:

• Incompatible with iodides, iron preparations, tannins, oxidizing agents

NURSING CONSIDERATIONS
Assess:

• Vital signs, B/P; check patients with cardiac disease more often, administer to conscious patients only

• Type of poisoning; do not administer if petroleum products or caustic substances have been ingested: kerosene, gasoline, lye, Drano

• Respiratory status before, during, after administration of emetic; check rate, rhythm, character; respiratory depression can occur rapidly with elderly or debilitated patients; record B/P, pulse; check for odor of alcohol on breath, clothes

Administer:

• Dopamine antagonists to reverse emetic effect of this drug

• Activated charcoal if this drug doesn't work; may begin lavage after 10-15 min

• Only clear solutions; do not expose to light or air

Evaluate:

• Therapeutic response: vomiting rapidly

---

apraclonidine HCl

(ap-raa-kloe′ni-deen)
Iopidine

Func. class.: Topical ophthalmic agent

Chem. class.: Selective α-adrenergic agonist

Action: Reduces intraocular pressure by reducing aqueous formation; exact mechanism of action unknown

Uses: Control elevations of intraocular pressure after laser iridotomy or trabeculoplasty

Dosage and routes

• *Adult:* Instill 1 gtt 1 hr before laser surgery, second gtt at completion of surgery

Available forms: Sol 1% apraclonidine HCl, 0.01% benzalkonium chloride

Side effects/adverse reactions:

EENT: Upper lid elevation, conjunctival blanching, mydriasis, burning, dryness, itching, blurred vision, conjunctival microhemorrhage, foreign body sensation, dry mouth, taste abnormalities, nasal dryness/burning

GI: Abdominal pain, diarrhea, cramps, emesis

CV: Bradycardia, palpitations, vasovagal attack, orthostatic episode

CNS: Insomnia, irritability, restlessness, headache, dream disturbances

OTHER: Shortness of breath, head cold sensation, sweaty palms, fatigue, paresthesia, pruritus

Contraindications: Hypersensitivity to this drug or clonidine, severe cardiovascular disease

Precautions: Pregnancy (C), lactation, children

NURSING CONSIDERATIONS
Assess:

• Cardiac status; watch for brady-

---

italics = common side effects   ***bold italic*** = life threatening reactions

cardia, palpitations, especially in cardiac disease (including hypertension)
• Vasovagal attack during laser surgery, primarily in individuals with history of such episodes
Perform/provide:
• Storage at room temperature, away from light
Evaluate:
Therapeutic response: absence of increased intraocular pressure
Teach patient/family
• Drug may cause burning, itching, blurring, dryness of eye area

---

ascorbic acid (vitamin C)

(a-skor'bic)
Ascorbic Acid, Ascorbicap, Ascorbic Acid Caplets, Cecon, Cenolate, Cetane, Cevalin, Cevi-Bid, Ce-Vi-Sol, C-Crystals, Cebid Timecelles, Dull-C, Flavorcee, N'íce Vitamin C Drops, Redoxon*, Vita-C

Func. class.: Vitamin C, water-soluble vitamin

Action: Needed for wound healing, collagen synthesis, antioxidant, carbohydrate metabolism
Uses: Vitamin C deficiency, scurvy, delayed wound and bone healing, chronic disease, urine acidification, before gastrectomy
Dosage and routes:
Scurvy
• *Adult:* PO/SC/IM/IV 100 mg-500 mg qd, then 50 mg or more qd
• *Child:* PO/SC/IM/IV 100-300 mg qd, then 35 mg or more qd
Wound healing/chronic disease/fracture
• *Adult:* SC/IM/IV/PO 200-500 mg qd

• *Child:* SC/IM/IV/PO 100-200 mg added doses
Urine acidification
• *Adult:* 4-12 g qd in divided doses
Available forms: Tabs 25, 50, 100, 250, 500, 1000, 1500 mg; tabs effervescent 1000 mg; tabs chewable 100, 250, 500 mg; tabs timed release 500, 750, 1000, 1500 mg; caps timed release 500 mg; crys 4 g/tsp; powd 4 g/tsp; liq 35 mg/0.6 ml; sol 100 mg/ml; syr 20 mg/ml, 500 mg/5 ml; inj SC, IM, IV 100, 250, 500 mg/ml
Side effects/adverse reactions:
CNS: Headache, insomnia, dizziness, fatigue, flushing
GI: Nausea, vomiting, diarrhea, anorexia, heartburn, cramps
GU: Polyuria, urine acidification, oxalate or urate renal stones
HEMA: **Hemolytic anemia in patients with G-6-PD**
Contraindications: None significant
Precautions: Gout, pregnancy (A)
Pharmacokinetics:
PO, INJ: Metabolized in liver, unused amounts excreted in urine (unchanged) and metabolites, crosses placenta, breast milk
Interactions/incompatibilities:
• Increased effects of salicylates, oral contraceptives
• Increased side effects of PAS, digitalis, sulfonamides
• Decreased effects of phenothiazines, disulfiram, amphetamines, heparin, coumarin (massive doses)
• Incompatible with aminophylline, bleomycin, chloramphenicol, chlordiazepoxide, chlorothiazide, estrogens (conjugated), dextran, erythromycin, hydrocortisone, nafcillin, phytonadione, sulfisoxazole, triflupromazine, Vit B_{12}, warfarin, $NaCo_3$

---

*Available in Canada only

A

Lab test interferences:
• *False positive:* negatives in glucose tests
• *False negative:* occult blood
NURSING CONSIDERATIONS
Assess:
• I&O ratio
• Ascorbic acid levels throughout treatment if continued deficiency is suspected
• Nutritional status: citrus fruits, vegetables
• Injection sites for inflammation
Administer:
• Undiluted by direct IV 100 mg over at least 1 min
• By IV INF diluted with D₅W, D₅NaCl, NS, LR, Ringer's, sodium lactate and given over 15 min
Evaluate:
• Therapeutic response: absence of anorexia, irritability, pallor, joint pain, hyperkeratosis, petechiae, poor wound healing
Teach patient/family:
• Necessary foods to be included in diet
• That if oral contraceptives are taken, increased levels of Vit C are needed
• That smoking decreases Vit C levels, not to exceed prescribed dose; increases will be excreted in urine, except time release

---

asparaginase (L-asparaginase)

(a-spar'a-gin-ase)
Elspar
Func. class.: Antineoplastic
Chem. class.: E. coli enzyme

Action: Indirectly inhibits protein synthesis in tumor cells; without amino acid, DNA, RNA synthesis is halted; asparagine, protein synthesis is halted; G₁ phase of cell cycle specific; a nonvesicant
Uses: Acute lymphocytic leukemia in combination with other antineoplastics
Dosage and routes:
In combination
• *Adult:* IV 1000 IU/kg/day × 10 days given over 30 min; IM 6000 IU/m²/day
Sole induction
• *Adult:* IV 200 IU/kg/day × 28 days
Available forms: Inj 10,000 IU
Side effects/adverse reactions:
*SYST: **Anaphylaxis, hypersensitivity***
*HEMA: **Thrombocytopenia, leukopenia, myelosuppression, anemia, decreased clotting factors***
*GI: Nausea, vomiting, anorexia, cramps, stomatitis, **hepatotoxicity, pancreatitis***
*GU: Urinary retention, **renal failure,** glycosuria, polyuria, azotemia, uric acid neuropathy*
INTEG: Rash, urticaria, chills, fever
ENDO: Hyperglycemia
*RESP: **Fibrosis, pulmonary infiltrate***
CV: Chest pain
*CNS: Neuritis, dizziness, headache, **coma,** depression, fatigue, confusion, hallucinations*
Contraindications: Hypersensitivity, infants, pregnancy (D), lactation, pancreatitis
Precautions: Renal disease, hepatic disease
Pharmacokinetics: Half-life 4-9 hr, terminal 1.4-1.8 hr
Interactions/incompatibilities:
• Decreased action of methotrexate
• Do not use with radiation
• Increased toxicity: vincristine, prednisone
• Synergism in combination with cytarabine, 6-azauridine

---

italics = common side effects   ***bold italic*** = life threatening reactions

• Considered incompatible with other drugs or sol

Lab test interferences:

Decrease: Thyroid function tests

NURSING CONSIDERATIONS

Assess:

• For signs and symptoms of pancreatitis (nausea, vomiting, severe abdominal pain), anaphylaxis (bronchospasm, dyspnea), cyanosis

• CBC, differential, platelet count weekly; withhold drug if WBC is <4000 or platelet count is <75,000; notify physician of these results

• Pulmonary function tests, chest x-ray studies before, during therapy; chest x-ray film should be obtained q2 wk during treatment

• Renal function studies: BUN, serum uric acid, ammonia urine CrCl, electrolytes before, during therapy

• I&O ratio; report fall in urine output of 30/ml/hr

• Monitor temperature q4h; may indicate beginning infection

• Liver function tests before, during therapy (bilirubin, AST, ALT, LDH) as needed or monthly

• RBC, Hct, Hgb, since these may be decreased

• Serum, urine glucose levels

• Bleeding: hematuria, guaiac, bruising or petechiae, mucosa or orifices q8h

• Dyspnea, rales, nonproductive cough, chest pain, tachypnea fatigue, increased pulse, pallor, lethargy, or swelling around eyes or lips; anaphylaxis may occur

• Food preferences; list likes, dislikes

• Yellowing of skin and sclera, dark urine, clay-colored stools, itchy skin, abdominal pain, fever, diarrhea

• Local irritation, pain, burning, discoloration at injection site

• Symptoms indicating severe allergic reaction: rash, pruritus, urticaria, purpuric skin lesions, itching, flushing, dyspnea

• Frequency of stools, characteristics: cramping, acidosis; signs of dehydration: rapid respirations, poor skin turgor, decreased urine output, dry skin, restlessness, weakness

Administer:

• After intradermal skin testing and desensitization, give 0.1 ml (2 IU) intradermally after reconstituting with 5 ml sterile H_2O or 0.9% NaCl for injection; then add 0.1 ml of reconstituted drug to 9.9 ml diluent (20 IU/ml); observe for 1 hr, check for wheal

• Allopurinol or sodium bicarbonate to reduce uric acid levels, alkalinization of urine

• IV infusion using 21-, 23-, 25-gauge needle; administer by slow IV infusion via Y-tube or 3-way stop cock of flowing D_5W or NS infusion over 30 min after diluting 10,000 IU/5 ml of sterile H_2O or 0.9% NaCl (no preservatives) (2000 IU/ml); use of filter may be necessary if fibers are present

• Transfusion for anemia

• Antispasmodic

Perform/provide:

• Deep-breathing exercises with patient 3-4 × day; place in semi-Fowler's position

• Increase fluid intake to 2-3 L/day to prevent urate deposits, calculi formation

• Diet low in purines: absence of organ meats (kidney, liver), dried beans, peas to maintain alkaline urine

• Rinsing of mouth 3-4 × day with water, club soda

---

* Available in Canada only

• Brushing of teeth 2-3 × day with soft brush or cotton-tipped applicators for stomatitis; use unwaxed dental floss

• Warm compresses at injection site for inflammation

• Nutritious diet with iron, vitamin supplements

• HOB raised to facilitate breathing

Evaluate:

• Therapeutic response: decreased exacerbations in A.L.L.

Teach patient/family:

• To report any complaints or side effects to nurse or physician

• To report any changes in breathing or coughing

Treatment of anaphylaxis:

Administer epinephrine, diphenhydramine, IV corticosteroids

---

aspirin
(as´pir-in)

Ancasal*, A.S.A., Aspergum, Aspirin*, Bayer, Bayer Children's Aspirin, Easprin, Ecotrin, Ecotrin Maximum Strength, 8-Hour Bayer Timed Release, Empirin, Entrophen*, Genprin, Maximum Bayer, Norwich Extra-Strength, Novasen*, Sal-Adult*, Sal-Infant*, St. Joseph Children's, Supasa*, Therapy Bayer, ZORprin

Func. class.: Nonnarcotic analgesic

Chem. class.: Salicylate

Action: Blocks pain impulses in CNS that occur in response to inhibition of prostaglandin synthesis; antipyretic action results from vasodilation of peripheral vessels. Decreases platelet aggregation.

Uses: Mild to moderate pain or fever including rheumatoid arthritis, osteoarthritis, thromboembolic disorders, transient ischemic attacks in men, rheumatic fever, postmyocardial infarction, prophylaxis of myocardial infarction.

Dosage and routes:

Arthritis

• *Adult:* PO 2.6-5.2 g/day in divided doses q4-6h

• *Child:* PO 90-130 mg/kg/day in divided doses q4-6h

Pain/fever

• *Adult:* PO/REC 325-650 mg q4h prn, not to exceed 4 g/day

• *Child:* PO/REC 40-100 mg/kg/day in divided doses q4-6h prn

Thromboembolic disorders

• *Adult:* PO 325-650 mg/day or bid

Transient ischemic attacks

• *Adult:* PO 650 mg qid or 325 mg qid

Available forms: Tabs 65, 81, 325, 500, 650, 975 mg; chewable tabs 81 mg; caps 325, 500 mg; tabs controlled-release 800 mg; tabs time-release 650 mg; supp 60, 120, 125, 130, 195, 200, 300, 325, 600, 650 mg, 1.2 g; cream; gum 227.5 mg

Side effects/adverse reactions:

HEMA: ***Thrombocytopenia, agranulocytosis, leukopenia, neutropenia, hemolytic anemia,*** increased pro-time, PTT, bleeding time

CNS: Stimulation, drowsiness, dizziness, confusion, ***convulsion,*** headache, flushing, hallucinations, ***coma***

*GI: Nausea, vomiting, **GI bleeding,*** diarrhea, heartburn, anorexia, ***hepatitis***

INTEG: Rash, urticaria, bruising

EENT: Tinnitus, hearing loss

CV: Rapid pulse, pulmonary edema

RESP: Wheezing, hyperpnea

ENDO: Hypoglycemia, hyponatremia, hypokalemia

Contraindications: Hypersensitivity to salicylates, tartrazine (FDC

---

italics = common side effects   ***bold italic*** = life threatening reactions

yellow dye #5), GI bleeding, bleeding disorders, children 12 yr, children with flulike symptoms, pregnancy (D), lactation, Vit K deficiency, peptic ulcer

Precautions: Anemia, hepatic disease, renal disease, Hodgkin's disease, pre/postoperatively

Pharmacokinetics: Well absorbed PO; enteric product and rectal product may be erratic

PO: Onset 15-30 min, peak 1-2 hr, duration 4-6 hr

REC: Onset slow, duration 4-6 hr; Metabolized by liver, inactive metabolites excreted by kidneys, crosses placenta, excreted in breast milk, half-life 1-3½ hr; up to 30 hrs in large doses

Interactions/incompatibilities:

• Decreased effects of aspirin: antacids, steroids, urinary alkalizers

• Increased bleeding: alcohol, heparin, valproic acid, plicamycin, cefamandole

• Increased effects of anticoagulants, insulin, methotrexate, thrombolytic agents, penicillins, phenytoin, valporic acid, oral hypoglycemics, sulfonamides

• Increased salicylate levels: urinary acidifiers

• Decreased effects of probenecid, spironolactone, sulfinpyrazone, sulfonylamides

• Toxic effects: PABA, furosemide, carbonic anhydrase inhibitors

• Decreased blood sugar levels: salicylates

• Gastric ulcer: steroids, antiinflammatories, nonsteroidal antiinflammatories

• Ototoxicity: vancomycin

Lab test interferences:

Increase: Coagulation studies, liver function studies, serum uric acid, amylase, CO_2, urinary protein

Decrease: Serum potassium, PBI, cholesterol

Interfere: Urine catecholamines, pregnancy test, urine glucose tests (Clinistix, Tes-Tape)

NURSING CONSIDERATIONS
Assess:

• Liver function studies: AST, ALT, bilirubin, creatinine if patient is on long-term therapy

• Renal function studies: BUN, urine creatinine if patient is on long-term therapy

• Blood studies: CBC, Hct, Hgb, pro-time if patient is on long-term therapy

• I&O ratio; decreasing output may indicate renal failure (long-term therapy)

• Hepatotoxicity: dark urine, clay-colored stools, yellowing of skin, sclera, itching, abdominal pain, fever, diarrhea if patient is on long-term therapy

• Allergic reactions: rash, urticaria; if these occur, drug may have to be discontinued

• Renal dysfunction: decreased urine output

• Ototoxicity: tinnitus, ringing, roaring in ears; audiometric testing needed before, after long-term therapy

• Visual changes: blurring, halos; corneal, retinal damage

• Edema in feet, ankles, legs

• Prior drug history; there are many drug interactions

• Pain: Location, duration, type, intensity, prior to dose and 1 hour after

• Musculoskeletal status: ROM prior to dose

• Fever; length of time and related symptoms

Administer:

• To patient crushed or whole; chewable tablets may be chewed

(do not crush enteric product)
• With food or milk to decrease gastric symptoms; give 30 min before or 2 hr after meals
• Antacids 1-2 hours of enteric products

Evaluate:
• Therapeutic response: decreased pain, inflammation, fever

Teach patient/family:
• To report any symptoms of hepatotoxicity, renal toxicity, visual changes, ototoxicity, allergic reactions, bleeding (long-term therapy)
• To take with 8 oz of water and sit upright for ½ hour after dose
• Not to exceed recommended dosage; acute poisoning may result
• To read label on other OTC drugs; many contain aspirin
• That the therapeutic response takes 2 wk (arthritis)
• To report tinnitus, confusion, diarrhea, sweating, hyperventilation
• To avoid alcohol ingestion; GI bleeding may occur
• That patients who have allergies may develop allergic reactions
• To avoid buffered or effervescent products
• Not to be given to children; Reye's syndrome may develop

Treatment of overdose: Lavage, activated charcoal, monitor electrolytes, VS

---

astemizole
(a-stem´-mi-zole)
Hismanal
Func. class.: Antihistamine
Chem. class.: H₁-histamine antagonist

Action: Acts on blood vessels, GI, respiratory system by competing with histamine for H₁-receptor site; decreases allergic response by blocking pharmacologic effects of histamine

Uses: Rhinitis, allergy symptoms

Dosage and routes:
• *Adult and child > 12 yr:* PO 10 mg qd; to reduce time to steady state may take 30 mg day 1, 20 mg day 2, followed by 10 mg daily
Available forms: Tabs 10 mg

Side effects/adverse reactions:
GU: Frequency, dysuria, urinary retention, impotence
*HEMA: **Hemolytic anemia, thrombocytopenia, leukopenia, agranulocytosis, pancytopenia***
RESP: Thickening of bronchial secretions, dry nose, throat
GI: Nausea, diarrhea, abdominal pain, vomiting, constipation
CNS: Headache, stimulation, drowsiness, sedation, fatigue, confusion, blurred vision, tinnitus, restlessness, tremors, paradoxical excitation in children or elderly
INTEG: Rash, eczema, photosensitivity, urticaria
CV: Hypotension, palpitations, bradycardia, tachycardia, ***dysrhythmias*** (rare)

Contraindications: Hypersensitivity, newborn or premature infants, lactation, severe hepatic disease

Precautions: Pregnancy (C), elderly, children, respiratory disease, narrow-angle glaucoma, prostatic hypertrophy, bladder neck obstruction, asthma, elderly

Pharmacokinetics:
PO: Peak 1-2 hr, 97% bound to plasma proteins; half-life is biphasic 3½ hr, 16-23 hr

Interactions/incompatibilities:
• Increased CNS depression: alcohol, other CNS depressants, procarbazine

---

italics = common side effects   ***bold italic*** = life threatening reactions

• Increased anticholinergic effects: MAOIs
• Decreased action of oral anticoagulants
• Serious CV reactions: ketoconazole, itraconazole, erythromycin
• Avoid use with antifungals, macrolide antibiotics

Lab test interferences:

False negative: Skin allergy tests

NURSING CONSIDERATIONS
Assess:
• I&O ratio: be alert for urinary retention, frequency, dysuria, especially elderly; drug should be discontinued if these occur
• CBC during long-term therapy
• Respiratory status: rate, rhythm, increase in bronchial secretions, wheezing, chest tightness

Administer:
• On empty stomach, 1 hr before or 2 hr after meals

Perform/provide:
• Hard candy, gum, frequent rinsing of mouth for dryness
• Storage in tight, light-resistant container

Evaluate:
• Therapeutic reponse: absence of running or congested nose or rashes

Teach patient/family:
• All aspects of drug use; to notify physician if confusion, sedation, hypotension occur
• To avoid driving or other hazardous activity if drowsiness occurs
• To avoid alcohol or other CNS depressants
• Not to exceed recommended dose; dysrrhythmias may occur

Treatment of overdose: Administer ipecac syrup or lavage, diazepam, vasopressors, barbiturates (short-acting)

atenolol
(a-ten'oh-lole)
Apo-Atenol*, Atenolol, Tenormin
Func. class.: Antihypertensive
Chem. class.: β-Blocker, β-1, 2 blocker (high doses)

Action: Competitively blocks stimulation of β-adrenergic receptor within vascular smooth muscle; produces negative chronotropic activity, positive inotropic activity (decreases rate of SA node discharge, increases recovery time), slows conduction of AV node, decreases heart rate, decreases O_2 consumption in myocardium; also decreases renin-aldosterone-angiotensin system at high doses, inhibits β-2 receptors in bronchial system at higher doses

Uses: Mild to moderate hypertension, prophylaxis of angina pectoris, suspected or known myocardial infarction

Dosage and routes:
• *Adult:* IV 5 mg, repeat in 10 min if initial dose is well tolerated, then start PO dose 10 min after last IV dose
• *Adult:* PO 50 mg qd, increasing q1-2 wk to 100 mg qd; may increase to 200 mg qd for angina

Available forms: Tabs 50, 100 mg

Side effects/adverse reactions:
*CV: **Profound hypotension, bradycardia, CHF,** cold extremities, postural hypotension, 2nd or 3rd degree heart block*
CNS: Insomnia, fatigue, dizziness, mental changes, memory loss, hallucinations, depression, lethargy, drowsiness, strange dreams, catatonia
GI: Nausea, diarrhea, vomiting,

mesenteric arterial thrombosis, ischemic colitis

INTEG: Rash, fever, alopecia

HEMA: **Agranulocytosis, thrombocytopenia, purpura**

EENT: Sore throat, dry burning eyes

GU: Impotence

ENDO: Increased hypoglycemic response to insulin

RESP: **Bronchospasm,** dyspnea, wheezing

Contraindications: Hypersensitivity to β-blockers, cardiogenic shock, 2nd or 3rd degree heart block, sinus bradycardia, CHF, cardiac failure

Precautions: Major surgery, pregnancy (C), lactation, diabetes mellitus, renal disease, thyroid disease, COPD, asthma, well-compensated heart failure

Pharmacokinetics:

PO: Peak 2-4 hr; half-life 6-7 hr, excreted unchanged in urine, protein binding 5%-15%

Interactions/incompatibilities:

• Increased hypotension, bradycardia: reserpine, hydralazine, methyldopa, prazosin, anticholinergics, digoxin

• Decreased antihypertensive effects: indomethacin

• Increased hypoglycemic effect: insulin

• Mutual inhibition: sympathomimetics (cough, cold preparations)

• Decreased bronchodilation: theophyllines, β₂ agonists

• Paradoxical hypertension: clonidine

• Incompatible with any other drug in sol or syringe

Lab test interferences:

Interference: Glucose/insulin tolerance tests

NURSING CONSIDERATIONS

Assess:

• I&O, weight daily

• B/P, pulse q4h; note rate, rhythm, quality

• Apical/radial pulse before administration; notify physician of any significant changes

• Baselines in renal, liver function tests before therapy begins

• Edema in feet, legs daily

• Skin turgor, dryness of mucous membranes for hydration status

Administer:

• PO ac, hs, tablet may be crushed or swallowed whole

• Reduced dosage in renal dysfunction

• IV undiluted by direct IV over 5 min or diluted in 10-50 ml of D₅W, Y₂NaCl, or NS and give as an infusion at prescribed rate

Perform/provide:

• Storage protected from light, moisture; placed in cool environment

Evaluate:

• Therapeutic response: decreased B/P after 1-2 wk

Teach patient/family:

• Not to discontinue drug abruptly; taper over 2 wk

• Not to use OTC products unless directed by physician

• To report bradycardia, dizziness, confusion, depression, fever

• To take pulse at home; advise when to notify physician

• To avoid alcohol, smoking, sodium intake

• To comply with weight control, dietary adjustments, modified exercise program

• To carry Medic Alert ID to identify drug that you are taking, allergies

• To avoid hazardous activities if dizziness is present

Treatment of overdose: Lavage, IV atropine for bradycardia, IV theophylline for bronchospasm, digitalis, O$_2$, diuretic for cardiac failure, hemodialysis

---

atovaquoné
(a-tove'-a-que-one)
Mepron
Func. class.: Antiprotozoal
Chem. class.: Aromatic diamide derivative, analog of ubiquinone

---

Action: Interferes with DNA/RNA synthesis in protozoa
Uses: *Pneumocystis carinii* infections not sensitive to trimethoprim/sulfamethoxazole
Dosage and routes:
• *Adult:* 750 mg with food 3× a day for 21 days
Available forms: TABS 250 mg
Side effects/adverse reactions:
CV: Hypotension
HEMA: Anemia, leukopenia
INTEG: Pruritus, urticaria, rash, oral monilia
GI: Nausea, vomiting, diarrhea, anorexia, increased AST and ALT, acute pancreatitis, constipation, abdominal pain
CNS: Dizziness, headache, anxiety
META: Hyperkalemia, hyperglycemia, hyponatremia
Contraindications: Hypersensitivity or history of developing life-threatening allergic reactions to any component of the formulation
Precautions: Blood dyscrasias, hepatic disease, diabetes mellitus, pregnancy (C), lactation, children, elderly
Pharmacokinetics: Excreted unchanged in feces (94%), highly protein bound
Interactions/incompatibilities:
Use caution when administering concurrently with other highly plasma protein–bound drugs with narrow therapeutic indices
NURSING CONSIDERATIONS
Assess:
• Blood studies, blood glucose, ACBC, platelets
• I&O ratio
• ECG for cardiac dysrhythmias, check B/P
• Liver studies: AST, ALT
• Signs of infection, anemia
• Bowel pattern before, during treatment
• Respiratory status: rate, character, wheezing, dyspnea
• Dizziness, confusion, hallucination
• Allergies before treatment, reaction of each medication; place allergies on chart; Kardex in bright red letters; notify all people giving drugs
Administer:
• With food because of increased absorption of the drug and higher plasma concentrations
Evaluate:
• Therapeutic response: decreased temperature, ability to breathe
Teach patient/family:
• To report sore throat, fever, fatigue; may indicate superimposed infection
• To take with food to increase plasma concentrations

---

atracurium besylate
(a-tra-cyoor'ee-um)
Tracrium
Func. class.: Neuromuscular blocker (nondepolarizing)
Chem. class.: Biquaternary ammonium ester

Action: Inhibits transmission of nerve impulses by binding with cholinergic receptor sites, antagonizing action of acetylcholine

Uses: Facilitation of endotracheal intubation, skeletal muscle relaxation during mechanical ventilation, surgery, or general anesthesia

Dosage and routes:

• *Adult:* IV BOL 0.4-0.5 mg/kg, then 0.08-0.10 mg/kg 20-45 min after 1st dose if needed for prolonged procedures

Available forms: Inj IV 10 mg/ml

Side effects/adverse reactions:

CV: Bradycardia, tachycardia, increase, decrease B/P

RESP: **Prolonged apnea, bronchospasm, cyanosis, respiratory depression**

EENT: Increased secretions

INTEG: Rash, flushing, pruritus, urticaria

Contraindications: Hypersensitivity

Precautions: Pregnancy (C), cardiac disease, lactation, children <2 yr, electrolyte imbalances, dehydration, neuromuscular disease, respiratory disease

Pharmacokinetics:

IV: Onset 2 min, duration 20-60 min; half-life 2 min, 29 min (terminal), excreted in urine, feces (metabolites), crosses placenta

Interactions/incompatibilities:

• Increased neuromuscular blockade: aminoglycosides, clindamycin, lincomycin, quinidine, local anesthetics, polymyxin antibiotics, lithium, narcotic analgesics, thiazides, enflurane, isoflurane

• Dysrhythmias: theophylline

• Do not mix with barbiturates or alkalies in solution or syringe

NURSING CONSIDERATIONS

Assess:

• For electrolyte imbalances (K, Mg), may lead to increased action of this drug

• Vital signs (B/P, pulse, respirations, airway) until fully recovered; rate, depth, pattern of respirations, strength of hand grip

• I&O ratio; check for urinary retention, frequency, hesitancy

• Recovery: decreased paralysis of face, diaphragm, leg, arm, rest of body

• Allergic reactions: rash, fever, respiratory distress, pruritus; drug should be discontinued

Administer:

• Using nerve stimulator by anesthesiologist to determine neuromuscular blockade

• Anticholinesterase to reverse neuromuscular blockade

• IV undiluted by direct IV over 5 min, or diluted in 10-50 ml of D_5W, ½ NaCl or NS and give as an infusion at prescribed rate

• By slow IV over 1-2 min (only by qualified person, usually an anesthesiologist); do not administer IM

• Only slightly discolored solution

Perform/provide:

• Storage in light-resistant area

• Reassurance if communication is difficult during recovery from neuromuscular blockade

Evaluate:

• Therapeutic response: paralysis of jaw, eyelid, head, neck, rest of body

Treatment of overdose: Edrophonium or neostigmine, atropine, monitor VS; may require mechanical ventilation

---

atropine sulfate

(a'troe-peen)

Func. class.: Anticholinergic parasympatholytic

Chem. class.: Belladonna alkaloid

Action: Blocks acetylcholine at

parasympathetic neuroeffector sites; increases cardiac output, heart rate by blocking cardiac vagal stimulation in heart; dries secretions by blocking vagus

Uses: Bradycardia, bradydysrhythmia, anticholinesterase insecticide poisoning, blocking cardiac vagal reflexes, decreasing secretions before surgery, antispasmodic with GU, biliary surgery, bronchodilator

Dosage and routes:

Bradycardia/bradydysrhythmias
• *Adult:* IV BOL 0.5-1 mg given q3-5 min, not to exceed 2 mg
• *Child:* IV BOL 0.01-0.03 mg/kg up to 0.4 mg or 0.3 mg/m²; may repeat q4-6h

Insecticide poisoning
• *Adult and child:* IM/IV 2 mg qh until muscarinic symptoms disappear, may need 6 mg qh

Presurgery
• *Adult:* SC/IM/IV 0.4-0.6 mg before anesthesia
• *Child:* SC 0.1-0.4 mg 30 min before surgery

Available forms: Inj 0.05, 0.1, 0.3, 0.4, 0.5, 0.8, 1 mg/ml, tabs 0.4 mg; tabs sol 0.4, 0.6 mg

Side effects/adverse reactions:

GU: Retention, hesitancy, impotence, dysuria

CNS: Headache, dizziness, involuntary movement, confusion, psychosis, anxiety, coma, flushing, drowsiness, insomnia, weakness

GI: Dry mouth, nausea, vomiting, abdominal pain, anorexia, constipation, paralytic ileus, abdominal distention, altered taste

CV: Hypotension, paradoxical bradycardia, angina, PVCs, hypertension, tachycardia, ectopic ventricular beats

INTEG: Rash, urticaria, contact dermatitis, dry skin, flushing

EENT: Blurred vision, photophobia, glaucoma, eye pain, pupil dilation, nasal congestion

MISC: Suppression of lactation, decreased sweating

Contraindications: Hypersensitivity to belladonna alkaloids, angle-closure glaucoma, GI obstructions, myasthenia gravis, thyrotoxicosis, ulcerative colitis, prostatic hypertrophy, tachycardia/tachydysrhythmias, asthma, acute hemorrhage, hepatic disease, myocardial ischemia

Precautions: Pregnancy (C), renal disease, lactation, CHF, tachydysrhythmias, hyperthyroidism, COPD, hepatic disease, child <6 yr, hypertension, elderly, intraabdominal infections, Down syndrome, spastic paralysis, gastric ulcer

Pharmacokinetics: Well absorbed PO, IM, SC; half-life 13-40 hours, excreted by kidneys unchanged (70%-90% in 24 hr); metabolized in liver, 40%-50% crosses placenta, excreted in breast milk

IV: Peak 2-4 min, duration 4-6 hours

IM/SC: Onset 15-50 min; peak 30 min, duration 4-6 hours

PO: Onset ½ hour; peak ½-1 hour; duration 4-6 hours

Interactions/incompatibilities:
• Decreases effect of atropine; antacids
• Decreased effects of phenothiazines
• Increased anticholinergic effects of anticholinergics, tricylic antidepressants, amantadine, MAOIs, quinidine
• Incompatible with amobarbital, ampicillin, chloramphenicol, chlortetracycline, cimetidine, epinephrine, heparin, isoproterenol, levarterenol, metaraminol, methicillin, methohexital, nitrofuran-

---

* Available in Canada only

toin, pentobarbital, promazine, thiopental, warfarin, NaCo₃ in sol or syringe

NURSING CONSIDERATIONS
Assess:
• I&O ratio; check for urinary retention, daily output
• ECG for ectopic ventricular beats, PVC, tachycardia
• For bowel sounds; check for constipation
• Respiratory status: rate, rhythm, cyanosis, wheezing, dyspnea, engorged neck veins
• Increased intraocular pressure: eye pain, nausea, vomiting, blurred vision, increased tearing
• Cardiac rate: rhythm, character, B/P continuously
• Allergic reaction: rash, urticaria

Administer:
• IV undiluted or diluted with 10 ml sterile H₂O, give at a rate of 0.6 mg/min, give through Y-tube or 3-way stopcock; do not add to IV solutions; may cause paradoxical bradycardia lasting 2 mins
• Increased bulk, water in diet if constipation occurs
• PO ½ hour ac
• IM; atropine flush may occur in children and is not harmful

Perform/provide:
• Sugarless hard candy, gum, frequent rinsing of mouth for dryness

Evaluate:
• Therapeutic response: decreased dysrhythmias, increased heart rate, secretions, GI, GU spasms, bronchodilation

Teach patient/family:
• To report blurred vision, chest pain, allergic reactions
• Not to perform strenuous activity in high temperatures; heat stroke may result
• To take as prescribed; not to skip doses

• Not to operate machinery if drowsiness occurs
• Not to take OTC products without approval of physician

Treatment of overdose: O₂, artificial ventilation, ECG; administer dopamine for circulatory depression; administer diazepam or thiopental for convulsions; assess need for antidysrhythmics

---

atropine sulfate (optic)
(a'troe-peen)
Atropine-Care Ophthalmic, Atropine Sulfate Ophthalmic, Atropine Sulfate S.O.P., Atropisol Ophthalmic, Isopto Atropine
Func. class.: Mydriatic
Chem. class.: Belladonna alkaloid

Action: Blocks response of iris sphincter muscle, muscle of accommodation of ciliary body to cholinergic stimulation, resulting in dilation, paralysis of accommodation
Uses: Iritis, cycloplegic refraction
Dosage and routes:
• *Adult:* INSTILL SOL 1-2 gtt of a 1% sol qd-tid for iritis or 1 hr before refracting (cycloplegic refraction); INSTILL OINT 2-3 ×/day
• *Child:* INSTILL SOL 1-2 gtts of a 0.5% sol qd-tid for iritis or bid × 1-3 days before exam (cycloplegic refraction); INSTILL OINT qd-bid 2-3 days before exam
Available forms: Oint 0.5%, 1%; sol 0.5%, 1%, 2%, 3%
Side effects/adverse reactions:
SYST: Tachycardia, confusion, fever, flushing, dry skin, dry mouth, abdominal discomfort, headache,

irritability (infants: bladder distention, irregular pulse, respiratory depression)

EENT: Photophobia, blurred vision, increased intraocular pressure, conjunctivitis

Contraindications: Hypersensitivity, infants <3 mo, open or narrow-angle glaucoma, conjunctivitis

Precautions: Elderly, pregnancy, lactation, Down syndrome

Pharmacokinetics:

INSTILL: Peak 30-40 min (mydriasis), 60-180 min (cycloplegia), duration 6-12 days

NURSING CONSIDERATIONS
Assess:

• Eye pain; discontinue use if pain occurs

Evaluate:

• Therapeutic response: decrease in inflammation (iritis) or cycloplegic refraction

Teach patient/family:

• To report change in vision; blurring or loss of sight; trouble breathing; sweating; flushing

• Method of instillation: pressure on lacrimal sac for 1 min; do not touch dropper to eye

• That blurred vision will decrease with repeated use of drug

• Not to do hazardous things until able to see

• To omit next instillation if side effects are present

• To wait 5 min to use other drops

• Not to blink more than usual

---

auranofin

(aur-an-oo-fin)

Ridaura

Func. class.: Gold salt

Chem. class.: Active gold compound (29%)

Action: Antiinflammatory action

unknown; may decrease phagocytosis, lysosomal activity or decrease prostaglandin synthesis; decreases concentration of rheumatoid factor, immunoglobulins

Uses: Rheumatoid arthritis

Dosage and routes:

• *Adult:* PO 6 mg qd or 3 mg bid, may increase to 9 mg/day after 3 mo

Available forms: Caps 3 mg

Side effects/adverse reactions:

*HEMA: **Thrombocytopenia, agranulocytosis, aplastic anemia, leukopenia, eosinophilia, neutropenia***

INTEG: Rash, pruritus, dermatitis, *exfoliative dermatitis,* urticaria, alopecia, photosensitivity

CNS: Dizziness, confusion, hallucinations, *seizures,* EEG abnormalities

GI: Diarrhea, abdominal cramping, stomatitis, nausea, vomiting, enterocolitis, anorexia, flatulence, metallic taste, dyspepsia, jaundice, increased AST, ALT, glossitis, gingivitis, melena, constipation

*GU: **Proteinuria, hematuria,*** increased BUN, creatinine, vaginitis

MISC: Iritis, corneal ulcers, gold deposits in ocular tissues

*RESP: **Interstitial pneumonitis, fibrosis,*** cough, dyspnea

Contraindications: Hypersensitivity to gold, necrotizing enterocolitis, bone marrow aplasia, child <6 yr, lactation, pulmonary fibrosis, exfoliative dermatitis, blood dyscrasias, recent radiation therapy, renal/hepatic disease, marked hypertension, uncontrolled CHF

Precautions: Elderly, CHF, diabetes mellitus, allergic conditions, ulcerative colitis, renal disease, liver disease, pregnancy (C)

Pharmacokinetics:

PO: Absorbed by GI tract, peak 2

hr, steady state 8-16 wk, excreted in urine, feces

Interactions/incompatibilities:
• Do not use with penicillamine or antimalarials
• May increase levels of phenytoin

Lab test interferences:
False positive: TB test

NURSING CONSIDERATIONS
Assess:
• Respiratory status: dyspnea, wheezing; if respiratory problems occur, drug should be discontinued
• I&O ratio
• Urine: hematuria, proteinuria, increased BUN, creatinine may require decrease in dosage
• Platelet counts qmo; drug should be discontinued if <100,000/mm³
• Hepatic test: ALT, AST, alk phosphatase
• Diarrhea stools; if severe, drug should be discontinued
• Allergy: rash, dermatitis, pruritus; drug should be discontinued if any of these occur
• Gold toxicity: decreased Hgb, WBC <4000/mm³, granulocytes <1500/mm³, platelets <150,000/mm³, severe diarrhea, stomatitis, hematuria, rash, itching, proteinuria

Administer:
• bid or may give as single dose qAM with food or drink

Evaluate:
• Therapeutic response: ability to move joints with less pain

Teach patient/family
• That drug must be taken as prescribed to be useful, to obtain lab work monthly
• That diarrhea is common, but if blood appears in stools or urine, notify physician at once; that patient should check for bruising, petechiae, bleeding gums
• To report abnormal skin conditions, stomatitis, fatigue, jaundice; may indicate blood dyscrasias
• To avoid exposure to sunlight or ultraviolet light; to use sunscreen to prevent burns
• That therapeutic effect may take 3-4 mo
• To use dilute hydrogen peroxide for mild stomatitis, avoid hot spicy foods, food with high acidic content; use soft toothbrush, rinse more frequently, floss daily
• That contraception should be used during treatment

---

aurothioglucose/gold sodium thiomalate
(aur-oh-thye-oh-gloo′kose)
Solganal/Myochrysine
Func. class.: Gold salts
Chem. class.: Active gold compound (50%)

Action: Antiinflammatory action unknown; may decrease phagocytosis, lysosomal activity, prostaglandin synthesis

Uses: Rheumatoid arthritis, psoriatic arthritis

Dosage and routes:
• *Adult:* IM 10 mg, then 25 mg q wk × 2-3 wk, then 50 mg/wk until total of 1 g is administered, then 25-50 mg q3-4 wk if there is improvement without toxicity (aurothioglucose) total of 800 mg-1 g
• *Adult:* IM 10 mg, then 25 mg after 1 wk, then 50 mg q wk for total of 14-20 doses, then 50 mg q2 wk × 4, then 50 mg q3 wk × 4, then 50 mg qmo for maintenance (gold sodium thiomalate)
• *Child 6-12 yr:* IM 1 mg/kg/wk × 20 wk, or ¼ of adult dose (aurothioglucose)
• *Child:* IM 1 mg/kg/wk × 20 wk, then q3-4 wk if improvement

---

without toxicity (gold sodium thiomalate) not to exceed 2.5 mg

Available forms: IM inj 50 mg/ml, 25 mg/ml

Side effects/adverse reactions:

EENT: Iritis, corneal ulcers

HEMA: ***Thrombocytopenia, agranulocytosis, aplastic anemia, leukopenia, eosinophilia, neutropenia***

INTEG: *Rash, pruritus, dermatitis,* urticaria, alopecia, photosensitivity, ***exfoliative dermatitis, angioedema***

GI: Stomatitis, nausea, vomiting, metallic taste, jaundice, ***hepatitis,*** diarrhea, cramping, flatulence

GU: *Proteinuria,* hematuria, ***nephrosis, tubular necrosis***

RESP: Interstitial pneumonitis, pharyngitis, ***pulmonary fibrosis***

CNS: *Dizziness,* EEG abnormalities, ***encephalitis,*** confusion, hallucinations

CV: Bradycardia, rapid pulse

SYST: ***Anaphylaxis***

Contraindications: Hypersensitivity to gold, systemic lupus erythematosus, uncontrolled diabetes mellitus, marked hypertension, recent radiation therapy, CHF, lactation, renal disease, liver disease

Precautions: Decreased tolerance in elderly, children, blood dyscrasias, pregnancy (C)

Pharmacokinetics:

IM: Peak 4-6 hr; half-life 3-27 days; excreted in urine, feces; half-life increases up to 168 days with 11th dose

Interactions/incompatibilities:

• Increased blood dyscrasias: antimalarials, cytotoxic agents, immunosuppressants, oxyphenbutazone, phenylbutazone, penicillamine

Lab test interferences:

False positive: TB test

NURSING CONSIDERATIONS

Assess:

• Respiratory status: dyspnea, wheezing; if respiratory problems occur, drug should be discontinued

• I&O ratio

• For pregnancy before administration; do not give in pregnancy

• Urine: hematuria, proteinuria, increased BUN, creatinine may require decrease in dosage

• Platelet counts qmo; drug should be discontinued if <100,000/mm^3

• Hepatic test: ALT, AST, alk phosphatase

• Diarrhea stools; if severe, drug should be discontinued

• Allergy: rash, dermatitis, pruritus; drug should be discontinued if any of these occur

• Gold toxicity: decreased Hgb, WBC <4000/mm^3, granulocytes <1500/mm^3, platelets <150,000/mm^3, severe diarrhea, stomatitis, hematuria, rash, itching, proteinuria

Administer:

• bid or may give as single dose qAM

• Deep IM, never IV

• Slowly, keep recumbent for 10 min after injection, monitor for transient reaction

Evaluate:

• Therapeutic response: ability to move joints with less pain

Teach patient/family

• That drug must be taken as prescribed to be useful

• To obtain lab work monthly

• That diarrhea is common, but if blood appears in stools or urine, notify physician at once; that patient should check for bruising, petechiae, bleeding gums

• To report skin conditions, stomatitis, fatigue, jaundice, which may indicate blood dyscrasias; re-

port fever, chills, which may indicate infection
• That therapeutic effect may take 3-4 months
• To use dilute hydrogen peroxide for mild stomatitis, avoid hot spicy foods or food with high acidic content; use soft toothbrush, rinse more frequently
• That contraception should be used during treatment
• To use sunscreen to prevent burns

---

azatadine maleate
(a-za'ta-deen)
Optimine
Func. class.: Antihistamine
Chem. class.: Piperidine H_1-receptor antagonist

Action: Acts on blood vessels, GI, respiratory system by competing with histamine for H_1-receptor site; decreases allergic response by blocking histamine
Uses: Allergy symptoms, rhinitis, chronic urticaria
Dosage and routes:
• *Adult:* PO 1-2 mg bid, not to exceed 4 mg/day
Available forms: Tabs 1 mg
Side effects/adverse reactions:
CNS: Dizziness, drowsiness, poor coordination, fatigue, anxiety, euphoria, confusion, paresthesia, neuritis, sweating, chills
CV: Hypotension, palpitations, tachycardia
RESP: Increased thick secretions, wheezing, chest tightness
*HEMA: **Thrombocytopenia, agranulocytosis, hemolytic anemia***
GI: Constipation, dry mouth, nausea, vomiting, anorexia, diarrhea
INTEG: Rash, urticaria, photosensitivity

GU: Retention, dysuria, frequency, impotence
EENT: Blurred vision, dilated pupils, tinnitus, nasal stuffiness, dry nose, throat, mouth
Contraindications: Hypersensitivity to H_1-receptor antagonist, acute asthma attack, lower respiratory tract disease, child <12 yr
Precautions: Increased intraocular pressure, renal disease, cardiac disease, bronchial asthma, seizure disorder, stenosed peptic ulcers, hyperthyroidism, prostatic hypertrophy, bladder neck obstruction, pregnancy (B), elderly
Pharmacokinetics:
PO: Peak 4 hr; metabolized in liver, excreted by kidneys, crosses placenta, crosses blood-brain barrier, minimally bound to plasma proteins, half-life 9-12 hr
Interactions/incompatibilities:
• Increased CNS depression: barbiturates, narcotics, hypnotics, tricyclic antidepressants, alcohol
• Decreased effect of oral anticoagulants, heparin
• Increased effect of azatadine: MAOIs
Lab test interferences:
False negative: Skin allergy tests
NURSING CONSIDERATIONS
Assess:
• I&O ratio; be alert for urinary retention, frequency, dysuria, especially elderly; drug should be discontinued if these occur
• CBC during long-term therapy
• Blood dyscrasias: thrombocytopenia, agranulocytosis; these occur rarely
• Respiratory status: rate, rhythm, increase or thickening in bronchial secretions, wheezing, chest tightness
Administer:
• With meals if GI symptoms oc-

---

italics = common side effects   ***bold italic*** = life threatening reactions

cur; absorption may slightly decrease

Perform/provide:
• Hard candy, gum, frequent rinsing of mouth for dryness
• Storage in tight container at room temperature

Evaluate:
• Therapeutic response: absence of running or congested nose; rash

Teach patient/family:
• All aspects of drug use; to notify physician if confusion, sedation, or hypotension occurs
• To avoid driving or other hazardous activities if drowsiness occurs
• To avoid concurrent use of alcohol or other CNS depressants

Treatment of overdose: Administer ipecac syrup or lavage, diazepam, vasopressors, barbiturates (short-acting)

---

azathioprine
(ay-za-thye'oh-preen)
Imuran
Func. class.: Immunosuppressant
Chem. class.: Purine analog

Action: Produces immunosuppression by inhibiting purine synthesis in cells

Uses: Renal transplants to prevent graft rejection, refractory rheumatoid arthritis, refractory ITP, glomerulonephritis, nephrotic syndrome, bone marrow transplant

Dosage and routes:
Prevention of rejection
• *Adult and child:* PO, IV 3-5 mg/kg/day, then maintenance (PO) of at least 1-2 mg/kg/day

Refractory rheumatoid arthritis
• *Adult:* PO 1/mg/kg/day, may increase dose after 2 mo by 0.5 mg/

kg/day, not to exceed 2.5 mg/kg/day

Available forms: Tabs 50 mg; inj IV 100 mg

Side effects/adverse reactions:
GI: Nausea, vomiting, stomatitis, esophagitis, *pancreatitis, hepatotoxicity, jaundice*
HEMA: Leukopenia, thrombocytopenia, anemia, pancytopenia
INTEG: Rash
MS: Arthralgia, muscle wasting

Contraindications: Hypersensitivity, pregnancy (D)

Precautions: Severe renal disease, severe hepatic disease

Pharmacokinetics: Metabolized in liver, excreted in urine (active metabolite), crosses placenta

Interactions/incompatibilities:
• Increased action of azathioprine: allopurinol
• Considered incompatible; do not admix with other drugs

NURSING CONSIDERATIONS
Assess:
• Blood studies: Hgb, WBC, platelets during treatment monthly; if leukocytes are <3000/mm³, drug should be discontinued
• Liver function studies: alk phosphatase, AST, ALT, bilirubin
• Hepatotoxicity: dark urine, jaundice, itching, light-colored stools; drug should be discontinued

Administer:
• IV after diluting 100 mg/10 ml of sterile H_2O for inj; rotate to dissolve; may further dilute with 50 ml or more saline or glucose in saline
• For several days before transplant surgery
• All medications PO if possible, avoiding IM injections, since bleeding may occur
• With meals to reduce GI upset

Evaluate:

• Therapeutic response: absence of graft rejection, immunosuppression in autoimmune disorders

Teach patient/family:

• That therapeutic response may take 3-4 mo in rheumatoid arthritis

• To report fever, rash, severe diarrhea, chills, sore throat, fatigue, since serious infections may occur

• To use contraceptive measures during treatment, for 12 wk after ending therapy

• To avoid crowds to reduce risk of infection

---

azithromycin

(ay-zi-thro-mye'sin)

Zithromax

Func. class.: Antibacterial

Chem. class.: Macrolide (azalide) antibiotic

Action: Binds to 50S ribosomal subunits of susceptible bacteria and suppresses protein synthesis; much greater spectrum of activity than erythromycin

Uses: Mild to moderate infections of the upper respiratory tract, lower respiratory tract; uncomplicated skin and skin structure infections caused by *M. catarrhalis, S. pneumoniae, S. pyogenes, S. aureus, S. agalactiae, H. influenzae, Clostridium, L. pneumophila;* nongonococcal urethritis or cervicitis due to *C. trachomatis*

Dosage and routes:

• *Adult:* PO 500 mg on day 1, then 250 mg qd on days 2-5 for a total dose of 1.5 g; may give a one-time dose of 1 g for chlamydial infections

Available forms: Caps 250

Side effects/adverse reactions:

INTEG: Rash, urticaria, pruritus, photosensitivity

CV: Palpitations, chest pain

CNS: Dizziness, headache, vertigo, somnolence

GI: Nausea, vomiting, diarrhea, **hepatotoxicity,** abdominal pain, stomatitis, heartburn, dyspepsia, flatulence, melena, **cholestatic jaundice**

GU: Vaginitis, moniliasis, nephritis

Contraindications: Hypersensitivity to azithromycin or erythromycin

Precautions: Pregnancy (C), lactation, hepatic, renal, cardiac disease, elderly, children <16 yrs

Pharmacokinetics: Peak 12 hr, duration 24 hr, half-life 11-57 hr, excreted in bile, feces, urine primarily as unchanged drug

Interactions/incompatibilities:

• Increased effects of oral anticoagulants, digoxin, theophylline, methylprednisolone, cyclosporine, bromocriptine, disopyramide, triazolam

• Decreased action of clindamycin

• Toxicity: carbamazepine, terfenadine

• Decreased absorption of azithromycin: food, aluminium, magnesium antacids

Lab test interferences:

False increase: 17-OHCS/17-KS, AST, ALT

Decrease: Folate assay

NURSING CONSIDERATIONS

Assess:

• I&O ratio; report hematuria, oliguria in renal disease

• Liver studies: AST, ALT

• Renal studies: urinalysis, protein, blood

• C&S before drug therapy; drug may be taken as soon as culture is taken; C&S may be repeated after treatment

---

italics = common side effects   ***bold italic*** = life threatening reactions

• Bowel pattern before, during treatment
• Skin eruptions, itching
• Respiratory status: rate, character, wheezing, tightness in chest; discontinue drug if these occur
• Allergies before treatment, reaction of each medication; place allergies on chart, notify all people giving drugs

Administer:
• Adequate intake of fluids (2 L) during diarrhea episodes

Perform/provide:
• Storage at room temperature

Evaluate:
• Therapeutic response: C&S negative for infection

Teach patient/family:
• To take with a full glass of water; do not take with food; take 1 hr before or 2 hr after meals; do not take with fruit juices
• To report sore throat, fever, fatigue; may indicate superimposed infection
• Not to take aluminum/magnesium-containing antacids simultaneously with this drug
• To notify nurse of diarrhea stools, dark urine, pale stools, yellow discoloration of eyes or skin, severe abdominal pain
• To take at evenly spaced intervals; complete dosage regimen

Treatment of overdose: Withdraw drug, maintain airway, administer epinephrine, aminophylline, O_2, IV corticosteroids

---

azlocillin sodium
(az-loe-sill'in)
Azlin
Func. class.: Broad-spectrum antibiotic
Chem. class.: Extended-spectrum penicillin

Action: Interferes with cell wall replication of susceptible organisms; the cell wall, rendered osmotically unstable, swells, bursts from osmotic pressure; a β-lactam antibiotic

Uses: Lower respiratory infections, skin, bone, bacterial septicemia, urinary tract infections, yaws; effective for gram-positive cocci *(S. aureus, S. pyogenes, S. faecalis)*, gram-positive bacilli *(C. perfringens, C. tetani)*, gram-negative bacilli *(Bacteroides, P. aeruginosa, E. coli)*, *H. influenzae, P. mirabilis, Pseudomonas*

Dosage and routes:
• *Adult:* IV 100-350 mg/kg/day in 4-6 divided doses, max 24 g
Cystic fibrosis
• *Child:* IV 75 mg/kg q4h max 24 g

Available forms: Powder for inj 2, 3, 4 g

Side effects/adverse reactions:
HEMA: Anemia, increased bleeding time, **bone marrow depression, granulocytopenia**
GI: Nausea, vomiting, diarrhea, increased AST, ALT, abdominal pain, glossitis, colitis
GU: Oliguria, proteinuria, hematuria, vaginitis, moniliasis, **glomerulonephritis**
CNS: Lethargy, hallucinations, anxiety, depression, twitching, **coma, convulsions**
META: Hypokalemia, alkalosis, hypernatremia

Contraindications: Hypersensitivity to penicillins

Precautions: Pregnancy (B), hypersensitivity to cephalosporins, neonates

Pharmacokinetics: Half-life 55-70 min, metabolized in liver, excreted in urine, bile, breast milk (small amount), crosses placenta

---

* Available in Canada only

Interactions/incompatibilities:
• Decreased antimicrobial effectiveness of azlocillin: tetracyclines, erythromycins
• Increased azlocillin concentrations: aspirin, probenecid
• Incompatible in sol with aminoglycosides, amphotericin B, chloramphenicol, lincomycin, oxytetracycline, polymyxin B, promethazine, tetracycline, Vit B with C

Lab test interferences:
False positive: Urine glucose, urine protein
Decrease: Uric acid

NURSING CONSIDERATIONS
Assess:
• I&O ratio; report hematuria, oliguria, since penicillin in high doses is nephrotoxic
• Any patient with compromised renal system, since drug is excreted slowly in poor renal system function; toxicity may occur rapidly
• Liver studies: AST, ALT
• Blood studies: WBC, RBC, H&H, bleeding time
• Renal studies: urinalysis, protein, blood
• Culture, sensitivity before drug therapy; drug may be taken as soon as culture is taken
• Bowel pattern before, during treatment
• Skin eruptions after administration of penicillin to 1 wk after discontinuing drug
• Respiratory status: rate, character, wheezing, tightness in chest
• Allergies before initiation of treatment; reaction of each medication; place allergies on chart in bright red

Administer:
• IV after reconstituting 1 g/10 ml of D₅W, NSS, or sterile water, shake. After further dilution in 50-100 ml of compatible solution, give

over 30 min; change IV site q48h
• After C&S completed
• Slowly (direct IV) over 5 min to prevent chest discomfort

Perform/provide:
• Adrenaline, suction, tracheostomy set, endotracheal intubation equipment on unit
• Adequate intake of fluids (2 L) during diarrhea episodes
• Scratch test to assess allergy after securing order from physician; usually done when penicillin is only drug of choice
• Storage in cool environment; solution is stable for 24 hr at room temperature

Evaluate:
• Therapeutic response: absence of fever, draining wounds

Teach patient/family:
• That culture may be taken after completed course of medication
• To report sore throat, fever, fatigue (may indicate superimposed infection)
• To wear or carry a Medic Alert ID if allergic to penicillins
• To notify nurse of diarrhea

Treatment of overdose: Withdraw drug, maintain airway, administer epinephrine, aminophylline, O₂, IV corticosteroids for anaphylaxis

---

aztreonam
(az-tree'oo nam)
Azactam
Func. class.: Misc antibiotic
Chem. class.: Monobactam

Action: Inhibits organisms by inhibiting bacterial cell wall synthesis, which causes death of organism (bactericidal)
Uses: Urinary tract infection; septicemia; skin, muscle, bone infec-

tion; and other infections caused by gram-negative organisms

Dosage and routes:

Urinary tract infections

• *Adult:* IV/IM 500 mg-1 g q8-12h

Systemic infections

Adult: IV/IM 1-2 g q8-12h

Severe systemic infections

Adult: IV/IM 2 g q6-8h; do not exceed 8 g/day

Continue treatment for 48 hr after negative culture or until patient is asymptomatic

Available forms: Powder for inj 500 mg, 1, 2 g

Side effects/adverse reactions:

HEMA: Anemia, increased bleeding time, *bone marrow depression, granulocytopenia*

GI:Nausea, vomiting, diarrhea, increased AST, ALT, abdominal pain, glossitis, colitis

CNS: Lethargy, hallucinations, anxiety, depression, twitching, *coma, convulsions,* malaise

EENT: Tinnitus, diplopia, nasal congestion

GU: Vaginal candidiasis, vaginitis, breast tenderness

Contraindications: Hypersensitivity to this drug, penicillins, cephalosporins

Precautions: Pregnancy (B), lactation, children, impaired renal, hepatic function, elderly

Pharmacokinetics:

IV: Peak immediate, trough 8 hr

IM: Peak 1 hr

Half-life: 1.7 hr; half-life prolonged in renal disease; protein binding 56%; metabolized by liver; excreted in urine; small amounts appear in breast milk, placenta

Interactions/incompatibilities:

• Decreased effect of both drugs: β-lactamase antibiotics (cefoxitin, imipenem)

• Incompatible with nafcillin, metronidazole, cephradine

• Increased nephrotoxicity: aminoglycosides

NURSING CONSIDERATIONS

Assess:

• Signs of bruising, bleeding, anemia

• Bowel pattern before, during treatment

• Respiratory status: rate, character, wheezing, tightness in chest

• I&O ratio; report hematuria, oliguria, since this drug in high doses is nephrotoxic

• Any patient with compromised renal system, since drug is excreted slowly in poor renal system function; toxicity may occur rapidly

• Liver studies: AST, ALT

• Blood studies: WBC, RBC, Hgb & Hct, bleeding time

• Renal studies: urinalysis, protein, blood

• Skin eruptions after administration of drug to 1 wk after discontinuing drug

• Allergies before initiation of treatment, reaction of medication; highlight allergies on chart

Administer:

• Direct IV after diluting with 6-10 ml sterile H_2O/15 ml drug; give over 3-5 min

• IV INF after diluting with 3 ml or more sterile H_2O/1 g drug; then dilute with 50-100 ml of D_5W, 0.9% NaCl solution; give over ½-1 hr, by Y-tube or 3-way stopcock; flush tubing before and after administration

• IM; dilute each g with at least 3 ml of 0.9% NaCl; give into large muscle

• Drug after C&S completed

Perform/provide:

• Adequate fluid intake (2 L) during diarrhea episodes

• Storage in refrigerator
Evaluate:
• Therapeutic response: absence of fever, purulent drainage, redness, inflammation
Teach patient/family:
• That culture may be taken after completed course of medication
• To report sore throat, fever, fatigue; could indicate superimposed infection

---

bacampicillin HCl
(ba-kam-pi-sill'in)
Penglobe,* Spectrobid
Func. class.: Broad-spectrum antibiotic
Chem. class.: Aminopenicillin

Action: Interferes with cell wall replication of susceptible organisms; the cell wall, rendered osmotically unstable, swells, bursts from osmotic pressure; drug is hydrolyzed to ampicillin during absorption

Uses: Respiratory tract infections, skin urinary tract infections; effective for gram-positive cocci *(S. faecalis, S. pneumoniae)*, gram-negative cocci *(N. gonorrhoeae)*, gram-negative bacilli *(E. coli, H. influenzae, P. mirabilis)*

Dosage and routes:
• *Adult:* PO 400-800 mg q12h
• *Child:* PO 25-50 mg/kg/day in divided doses q12h
Available forms: Tabs 400 mg; powder for oral susp 125 mg/5 ml (equivalent to 87.5 mg ampicillin)
Side effects/adverse reactions:
HEMA: Anemia, increased bleeding time, **bone marrow depression, granulocytopenia**
GI: Nausea, vomiting, diarrhea, increased AST, ALT, abdominal pain, glossitis, colitis

GU: Oliguria, proteinuria, hematuria, *vaginitis, moniliasis,* **glomerulonephritis**
CNS: Lethargy, hallucinations, anxiety, depression, twitching, **coma, convulsions**
Contraindications: Hypersensitivity to penicillins; neonates
Precautions: Pregnancy (B), hypersensitivity to cephalosporins
Pharmacokinetics:
PO: Peak 30-60 min, duration 5-6 hr, half-life ½-1 hr, metabolized in liver, excreted in urine
Interactions/incompatibilities:
• Decreased antimicrobial effectiveness of bacampicillin: tetracyclines, erythromycins
• Increased bacampicillin concentrations: aspirin, probenecid
• Do not give with disulfiram
Lab test interferences:
False positive: Urine glucose, urine protein
Decrease: Uric acid
NURSING CONSIDERATIONS
Assess:
• I&O ratio; report hematuria, oliguria, since penicillin in high doses is nephrotoxic
• Any patient with compromised renal system, since drug is excreted slowly in poor renal system function; toxicity may occur rapidly
• Liver studies: AST, ALT
• Blood studies: WBC, RBC, H&H, bleeding time
• Renal studies: urinalysis, protein, blood
• Culture, sensitivity before drug therapy; drug may be given as soon as culture is taken
• Bowel pattern before, during treatment
• Skin eruptions after administration of penicillin to 1 wk after discontinuing drug
• Respiratory status: rate, charac-

---

italics = common side effects   ***bold italic*** = life threatening reactions

ter, wheezing, tightness in chest
• Allergies before initiation of treatment; reaction of each medication; report allergies on chart in bright red

Administer:
• After C&S completed
• Oral susp 1 hr before or 2 hr after meals

Perform/provide:
• Adrenaline, suction, tracheostomy set, endotracheal intubation equipment on unit
• Adequate intake of fluids (2 L) during diarrhea episodes
• Scratch test to assess allergy after securing order from physician; usually done when penicillin is only drug of choice
• Storage in dry tight container, oral suspension refrigerated for 2 wk or at room temperature for 1 wk

Evaluate:
• Therapeutic response: absence of temperature, draining wounds

Teach patient/family:
• Aspects of drug therapy: culture may be taken after completed course of medication; patient must complete course of therapy
• To report sore throat, fever, fatigue (may indicate superimposed infection)
• To wear or carry a Medic Alert ID if allergic to penicillins
• To notify nurse of diarrhea
• That drug should be taken on an empty stomach, with a full glass of water

Treatment of overdose: Withdraw drug, maintain airway, administer epinephrine, aminophylline, O$_2$, IV corticosteroids for anaphylaxis

---

bacitracin
(bass-i-tray'sin)
Bacitracin Sterile, Bacitracin U.S.P.

Func. class.: Antibacterial
Chem. class.: Bacillus subtilis derivative

Action: Inhibits bacterial cell wall synthesis, interfering with osmotic pressure within cell

Uses: Staphylococcal pneumonia, empyema, pseudomembranous colitis

Dosage and routes:
• *Infants >2.5 kg:* IM 1,000 U/kg/day in divided doses q8-12h
• *Infants <2.5 kg:* IM 900 U/kg/day in divided doses q8-12h
• *Adults:* 20,000-25,000 U q6h × 7-10 days

Available forms: Inj IM 10,000, 50,000 U

Side effects/adverse reactions:
INTEG: Rash, pain at injection site
GI: Nausea, vomiting, diarrhea
GU: Proteinuria, casts, azotemia

Contraindications: Hypersensitivity, severe renal disease

Precautions: Pregnancy (C)

Pharmacokinetics: Peak 1-2 hr, duration >12 hr, metabolized in liver, excreted in urine

Interactions/incompatibilities:
• Increased nephrotoxicity, neurotoxicity: aminoglycosides, polymyxin
• Increased neuromuscular blockage: nondepolarizing skeletal muscle relaxants, anesthetics

NURSING CONSIDERATIONS
Assess:
• I&O ratio; report oliguria, change in urinary output; high doses are nephrotoxic
• Any patient with compromised renal system; drug is excreted

---

slowly in poor renal system function; toxicity may occur rapidly
• Renal studies: urinalysis, protein, blood, BUN, creatinine, urine pH (keep at 6.0)
• C&S before drug therapy; drug may be taken as soon as culture is taken; repeat C&S after treatment
• Bowel pattern before, during treatment; if severe diarrhea occurs, drug should be discontinued
• Skin eruptions, itching: rash, urticaria, erythema
• Respiratory status: rate, character, wheezing, tightness in chest, dyspnea on exertion
• Allergies before treatment, reaction of each medication; report allergies on chart, Kardex in bright red; notify all people giving drugs
Administer:
• After reconstituting with NS
• IM in deep muscle mass; rotate injection site; do not give IV/SC
Perform/provide:
• Storage in refrigerator; protect from direct sunlight
• Adrenalin, suction, tracheostomy set, endotracheal intubation equipment on unit
• Adequate intake of fluids (2 L) during diarrhea episodes
Evaluate:
• Therapeutic response: absence of fever, cough, dyspnea, malaise
Teach patient/family:
• To report sore throat, fever, fatigue; may indicate superimposed infection

bacitracin (ophthalmic)
(bass-i-tray′sin)
AK-Tracin, Bacitracin Ophthalmic
Func. class.: Antiinfective

Action: Inhibits cell wall synthesis in bacteria
Uses: Infection of eye
Dosage and routes:
• *Adult and child:* Apply to conjunctival sac bid-qid until desired response
Available forms: Oint 500 U/g
Side effects/adverse reactions:
EENT: Poor corneal wound healing, visual haze (temporary), overgrowth of nonsusceptible organisms
Contraindications: Hypersensitivity
Precautions: Antibiotic hypersensitivity, pregnancy (C)
NURSING CONSIDERATIONS
Assess:
• Allergy: itching, lacrimation, redness, swelling
Administer:
• After washing hands, cleanse crusts or discharge from eye before application
Perform/provide:
• Storage at room temperature
Evaluate:
• Therapeutic response: absence of redness, inflammation, tearing
Teach patient/family:
• To use drug exactly as prescribed
• Not to use eye makeup, towels, washcloths, eye medication of others; reinfection may occur
• That drug container tip should not be touched to eye
• To report itching, increased redness, burning, stinging, swelling; drug should be discontinued

italics = common side effects   ***bold italic*** = life threatening reactions

• That drug may cause blurred vision when ointment is applied

---

bacitracin (topical)
(bass-i-tray'sin)
Baciguent, Bacitin*, Bacitracin
Func. class.: Local antiinfective
Chem. class.: Antibacterial

Action: Interferes with bacterial cell wall function by inhibiting protein synthesis
Uses: Topical staphylococci, streptococci
Dosage and routes:
• *Adult and child:* TOP bid-qid or more often if needed
Available forms include: Oint 500 U/g
Side effects/adverse reactions:
INTEG: Rash, urticaria, stinging, burning, contact dermatitis
Contraindications: Hypersensitivity
Precautions: Pregnancy (C), lactation
NURSING CONSIDERATIONS
Assess:
• Allergic reaction: burning, stinging, swelling, redness
• For systemic effects and superimposed infections
Administer:
• After C&S is obtained, if lesion is weeping
• Enough medication to cover lesions completely
• After cleansing with soap, water before each application, dry well (as ordered)
Perform/provide:
• Storage at room temperature in dry place
Evaluate:
• Therapeutic response: decrease in size, number of lesions

Teach patient/family:
• To use medical asepsis (hand washing) before, after each application to prevent further infection
• To apply with glove or sterile swab to prevent further infection
• To avoid use of OTC creams, ointments, lotions unless directed by physician
• To watch for superimposed infections with long-term use or allergic reaction

---

baclofen
(bak'loe-fen)
Baclofen, Lioresal, Lioresal DS, Lioresal Intrathecal
Func. class.: Skeletal muscle relaxant, central acting
Chem. class.: GABA chlorophenyl derivative

Action: Inhibits synaptic responses in CNS by decreasing GABA, which decreases neurotransmitter function; decreases frequency, severity of muscle spasms
Uses: Spinal cord injury, spasticity in multiple sclerosis
Dosage and routes:
• *Adult:* PO 5 mg tid × 3 days, then 10 mg tid × 3 days, then 15 mg tid × 3 days, then 20 mg tid × 3 days, then titrated to response, not to exceed 80 mg/day
• Intrathecal: use implantable intrathecal INF pump. Use screening trial of 3 separate BOL doses if needed (50 µg/ml, 75 µg/1.5 ml, 100 µg/2 ml). Initial: double screening dose that produced result and give over 24 hr: increase by 10%-30% q24hr only. Maintenance: 12-1500 µg/day
Available forms: Tabs 10, 20 mg, 10 mg/20 ml (500 µg/ml), 10 mg/5 ml (2000 µg/ml)

Side effects/adverse reactions:

CNS: Dizziness, weakness, fatigue, drowsiness, headache, disorientation, insomnia, paresthesias, tremors

EENT: Nasal congestion, blurred vision, mydriasis, tinnitus

CV: Hypotension, chest pain, palpitations, edema

GI: Nausea, constipation, vomiting, increased AST, alk phosphatase, abdominal pain, dry mouth, anorexia

GU: Urinary frequency

INTEG: Rash, pruritus

Contraindications: Hypersensitivity

Precautions: Peptic ulcer disease, renal disease, hepatic disease, stroke, seizure disorder, diabetes mellitus, pregnancy (C), elderly

Pharmacokinetics:

PO: Peak 2-3 hr, duration >8 hr, half-life 2½-4 hr, partially metabolized in liver,˙ excreted in urine (unchanged)

INTRATHECAL: CSF levels with plasma levels 100 times oral route

Interactions/incompatibilities:

• Increased CNS depression: alcohol, tricyclic antidepressants, narcotics, barbiturates, sedatives, hypnotics

Lab test interferences:

Increase: AST, alk phosphatase, blood glucose

NURSING CONSIDERATIONS
Assess:

• B/P, weight, blood sugar, and hepatic function periodically

• For increased seizure activity in epilepsy patient; this drug decreases seizure threshold

• I&O ratio; check for urinary retention, frequency, hesitancy

• ECG in epileptic patients; poor seizure control has occurred in patients taking this drug

• Allergic reactions: rash, fever, respiratory distress

• Severe weakness, numbness in extremities

• Psychologic dependency: increased need for medication, more frequent requests for medication, increased pain

• CNS depression: dizziness, drowsiness, psychiatric symptoms

• Dosage, as individual titration is required

Administer:

• With meals for GI symptoms

• Gum, frequent sips of water for dry mouth

Perform/provide:

• Storage in tight container at room temperature

• Assistance with ambulation if dizziness or drowsiness occurs

Evaluate:

• Therapeutic response: decreased pain, spasticity

Teach patient/family:

• Not to discontinue medication quickly; hallucinations, spasticity, tachycardia will occur; drug should be tapered off over 1-2 wk

• Not to take with alcohol, other CNS depressants

• To avoid altering activities while taking this drug

• To avoid hazardous activities if drowsiness or dizziness occurs

• To avoid using OTC medication: cough preparations, antihistamines, unless directed by physician

• To increase fluid intake >2L/day

Treatment of overdose: Induce emesis of conscious patient, lavage, dialysis

---

italics = common side effects   ***bold italic*** = life threatening reactions

beclomethasone dipropionate
(be-kloe-meth'a-sone)
Beclovent, Vanceril
Func. class.: Corticosteroid, synthetic
Chem. class.: Glucocorticoid

Action: Prevents inflammation by depression of migration of polymorphonuclear leukocytes, fibroblasts, reversal of increased capillary permeability and lysosomal stabilization; does not suppress hypothalamus and pituitary function
Uses: Chronic asthma, rhinitis
Dosage and routes:
• *Adult:* INH 2-4 puffs tid-qid, not to exceed 20 inhalations/day
• *Child:* 6-12 yr: INH 1-2 puffs tid-qid, not to exceed 10 inhalations/day
Available forms: Aerosol 42 μg/actuation
Side effects/adverse reactions:
*RESP: **Bronchospasm***
GI: Dry mouth
EENT: Hoarseness, candidal infections of oral cavity, sore throat
Contraindications: Hypersensitivity, status asthmaticus (primary treatment), nonasthmatic bronchial disease, bacterial, fungal, or viral infections of mouth, throat, or lungs, children < 3 yr
Precautions: Nasal disease/surgery, pregnancy (C)
Pharmacokinetics:
INH: Onset 10 min, excreted in feces (metabolites), half-life 3-15 hr, crosses placenta, metabolized in lungs, liver, GI system
NURSING CONSIDERATIONS
Assess:
• Adrenal function periodically for HPA axis suppression

Administer:
• INH with water to decrease possibility of fungal infections
• Titrated dose, use lowest effective dose
Perform/provide:
• Gum, rinsing of mouth for dry mouth
Evaluate:
• Therapeutic response: decreased dyspnea, wheezing, dry rales on auscultation
Teach patient/family:
• That ID as steroid user should be carried
• To notify physician if therapeutic response decreases; dosage adjustment may be needed
• Proper administration technique
• To wash inhaler with warm water and dry after each use
• All aspects of drug usage including cushingoid symptoms
• Symptoms of adrenal insufficiency: nausea, anorexia, fatigue, dizziness, dyspnea, weakness, joint pain, depression
• To keep drug out of children's reach

beclomethasone dipropionate (nasal)
(be-kloe-meth'a-sone)
Beconase AQ Nasal, Beconase Inhalation, Vancenase AQ Nasal, Vancenase Nasal
Func. class.: Synthetic corticosteroid
Chem. class.: Beclomethasone diester

Action: Antiinflammatory, vasoconstrictive properties in nasal passages
Uses: Seasonal or perennial rhinitis
Dosage and routes:
• *Adult and child >12 yr:* IN-

STILL 1-2 sprays in each nostril bid-qid

Available forms: Aero 42 μg/spray

Side effects/adverse reactions:

EENT: Dryness, nasal irritation, burning, sneezing, secretions with blood, nasal ulcerations, **perforation of nasal septum,** Candida infection, earache, hoarseness

ENDO: Adrenal suppression

INTEG: Rash, urticaria, pruritus

CNS: Headache, paresthesia

RESP: Acute status asthmaticus

Contraindications: Hypersensitivity, systemic corticosteroid therapy

Precautions: Pregnancy (C), lactation, children <12, nasal ulcers, recurrent epistaxis respiration

Pharmacokinetics:

INSTILL: Readily absorbed; peak concentration, other data have not been determined

NURSING CONSIDERATIONS

Assess:

• Adrenal function periodically for HPA axis suppression

• Adrenal suppression: 17-KS, plasma cortisol for decreased levels

• Nasal passages during long-term treatment for changes in mucus

Administer:

• After cleaning aerosol top daily with warm water, dry thoroughly

Perform/provide:

• Storage in cool environment; do not puncture or incinerate container

Evaluate:

• Therapeutic response: decrease in runny nose

Teach patient/family:

• To clear nasal passages if sneezing attack occurs, repeat dose

• To continue using product even if mild nasal bleeding occurs; is usually transient

• Method of installation after providing written instructions from manufacturer

• To clear nasal passages before administration; use decongestant if needed; shake inhaler, invert, tilt head backward, insert nozzle into nostril, away from septum; hold other nostril closed and depress activator, inhale through nose, exhale through mouth

---

belladonna alkaloids

(bell-a-don'a)

Bellafoline

Func. class.: Gastrointestinal anticholinergic

Chem. class.: Belladonna alkaloid

Action: Inhibits muscarinic actions of acetylcholine at postganglionic parasympathetic neuron effector sites

Uses: Treatment of peptic ulcer disease, irritable bowel syndrome in combination with other drugs; for other GI disorders

Dosage and routes:

• *Adult:* PO 0.25-0.5 mg tid; SC 0.125-0.5 mg qd or bid

• *Child >6 yr:* PO 0.125-0.25 mg tid

Available forms: Tabs 0.25 mg; inj SC 0.5 mg/ml

Side effects/adverse reactions:

CNS: Confusion, stimulation in elderly, headache, insomnia, dizziness, drowsiness, anxiety, weakness, hallucination

GI: Dry mouth, constipation, paralytic ileus, heartburn, nausea, vomiting, dysphagia, absence of taste

GU: Hesitancy, retention, impotence

CV: Palpitations, tachycardia

EENT: Blurred vision, photophobia, mydriasis, cycloplegia, increased ocular tension

---

italics = common side effects   ***bold italic*** = life threatening reactions

INTEG: Urticaria, rash, pruritus, anhidrosis, fever, allergic reactions, flushing

Contraindications: Hypersensitivity to anticholinergics, narrow-angle glaucoma, GI obstruction, myasthenia gravis, paralytic ileus, GI atony, toxic megacolon

Precautions: Hyperthyroidism, coronary artery disease, dysrhythmias, CHF, ulcerative colitis, hypertension, hiatal hernia, hepatic disease, renal disease, pregnancy (C), urinary obstruction

Pharmacokinetics:
PO: Duration 4-6 hr; metabolized by liver, excreted in urine, half-life 13-38 hr

Interactions/incompatibilities:
• Increased anticholinergic effect: amantadine, tricyclic antidepressants, MAOIs
• Increased effect of nitrofurantoin
• Decreased effect of phenothiazines, levodopa

NURSING CONSIDERATIONS
Assess:
• VS, cardiac status: checking for dysrhythmias, increased rate, palpitations, flushing
• I&O ratio; check for urinary retention or hesitancy
• GI complaints: pain, bleeding (frank or occult), nausea, vomiting, anorexia, constipation

Administer:
• ½-1 hr ac for better absorption
• Decreased dose to elderly patients; their metabolism may be slowed
• Gum, hard candy, frequent rinsing of mouth for dryness of oral cavity

Perform/provide:
• Storage in tight container protected from light
• Increased fluids, bulk, exercise to decrease constipation

Evaluate:
• Therapeutic response: absence of epigastric pain, bleeding, nausea, vomiting

Teach patient/family:
• To avoid driving or other hazardous activities until stabilized on medication
• To avoid alcohol or other CNS depressants; will enhance sedating properties of this drug
• To avoid hot environments; stroke may occur; drug suppresses perspiration
• To use sunglasses when outside to prevent photophobia

---

benazepril
(ben-a-ze′prel)
Lotensin
Func. class.: Antihypertensive
Chem. class.: Angiotensin-converting enzyme (ACE) inhibitor

Action: Selectively suppresses renin-angiotensin-aldosterone system; inhibits ACE, prevents conversion of angiotensin I to angiotensin II; results in dilation of arterial, venous vessels

Uses: Hypertension, alone or in combination with thiazide diuretics

Dosage and routes:
• *Adult:* PO 10 mg qd initially, then 20-40 mg/day divided bid or qd
Renal impairment: 5 mg qd with Ccr <30 ml/min/1.73 m², increase as needed to maximum of 40 mg/day

Available forms: Tabs 5, 10, 20, 40 mg

Side effects/adverse reactions:
CV: Hypotension, postural hypotension, syncope, palpitations, angina
GU: Increased BUN, creatinine, de-

creased libido, impotence, urinary
tract infection
*HEMA: **Neutropenia, agranulocytosis***
*INTEG: **Angioedema,** rash, flushing, sweating*
RESP: Cough, asthma, bronchitis,
dyspnea, sinusitis
META: Hyperkalemia, hyponatremia
GI: Nausea, constipation, vomiting, gastritis, melena
CNS: Anxiety, hypertonia, insomnia, paresthesia, headache, dizziness, fatigue
MS: Arthralgia, arthritis, myalgia
Contraindications: Hypersensitivity to ACE inhibitors, pregnancy
(D), lactation, children
Precautions: Impaired renal, liver
function, dialysis patients, hypovolemia, blood dyscrasias, CHF,
COPD, asthma, elderly, bilateral
renal artery stenosis
Pharmacokinetics:
PO: Peak ½-1 hr, serum protein
binding 97%, half-life 10-11 hr,
metabolized by liver (metabolites),
excreted in urine
Interactions/incompatibilities:
• Increased hypotension: diuretics,
other antihypertensives, ganglionic
blockers, adrenergic blockers
• Increased toxicity: vasodilators,
hydralazine, prazosin, potassium-sparing diuretics, sympathomimetics, potassium supplements
• Decreased absorption: antacids
• Decreased antihypertensive effect: indomethacin
• Increased serum levels of digoxin, lithium
• Increased hypersensitivity: allopurinol
Lab test interferences:
False positive: Urine acetone
NURSING CONSIDERATIONS
Assess:

• Blood studies: neutrophils, decreased platelets
• B/P, orthostatic hypotension,
syncope
• Renal studies: protein, BUN, creatinine; watch for increased levels
that may indicate nephrotic syndrome
• Baselines in renal, liver function
tests before therapy begins
• Potassium levels, although hyperkalemia rarely occurs
• Dipstick of urine for protein qd
in first morning specimen; if protein is increased, a 24 hr urinary
protein should be collected
• Edema in feet, legs daily
• Allergic reactions: rash, fever,
pruritus, urticaria; drug should be
discontinued if antihistamines fail
to help
• Renal symptoms: polyuria, oliguria, frequency, dysuria
Administer:
• IV infusion of 0.9% NaCl (as ordered) to expand fluid volume if
severe hypotension occurs
Perform/provide:
• Storage in tight container at 86°
F (30° C) or less
• Supine or Trendelenburg position
for severe hypotension
Evaluate:
• Therapeutic response: decrease in
B/P
Teach patient/family:
• Not to discontinue drug abruptly
• Not to use OTC products (cough,
cold, allergy) unless directed by
physician; do not use salt substitutes containing potassium without
consulting physician
• Importance of complying with
dosage schedule, even if feeling
better
• To rise slowly to sitting or standing position to minimize orthostatic
hypotension

italics = common side effects   ***bold italic*** = life threatening reactions

• To notify physician of mouth sores, sore throat, fever, swelling of hands or feet, irregular heartbeat, chest pain
• To report excessive perspiration, dehydration, vomiting, diarrhea; may lead to fall in B/P
• That drug may cause dizziness, fainting, light-headedness; may occur during 1st few days of therapy
• That drug may cause skin rash or impaired perspiration
• How to take B/P, and normal readings for age group
Treatment of overdose: 0.9% NaCl IV INF, hemodialysis

---

benzalkonium chloride

(benz-al-koe′nee-um)
Benasept, Benza, Benzachlor-50*, Benzalkonium Chloride, Germicin, Ionax Scrub*, Sabol Shampoo*, Zephiran, Zephiran Chloride*

Func. class.: Disinfectant
Chem. class.: Quaternary ammonium cationic surfactant

Action: Inhibits and destroys organisms by enzyme inactivation (bactericidal/bacteriostatic)
Uses: Irrigate eye, vagina, body cavities, disinfection of skin before surgery
Dosage and routes:
• *Adult and child:* TOP 1:750 for minor wounds, disinfection before surgery; 1:3000-20,000 deep infected wounds; 1:2000-5000 vaginal irrigation; 1:5000-10,000 denuded skin, eye, mucous membrane irrigation; 1:5000-20,000 bladder, urethral irrigation
Available forms: Top sol 0.1%, 0.13%, 17%, 17.5%, 50%; tinct 0.13%

Side effects/adverse reactions:
CNS: Confusion, restlessness
INTEG: Irritation, contact dermatitis, hypersensitivity, rash, burning
GI: Nausea, vomiting
RESP: Dyspnea, *respiratory paralysis, coma* (if ingested)
Contraindications: Hypersensitivity, occlusive dressing, casts/traction
Interactions/incompatibilities:
• Decreased action of benzalkonium: soap
• Not to be used with fluorescein, nitrates, lanolin, potassium permanganate, kaolin, zinc sulfate, zinc oxide, caramel, aluminum, iodine, peroxide, yellow oxide of mercury, citrates, sulfonamides

Administer:
• After diluting with sterile water for injection for irrigating wounds
• To ⅓ of body or less to avoid chilling
Perform/provide:
• Rust tablets for cleaning metal objects, or instrument will rust
• Wet dressings using clear solution only; discontinue if necrosis occurs
Evaluate:
• Area of body involved: irritation, rash, breaks, dryness, scales, discharge
Teach patient/family:
• To store at room temperature no longer than 1 wk
• To use applicator, insert high into vagina, notify physician of itching, discharge, burning
Treatment of ingestion: Administer milk, soap solution, gastric lavage, supportive care

---

B

benzocaine (oral)

(ben-zoe-kane)

Anbesol Maximum Strength, Baby Anbesol, Children's Chloraseptic, Medamint, Orabase Baby, Oracin, Ora-Jel, Oratect, Spec-T Anesthetic, T-Caine, Tyrobenz

Func. class.: Topical local anesthetic

Chem. class.: Ester

Action: Inhibits conduction of nerve impulses from sensory nerves

Uses: Oral irritation, sore throat, toothache, cold sore, canker sore, sunburn, minor cuts, insect bites, pain, itching

Dosage and routes:

• *Adult and child >12 yr:* TOP apply to affected area; LOZ suck as needed

Available forms: Cream 1%, 5%; lotion 0.5%, 8%; oint 2%, 5%, 20%; sol 2.1%, 2.5%, 6.3%, 20%; lozenges 3, 5, 6.25, 10 mg; topical aerosol 20%; gel 6.3%, 7.5%, 10%, 20%

Side effects/adverse reactions:

EENT: Itching, irritation in ear

INTEG: Rash, urticaria

Contraindications: Hypersensitivity

Precautions: Pregnancy (C)

Pharmacokinetics:

TOP: Peak 1 min, duration ½-1 hr

Administer:

• To gums as needed for teething pain

• Lozenges for temporary sore throat pain

Perform/provide:

• Storage in tight, light-resistant container; do not freeze, puncture, or incinerate aerosol container

Evaluate:

• Affected area for redness, swelling, pain

Teach patient/family:

• To avoid contact with eyes

• Not to use for prolonged periods: use for <1 wk; if condition remains, physician should be contacted

benzonatate

(ben-zoe'na-tate)

Tessalon Perles

Func. class.: Antitussive, non-narcotic

Chem. class.: Tetracaine derivative

Action: Inhibits cough reflex by anesthetizing stretch receptors in respiratory system, direct action on cough center in medulla

Uses: Nonproductive cough

Dosage and routes:

• *Adult and child:* PO 100 mg tid, not to exceed 600 mg/day

• *Child <10 yr:* PO 8 mg/kg in 3-6 divided doses

Available forms: Perles 100 mg

Side effects/adverse reactions:

CNS: Dizziness, drowsiness, headache

GI: Nausea, constipation, upset stomach

EENT: Nasal congestion, burning eyes

CV: Increased B/P, chest tightness, numbness

INTEG: Urticaria, rash, pruritus

Contraindications: Hypersensitivity

Precautions: Pregnancy (C), lactation

Pharmacokinetics:

PO: Onset 15-20 min, duration 3-8 hr, metabolized by liver, excreted in urine

---

italics = common side effects   ***bold italic*** = life threatening reactions

NURSING CONSIDERATIONS
Assess:
• Cough: type, frequency, character including sputum

Perform/provide:
• Storage in tight, light-resistant containers
• Increased fluids, bulk, exercise to decrease constipation, liquefy sputum
• Chest percussion to bring up secretion if needed

Evaluate:
• Therapeutic response: absence of cough

Teach patient/family:
• To avoid driving, other hazardous activities until patient is stabilized on this medication
• Not to chew or break capsules; will anesthetize mouth
• To avoid smoking, smoke-filled rooms, perfumes, dust, environmental pollutants, cleaners

---

benzoyl peroxide
(ben'zoe-ill per-ox'ide)
Acne-10, Acne-Aid, Ben-Aqua-5, Ben-Aqua-10, Benoxyl 5, Benoxyl 10, Benzoyl Peroxide, Benzac AC, Benzac W Wash 5, Benzac W Wash 10, Benzac W 2½, Benzac W 5, Benzac 5, Benzac 10, Benzac W 10, 5-Benzagel, 10-Benzagel, Brevoxil, Clear By Design, Clearasil 10%, Clearasil Maximum Strength Acne Treatment, Cuticura Acne, Del Aqua-5, Del Aqua-10, Desquam-E, Desquam-X2.5, Desquam-X5, Desquam-X10, Desquam-X5 Wash, Desquam-X10 Wash, Dry and Clear, Dry and Clear Double Strength, Fostex 5% BPO, Fostex 10% BPO, Fostex 10% BPO Wash, Fostex 10% BPO Tinted, Luroxide, Oxy 5, Oxy 5 Tinted, Oxy 10, Oxy 10 Cover, Oxy 10 Wash, Pan Oxyl 5, Pan Oxyl 10, Pan Oxyl AQ 2½, Pan Oxyl AQ 5, Pan Oxyl AQ 10, Persa-Gel, Persa Gel W 5%, Persa Gel W 10%, pHisoAc BP, Propa P.H. Liquid Acne Soap, Theroxide, Theroxide Wash, Vanoxide, Xerac BP10, Xerac BP5, Zeroxin-5, Zeroxin-10
Func. class.: Antiacne medication

Action: Antibacterial activity, especially against predominant bacteria causing acne

Uses: Mild-moderate acne

Dosage and routes:
• *Adult and child:* TOP apply to affected area qd or bid

Available forms: Topical cleansers, lotions, creams, sticks, pads, gels, bars

---

Side effects/adverse reactions:

INTEG: Local skin irritation; stinging; warmth (dryness); scaling; erythema; edema; allergic, contact dermatitis

Contraindications: Hypersensitivity to benzoic acid derivatives

Precautions: Pregnancy (C), lactation, children <12 yr

Pharmacokinetics:

TOP: 50% absorbed through skin, metabolized to benzoic acid, excreted in urine as benzoate

Interaction/incompatibilities:

• Skin irritation: tretinoin

NURSING CONSIDERATIONS

Assess:

• Area of body involved, including time involved, what helps or aggravates condition

• Allergic reaction: rash, irritation, scaling, dermatitis; discontinue use

Administer:

• Then wash hands immediately to avoid irritation

Perform/provide:

• Storage at room temperature

Evaluate:

• Therapeutic response: decreased amount of acne on body

Teach patient/family:

• To avoid application on normal skin or getting cream in eyes, nose, or other mucous membranes

• To discontinue use if rash or irritation develops

• That transitory warmth or stinging may develop over area treated

• To expect dryness, peeling of area treated

• To avoid contact with hair or clothing; they may stain

• That cosmetics may be used over drug

• That dryness and peeling can be expected

benzquinamide HCl 171

benzquinamide HCl

(benz-kwin'a-mide)

Emete-Con

Func. class.: Antiemetic

Chem. class.: Benzoquinolize amide

Action: Acts centrally by blocking chemoreceptor trigger zone, which in turn acts on vomiting center

Uses: To inhibit nausea, vomiting associated with anesthetic, surgery

Dosage and routes:

• *Adult:* IM 50 mg or 0.5-1 mg/kg, may be repeated in 1 hr, then q3-4 hr prn; IV 25 mg or 0.2-0.4 mg/kg as a one-time dose

Available forms: Inj 50 mg/vial

Side effects/adverse reactions:

CNS: Drowsiness, fatigue, restlessness, tremor, headache, stimulation, dizziness, insomnia, twitching, excitement, nervousness, extrapyramidal symptoms

GI: Nausea, anorexia

CV: **Premature atrial** or **ventricular contractions, atrial fibrillation,** hypertension, hypotension

INTEG: Rash, urticaria, fever, chills, flushing, hives, shivering, sweating, temperature

EENT: Dry mouth, blurred vision, hiccups, salivation

Contraindications: Hypersensitivity, hypertension

Precautions: Children, pregnancy (C), lactation, elderly

Pharmacokinetics:

IM/IV: Onset 15 min, duration 3-4 hr, metabolized by liver, excreted in urine, feces, half-life 40 min

Interactions/incompatibilities:

• Incompatible with chlordiazepoxide, diazepam, pentobarbital, phenobarbital, secobarbital, thiopental, NaCl sol

italics = common side effects   ***bold italic*** = life threatening reactions

NURSING CONSIDERATIONS
Assess:
• Vital signs, B/P; check patients with cardiac disease more often; hypotension, hypertension, dysrhythmias may occur
• Observe for drowsiness; instruct patient not to drive, operate machinery

Administer:
• After reconstituting 50 mg of drug with 2.2 ml sterile water for injection to a concentration of 25 mg/ml; do not use NaCl. Direct IV 25 mg over ½-1 min by Y-tube or 3-way stopcock
• Reduced dosage if patient is receiving pressor drugs

Perform/provide:
• Storage of injection before, after reconstitution in light-resistant container, single-dose container

Evaluate:
• Therapeutic response: absence of nausea, vomiting

Treatment of overdose:
• Supportive care; atropine may be helpful

---

benztropine mesylate
(benz'troe-peen)
Benztropine mesylate, Cogentin
Func. class.: Cholinergic blocker
Chem. class.: Tertiary amine

Action: Blockade of central acetylcholine receptors
Uses: Parkinson symptoms, extrapyramidal symptoms associated with neuroleptic drugs

Dosage and routes:
Drug-induced extrapyramidal symptoms
• *Adult:* IM/IV 1-4 mg 1-2 × /day; give PO dose as soon as possible;

PO 1-2 mg bid/tid, increase by 0.5 mg q5-6 days
Parkinson symptoms
• *Adult:* PO 0.5-1 mg qd, increased 0.5 mg q5-6 days titrated to patient response
Available forms: Tabs 0.5, 1, 2 mg; inj IM, IV 1 mg/ml

Side effects/adverse reactions:
MS: Muscular weakness, cramping
INTEG: Rash, urticaria, dermatoses
MISC: Increased temperature, flushing, decreased sweating, hyperthermia, heat stroke, numbness of fingers
CNS: Confusion, anxiety, restlessness, irritability, delusions, hallucinations, headache, sedation, depression, incoherence, dizziness, memory loss
EENT: Blurred vision, photophobia, dilated pupils, difficulty swallowing, dry eyes, mydriasis, increased intraocular tension, angle-closure glaucoma
CV: Palpitations, tachycardia, hypotension, bradycardia
GI: Dryness of mouth, constipation, nausea, vomiting, abdominal distress, *paralytic ileus,* epigastric distress
GU: Hesitancy, retention, dysuria

Contraindications: Hypersensitivity, narrow-angle glaucoma, myasthenia gravis, GI/GU obstruction, child <3 yr, peptic ulcer, megacolon, prostate hypertrophy
Precautions: Pregnancy (C), elderly, lactation, tachycardia, liver, kidney disease, drug abuse history, dysrhythmias, hypotension, hypertension, psychiatric patients, children

Pharmacokinetics:
IM/IV: Onset 15 min, duration 6-10 hr
PO: Onset 1 hr, duration 6-10 hr

Interactions/incompatibilities:
• Increased anticholinergic effect: antihistamines, phenothiazines, amantadine
• Decreased effect of levodopa
• Increased schizophrenic symptoms: haloperidol
• Incompatibilities: unknown

NURSING CONSIDERATIONS
Assess:
• I&O ratio; retention commonly causes decreased urinary output
• Parkinsonism, extrapyramidal symptoms: shuffling gait, muscle rigidity, involuntary movements
• Urinary hesitancy, retention; palpate bladder if retention occurs
• Constipation; increase fluids, bulk, exercise if this occurs
• For tolerance over long-term therapy; dose may have to be increased or changed
• Mental status: affect, mood, CNS depression, worsening of mental symptoms during early therapy
• Use caution in hot weather; drug may increase susceptibility to stroke

Administer:
• With or after meals to prevent GI upset; may give with fluids other than water
• At hs to avoid daytime drowsiness in patient with parkinsonism
• Undiluted IV (1 mg = 1 ml) dose at a rate of ≤1 mg/> 1 min; keep in bed for at least 1 hr after dose

Perform/provide:
• Storage at room temperature
• Hard candy, frequent drinks, gum to relieve dry mouth

Evaluate:
• Therapeutic response: absence of involuntary movements

Teach patient/family:
• Not to discontinue this drug abruptly; to taper off over 1 wk
• To avoid driving or other hazardous activities; drowsiness may occur
• To avoid OTC medication: cough, cold preparations with alcohol, antihistamines unless directed by physician

---

bepridil HCl
(beh'prih-dill)
Vascor
Func. class.: Calcium channel blocker type 4

Action: Inhibits calcium ion influx across cell membrane during cardiac depolarization; produces relaxation of coronary vascular smooth muscle, dilates coronary arteries, decreases SA/AV node conduction, dilates peripheral arteries
Uses: Chronic stable angina, used alone or in combination with propranolol
Dosage and routes:
Angina
Adult: 200-450 mg qd
Available forms: Tabs, film-coated, 200, 300, 400 mg
Side effects/adverse reactions:
CV: Dysrhythmia, edema, CHF, bradycardia, hypotension, palpitations, AV block
GI: Nausea, vomiting, diarrhea, gastric upset, constipation, increased liver function studies
GU: Nocturia, polyuria
CNS: Headache, fatigue, drowsiness, dizziness, anxiety, depression, weakness, insomnia, confusion, light-headedness, nervousness
Contraindications: Sick sinus syndrome, 2nd or 3rd degree heart block, Wolff-Parkinson-White syndrome, hypotension less than 90 mm Hg systolic, cardiogenic

---

shock, history of serious ventricular arrhythmias

Precautions: CHF, hypotension, hepatic injury, pregnancy (C), lactation, children, renal disease, Idiopathic hypertropic subaortic stenosis (IHSS), concomitant β-blocker therapy

Pharmacokinetics: Peak 2-3 hr, 99% plasma protein bound, half-life 42 hr; completely metabolized in the liver and excreted in urine and feces

Interactions/incompatibilities:
• Increased effects: β-blockers
• Decreased effects of lithium, rifampin
• Increased levels of digoxin

Lab test interferences:
Increase: Liver function tests, aminotransferase, CPK, LDH

NURSING CONSIDERATIONS
Assess:
• Cardiac status: B/P, pulse, respiration, ECG intervals (PR, QRS, QT), dysrhythmias

Administer:
• Before meals, hs

Evaluate:
• Therapeutic response: decreased anginal pain, decreased B/P

Teach patient/family:
• How to take pulse before taking drug; record or graph should be kept
• To avoid hazardous activities until stabilized on drug, dizziness no longer a problem
• To limit caffeine consumption
• To avoid OTC drugs unless directed by a physician
• Importance of patient compliance with all areas of medical regimen: diet, exercise, stress reduction, drug therapy

Treatment of overdose: Defibrillation, atropine for AV block, vasopressor for hypotension

beractant
(bear-ac´-tant)
Survanta
Func. class.: Natural lung surfactant

Action: Replenishes surfactant and restores surface activity to the lungs in premature infants

Uses: Prevention and treatment (rescue) of respiratory distress syndrome in premature infants

Dosage and routes:
INTRATRACHEAL INSTILL: 4 doses can be administered in the 1st 48 hrs of life; give doses no more frequently than q6h; each dose is 100 mg of phospholipids/kg birth weight (4 ml/kg)

Available forms: Susp 25 mg phospholipids/ml in 0.9% NaCl in single-use vials containing 8 ml susp

Side effects/adverse reactions:
Concurrent illnesses that have occurred during treatment are in bold
*RESP: **Pulmonary air leaks, pulmonary interstitial emphysema, apnea, pulmonary hemorrhage***
*SYST: **Patent ductus arteriosus, intracranial hemorrhage, severe intracranial hemorrhage, necrotizing entercolitis, posttreatment sepsis, posttreatment infection,*** bradycardia, oxygen desaturation, pallor, vasoconstriction, hypotension, hypertension

Precautions: Bradycardia, rales, infections

Pharmacokinetics: Becomes lung associated within hours of administration

NURSING CONSIDERATIONS
Assess:
• Respiratory rate, rhythm, character, chest expansion, color, transcutaneous saturation, ABGs

• Endotracheal tube placement before dosing; for apnea after endotracheal administration

• Reflux of drug into the endotracheal tube during administration; stop drug administration if this occurs, and if needed, increase peak inspiratory pressure on the ventilator by 4-5 cm H₂O until tube is cleared

• Infant for repeat dosing using radiographic confirmation of RDS; repeat doses should be given as above; ventilator settings for repeat doses FIO₂ were decreased by 0.2 or amount to prevent cyanosis; ventilator rate of 30/min; inspiratory time <1 sec; if infant's pretreatment rate was >30, it was left unchanged during dosing; resume usual ventilator management after dosing

Administer:

• After suctioning

• By endotracheal administration only by persons trained in neonatal intubation and ventilation

• After using a No. 5 Fr end-hole catheter inserted into the endotracheal tube with the tip protruding just beyond the end of the endotracheal tube; shorten the catheter before insertion; do not insert the drug into the mainstem bronchus

• Divide each dose into quarters and administer with infant in different positions

• Determine the dosing by weight of infant; slowly withdraw the contents into the plastic syringe through a 20G needle; do not filter or shake; attach the premeasured No. 5 Fr catheter to syringe; fill with drug and discard excess through the catheter so only dose to be given remains in syringe

• For prevention dosing, stabilize, weigh, and intubate the infant; give

drug within 15 min of birth if possible; position infant and inject the first quarter-dose through catheter over 2-3 sec; remove catheter and manually ventilate with O₂ to prevent cyanosis (60 bpm) and sufficient positive pressure to promote adequate air exchange and chest wall excursion

• For rescue dosing, give dosing as soon as infant is placed on ventilator after birth; immediately before administering dose, change ventilator settings to 60/min, inspiratory time 0.5 sec, FIO₂ 1; position infant and inject first quarter through catheter over 2-3 sec; remove catheter; return to mechanical ventilator

• Ventilate infant for >30 sec or until stable after prevention or rescue strategy; resposition for next dose; same procedure for subsequent dosing; do not suction for at least 1 hr after dosing unless airway obstruction is evident; resume ventilator therapy after dosing

Perform/provide:

• Reduction in peak venilator inspiratory pressures immediately if chest expansion improves substantially after dose

• Reduction in FIo₂ in small, repeated steps when infant becomes pink and transcutaneous oxygen saturation is in excess of 95%; oxygen saturation should remain between 90% and 95%

• Suctioning of all infants before administration to prevent mucus plugging; if endotracheal tube obstruction is suspected, remove the obstruction and replace tube immediately

• Storage in refrigeration; protect from light, warm to room temperature for >20 min or warm in hand >8 min before giving; do not use artificial warming methods; enter a vial only once; unopened, unused vials that have been warmed to room temperature may be rerefrigerated within 8 hr of warming; do not warm and return to refrigerator more than once

Evaluate:

• Therapeutic response: significant improvement in respiratory status

---

betamethasone/beta-methasone sodium phosphate/betameth-asone disodium phosphate/betametha-sone acetate/beta-methasone sodium phosphate

(bay-ta-meth'a-sone)

Betnelan, Celestone/Alphatrex, Betamethasone Dipropionate, Diprosone, Maxivate, Teladar/Diprolene, Diprolene AF/Betamethasone Sodium Phosphate, Celestone Phosphate, Cel-U-Jec, Selestoject

Func. class.: Corticosteroid, synthetic

Chem. class.: Glucocorticoid, long-acting

Action: Decreases inflammation by suppression of migration of polymorphonuclear leukocytes, fibroblasts, reversal of increased capillary permeability and lysosomal stabilization

Uses: Immunosupression, severe inflammation, prevention of neonatal respiratory distress syndrome (by administration to mother)

Dosage and routes:

• *Adult:* PO 0.6-7.2 mg qd; IM/IV 0.6-7.2 mg qd in joint or soft tissue (sodium phosphate)

• *Pregnant adult:* IM 12 mg 36-48 hr, before premature delivery, then same dose in 24 hr (betamethasone acetate)

Available forms: Tabs 0.6 mg; syr 0.6 mg/5 ml; inj 3, 4 mg/ml

Side effects/adverse reactions:

INTEG: Acne, poor wound healing, ecchymosis, bruising, petechiae

CNS: Depression, flushing, sweating, headache, ecchymosis, bruising, mood changes

*CV: Hypertension, **circulatory collapse, thrombophlebitis, embolism,** tachycardia, **necrotizing angiitis, CHF***

*HEMA: **Thrombocytopenia***

MS: Fractures, osteoporosis, weakness

*GI: Diarrhea, nausea, abdominal distention, **GI hemorrhage,** increased appetite, **pancreatitis***

EENT: Fungal infections, increased intraocular pressure, blurred vision

Contraindications: Psychosis, hypersensitivity, idiopathic thrombocytopenia, acute glomerulonephritis, amebiasis, fungal infections, nonasthmatic bronchial disease, child <2 yr, AIDS, TB

Precautions: Pregnancy (C), diabetes mellitus, glaucoma, osteoporosis, seizure disorders, ulcerative colitis, CHF, myasthenia gravis, renal disease, esophagitis, peptic ulcer

Pharmacokinetics:

PO: Onset 1-2 hr, peak 1 hr, duration 3 days

IM/IV: Onset 10 min, peak 4-8 hr, duration 1-1½ days

Metabolized in liver, excreted in urine as steroids, crosses placenta

Interactions/incompatibilities:

• Decreased action of betamethasone: cholestyramine, colestipol, barbiturates, rifampin, ephedrine, phenytoin, theophylline

• Decreased effects of anticoagu-

lants, anticonvulsants, antidiabetics, ambenonium, neostigmine, isoniazid, toxoids, vaccines, anticholinesterases, salicylates, somatrem
• Increased side effects: alcohol, salicylates, indomethacin, amphotericin B, digitalis, cyclosporine, diuretics
• Increased action of betamethasone: salicylates, estrogens, indomethacin, oral contraceptives, ketoconazole, macrolide antibiotics

Lab test interferences:
Increase: Cholesterol, sodium, blood glucose, uric acid, calcium, urine glucose
Decrease: Calcium, potassium, T$_4$, T$_3$, thyroid ^{131}I uptake test, urine 17-OHCS, 17-KS, PBI
False negative: Skin allergy tests

NURSING CONSIDERATIONS
Assess:
• Potassium, blood sugar, urine glucose while on long-term therapy; hypokalemia and hyperglycemia
• Weight daily; notify physician of weekly gain >5 lb
• B/P q4h, pulse; notify physician if chest pain occurs
• I&O ratio; be alert for decreasing urinary output and increasing edema
• Plasma cortisol levels during long-term therapy (normal level: 138-635 nmol/L SI units when drawn at 8 AM)

Administer:
• IV, only sodium phosphate product; give > 1 min; may be given by IV INF in compatible sol
• After shaking suspension (parenteral)
• Titrated dose; use lowest effective dose
• IM injection deeply in large mass, rotate sites, avoid deltoid, use 21G needle
• In one dose in AM to prevent adrenal suppression, avoid SC administration; may damage tissue
• With food or milk to decrease GI symptoms

Perform/provide:
• Assistance with ambulation in patient with bone tissue disease to prevent fractures

Evaluate:
• Therapeutic response: ease of respirations, decreased inflammation
• Infection: increased temperature, WBC even after withdrawal of medication; drug masks infection symptoms
• Potassium depletion: paresthesias, fatigue, nausea, vomiting, depression, polyuria, dysrhythmias, weakness
• Edema, hypertension, cardiac symptoms
• Mental status: affect, mood, behavioral changes, aggression

Teach patient/family:
• That ID as steroid user should be carried
• To notify physician if therapeutic response decreases; dosage adjustment may be needed
• Not to discontinue abruptly; adrenal crisis can result
• To avoid OTC products: salicylates, alcohol in cough products, cold preparations unless directed by physician
• All aspects of drug usage including cushingoid symptoms
• Symptoms of adrenal insufficiency: nausea, anorexia, fatigue, dizziness, dyspnea, weakness, joint pain

italics = common side effects   ***bold italic*** = life threatening reactions

betamethasone benzoate

(bay-ta-meth'a-sone)
Benisone, Uticort
Func. class.: Topical corticosteroid
Chem. class.: Synthetic fluorinated agent, group III potency

Action: Antipruritic, antiinflammatory
Uses: Psoriasis, eczema, contact dermatitis, pruritus
Dosage and routes:
• *Adult and child:* Apply to affected area qid
Available forms: Oint 0.025%; cream 0.025%; lotion 0.025%; gel 0.025%
Side effects/adverse reactions:
INTEG: Burning, dryness, itching, irritation, acne, folliculitis, hypertrichosis, perioral dermatitis, hypopigmentation, atrophy, striae, miliaria, allergic contact dermatitis, secondary infection
Contraindications: Hypersensitivity to corticosteroids, fungal infections
Precautions: Pregnancy (C), lactation, viral infections, bacterial infections
NURSING CONSIDERATIONS
Assess:
• Temperature; if fever develops, drug should be discontinued
• For systemic absorption: increased temperature, inflammation, irritation
Administer:
• Only to affected areas; do not get in eyes
• Medication, then cover with occlusive dressing (only if prescribed), seal to normal skin, change q12h; systemic absorption may occur

• Only to dermatoses; do not use on weeping, denuded, or infected area
Perform/provide:
• Cleansing before application of drug
• Treatment for a few days after area has cleared
• Storage at room temperature
Evaluate:
• Therapeutic response: absence of severe itching, patches on skin, flaking
Teach patient/family:
• To avoid sunlight on affected area; burns may occur

betamethasone valerate

(bay-ta-meth'a-sone)
Beta Cort,* Betaderm,* Betamethasone Valerate, Betatrex, Beta-Val, Valisone, Valisone Reduced Strength
Func. class.: Topical corticosteroid
Chem. class.: Synthetic fluorinated agent

Action: Possesses antipruritic, antiinflammatory actions
Uses: Psoriasis, eczema, contact dermatitis, pruritus
Dosage and routes:
• *Adult and child:* Apply to affected area qid
Available forms: Oint 0.1%; cream 0.01%, 0.1%; lotion 0.1%
Side effects/adverse reactions:
INTEG: Burning, dryness, itching, irritation, acne, folliculitis, hypertrichosis, perioral dermatitis, hypopigmentation, atrophy, striae, miliaria, allergic contact dermatitis, secondary infection
Contraindications: Hypersensitiv-

ity to corticosteroids, fungal infections

Precautions: Pregnancy (C), lactation, viral infections, bacterial infections

NURSING CONSIDERATIONS
Assess:
• Temperature; if fever develops, drug should be discontinued
• For systemic absorption: increased temperature, inflammation, irritation

Administer:
• Only to affected areas; do not get in eyes
• Medication, then cover with occlusive dressing (only if prescribed), seal to normal skin, change q12h; systemic absorption may occur
• Only to dermatoses; do not use on weeping, denuded, or infected area

Perform/provide:
• Cleansing before applying drug
• Treatment for a few days after area has cleared
• Storage at room temperature

Evaluate:
• Therapeutic response: absence of severe itching, patches on skin, flaking

Teach patient/family:
• To avoid sunlight on affected area; burns may occur

---

bethanechol chloride
(be-than'e-kile)
Bethanechol Chloride, Duvoid, Myotonachol, Urecholine
Func. class.: Cholinergic stimulant
Chem. class.: Synthetic choline ester

Action: Stimulates muscarinic ACh receptors directly; mimics ef-

fects of parasympathetic nervous system stimulation; stimulates gastric motility, stimulates micturition

Uses: Urinary retention (postoperative, postpartum), neurogenic atony of bladder with retention

Dosage and routes:
• *Adult:* PO 10-50 mg bid-qid; SC 2.5-10 mg tid-qid prn
Test dose
• *Adult:* SC 2.5 mg repeated 15-30 min intervals × 4 doses to determine effective dose

Available forms: Tabs 5, 10, 25, 50 mg; inj SC 5 mg/ml

Side effects/adverse reactions:
INTEG: Rash, urticaria, flushing, increased sweating
CNS: Dizziness
GI: Nausea, bloody diarrhea, belching, vomiting, cramps, fecal incontinence
CV: Hypotension, bradycardia, orthostatic hypotension, reflex tachycardia, **cardiac arrest, circulatory collapse**
GU: Urgency
RESP: **Acute asthma, dyspnea**
EENT: Miosis, increased salivation, lacrimation, blurred vision

Contraindications: Hypersensitivity, severe bradycardia, asthma, severe hypotension, hyperthyroidism, peptic ulcer, parkinsonism, seizure disorders, CAD, coronary occlusion, mechanical obstruction, peritonitis, recent urinary or GI surgery

Precautions: Hypertension, pregnancy (C), lactation, child <8 yr, urinary retention

Pharmacokinetics:
PO: Onset 30-90 min, duration 1-6 hr
SC: Onset 5-15 min, duration 2 hr, excreted by kidneys

Interactions/incompatibilities:
• Increased action of bethanechol: other cholinergics

---

italics = common side effects   ***bold italic*** = life threatening reactions

• Hypotension: ganglionic blockers
• Decreased action of bethanechol: procainamide, quinidine

Lab test interferences:
Increase: AST, lipase/amylase, bilirubin, BSP

NURSING CONSIDERATIONS
Assess:
• B/P, pulse; observe after parenteral dose for 1 hr
• I&O ratio; check for urinary retention or incontinence
• Bradycardia, hypotension, bronchospasm, headache, dizziness, convulsions, respiratory depression; drug should be discontinued if toxicity occurs

Administer:
• Parenteral dose by SC route; use of IM, IV may result in cardiac arrest
• Only with atropine sulfate available for cholinergic crisis
• Only after all other cholinergics have been discontinued
• Increased doses if tolerance occurs
• To avoid nausea and vomiting, take on an empty stomach

Perform/provide:
• Storage at room temperature
• Bedpan/urinal if given for urinary retention
• Use of rectal tube if ordered, to increase passage of gas when used for abdominal distention

Evaluate:
• Therapeutic response: absence of urinary retention, abdominal distention

Teach patient/family:
• To take drug exactly as prescribed
• To make position changes slowly; orthostatic hypotension may occur
Treatment of overdose: Administer atropine 0.6-1.2 mg IV or IM (adult)

---

biperiden HCl, biperiden lactate
(bye-per′i-den)
Akineton
Func. class.: Cholinergic blocker

Action: Centrally acting competitive anticholinergic
Uses: Parkinson symptoms, extrapyramidal symptoms secondary to neuroleptic drug therapy

Dosage and routes:
Extrapyramidal symptoms
• *Adult:* PO 2 mg 1-3 times a day; IM/IV 2 mg q30min, if needed, not to exceed 8 mg/24 hr
Parkinson symptoms
• *Adult:* PO 2 mg tid-qid max 16 mg/24 hr
Available forms: Tabs 2 mg; inj IM/IV 5 mg/ml (lactate)

Side effects/adverse reactions:
CNS: Confusion, anxiety, restlessness, irritability, delusions, hallucinations, headache, sedation, depression, incoherence, dizziness, euphoria, tremors, memory loss
EENT: Blurred vision, photophobia, dilated pupils, difficulty swallowing, mydriasis, increased intraocular tension, angle-closure glaucoma
CV: Palpitations, tachycardia, postural hypotension, bradycardia
GI: Dryness of mouth, constipation, nausea, vomiting, abdominal distress, *paralytic ileus*
GU: Hesitancy, retention, dysuria
MS: Weakness, cramping
INTEG: Rash, urticaria, dermatoses
MISC: Increased temperature, flushing, decreased sweating, hyperthermia, heat stroke, numbness of fingers

---

* Available in Canada only

Contraindications: Hypersensitivity, narrow-angle glaucoma, myasthenia gravis, GI/GU obstruction, megacolon, stenosing peptic ulcers, prostatic hypertrophy

Precautions: Pregnancy (C), elderly, lactation, tachycardia, dysrhythmias, liver, kidney disease, drug abuse, hypotension, hypertension, psychiatric patients, children

Pharmacokinetics:

IM/IV: Onset 15 min, duration 6-10 hr

PO: Onset 1 hr, duration 6-10 hr

Interactions/incompatibilities:

• Increased levels of digoxin, levodopa

• Increased schizophrenic symptoms: haloperidol

• Increased anticholinergic effect: antihistamines, phenothiazines, amantadine

• Incompatibilities are unknown

NURSING CONSIDERATIONS

Assess:

• I&O ratio; retention commonly causes decreased urinary output

• Parkinsonism, extrapyramidal symptoms: shuffling gait, muscle rigidity, involuntary movements

• Urinary hesitancy, retention; palpate bladder if retention occurs

• Constipation; increase fluids, bulk, exercise if this occurs

• For tolerance over long-term therapy; dose may have to be increased or changed

• Mental status: affect, mood, CNS depression, worsening of mental symptoms during early therapy

Administer:

• Parenteral dose with patient recumbent to prevent postural hypotension, give undiluted 2 mg or less/>1 min

• With or after meals to prevent GI upset; may give with fluids other than water

• At hs to avoid daytime drowsiness in patient with parkinsonism

Perform/provide:

• Storage at room temperature

• Hard candy, frequent drinks, gum to relieve dry mouth

Evaluate:

• Therapeutic response: absence of involuntary movements

Teach patient/family:

• Use caution in hot weather; drug may increase susceptibility to stroke

• Not to discontinue this drug abruptly; to taper off over 1 wk

• To avoid driving or other hazardous activities; drowsiness may occur

• To avoid OTC medication: cough, cold preparations with alcohol, antihistamines unless directed by physician

---

bisacodyl

(bis-a-koe′dill)

Apo-Bisacodyl,* Bisacodyl, Bisacodyl Uniserts, Bisco-Lax, Dulcagen, Dulcolax, Fleet Bisacodyl

Func. class.: Laxative, stimulant

Chem. class.: Diphenylmethane

Action: Acts directly on intestine by increasing motor activity; thought to irritate colonic intramural plexus

Uses: Short-term treatment of constipation, bowel or rectal preparation for surgery, examination

Dosage and routes:

• *Adult:* PO 10-15 mg in PM or AM; may use up to 30 mg for bowel or rectal preparation; REC 10 mg; ENEMA 1.25 oz

• *Child >3 yr:* PO 5-10 mg

---

italics = common side effects   ***bold italic*** = life threatening reactions

- *Child >2 yr:* REC 10 mg
- *Child <2 yr:* REC 5 mg
- *Child <6 yr:* ENEMA ½ contents of micro enema

Available forms: Enteric coated tabs 5 mg; rec supp 10 mg

Side effects/adverse reactions:

CNS: Muscle weakness

GI: Nausea, vomiting, anorexia, cramps, diarrhea, rectal burning (suppositories)

META: Protein-losing enteropathy, alkalosis, hypokalemia, *tetany,* electrolyte, fluid imbalances

Contraindications: Hypersensitivity, rectal fissures, abdominal pain, nausea, vomiting, appendicitis, acute surgical abdomen, ulcerated hemorrhoids, acute hepatitis, fecal impaction, intestinal/biliary tract obstruction

Precautions: Pregnancy (C)

Pharmacokinetics:

PO: Onset 6-10 min; acts within 6-12 hr

REC: Onset 15-16 min

Metabolized by liver; excreted in urine, bile, feces, breast milk

Interactions/incompatibilities:

- Gastric irritation: antacids, milk, H$_2$ blockers

NURSING CONSIDERATIONS

Assess:

- Blood, urine electrolytes if drug is used often by patient
- I&O ratio to identify fluid loss
- Cause of constipation; identify whether fluids, bulk, or exercise missing from life-style
- Cramping, rectal bleeding, nausea, vomiting; if these symptoms occur, drug should be discontinued

Administer:

- Alone only with water for better absorption; do not take within 1 hr of other drugs or within 1 hr of antacids, milk, or cimetidine
- In AM or PM (oral dose)

Evaluate:

- Therapeutic response: decrease in constipation

Teach patient/family:

- To swallow tabs whole; do not chew
- Not to use laxatives for long-term therapy; bowel tone will be lost
- That normal bowel movements do not always occur daily
- Not to use in presence of abdominal pain, nausea, vomiting
- To notify physician if constipation is unrelieved or if symptoms of electrolyte imbalance occur: muscle cramps, pain, weakness, dizziness

---

bismuth subsalicylate

(bis-meth)

Pepto-Bismol, Pepto-Bismol Maximum Strength

Func. class.: Antidiarrheal

Chem. class.: Salicylate

Action: Inhibits prostaglandin synthesis responsible for GI hypermotility; stimulates absorption of fluid and electrolytes

Uses: Diarrhea (cause undetermined), prevention of diarrhea when traveling

Dosage and routes:

- *Adult:* PO 30 ml or 2 tabs q30-60 min, not to exceed 8 doses for >2 days
- *Child 10-14 yr:* PO 15 ml

Available forms: Chewable tabs 262 mg; susp 262 mg/15 ml

Side effects/adverse reactions:

HEMA: Increased bleeding time

GI: Increased fecal impaction (high doses), dark stools

CNS: Confusion, twitching

EENT: Hearing loss, tinnitus, metallic taste, blue gums

Contraindications: Child <3 yr

Precautions: Anticoagulant therapy

Pharmacokinetics:

PO: Onset 1 hr, peak 2 hr, duration 4 hr

Interactions/incompatibilities:

• Increased side effects: alcohol, aminosalicyclic acid, carbonic anhydrase inhibitors
• Increased action of bismuth: ammonium chloride
• Decreased action of bismuth: antacids, corticosteroids
• Decreased action of uricosurics, indomethacin, antidiabetics, tetracyclines

Lab test interferences:

Interfere: Radiographic studies of GI system

NURSING CONSIDERATIONS

Assess:

• Skin turgor; shift if dehydration is suspected
• Electrolytes (K, Na, Cl) if diarrhea is severe or continues long term
• Bowel pattern before drug therapy, after treatment

Administer:

• But stop use if symptoms do not improve within 2 days or become worse, or if diarrhea is accompanied by high fever
• Increased fluids to rehydrate the patient

Evaluate:

• Therapeutic response: decreased diarrhea or absence of diarrhea when traveling

Teach patient/family:

• To chew or dissolve in mouth; do not swallow whole; shake liquid before using
• To avoid other salicylates unless directed by physician; not to give to children, possibility of Reye's syndrome
• That stools may turn gray; tongue

may darken; impaction may occur in debilitated patients

---

bisoprolol

(bis-o-prole'-lole)

Zebeta

Func. class.: Antihypertensive

Chem. class.: β₁-blocker

Action: Preferentially and competitively blocks stimulation of β₁-adrenergic receptor within cardiac muscle; produces negative chronotropic and inotropic activity (decreases rate of SA node discharge, increases recovery time), slows conduction of AV node, decreases heart rate, which decreases O_2 consumption in myocardium; decreases renin-aldosterone-angiotensin system; inhibits β₂ receptors in bronchial and vascular smooth muscle at high doses

Uses: Mild to moderate hypertension

Dosage and routes:

Hypertension

• *Adult:* PO 2.5–5.0 mg once daily; may increase if necessary to 20 mg once daily; may need to reduce dose in presence of renal or hepatic impairment

Available forms: Tabs 5, 10 mg

Side effects/adverse reactions:

MS: Joint pain, arthralgia

MISC: Facial swelling, weight gain, decreased exercise tolerance

CV: Ventricular dysrhythmias, **profound hypotension**, bradycardia, **CHF**, cold extremities, postural hypotension, **2nd or 3rd degree heart block**

CNS: Vertigo, headache, insomnia, fatigue, dizziness, mental changes, memory loss, hallucinations, depression, lethargy, drowsiness,

---

italics = common side effects   ***bold italic*** = life threatening reactions

strange dreams, catatonia, peripheral neuropathy

GI: Nausea, diarrhea, vomiting, mesenteric arterial thrombosis, ischemic colitis, flatulence, gastritis, gastric pain

INTEG: Rash, fever, alopecia, pruritus, sweating

HEMA: Agranulocytosis, thrombocytopenia, purpura, eosinophilia

EENT: Sore throat, dry burning eyes

GU: Impotence, decreased libido

ENDO: Increased hypoglycemic response to insulin

RESP: Bronchospasm, dyspnea, wheezing, cough, nasal stuffiness

Contraindications: Hypersensitivity to β-blockers, cardiogenic shock, heart block (2nd, 3rd degree), sinus bradycardia, CHF, cardiac failure

Precautions: Major surgery, pregnancy (B), lactation, children, diabetes mellitus, renal or hepatic disease, thyroid disease, COPD, asthma, well-compensated heart failure, aortic or mitral valve disease, peripheral vascular disease, myasthenia gravis

Pharmacokinetics:

PO: Peak 2-4 hr; half-life 9-12 hr, 50% excreted unchanged in urine, protein binding 30%; metabolized in liver to inactive metabolites

Interactions/incompatibilities:

• Increased hypotension, bradycardia: reserpine, hydralazine, methyldopa, quinidine, prazosin

• Decreased antihypertensive effects: indomethacin, nonsteroidal antiinflammatories, barbiturates, cholestyramine, colestipol, penicillins, salicylates

• Increased hypoglycemic effect: insulin

• Decreased bronchodilation: theophylline

• Decreased hypoglycemic effect of sulfonylureas

Lab test interferences:

Increase: AST and ALT

Interference: Glucose/insulin tolerance tests

NURSING CONSIDERATIONS

Assess:

• B/P during beginning treatment, periodically thereafter: pulse q4h: note rate, rhythm, quality

• Apical/radial pulse before administration; notify physician of any significant changes (pulse <60 bpm)

• Baselines in renal, liver function tests before therapy begins

• Edema in feet, legs daily

• Skin turgor, dryness of mucous membranes for hydration status, especially elderly

Administer:

• PO ac, hs tablet may be crushed or swallowed whole

• Reduced dosage in renal and hepatic dysfunction

Perform/provide:

• Storage protected from light, moisture; placed in cool environment

Evaluate:

• Therapeutic response: decreased B/P after 1-2 wk

Teach patient/family:

• Not to discontinue drug abruptly, taper over 2 wk, may cause precipitate angina

• Not to use OTC products containing α-adrenergic stimulants (such as nasal decongestants, OTC cold preparations) unless directed by physician

• To report bradycardia, dizziness, confusion, depression, fever

• To take pulse at home; advise when to notify physician

• To avoid alcohol, smoking, sodium intake

---

*Available in Canada only

• To comply with weight control, dietary adjustments, modified exercise program
• To carry Medic Alert ID to identify drug taking, allergies
• To avoid hazardous activities if dizziness is present
• To report symptoms of CHF: difficult breathing, especially on exertion or when lying down, night cough, swelling of extremities
Treatment of overdose: Lavage, IV atropine for bradycardia, IV theophylline for bronchospasm, digitalis, O_2, diuretic for cardiac failure, hemodialysis, IV glucose for hyperglycemia, IV diazepam (or phenytoin) for seizures

---

bitolterol mesylate

(bye-tole'-ter-ol)
Tornalate
Func. class.: Adrenergic β_2-agonist
Chem. class.: Acid ester of colterol

Action: Causes bronchodilation by action on β_2 receptors with increased synthesis of cAMP; relaxes bronchial smooth muscle; inhibits mast cell degranulation; stimulates cilia to remove secretions with very little effect on heart rate
Uses: Asthma, bronchospasm
Dosage and routes:
• *Adult and child >12 yr:* INH 2 puffs, wait 1-3 min before 3rd puff if needed, not to exceed 3 INH q6h or 2 INH q4h
Available forms: Aerosol 0.37 mg/actuation, 0.02% neb sol
Side effects/adverse reactions:
CNS: Tremors, anxiety, insomnia, headache, dizziness, stimulation, restlessness, hallucinations

EENT: Dry nose, irritation of nose and throat
CV: Palpitations, tachycardia, hypertension, angina, hypotension
GI: Heartburn, nausea, vomiting, anorexia
MS: Muscle cramps
*RESP: **Bronchospasm**,* dyspnea
Contraindications: Hypersensitivity to sympathomimetics
Precautions: Lactation, pregnancy (C), cardiac disorders, hyperthyroidism, diabetes mellitus
Pharmacokinetics:
INH: Onset 3 min, peak ½-1 hr, duration 5-8 hr
Interactions/incompatibilities:
• Increased action of aerosol bronchodilators
• Increased action of bitolterol: tricyclic antidepressants, MAOIs
• May inhibit action when used with other β-blockers
NURSING CONSIDERATIONS
Assess:
• Respiratory function: vital capacity, forced expiratory volume, ABGs
Administer:
• After shaking, exhale, place mouthpiece in mouth, inhale slowly, hold breath, remove, exhale slowly
• Gum, sips of water for dry mouth
Perform/provide:
• Storage in light-resistant container, do not expose to temperatures over 86° F (30° C)
Evaluate:
• Therapeutic response: absence of dyspnea, wheezing over 1 hr
Teach patient/family:
• Not to use OTC medications; extra stimulation may occur
• To use inhaler; review package insert with patient
• To avoid getting aerosol in eyes

---

italics = common side effects   ***bold italic*** = life threatening reactions

• To wash inhaler in warm water and dry qd
• On all aspects of drug; avoid smoking, smoke-filled rooms, persons with respiratory infections
Treatment of overdose: Administer a β_2 adrenergic blocker

---

bleomycin sulfate
(blee-oh-mye'sin)
Blenoxane
Func. class.: Antineoplastic, antibiotic
Chem. class.: Glycopeptide

Action: Inhibits synthesis of DNA, RNA, protein; derived from *Streptomyces verticillus;* replication is decreased by binding to DNA, which causes strand splitting; phase specific in the G_2 and M phases; a nonvesicant

Uses: Cancer of head, neck, penis, cervix, vulva of squamous cell origin, Hodgkin's disease, lymphosarcoma, reticulum cell sarcoma, testicular carcinoma

Dosage and routes:
• *Adult:* SC/IV/IM 0.25-0.5 U/kg 1-2 × /wk or 10-20 U/m², then 1 U/day or 5 U/wk; may also be given intraarterially; do not exceed total dose, 400 U in lifetime
Available forms: Inj IV, SC, IM, IA, intralesional, intracavity 5 units

Side effects/adverse reactions:
*SYST: **Anaphylaxis***
GI: Nausea, vomiting, anorexia, stomatitis, weight loss
INTEG: Rash, hyperkeratosis, nail changes, alopecia, fever and chills
*RESP: **Fibrosis**, pneumonitis, wheezing, **pulmonary toxicity***
CNS: Fever, chills
IDIOSYNCRATIC REACTION: Hypotension, confusion, fever, chills, wheezing

Contraindications: Hypersensitivity
Precautions: Renal, hepatic, respiratory disease, pregnancy (D)
Pharmacokinetics: Half-life 2 hr when CrCl >35 ml/min half-life is increased in lower clearance, metabolized in liver, 50% excreted in urine (unchanged)

Interactions/incompatibilities:
• Increased toxicity: other antineoplastics or radiation therapy
• Decreased serum digoxin levels: digoxin
• Incompatible with aminophylline, diazepam, furosemide, amino acid sol, Vit C

NURSING CONSIDERATIONS
Assess:
• IM test dose
• Pulmonary function tests: chest x-ray film before and during therapy; should be obtained q2wk during treatment
• Temperature q4h; fever may indicate beginning infection
• Serum creatinine
• Dyspnea, rales, unproductive cough, chest pain, tachypnea, fatigue, increased pulse, pallor, lethargy
• Food preferences; list likes, dislikes
• Effects of alopecia and skin color on body image; discuss feelings about body changes
• Buccal cavity q8h for dryness, sores, ulceration, white patches, oral pain, bleeding, dysphagia
• Local irritation, pain, burning, discoloration at injection site
• Symptoms indicating severe allergic reaction: rash, pruritus, urticaria, purpuric skin lesions, itching, flushing
• Storage for 2 wk after reconstituting at room temperature; discard unused portions

---

*Available in Canada only

Administer:

• IM/SC after reconstituting 5 U/ 1-5 ml sterile H_2O, D_5W, 0.9% NaCl, or bacteriostatic water for inj; do not use products containing benzyl alcohol when giving to neonates

• Direct IV after reconstituting 15 U or less/5 ml or more of D_5W or 0.9% NaCl; after further diluting with 50-100 ml D_5W or 0.9% NaCl, give 15 U or less/10 min through Y-tube or 3-way stopcock

• Two test doses 2-5 U before initial dose; monitor for anaphylaxis

• Antiemetic 30-60 min before giving drug to prevent vomiting, continue antiemetics 6-10 hr after treatment

• Topical or systemic analgesics for pain of stomatitis as ordered; antihistamines and antipyretics for fever and chills

• Intraarterial/IV injections over >10 min

Perform/provide:

• Deep breathing exercises with patient tid-qid; place in semi-Fowler's position

• Liquid diet: carbonated beverage; gelatin may be added if patient is not nauseated or vomiting

• Rinsing of mouth tid-qid with water, club soda; brushing of teeth with baking soda bid-tid with soft brush or cotton-tipped applicators for stomatitis; use unwaxed dental floss

• HOB raised to facilitate breathing

Evaluate:

• Therapeutic response: decrease in size of tumor

Teach patient/family:

• To report any complaints, side effects to nurse or physician

• To report any changes in breathing, coughing, fever

• That hair may be lost during treatment and wig or hairpiece may make patient feel better; tell patient that new hair may be different in color, texture

• To avoid foods with citric acid, hot or rough texture

• To report any bleeding, white spots, ulcerations in mouth; to examine mouth qd and report symptoms

---

bretylium tosylate
(bre-til′ee-um)
Bretylate,* Bretylium Tosylate, Bretylol
Func. class.: Antidysrhythmic (Class III)
Chem. class.: Quaternary ammonium compound

Action: After a transient release of norepinephrine, inhibits further release by postganglionic nerve endings; prolongs action, potential duration and effective refractory period

Uses: Serious ventricular tachycardia, cardioversion, ventricular fibrillation; for short-term use only

Dosage and routes:

Severe ventricular fibrillation

• *Adult:* IV BOL 5 mg/kg, increase to 10 mg/kg repeated q15 min, up to 30 mg/kg; IV INF 1-2 mg/min or give 5-10 mg/kg over 10 min q6h (maintenance)

Ventricular dysrhythmias

• *Adult:* IV INF 500 mg diluted in 50 ml D_5W or NS, infuse over 10-30 min, may repeat in 1 hr, maintain with 1-2 mg/min or 5-10 mg/ kg over 10-30 min q6h; IM 5-10 mg/kg undiluted; repeat in 1-2 hr if needed; maintain with same dose q6-8h

Available forms: Inj IV 50 mg/ml; 1, 2, 4 mg/ml prefilled syringes

---

italics = common side effects   ***bold italic*** = life threatening reactions

Side effects/adverse reactions:
CNS: Syncope, dizziness, confusion, psychosis, anxiety
GI: Nausea, vomiting
CV: Hypotension, postural hypotension, bradycardia, angina, PVCs, substernal pressure, transient hypertension, precipitation of angina
*RESP: **Respiratory depression***
Contraindications: Hypersensitivity, digitalis toxicity, aortic stenosis, pulmonary hypertension, children
Precautions: Renal disease, pregnancy (C), lactation, children
Pharmacokinetics: Well absorbed by IM/IV routes
IV: Onset 5 min; duration 6-24 hr
IM: Onset ½-2 hr, duration 6-24 hr Half-life 4-17 hr, excreted unchanged by kidneys (70%-80% in 24 hr), not metabolized
Interactions/incompatibilities:
• Increased or decreased effects of bretylium: quinidine, procainamide, propranolol, other antidysrhythmics
• Hypotension: antihypertensives
• Toxicity: digitalis
• Incompatible with phenytoin
Lab test interferences:
Decrease: Urinary epinephrine, urinary norepinephrine, urinary VMA epinephrine
NURSING CONSIDERATIONS
Assess:
• ECG continuously to determine drug effectiveness, PVCs or other dysrhythmias
• IV inf rate to avoid causing nausea, vomiting
• For dehydration or hypovolemia
• B/P continuously for hypotension, hypertension; orthostatic hypotension; keep supine until hypotension subsides
• I&O ratio

• If systolic B/P <75 mm HG; notify physician
• For rebound hypertension after 1-2 hr
• Cardiac status: rate, rhythm, character, continuously
Administer:
• IV direct undiluted over 15-30 sec (ventricular fibrillation); may repeat in 15-30 mins, not to exceed 30 mg/kg/24 hour.
• IV INT INF by diluting 500 mg of drug/50 ml or more D₅W, 0.9% NaCl, D₅/0.45%, D₅/0.9% NaCl, D₅/Lr, LRONS, give over 15-30 min
• IV cont INF by diluting further; give at 1-2 mg diluted sol/min via infusion pump
• IM inj, rotate sites, inject <5 ml in any one site to prevent tissue necrosis, may repeat 1-2 hour
• Reduced dosage slowly with ECG monitoring, discontinue over 3-5 days, maintain on oral dysrhythmic
Perform/provide:
• Place patient in supine position unless otherwise ordered; assist with ambulation
• Have suction equipment available
Evaluate:
• Therapeutic response: absence of ventricular tachycardia, fibrillation
Teach patient/family:
• To make position changes slowly; orthostatic hypotension may occur
Treatment of overdose: O₂, artificial ventilation, ECG; administer dopamine for circulatory depression; administer diazepam or thiopental for convulsions

bromocriptine mesylate

(broe-moe-krip′teen)
Parlodel

Func. class.: Dopamine receptor agonist; ovulation stimulant
Chem. class.: Ergot alkaloid derivative

Action: Inhibits prolactin release by activating postsynaptic dopamine receptors; activation of striatal dopamine receptors may be reason for improvement in Parkinson's disease

Uses: Female infertility, Parkinson's disease, prevention of postpartum lactation, amenorrhea caused by hyperprolactinemia, acromegaly

Dosage and routes:

Hyperprolactinemic indications

• *Adult:* PO 1.25-2.5 mg with meals; may increase by 2.5 mg q3-7 days, usual 5-7.5 mg

Acromegaly

• *Adult:* PO 1.25-2.5 mg × 3 days hs; may increase by 1.25-2.5 mg q3-7 days; usual range 20-30 mg/day, max 100 mg/day

Postpartum lactation

• *Adult:* PO 2.5 mg qd-tid with meal × 14 or 21 days

Parkinson's disease

• *Adult:* PO 1.25 mg bid with meals, may increase q2-4 wk by 2.5 mg/day, not to exceed 100 mg qd

Available forms: Caps 5 mg; tabs 2.5 mg

Side effects/adverse reactions:

EENT: Blurred vision, diplopia, burning eyes, nasal congestion

CNS: Headache, depression, restlessness, anxiety, nervousness, confusion, ***convulsions,*** hallucinations, dizziness, fatigue, drowsiness, abnormal involuntary movements, psychosis

GU: Frequency, retention, incontinence, diuresis

GI: Nausea, vomiting, anorexia, cramps, constipation, diarrhea, dry mouth, GI hemorrhage

INTEG: Rash on face, arms, alopecia

CV: Orthostatic hypotension, decreased B/P, palpitation, extra systole, ***shock,*** dysrhythmias, bradycardia

Contraindications: Hypersensitivity to ergot, severe ischemic disease, pregnancy (D), severe peripheral vascular disease

Precautions: Lactation, hepatic disease, renal disease, children, pituitary tumors

Pharmacokinetics:

PO: Peak 1-3 hr, duration 4-8 hr, 90%-96% protein bound, half-life 3 hr, metabolized by liver (inactive metabolites), 85%-98% of dose excreted in feces

Interactions/incompatibilities:

• Decreased action of bromocriptine: phenothiazines, imipramine, haloperidol, droperidol, amitriptyline

• Increased action of antihypertensives

Lab test interferences:

Increase: Growth hormone, AST/ALT, CPK, BUN, uric acid, alk phosphatase, GGTP

NURSING CONSIDERATIONS

Assess:

• B/P; establish baseline, compare with other reading; this drug decreases B/P

Administer:

• With meal to prevent GI symptoms

• At hs so dizziness, orthostatic hypotension do not occur

---

italics = common side effects   ***bold italic*** = life threatening reactions

Perform/provide:
• Storage at room temperature in tight container
Evaluate:
• Therapeutic response (Parkinson's disease): decreased dyskinesia, decreased slow movements, decreased drooling
Teach patient/family:
• To change position slowly, to prevent orthostatic hypotension
• To use contraceptives during treatment with this drug; pregnancy may occur; to use methods other than oral contraceptives
• That therapeutic effect for Parkinson's disease may take 2 mo: galactorrhea, amenorrhea
• To avoid hazardous activity if dizziness occurs

---

brompheniramine maleate

(brome-fen-ir′a-meen)
Bromphen, Brompheniramine, Codimal-A, Cophene-B, Dehist, Diamine T.D., Dimetane, Dimetane Extentabs, Histaject, ND Stat, Nasahist-B, Oraminic II, Veltane

Func. class.: Antihistamine
Chem. class.: Alkylamine, H_1-receptor antagonist

Action: Acts on blood vessels, GI, respiratory system by competing with histamine for H_1-receptor site; decreases allergic response by blocking histamine
Uses: Allergy symptoms, rhinitis
Dosage and routes:
• *Adult:* PO 4-8 mg tid-qid, not to exceed 36 mg/day; TIME REL 8-12 mg bid-tid, not to exceed 36 mg/day; IM/IV/SC 5-20 mg q6-12h, not to exceed 40 mg/day
• *Child >6 yr:* PO 2 mg tid-qid,

not to exceed 12 mg/day; IM/IV/SC 0.5 mg/kg/day divided tid or qid
• *Child <6 yr:* Only as directed by physician
Available forms: Tabs 4 mg; tabs, time rel 8, 12 mg; elix 2 mg/5 ml; inj IM/SC/IV 10, 100 mg/ml
Side effects/adverse reactions:
CNS: Dizziness, drowsiness, poor coordination, fatigue, anxiety, euphoria, confusion, paresthesia, neuritis
CV: Hypotension, palpitations, tachycardia
RESP: Increased thick secretions, wheezing, chest tightness
*HEMA: **Thrombocytopenia, agranulocytosis, hemolytic anemia***
GI: Dry mouth, nausea, vomiting, anorexia, constipation, diarrhea
INTEG: Photosensitivity
GU: Retention, dysuria, frequency, impotence
EENT: Blurred vision, dilated pupils, tinnitus, nasal stuffiness, dry nose, throat, mouth
Contraindications: Hypersensitivity to H_1-receptor antagonists, acute asthma attack, lower respiratory tract disease, child <6 yr
Precautions: Increased intraocular pressure, renal disease, cardiac disease, hypertension, bronchial asthma, seizure disorder, stenosed peptic ulcers, hyperthyroidism, prostatic hypertrophy, bladder neck obstruction, pregnancy (C)
Pharmacokinetics:
PO: Peak 2-5 hr, duration to 48 hr; metabolized in liver, excreted by kidneys, excreted in breast milk, half-life 12-34 hr
Interactions/incompatibilities:
• Increased CNS depression: barbiturates, narcotics, hypnotics, tricyclic antidepressants, alcohol

• Decreased effect of oral antico-agulants, heparin
• Increased drying effect: MAOIs
• Incompatible with aminophyl-line, insulins, pentobarbital
Lab test interferences:
False negative: Skin allergy tests
NURSING CONSIDERATIONS
Assess:
• I&O ratio; be alert for urinary re-tention, frequency, dysuria; drug should be discontinued if these occur
• CBC during long-term therapy
• Blood dyscrasias: thrombocyto-penia, agranulocytosis (rare)
• Respiratory status: rate, rhythm, increase in bronchial secretions, wheezing, chest tightness
Administer:
• Direct IV undiluted or diluted with 10 ml 0.9% NaCl, given over 1 min or more
• IV INF by diluting in D₅W, 0.9% NaCl given at prescribed rate
• With meals if GI symptoms oc-cur; absorption may slightly de-crease
Perform/provide:
• Hard candy, gum, frequent rins-ing of mouth for dryness
• Storage in tight container at room temperature
Evaluate:
• Therapeutic response: absence of running or congested nose or rashes
Teach patient/family:
• Not to crush or chew sustained release forms
• All aspects of drug use; to notify physician if confusion/sedation/hypotension occurs
• To avoid driving or other hazard-ous activities if drowsiness occurs
• To avoid use of alcohol or other CNS depressants while taking drug
Treatment of overdose: Admin-ister ipecac syrup or lavage, diaz-

epam, vasopressors, barbiturates (short-acting)

B

buclizine HCl
(byoo'kli-zeen)
Bucladin-S, Softabs
Func. class.: Antiemetic, antihistamine, anticholiner-gic
Chem. class.: H₁-receptor antagonist (piperazine)

Action: Acts centrally by blocking chemoreceptor trigger zone, which in turn acts on vomiting center
Uses: Motion sickness, dizziness, nausea, vomiting
Dosage and routes:
• *Adult:* PO 25-50 mg prn ½ hr before travel; may be repeated q4-6h prn
Available forms: Tabs 50 mg
Side effects/adverse reactions:
CNS: Drowsiness, dizziness, fa-tigue, restlessness, headache, in-somnia
GI: Nausea, anorexia, bitterness
EENT: Dry mouth, blurred vision
Contraindications: Hypersensitiv-ity to cyclizines, shock
Precautions: Children, narrow-angle glaucoma, lactation, pros-tatic hypertrophy, elderly, preg-nancy (C)
Pharmacokinetics:
PO: Duration 4-6 hr; other phar-macokinetics not known
NURSING CONSIDERATIONS
Assess:
• VS, B/P
• Signs of toxicity of other drugs or masking of symptoms of disease: brain tumor, intestinal obstruction
• Drowsiness, dizziness
Administer:
• Tablets may be swallowed whole, chewed, or allowed to dissolve

italics = common side effects   ***bold italic*** = life threatening reactions

Evaluate:
• Therapeutic response: absence of dizziness, nausea, vomiting
Teach patient/family:
• To avoid hazardous activities or activities requiring alertness; dizziness may occur; instruct patient to request assistance with ambulation
• To avoid alcohol, other depressants

---

bumetanide
(byoo-met'a-nide)
Bumex
Func. class.: Loop diuretic
Chem. class.: Sulfonamide derivative

Action: Acts on ascending loop of Henle by increasing excretion of chloride, sodium
Uses: Edema in CHF, liver disease, renal disease (nephrotic syndrome), pulmonary edema, ascites (nephrotic syndrome), hypertension, anasarca
Dosage and routes:
• *Adult:* PO 0.5-2.0 mg qd; may give 2nd or 3rd dose at 4-5 hr intervals, not to exceed 20 mg/day; may be given on alternate days or intermittently; IV/IM 0.5-1.0 mg/day; may give 2nd or 3rd dose at 2-3 hr intervals, not to exceed 20 mg/day
• *Child:* PO, IM, IV 0.02-0.1 mg/kg q12hr
Available forms: Tabs 0.5, 1, 2 mg; inj IV, IM 0.25 mg/ml
Side effects/adverse reactions:
GU: Polyuria, **renal failure,** glycosuria
ELECT: Hypokalemia, hypochloremic alkalosis, hypomagnesemia, hyperuricemia, hypocalcemia, hyponatremia, hyperglycemia

CNS: Headache, fatigue, weakness, vertigo
GI: Nausea, diarrhea, dry mouth, vomiting, anorexia, cramps, upset stomach, abdominal pain, *acute pancreatitis, jaundice*
EENT: **Loss of hearing,** ear pain, tinnitus, blurred vision
INTEG: Rash, pruritus, purpura, **Stevens-Johnson syndrome,** sweating, photosensitivity
MS: Muscular cramps, arthritis, stiffness, tenderness
ENDO: Hyperglycemia
HEMA: **Thrombocytopenia, agranulocytosis, neutropenia**
CV: **Chest pain,** hypotension, **circulatory collapse,** ECG changes
Contraindications: Hypersensitivity to sulfonamides, anuria, hepatic coma, hypovolemia, lactation
Precautions: Dehydration, ascites, severe renal disease, pregnancy (C), hepatic cirrhosis
Pharmacokinetics:
PO: Onset ½-1 hr, duration 4 hr
IM: Onset 40 min, duration 4 hr
IV: Onset 5 min, duration 2-3 hr, Excreted by kidneys, crosses placenta, excreted by breast milk
Interactions/incompatibilities:
• Decreased diuretic effect: indomethacin, NSAIDs
• Ototoxicity: cisplatin, aminoglycosides, vancomycin
• Increased effect: antihypertensives
• Increased toxicity: lithium, nondepolarizing skeletal muscle relaxants, digitalis
• Decreased effects of antidiabetics
• Incompatible with dobutamine, milrinone
NURSING CONSIDERATIONS
Assess:
• Hearing with high IV doses
• Weight, I&O daily to determine

---

fluid loss; effect of drug may be decreased if used qd
• Rate, depth, rhythm of respiration, effect of exertion
• B/P lying, standing; postural hypotension may occur
• Electrolytes: potassium, sodium, chloride; include BUN, blood sugar, CBC, serum creatinine, blood pH, ABGs, uric acid, calcium, magnesium
• Glucose in urine if patient is diabetic
• Improvement in edema of feet, legs, sacral area daily if medication is being used in CHF
• Improvement in CVP q8h
• Signs of metabolic alkalosis: drowsiness, restlessness
• Signs of hypokalemia: postural hypotension, malaise, fatigue, tachycardia, leg cramps, weakness
• Rashes, temperature elevation qd
• Confusion, especially in elderly; take safety precautions if needed
Administer:
• Direct IV undiluted over at least 1 min through Y-tube or 3-way stopcock or heplock
• INT IV after dilution in LR, D₅W, 0.9% NaCl (rarely given by this method)
• In AM to avoid interference with sleep if using drug as a diuretic
• Potassium replacement if potassium is less than 3.0
• With food if nausea occurs; absorption may be decreased slightly
Evaluate:
• Therapeutic response: decreased edema, B/P
Teach patient/family:
• To increase fluid intake to 2-3 L/ day unless contraindicated, to take Vit K supplement, to rise slowly from lying or sitting position
• Adverse reactions: muscle cramps, weakness, nausea, dizziness
• To take with food or milk for GI symptoms
• To take early in day to prevent nocturia
• To use sunscreen to prevent photosensitivity
Treatment of overdose: Lavage if taken orally; monitor electrolytes; administer dextrose in saline; monitor hydration, CV, renal status

---

bupivacaine HCl
(byoop-a-va′caine)
Bupivacaine HCl, Marcaine HCl, Marcaine Spinal, Sensorcaine
Func. class.: Local anesthetic
Chem. class.: Amide

Action: Competes with calcium for sites in nerve membrane that control sodium transport across cell membrane; decreases rise of depolarization phase of action potential
Uses: Epidural anesthesia, peripheral nerve block, caudal anesthesia
Dosage and routes:
Varies with route of anesthesia
Available forms: Inj 0.25%, 0.5%, 0.75%; inj with epinephrine 0.25%, 0.5%, 0.75%
Side effects/adverse reactions:
CNS: Anxiety, restlessness, *convulsions, loss of consciousness,* drowsiness, disorientation, tremors, shivering
CV: Myocardial depression, cardiac arrest, dysrhythmias, bradycardia, hypotension, hypertension, fetal bradycardia
GI: Nausea, vomiting
EENT: Blurred vision, tinnitus, pupil constriction
INTEG: Rash, urticaria, allergic re-

---

italics = common side effects   ***bold italic*** = life threatening reactions

actions, edema, burning, skin discoloration at injection site, tissue necrosis

*RESP: **Status asthmaticus, respiratory arrest, anaphylaxis***

Contraindications: Hypersensitivity, child <12 yr, elderly, severe liver disease

Precautions: Elderly, severe drug allergies, pregnancy (C)

Pharmacokinetics: Onset 4-17 min, duration 4-8 hr; excreted in urine (metabolites); metabolized by liver

Interactions/incompatibilities:
- Dysrhythmias: epinephrine, halothane, enflurane
- Hypertension: MAOIs, tricyclic antidepressants, phenothiazines
- Decreased action of bupivacaine: chloroprocaine

NURSING CONSIDERATIONS
Assess:
- B/P, pulse, respiration during treatment
- Fetal heart tones if drug is used during labor
- Allergic reactions: rash, urticaria, itching
- Cardiac status: ECG for dysrhythmias, pulse, B/P during anesthesia

Administer:
- Only with crash cart, resuscitative equipment nearby
- Only drugs without preservatives for epidural or caudal anesthesia

Perform/provide:
- Use of new solution, discard unused portions

Evaluate:
- Therapeutic response: anesthesia necessary for procedure

Treatment of overdose: Airway, O_2, vasopressor, IV fluids, anticonvulsants for seizures

---

buprenorphine HCl
(byoo-preen′or-feen)
Buprenex
Func. class.: Narcotic analgesic
Chem. class.: Opiate, thebaine derivative

Controlled Substance Schedule V
Action: Depresses pain impulse transmission at the spinal cord level by interacting with opioid receptors
Uses: Moderate to severe pain
Dosage and routes:
- *Adult:* IM/IV 0.3-0.6 mg q6h prn, reduce dosage in elderly
Available forms: Inj IM, IV 1, 2 mg/ml, 0.3 mg/ml (1 ml vials)
Side effects/adverse reactions:
CNS: Drowsiness, dizziness, confusion, headache, sedation, euphoria
GI: Nausea, vomiting, anorexia, constipation, cramps
GU: Increased urinary output, dysuria
INTEG: Rash, urticaria, bruising, flushing, diaphoresis, pruritus
EENT: Tinnitus, blurred vision, miosis, diplopia
CV: Palpitations, bradycardia, change in B/P
*RESP: **Respiratory depression***
Contraindications: Hypersensitivity, addiction (narcotic)
Precautions: Addictive personality, pregnancy (C), lactation, increased intracranial pressure, MI (acute), severe heart disease, respiratory depression, hepatic disease, renal disease
Pharmacokinetics:
IM: Onset 10-30 min, peak ½ hr, duration 3-4 hr
IV: Onset 1 min, peak 5 min, duration 2-5 hr

REC: Onset slow, duration 4-6 hr; metabolized by liver; excreted by kidneys; crosses placenta; excreted in breast milk; half-life 2½-3½ hr; 96% bound to plasma proteins

Interactions/incompatibilities:

• Effects may be increased with other CNS depressants: alcohol, narcotics, sedative/hypnotics, antipsychotics, skeletal muscle relaxants

• Incompatible with diazepam, lorazepam, alcohol sol

NURSING CONSIDERATIONS
Assess:

• I&O ratio; check for decreasing output; may indicate urinary retention

• CNS changes, dizziness, drowsiness, hallucinations, euphoria, LOC, pupil reaction

• Allergic reactions: rash, urticaria

• Respiratory dysfunction: respiratory depression, character, rate, rhythm; notify physician if respirations are <12/min

• Need for pain medication, physical dependence

Administer:

• IV undiluted over 3-5 min, titrate to patient response

• With antiemetic if nausea, vomiting occur

• When pain is beginning to return; determine dosage interval by patient response

Perform/provide:

• Assistance with ambulation

• Safety measures: side rails

Evaluate:

• Therapeutic response: decrease in pain, absence of grimacing

Teach patient/family:

• To report any symptoms of CNS changes, allergic reactions

• That physical dependency may result when used for extended periods

italics = common side effects

Treatment of overdose: Naloxone HCl (Narcan) 0.2-0.8 mg IV, O₂, IV fluids, vasopressors

bupropion
(byoo-proe′ pee-on)
Wellbutrin
Func. class.: Misc. antidepressant

Action: Inhibits reuptake of dopamine, serotonin, norepinephrine
Uses: Depression
Dosage and routes:
Adult: PO 100 mg bid initially, then increase after 3 days to 100 mg tid if needed; may increase after 1 month to 150 mg tid
Available forms: 75, 100 mg
Side effects/adverse reactions:
*CNS: Headache, agitation, confusion, **seizures**, akathisia, delusions, insomnia, sedation, tremors*
CV: Dysrhythmias, hypertension, palpitations, tachycardia, hypotension
GI: Nausea, vomiting, dry mouth, increased appetite, constipation
GU: Impotence, frequency, retention
INTEG: Rash, pruritus, sweating
EENT: Blurred vision, auditory disturbance
Contraindications: Hypersensitivity, seizure disorder, eating disorders
Precautions: Renal and hepatic disease, recent MI, cranial trauma, pregnancy (B), lactation, children
Pharmacokinetics: Onset 2-4 wk, half-life 12-14 hr; metabolized by liver
Interactions/incompatibilities:
• Increased adverse reactions: levodopa, MAOIs, phenothiazines, tricyclic antidepressants, benzodiazepines, alcohol

bold italic = life threatening reactions

NURSING CONSIDERATIONS
Assess:
• Blood studies: CBC, leukocytes, differential, cardiac enzymes if patient is on long-term therapy
• Liver function tests before, during therapy: bilirubin, AST, ALT
• ECG: watch for flattening of T wave, bundle branch block, AV block, dysrhythmias in cardiac patients
• Mental status: mood sensorium, affect, suicidal tendencies, increase in psychiatric symptoms
• EPS primarily in elderly: akathisia
• Withdrawal symptoms: headache, nausea, vomiting, muscle pain, weakness if drug is discontinued abruptly
• Alcohol consumption: if alcohol is consumed, hold dose until morning

Administer:
• Increased fluids, bulk in diet if constipation occurs
• With food or milk for GI symptoms
• Gum, hard candy, or frequent sips of water for dry mouth

Perform/provide:
• Assistance with ambulation during beginning therapy, since sedation occurs
• Safety measures, including side rails, primarily in elderly
• Checking to see PO medication is swallowed

Evaluate:
• Therapeutic response: decreased depression, ability to function in daily activities, ability to sleep throughout the night

Teach patient/family:
• Therapeutic effects may take 2-4 wk
• To use caution in driving or other activities requiring alertness; sedation and blurred vision may occur
• To avoid alcohol ingestion, other CNS depressants
• Not to discontinue medication quickly after long-term use; may cause nausea, headache, malaise

Treatment of overdose: ECG monitoring; induce emesis, lavage, activated charcoal; administer anticonvulsant

buspirone HCl
(byoo-spear′own)
BuSpar
Func. class.: Antianxiety agent
Chem. class.: Azaspirodeca-nedione

Action: Acts by inhibiting the action of serotonin (5-HT)
Uses: Management and short-term relief of anxiety disorders
Dosage and routes:
• *Adult:* PO 5 mg tid; may increase by 5 mg/day q2-3d, not to exceed 60 mg/day
Available forms: Tabs 5, 10 mg
Side effects/adverse reactions:
CNS: Dizziness, headache, depression, stimulation, insomnia, nervousness, light-headedness, numbness, paresthesia, incoordination, tremors, excitement, involuntary movements, confusion, akathisia
GI: Nausea, dry mouth, diarrhea, constipation, flatulence, increased appetite, rectal bleeding
CV: Tachycardia, palpitations, hypotension, hypertension, *CVA, CHF, MI*
EENT: Sore throat, tinnitus, blurred vision, nasal congestion, red, itching eyes, change in taste, smell
*GU: Frequency, hesitancy, menstrual irregularity, change in libido

MS: Pain, weakness, muscle cramps, spasms
RESP: Hyperventilation, chest congestion, shortness of breath
INTEG: Rash, edema, pruritus, alopecia, dry skin
MISC: Sweating, fatigue, weight gain, fever

Contraindications: Hypersensitivity, child <18 yr

Precautions: Pregnancy (B), lactation, elderly, impaired hepatic/renal function

Interactions/incompatibilities:
• Increased B/P: MAOIs; do not use together
• Increased effects: psychotropic drugs, alcohol (avoid use)
• Increased ALT: trazodone

NURSING CONSIDERATIONS
Assess:
• B/P (lying, standing), pulse; if systolic B/P drops 20 mm Hg, hold drug, notify physician
• Blood studies: CBC during long-term therapy; blood dyscrasias have occurred rarely
• Hepatic studies: AST, ALT, bilirubin, creatinine, LDH, alk phosphatase
• I&O; may indicate renal dysfunction
• Mental status: mood, sensorium, affect, sleeping pattern, drowsiness, dizziness
• Suicidal tendencies

Administer:
• With food or milk for GI symptoms
• Crushed if patient unable to swallow medication whole
• Sugarless gum, hard candy, frequent sips of water for dry mouth

Perform/provide:
• Assistance with ambulation during beginning therapy; drowsiness, dizziness occur

• Safety measures, including side rails, if drowsiness occurs
• Check to see PO medication swallowed

Evaluate:
• Therapeutic response: decreased anxiety, restlessness, sleeplessness

Teach patient/family:
• That drug may be taken with food
• To avoid OTC preparations unless approved by physician
• To avoid driving, activities requiring alertness, since drowsiness may occur
• To avoid alcohol ingestion or other psychotropic medications, unless prescribed by physician
• Not to discontinue medication abruptly after long-term use
• To rise slowly or fainting may occur, especially elderly
• That drowsiness may worsen at beginning of treatment
• That 1-2 wk of therapy may be required before therapeutic effects occur

Treatment of overdose: Gastric lavage, VS, supportive care

---

busulfan
(byoo-sul'fan)
Myleran
Func. class.: Antineoplastic alkylating agent
Chem. class.: Nitrosurea

Action: Changes essential cellular ions to covalent bonding with resultant alkylation; this interferes with normal biologic function of DNA; activity is not phase specific; action is due to myelosuppression
Uses: Chronic myelocytic leukemia

Dosage and routes:
• *Adult:* PO 4-12 mg/day initially until WBC levels fall to 10,000/

---

italics = common side effects   ***bold italic*** = life threatening reactions

mm³, then drug is stopped until WBC levels raise over 50,000/mm³, then 1-3 mg/day
• *Child:* PO 0.06-0.12 mg/kg or 1.8-4.6 mg/m² day; dose is titrated to maintain WBC levels at 20,000/mm³

Available forms: Tab 2 mg

Side effects/adverse reactions:

*HEMA: **Thrombocytopenia, leukopenia, pancytopenia, severe bone marrow depression***

GI: Nausea, vomiting, *diarrhea, weight loss*

GU: Impotence, sterility, amenorrhea, gynecomastia, *renal toxicity,* hyperuremia, adrenal insufficiency-like syndrome

INTEG: Dermatitis, hyperpigmentation, alopecia

*RESP: **Irreversible pulmonary fibrosis,** pneumonitis*

*OTHER: **Chromosomal aberrations***

Contraindications: Radiation, chemotherapy, lactation, pregnancy (3rd trimester) (D), "blastic" phase of chronic myelocytic leukemia, hypersensitivity

Precautions: Childbearing age men and women, leukopenia, thrombocytopenia, anemia, hepatotoxicity, renal toxicity

Pharmacokinetics: Well absorbed orally; excreted in urine; crosses placenta; excreted in breast milk

Interactions/incompatibilities:
Increased toxicity: other antineoplastics or radiation

NURSING CONSIDERATIONS
Assess:
• CBC, differential, platelet count weekly; withhold drug if WBC is <4000 or platelet count is <75,000; notify physician of results
• Pulmonary function tests, chest x-ray films before, during therapy;

chest film should be obtained q2wk during treatment
• Renal function studies: BUN, serum uric acid, urine CrCl before, during therapy
• I&O ratio; report fall in urine output of 30 ml/hr
• Monitor for cold, fever, sore throat (may indicate beginning infection)
• For decreased hyperuricemia
• Bleeding: hematuria, guaiac, bruising or petechiae, mucosa or orifices q8h, no rectal temps
• Dyspnea, rales, unproductive cough, chest pain, tachypnea
• Food preferences; list likes, dislikes
• Edema in feet, joint, stomach pain, shaking
• Inflammation of mucosa, breaks in skin; use viscous xylocaine for oral pain

Administer:
• Antacid before oral agent, give drug after evening meal, before bedtime
• Antiemetic 30-60 min before giving drug to prevent vomiting
• Allopurinol or sodium bicarbonate to maintain uric acid levels, alkalinization of urine
• Antibiotics for prophylaxis of infection

Perform/provide:
• Comprehensive oral hygiene
• Strict medical asepsis, protective isolation if WBC levels are low
• Deep breathing exercises with patient tid-qid; place in semi-Fowler's position for pulmonary reactions
• Increase fluid intake to 2-3 L/day to prevent urate deposits, calculi formation
• Diet low in purines: organ meats (kidney, liver), dried beans, peas to maintain alkaline urine
• Storage in tight container

Evaluate:
• Therapeutic response: decreased exacerbations of chronic myelocytic leukemia

Teach patient/family:
• About protective isolation precautions
• To avoid use of products containing aspirin or ibuprofen, razors, commercial mouthwash
• To report signs of anemia, (fatigue, headache, irritability, faintness, shortness of breath)
• To report symptoms of bleeding (hematuria, tarry stools)
• That impotence or amenorrhea can occur, are reversible after discontinuing treatment
• To report any changes in breathing or coughing even several months after treatment

---

butoconazole nitrate
(byoo'toe-kone-a-zole)
Femstat
Func. class.: Local antiinfective
Chem. class.: Antifungal

Action: Binds sterols in fungal cell membrane, which increases permeability
Uses: Vulvovaginal infections caused by *Candida*
Dosage and routes:
• *Adult:* INTRA VAG 1 applicatorful hs × 3 days (nonpregnant), 6 days (2nd/3rd trimester pregnancy)
Available forms: Vaginal cream 2%
Side effects/adverse reactions:
GU: Rash, stinging, burning, vulvovaginal itching, soreness, swelling, discharge, finger itching
Contraindications: Hypersensitivity
Precautions: Pregnancy (C), lactation

NURSING CONSIDERATIONS
Assess:
• Allergic reaction: burning, stinging, itching, discharge, soreness
Administer:
• 1 applicatorful every night into vagina
Perform/provide:
• Storage at room temperature in dry place
Evaluate:
• Therapeutic response: decrease in itching or white discharge
Teach patient/family:
• To use medical asepsis (hand washing) before, after each application
• That increased dreaming may occur
• To apply with applicator only
• To avoid use of any other vaginal product unless directed by physician; sanitary napkin may prevent soiling of undergarments
• To abstain from sexual intercourse until treatment is completed
• To notify physician if symptoms persist

---

butorphanol tartrate
(byoo-tor'fa-nole)
Stadol
Func. class.: Narcotic analgesics
Chem. class.: Opiate

Action: Depresses pain impulse transmission at the spinal cord level by interacting with opioid receptors
Uses: Moderate to severe pain
Dosage and routes:
• *Adult:* IM 1-4 mg q3-4h prn; IV 0.5-2 mg q3-4h prn
Available forms: Inj IM, IV 1, 2 mg/ml
Side effects/adverse reactions:
CNS: Drowsiness, dizziness, con-

italics = common side effects   ***bold italic*** = life threatening reactions

fusion, headache, sedation, euphoria, weakness, hallucinations
GI: Nausea, vomiting, anorexia, constipation, cramps
GU: Increased urinary output, dysuria, urinary retention
INTEG: Rash, urticaria, bruising, flushing, diaphoresis, pruritus
EENT: Tinnitus, blurred vision, miosis, diplopia
CV: Palpitations, bradycardia, change in B/P
*RESP: **Respiratory depression,** pulmonary hypertension*

Contraindications: Hypersensitivity, addiction (narcotic), CHF, myocardial infarction

Precautions: Addictive personality, pregnancy (B), lactation, increased intracranial pressure, respiratory depression, hepatic disease, renal disease, child <18 yr

Pharmacokinetics:
IM: Onset 10-30 min, peak ½ hr, duration 3-4 hr
IV: Onset 1 min, peak 5 min, duration 2-4 hr
REC: Onset slow, duration 4-6 hr; metabolized by liver; excreted by kidneys; crosses placenta; excreted in breast milk; half-life 2½-3½ hr

Interactions/incompatibilities:
• Effects may be increased with other CNS depressants: alcohol, narcotics, sedative/hypnotics, antipsychotics, skeletal muscle relaxants
• Incompatible with barbiturates

Lab test interferences:
Increase: Amylase

NURSING CONSIDERATIONS
Assess:
• I&O ratio; check for decreasing output; may indicate urinary retention
• For withdrawal symptoms in narcotic dependent patients: pulmonary embolus, vascular occlusion, abscesses, ulcerations
• CNS changes: dizziness, drowsiness, hallucinations, euphoria, LOC, pupil reaction
• Allergic reactions: rash, urticaria
• Respiratory dysfunction: respiratory depression, character, rate, rhythm; notify physician if respirations are <10/min
• Need for pain medication, physical dependence

Administer:
• IV undiluted at a rate of ≤2 mg/>3-5 min, titrate to patient response
• IM deeply in large muscle mass
• With antiemetic if nausea, vomiting occur
• When pain is beginning to return; determine dosage interval by patient response

Perform/provide:
• Storage in light-resistant area at room temperature
• Assistance with ambulation
• Safety measures: side rails, nightlight, call bell within easy reach, especially elderly

Evaluate:
• Therapeutic response: decrease in pain

Teach patient/family:
• To report any symptoms of CNS changes, allergic reactions
• That physical dependency may result when used for extended periods
• That withdrawal symptoms may occur: nausea, vomiting, cramps, fever, faintness, anorexia

Treatment of overdose: Naloxone HCl (Narcan) 0.2-0.8 mg IV, O₂, IV fluids, vasopressors

caffeine
(kaf-een)
Caffedrine, Caffeine, Citrated Caffeine, Dexitac, Nō-Dōz, Quick Pep, Tirend, Vivarin
Func. class.: Analeptic
Chem. class.: Xanthine

Action: Increases calcium permeability in sarcoplasmic reticulum; promotes accumulation of cAMP; competitively blocks adenosine receptors

Uses: Mild CNS stimulation in combination with analgesics, diuretics for tension and fluid retention associated with menstruation

Dosage and routes:
• *Adult:* PO 100-200 mg q4h prn; IM 500 mg; timed rel 200-250 mg q4-6h
Available forms: Tabs 65, 100, 150, 200 mg; time rel caps 200, 250 mg; inj 250 mg/ml, time rel tabs 200 mg

Side effects/adverse reactions:
CNS: Hyperactivity, insomnia, restlessness, talkativeness, dizziness, headache, *stimulation,* irritability, aggressiveness, tremors, twitching, mild delirium, tinnitus, scintillating scotoma
HEMA: Hypoglycemia
GI: Nausea, vomiting, anorexia, gastric irritation, diarrhea
GU: Diuresis
CV: Tachycardia, extrasystole, dysrhythmias, palpitations
INTEG: Hyperesthesia

Contraindications: Hypersensitivity

Precautions: Dysrhythmias, Gilles de la Tourette's disorder, pregnancy (B), lactation, renal, psychologic disorders, depression, ulcers, diabetes mellitus

Pharmacokinetics:
PO: Onset 15 min, peak ½-1 hr, metabolized by liver, less than 5% excreted unchanged by kidneys, crosses placenta, breast milk, half-life 3-4 hr

Interactions/incompatibilities:
• Increased effect of caffeine: oral contraceptives, cimetidine, disulfiram, ciprofloxacin, endoxacin, phenyl propanolamine

Lab test interferences:
Increase: Urinary cathecholamines
False positive: Serum urate

NURSING CONSIDERATIONS
Assess:
• VS, B/P
• Mental status: mood, sensorium, affect, stimulation, insomnia, irritability
• Tolerance or dependency: an increased amount may be used to get same effect
• Overdose: pain, fever, dehydration, insomnia, hyperactivity

Evaluate:
• Therapeutic response: increased CNS stimulation, decreased drowsiness

Teach patient/family:
• To decrease other caffeine consumption (coffee, tea, cola, chocolate), which may increase irritability, stimulation
• To taper off drug over several weeks if used long-term

Treatment of overdose: Lavage, activated charcoal, monitor electrolytes, VS, administer anticonvulsants if needed

calcifediol
(kal-si-fe-dye'ole)
Calderol
Func. class.: Vit D analog
Chem. class.: Sterol

Action: Increases intestinal absorp-

---

tion of calcium for bones; increases renal tubular absorption of phosphate; increases mobilization of calcium from bones, bone resorption

Uses: Metabolic bone disease with chronic renal failure, osteopenia, osteomalacia, hypocalcemia

Dosage and routes:

• *Adult:* PO 300-350 µg qwk divided into qd or qod doses; may increase q4wk

Available forms: Caps 20, 50 µg

Side effects/adverse reactions:

EENT: Tinnitus, conjunctivitis, photophobia, rhinorrhea

CNS: Drowsiness, headache, vertigo, fever, lethargy

GI: Nausea, diarrhea, vomiting, jaundice, anorexia, dry mouth, constipation, cramps, metallic taste

MS: Myalgia, arthralgia, decreased bone development

GU: Polyuria, hypercalciuria, hyperphosphatemia, hematuria

CV: dysrhythmias

Contraindications: Hypersensitivity, hyperphosphatemia, hypercalcemia, Vit D toxicity

Precautions: Pregnancy (C), renal calculi, lactation, CV disease

Pharmacokinetics:

PO: Peak 4 hr, duration 15-20 days; half-life 12-22 days

Interactions/incompatibilities:

• Decreased absorption of calcifediol: cholestyramine, colestipol HCl, mineral oil, fat-soluble vitamins

• Hypercalcemia: thiazide diuretics

• Cardiac dysrhythmias: cardiac glycosides

• Decreased effect of this drug: corticosteroids

Lab test interferences:

False increase: Cholesterol

NURSING CONSIDERATIONS

Assess:

• BUN, urinary calcium, AST,

ALT, cholesterol, creatinine, uric acid, chloride, magnesium, electrolytes, urine pH, phosphate; may increase; calcium should be kept at 9-10 mg/dl, vitamin D 50-135 IU/dl, phosphate 70 mg/dl

• Alk phosphatase; may be decreased

• For increased blood level, since toxic reactions may occur rapidly

• For dry mouth, metallic taste, polyuria, bone pain, muscle weakness, headache, fatigue, tinnitus, change in LOC, irregular pulse, dysrhythmias, increased respirations, anorexia, nausea, vomiting, cramps, diarrhea, constipation; may indicate hypercalcemia

• Renal status: decreased urinary output (oliguria, anuria), edema in extremities, weight gain 5 lb, periorbital edema

• Nutritional status, diet for sources of vitamin D (milk, some seafood), calcium (dairy products, dark green vegetables), phosphates (dairy products)

Administer:

• PO may be increased q4wk depending on blood level

Perform/provide:

• Storage in tight, light-resistant containers at room temperature

• Restriction of sodium, potassium if required

• Restriction of fluids if required for chronic renal failure

Evaluate:

• Therapeutic response: calcium levels 9-10 mg/dl, decreasing symptoms of bone disease

Teach patient/family:

• The symptoms of hypercalcemia

• About foods rich in calcium

calcitonin (human)

(kal-si-toe'nin)

Cibacalcin

Func. class.: Parathyroid agents (calcium regulator)

Chem. class.: Polypeptide hormone

Action: Decreases bone resorption, blood calcium levels; increases deposits of calcium in bones

Uses: Paget's disease

Dosage and routes:

Paget's disease

• *Adult:* SC 0.5 mg/day initially; may require 0.5 mg bid × 6 mo, then decrease until symptoms reappear

Available forms: Inj (SC) 0.5 mg/vial

Side effects/adverse reactions:

INTEG: Rash, flushing, pruritus of ear lobes, edema of feet

CNS: Headache, tetany, chills, weakness, dizziness

GU: Diuresis

GI: Nausea, diarrhea, vomiting, anorexia, abdominal pain, salty taste, epigastric pain

MS: Swelling, tingling of hands

CV: Chest pressure

RESP: Dyspnea

Contraindications: Hypersensitivity

Precautions: Renal disease, children, lactation, osteogenic sarcoma, pregnancy (C)

Pharmacokinetics:

IM/SC: Onset 15 min, peak 4 hr, duration 8-24 hr; metabolized by kidneys, excreted as inactive metabolites

NURSING CONSIDERATIONS

Assess:

• GI symptoms, polyuria, flushing, head swelling, tingling, headache; may indicate hypercalcemia

• Nutritional status; diet for sources of vitamin D (milk, some seafood), calcium (dairy products, dark green vegetables), phosphates

• BUN, creatinine, uric acid, chloride, electrolytes, urine pH, urinary calcium, magnesium, phosphate, urinalysis (calcium should be kept at 9-10 mg/dl, Vit D 50-135 IU/dl), alk phosphatase baseline and q3-6mo

• Increased drug level, since toxic reactions occur rapidly; have calcium chloride on hand if calcium level drops too low; check for tetany

• Urine for sediment

Administer:

• By SC route only; rotate injection sites; use within 6 hr of reconstitution; give hs to minimize nausea, vomiting

Perform/provide:

• Store at <77° F (25° C); protect from light

Evaluate:

• Therapeutic response: calcium levels 9-10 mg/dl, decreasing symptoms of Paget's disease

Teach patient/family:

• Method of injection if patient will be responsible for self-medication

calcitonin (salmon)

(kal-si-toe'nin)

Calcimar, Miacalcin

Func. class.: Parathyroid agents (calcium regulator)

Chem. class.: Polypeptide hormone

Action: Decreases bone resorption, blood calcium levels; increases deposits of calcium in bones

Uses: Hypercalcemia, postmenopausal osteoporosis, Paget's disease

---

italics = common side effects   ***bold italic*** = life threatening reactions

Dosage and routes:
Osteoporosis/Paget's disease
• *Adult:* SC/IM 100 IU qd, maintenance for Paget's disease 50-100 IU qd or qod
Hypercalcemia
• *Adult:* IM 4-8 IU/kg q6-12h
Available forms: Inj SC/IM 200 MRC units/ml, 100 IU/ml
Side effects/adverse reactions:
INTEG: Rash, pruritus of ear lobes, edema of feet
CNS: Headache, flushing, *tetany*, chills, weakness, dizziness
GU: Diuresis
GI: Nausea, diarrhea, vomiting, anorexia, abdominal pain, salty taste
MS: Swelling, tingling of hands
Contraindications: Hypersensitivity, children, lactation
Precautions: Renal disease, osteoporosis, pernicious anemia, Zollinger-Ellison syndrome, pregnancy (C)
Pharmacokinetics:
IM/SC: Onset 15 min, peak 4 hr, duration 8-24 hr; metabolized by kidneys, excreted as inactive metabolites

NURSING CONSIDERATIONS
Assess:
• BUN, creatinine, uric acid, chloride, electrolytes, urine pH, urinary calcium, magnesium, phosphatase, urinalysis, calcitonin antibody formation (calcium should be kept at 9-10 mg/dl, Vit D 50-135 IU/dl), alk phosphatase
• Increased level, since toxic reactions may occur rapidly
• Urine for sediment and casts
• History of allergies
• GI symptoms, polyuria, flushing, head swelling, tingling, headache; may indicate hypercalcemia
• Nutritional status; diet for sources of Vit D (milk, some seafood), cal-cium (dairy products, dark green vegetables), phosphates
• Systemic allergic reaction to drug: skin test before 1st dose
Administer:
• After test dose of 10 IU/ml, 0.1 ml intradermally; watch 15 min; give only with epinephrine and emergency meds available
• IM injection in deep muscle mass slowly; rotate sites
Perform/provide:
• Storage in light-resistant area; refrigerate
• Restriction of sodium, potassium if required
Evaluate:
• Therapeutic response: calcium 9-10 mg/dl, decreasing symptoms of bone disease
Teach patient/family:
• To avoid OTC products
• To administer drug SC if patient will be responsible for self-medication
• Report difficulty swallowing or change in side effects immediately to physician

calcitriol (1,25-Dihydroxycholecalciferol)
(kal-si-tyre'ole)
Calcimar, Rocaltrol
Func. class.: Parathyroid agents (calcium regulator)
Chem. class.: Vitamin D hormone

Action: Increases intestinal absorption of calcium, provides calcium for bones, increases renal tubular resorption of phosphate
Uses: Hypocalcemia in chronic renal disease, hypoparathyroidism, pseudohypoparathyroidism
Dosage and routes:
Hypocalcemia

• *Adult:* PO 0.25 µg qd, may increase by 0.25 µg/day q4-8wk, maintenance 0.25 µg qod-1 µg qd

Hypoparathyroidism/pseudohypoparathyroidism

• *Adult and child >1 yr:* PO 0.25 µg qd, may be increased q2-4wk; maintenance 0.25-2 µg qd

Available forms: Caps 0.25, 0.5 µg

Side effects/adverse reactions:

CNS: Drowsiness, headache, vertigo, fever, lethargy

GI: Nausea, diarrhea, vomiting, jaundice, anorexia, dry mouth, constipation, cramps, metallic taste

MS: Myalgia, arthralgia, decreased bone development

GU: Polyuria, hypercalciuria, hyperphosphatemia, hematuria

Contraindications: Hypersensitivity, hyperphosphatemia, hypercalcemia, Vit D toxicity

Precautions: Pregnancy (C), renal calculi, lactation, CV disease

Pharmacokinetics:

PO: Peak 4 hr, duration 15-20 days, half-life 3-6 hr

Interactions/incompatibilities:

• Decreased absorption of calcitriol: cholestyramine, mineral oil

• Hypercalcemia: thiazide diuretics, calcium supplement

• Cardiac dysrhythmias: cardiac glycosides, verapamil

• Decreased effect of calcifediol: barbiturates, phenytoin, corticosteroids

Lab test interferences:

False increase: Cholesterol

NURSING CONSIDERATIONS

Assess:

• BUN, urinary calcium, AST, ALT, cholesterol, creatinine, albumin, uric acid, chloride, magnesium, electrolytes, urine pH, phosphate; may increase calcium, should be kept at 9-10 mg/dl, Vit D 50-135 IU/dl, phosphate 70 mg/dl

• Alk phosphatase; may be decreased

• For increased drug level, since toxic reactions may occur rapidly

• For dry mouth, metallic taste, polyuria, bone pain, muscle weakness, headache, fatigue, change in LOC, dysrhythmias, increased respirations, anorexia, nausea, vomiting, cramps, diarrhea, constipation; may indicate hypercalcemia

• Renal status: decreased urinary output (oliguria, anuria), edema in extremities, weight gain 5-7 lb, periorbital edema

• Nutritional status, diet for sources of vitamin D (milk, some seafood), calcium (dairy products, dark green vegetables), phosphates (dairy products) must be avoided

Perform/provide:

• Storage protected from light, heat, moisture

• Restriction of sodium, potassium if required

• Restriction of fluids if required for chronic renal failure

Evaluate:

• Therapeutic response: calcium 9-10 mg/dl, decreasing symptoms of hypocalcemia, hypoparathyroidism

Teach patient/family:

• The symptoms of hypercalcemia

• About foods rich in calcium

• To avoid products with sodium: cured meats, dairy products, cold cuts, olives, beets, pickles, soups, meat tenderizers in chronic renal failure

• To avoid products with potassium: oranges, bananas, dried fruit, peas, dark green leafy vegetables, milk, melons, beans in chronic renal failure

• To avoid OTC products contain-

---

ing calcium, potassium, or sodium in chronic renal failure
• To avoid all preparations containing Vit D
• To monitor weight weekly

---

calcium carbonate

Alka-Mints, Amitone, Cal Carb-HD, Calci-Chew, Calci-Mix, Calciday 667, Calcium 600, Calcium Carbonate, Cal-Guard, Cal-Plus, Caltrate 600, Caltrate Jr., Chooz, Dicarbosil, Equilet, Gelcalc 600, Mallamint, Nephro-Calci, Os-Cal 500, Oystercal 500, Oysco 500, Oyst-Cal 500, Oyster Shell Calcium 500, Rolaids Calcium Rich, Tums, Tums E-X Extra Strength, Tums Extra Strength

Func. class.: Antacid, calcium supplement
Chem. class.: Calcium product

Action: Neutralizes gastric acidity
Uses: Antacid, calcium supplement; not suitable for chronic therapy

Dosage and routes:
• *Adult:* PO 1 g 4-6 × /day, chewed with water; SUSP 1 g 1 hr pc, hs
Available forms: Chewable tabs 350, 420, 500, 750 mg; tabs 650 mg; gum 500 mg; susp 1 g/5 ml
Side effects/adverse reactions:
GI: Constipation, anorexia, *obstruction,* nausea, vomiting, flatulence, diarrhea, rebound hyperacidity, eructation
CV: Hemorrhage, rebound hypertension
META: Hypercalcemia, metabolic alkalosis
GU: Renal dysfunction, renal stones, *renal failure*
Contraindications: Hypersensitiv-

ity, hypercalcemia, hyperparathyroidism, bone tumors
Precautions: Elderly, fluid restriction, decreased GI motility, GI obstruction, dehydration, renal disease, pregnancy (C)
Pharmacokinetics:
PO: Onset 3 min, excreted in feces
Interactions/incompatibilities:
• Increased plasma levels of quinidine, amphetamines
• Decreased levels of salicylates, calcium channel blockers, ketoconazole, tetracyclines, iron salts
• Hypercalcemia: thiazide diuretics
NURSING CONSIDERATIONS
Assess:
• Ca^+ (serum, urine), Ca^+ should be 8.5-10.5 mg/dl, urine Ca^+ should be 150 mg/day, monitor weekly
• Milk-alkali syndrome: nausea, vomiting, disorientation, headache
• Constipation; increase bulk in the diet if needed
• Hypercalcemia: headache, nausea, vomiting, confusion
Administer:
• As antacid 1 hr pc and hs
• As supplement 1½ hr pc and hs
• Only with regular tablets or capsules; do not give with enteric-coated tablets
• Laxatives or stool softeners if constipation occurs
Evaluate:
• Therapeutic response: absence of pain, decreased acidity
Teach patient/family:
• To increase fluids to 2 L unless contraindicated
• Not to switch antacids unless directed by physician

---

*Available in Canada only

C

calcium chloride/calcium gluceptate/calcium gluconate/calcium lactate

Func. class.: Electrolyte replacement—calcium product

Action: Cation needed for maintenance of nervous, muscular, skeletal, enzyme reactions, normal cardiac contractility, coagulation of blood; affects secretory activity of endocrine, exocrine glands

Uses: Prevention and treatment of hypocalcemia, hypermagnesemia, hypoparathyroidism, neonatal tetany, cardiac toxicity caused by hyperkalemia, lead colic, hyperphosphatemia, Vit D deficiency

Dosage and routes:
Calcium chloride
• *Adult:* IV 500 mg-1 g q1-3 days as indicated by serum calcium levels, give at <1 ml/min; IAV 200-800 mg injected in ventricle of heart
• *Child:* IV 25 mg/kg over several min

Calcium gluceptate
• *Adult:* IV 5-20 ml; IM 2-5 ml
• *Newborn:* 0.5 ml/100 ml of blood transfused

Calcium gluconate
• *Adult:* PO 0.5-2 g bid-qid; IV 0.5-2 g at 0.5 ml/min (10% solution)
• *Child:* PO/IV 500 mg/kg/day in divided doses

Calcium lactate
• *Adult:* PO 325 mg-1.3 g tid with meals
• *Child:* PO 500 mg/kg/day in divided doses

Available forms: Many; check product listings

Side effects/adverse reactions:
INTEG: Pain, burning at IV site, severe venous thrombosis, necrosis, extravasation

Hypercalcemia: Drowsiness, lethargy, muscle weakness, headache, constipation, ***coma***, anorexia, nausea, vomiting, polyuria, thirst
CV: Shortened Q-T, heart block, hypotension, bradycardia, dysrthymias, ***cardiac arrest***
GI: Vomiting, nausea, constipation
Contraindications: Hypercalcemia, digitalis toxicity, ventricular fibrillation, renal calculi

Precautions: Pregnancy (C), lactation, children, renal disease, respiratory disease, cor pulmonale, digitalized patient, respiratory failure

Interactions/incompatibilities:
• Increased dysrhythmias: digitalis glycosides
• Decreased action: calcium channel blockers
• Incompatible with amphotericin B, cephalothin, chlorpheniramine, chlortetracycline, digoxin, digitoxin, epinephrine, tetracycline, warfarin, $NaCo_3$, carbonate, phosphate, sulfate

Lab test interferences:
Increase: 11-OCHS
False decrease: Magnesium
Decrease: 17-OHCS

NURSING CONSIDERATIONS
Assess:
• ECG for decreased QT and T wave inversion: hypercalcemia, drug should be reduced or discontinued
• Calcium levels during treatment (8.5-1.5 g/dl is normal level)
• Cardiac status: rate, rhythm, CVP, (PWP, PAWP if being monitored directly)
Administer:
• IV undiluted or diluted with equal amounts of NS for inj to a 5% sol, give 0.5-1 ml/min

---

italics = common side effects   ***bold italic*** = life threatening reactions

• Through small-bore needle into large vein; if extravasation occurs, necrosis will result (IV); IM injection may cause severe burning, necrosis, and tissue sloughing; warm sol to body temp before administering
• PO with or following meals to enhance absorption

Perform/provide:
• Seizure precautions: padded side rails, decreased stimuli, (noise, light); place airway suction equipment, padded mouth gag if Ca levels are low
• Store at room temperature

Evaluate:
• Therapeutic response: decreased twitching, paresthesias, muscle spasms, absence of tremors, convulsions, dysrhythmias, dyspnea, laryngospasm, negative Chvostek's sign, negative Trousseau's sign

Teach patient/family:
• To remain recumbent ½ hr after IV dose
• To add food high in Vit D content
• To add calcium-rich foods to diet: dairy products, shellfish, dark green leafy vegetables; decrease oxalate-rich and zinc-rich foods: nuts, legumes, chocolate, spinach, soy
• To prevent injuries, avoid immobilization

---

calcium polycarbophil
(pol-i-kar'boe-fil)
Fiber Norm, Mitrolan
Func. class.: Laxative
Chem. class.: Bulk-forming

Action: Attracts water, expands in intestine to increase peristalsis; also absorbs excess water in stool; decreases diarrhea

Uses: Constipation, irritable bowel syndrome (diarrhea), acute, non-specific diarrhea

Dosage and routes:
• *Adult:* PO 1 g qd-qid prn, not to exceed 6 g/24 hr
• *Child 6-12 yr:* PO 500 mg bid prn, not to exceed 3 g/24 hr
• *Child 3-6 yr:* PO 500 mg bid prn, not to exceed 1.5 g/24 hr

Available forms: Chew tab 500, 625, 1250 mg

Side effects/adverse reactions:
GI: Obstruction, abdominal distention, laxative dependency, flatus

Contraindications: Hypersensitivity, GI obstruction

Precautions: Pregnancy (C)

Pharmacokinetics:
PO: Onset 12-24 min, peak 1-3 days

NURSING CONSIDERATIONS
Assess:
• Blood, urine electrolytes if used often
• I&O ratio to identify fluid loss
• Cause of constipation; identify whether fluids, bulk, or exercise is missing from life-style
• Cramping, rectal bleeding, nausea, vomiting; if these symptoms occur, drug should be discontinued

Administer:
• Alone for better absorption; do not take within 1 hr of other drugs
• In morning or evening (oral dose)

Evaluate:
• Therapeutic response: decreased constipation

Teach patient/family:
• Not to use laxatives for long-term therapy; bowel tone will be lost
• That normal bowel movements do not always occur daily
• Not to use in presence of abdominal pain, nausea, vomiting
• To notify physician if constipation unrelieved or if symptoms of

---

*Available in Canada only

electrolyte imbalance occur: muscle cramps, pain, weakness, dizziness
• To chew thoroughly and follow with water

---

capreomycin sulfate
(kap-ree-oh-mye'sin)
Capastat Sulfate
Func. class.: Antitubercular
Chem. class.: *S. capreolus* polypeptide antibiotic

Action: Inhibits RNA synthesis, decreases tubercle bacilli replication

Uses: Pulmonary tuberculosis as adjunct

Dosage and routes:
• *Adult:* IM 1 g qd × 2-4 mo, then 1 g 2-3 × /wk × 18-24 mo, not to exceed 20 mg/kg/day, must be given with another antitubercular medication

Available forms: Powder for inj 1 g/10 ml vial

Side effects/adverse reactions:
INTEG: Pain, irritation, sterile abscess at injection site, rash, urticaria
CNS: Vertigo, fever, headache
EENT: Tinnitus, *deafness, ototoxicity*
GU: Proteinuria, decreased CrCl, increased BUN, serum Cr, *tubular necrosis,* hypokalemia, alkalosis, *hematuria, albuminuria, nephrotoxicity*
HEMA: Eosinophilia, leukocytosis, leukopenia

Contraindications: Hypersensitivity

Precautions: Renal disease, hearing impairment, allergy history, hepatic disease, pregnancy (C)

Pharmacokinetics:
IM: Peak 1-2 hr, half-life 4-6 hr; excreted in urine unchanged

Interactions/incompatibilities:
• Increased renal toxicity: aminoglycosides, polymyxin, colistin, vancomycin
• Increased neuroblocking action: phenothiazine, tubocurarine, neostigmine

NURSING CONSIDERATIONS
Assess:
• Liver studies qwk: ALT, AST, bilirubin; potassium
• Renal status: before; qwk: BUN, creatinine, output, sp gr, urinalysis
• Blood levels of drug
• Audiometric testing before, during, after treatment
• Ototoxicity: tinnitus, vertigo, change in hearing
• Hepatic status: decreased appetite, jaundice, dark urine, fatigue

Administer:
• After reconstituting with NS or sterile water for injection, wait 2-3 min before giving
• With other antituberculars
• IM in large muscle mass; rotate sites
• Reduced dosage in renal impairment; if BUN >20 mg/dl, drug should be decreased or discontinued

Evaluate:
• Therapeutic response: decreased dyspnea, fatigue

Teach patient/family:
• That compliance with dosage schedule, duration is necessary
• Side effects, adverse reactions: hearing loss, change in urine or urinary habits

---

captopril
(kap'toe-pril)
Capoten
Func. class.: Antihypertensive
Chem. class.: Angiotensin-converting enzyme inhibitor

Action: Selectively suppresses

---

renin-angiotensin-aldosterone system; inhibits ACE; prevents conversion of angiotensin I to angiotensin II; results in dilation of arterial, venous vessels

Uses: Hypertension, heart failure not responsive to conventional therapy

Dosage and routes:
Malignant hypertension
• *Adult:* PO 25 mg increasing q2h until desired response, not to exceed 450 mg/day

Hypertension
• *Initial dose:* 12.5 mg 2-3 × daily; may increase to 50 mg bid-tid at 1-2 wk intervals; usual range: 25-150 mg bid-tid; max 450 mg

CHF
• *Adult:* PO 12.5 mg 2-3 × daily given with a diuretic; may increase to 50 mg bid-tid; after 14 days, may increase to 150 mg tid if needed

Available forms: Tabs 12.5, 25, 37.5, 50, 100 mg

Side effects/adverse reactions:
CV: Hypotension, postural hypotension
GU: Impotence, dysuria, nocturia, proteinuria, *nephrotic syndrome, acute reversible renal failure,* polyuria, oliguria, frequency
HEMA: Neutropenia
INT: Rash, *angioedema*
RESP: Bronchospasm, dyspnea, cough
META: Hyperkalemia
GI: Loss of taste
CNS: Fever, chills

Contraindications: Hypersensitivity, pregnancy (C), lactation, heart block, children, K-sparing diuretics, bilateral renal artery stenosis

Precautions: Dialysis patients, hypovolemia, leukemia, scleroderma, lupus erythematosus, blood dyscrasias, CHF, diabetes mellitus, renal disease, thyroid disease, COPD, asthma

Pharmacokinetics:
PO: Peak 1 hr; duration 2-6 hr; half-life 6-7 hr; metabolized by liver (metabolites), excreted in urine; crosses placenta; excreted in breast milk

Interactions/incompatibilities:
• Increased hypotension: diuretics, other antihypertensives, ganglionic blockers, adrenergic blockers
• Do not use with potassium-sparing diuretics, sympathomimetics, potassium supplements

Lab test interferences:
False positive: Urine acetone

NURSING CONSIDERATIONS
Assess:
• Blood studies: neutrophils, decreased platelets
• B/P
• Renal studies: protein, BUN, creatinine; watch for increased levels that may indicate nephrotic syndrome
• Baselines in renal, liver function tests before therapy begins
• K levels, although hyperkalemia rarely occurs
• Dipstick of urine for protein qd in first morning specimen; if protein is increased, a 24-hr urinary protein should be collected
• Edema in feet, legs daily
• Allergic reaction: rash, fever, pruritus, urticaria; drug should be discontinued if antihistamines fail to help
• Symptoms of CHF: edema, dyspnea, wet rales, B/P
• Renal symptoms: polyuria, oliguria, frequency

Administer:
• IV infusion of 0.9% NaCl (as ordered) to expand fluid volume if severe hypotension occurs

Perform/provide:
• Storage in tight container at 86°
F (30° C) or less
• Supine or Trendelenburg position
for severe hypotension
Evaluate:
• Therapeutic response: decrease in
B/P in hypertension, decreased
B/P, edema, moist rales (CHF)
Teach patient/family:
• To administer 1 hr before meals
• Not to discontinue drug abruptly
• Not to use OTC (cough, cold, or
allergy) products unless directed by
physician
• To avoid sunlight or wear sun-
screen if in sunlight; photosensitiv-
ity may occur
• To comply with dosage schedule,
even if feeling better
• To rise slowly to sitting or standing position to minimize orthostatic
hypotension
• To notify physician of mouth
sores, sore throat, fever, swelling
of hands or feet, irregular heartbeat, chest pain, signs of angioedema
• That excessive perspiration, dehydration, vomiting; diarrhea may
lead to fall in blood pressure—consult physician if these occur
• That dizziness, fainting, light-
headedness may occur during 1st
few days of therapy
• That skin rash or impaired perspiration may occur
• How to take B/P
Treatment of overdose: 0.9% Na
Ca IV/INF hemodialysis

---

carbachol
(kar'ba-kole)
Miostat
Func. class.: Miotic, cholinergic

Action: Contracts sphincter muscle
of iris; causes spasms of ciliary
muscle, deepening of anterior
chamber
Uses: Miosis in ocular surgery,
glaucoma (open-angle, narrow-
angle)
Dosage and routes:
Ocular surgery
• *Adult:* INSTILL 0.5 ml (intraocular) of 0.01% solution in anterior chamber of eye (done by
physician) for miosis during surgery
Glaucoma
• *Adult:* INSTILL 1-2 gtt (topical)
of 0.75%-3% solution into eye bid-
tid
Available forms: 0.75%, 1.5%,
2.25%, 3.0% sol for topical use;
sol, powders for preparing sol for
inj
Side effects/adverse reactions:
*CV: **Marked hypotension,** bradycardia, headache
GI: Nausea, vomiting, abdominal
discomfort, diarrhea, salivation
EENT: Blurred vision, varying degrees of myopia, decreased visual
acuity in dim light, slight conjunctival hyperemia, altered distance
vision, decreased night vision, eye
ache
RESP: Asthma attacks
Contraindications: Hypersensitivity; when miosis is undesirable;
corneal abrasions
Precautions: Bradycardia, CAD,
hyperthyroidism, asthma, pregnancy, obstruction of GI or urinary
tract, peptic ulcer, parkinsonism,
epilepsy, peritonitis
Pharmacokinetics:
INSTILL/OINT: Miosis onset 10-20
min, duration 4-8 hr; decreased
IOP onset 4 hr; duration 8 hr
NURSING CONSIDERATIONS
Assess:
• Heart, respiratory rate, B/P

---

italics = common side effects   ***bold italic*** = life threatening reactions

Perform/provide:
• Use of reconstituted solution immediately, discard unused potion

Evaluate:
• Therapeutic response: decreasing intraocular pressure, miosis during ocular surgery

Teach patient/family:
• To report change in vision, blurring or loss of sight, trouble breathing, sweating, flushing
• Method of instillation, including pressure on lacrimal sac for 1 min, and not to touch dropper to eye
• That long-term therapy may be required in glaucoma
• That blurred vision will decrease with repeated use of drug
• Not to drive during first few days of treatment

---

carbamazepine
(kar-ba-maz′e-peen)
Apo-Carbamazepine,*   Epitol,
Mazepine,* Tegretol
Func. class.: Anticonvulsant
Chem. class.: Iminostilbene derivative

Action: Inhibits nerve impulses by limiting influx of sodium ions across cell membrane in motor cortex

Uses: Tonic-clonic, complex-partial, mixed seizures; trigeminal neuralgia

Dosage and routes:
Seizures
• *Adult and child >12 yr:* PO 200 mg bid, may be increased by 200 mg/day in divided doses q6-8h; maintenance 800-1200 mg/1 qd maximum 1200 mg/day; adjustment is needed to minimum dose to control seizures

• *Child <12 yr:* PO 10-20 mg/kg/day in 2-3 divided doses
Trigeminal neuralgia
• *Adult:* PO 100 mg bid, may increase 100 mg q12h until pain subsides, not to exceed 1.2 g/day; maintenance is 200-400 mg bid
Available forms: Tabs, chewable 100 mg; tabs 200 mg

Side effects/adverse reactions:
*HEMA: **Thrombocytopenia, agranulocytosis, leukocytosis, neutropenia, aplastic anemia, eosinophilia,** increased pro-time*
*CNS: Drowsiness, dizziness, confusion, fatigue, **paralysis,** headache, hallucinations*
*GI: Nausea, constipation, diarrhea, anorexia, vomiting, abdominal pain, stomatitis, glossitis, increased liver enzymes, **hepatitis***
*INTEG: Rash, **Stevens-Johnson syndrome,** urticaria*
EENT: Tinnitus, dry mouth, blurred vision, diplopia, nystagmus, conjunctivitis
*CV: **Hypertension, CHF,** hypotension, aggravation of cardiac artery disease*
RESP: Pulmonary hypersensitivity (fever, dyspnea, pneumonitis)
GU: Frequency, retention, albuminuria, glycosuria, impotence

Contraindications: Hypersensitivity to carbamazepine or tricyclic antidepressants, bone marrow depression, concomitant use of MAOIs

Precautions: Glaucoma, hepatic disease, renal disease, cardiac disease, psychosis, pregnancy (C), lactation, child <6 yr

Pharmacokinetics:
PO: Onset slow, peak 4-8 hr; metabolized by liver; excreted in urine, feces; crosses placenta; excreted in breast milk; half-life 14-16 hr

---

Interactions/incompatibilities:
• Toxicity: troleandomycin, erythromycin, cimetidine, isoniazid, propoxyphene, lithium
• Decreased effects of phenobarbital, phenytoin, primidone
• Increased effects of vasopressin, lypressin, desmopressin

Lab test interferences:
Decrease: Thyroid function tests

NURSING CONSIDERATIONS
Assess:
• Renal studies: urinalysis, BUN, urine creatinine q3mo
• Blood studies: RBC, Hct, Hgb, reticulocyte counts qwk for 4 wk then qmo; if myelosupression occurs, drug should be discontinued
• Hepatic studies: ALT, AST, bilirubin
• Drug levels during initial treatment; should remain at 3-9 μg/ml; anorexia may indicate increased blood levels
• Description of seizures
• Mental status: mood, sensorium, affect, behavioral changes; if mental status changes, notify physician
• Eye problems: need for ophthalmic examinations before, during, after treatment (slit lamp, fundoscopy, tonometry)
• Allergic reaction: purpura, red raised rash; if these occur, drug should be discontinued
• Blood dyscrasias: fever, sore throat, bruising, rash, jaundice
• Toxicity: bone marrow depression, nausea, vomiting, ataxia, diplopia, cardiovascular collapse, Stevens-Johnson syndrome

Administer:
• With food, milk to decrease GI symptoms
• Chewable tablets; tell patient to chew tablet, not swallow it whole

Perform/provide:
• Storage at room temperature

• Hard candy, frequent rinsing of mouth, gum for dry mouth
• Assistance with ambulation during early part of treatment; dizziness occurs

Evaluate:
• Therapeutic response: decreased seizure activity, document on patient's chart

Teach patient/family:
• To carry Medic-Alert ID stating patient's name, drugs taken, condition, physician's name, phone number
• To avoid driving, other activities that require alertness
• To avoid alcohol ingestion; convulsions may result
• Not to discontinue medication quickly after long-term use
• That urine may turn pink to brown

Treatment of overdose: Lavage, VS

---

carbamide peroxide (otic)

(kar'ba-mide per-ox'ide)
Auro Ear Drops, Debrox, Murine Ear Drops
Func. class.: Otic
Chem. class.: Urea compound, hydrogen peroxide

Action: Foaming action facilitates removal of impacted cerumen
Uses: Impacted cerumen, prevention of ceruminosis

Dosage and routes:
• *Adult and child:* INSTILL 5-10 gtts bid × 3-4 days
Available forms: Sol 6.5%

Side effects/adverse reactions:
EENT: Itching, irritation in ear, redness

Contraindications: Hypersensitiv-

---

italics = common side effects   ***bold italic*** = life threatening reactions

ity, otic surgery, perforated eardrum
Precautions: Pregnancy (C)
NURSING CONSIDERATIONS
Administer:
• Drug, then irrigate to remove cerumen
• By allowing drops to enter ear canal; do not touch dropper to ear
Evaluate:
• Therapeutic response: loosened cerumen, ability to hear better
Teach patient/family:
• Method of instillation, using aseptic technique
• Do not use for more than 4 days

---

carbarsone
(kar-bar′sone)
Func. class.: Amebicide
Chem. class.: Pentavalent organic arsenic

Action: Organism death occurs in intestinal lumen by inhibition of sulfhydryl enzymes
Uses: Intestinal amebiasis
Dosage and routes:
• *Adult:* PO 250 mg bid-tid × 10 days; REC 2 g/200 ml warm 2% NaHCO₃ sol, qod × 5 doses
• *Child:* PO 75 mg/kg/day in 3 divided doses × 10 days
Available forms: Caps 250 mg; powder
Side effects/adverse reactions:
RESP: Congestion
HEMA: **Agranulocytosis, aplastic anemia**
INTEG: Rash, pruritus, **exfoliative dermatitis**
CNS: Neuritis, **convulsion, hemorrhagic encephalitis, coma**
EENT: Blurred vision, sore throat, retinal edema
GI: Nausea, vomiting, diarrhea, epigastric distress, anorexia, con-

stipation, abdominal cramps, irritation, hepatomegaly, jaundice, **hepatitis, gastric necrosis,** weight decrease
GU: Polyuria, albuminuria, **nephrotoxicity**
CV: Tachycardia, hypotension, edema
Contraindications: Hypersensitivity to this drug or arsenic, renal disease, hepatic disease, contracted visual or color fields
Precautions: Pregnancy (D), elderly
Pharmacokinetics:
PO: Slowly excreted by kidneys, accumulation may occur
NURSING CONSIDERATIONS
Assess:
• Stools during entire treatment; should be clear at end of therapy; stools must be clear for 1 yr before patient is considered cured
• ECG before, during, after therapy; be aware that T wave inversion occurs
• Vision by ophthalmologic exam during, after therapy; vision problems often occur
• I&O; stools for number, frequency, character
• Blood studies: CBC as dyscrasias occur
• Allergic reaction: fever, rash, itching, chills; drug should be discontinued if these occur
• Nephrotoxicity: polyuria, albuminuria, hematuria
• Arsenic toxicity: sore throat, edema, pruritus, nausea, vomiting, dizziness, anorexia, epigastric pain, weight decrease, gastritis, hepatitis, visual problems, convulsions, polyuria, agranulocytosis
• Superimposed infection: fever, monilial growth, fatigue, malaise
• Tachycardia, decreasing B/P, GI

symptoms, weakness, neuromuscular symptoms

• Diarrhea for 2-3 days

Administer:

• Dimercaprol for arsenic toxicity as ordered

• PO after meals to avoid GI symptoms

Perform/provide:

• Storage in tight container

Evaluate:

• Therapeutic response: decreasing diarrhea, absence of amebiasis on culture

Teach patient/family:

• To report any side effects

• Proper hygiene after BM: handwashing technique

• To avoid contact of drug with eyes, mouth, nose, other mucous membranes

• Need for compliance with dosage schedule, duration of treatment

Treatment of overdose: Administer dimercaprol, gastric lavage, O_2, IV fluids

---

carbidopa-levodopa
(lee-voe-doe′pa) (kar-bi-doe′pa)
Carbidopa/Levodopa, Sinemet
Func. class.: Antiparkinson agent
Chem. class.: Catecholamine

Action: Decarboxylation of levodopa to periphery is inhibited by carbidopa; more levodopa is made available for transport to brain and conversion to dopamine in the brain

Uses: Parkinsonism resulting from carbon monoxide, chronic manganese intoxication, cerebral arteriosclerosis

Dosage and routes:

• *Adult:* PO 3-6 tabs of 25 mg carbidopa/250 mg levodopa qd in divided doses, not to exceed 8 tabs/day *Sus. Rel:* 1 tablet BID at intervals of not less than 6 hrs usual: 2-8 tabs/day at intervals of 4-8 hr

Available forms: Tabs 10/100, 25/100, 25 mg carbidopa/250 mg levodopa Sus Rel tab: 50 mg/200 mg carbidopa/levodopa

Side effects/adverse reactions:

HEMA: **Hemolytic anemia, leukopenia, agranulocytosis**

CNS: Involuntary choreiform movements, hand tremors, fatigue, headache, anxiety, twitching, numbness, weakness, confusion, agitation, insomnia, nightmares, psychosis, hallucination, hypomania, severe depression, dizziness

GI: Nausea, vomiting, anorexia, abdominal distress, dry mouth, flatulence, dysphagia, bitter taste, diarrhea, constipation

INTEG: Rash, sweating, alopecia

CV: Orthostatic hypotension, tachycardia, hypertension, palpitation

EENT: Blurred vision, diplopia, dilated pupils

MISC: Urinary retention, incontinence, weight change, dark urine

Contraindications: Hypersensitivity, narrow-angle glaucoma, undiagnosed skin lesions

Precautions: Renal disease, cardiac disease, hepatic disease, respiratory disease, MI with dysrhythmias, convulsions, peptic ulcer, pregnancy (C)

Pharmacokinetics:

PO: Peak 1-3 hr, excreted in urine (metabolites)

Interactions/incompatibilities:

• Hypertensive crisis: MAOIs, furazolidone

• Decreased effects of levodopa: anticholinergics, hydantoins, methionine, papaverine, pyridoxine, tricyclics, benzodiazepines

italics = common side effects   ***bold italic*** = life threatening reactions

• Increased effects of levodopa: antacids, metoclopramide
Lab test interferences:
False positive: Urine ketones
False negative: Urine glucose
False increase: Uric acid, urine protein
Decrease: VMA, BUN, creatinine
NURSING CONSIDERATIONS
Assess:
• B/P, respiration
• Mental status: affect, mood, behavioral changes, depression, complete suicide assessment
Administer:
• Drug until NPO before surgery
• Adjust dosage depending on patient response
• With meals; limit protein taken with drug
• Only after MAOIs have been discontinued for 2 wk; if previously on levodopa, discontinue for at least 8 hr before change to levodopa-carbidopa
Perform/provide:
• Assistance with ambulation during beginning therapy
• Testing for diabetes mellitus, acromegaly if on long-term therapy
Evaluate:
• Therapeutic response: decrease in akathisia, improved mood
Teach patient/family:
• To change positions slowly to prevent orthostatic hypotension
• To report side effects: twitching, eye spasms; indicate overdose
• To use drug exactly as prescribed; if drug is discontinued abruptly, parkinsonian crisis may occur; physician may recommend drug-free holidays
• That urine, sweat may darken
• To use physical activities to maintain mobility and lessen spasms

• That improvement may not occur for 3-4 months

carboplatin
(kar-boe′-pla-tin)
Paraplatin
Func. class.: Antineoplastic alkylating agent
Chem. class.: Platinum coordination compound

Action: Produces interstrand DNA cross-links and to a lesser extent DNA-protein cross-links; activity is not cell cycle phase specific
Uses: Palliative treatment of ovarian carcinoma recurrent after treatment with other antineoplastic agents, including cisplatin
Dosage and routes (single agent):
• *Adult:* IV INF 360 mg/m² given over >15 min on day 1 q4wk; do not repeat single intermittent courses until neutrophil count is >2,000/mm³ and platelet count is >100,000/mm³
Available forms: Inj 50, 150, 450 mg/vial
Side effects/adverse reactions:
EENT: Tinnitus, hearing loss, *vestibular toxicity*
HEMA: **Thrombocytopenia, leukopenia, pancytopenia, neutropenia,** anemia, bleeding
CV: Cardiac abnormalities
GI: Severe nausea, vomiting, diarrhea, weight loss
GU: **Renal tubular damage,** renal insufficiency, impotence, sterility, amenorrhea, gynecomastia
INTEG: Alopecia, dermatitis, rash, erythema, pruritus, urticaria
CNS: **Convulsions, central neurotoxicity,** peripheral neuropathy
RESP: Mucositis
META: Hypomagnesemia, hypocal-

cemia, hypokalemia, hyponatremia, hyperuremia

Contraindications: Hypersensitivity to this drug, platinum products, mannitol; severe bone marrow depression, significant bleeding, pregnancy (D)

Precautions: Radiation therapy with 1 mo, chemotherapy within 1 mo, lactation, liver disease

Pharmacokinetics: Initial half-life 1-2 hr, postdistribution half-life 2½-6 hr, not bound to plasma proteins, excreted by the kidneys

Interactions/incompatibilities:
• Increased nephrotoxicity or ototoxicity: aminoglycosides
• Considered incompatible with any other drug in syringe or sol

NURSING CONSIDERATIONS
Assess:
• CBC, differential, platelet count weekly; withhold drug if WBC count is <4000/mm³ or platelet count is <100,000/mm³; notify physician of results
• Renal function studies: BUN, creatinine, serum uric acid, urine CrCl before and during therapy
• I&O ratio; report fall in urine output to <30 ml/hr
• Monitor temperature q4h (may indicate beginning of infection)
• Liver function tests before and during therapy (bilirubin, AST, ALT, LDH) as needed or monthly
• Bleeding: hematuria, stool guaiac, bruising or petechiae, mucosa or orifices q8h
• Dyspnea, rales, unproductive cough, chest pain, tachypnea
• Food preferences; list likes, dislikes
• Effects of alopecia on body image; discuss feelings about body changes
• Yellowing of skin, sclera, dark urine, clay-colored stools, itchy

skin, abdominal pain, fever, diarrhea
• Edema in feet, joint pain, stomach pain, shaking
• Inflammation of mucosa, breaks in skin

Administer:
• IV after diluting 10 mg/ml of sterile water for inj, D₅W, NS (10 mg/ml); then further dilute with the same sol 1-4 mg/ml; give over 15 min or more (INT INF)
• IV INF over 5-6 hr; do not use needles or IV administration sets containing aluminum, may cause precipitate
• Antiemetic 30-60 min before giving drug to prevent vomiting, and PRN
• Allopurinol or sodium bicarbonate to maintain uric acid levels, alkalinization of urine
• Antibiotics for prophylaxis of infection
• Diuretic (furosemide 40 mg IV) after infusion

Perform/provide:
• Storage protected from light at room temperature; reconstituted solutions are stable for 8 hr at room temperature
• Deep-breathing exercises with patient tid-qid; place in semi-Fowler's position
• Increase fluid intake to 2-3 L/day to prevent urate deposits and calculi formation and to speed elimination of drug
• Diet low in purines: organ meats (kidney, liver), dried beans, peas to maintain alkaline urine

Evaluate:
• Therapeutic response: decreasing size of tumor; spread of malignancy

Teach patient/family:
• To report any complaints or side effects to nurse or physician
• That impotence or amenorrhea

---

italics = common side effects   ***bold italic*** = life threatening reactions

can occur; reversible after treatment is discontinued
• To report any changes in breathing or coughing
• That hair may be lost during treatment; a wig or hairpiece may make patient feel better; new hair may be different in color, texture

---

carboprost tromethamine

(kar'boe-prost)
Prostin/15M
Func. class.: Oxytocic
Chem. class.: Prostaglandin

Action: Stimulates uterine contractions, causing complete abortion in approximately 16 hr
Uses: Abortion between 13-20 wk gestation
Dosage and routes:
• *Adult:* IM 250 μg, then 250 μg q1½-3½ hr, may increase to 500 μg if no response, not to exceed 12 mg total dose
Available forms: Inj IM 250 μg/ml carboprost, 83 μg/ml tromethamine
Side effects/adverse reactions:
CNS: Fever, chills, headache
GI: Nausea, vomiting, diarrhea
Contraindications: Hypersensitivity, severe hepatic disease, severe renal disease, PID, respiratory disease, cardiac disease
Precautions: Asthma, anemia, jaundice, diabetes mellitus, convulsive disorders, past uterine surgery, pregnancy (C)
Pharmacokinetics: Onset: 15 min, peak 2 hr; metabolized in lungs, liver; excreted in urine (metabolites)

NURSING CONSIDERATIONS
Assess:
• B/P, pulse; watch for change that may indicate hemorrhage

• Respiratory rate, rhythm, depth; notify physician of abnormalities
• For length, duration of contraction; notify physician of contractions lasting over 1 min or absence of contractions
• For incomplete abortion, pregnancy must be terminated by another method; drug is teratogenic
Administer:
• IM in deep muscle mass; rotate injection sites if additional doses are given
• Having crash cart available on unit
Perform/provide:
• Emotional support before and after the abortion
Evaluate:
• Therapeutic response: expulsion of fetus
Teach patient/family:
• To report increased blood loss, abdominal cramps, increased temperature or foul-smelling lochia
• Methods of comfort control and pain control

---

carisoprodol

(kar-eye-soe-proe'dole)
Carisoprodol, Rela, Soma, Soprodol
Func. class.: Skeletal muscle relaxant, central acting
Chem. class.: Meprobamate congener

Action: Depresses CNS by blocking interneuronal activity in descending reticular formation, spinal cord, producing sedation
Uses: Relieving pain, stiffness in musculoskeletal disorders
Dosage and routes:
• *Adult and child >12 yr:* PO 350 mg tid, hs
Available forms: Tabs 350 mg

Side effects/adverse reactions:
CNS: Dizziness, weakness, drowsiness, headache, tremor, depression, insomnia, ataxia, irritability
EENT: Diplopia, temporary loss of vision
CV: Postural hypotension, tachycardia
GI: Nausea, vomiting, hiccups, epigastric discomfort
INTEG: Rash, pruritus, fever, facial flushing
Contraindications: Hypersensitivity, child <12 yr, intermittent porphyria
Precautions: Renal disease, hepatic disease, addictive personality, pregnancy (C), elderly
Pharmacokinetics:
PO: Onset ½ hr, duration 4-6 hr; metabolized by liver; excreted in urine; crosses placenta; excreted in breast milk (large amounts); half-life 8 hr
Interactions/incompatibilities:
• Increased CNS depression: alcohol, tricyclic antidepressants, narcotics, barbiturates, sedatives, hypnotics
NURSING CONSIDERATIONS
Assess:
• Blood studies: CBC, WBC, differential; blood dyscrasias may occur
• Liver function studies: AST, ALT, alk phosphatase; hepatitis may occur
• ECG in epileptic patients; poor seizure control has occurred with patients taking this drug
• Idiosyncratic reaction, anaphylaxis within a few min or hr of first to fourth dose
• Allergic reactions: rash, fever, respiratory distress
• Severe weakness, numbness in extremities
• Psychologic dependency: increased need for medication, more frequent requests for medication, increased pain
• CNS depression: dizziness, drowsiness, psychiatric symptoms
Administer:
• With meals for GI symptoms
Perform/provide:
• Storage in tight container at room temperature
• Assistance with ambulation if dizziness, drowsiness occurs, especially elderly
Evaluate:
• Therapeutic response: decreased pain, spasticity
Teach patient/family:
• Not to discontinue the medication quickly; insomnia, nausea, headache, spasticity, tachycardia will occur; drug should be tapered off over 1-2 wk
• Not to take with alcohol, other CNS depressants
• To avoid altering activities while taking this drug
• To avoid hazardous activities if drowsiness, dizziness occurs
• To avoid using OTC medication: cough preparations, antihistamines, unless directed by physician
Treatment of overdose: Induce emesis of conscious patient, lavage, dialysis

---

carmustine (BCNU)
(kar-mus'teen)
BiCNU
Func. class.: Antineoplastic alkylating agent
Chem. class.: Nitrosourea

Action: Alkylates DNA, RNA; is able to inhibit enzymes that allow synthesis of amino acids in proteins; activity is not cell cycle phase specific

---

italics = common side effects   ***bold italic*** = life threatening reactions

Uses: Brain tumors such as glioblastoma, medulloblastoma, astrocytoma; multiple myeloma, Hodgkin's disease, other lymphomas, GI, breast, bronchogenic and renal carcinomas

Dosage and routes:
• *Adult:* IV 75-100 mg/m² over 1-2 hr × 2 days or 200 mg/m² × 1 dose q6-8wk; if leukocytes fall below 2000 or platelets below 75,000, only 50% of dose should be given

Available forms: Inj IV 100 mg; powder

Side effects/adverse reactions:
HEMA: Thrombocytopenia, leukopenia, myelosuppression, anemia
GI: Nausea, vomiting, anorexia, stomatitis, hepatotoxicity
GU: Azotemia, renal failure
INTEG: Burning, hyperpigmentation at injection site
RESP: Fibrosis, pulmonary infiltrate

Contraindications: Hypersensitivity, leukopenia, thrombocytopenia
Precautions: Pregnancy (D)
Pharmacokinetics: Degraded within 15 min; crosses blood-brain barrier; 70% excreted in urine within 96 hr; 10% excreted as CO_2; fate of 20% is unknown

Interactions/incompatibilities:
• Increased toxicity: other antineoplastics, or radiation
• Enhanced action: Vit A or caffeine
• Increased toxicity: cimetidine, other antineoplastics or radiation
• Considered incompatible with any other drug in syringe or sol

NURSING CONSIDERATIONS
Assess:
• CBC, differential, platelet count weekly; withhold drug if WBC is <4000 or platelet count is <75,000; notify physician of results
• Liver function tests: AST, ALT, bilirubin
• Pulmonary function tests, chest x-ray films before, during therapy; chest film should be obtained q2wk during treatment
• Renal function studies: BUN, serum uric acid, urine CrCl before, during therapy
• I&O ratio; report fall in urine output of 30 ml/hr
• Monitor for cold, cough, fever (may indicate beginning infection)
• Bleeding: hematuria, guaiac, bruising or petechiae, mucosa or orifices q8h
• Dyspnea, rales, unproductive cough, chest pain, tachypnea
• Food preferences; list likes, dislikes
• Inflammation of mucosa, breaks in skin

Administer:
• IV after diluting 100 mg drug/3 ml ethyl alcohol (provided); then further dilute 27 ml sterile H_2O for INJ; then dilute with 100-500 ml 0.9% NaCl or D_5W, give over 1 hr or more, reduce rate if discomfort is felt
• Antiemetic 30-60 min before giving drug to prevent vomiting
• Antibiotics for prophylaxis of infection

Perform/provide:
• Storage in refrigerator
• Strict medical asepsis, protective isolation if WBC levels are low
• Special skin care
• Deep-breathing exercises with patient tid-qid; place in semi-Fowler's position
• Increase fluid intake to 2-3 L/day to prevent urate deposits, calculi formation
• Rinsing of mouth tid-qid with

water or club soda; brushing of teeth bid-tid with soft brush or cotton-tipped applicators for stomatitis; use unwaxed dental floss, use viscous lidocaine (Xylocaine)

• Warm compresses at injection site for inflammation; reduce flow rate if patient complains of burning at injection site

Evaluate:

• Therapeutic response: decreasing size of tumor, spread of malignancy

Teach patient/family:

• Protective isolation precautions

• To report any changes in breathing or coughing

• To avoid foods with citric acid, hot or rough texture

• To report any bleeding, white spots, or ulceration in mouth to physician; tell patient to examine mouth qd

• To avoid use of aspirin, ibuprofen; razors, commercial mouthwash

• To report signs of anemia (fatigue, irritability, shortness of breath, faintness)

• To report signs of infection (sore throat, fever)

---

carteolol

(kar-tee'oe-lole)
Cartrol, Ocupress

Func. class.: Antihypertensive
Chem. class.: Nonselective β-blocker

Action: Produces fall in B/P without reflex tachycardia or significant reduction in heart rate through mixture of α-blocking, β-blocking effects and intrinsic sympathomimetic activity; elevated plasma renins are reduced

Uses: Mild to moderate hypertension

Dosage and routes:

• *Adult:* PO 2.5 mg tid initially, may gradually increase to desired response

Available forms: Tabs 2.5, 5, 10 mg

Side effects/adverse reactions:

CV: Orthostatic hypotension, **bradycardia, CHF, chest pain, ventricular dysrhythmias, AV block, peripheral vascular insufficiency,** palpitations

CNS: Dizziness, mental changes, drowsiness, fatigue, headache, catatonia, depression, anxiety, nightmares, paresthesia, lethargy, insominia, decreased concentration

GI: Nausea, vomiting, diarrhea, dry mouth, flatulence, constipation, anorexia

INTEG: Rash, alopecia, urticaria, pruritus, fever

HEMA: **Agranulocytosis, thrombocytopenic purpura (rare)**

EENT: Tinnitus, visual changes, sore throat, double vision, dry burning eyes

GU: Impotence, dysuria, ejaculatory failure, urinary retention

RESP: **Bronchospasm,** dyspnea, wheezing, nasal stuffiness, pharyngitis

MS: Joint pain, arthralgia, muscle cramps, pain

OTHER: Facial swelling, decreased exercise tolerance, weight change, Raynaud's disease

Contraindications: Hypersensitivity to β-blockers, cardiogenic shock, heart block (2nd or 3rd degree), sinus bradycardia, CHF, bronchial asthma

Precautions: Major surgery, pregnancy (C), lactation, diabetes mellitus, renal disease, thyroid disease, COPD, well-compensated heart failure, nonallergic bronchospasm

---

italics = common side effects   ***bold italic*** = life threatening reactions

Pharmacokinetics:
PO: Onset 1-2 hr, peak 2-4 hr, duration 8-12 hr, half-life 6-8 hr; metabolized by liver (metabolites inactive); excreted in urine, bile; crosses placenta; excreted in breast milk

Interactions/incompatibilities:
• Increased hypotension: diuretics, other antihypertensives, halothane, nitroglycerin, prazosin
• Decreased β-blocker effects: sympathomimetics, nonsteroidal antiinflammatory agents, salicylates
• Increased hypoglycemia effect: insulin
• Increased effects of lidocaine
• Decreased bronchodilating effects of theophylline β-agonists

Lab test interferences:
False increase: Urinary catecholamines
Interference: Glucose, insulin tolerance tests

NURSING CONSIDERATIONS
Assess:
• I&O, weight daily
• B/P, pulse q4h; note rate, rhythm, quality
• Apical/radial pulse before administration; notify physician of any significant changes
• Baselines in renal, liver function tests before therapy begins
• Edema in feet, legs daily
• Skin turgor, dryness of mucous membranes for hydration status

Administer:
• PO: ac, hs; tablet may be crushed or swallowed whole
• Reduced dosage in renal dysfunction

Perform/provide:
• Storage in dry area at room temperature; do not freeze

Evaluate:
• Therapeutic response: decreased B/P after 1-2 wk

Teach patient/family:
• Not to discontinue drug abruptly; taper over 2 wk or may precipitate angina
• Not to use OTC products containing α-adrenergic stimulants (nasal decongestants, OTC cold preparations) unless directed by physician
• To report bradycardia, dizziness, confusion, depression, fever
• To take pulse at home, advise when to notify physician
• To avoid alcohol, smoking, sodium intake
• To comply with weight control, dietary adjustments, modified exercise program
• To carry Medic Alert ID to identify drug being taken, allergies
• To avoid hazardous activities if dizziness is present
• To report symptoms of CHF: difficult breathing, especially on exertion or when lying down, night cough, swelling of extremities
• To take medication hs to minimize orthostatic hypotension
• To wear support hose to minimize effects of orthostatic hypotension

Treatment of overdose: Lavage, IV atropine for bradycardia, IV theophylline for bronchospasm, digitalis, O₂, diuretic for cardiac failure; hemodialysis is useful for removal; administer vasopressor (norepinephrine) for hypotension, isoproterenol for heart block

---

cascara sagrada/cascara sagrada aromatic fluid extract/ cascara sagrada fluid extract
(kas-kar′a)
Func. class.: Laxative
Chem. class.: Anthraquinone

Action: Direct chemical irritation

in colon; increases propulsion of stool

Uses: Constipation; bowel or rectal preparation for surgery or examination

Dosage and routes:
• *Adult:* PO 325 mg hs; FLUID 1 ml qd; AROMATIC FLUID 5 ml qd
• *Child 2-12 yr:* PO/FLUID/AROMATIC FLUID ½ adult dose
• *Child <2 yr:* PO/FLUID/AROMATIC FLUID ¼ adult dose
Available forms: Powder, tabs 325 mg; oral sol

Side effects/adverse reactions:
GI: Nausea, vomiting, anorexia, cramps, diarrhea
META: Hypocalcemia, enteropathy, alkalosis, hypokalemia, *tetany*

Contraindications: Hypersensitivity, GI bleeding, obstruction, CHF, lactation, abdominal pain, nausea/vomiting, appendicitis, acute surgical abdomen, alcoholics (aromatic form)

Precautions: Pregnancy (C)

Pharmacokinetics:
PO: Peak 6-12 hr; metabolized by liver; excreted by kidneys, in feces

Interactions/incompatibilities:
• Decreased absorption: antibiotics, digitalis, nitrofurantoin, salicylates, tetracyclines, oral anticoagulants

NURSING CONSIDERATIONS
Assess:
• Blood, urine electrolytes if drug is used often by patient
• I&O ratio to identify fluid loss
• Cause of constipation; identify whether fluids, bulk, or exercise missing from life-style
• Cramping, rectal bleeding, nausea, vomiting; if these symptoms occur, drug should be discontinued

Administer:
• Alone for better absorption; do not take within 1 hr of other drugs or within 1 hr of antacids, milk
• In morning or evening (oral dose)

Evaluate:
• Therapeutic response: decrease in constipation

Teach patient/family:
• To swallow tabs whole; do not chew
• Not to use laxatives for long-term therapy; bowel tone will be lost
• That normal bowel movements do not always occur daily
• Not to use in presence of abdominal pain, nausea, vomiting
• To notify physician if constipation unrelieved or if symptoms of electrolyte imbalance occur: muscle cramps, pain, weakness, dizziness

---

castor oil
Alphamul, Emulsoil, Fleet Castor Oil, Kelloff's Castor Oil, Neoloid, Purge
Func. class.: Laxative

Action: Directly acts on intestine by increasing motor activity; thought to irritate colonic intramural plexus

Uses: Bowel, rectal preparation for surgery or examination

Dosage and routes:
• *Adult:* PO LIQ 15-60 ml
• *Child >2 yr:* LIQ 5-15 ml
• *Child <2 yr:* LIQ 1.25-7.5 ml
• *Infants:* LIQ 1-4 ml
Available forms: Liq 36.4%, 60%, 64%, 95%; caps 0.62 ml/cap

Side effects/adverse reactions:
GI: Nausea, vomiting, anorexia, cramps, diarrhea, rebound constipation, colon irritation, flatus
META: Alkalosis, hypokalemia, electrolytes, fluid imbalance

Contraindications: Hypersensitiv-

---

ity, fecal impaction, GI bleeding, pregnancy (X), lactation, abdominal pain, nausea/vomiting, appendicitis, acute surgical abdomen

Pharmacokinetics:

PO: Peak 2-3 hr; excreted in breast milk

NURSING CONSIDERATIONS

Assess:

• Blood, urine electrolytes if drug is used often by patient

• I&O ratio to identify fluid loss

• Cause of constipation; identify whether fluids, bulk, or exercise missing from life-style

• Cramping, rectal bleeding, nausea, vomiting; if these symptoms occur, drug should be discontinued

Administer:

• Alone for better absorption; do not take within 1 hr of other drugs or within 1 hr of antacids, milk

• In morning or evening (oral dose)

Perform/provide:

• Storage in cool environment, do not freeze

Evaluate:

• Therapeutic response: decrease in constipation

Teach patient/family:

• To swallow tabs whole; do not chew

• Not to use laxatives for long-term therapy; bowel tone will be lost

• That normal bowel movements do not always occur daily

• Not to use in presence of abdominal pain, nausea, vomiting

• To notify physician if constipation unrelieved or if symptoms of electrolyte imbalance occur: muscle cramps, pain, weakness, dizziness, severe thirst

• To keep out of children's reach

cefaclor

(sef′a-klor)

Ceclor

Func. class.: Antibiotic

Chem. class.: Cephalosporin (2nd generation)

Action: Inhibits bacterial cell wall synthesis, which renders cell wall osmotically unstable, leading to cell death

Uses: Gram-negative bacilli: *H. influenzae, E. coli, P. mirabilis, Klebsiella;* gram-positive organisms: *S. pneumoniae, S. pyogenes, S. aureus;* upper and lower respiratory tract, urinary tract, skin infections, otitis media

Dosage and routes:

• *Adult:* PO 250-500 mg q8h, not to exceed 4 g/day

• *Child >1 mo:* PO 20-40 mg/kg/qd in divided doses q8h, not to exceed 1 g/day

Available forms: Caps 250, 500 mg; oral susp 125, 250 mg/5 ml

Side effects/adverse reactions:

CNS: Headache, dizziness, weakness, paresthesia, fever, chills

GI: Nausea, vomiting, *diarrhea, anorexia,* pain, glossitis, bleeding, increased AST, ALT, bilirubin, LDH, alk phosphatase, abdominal pain

GU: Proteinuria, vaginitis, pruritus, candidiasis, increased BUN, ***nephrotoxicity, renal failure***

HEMA: ***Leukopenia, thrombocytopenia, agranulocytosis,*** anemia, ***neutropenia, lymphocytosis, eosinophilia, pancytopenia, hemolytic anemia***

INTEG: Rash, urticaria, dermatitis, ***anaphylaxis***

RESP: Dyspnea

Contraindications: Hypersensitivity to cephalosporins, infants <1 mo

Precautions: Hypersensitivity to penicillins, pregnancy (B), lactation, renal disease

Pharmacokinetics: Peak ½-1 hr, half-life 36-54 min; 25% bound by plasma proteins; 60%-85% eliminated unchanged in urine in 8 hr; crosses placenta; excreted in breast milk

Interactions/incompatibilities:
• Decreased effects: tetracyclines, erythromycins
• Increased toxicity: aminoglycosides, furosemide, probenecid, sulfinpyrazone, colistin, ethacrynic acid, vancomycin

Lab test interferences:
Increase (false): Creatinine (serum urine), urinary 17-KS
False positive: Urinary protein, direct Coombs' test, urine glucose
Interference: Cross-matching

NURSING CONSIDERATIONS
Assess:
• Sensitivity to penicillins and other cephalosporins
  Nephrotoxicity: increased BUN, creatinine
• I&O daily
• Blood studies: AST, ALT, CBC, Hct, bilirubin, LDH, alk phosphatase, Coombs' test monthly if patient is on long-term therapy
• Electrolytes: K, Na, Cl monthly if patient is on long-term therapy
• Bowel pattern qd; if severe diarrhea occurs, drug should be discontinued; may indicate pseudomembranous colitis
• Urine output; if decreasing, notify physician (may indicate nephrotoxicity)
• Allergic reactions: rash, urticaria, pruritus, chills, fever, joint pain; angioedema may occur a few days after therapy begins
• Bleeding: ecchymosis, bleeding gums, hematuria, stool guaiac daily
• Overgrowth of infection: perineal itching, fever, malaise, redness, pain, swelling, drainage, rash, diarrhea, change in cough, sputum

Administer:
• For 10-14 days to ensure organism death, prevent superimposed infection
• With food if needed for GI symptoms
• After C&S completed

Evaluate:
• Therapeutic response: decreased symptoms of infection

Teach patient/family:
• If diabetic, to use Clinistix or Ketodiastix, blood glucose level
• Not to drink alcohol or meds with alcohol: reaction may occur
• To use yogurt or buttermilk to maintain intestinal flora, decrease diarrhea
• To take all medication prescribed for length of time ordered
• To report sore throat, bruising, bleeding, joint pain; may indicate blood dyscrasias (rare)

Treatment of overdose: Epinephrine, antihistamines, resuscitate if needed (anaphylaxis)

---

cefadroxil
(sef-a-drox′ill)
Cefadroxil, Duricef, Ultracef
Func. class.: Antibiotic
Chem. class.: Cephalosporin
(1st generation)

Action: Inhibits bacterial cell wall synthesis, rendering cell wall osmotically unstable, leading to cell death

Uses: Gram-negative bacilli: *E. coli, P. mirabilis, Klebsiella (UTI only);* gram-positive organisms: *S.*

---

italics = common side effects   ***bold italic*** = life threatening reactions

pneumoniae, S. pyogenes, S. aureus; upper, lower respiratory tract, urinary tract, skin infections, otitis media; tonsillitis; particularly for UTI.

Dosage and routes:
• *Adult:* PO 1-2 g qd or q12h, give a loading dose of 1 g initially; dosage reduction indicated in renal impairment (CrCl < 50 ml/min)
• *Child:* 30 mg/kg/day
Available forms: Caps 500 mg; tabs 1 g; oral susp 125, 250, 500 mg/5 ml

Side effects/adverse reactions:
CNS: Headache, dizziness, weakness, paresthesia, fever, chills
GI: Nausea, vomiting, *diarrhea, anorexia,* pain, glossitis, bleeding, increased AST, ALT, bilirubin, LDH, alk phosphatase, abdominal pain, *pseudomembranous colitis*
GU: Proteinuria, vaginitis, pruritus, candidiasis, increased BUN, *nephrotoxicity, renal failure*
HEMA: Leukopenia, thrombocytopenia, agranulocytosis, anemia, *neutropenia, lymphocytosis, eosinophilia, pancytopenia, hemolytic anemia*
INTEG: Rash, urticaria, dermatitis, *anaphylaxis*
RESP: Dyspnea

Contraindications: Hypersensitivity to cephalosporins, infants <1 mo
Precautions: Hypersensitivity to penicillins, pregnancy (B), lactation, renal disease
Pharmacokinetics: Peak 1-1½ hr, half-life 1-2 hr; 20% bound by plasma proteins; crosses placenta; excreted in breast milk
Interactions/incompatibilities:
• Decreased effects: tetracyclines, erythromycins
• Increased toxicity: aminoglycosides, furosemide, probenecid, sulfinpyrazone, colistin, ethacrynic acid, vancomycin

Lab test interferences:
Increase (false): Creatinine (serum urine), urinary 17-KS
False positive: Urinary protein, direct Coombs' test, urine glucose
Interference: Cross-matching

NURSING CONSIDERATIONS
Assess:
• Sensitivity to penicillin and other cephalosporins
• Nephrotoxicity: increased BUN, creatinine
• I&O daily
• Blood studies: AST, ALT, CBC, Hct, bilirubin, LDH, alk phosphatase, Coombs' test monthly if patient is on long-term therapy
• Electrolytes: K, Na, Cl monthly if patient is on long-term therapy
• Bowel pattern qd; if severe diarrhea occurs, drug should be discontinued; may indicate pseudomembranous colitis
• Urine output; if decreasing, notify physician; may indicate nephrotoxicity
• Allergic reactions: rash, urticaria, pruritus, chills, fever, joint pain; angioedema; may occur few days after therapy begins
• Bleeding: ecchymosis, bleeding gums, hematuria, stool guaiac daily
• Overgrowth of infection: perineal itching, fever, malaise, redness, pain, swelling, drainage, rash, diarrhea, change in cough, sputum
Administer:
• For 10-14 days to ensure organism death, prevent superimposed infection
• With food if needed for GI symptoms
• After C&S completed
Evaluate:
• Therapeutic response: decreased symptoms of infection

Teach patient/family:
• If diabetic to use Clinistix or Ketodiastix, blood glucose level
• Not to drink alcohol or use meds with alcohol: reaction may occur
• To use yogurt or buttermilk to maintain intestinal flora, decrease diarrhea
• To take all medication prescribed for length of time ordered
• To report sore throat, bruising, bleeding, joint pain; may indicate blood dyscrasias (rare)
Treatment of overdose: Epinephrine, antihistamines; resuscitate if needed (anaphylaxis)

---

cefamandole nafate
(sef-a-man'dole)
Mandol
Func. class.: Antibiotic
Chem. class.: Cephalosporin (2nd generation)

Action: Inhibits bacterial cell wall synthesis, rendering cell wall osmotically unstable, leading to cell death

Uses: Gram-negative bacilli: *H. influenzae, E. coli, P. mirabilis, Klebsiella;* gram-positive organisms: *S. pneumoniae, S. pyogenes, S. aureus;* upper, lower respiratory tract, urinary tract, skin infections, peritonitis, septicemia, surgical prophylaxis

Dosage and routes:
• *Adult:* IM/IV 500 mg-1 g q4-8h; may give up to 2 g q4h for severe infections
• *Child >1 mo:* IM/IV 50-100 mg/kg/day in divided doses q4-8h, not to exceed adult dose
• Dosage reduction indicated in renal impairment (CrCl < 5 ml/min)
Available forms: Inj IM, IV 500 mg, 1, 2, 10 g; IV 1, 2 g

Side effects/adverse reactions:
CNS: Headache, dizziness, weakness, paresthesia, fever, chills
GI: Nausea, vomiting, diarrhea, anorexia, pain, glossitis, bleeding, increased AST, ALT, bilirubin, LDH, alk phosphatase, abdominal pain
GU: Proteinuria, vaginitis, pruritus, candidiasis, increased BUN, ***nephrotoxicity, renal failure***
*HEMA: **Leukopenia, thrombocytopenia, agranulocytosis,** anemia, **neutropenia, lymphocytosis, eosinophilia, pancytopenia, hemolytic anemia,** bleeding, **hypoprothrombinemia***
INTEG: Rash, urticaria, dermatitis, *anaphylaxis*
RESP: Dyspnea
Contraindications: Hypersensitivity to cephalosporins, infants <1 mo
Precautions: Hypersensitivity to penicillins, pregnancy, lactation, renal disease
Pharmacokinetics: Peak 1-1½ hr, half-life ½-1 hr; 60%-75% bound by plasma proteins; crosses placenta; excreted in breast milk
Interactions/incompatibilities:
• Incompatible with tetracyclines, erythromycins, calcium chloride, magnesium salts, aminoglycosides, cimetidine
• Decreased effects: tetracyclines, erythromycins
• Increased toxicity: aminoglycosides, furosemide, probenecid, sulfinpyrazone, colistin, ethacrynic acid, vancomycin
• Disulfiram reaction: disulfiram
Lab test interferences:
Increase (false): Urinary 17-KS
False positive: Urinary protein, direct Coombs', urine glucose
Interference: Cross-matching

---

italics = common side effects   ***bold italic*** = life threatening reactions

NURSING CONSIDERATIONS
Assess:
• Sensitivity to penicillin or other cephalosporins
• Nephrotoxicity: increased BUN, creatinine
• I&O daily
• Blood studies: AST, ALT, CBC, Hct, bilirubin, LDH, alk phosphatase, Coombs' test, pro-time monthly if patient is on long-term therapy
• Electrolytes: K, Na, Cl monthly if patient is on long-term therapy
• Bowel pattern qd; if severe diarrhea occurs, drug should be discontinued; may indicate pseudomembranous colitis
• IV site for extravasation or phlebitis, change site q72h
• Urine output: if decreasing, notify physician; may indicate nephrotoxicity
• Allergic reactions: rash, urticaria, pruritus, chills, fever, joint pain, angioedema; may occur few days after therapy begins
• Bleeding: ecchymosis, bleeding gums, hematuria, stool guaiac daily
• Overgrowth of infection: perineal itching, fever, malaise, redness, pain, swelling, drainage, rash, diarrhea, change in cough, sputum
Administer:
• IV; check often for irritation, extravasation; dilute 1 g or less of drug/10 ml or more normal saline or sterile H_2O for inj; run over 3-5 min; may be further diluted with 100 ml of compatible sol and run over 15-30 min via Y-tube or 3-way stopcock; may also be diluted in 1 L compatible sol, run over prescribed rate
• For 10-14 days to ensure organism death, prevent superimposed infection
• After C&S completed

Evaluate:
• Therapeutic response: decreased symptoms of infection
Teach patient/family:
• If diabetic, to use Clinistix or Ketodiastix, blood glucose level
• Not to drink alcohol or meds with alcohol: reaction may occur
• To report sore throat, bruising, bleeding, joint pain; may indicate blood dyscrasias (rare)
Treatment of overdose: Epinephrine, antihistamines, resuscitate if needed (anaphylaxis)

---

cefazolin sodium
(sef-a'zoe-lin)
Ancef, Cefazolin Sodium, Kefzol, Zolicef
Func. class.: Antibiotic
Chem. class.: Cephalosporin (1st generation)

Action: Inhibits bacterial cell wall synthesis, rendering cell wall osmotically unstable, leading to cell death
Uses: Gram-negative bacilli: *H. influenzae, E. coli, P. mirabilis, Klebsiella;* gram-positive organisms: *S. pneumoniae, S. pyogenes, S. aureus;* upper, lower respiratory tract, urinary tract, skin infections, bone, joint, biliary, genital infections, endocarditis, surgical prophylaxis, septicemia
Dosage and routes:
Life-threatening infections
• *Adult:* IM/IV 1-1.5 g q6h
• *Child >1 mo:* IM/IV 100 mg/kg in 3-4 equal doses
Mild/moderate infections
• *Adult:* IM/IV 250-500 mg q8h
• *Child >1 mo:* IM/IV 25-50 mg/kg in 3-4 equal doses
• Dosage reduction indicated in re-

---

nal impairment (CrCl < 54 ml/min)

Available forms: Inj IM, IV, 250, 500 mg, 1, 5, 10 g

Side effects/adverse reactions:

CNS: Headache, dizziness, weakness, paresthesia, fever, chills

GI: Nausea, vomiting, *diarrhea, anorexia,* pain, glossitis, bleeding, increased AST, ALT, bilirubin, LDH, alk phosphatase, abdominal pain, oral candidiasis

GU: Proteinuria, vaginitis, pruritus, candidiasis, increased BUN, *nephrotoxicity, renal failure*

HEMA: Leukopenia, thrombocytopenia, agranulocytosis, anemia, *neutropenia, lymphocytosis, eosinophilia, pancytopenia, hemolytic anemia*

INTEG: Rash, urticaria, dermatitis, *anaphylaxis*

Contraindications: Hypersensitivity to cephalosporins, infants <1 mo

Precautions: Hypersensitivity to penicillins, pregnancy (B), lactation, renal disease

Pharmacokinetics

IM: Peak ½-2 hr, half-life 1½-2¼ hr

IV: Peak 10 min; eliminated unchanged in urine; 70% to 86% protein bound

Interactions/incompatibilities:

• Incompatible with tetracyclines, erythromycins, calcium salts, magnesium salts, barbiturates, aminoglycosides, Vit C, Vit B with C, bleomycin, colistimethate, lidocaine

• Decreased effects: tetracyclines, erythromycins

• Increased toxicity: aminoglycosides, furosemide, probenecid, sulfinpyrazone, colistin, ethacrynic acid

Lab test interferences:

Increase (false): Urinary 17-KS

False positive: urinary protein, direct Coombs' test, urine glucose

Interference: Cross-matching

NURSING CONSIDERATIONS

Assess:

• Sensitivity to penicillin or other cephalosporins

• Nephrotoxicity: increased BUN, creatinine

• I&O daily

• Blood studies: AST, ALT, CBC, Hct, alk phosphatase, bilirubin, LDH, Coombs' test monthly if patient is on long-term therapy

• Electrolytes: K, Na, Cl monthly if patient is on long-term therapy

• Bowel pattern qd; if severe diarrhea occurs, drug should be discontinued; may indicate pseudomembranous colitis

• IV site for extravasation or phlebitis, change site q72h

• Urine output, if decreasing, notify physician; may indicate nephrotoxicity

• Allergic reactions: rash, urticaria, pruritus, chills, fever, joint pain, angioedema; may occur few days after therapy begins

• Bleeding: ecchymosis, bleeding gums, hematuria, stool guaiac daily

• Overgrowth of infection: perineal itching, fever, malaise, redness, pain, swelling, drainage, rash, diarrhea, change in cough, sputum

Administer:

• IV; check for irritation, extravasation often; dilute in 10 ml sterile H₂O for inj and run over 3-5 min; may be further diluted with 50-100 ml of N$_s$, D$_5$W sol and run over ½-1 hr by Y-tube or 3-way stopcock

• For 10-14 days to ensure organism death, prevent superimposed infection

• After C&S completed

---

italics = common side effects   ***bold italic*** = life threatening reactions

Evaluate:
• Therapeutic response: decreased fever, malaise, chills
Teach patient/family:
• If diabetic, to use Clinistix or Ketodiastix, blood glucose level
• Not to use alcohol or meds with alcohol: reaction may occur
Treatment of overdose: Epinephrine, antihistamines, resuscitate if needed (anaphylaxis)

---

cefixime
(sef-ix'ime)
Suprax
Func. class.: Broad-spectrum antibiotic
Chem. class.: Cephalosporin (3rd generation)

Action: Inhibits bacterial cell wall synthesis, rendering cell wall osmotically unstable, leading to cell death
Uses: Uncomplicated UTI *(E. coli, P. mirabilis),* pharyngitis and tonsillitis *(S. pyogenes),* otitis media *(H. influenzae), M. catarrhalis,* acute bronchitis, and acute exacerbations of chronic bronchitis *(S. pneumoniae, H. influenzae)*
Dosage and routes:
• *Adult:* PO 400 mg qd as a single dose or 200 mg q12h
• *Child >50 kg or >12 yrs:* PO use adult dosage
• *Child: <50 kg or <12 years:* PO 8 mg/kg/day as a single dose or 4 mg/kg q12h
•*Available forms:* Tabs 200, 400 g; powder for oral susp 100 mg/5 ml
Side effects/adverse reactions:
CNS: Headache, dizziness, paresthesia, fever, chills, lethargy, fatigue, confusion
GI: Nausea, vomiting, diarrhea, anorexia, pain, glossitis, bleeding, increased AST, ALT, bilirubin, LDH, alk phosphatase, heartburn, dysgeusia, flatulence
GU: Proteinuria, vaginitis, pruritus, increased BUN, *nephrotoxicity, renal failure,* pyuria, dysuria
HEMA: Leukopenia, thrombocytopenia, agranulocytosis, anemia, *neutropenia, lymphocytosis, eosinophilia, pancytopenia, hemolytic anemia*
INTEG: Rash, urticaria, *exfoliative dermatitis, anaphylaxis*
RESP: Bronchospasm, dyspnea, tight chest
Contraindications: Hypersensitivity to cephalosporins, infants <6 mo
Precautions: Hypersensitivity to penicillins, pregnancy (B), lactation, renal disease
Pharmacokinetics:
PO: Peak 1 hr
Half-life 3-4 hr, 65% bound by plasma proteins, 50% eliminated unchanged in urine; crosses placenta; excreted in breast milk
Interactions/incompatibilities:
• Decreased bactericidal effects: tetracyclines, erythromycins, chloramphenicol
• Increased renal toxicity: aminoglycosides, furosemide, colistin, ethacrynic acid, vancomycin
Lab test interferences:
Increase (false): Urinary 17-KS
False positive: Urinary protein, direct Coombs', urine glucose
Interference: Cross-matching
NURSING CONSIDERATIONS
Assess:
• Sensitivity to penicillin or other cephalosporins
• Nephrotoxicity: increased BUN, creatinine
• I&O daily
• Blood studies: AST, ALT, CBC, Hct, bilirubin, LDH, alk phospha-

---

tase; Coombs' test monthly if patient is on long-term therapy

• Bowel pattern qd; if severe diarrhea occurs, drug should be discontinued (may indicate pseudomembranous colitis)

• Urine output: if decreasing, notify physician (may indicate nephrotoxicity)

• Allergic reactions: rash, urticaria, pruritus, chills, fever, joint pain, angioedema; may occur a few days after therapy begins

• Bleeding: ecchymosis, bleeding, itching, fever, malaise, redness, pain, swelling, drainage, rash, diarrhea, change in cough, sputum

Administer:

• For 10-14 days to ensure organism death, prevent superimposed infection

• After C&S completed

Evaluate:

• Therapeutic response: decreased fever, malaise, chills

Teach patient/family:

• To report sore throat, bruising, bleeding, joint pain (may indicate blood dyscrasias [rare])

• If diabetic, to use Clinistix or Ketodiastix, blood glucose level

• Not to use alcohol or meds with alcohol or reaction may occur

Treatment of overdose: Epinephrine, antihistamines, resuscitate if needed (anaphylaxis)

---

cefmetazole

(sef-met'a-zole)

Zefazone

Func. class.: Broad-spectrum antibiotic

Chem. class.: Cephalosporin (2nd generation)

Action: Inhibits bacterial cell wall synthesis, rendering cell wall os-

motically unstable, leading to cell death

Uses: Gram-negative bacilli: *H. influenzae, E. coli, Proteus, Klebsiella, B. fragilis;* gram-positive organisms: *S. pneumoniae, S. pyogenes, S. aureus;* anaerobes, including *Clostridium;* infections of lower respiratory tract, urinary tract, skin, bone; septicemia; intraabdominal infections

Dosage and routes:

• *Adult:* IV 1-8 g divided q6-12h × 5-14 days

Available forms: Powder for inj 1, 2 gm/vial

Side effects/adverse reactions:

CNS: Headache, dizziness, paresthesia, fever, chills, lethargy, fatigue, confusion

GI: Nausea, vomiting, diarrhea, anorexia, pain, glossitis, bleeding, increased AST, ALT, bilirubin, LDH, alk phosphatase, heartburn, flatulence

GU: Proteinuria, vaginitis, pruritus, candidiasis, increased BUN, *nephrotoxicity, renal failure*

HEMA: Leukopenia, thrombocytopenia, agranulocytosis, anemia, *neutropenia, lymphocytosis, eosinophilia, pancytopenia, hemolytic anemia*

INTEG: Rash, urticaria, *exfoliative dermatitis,* thrombophlebitis *angioedema,* erythema, pruritus

SYST: Anaphylaxis

Contraindications: Hypersensitivity to cephalosporins, infants <1 mo

Precautions: Hypersensitivity to penicillins, pregnancy (B), lactation, renal disease

Pharmacokinetics:

IM: Peak 30-45 min; 68% bound by plasma proteins; excreted by kidneys; half-life 1-3 hr

---

italics = common side effects   ***bold italic*** = life threatening reactions

Interactions/incompatibilities:
• Incompatible with aminoglycosides
• Decreased bactericidal effects: tetracyclines, erythromycins, chloramphenicol
• Increased renal toxicity and ototoxicity: aminoglycosides, furosemide, colistin, ethacrynic acid, vancomycin
• Increased plasma level of cefmetazole

Lab test interferences:
Increase (false): Creatinine (serum urine), urinary 17-KS
False positive: Urinary protein, direct Coombs' test, urine glucose
Interference: Cross-matching

NURSING CONSIDERATIONS
Assess:
• Sensitivity to penicillin and other cephalosporins
• Nephrotoxicity: increased BUN, creatinine
• I&O daily
• Blood studies: AST, ALT, CBC, Hct, bilirubin, LDH, alk phosphatase, Coombs' test monthly if patient is on long-term therapy
• Electrolytes: K, Na, Cl monthly if patient is on long-term therapy
• Bowel pattern qd; if severe diarrhea occurs, drug should be discontinued (may indicate pseudomembranous colitis)
• IV site for extravasation or phlebitis; change site q72h
• Urine output; if decreasing, notify physician (may indicate nephrotoxicity)
• Allergic reactions: rash, urticaria, pruritis, chills, fever, joint pain, 7-10 days after therapy begins
• Bleeding: ecchymosis, bleeding gums, hematuria, stool guaiac daily
• Overgrowth of infection: perineal itching, fever, malaise, redness,

pain, swelling, drainage, rash, diarrhea, change in cough, sputum
Administer:
• IV after diluting 3.7 or 10 ml sterile H_2O for inj. 2 gm/7 or 15 ml, shake, let stand until clear, run over 3-5 min; may be further diluted in 50-100 ml of D_5W, NS, LR to 1-20 mg/ml and run over ½-1 hr by Y-tube or 3-way stopcock
• For 10-14 days to ensure organism death, prevent superimposed infection
• After C&S completed
Evaluate:
• Therapeutic response: decreased fever, malaise, chills
Teach patient/family:
• If diabetic, to use Clinistix or Ketodiastix, blood glucose level
• Not to use alcohol or meds with alcohol or reaction may occur
• To report sore throat, bruising, bleeding, joint pain (may indicate blood dyscrasias [rare])
Treatment of overdose: Epinephrine, antihistamines, resuscitate if needed (anaphylaxis)

---

cefonicid sodium
(se-fon'i-sid)
Monocid
Func. class.: Antibiotic
Chem. class.: Cephalosporin
(2nd generation)

Action: Inhibits bacterial cell wall synthesis, rendering cell wall osmotically unstable, leading to cell death
Uses: Gram-negative bacilli: *H. influenzae, E. coli, P. mirabilis, Klebsiella;* gram-positive organisms: *S. pneumoniae, S. pyogenes, S. aureus;* lower respiratory tract, urinary tract, skin infections, otitis media, peritonitis, septicemia

Dosage and routes:
Life-threatening infections
• *Adult:* IM/IV BOL or INF 1-2 g/ 24 hr; divide in two doses if giving 2 g
• Dosage reduction indicated in renal impairment
Available forms: Inj IM, IV, 500 mg, 1, 10 g
Side effects/adverse reactions:
CNS: Headache, dizziness, weakness, paresthesia, fever, chills
GI: Nausea, vomiting, diarrhea, anorexia, pain, glossitis, bleeding, increased AST, ALT, bilirubin, LDH, alk phosphatase, abdominal pain
GU: Proteinuria, vaginitis, pruritus, candidiasis, increased BUN, *nephrotoxicity, renal failure*
HEMA: Leukopenia, thrombocytopenia, agranulocytosis, anemia, *neutropenia, lymphocytosis, eosinophilia, pancytopenia, hemolytic anemia*
INTEG: Rash, urticaria, dermatitis, *anaphylaxis*
Contraindications: Hypersensitivity to cephalosporins, infants <1 mo
Precautions: Hypersensitivity to penicillins, pregnancy (B), lactation, renal disease
Pharmacokinetics:
IV: Onset 5 min
IM: Peak 1 hr
Half-life 4½ hr; excreted in breast milk; 98% protein bound
Interactions/incompatibilities:
• Incompatible with aminoglycosides
• Decreased effects: tetracyclines, erythromycins
• Increased toxicity: aminoglycosides, furosemide, probenecid, sulfinpyrazone, colistin, ethacrynic acid, vancomycin, other cephalosporins

Lab test interferences:
Increase (false): Urinary 17-KS
False positive: Urinary protein, direct Coombs' test, urine glucose
Interference: Cross-matching
NURSING CONSIDERATIONS
Assess:
• Sensitivity to penicillin and other cephalosporins
• Nephrotoxicity: increased BUN, creatinine
• I&O daily
• Blood studies: AST, ALT, CBC, Hct, bilirubin, LDH, alk phosphatase, Coombs' test monthly if patient is on long-term therapy
• Electrolytes: K, Na, Cl monthly if patient is on long-term therapy
• Bowel pattern qd; if severe diarrhea occurs, drug should be discontinued; may indicate pseudomembranous colitis
• Urine output; if decreasing, notify physician; may indicate nephrotoxicity
• Allergic reactions: rash, urticaria, pruritus, chills, fever, joint pain, angioedema; may occur few days after therapy begins
• Bleeding: ecchymosis, bleeding gums, hematuria, stool guaiac daily
• Overgrowth of infection: perineal itching, fever, malaise, redness, pain, swelling, drainage, rash, diarrhea, change in cough, sputum
Administer:
• IV direct dilute 0.5 g/2 ml or 1 g/2.5 ml sterile H_2O for inj. and give by Y-tube or 3-way stopcock over 3-5 min
• IV INT may be further diluted in 50-100 ml D_5W, NS and given over 30 min; slight yellowing of sol does not affect potency
• IV; check for irritation, extravasation often
• For 10-14 days to ensure or-

---

italics = common side effects   ***bold italic*** = life threatening reactions

ganism death, prevent superimposed infection
• After C&S completed
Evaluate:
• Therapeutic response: decreased symptoms of infection
Teach patient/family:
• If diabetic, to use Clinistix or Ketodiastix, blood glucose level
• Not to use alcohol or meds with alcohol or reaction may occur
• To report sore throat, bruising, bleeding, joint pain; may indicate blood dyscrasias (rare)
Treatment of overdose: Epinephrine, antihistamines, resuscitate if needed (anaphylaxis)

---

cefoperazone sodium
(sef-oh-per′a-zone)
Cefobid
Func. class.: Antibiotic, broad-spectrum
Chem. class.: Cephalosporin (3rd generation)

Action: Inhibits bacterial cell wall synthesis, rendering cell wall osmotically unstable, leading to cell death
Uses: Gram-negative bacilli: *H. influenzae, E. coli, P. mirabilis, Klebsiella, Enterobacter, Serratia, Citrobacter, Providencia, P. aeruginosa;* lower respiratory tract, urinary tract, skin, bone infections, bacterial septicemia, peritonitis, pelvic inflammatory disease (PID)
Dosage and routes:
Mild/moderate infections
• *Adult:* IM/IV 1-2 g q12h
Severe infections
• *Adult:* IM/IV 6-12 g/day divided in 2-4 equal doses
Available forms: Inj IM, IV, 1, 2 g

Side effects/adverse reactions:
CNS: Headache, dizziness, weakness, paresthesia, fever, chills
GI: Nausea, vomiting, diarrhea, anorexia, pain, glossitis, bleeding, increased AST, ALT, bilirubin, LDH, alk phosphatase, abdominal pain, pseudomembranous colitis
GU: Proteinuria, vaginitis, pruritus, candidiasis, increased BUN, ***nephrotoxicity, renal failure***
*HEMA: **Leukopenia, thrombocytopenia, agranulocytosis,** anemia, **neutropenia, lymphocytosis, eosinophilia, pancytopenia, hemolytic anemia, bleeding, hypoprothrombinemia***
INTEG: Rash, urticaria, dermatitis, ***anaphylaxis***
RESP: Dyspnea
Contraindications: Hypersensitivity to cephalosporins, infants <1 mo
Precautions: Hypersensitivity to penicillins, pregnancy (B), lactation, renal disease
Pharmacokinetics:
IV: Onset 5 min, peak 5-20 min, duration 6-8 hr
IM: Peak 1-2 hr, duration 6-8 hr
Half-life 2 hr; 70%-75% is eliminated unchanged in bile; 20%-30% unchanged in urine; excreted in breast milk (small amounts)
Interactions/incompatibilities:
• Incompatible mix with aminoglycosides, labetalol, perphenazine
• Decreased effects: tetracyclines, erythromycins
• Increased toxicity: aminoglycosides, furosemide, probenecid, sulfinpyrazone, colistin, ethacrynic acid, vancomycin
• Disulfiram-like reactions if alcohol ingested within 24-72 hr of cefoperazone administration
Lab test interferences:
Increase (false): Urinary 17-KS

False positive: Urinary protein, direct Coombs' test, urine glucose
Interference: Cross-matching
NURSING CONSIDERATIONS
Assess:
• Sensitivity to penicillin or other cephalosporins
• Nephrotoxicity: increased BUN, creatinine
• I&O daily
• Blood studies: AST, ALT, CBC, Hct, bilirubin, LDH, alk phosphatase, Coombs' test pro-time monthly if patient is on long-term therapy
• Electrolytes: K, Na, Cl monthly if patient is on long-term therapy
• Bowel pattern qd; if severe diarrhea occurs, drug should be discontinued; may indicate pseudomembranous colitis
• IV site for extravasation or phlebitis, change site q72h
• Urine output, if decreasing, notify physician; may indicate nephrotoxicity
• Allergic reactions: rash, urticaria, pruritus, chills, fever, joint pain, angioedema; may occur few days after therapy begins
• Bleeding: ecchymosis, bleeding gums, hematuria, stool guaiac daily
• Overgrowth of infection: perineal itching, fever, malaise, redness, pain, swelling, drainage, rash, diarrhea, change in cough, sputum
Administer:
• IV after diluting 1 g/ml sterile H₂O for inj, or 0.9% NaCl; shake, give over 3-5 min; each g may be further diluted with 20-40 ml D₅W, NS given over 30 min or as a cont inf over 6-24 hr to a concentration of no greater than 25 mg/ml
• IM for concentration of >250 mg/ml, dilute in sterile water, then lidocaine, inject deeply
• For 10-14 days to ensure organism death, prevent superimposed infection
• After C&S completed
Evaluate:
• Therapeutic response: decreased symptoms of infection
Teach patient/family:
• Not to drink alcohol during or for 3 days after use
• To report sore throat, bruising, bleeding, joint pain; may indicate blood dyscrasias (rare)
Treatment of overdose: Epinephrine, antihistamines, resuscitate if needed (anaphylaxis)

ceforanide
(sef-or-aa-nide)
Precef
Func. class.: Antibiotic, broad-spectrum
Chem. class.: Cephalosporin (2nd generation)

Action: Inhibits bacterial cell wall synthesis, rendering cell wall osmotically unstable leading to cell death
Uses: Gram-negative bacilli: *H. influenzae, E. coli, P. mirabilis, Klebsiella;* gram-positive organisms: *S. pneumoniae, S. aureus;* lower respiratory tract, urinary tract, skin, bone infections, septicemia, endocarditis
Dosage and routes:
• *Adult:* IM/IV 0.5-1 g q12h
• *Child:* IM/IV 20-40 mg/kg/day in 2 equal doses q12h
• Dosage reduction indicated in renal impairment (CrCl < 59 ml/min)
Available forms: Powder for inj IM, IV 500 mg, 1, 10 g
Side effects/adverse reactions:
CNS: Headache, dizziness, weakness, paresthesia, fever, chills

GI: Nausea, vomiting, diarrhea, *anorexia,* pain, glossitis, bleeding, increased AST, ALT, bilirubin, LDH, alk phosphatase, abdominal pain

GU: Proteinuria, vaginitis, pruritus, increased BUN, *nephrotoxicity, renal failure*

HEMA: Leukopenia, thrombocytopenia, agranulocytosis, anemia, *neutropenia, lymphocytosis, eosinophilia, pancytopenia, hemolytic anemia*

INTEG: Rash, urticaria, dermatitis, *anaphylaxis*

RESP: Dyspnea

Contraindications: Hypersensitivity to cephalosporins, infants <1 mo

Precautions: Hypersensitivity to penicillins, pregnancy (B), lactation, renal disease

Pharmacokinetics:

IV: Peak 2 hr

IM: Peak 1 hr

Half-life 2½-3 hr; 80% is bound by plasma proteins; 90% is eliminated unchanged in urine; crosses placenta; excreted in breast milk

Interactions/incompatibilities:
• Incompatible with aminoglycosides
• Decreased effects: tetracyclines, erythromycins
• Increased toxicity: aminoglycosides, furosemide, probenecid, sulfinpyrazone, colistin, ethacrynic acid, vancomycin

Lab test interferences:

Increase (false): Urinary 17-KS

False positive: Urinary protein, direct Coombs' test, urine glucose

Interference: Cross-matching

NURSING CONSIDERATIONS

Assess:
• Sensitivity to penicillin or other cephalosporins

• Nephrotoxicity: increased BUN, creatinine
• I&O daily
• Blood studies: AST, ALT, CBC, Hct, bilirubin, LDH alk phosphatase, Coombs' test monthly if patient is on long-term therapy
• Electrolytes: K, Na, Cl monthly if patient is on long-term therapy
• Urine output: if decreasing, notify physician; may indicate nephrotoxicity
• Allergic reactions: rash, urticaria, pruritus, chills, fever, joint pain, angioedema; may occur few days after therapy begins
• Bleeding: ecchymosis, bleeding gums, hematuria, stool guaiac daily
• Overgrowth of infection: perineal itching, fever, malaise, redness, pain, swelling, drainage, rash, diarrhea, change in cough, sputum
• Bowel pattern qd; if severe diarrhea occurs, drug should be discontinued; may indicate pseudomembranous colitis
• IV site for extravasation or phlebitis; change site q72h

Administer:
• IV direct after diluting 0.5 g/5 ml NS or sterile H_2O for inj; give over 3-5 min
• IV INF may be further diluted in 50-100 ml D_5W, NS and given over 30 min
• For 10-14 days to ensure organism death, prevent superimposed infection
• After C&S completed

Evaluate:
• Therapeutic response: decreased symptoms of infection

Teach patient/family:
• If diabetic, to use Clinistix, Ketodiastix, blood glucose level
• Not to drink alcohol or meds with alcohol, as reaction may occur
• To report sore throat, bruising,

bleeding, joint pain; may indicate blood dyscrasias (rare)
Treatment of overdose: Epinephrine, antihistamines; resuscitate if needed (anaphylaxis)

---

cefotaxime sodium
(sef-oh-taks'eem)
Claforan
Func. class.: Antibiotic, broad-spectrum
Chem. class.: Cephalosporin (3rd generation)

Action: Inhibits bacterial cell wall synthesis, rendering cell wall osmotically unstable, leading to cell death
Uses: Gram-negative organisms: *H. influenzae, E. coli, N. gonorrhoeae, N. meningitidis, P. mirabilis, Klebsiella, Citrobacter, Serratia, Salmonella, Shigella,* gram-positive organisms: *S. pneumoniae, S. pyogenes, S. aureus,* lower serious respiratory tract, urinary tract, skin, bone, gonococcal infections, bacteremia, septicemia, meningitis
Dosage and routes:
• *Adult:* IM/IV 1 g q8-12h
Severe infections
• *Adult:* IM/IV 2 g q4h, not to exceed 12 g/day
• Uncomplicated gonorrhea, 1 g IM
• Dosage reduction indicated for severe renal impairment (CrCl < 10 ml/min)
Available forms: Powder for inj IM, IV, 1, 2, 10 g, frozen inj/IV 20, 40 mg/ml
Side effects/adverse reactions:
CNS: Headache, dizziness, weakness, paresthesia, fever, chills
GI: Nausea, vomiting, diarrhea, anorexia, pain, glossitis, bleeding,

increased AST, ALT, bilirubin, LDH, alk phosphatase, abdominal pain
GU: Proteinuria, vaginitis, pruritus, candidiasis, increased BUN, ***nephrotoxicity, renal failure***
*HEMA: **Leukopenia, thrombocytopenia, agranulocytosis,** anemia, **neutropenia, lymphocytosis, eosinophilia, pancytopenia, hemolytic anemia***
INTEG: Rash, urticaria, dermatitis, ***anaphylaxis,*** pain, induration (IM), inflammation (IV)
Contraindications: Hypersensitivity to cephalosporins, infants <1 mo
Precautions: Hypersensitivity to penicillins, pregnancy (B), lactation, renal disease
Pharmacokinetics:
IV: Onset 5 min
IM: Onset 30 min
Half-life 1 hr; 35%-65% is bound by plasma proteins; 40%-65% is eliminated unchanged in urine in 24 hr; 25% metabolized to active metabolites; excreted in breast milk (small amounts)
Interactions/incompatibilities:
• Incompatible with aminoglycosides, aminophylline, HCO₃, erythromycins
• Decreased effects: tetracyclines, erythromycins
• Increased toxicity: aminoglycosides, furosemide, probenecid, sulfinpyrazone, colistin, ethacrynic acid, vancomycin
Lab test interferences:
Increase (false): Urinary 17-KS
False positive: Urinary protein, direct Coombs' test, urine glucose
Interference: Cross-matching
NURSING CONSIDERATIONS
Assess:
• Sensitivity to penicillin or other cephalosporins

---

italics = common side effects   ***bold italic*** = life threatening reactions

• Nephrotoxicity: increased BUN, creatinine
• I&O daily
• Blood studies: AST, ALT, CBC, Hct, bilirubin, LDH, alk phosphatase, Coombs' test monthly if patient is on long-term therapy
• Electrolytes: K, Na, Cl monthly if the patient is on long-term therapy
• Bowel pattern qd; if severe diarrhea occurs, drug should be discontinued; may indicate pseudomembranous colitis
• IV site for extravasation or phlebitis; change site q72h
• Urine output; if decreasing, notify physician; may indicate nephrotoxicity
• Allergic reactions: rash, urticaria, pruritis, chills, fever, joint pain, angioedema; may occur few days after therapy begins
• Bleeding: ecchymosis, bleeding gums, hematuria, stool guaiac daily
• Overgrowth of infection: perineal itching, fever, malaise, redness, pain, swelling, drainage, rash, diarrhea, change in cough, sputum
Administer:
• IV after diluting 1g/10 ml D₅W, NS, sterile H₂O for inj and give over 3-5 min by Y-tube or 3-way stopcock; may be diluted further with 50-100 ml of normal saline or D₅W; run over ½-1 hr; discontinue primary inf during administration; or may be diluted in larger vol of sol and given as a cont inf over 6-24 hr
• For 10-14 days to ensure organism death, prevent superimposed infection
• After C&S completed
Evaluate:
• Therapeutic response: decreased symptoms of infection

Teach patient/family:
• To report sore throat, bruising, bleeding, joint pain; may indicate blood dyscrasias (rare)
• If diabetic, to use Clinistix or Ketodiastix, blood gluose level
• Not to use alcohol or meds with alcohol or reaction may occur
Treatment of overdose: Epinephrine, antihistamines; resuscitate if needed (anaphylaxis)

cefotetan disodium
(sef'oh-tee-tan)
Cefotan
Func. class.: Antibiotic, broad spectrum
Chem. class.: Cephalosporin (2nd generation)

Action: Inhibits bacterial cell wall synthesis, which renders cell osmotically unstable, leading to cell death
Uses: Gram-negative organisms: *H. influenzae, E. coli, E. aerogenes, P. mirabilis, Klebsiella, Citrobacter, Enterobacter, Salmonella, Shigella, Acinetobacter, B. fragilis, Neisseria, Serratia;* grampositive organisms: *S. pneumoniae, S. pyogenes, S. aureus;* upper, lower, serious respiratory tract, urinary tract, skin, gonococcal, intraabdominal infections, septicemia, meningitis
Dosages and routes:
• *Adult:* IV/IM 1-2g q12h × 5-10 days
Perioperative prophylaxis
• *Adult:* IV 1-2 g ½-1 hr before surgery
Available forms: Inj (IV, IM)
Side effects/adverse reactions:
CNS: Headache, dizziness, weakness, paresthesia, fever, chills
GI: Nausea, vomiting, diarrhea,

anorexia, pain, glossitis, bleeding, increased AST, ALT, bilirubin, LDH, alk phosphatase, *pseudomembranous colitis*

GU: Proteinuria, vaginitis, pruritus, candidiasis, increased BUN, *nephrotoxicity, renal failure*

HEMA: **Leukopenia, thrombocytopenia, agranulocytosis,** anemia, **neutropenia, lymphocytosis, eosinophilia, pancytopenia, hemolytic anemia**

INTEG: Rash, urticaria, dermatitis

RESP: Dyspnea, **anaphylaxis**

Contraindications: Hypersensitivity to cephalosporins; children

Precautions: Hypersensitivity to penicillins, pregnancy (B), lactation, renal disease

Pharmacokinetics:

IV/IM: Peak 1½-3 hr; half-life 3-5 hr, 70%-90% bound by plasma proteins, 50%-80% eliminated unchanged in urine, crosses placenta, excreted in milk

Interactions/incompatibilities:

• Incompatible with tetracyclines, erythromycins, aminoglycosides, heparin, doxapram

• Increased toxicity: aminoglycosides

Lab test interferences:

Increase (false): Urinary 17-KS

False positive: Urinary protein, direct Coombs' test, urine glucose

Interference: Cross-matching

NURSING CONSIDERATIONS

Assess:

• Sensitivity to penicillin or other cephalosporins

• Nephrotoxicity: increased BUN, creatinine

• I&O daily

• Blood studies: AST, ALT, CBC, Hct, bilirubin, LDH, alk phosphatase, Coombs' test monthly if patient is on long-term therapy

• Electrolytes: K, Na, Cl monthly if patient is on long-term therapy

• Bowel pattern qd; if severe diarrhea occurs, drug should be discontinued; may indicate pseudomembranous colitis

• IV site for extravasation, phlebitis, change site q72h

• Urine output: if decreasing, notify physician; may indicate nephrotoxicity

• Allergic reactions: rash, urticaria, pruritus, chills, fever; may occur a few days after therapy begins

• Bleeding: ecchymosis, bleeding gums, hematuria, stool guaiac daily

• Overgrowth of infection: perineal itching, fever, malaise, redness, swelling, drainage, rash, diarrhea, change in cough, sputum

Administer:

• IV direct after diluting 1 g/10 ml sterile H_2O for inj and give over 3-5 min; may be diluted further with 50-100 ml of normal saline or D_5W shake; run over ½-1 hr by Y-tube or 3-way stopcock discontinue primary inf during administration

• For 5-10 days to ensure organism death, prevent superimposed infection

• After C&S is taken

Evaluate:

• Therapeutic response: decreased symptoms of infection

Teach patient/family:

• To report sore throat, bruising, bleeding, joint pain; may indicate blood dyscrasias

• To report severe diarrhea; may indicate pseudomembranous colitis

• To avoid use of alcohol during and for 3 days after use

Treatment of overdose: Epinephrine, antihistamines; resuscitate if needed (anaphylaxis)

---

italics = common side effects   ***bold italic*** = life threatening reactions

cefoxitin sodium

(se-fox'i-tin)

Mefoxin

Func. class.: Antibiotic, broad-spectrum

Chem. class.: Cephamycin (2nd generation)

Action: Inhibits bacterial cell wall synthesis, rendering cell wall osmotically unstable, leading to cell death

Uses: Gram-negative bacilli: *H. influenzae, E. coli, Proteus, Klebsiella, B. fragilis, N. gonorrhoeae;* gram-positive organisms: *S. pneumoniae, S. pyogenes, S. aureus;* anaerobes including *Clostridium,* lower respiratory tract, urinary tract, skin, bone, gonococcal infections, septicemia, peritonitis

Dosage and routes:
• *Adult:* IM/IV 1-2 g q6-8h
• Dosage reduction indicated in renal impairment (CrCl <50 ml/min)
• Uncomplicated gonorrhea 2 g IM as single dose with 1 g PO probenecid at same time

Severe infections
• *Adult:* IM/IV 2 g q4h

Available forms: Powder for inj IM, IV 1, 2, 10 g

Side effects/adverse reactions:
CNS: Headache, dizziness, weakness, paresthesia, fever, chills
GI: Nausea, vomiting, diarrhea, anorexia, pain, glossitis, bleeding, increased AST, ALT, bilirubin, LDH, alk phosphatase, abdominal pain
GU: Proteinuria, vaginitis, pruritus, candidiasis, increased BUN, *nephrotoxicity, renal failure*
HEMA: Leukopenia, thrombocytopenia, agranulocytosis, anemia, *neutropenia, lymphocytosis, eosinophilia, pancytopenia, hemolytic anemia*
INTEG: Rash, urticaria, dermatitis, thrombophlebitis
SYST: Anaphylaxis

Contraindications: Hypersensitivity to cephalosporins; infants <1 mo

Precautions: Hypersensitivity to penicillins, pregnancy (B), lactation, renal disease

Pharmacokinetics:
IV: Peak 3 min
IM: Peak 15-60 min
Half-life 1 hr, 55%-75% bound by plasma proteins, 90%-100% eliminated unchanged in urine; crosses placenta, blood-brain barrier, eliminated in milk, not metabolized

Interactions/incompatibilities:
• Incompatible with aminoglycosides
• Decreased effects: tetracyclines, erythromycins
• Increased toxicity: aminoglycosides, furosemide, probenecid, sulfinpyrazone, colistin, ethacrynic acid, vancomycin

Lab test interferences:
Increase (false): Creatinine (serum urine), urinary 17-KS
False positive: Urinary protein, direct Coombs' test, urine glucose
Interference: Cross-matching

NURSING CONSIDERATIONS
Assess:
• Sensitivity to penicillin or other cephalosporins
• Nephrotoxicity: increased BUN, creatinine
• I&O daily
• Blood studies: AST, ALT, CBC, Hct, bilirubin, LDH, alk phosphatase, Coombs' test monthly if patient is on long-term therapy
• Electrolytes: K, Na, Cl monthly if patient is on long-term therapy

---

*Available in Canada only

• Bowel pattern qd; if severe diarrhea occurs, drug should be discontinued (may indicate pseudomembranous colitis)
• IV site for extravasation or phlebitis; change site q72h
• Urine output; if decreasing, notify physician; may indicate nephrotoxicity
• Allergic reactions: rash, urticaria, pruritus, chills, fever, joint pain, angioedema; may occur few days after therapy begins
• Bleeding: ecchymosis, bleeding gums, hematuria, stool guaiac daily
• Overgrowth of infection: perineal itching, fever, malaise, redness, pain, swelling, drainage, rash, diarrhea, change in cough, sputum
Administer:
• IV after diluting 1 g or less/10 ml or more D₅W, NS and give over 3-5 min; may be diluted further with 50-100 ml of normal saline or D₅W; run over ½-1 hr by Y-tube or 3-way stopcock; discontinue primary inf during administration; by cont inf at prescribed rate
• For 10-14 days to ensure organism death, prevent superimposed infection
• After C&S completed
Evaluate:
• Therapeutic response: decreased symptoms of infection
Teach patient/family:
• If diabetic, to use Clinistix or Ketodiastix, blood glucose level
• Not to use alcohol or meds with alcohol or reaction can occur
• To report severe diarrhea; may indicate pseudomembranous colitis
• To report sore throat, bruising, bleeding, joint pain; may indicate blood dyscrasias (rare)
Treatment of overdose: Epinephrine, antihistamines; resuscitate if needed (anaphylaxis)

cefpodoxime
(sef-pod'-ox-ime)
Vantin
Func. class.: Antibiotic
Chem. class.: Cephalosporin
(2nd generation)

Action: Inhibits bacterial cell synthesis, which renders cell wall osmotically unstable
Uses: Gram-negative bacilli: *N. gonorrhoeae, H. influenzae, E. coli, P. mirabilis, Klebsiella;* gram-positive organisms: *S. pneumoniae, S. pyogenes, S. aureus;* upper and lower respiratory tract, urinary tract, skin infections, otitis media, sexually transmitted diseases
Dosage and routes:
• *Adult (>13 years of age):* pneumonia: 200 mg q12h for 14 days; uncomplicated gonorrhea: 200 mg single dose; skin and skin structure: 40 mg q12h for 7-14 days; pharyngitis and tonsillitis: 100 mg q12h for 10 days; uncomplicated UTI: 100 mg q12h for 7 days; dosing interval increased in presence of severe renal impairment
• *Child (6 mo-12 yrs):* acute otitis media: 5 mg/kg q12h for 14 days; uncomplicated gonorrhea: 200 mg single dose; skin and skin structure: 400 mg q12h for 7-14 days; pharyngitis and tonsillitis: 100 mg q12h (max 200 mg/dose or 400 mg/day) for 10 days; pharyngitis/tonsillitis: 5 mg/kg q12h (max 100 mg/dose or 200 mg/day) for 10 days
Available forms: Tabs 100, 200 mg; granules for suspension 50 mg/5 ml and 100 mg/5 ml
Side effects/adverse reactions:
CNS: Headache, dizziness, lethargy, fatigue, paresthesia, fever, chills

---

italics = common side effects ***bold italic*** = life threatening reactions

GI: Nausea, vomiting, diarrhea, anorexia, pain, glossitis, bleeding, increased AST, ALT, bilirubin, LDH, alk phosphatase

GU: Proteinuria, vaginitis, pruritus, candidiasis, increased BUN, nephrotoxicity, renal failure

HEMA: Leukopenia, thrombocytopenia, agranulocytosis, anemia, neutropenia, lymphocytosis, eosinophilia, pancytopenia, hemolytic anemia

INTEG: Rash, urticaria, dermatitis, anaphylaxis

RESP: Dyspnea

Contraindications: Hypersensitivity to cephalosporins; infants

Precautions: Hypersensitivity to penicillins, pregnancy (B), lactation, renal disease

Pharmacokinetics:
Half-life 2-3 min; 25% bound by plasma proteins; 30% eliminated unchanged in urine in 8 hr; crosses placenta; excreted in breast milk

Interactions/incompatibilities:
• Increased toxicity: aminoglycosides, probenecid, colistin, vancomycin

Lab test interferences:
False increase: Creatinine (serum urine), urinary 17-KS
False positive: Urinary protein, direct Coombs' test, urine glucose
Interference: Cross-matching

NURSING CONSIDERATIONS
Assess:
• Sensitivity to penicillins and other cephalosporins
• Nephrotoxicity: increased BUN, creatinine
• I&O daily
• Blood studies: AST, ALT, CBC, Hct, bilirubin, LDH, alk phosphatase, Coombs' test monthly if patient is on long-term therapy
• Electrolytes: K, Na, Cl monthly if patient is on long-term therapy

• Bowel pattern qd; if severe diarrhea occurs, drug should be discontinued; may indicate pseudomembranous colitis
• Urine output; if decreasing, notify physician (may indicate nephrotoxicity)
• Allergic reactions: rash, urticaria, pruritus, chills, fever, joint pain; angioedema may occur a few days after therapy begins
• Bleeding: ecchymosis, bleeding gums, hematuria, stool guaiac daily
• Overgrowth of infection: perineal itching, fever, malaise, redness, pain, swelling, drainage, rash, diarrhea, change in cough, sputum
Administer:
• For 10-14 days to ensure organism death, prevent superimposed infection
• With food to enhance absorption
• After C&S completed
Evaluate:
• Therapeutic response: decreased symptoms of infection
Teach patient/family:
• If diabetic, to use Keto-Diastix, blood glucose level monitor to identify level
• Not to drink alcohol or meds with alcohol or reaction may occur
• To use yogurt or buttermilk to maintain intestinal flora, decrease diarrhea
• To take all med prescribed for length of time ordered
• To report sore throat, bruising, bleeding, joint pain; may indicate blood dyscrasias (rare)
Treatment of overdose: Epinephrine, antihistamines; resuscitate if needed (anaphylaxis)

cefprozil monohydrate

(sef-pro'zil)
Cefzil
Func. class.: Antibiotic, broad spectrum
Chem. class.: Cephalosporin

Action: Inhibits bacterial cell wall synthesis, which renders cell wall osmotically unstable, leading to cell death

Uses: Pharyngitis/tonsillitis, otitis media, secondary bacterial infection of acute bronchitis, and acute bacterial exacerbation of chronic bronchitis and uncomplicated skin and skin structure infections

Dosage and routes:
Upper respiratory infections
• *Adult:* PO 500 mg qd × 10 days
Otitis media
• *Child:* (6 mo-12 yr) PO 15mg/kg q12h × 10 days
Lower respiratory infections
• *Adult:* PO 500 mg bid × 10 days
Skin/skin structure infections
• *Adult:* PO 250-500 mg q12h × 10 days
Available forms: Tabs 250, 500 mg; susp. 125, 250 mg/5ml

Side effects/adverse reactions:
CNS: Dizziness, headache, weakness, paresthesia, fever, chills
*GU: **Nephrotoxicity, proteinuria, increased BUN, renal failure, hematuria,** vaginitis, genitoanal pruritus, candidiasis*
GI: Diarrhea, nausea, vomiting, pain, glossitis, anorexia, bleeding, increased AST, ALT, bilirubin, LDH, alk phosphatse, abdominal pain, **pseudomembranous colitis,** flatulence
*HEMA: **Leukopenia, thrombocytopenia, agranulocytosis, anemia,** neutropenia, lymphocytosis, eosinophilia, pancytopenia, hemolytic anemia*
INTEG: Rash, urticaria, dermatitis
*RESP: **Anaphylaxis,** dyspnea*

Contraindications: Hypersensitivity to cephalosporins

Precautions: Pregnancy (B), lactation, elderly, hypersensitivity to penicillins, renal disease

Pharmacokinetics:
PO: Peak 6-10 hr; plasma protein binding 99%; elimination half-life 25 hr; extensively metabolized to an active metabolite

Interactions/incompatibilities:
• Decreased effects of: tetracyclines, erythromycins, chloramphenicol
• Increased toxicity of: aminoglycosides, probenecid, sulfinpyrazone, colistin

Lab test interferences:
Increase (false): Urinary 17-KS
False positive: Urinary protein, direct Coombs' test, urine glucose
Interference: Cross-matching

NURSING CONSIDERATIONS
Assess:
• Sensitivity to penicillin or other cephalosporins
• Nephrotoxicity: increased BUN, creatinine
• I&O daily
• Blood studies: AST, ALT, CBC, Hct, bilirubin, LDH, alk phosphatase, Coombs' test monthly, bowel pattern qd; if severe diarrhea occurs, drug should be discontinued; may indicate pseudomembranous colitis
• Urine output; if decreasing, notify physician; may indicate nephrotoxicity
• Allergic reactions: rash, urticaria, pruritus, chills, fever, joint pain, angioedema; may occur few days after therapy begins

---

italics = common side effects   ***bold italic*** = life threatening reactions

• Bleeding: ecchymosis, bleeding gums, hematuria, stool guaiac daily
• Overgrowth of infection: perineal itching, fever, malaise, redness, pain, swelling, drainage, rash, diarrhea, change in cough, sputum

Administer:
• For 10-14 days to ensure organism death, prevent superimposed infection
• After C&S is taken

Evaluate:
• Therapeutic response: negative C&S

Teach patient/family:
• Not to use alcohol or meds with alcohol or reaction may occur
• To report severe diarrhea; may indicate pseudomembranous colitis
• To report sore throat, bruising, bleeding, joint pain; may indicate blood dyscrasias (rare)

Treatment of overdose: Epinephrine, antihistamines; resuscitate if needed (anaphylaxis)

---

ceftazidime

(sef'tay-zi-deem)
Ceptaz, Fortaz, Pentacef, Tazicef, Tazidime
Func. class.: Antibiotic, broad-spectrum
Chem. class.: Cephalosporin (3rd generation)

Action: Inhibits bacterial cell wall synthesis, which renders cell osmotically unstable

Uses: Gram-negative organisms: *H. influenzae, E. coli, E. aerogenes, P. aeruginosa mirabilis, Klebsiella, Citrobacter, Enterobacter, Salmonella, Shigella, Acinetobacter, B. fragilis, Neisseria, Serratia;* gram-positive organisms: *S. pneumoniae, S. pyogenes, S. aureus;* upper, lower, serious respiratory tract, urinary tract, skin, gonococcal, intraabdominal infections; septicemia, meningitis

Dosage and routes:
• *Adult:* IV/IM 1 g q8-12h × 5-10 days
• *Children:* IV 30-50 mg/kg/day, not to exceed 6 g/day
• *Neonates:* IV 30 mg/kg q12h

Available forms: Inj (IV, IM), 1, 2 g

Side effects/adverse reactions:
CNS: Headache, dizziness, weakness, paresthesia, fever, chills
GI: Nausea, vomiting, diarrhea, anorexia, pain, glossitis, bleeding, increased AST, ALT, bilirubin, LDH, alk phosphatase
GU: Proteinuria, vaginitis, pruritus, candidiasis, increased BUN, *nephrotoxicity, renal failure*
HEMA: Leukopenia, thrombocytopenia, agranulocytosis, anemia, *neutropenia, lymphocytosis, eosinophilia, pancytopenia, hemolytic anemia*
INTEG: Rash, urticaria, dermatitis, *anaphylaxis*
RESP: Dyspnea

Contraindications: Hypersensitivity to cephalosporins, children

Precautions: Hypersensitivity to penicillins, pregnancy (B), lactation, renal disease

Pharmacokinetics:
IV/IM: Peak 1 hr, half-life ½-1 hr, 90% bound by plasma proteins, 80% eliminated unchanged in urine, crosses placenta, excreted in breast milk

Interactions/incompatibilities:
• Incompatible with aminoglycosides
• Increased toxicity: aminoglycosides

Lab test interferences:
Increase (false): Urinary 17-KS
False positive: Urinary protein, di-

---

rect Coombs' test, urine glucose
Interference: Cross-matching
NURSING CONSIDERATIONS
Assess:
• Sensitivity to penicillin or other cephalosporins
• Nephrotoxicity: increased BUN, creatinine
• I&O daily
• Blood studies: AST, ALT, CBC, Hct, bilirubin, LDH, alk phosphatase, Coombs' test monthly if patient is on long-term therapy
• Electrolytes: K, Na, Cl monthly if patient is on long-term therapy
• Bowel pattern qd; if severe diarrhea occurs, drug should be discontinued; may indicate pseudomembranous colitis
• IV site for extravasation, phlebitis, change site q72h
• Urine output: if decreasing, notify physician; may indicate nephrotoxicity
• Allergic reactions: rash, urticaria, pruritus, chills, fever; may occur a few days after therapy begins
• Bleeding: ecchymosis, bleeding gums, hematuria, stool guaiac daily
• Overgrowth of infection: perineal itching, fever, malaise, redness, swelling, drainage, rash, diarrhea, change in cough, sputum
Administer:
• IV after diluting 1 g/10 ml sterile H$_2$O for inj, shake, invert needle, push plunger, insert needle through stopper and keep in sol, expel bubbles and give over 3-5 min; may be diluted further with 50-100 ml of normal saline or D$_5$W; run over ½-1 hr give through Y-tube, or 3-way stopcock, discontinue primary inf during administration
• For 5-10 days to ensure organism death, prevent superimposed infection
• After C&S is taken

Evaluate:
• Therapeutic response: decreased symptoms of infection
Teach patient/family:
• To report sore throat, bruising, bleeding, joint pain; may indicate blood dyscrasias
• To report severe diarrhea; may indicate pseudomembranous colitis
• If diabetic, to use Clinistix or Ketodiastix, blood glucose level
• Not to use alcohol or meds with alcohol or reaction may occur
Treatment of overdose: Epinephrine, antihistamines; resuscitate if needed (anaphylaxis)

---

ceftizoxime sodium
(sef-ti-zox'eem)
Cefizox
Func. class.: Antibiotic, broad-spectrum
Chem. class.: Cephalosporin (3rd generation)

Action: Inhibits bacterial cell wall synthesis, which renders cell wall osmotically unstable, leading to cell death
Uses: Gram-negative organisms: *H. influenzae, E. coli, E. aerogenes, P. mirabilis, Klebsiella, Enterobacter;* gram-positive organisms: *S. pneumoniae, S. pyogenes, S. aureus;* lower serious respiratory tract, urinary tract, skin, intraabdominal infections, septicemia, meningitis, bone, joint infections, pelvic inflammatory disease (PID) caused by *N. gonorrhoeae*
Dosage and routes:
• *Adult:* IM/IV 1-2 g q8-12h, may give up to 2g q4h in life-threatening infections.
Pelvic Inflammatory Disease (PID)
• *Adult* IV 2 g q8h, may increase to 2 g q4h in severe infections

---

italics = common side effects   ***bold italic*** = life threatening reactions

Available forms: Inj 500 mg, 1, 2 g/100 ml piggyback, 50 ml/5% D

Side effects/adverse reactions:

CNS: Headache, dizziness, paresthesia, fever

GI: Nausea, vomiting, diarrhea, anorexia, pain, glossitis, bleeding, increased AST, ALT, bilirubin, LDH, alk phosphatase, abdominal pain, *pseudomembranous colitis*

GU: Proteinuria, vaginitis, pruritus, candidiasis

HEMA: Leukopenia, thrombocytopenia, agranulocytosis, anemia, *neutropenia, eosinophilia, hemolytic anemia*

INTEG: Rash, urticaria, dermatitis

RESP: Dyspnea, *anaphylaxis*

Contraindications: Hypersensitivity to cephalosporins, infants <1 mo

Precautions: Hypersensitivity to penicillins, pregnancy (B), lactation, renal disease

Pharmacokinetics:

IV: Onset 5 min

IM: Peak 1 hr

Half-life 5-8 hr; 90% bound by plasma proteins; 36%-60% is eliminated unchanged in urine; crosses placenta; excreted in milk

Interactions/incompatibilities:

• Incompatible with aminoglycosides

• Decreased effects: tetracyclines, erythromycins

• Increased toxicity: aminoglycosides, furosemide, probenecid, sulfinpyrazone, colistin, ethacrynic acid

Lab test interferences:

Increase (false): Urinary 17-KS

False positive: Urinary protein, direct Coombs' test, urine glucose

Interference: Cross-matching

NURSING CONSIDERATIONS

Assess:

• Sensitivity to penicillin or other cephalosporins

• Nephrotoxicity: increased BUN, creatinine

• I&O daily

• Blood studies: AST, ALT, CBC, Hct, bilirubin, LDH, alk phosphatase, Coombs' test monthly if patient is on long-term therapy

• Electrolytes: K, Na, Cl monthly if patient is on long-term therapy

• Bowel pattern qd; if severe diarrhea occurs, drug should be discontinued; may indicate pseudomembranous colitis

• IV site for extravasation, phlebitis; change site q72h

• Allergic reactions: rash, urticaria, pruritus, chills, fever, joint pain, angioedema; may occur few days after therapy begins

• Bleeding: ecchymosis, bleeding gums, hematuria, stool guaiac daily

• Overgrowth of infection: perineal itching, fever, malaise, redness, pain, swelling, drainage, rash, diarrhea, change in cough, sputum

Administer:

• IV after diluting 1 g/10 ml sterile water, shake and give over 3-5 min; may be diluted further with 50-100 ml of normal saline or D₅W give through Y-tube or 3-way stopcock; run over ½-1 hr

• For 10-14 days to ensure organism death, prevent superimposed infection

• After C&S

Evaluate:

• Therapeutic response: decreased symptoms of infection

Teach patient/family:

• If diabetic, to use Clinistix or Ketodiastix, blood glucose level

• Not to use alcohol or meds with alcohol or reaction can occur

• To report sore throat, bruising, bleeding, joint pain; may indicate blood dyscrasias (rare)

Treatment of overdose: Epinephrine, antihistamines; resuscitate if needed (anaphylaxis)

ceftriaxone sodium
(sef-try-ax'-one)
Rocephin
Func. class.: Antibiotic, broad spectrum
Chem. class.: Cephalosporin (3rd generation)

Action: Inhibits bacterial cell wall synthesis, which renders cell wall osmotically unstable, leading to cell death

Uses: Gram-negative organisms: *H. influenzae, E. coli, E. aerogenes, P. mirabilis, Klebsiella, Citrobacter, Enterobacter, Salmonella, Shigella, Acinetobacter, B. fragilis, Neisseria, Serratia;* gram-positive organisms: *S. pneumoniae, S. pyogenes, S. aureus;* lower serious respiratory tract, urinary tract, skin, gonococcal, intraabdominal infections, septicemia, meningitis, bone, joint infections

Dosage and routes:
• *Adult:* IM/IV 1-2 g qd or in two equal doses
• *Child:* IM/IV 50-75 mg/kg/day in equal doses q12h
Uncomplicated gonorrhea
• 250 mg IM as single dose
• Dosage reduction may be indicated in severe renal impairment (CrCl < 10 ml/min)
Meningitis
• *Adult and child:* IM/IV 100 mg/kg/day in equal doses q12h
Surgical prophylaxis
• Adult: IV 1 g ½-2 hr preop
Available forms: Inj IM, IV 250, 500 mg, 1, 2, 10 g
Side effects/adverse reactions:
CNS: Headache, dizziness, weakness, paresthesia, fever, chills

GI: Nausea, vomiting, diarrhea, anorexia, pain, glossitis, bleeding, increased AST, ALT, bilirubin, LDH, alk phosphatase, abdominal pain, *pseudomembranous colitis*
GU: Proteinuria, vaginitis, pruritus, candidiasis, increased BUN, ***nephrotoxicity, renal failure***
*HEMA: **Leukopenia, thrombocytopenia, agranulocytosis,** anemia, **neutropenia, lymphocytosis, eosinophilia, pancytopenia, hemolytic anemia***
INTEG: Rash, urticaria, dermatitis
RESP: Dyspnea, ***anaphylaxis***
Contraindications: Hypersensitivity to cephalosporins, infants <1 mo
Precautions: Hypersensitivity to penicillins, pregnancy (B), lactation, renal disease
Pharmacokinetics:
IV: Onset 5 min
IM: Peak 1 hr
Half-life 5-8 hr, 90% bound by plasma proteins; 35%-60% is eliminated unchanged in urine; crosses placenta; excreted in milk
Interactions/incompatibilities:
• Incompatible with erythromycins, aminoglycosides
• Decreased effects: tetracyclines, erythromycins
• Increased toxicity: aminoglycosides, furosemide, probenecid, sulfinpyrazone, colistin, ethacrynic acid
Lab test interferences:
Increase (false): Urinary 17-KS
False positive: Urinary protein, direct Coombs' test, urine glucose
Interference: Cross-matching
NURSING CONSIDERATIONS
Assess:
• Sensitivity to penicillin or other cephalosporins
• Nephrotoxicity: increased BUN, creatinine

---

italics = common side effects   ***bold italic*** = life threatening reactions

• I&O daily
• Blood studies: AST, ALT, CBC, Hct, bilirubin, LDH, alk phosphatase, Coombs' test monthly if patient is on long-term therapy
• Electrolytes: K, Na, Cl monthly if patient is on long-term therapy
• Bowel pattern qd; if severe diarrhea occurs, drug should be discontinued; may indicate pseudomembranous colitis
• IV site for extravasation, phlebitis; change site q72h
• Urine output; if decreasing, notify physician; may indicate nephrotoxicity
• Allergic reactions: rash, urticaria, pruritus, chills, fever, joint pain, angioedema; may occur few days after therapy begins
• Bleeding: ecchymosis, bleeding gums, hematuria, stool guaiac daily
• Overgrowth of infection: perineal itching, fever, malaise, redness, pain, swelling, drainage, rash, diarrhea, change in cough, sputum

Administer:
• For 10-14 days to ensure organism death, prevent superimposed infection
• IV after diluting 250 mg/2.4 ml of D₅W, H₂O for inj, 0.9% NaCl; may be further diluted with 50-100 ml of NS, D₅W, D₁₀W shake; run over ½-1 hr
• After C&S

Evaluate:
• Therapeutic response: decreased symptoms of infection

Teach patient/family:
• If diabetic, to use Clinistix or Ketodiastix, blood glucose level
• Not to use alcohol or meds with alcohol or reaction may occur
• To report severe diarrhea; may indicate pseudomembranous colitis
• To report sore throat, bruising,

bleeding, joint pain; may indicate blood dyscrasias (rare)

Treatment of overdose: Epinephrine, antihistamines; resuscitate if needed (anaphylaxis)

cefuroxime axetil

(sef-fyoor-ox′eem)
Ceftin
Func. class.: Antibiotic, broad-spectrum
Chem. class.: Cephalosporin (2nd generation)

Action: Inhibits bacterial cell wall synthesis, rendering cell wall osmotically unstable

Uses: Gram-negative bacilli (*H. influenzae, E. coli, Neisseria, P. mirabilis, Klebsiella*); gram-positive organisms (*S. pneumoniae, S. pyogenes, S. aureus*); serious lower respiratory tract, urinary tract, skin, gonococcal infections; septicemia; meningitis

Dosage and routes:
• *Adult and child:* PO 250 mg q12h; may increase to 500 mg q12h in serious infections

Urinary tract infections
• *Adult:* PO 125 mg q12h; may increase to 250 q12h if needed

Otitis media
• Child <2 yr: PO 125 mg bid
• Child >2 yr: PO 250 mg bid

Available forms: Tabs 125, 250, 500 mg

Side effects/adverse reactions:
CNS: Headache, dizziness, weakness, paresthesia, fever, chills
GI: Nausea, vomiting, diarrhea, anorexia, pain, glossitis, bleeding, increased AST, ALT, bilirubin, LDH, alk phosphatase, abdominal pain, ***pseudomembranous colitis***
GU: Proteinuria, vaginitis, pruritus,

candidiasis, increased BUN, *nephrotoxicity, renal failure*
HEMA: **Leukopenia, thrombocytopenia, agranulocytosis,** anemia, **neutropenia, lymphocytosis, eosinophilia, pancytopenia, hemolytic anemia**
INTEG: Rash, urticaria, dermatitis
RESP: **Anaphylaxis**
Contraindications: Hypersensitivity to cephalosporins, infants <1 mo
Precautions: Hypersensitivity to penicillins, pregnancy (B), lactation, renal disease
Pharmacokinetics:
65% excreted unchanged in urine, half-life 1-2 hr in normal renal function
Interactions/incompatibilities:
• Decreased effects: tetracyclines, erythromycins
• Increased side effects: aminoglycosides, furosemide, probenecid, sulfinpyrazone, colistin, ethacrynic acid
Lab test interferences:
Increase (false): Creatinine (serum urine), urinary 17-KS
False positive: Urinary protein, direct Coombs' test, urine glucose
Interferences: Cross-matching
NURSING CONSIDERATIONS
Assess:
• Sensitivity to penicillin or other cephalosporins
• Nephrotoxicity: increased BUN, creatinine
• I&O daily
• Blood studies: AST, ALT, CBC, Hct, bilirubin, LDH, alk phosphatase, Coombs' test monthly if patient is on long-term therapy
• Electrolytes: K, Na, Cl monthly if patient is on long-term therapy
• Bowel pattern qd; if severe diarrhea occurs, drug should be discontinued; may indicate pseudomembranous colitis
• IV site for extravasation, phlebitis; change site q72h
• Urine output: if decreasing, notify physician; may indicate nephrotoxicity
• Allergic reactions: rash, urticaria, pruritus, chills, fever, joint pain, angioedema; may occur a few days after therapy begins
• Bleeding: ecchymosis, bleeding gums, hematuria, stool guaiac daily
• Overgrowth of infection: perineal itching, fever, malaise, redness, pain, swelling, drainage, rash, diarrhea, change in cough, sputum
Administer:
• For 10-14 days to ensure organism death, prevent superimposed infection
• With food if needed for GI symptoms
• After C&S
Evaluate:
• Therapeutic response: decreased symptoms of infection
Teach patient/family:
• To use yogurt or buttermilk to maintain intestinal flora, decrease diarrhea
• To take all medication prescribed for length of time ordered
• To report sore throat, bruising, bleeding, joint pain; may indicate blood dyscrasias (rare)
• If diabetic, to use Clinistix or Ketodiastix, blood glucose level
• Not to use alcohol or meds with alcohol or reaction may occur
Treatment of overdose: Epinephrine, antihistamine; resuscitate if needed (anaphylaxis)

italics = common side effects   ***bold italic*** = life threatening reactions

cefuroxime sodium

(se-fyoor-ox′eem)
Zinacef, Kefurox

Func. class.: Antibiotic, broad spectrum
Chem. class.: Cephalosporin (2nd generation)

Action: Inhibits bacterial cell wall synthesis, rendering cell wall osmotically unstable, leading to cell death

Uses: Gram-negative organisms: *H. influenzae, E. coli, Neisseria, P. mirabilis, Klebsiella;* gram-positive organisms: *S. pneumoniae, S. pyogenes, S. aureus;* serious lower respiratory tract, urinary tract, skin, gonococcal infections, septicemia, meningitis

Dosage and routes:
• *Adult:* IM/IV 750 mg-1.5 g q8h for 5-10 days
Surgical prophylaxis
• *Adult:* IV 1.5 g ½-1 hr preop
Severe infections
• *Adult:* IM/IV 1.5 g q6h; may give up to 3 g q8h for bacterial meningitis
• *Child >3 mo:* IM/IV 50-100 mg/kg/day; may give up to 200-240 mg/kg/day IV in divided doses for bacterial meningitis
• Dosage reduction indicated in severe renal impairment (CrCl < 20 ml/min)
• *Uncomplicated gonorrhea:* 1.5 g IM as single dose with oral probenecid
Available forms: Inj IM, IV 750 mg, 1.5 g, powder

Side effects/adverse reactions:
CNS: Headache, dizziness, weakness, paresthesia, fever, chills
GI: Nausea, vomiting, diarrhea, anorexia, pain, glossitis, bleeding, increased AST, ALT, bilirubin, LDH, alk phosphatase, abdominal pain, *pseudomembranous colitis*
GU: Proteinuria, vaginitis, pruritus, candidiasis, increased BUN, *nephrotoxicity, renal failure*
HEMA: Leukopenia, thrombocytopenia, agranulocytosis, anemia, *neutropenia, lymphocytosis, eosinophilia, pancytopenia, hemolytic anemia*
INTEG: Rash, urticaria, dermatitis
RESP: Dyspnea, *anaphylaxis*

Contraindications: Hypersensitivity to cephalosporins, infants <1 mo

Precautions: Hypersensitivity to penicillins, pregnancy (B), lactation, renal disease

Pharmacokinetics:
IV: Peak 3 min
IM: Peak 15-60 min
Half-life 1-2 hr; 33%-50% bound by plasma proteins; 70%-100% eliminated unchanged in urine; crosses placenta; blood-brain barrier; excreted in breast milk; not metabolized

Interactions/incompatibilities:
• Incompatible with aminoglycosides
• Decreased effects: tetracyclines, erythromycins
• Increased toxicity: aminoglycosides, furosemide, probenecid, sulfinpyrazone, colistin, ethacrynic acid, vancomycin

Lab test interferences:
Increase (false): Urinary 17-KS
False positive: Urinary protein, direct Coombs' test, urine glucose
Interference: Cross-matching

NURSING CONSIDERATIONS
Assess:
• Sensitivity to penicillin or other cephalosporins
• Nephrotoxicity: increased BUN, creatinine

- I&O daily
- Blood studies: AST, ALT, CBC, Hct, bilirubin, LDH, alk phosphatase, Coombs' test monthly if patient is on long-term therapy
- Electrolytes: K, Na, Cl monthly if patient is on long-term therapy
- Bowel pattern qd; if severe diarrhea occurs, drug should be discontinued; may indicate pseudomembranous colitis
- IV site for extravasation, phlebitis; change site q72h
- Urine output: if decreasing, notify physician; may indicate nephrotoxicity
- Allergic reactions: rash, urticaria, pruritus, chills, fever, joint pain, angioedema; may occur few days after therapy begins
- Bleeding: ecchymosis, bleeding gums, hematuria, stool guaiac daily
- Overgrowth of infection: perineal itching, fever, malaise, redness, pain, swelling, drainage, rash, diarrhea, change in cough, sputum

Administer:
- IV after diluting 750 mg/9 ml of sterile H_2O for Inj, NS, D_5W, shake and give over 3-5 min; may be further diluted with 100 ml of compatible sol; run over ½ hr; may also be given by continuous infusion added to 500-1000 ml given over 6-24 hr
- For 10-14 days to ensure organism death, prevent superimposed infection
- After C&S

Evaluate:
- Therapeutic response: decreased symptoms of infection

Teach patient/family:
- To report severe diarrhea; may indicate pseudomembranous colitis
- If diabetic, to use Clinistix or Ketodiastix, blood glucose level

- Not to use alcohol or meds with alcohol or reaction can occur
- To report sore throat, bruising, bleeding, joint pain; may indicate blood dyscrasias (rare)

Treatment of overdose: Epinephrine, antihistamines; resuscitate if needed (anaphylaxis)

---

cellulose sodium phosphate
Calcibind, Calcisorb*

Func. class.: Antihypercalcemia
Chem. class.: Phosphorylated cellulose

Action: Decreases hypercalcium by binding with calcium in bowel; facilitates excretion of calcium

Uses: Absorptive hypercalciuria type I with recurrent calcium oxalate or phosphate renal stones

Dosage and routes:
- *Adult:* PO 15 g/day divided between each meal, then 10 g/day when urine Ca <150 mg/day

Available forms: Powder 2.5 g packets

Side effects/adverse reactions:
GU: Hypomagnesuria, hyperoxaluria
GI: Nausea, anorexia, diarrhea, dyspepsia

Contraindications: Hypersensitivity, hyperparathyroidism, hypomagnesemia, enteric hyperoxaluria, bone disease, hypocalcemia

Precautions: CHF, ascites, liver disease, pregnancy (C), children, elderly

Pharmacokinetics:
Not known

Interactions/incompatibilities:
- Decreased action of cellulose: magnesium preparations

NURSING CONSIDERATIONS
Assess:
• Calcium levels (serum, urinary) throughout treatment (therapeutic values: 2.3-2.8 mmol/L, serum; <3.75 mmol/24 hr, urine)
Administer:
• Powder with water, juice; take within 30 min of meals
• Increase fluids to 3 L/day; urinary output should be >2 L/day
Evaluate:
• Therapeutic response: absence of renal stone formation
Teach patient/family:
• To decrease calcium in diet: dairy products; decrease sodium, citrus fruits in diet; increased excretion of drug will occur; decrease oxalate (chocolate, tea, spinach)
• To increase fluid intake to 3 L/day

---

cephalexin
(sef-a-lex'in)
Keftab, Biocef, Cefanex, Cephalexin, Ceporex,* Keflet, Keflex, Novolexin,* Zartan

Func. class.: Antibiotic
Chem. class.: Cephalosporin (1st generation)

Action: Inhibits bacterial cell wall synthesis, rendering cell wall osmotically unstable, leading to cell death
Uses: Gram-negative bacilli: *H. influenzae, E. coli, P. mirabilis, Klebsiella;* gram-positive organisms: *S. pneumoniae, S. pyogenes, S. aureus;* upper, lower respiratory tract, urinary tract, skin, bone infections, otitis media
Dosage and routes:
• *Adult:* PO 250-500 mg q6h
• *Child:* PO 25-50 mg/kg/day in 4 equal doses

Moderate skin infections
500 mg q12h
Severe infections
• *Adult:* PO 500 mg-1 g q6h
• *Child:* PO 50-100 mg/kg/day in 4 equal doses
• Dosage reduction indicated in renal impairment (CrCl < 50 ml/min)
Available forms: Caps 250, 500 mg; tabs 250, 500, 1000 mg; pulvules 250 mg; oral susp 125, 250 mg/5 ml; pediatric susp 100 mg/5 ml
Side effects/adverse reactions:
CNS: Headache, dizziness, weakness, paresthesia, fever, chills
GI: Nausea, vomiting, diarrhea, anorexia, pain, glossitis, bleeding, increased AST, ALT, bilirubin, LDH, alk phosphatase, abdominal pain, *pseudomembranous colitis*
GU: Proteinuria, vaginitis, pruritus, candidiasis, increased BUN, *nephrotoxicity, renal failure*
HEMA: Leukopenia, thrombocytopenia, agranulocytosis, anemia, *neutropenia, lymphocytosis, eosinophilia, pancytopenia, hemolytic anemia*
INTEG: Rash, urticaria, dermatitis
RESP: Dyspnea, *anaphylaxis*
Contraindications: Hypersensitivity to cephalosporins, infants <1 mo.
Precautions: Hypersensitivity to penicillins, pregnancy (B), lactation, renal disease
Pharmacokinetics:
PO: Peak 1 hr, duration 6-8 hr, half-life 30-72 min; 5%-15% bound by plasma proteins; 90%-100% eliminated unchanged in urine; crosses placenta; excreted in breast milk
Interactions/incompatibilities:
• Decreased effects: tetracyclines, erythromycins
• Increased toxicity: aminoglyco-

sides, furosemide, probenecid, sulfinpyrazone, colistin, ethacrynic acid, vancomycin

Lab test interferences:

Increase (false): Creatinine (serum urine), urinary 17-KS

False positive: Urinary protein, direct Coombs' test, urine glucose

Interference: Cross-matching

NURSING CONSIDERATIONS

Assess:

• Sensitivity to penicillin or other cephalosporins

• Nephrotoxicity: increased BUN, creatinine

• I&O daily

• Blood studies: AST, ALT, CBC, Hct, bilirubin, LDH, alk phosphatase, Coombs' test monthly if patient is on long-term therapy

• Electrolytes: K, Na, Cl monthly if patient is on long-term therapy

• Bowel pattern qd; if severe diarrhea occurs, drug should be discontinued; may indicate pseudomembranous colitis

• Urine output: if decreasing, notify physician; may indicate nephrotoxicity

• Allergic reactions: rash, urticaria, pruritus, chills, fever, joint pain, angioedema; may occur few days after therapy begins

• Bleeding: ecchymosis, bleeding gums, hematuria, stool guaiac daily

• Overgrowth of infection: perineal itching, fever, malaise, redness, pain, swelling, drainage, rash, diarrhea, change in cough, sputum

Administer:

• For 10-14 days to ensure organism death, prevent superimposed infection

• With food if needed for GI symptoms

• After C&S

Evaluate:

• Therapeutic response: decreased symptoms of infection

Teach patient/family:

• If diabetic, to use Clinistix or Ketodiastix, blood glucose level

• Not to use alcohol or meds with alcohol or reaction may occur

• To use yogurt or buttermilk to maintain intestinal flora, decrease diarrhea

• To take all medication prescribed for length of time ordered

• To report sore throat, bruising, bleeding, joint pain; may indicate blood dyscrasias (rare)

• To report severe diarrhea; may indicate pseudomembranous colitis

Treatment of overdose: Epinephrine, antihistamines, resuscitate if needed (anaphylaxis)

---

cephalothin sodium

(sef-a'loe-thin)

Cephalothin Sodium, Ceporacin,* Keflin, Neutral

Func. class.: Broad-spectrum antibiotic

Chem. class.: Cephalosporin (1st generation)

Action: Inhibits bacterial cell wall synthesis, rendering cell wall osmotically unstable and leading to cell death by binding to the cell wall membrane

Uses: Gram-negative bacilli: *H. influenzae, E. coli, P. mirabilis, Klebsiella, Salmonella, Shigella*; gram-positive organisms: *S. pneumoniae, S. pyogenes, S. aureus*; lower respiratory tract, urinary tract, skin and bone infections; septicemia, endocarditis, bacterial peritonitis

Dosage and routes:

• *Adult:* IM/IV 500 mg-1 g q4-6h

• *Child:* IM/IV 14-27 mg/kg q4h or 20-40 mg/kg q6h

• Dosage reduction indicated in re-

---

italics = common side effects   ***bold italic*** = life threatening reactions

nal impairment (CrCl 50 ml/min)
Uncomplicated gonorrhea
• 2 g IM as single dose
Severe infections
• *Adult:* IM/IV 1-2 g q4h
Available forms: Powder for inj
IM, IV 1, 2, 4, 10, 20 g; frozen IV
20, 30, 40 mg/ml
Side effects/adverse reactions:
CNS: Headache, dizziness, weakness, paresthesia, fever, chills
GI: Nausea, vomiting, diarrhea, anorexia, pain, glossitis, bleeding; increased AST, ALT, bilirubin, LDH, alk phosphatase; abdominal pain, *pseudomembranous colitis*
GU: Proteinuria, vaginitis, pruritus, candidiasis, increased BUN, *nephrotoxicity, renal failure*
HEMA: Leukopenia, thrombocytopenia, agranulocytosis, anemia, *neutropenia, lymphocytosis, eosinophilia, pancytopenia, hemolytic anemia*
INTEG: Rash, urticaria, dermatitis
RESP: Dyspnea, *anaphylaxis*
Contraindications: Hypersensitivity to cephalosporins
Precautions: Hypersensitivity to penicillins, pregnancy (B), lactation, renal disease
Pharmacokinetics: Well absorbed (IM)
IV: Peak 15 min
IM: Peak 30 min
Half-life ½-1 hr, 65%-80% bound by plasma proteins, 50%-75% eliminated unchanged in urine in 8 hr; crosses placenta, excreted in breast milk, deacetylated in kidneys, liver
Interactions/incompatibilities:
• Incompatible in sol with tetracyclines, erythromycins, calcium chloride, magnesium salts, aminoglycosides, barbiturates, aminophylline heparin, levarterenol, metaraminol, methylprednisolone, met-

oclopramide, penicillin G, phenytoin, phytonadione, polymyxin B, prochlorperazine, succinylcholine, thiopental, warfarin
• Decreased effects: Tetracyclines, erythromycins
• Increased toxicity: Aminoglycosides, furosemide, probenecid, sulfinpyrazone, colistin, ethacrynic acid, vancomycin
Lab test interferences:
False increase: Creatinine (serum, urine), urinary 17-KS
False positive: Urinary protein, direct Coombs', urine glucose, Clinitest
Interference: Crossmatching
NURSING CONSIDERATIONS
Assess:
• Infection: fever, wound drainage, sputum, malaise
• Nephrotoxicity: increased BUN, creatinine
• Sensitivity to penicillin, other cephalosporins
• Blood studies: AST, ALT, CBC
• Hct, bilirubin, LDH, alk phosphatase, Coombs' test monthly if patient is on long-term therapy
• Electrolytes: K, Na, Cl monthly if patient is on long-term therapy
• Bowel pattern qd; if severe diarrhea occurs, drug should be discontinued; may indicate pseudomembranous colitis
• IV site for extravasation, phlebitis; change site q72h
• I&O daily and weight; if output is decreasing, notify physician; may indicate nephrotoxicity
• Allergic reactions: rash, urticaria, pruritus, chills, fever, wheezing, joint pain, angioedema; may occur few days after therapy begins; keep resuscitation equipment and epinephrine on unit
• Bleeding: ecchymosis, bleeding gums, hematuria, stool guaiac daily

- Overgrowth of infection: perineal itching, fever, malaise, redness, pain, swelling, drainage, rash, diarrhea, change in cough, sputum
Administer:
- Clear solution; do not give cloudy sol
- IV after diluting 1 g or less/10 ml or more of sterile H_2O for inj; give over 3-5 min; may be further diluted with 50 ml D_5W, NS by Y-tube or 3-way stopcock; run over 15-30 min; discontinue primary IV during administration; may also be given by continuous infusion
- IM after reconstituting with 4 ml sterile H_2O for inj/1 gm vial
- For 10-14 days to ensure organism death, prevent superimposed infection after C&S
- Insert IM in deep muscle mass, massage
Evaluate:
- Therapeutic response: decreased symptoms of infection
Teach patient/family:
- If diabetic, to use Clinistix or Ketodiastix for blood glucose level
- Not to use alcohol or meds with alcohol, or reaction can occur
- To report sore throat, bruising, bleeding, joint pain; may indicate blood dyscrasias (rare)
- To report severe diarrhea; may indicate pseudomembranous colitis
- To report furry tongue, loose, foul-smelling stools; vaginal itching may indicate superinfection
Treatment of overdose: Epinephrine, antihistamines; resuscitate if needed (anaphylaxis)

cephapirin sodium
(sef-a-pye′rin)
Cefadyl, Cephaprin Sodium
Func. class.: Antibiotic, broad spectrum
Chem. class.: Cephalosporin (1st generation)

Action: Inhibits bacterial cell wall synthesis, rendering cell wall osmotically unstable, leading to cell death
Uses: Gram-negative bacilli: *H. influenzae, E. coli, P. mirabilis, Klebsiella;* gram-positive organisms: *S. pneumoniae, S. viridans, S. aureus;* lower respiratory tract, urinary tract, skin infections, septicemia, endocarditis, bacterial peritonitis
Dosage and routes:
- *Adult:* IM/IV 500 mg-1 g q4-6h
- *Child:* IM/IV 20-30 mg/kg, q6h
- Dosage reduction indicated in renal impairment (CrCl < 50 ml/min)
Available forms: Powder for inj IM, IV 500 mg, 1, 2, 20 g; IV only 1, 2, 4 g
Side effects/adverse reactions:
CNS: Headache, dizziness, weakness, paresthesia, fever, chills
GI: Nausea, vomiting, diarrhea, anorexia, pain, glossitis, bleeding, increased AST, ALT, bilirubin, LDH, alk phosphatase, abdominal pain, **pseudomembranous colitis**
GU: Proteinuria, vaginitis, pruritus, candidiasis, increased BUN, **nephrotoxicity, renal failure**
HEMA: Leukopenia, thrombocytopenia, agranulocytosis, anemia, **neutropenia, lymphocytosis, eosinophilia, pancytopenia, hemolytic anemia**
INTEG: Rash, urticaria, dermatitis

RESP: Dyspnea, **anaphylaxis**

Contraindications: Hypersensitivity to cephalosporins, infants <1 mo

Precautions: Hypersensitivity to penicillins, pregnancy (B), lactation, renal disease

Pharmacokinetics:

IV: Peak 5 min

IM: Peak 30 min

Half-life 21-47 min; 44%-50% bound by plasma proteins; 40%-70% eliminated unchanged in urine; crosses placenta; excreted in breast milk; metabolized in liver

Interactions/incompatibilities:

• Tetracyclines, aminoglycosides, aminophylline, epinephrine, levarterenol, mannitol, phenytoin, thiopental

• Decreased effects: tetracyclines, erythromycins

• Increased toxicity: aminoglycosides, furosemide, probenecid, sulfinpyrazone, colistin, ethacrynic acid

Lab test interferences:

Increase (false:) Creatinine (serum urine), urinary 17-KS

False positive: Urinary protein, direct Coombs' test, urine glucose

Interference: Cross-matching

NURSING CONSIDERATIONS

Assess:

• Sensitivity to penicillin or other cephalosporins

• Nephrotoxicity: increased BUN, creatinine

• I&O daily

• Blood studies: AST, ALT, CBC, Hct, bilirubin, LDH, alk phosphatase, Coombs' test monthly if patient is on long-term therapy

• Electrolytes: K, Na, Cl monthly if patient is on long-term therapy

• Bowel pattern qd; if severe diarrhea occurs, drug should be discontinued; may indicate pseudomembranous colitis

• IV site for extravasation, phlebitis; change site q72h

• Urine output: if decreasing, notify physician; may indicate nephrotoxicity

• Allergic reactions: rash, urticaria, pruritus, chills, fever, joint pain, angioedema; may occur few days after therapy begins

• Bleeding: ecchymosis, bleeding gums, hematuria, stool guaiac daily

• Overgrowth of infection: perineal itching, fever, malaise, redness, pain, swelling, drainage, rash, diarrhea, change in cough, sputum

Administer:

• IV after diluting 1 g or less/10 ml or more normal saline, D₅W, or bacteriostatic H₂O for inj; give 1 g or less/5 min or more; may be further diluted in 50-100 ml of D₅W, NS; run over 15 min; discontinue primary inf during administration; may also be given by continuous infusion

• For 10-14 days to ensure organism death, prevent superimposed infection

• After C&S

Evaluate:

• Therapeutic response: decreased symptoms of infection

Teach patient/family:

• If diabetic, to use Clinistix or Ketodiastix, blood glucose level

• Not to use alcohol or meds with alcohol or reaction may occur

• To report severe diarrhea; may indicate pseudomembranous colitis

• To report sore throat, bruising, bleeding, joint pain; may indicate blood dyscrasias (rare)

Treatment of overdose: Epinephrine, antihistamines; resuscitate if needed (anaphylaxis)

---

cephradine
(sef'ra-deen)
Cephradine, Velosef
Func. class.: Antibiotic
Chem. class.: Cephalosporin
(1st generation)

Action: Inhibits bacterial cell wall synthesis, rendering cell wall osmotically unstable, leading to cell death

Uses: Gram-negative bacilli: *H. influenzae, E. coli, P. mirabilis, Klebsiella;* gram-positive organisms: *S. pneumoniae, S. pyogenes, S. aureus;* serious respiratory tract, urinary tract, skin infections, otitis media

Dosage and routes:
• *Adult:* IM/IV 500 mg-1 g q4-6h not to exceed 8 g/day; PO 250 mg-1 g q6-12h
• *Child >1 yr.:* IM/IV 12-25 mg/kg q6h; PO 6-12 mg/kg q6h
Available forms: Powder for inj IM, IV 250, 500 mg, 1 g; caps 250, 500 mg; oral susp 125, 250 mg/5 ml

Side effects/adverse reactions:
CNS: Headache, dizziness, weakness, paresthesia, fever, chills
GI: Nausea, vomiting, diarrhea, anorexia, pain, glossitis, bleeding, increased AST, ALT, bilirubin, LDH, alk phosphatase, abdominal pain, *pseudomembranous colitis*
GU: Proteinuria, vaginitis, pruritus, candidiasis, increased BUN, *nephrotoxicity, renal failure*
HEMA: Leukopenia, thrombocytopenia, agranulocytosis, anemia, *neutropenia, lymphocytosis, eosinophilia, pancytopenia, hemolytic anemia*
INTEG: Rash, urticaria, dermatitis
RESP: Dyspnea, *anaphylaxis*

Contraindications: Hypersensitivity to cephalosporins, infants <1 mo
Precautions: Hypersensitivity to penicillins, pregnancy (B), lactation, renal disease
Pharmacokinetics:
PO: Peak 1 hr
IV: Peak 5 min
IM: Peak 1 hr
Half-life 0.75-1.5 h; 20% bound by plasma proteins; 80%-90% eliminated unchanged in urine; crosses placenta; excreted in breast milk
Interactions/incompatibilities:
• Incompatible with tetracyclines, erythromycins, calcium salts, magnesium salts, aminoglycosides, epinephrine, lidocaine, all antibiotics, Ringer's sol
• Decreased effects: tetracyclines, erythromycins
• Increased toxicity: aminoglycosides, furosemide, probenecid, sulfinpyrazone, colistin, ethacrynic acid, vancomycin
Lab test interferences:
Increase (false): Creatinine (serum urine), urinary 17-KS
False positive: Urinary protein, direct Coombs' test, urine glucose
Interference: Cross-matching
NURSING CONSIDERATIONS
Assess:
• Sensitivity to penicillin or other cephalosporins
• Nephrotoxicity: increased BUN, creatinine
• I&O daily
• Blood studies: AST, ALT, CBC, Hct, bilirubin, LDH, alk phosphatase, Coombs' test monthly if patient is on long-term therapy
• Electrolytes: K, Na, Cl monthly if patient is on long-term therapy
• Bowel pattern qd; if severe diarrhea occurs, drug should be dis-

continued; may indicate pseudo-membranous colitis

• IV site for extravasation, phlebitis; change site q72h

• Urine output: if decreasing, notify physician; may indicate nephrotoxicity

• Allergic reactions: rash, urticaria, pruritus, chills, fever, joint pain, angioedema; may occur few days after therapy begins

• Bleeding: ecchymosis, bleeding gums, hematuria, stool guaiac daily

• Overgrowth of infection: perineal itching, fever, malaise, redness, pain, swelling, drainage, rash, diarrhea, change in cough, sputum

Administer:

• IV after diluting 500 mg or less/ 5 ml or more sterile H_2O for inj; give over 3-5 min; may be further diluted 500 mg or less/10-20 ml D_5W, NS give through Y-tube or 3-way stopcock, run over ½-1 hr

• For 10-14 days to ensure organism death, prevent superimposed infection

• With food if needed for GI symptoms

• After C&S

Evaluate:

• Therapeutic response: decreased symptoms of infection

Teach patient/family:

• If diabetic, to use Clinistix or Ketodiastix, blood glucose level

• Not to use alcohol or meds with alcohol or reaction can occur

• To use yogurt or buttermilk to maintain intestinal flora, decrease diarrhea

• To take all medication prescribed for length of time ordered

• To report sore throat, bruising, bleeding, joint pain; may indicate blood dyscrasias (rare)

Treatment of overdose: Epineph-

rine, antihistamines, resuscitate if needed (anaphylaxis)

chenodiol
(kee-noe-dye'ole)
Chenix
Func. class.: Antilithic
Chem. class.: Chenodeoxycholic acid

Action: Suppresses synthesis of cholesterol, cholic acid, replacing cholic acid with drug metabolite, which leads to the degradation of gallstones

Uses: Dissolving gallstones instead of surgery; drug has no effect on radiopaque, calcified gallstones or bile pigment stones

Dosage and routes:

• *Adult:* PO 250 mg bid × 2 wk, then increased by 250 mg/day, not to exceed 16 mg/kg/day × 24 mo

Available forms: Tabs 250 mg

Side effects/adverse reactions:

*HEMA: **Leukopenia***

GI: Diarrhea, fecal urgency, heartburn, nausea, cramps, increased ALT, AST, LDH, vomiting, dysphagia, absence of taste, ***hepatotoxicity,*** flatulence, dyspepsia

Contraindications: Hypersensitivity, hepatic disease, bile duct obstruction, biliary GI fistula, pregnancy (X)

Precautions: Lactation, children, atherosclerosis, elderly

Pharmacokinetics: Metabolized by liver; excreted in feces (metabolite/unchanged drug); crosses placenta

Interactions/incompatibilities:

• Decreased action of chenodiol: cholestyramine, colestipol, aluminum antacids, estrogens, clofibrate

NURSING CONSIDERATIONS

Assess:

• Vital signs, cardiac status: check-

ing for dysrhythmias, increased rate, palpitations
• I&O ratio; check for urinary retention or hesitancy, especially elderly
• Oral cholecystogram or ultrasonogram q6-9mo
• GI complaints: nausea, vomiting, anorexia, diarrhea; if diarrhea is severe, dosage may have to be decreased

Administer:
• With meals for better absorption
• Antidiarrheals if diarrhea occurs

Perform/provide:
• Storage at room temperature
• Increased fluids, bulk, exercise to patient's life-style to decrease constipation

Evaluate:
• Therapeutic response: absence of pain (epigastric), gallstones on diagnostic testing

Teach patient/family:
• That stone dissolution may take 6-24 mo; therapy is discontinued in 18 mo if gallstones are still intact
• To notify physician if pregnancy is suspected; birth defects may occur

---

chloral hydrate
(klor-al hye′drate)
Aquachloral Supprettes, Chloral Hydrate, Noctec, Novochlorhydrate*
Func. class.: Sedative-hypnotic
Chem. class.: Chloral derivative

Controlled Substance Schedule IV (USA), Schedule F (Canada)
Action: Reduction product trichloroethanol produces mild cerebral depression, which causes sleep
Uses: Sedation, insomnia

Dosage and routes:
Sedation
• *Adult:* PO/REC 250 mg tid pc
• *Child:* PO 8 mg/kg tid, not to exceed 500 mg tid
Insomnia
• *Adult:* PO/REC 500 mg-1g ½ hr before hs
• *Child:* PO/REC 50 mg/kg in one dose
Available forms: Caps 250, 500 mg; syr 250, 500 mg/5 ml; supp 325, 500, 650 mg

Side effects/adverse reactions:
*HEMA: **Eosinophilia, leukopenia***
CNS: Drowsiness, dizziness, stimulation, nightmares, ataxia, hangover (rare), light-headedness, headache, paranoia
GI: Nausea, vomiting, flatulence, diarrhea, unpleasant taste, ***gastric necrosis***
INTEG: Rash, urticaria, angioedema, fever, purpura, eczema
CV: Hypotension, dysrhythmias
*RESP: **Depression***

Contraindications: Hypersensitivity to this drug or triclofos, severe renal disease, severe hepatic disease, GI disorders (oral forms), gastritis

Precautions: Severe cardiac disease, depression, suicidal individuals, asthma, intermittent porphyria, pregnancy (C), lactation, elderly

Pharmacokinetics:
PO: Onset 30 min-1 hr, duration 4-8 hr
REC: Onset slow, duration 4-6 hr; metabolized by liver; excreted by kidneys (inactive metabolite) and feces; crosses placenta; excreted in breast milk; metabolite is highly protein bound

Interactions/incompatibilities:
• Increased action: oral anticoagulants, furosemide

---

italics = common side effects   ***bold italic*** = life threatening reactions

• Increased action of both drugs: alcohol, CNS depressants

Lab test interferences:
Interferences: Urine catecholamines, urinary 17-OHCS
False Positive: Urine glucose (copper sulfate test)

NURSING CONSIDERATIONS
Assess:
• Blood studies: Hct, Hgb, RBCs, serum folate (if on long-term therapy), pro-time in patients receiving anticoagulants
• Mental status: mood, sensorium, affect, memory (long, short)
• Physical dependency: more frequent requests for medication, shakes, anxiety, pinpoint pupils
• Respiratory dysfunction: respiratory depression, character, rate, rhythm; hold drug if respirations are <10/min or if pupils are dilated (rare)
• Blood dyscrasias: fever, sore throat, bruising, rash, jaundice, epistaxis (rare)
• Previous history of substance abuse, cardiac disease, or gastritis

Administer:
• After removal of cigarettes, to prevent fires
• After trying conservative measures for insomnia
• ½-1 hr before hs for sleeplessness
• On empty stomach with full glass of water or juice for best absorption and to decrease corrosion (do not chew); after meals to decrease GI symptoms if using for sedation

Perform/provide:
• Assistance with ambulation after receiving dose, especially elderly
• Safety measure: side rails, nightlight, call bell within easy reach
• Checking to see PO medication swallowed
• Storage in dark container, suppositories in refrigerator

Evaluate:
• Therapeutic response: ability to sleep at night, decreased amount of early morning awakening if taking drug for insomnia

Teach patient/family:
• To avoid driving or other activities requiring alertness
• To avoid alcohol ingestion or CNS depressants; serious CNS depression may result
• Not to discontinue medication quickly after long-term use; drug should be tapered over 1-2 wk
• That effects may take 2 nights for benefits to be noticed
• Alternate measures to improve sleep (reading, exercise several hours before hs, warm bath, warm milk, TV, self-hypnosis, deep breathing)

Treatment of overdose: Lavage, activated charcoal; monitor electrolytes, vital signs

---

chlorambucil
(klor-am′byoo-sil)
Leukeran
Func. class.: Antineoplastic alkylating agent
Chem. class.: Nitrogen mustard

Action: Alkylates DNA, RNA; inhibits enzymes that allow synthesis of amino acids in proteins; activity is not cell cycle phase specific

Uses: Chronic lymphocytic leukemia, Hodgkin's disease, other lymphomas, macroglobulinemia, nephrotic syndrome, breast carcinoma, choreocarcinoma, ovarian carcinoma

Dosage and routes:
• *Adult:* PO 0.1-0.2 mg/kg/day for 3-6 wk initially, then 2-6 mg/day; maintenance 0.2 mg/kg for

---

2-4 wk; course may be repeated at 2-4 wk intervals

• *Child:* PO 0.1-0.2 mg/kg/day in divided doses or 4.5 mg/m²/day as 1 dose or in divided doses

Available forms: Tabs 2 mg

Side effects/adverse reactions:

CNS: **Convulsions in children**

HEMA: **Thrombocytopenia, leukopenia, pancytopenia** (prolonged use), **permanent bone marrow depression**

GI: *Nausea, vomiting, diarrhea, weight loss,* hepatoxicity, jaundice

GU: Hyperuremia

INTEG: Alopecia (rare), dermatitis, rash

RESP: **Fibrosis, pneumonitis**

Contraindications: Radiation therapy within 1 mo, chemotherapy within 1 mo, thrombocytopenia, smallpox vaccination, pregnancy (1st trimester) (D)

Precautions: *Pneumococcus* vaccination

Pharmacokinetics: Well absorbed orally; metabolized in liver; excreted in urine; half-life 2 hr

Interactions/incompatibilities:

• Increased toxicity: other antineoplastics, or radiation

NURSING CONSIDERATIONS

Assess:

• Bleeding: hematuria, guaiac, bruising or petechiae, mucosa or orifices q8h

• Food preferences; list likes, dislikes

• Yellowing of skin, sclera, dark urine, clay-colored stools, itchy skin, abdominal pain, fever, diarrhea

• Dyspnea, rales, unproductive cough, chest pain, tachypnea

• Effects of alopecia on body image; discuss feelings about body changes (rare)

• CBC, differential, platelet count

weekly; withhold drug if WBC is <4000 or platelet count is <75,000; notify physician of results

• Pulmonary functions test, chest x-ray films before, during therapy; chest film should be obtained q2wk during treatment

• Renal function studies: BUN, serum uric acid, urine CrCl before, during therapy

• I&O ratio; report fall in urine output of 30 ml/hr

• Monitor temperature q4h (may indicate beginning infection)

• Liver function tests before, during therapy (bilirubin, AST, ALT, LDH) as needed or monthly

Administer:

• Antacid before oral agent; give drug 2 hr after evening meal, before bedtime

• Antiemetic 30-60 min before giving drug to prevent vomiting

• Allopurinol or sodium bicarbonate to maintain uric acid levels, alkalinization of urine

• Antibiotics for prophylaxis of infection

Perform/provide:

• Storage in tight container

• Strict medical asepsis, protective isolation if WBC levels are low

• Increase fluid intake to 2-3 L/day to prevent urate deposits, calculi formation

• Diet low in purines: organ meats (kidney, liver), dried beans, peas to maintain alkaline urine

Evaluate:

• Therapeutic response: decreased size of tumor, spread of malignancy

Teach patient/family:

• To report signs of infection: increased temperature, sore throat, flu symptoms

• To report signs of anemia: fa-

italics = common side effects   ***bold italic*** = life threatening reactions

tigue, headache, faintness, short-ness of breath, irritability
• To report bleeding; avoid use of razors or commercial mouthwash
• To avoid use of aspirin products or ibuprofen
• About protective isolation precautions
• To report any changes in breathing or coughing
• That hair may be lost during treatment; a wig or hairpiece may make patient feel better; new hair may be different in color, texture (rare)

---

chloramphenicol/ chloramphenicol palmitate/ chloramphenicol sodium succinate

Chloramphenicol, Chloramphenicol Sodium Succinate, Chloromycetin Kapseals, Chloromycetin Sodium Succinate, Chloromycetin Palmitate, Novochlorocap*

Func. class.: Antibacterial/ anti-rickettsial
Chem. class.: Dichloroacetic acid derivative

Action: Binds to 50S ribosomal subunit, which interferes with or inhibits protein synthesis
Uses: Infections caused by *H. influenzae, S. typhi, Rickettsia, Neisseria,* mycoplasma
Dosage and routes:
• *Adult and child:* PO/IV 50-100 mg/kg/day in divided doses q6h, not to exceed 100 mg/kg/day
• *Premature infants and neonates:* IV/PO 25 mg/kg/day in divided doses q6h

Available forms: Inj (IV) 1 g; caps 250, 500 mg; oral susp 150 mg/5 ml
Side effects/adverse reactions:
*HEMA: **Anemia, bone marrow depression, thrombocytopenia, aplastic anemia, granulocytopenia, leukopenia** (rare)*
EENT: Optic neuritis, blindness
GI: Nausea, vomiting, diarrhea, abdominal pain, xerostomia, glossitis, colitis, pruritus ani
INTEG: Itching, urticaria, contact dermatitis, rash
*CV: **Gray syndrome in newborns: failure to feed, pallid, cyanosis, abdominal distention, irregular respiration, vasomotor collapse***
CNS: Headache, *depression,* confusion
Contraindications: Hypersensitivity, severe renal disease, severe hepatic disease, minor infections
Precautions: Hepatic disease, renal disease, infants, children, bone marrow depression (drug-induced), pregnancy (C), lactation
Pharmacokinetics:
PO/IV: Peak 1-2 hr, duration 8 hr, half-life 1½-4 hr; conjugated in liver; excreted in urine (up to 15% as free drug), breast milk, feces; crosses placenta
Interactions/incompatibilities:
• Increased action of: dicumarol, phenytoin, tolbutamide, chlorpropamide, phenobarbital
• Increased prothrombin time: anticoagulants
• Decreased action of iron, Vit B$_{12}$, folic acid, penicillins
• Incompatible with ampicillin, amobarbital, carbenicillin, chlorpromazine, digitoxin, erythromycins, glycopyrrolate, hydrocortisone, hydroxyzine, metoclopramide, oxacillin, pentobarbital, phenytoin, polymyxin B, procaine,

prochlorperazine, promazine, promethazine, thiopental, tripelennamine, vancomycin, warfarin
• Avoid use with myelosuppressive drugs

NURSING CONSIDERATIONS
Assess:
• Signs of infections, anemia
• Any patient with compromised renal system; drug is excreted slowly in poor renal system function; toxicity may occur rapidly
• Liver studies: AST, ALT
• Blood studies: WBC, RBC, Hct, Hgb, platelets, serum iron, reticulocytes; drug should be discontinued if bone marrow depression occurs
• Renal studies: urinalysis, protein, blood, BUN, creatinine
• C&S before drug therapy; may be given as soon as culture is taken
• Drug level in impaired hepatic, renal systems
• Bowel pattern before, during treatment
• Skin eruptions, itching, dermatitis after administration
• Respiratory status: rate, character, wheezing, tightness in chest
• Allergies before treatment, reaction of each medication; place allergies on chart, Kardex in bright red letters; notify all people giving drugs
• Neonates for beginning gray syndrome: cyanosis, abdominal distention, irregular respiration, failure to feed; drug should be discontinued immediately

Administer:
• IV after diluting 1 g/10 ml of sterile H_2O for inj or D_5W (10% sol); give over >1 min; may be further diluted in 50-100 ml of D_5W; give through Y-tube, 3-way stopcock, or additive inf set; run over ½-1 hr

• Oral form on empty stomach with full glass of water

Perform/provide:
• Storage of capsules in tight container at room temperature, reconstituted solution at room temperature for up to 30 days
• Adrenalin, suction, tracheostomy set, endotracheal intubation equipment on unit
• Adequate intake of fluids (2 L) during diarrhea episodes

Evaluate:
• Therapeutic response: decreased symptoms of infection

Teach patient/family:
• Aspects of drug therapy: need to complete entire course of medication to ensure organism death (10-14 days); culture may be taken after complete course of medication
• To report sore throat, fever, fatigue, unusual bleeding, bruising; could indicate bone marrow depression (may occur weeks or months after termination of drug)
• That drug must be taken in equal intervals around clock to maintain blood levels

Treatment of overdose: Withdraw drug, maintain airway, administer epinephrine, aminophylline, O_2, IV corticosteroids

---

chloramphenicol (ophthalmic)
(klor-am-fen′i-kole)
AK-Chlor, Chloramphenicol, Chloramphenicol Ophthalmic, Chloromycetin Ophthalmic, Chloroptic, Chloroptic S.O.P., Fenicol,* Isopto Fenical,* Pentamycin*
Func. class.: Antiinfective

Action: Inhibits bacterial protein synthesis
Uses: Infection of eye

---

italics = common side effects   ***bold italic*** = life threatening reactions

Dosage and routes:
• *Adult and child:* INSTILL 2 gtts in eye qd-qid until desired response; TOP apply oint to conjunctival sac q3-6h as needed or hs if using gtts also
Available forms: Oint 1%; sol 0.25, 0.5%, 25 mg

Side effects/adverse reactions:
EENT: Poor corneal wound healing, temporary visual haze, overgrowth of nonsusceptible organisms

Contraindications: Hypersensitivity

Precautions: Antibiotic hypersensitivity, pregnancy (C)

NURSING CONSIDERATIONS
Assess:
• Allergy: itching, lacrimation, redness, swelling

Administer:
• After washing hands, cleanse crusts or discharge from eye before application
• Apply pressure to lacrimal sac for 1 min to prevent systemic absorption

Perform/provide:
• Storage at room temperature; protect from light

Evaluate:
• Therapeutic response: absence of redness, inflammation, tearing

Teach patient/family:
• To use drug exactly as prescribed
• Not to use eye makeup, towels, washcloths, eye medication of others; reinfection may occur
• That drug container tip should not touch eye
• To report itching, increased redness, burning, stinging, swelling; drug should be discontinued
• That drug may cause blurred vision when ointment is applied
• That prolonged or frequent use may lead to serious reactions: hypersensitivity, bone marrow depression

---

chloramphenicol (otic)
(klor-am-fen'i-kole)
Chloromycetin Otic, Sopamycetin*
Func. class.: Otic, broad-spectrum antibiotic
Chem. class.: Antibacterial

Action: Inhibits protein synthesis in susceptible gram-positive, gram-negative microorganisms

Uses: Ear infection (external)

Dosage and routes:
• *Adult and child:* INSTILL 2-3 gtts tid
Available forms: Sol 0.5%

Side effects/adverse reactions:
EENT: Itching, irritation in ear
INTEG: Rash, urticaria, contact dermatitis, burning, *angioedema*
HEMA: Bone marrow hypoplasia, aplastic anemia

Contraindications: Hypersensitivity, perforated eardrum

Precautions: Inner ear infections

NURSING CONSIDERATIONS
Assess:
• For redness, swelling, pain in ear, which indicates superimposed infection

Administer:
• After removing impacted cerumen by irrigation
• After cleaning stopper with alcohol
• After restraining child if necessary
• Warming solution to body temperature; do not warm above body temperature; loss of potency will occur

Perform/provide:
• Storage at room temperature, protection from light

Evaluate:
• Therapeutic response: decreased ear pain
Teach patient/family:
• Method of instillation, using aseptic technique, including not touching dropper to ear
• That dizziness may occur after instillation

chloramphenicol (topical)
(klor-am-fen'i-kole)
Chloromycetin
Func. class.: Local antiinfective
Chem. class.: Antibacterial

Action: Interferes with bacterial protein synthesis
Uses: Skin infections (bacterial)
Dosage and routes:
• *Adult and child:* TOP apply to affected area bid-qid
Available forms: Cream 1%
Side effects/adverse reactions:
HEMA: Blood dyscrasias
INTEG: Rash, urticaria, stinging, burning, vesicular, maculopapular dermatitis, *angioedema*
Contraindications: Hypersensitivity
Precautions: Pregnancy (C), lactation
NURSING CONSIDERATIONS
Assess:
• Allergic reaction: burning, stinging, swelling, redness
• Signs and symptoms of blood dyscrasias
Administer:
• Enough medication to cover lesions completely
• After cleansing with soap, water before each application; dry well
Perform/provide:
• Storage at room temperature in dry place; protect from light

Evaluate:
• Therapeutic response: decrease in size, number of lesions
Teach patient/family:
• To use medical asepsis (hand washing) before, after each application to prevent further infection
• To apply with glove to prevent further infection
• To avoid use of OTC creams, ointments, lotions unless directed by physician
• To notify physician if conditions worsen or if rash or irritation develops
• To watch for superimposed infections with diarrhea

chlordiazepoxide HCl
(klor-dye-az-e-pox'ide)
Chlordiazepoxide HCl, Libritabs, Librium, Medilium,* Mitran, Novopoxide,* Resposans-10, Solium*
Func. class.: Antianxiety
Chem. class.: Benzodiazepine

Controlled Substance Schedule IV
Action: Potentiates the actions of GABA, especially in the limbic system, reticular formation
Uses: Short-term management of anxiety, acute alcohol withdrawal, preoperatively for relaxation
Dosage and routes:
Mild anxiety
• *Adult:* PO 5-10 mg tid-qid
• *Child >6 yr:* 5 mg bid-qid, not to exceed 10 mg bid-tid
Severe anxiety
• *Adult:* PO 20-25 mg tid-qid
Preoperatively
• *Adult:* PO 5-10 mg tid-qid on day before surgery; IM 50-100 mg 1 hr before surgery
Alcohol withdrawal

---

italics = common side effects   ***bold italic*** = life threatening reactions

• *Adult:* PO/IM/IV 50-100 mg, not to exceed 300 mg/day

Available forms: Caps 5, 10, 25 mg; tabs 5, 10, 25 mg; powder for IM inj 100 mg

Side effects/adverse reactions:

CNS: Dizziness, drowsiness, confusion, headache, anxiety, tremors, stimulation, fatigue, depression, insomnia, hallucinations

GI: Constipation, dry mouth, nausea, vomiting, anorexia, diarrhea

INTEG: Rash, dermatitis, itching

*CV: Orthostatic hypotension, **ECG changes, tachycardia,*** hypotension

EENT: Blurred vision, tinnitus, mydriasis

Contraindications: Hypersensitivity to benzodiazepines, narrow-angle glaucoma, psychosis, pregnancy (D), child <18 yr

Precautions: Elderly, debilitated, hepatic disease, renal disease

Pharmacokinetics:

PO: Onset 30 min, peak ½ hr, duration 4-6 hr; metabolized by liver, excreted by kidneys; crosses placenta, breast milk; half-life 5-30 hr

Interactions/incompatibilities:

• Decreased effects of chlordiazepoxide: oral contraceptives, rifampin, valproic acid

• Increased effects of chlordiazepoxide: CNS depressants, alcohol, cimetidine, disulfiram, oral contraceptives

• Incompatible with Vit C, benzquinamide, heparin, pentobarbital, phenytoin, promethazine, Ringer's inj, 0.9% NaCl

Lab test interferences:

Increase: AST/ALT, serum bilirubin

False increase: 17-OHCS

Decrease: RAIU

NURSING CONSIDERATIONS

Assess:

• B/P (lying, standing), pulse; if systolic B/P drops 20 mm Hg, hold drug, notify physician

• Blood studies: CBC during long-term therapy; blood dyscrasias have occurred rarely

• Hepatic studies: AST, ALT, bilirubin, creatinine, LDH, alk phosphatase

• I&O; may indicate renal dysfunction

• For ataxia, oversedation in elderly, debilitated patients

• Mental status: mood, sensorium, affect, sleeping pattern, drowsiness, dizziness

• Physical dependency, withdrawal symptoms: headache, nausea, vomiting, muscle pain, weakness after long-term use

• Suicidal tendencies, paradoxical reactions such as excitement, stimulation, and acute rage

Administer:

• By IV 5 ml saline/100 mg of powder; agitate ample gently; give through Y-tube or 3-way stopcock; give 100 mg or less over ≥1 min; do not use IM diluent for IV use

• With food or milk for GI symptoms

• Crushed if patient is unable to swallow medication whole

• Sugarless gum, hard candy, frequent sips of water for dry mouth

Perform/provide:

• Assistance with ambulation during beginning therapy, since drowsiness/dizziness occurs

• Safety measure, including side rails

• Check to see PO medication has been swallowed

Evaluate:

• Therapeutic response: decreased anxiety, restlessness, sleeplessness

Teach patient/family:

• That drug may be taken with food

• Not to be used for everyday stress

or used longer than 4 mo, unless directed by physician
• Not to take more than prescribed amount; may be habit-forming
• To avoid OTC preparations unless approved by physician
• To avoid driving, activities that require alertness; drowsiness may occur
• To avoid alcohol ingestion or other psychotropic medications, unless prescribed by physician
• Not to discontinue medication abruptly after long-term use; may precipitate convulsions
• To rise slowly or fainting may occur, especially elderly
• That drowsiness may worsen at beginning of treatment
Treatment of overdose: Lavage, VS, supportive care

---

chloroprocaine HCl
(klor'-oh-pro-kane)
Nesacaine, Nesacaine-MPF
Func. class.: Local anesthetic
Chem. class.: Ester

Action: Competes with calcium for sites in nerve membrane that control sodium transport across cell membrane; decreases rise of depolarization phase of action potential
Uses: Epidural anesthesia, peripheral nerve block, caudal anesthesia, infiltration block
Dosage and routes:
Varies depending on route of anesthesia
Available forms: Inj 1%, 2%, 3%
Side effects/adverse reactions:
CNS: Anxiety, restlessness, *convulsions, loss of consciousness,* drowsiness, disorientation, tremors, shivering
CV: Myocardial depression, cardiac arrest, dysrhythmias, brady-

cardia, hypotension, hypertension, fetal bradycardia
GI: Nausea, vomiting
EENT: Blurred vision, tinnitus, pupil constriction
INTEG: Rash, urticaria, allergic reactions, edema, burning, skin discoloration at injection site, tissue necrosis
RESP: Status asthmaticus, respiratory arrest, anaphylaxis
Contraindications: Hypersensitivity, child <12 yr, elderly, severe liver disease
Precautions: Elderly, severe drug allergies, pregnancy (C)
Pharmacokinetics: Duration ½-1 hr; metabolized by liver; excreted in urine (metabolites)
Interactions/incompatibilities:
• Dysrhythmias: epinephrine, halothane, enflurane
• Hypertension: MAOIs, tricyclic antidepressants, phenothiazines
NURSING CONSIDERATIONS
Assess:
• B/P, pulse, respiration during treatment
• Fetal heart tones if drug is used during labor
• Allergic reactions: rash, urticaria, itching
• Cardiac status: ECG for dysrhythmias, pulse, B/P during anesthesia
Administer:
• Only with crash cart, resuscitative equipment nearby
• Only drugs without preservatives for epidural or caudal anesthesia
Perform/provide:
• Use of new solution; discard unused portions
Evaluate:
• Therapeutic response: anesthesia necessary for procedure
Treatment of overdose: Airway,

---

italics = common side effects   ***bold italic*** = life threatening reactions

O$_2$, vasopressor, IV fluids, anticonvulsants for seizures

---

chloroquine HCl/ chloroquine phosphate

(klor'oh-kwin)

Aralen HCl, Aralen Phosphate, Chloroquine Phosphate, Novochloroquine*

Func. class.: Antimalarial
Chem. class.: Synthetic 4-aminoquinoline derivative

Action: Inhibits parasite replications, transcription of DNA to RNA by forming complexes with DNA of parasite

Uses: Malaria caused by *Plasmodium vivax, P. malariae, P. ovale, P. falciparum* (some strains), amebiasis

Dosage and routes:
Malaria suppression
• *Adult and child:* PO 5 mg/kg/wk on same day of week, not to exceed 500 mg; treatment should begin 1-2 wk before exposure and for 8 wk after; if treatment begins after exposure, 600 mg for adult and 10 mg/kg for children in 2 divided doses 6 hr apart

Extraintestinal amebiasis
• *Adult:* IM 200-250 mg qd (HCl) up to 12 days, then 1 g (phosphate) qd × 2 days, then 500 mg qd × 2-3 wk
• *Child:* IM/PO 10 mg/kg qd (HCl) × 2-3 wk, not to exceed 300 mg/day

Available forms: Tabs 250, 500 mg; inj IM 50 mg/ml

Side effects/adverse reactions:
CV: Hypotension, heart block, asystole with syncope, ECG changes

INTEG: Pruritus, pigmentary changes, skin eruptions, lichen planuslike eruptions, eczema, *exfoliative dermatitis*

CNS: Headache, stimulation, fatigue, *convulsion,* psychosis

EENT: Blurred vision, corneal changes, retinal changes, difficulty focusing, tinnitus, vertigo, deafness, photophobia, corneal edema

GI: Nausea, vomiting, anorexia, diarrhea, cramps

HEMA: Thrombocytopenia, agranulocytosis, hemolytic anemia, leukopenia

Contraindications: Hypersensitivity, retinal field changes, porphyria

Precautions: Pregnancy (C), children, blood dyscrasias, severe GI disease, neurologic disease, alcoholism, hepatic disease, G-6-PD deficiency, psoriasis, eczema, lactation, porphyria

Pharmacokinetics:
PO: Peak 1-6 hr, half-life 3-5 days; metabolized in the liver; excreted in urine, feces, breast milk; crosses placenta

Interactions/incompatibilities:
• Decreased action of chloroquine: magnesium aluminum compounds, kaolin
• Reduced oral clearance and metabolism of chloroquine: cimetidine

NURSING CONSIDERATIONS
Assess:
• Ophthalmic test if long-term treatment or drug dosage >150 mg/day
• Liver studies qwk: AST, ALT, bilirubin
• Blood studies: CBC, since blood dyscrasias occur
• For decreased reflexes: knee, ankle
• ECG during therapy
• Watch for depression of T waves, widening of QRS complex

---

* Available in Canada only

• Allergic reactions: pruritus, rash, urticaria
• Blood dyscrasias: malaise, fever, bruising, bleeding (rare)
• For ototoxicity (tinnitus, vertigo, change in hearing); audiometric testing should be done before, after treatment
• For toxicity: blurring vision; difficulty focusing; headache; dizziness; knee, ankle reflexes; drug should be discontinued immediately

Administer:
• Before or after meals at same time each day to maintain drug level
• IM after aspirating to avoid injection into blood system, which may cause hypotension, asystole, heart block; rotate injection sites

Perform/provide:
• Storage in tight, light-resistant containers at room temperature; injection should be kept in cool environment

Evaluate:
• Therapeutic response: decreased symptoms of infection

Teach patient/family:
• To use sunglasses in bright sunlight to decrease photophobia
• That urine may turn rust or brown color
• To report hearing, visual problems, fever, fatigue, bruising, bleeding, which may indicate blood dyscrasias

Treatment of overdose: Induce vomiting, gastric lavage, administer barbiturate (ultrashort-acting), vasopressin; tracheostomy may be necessary

chlorothiazide
(klor-oh-thye′a-zide)
Diachlor, Diuril, Diuril Sodium
Func. class.: Diuretic
Chem. class.: Thiazide; sulfonamide derivative

Action: Acts on distal tubule by increasing excretion of water, sodium, chloride, potassium, magnesium

Uses: Edema, hypertension, diuresis

Dosage and routes:
Edema, hypertension
• *Adult:* PO/IV 500 mg-2 g qd in 2 divided doses
Diuresis
• *Child >6 mo:* PO 20 mg/kg/day in 2 divided doses

Available forms: Tabs 250, 500 mg; oral susp 250 mg/5 ml; inj 500 mg

Side effects/adverse reactions:
CNS: Drowsiness, paresthesia, anxiety, depression, headache, *dizziness, fatigue, weakness*
CV: Irregular pulse, orthostatic hypotension, palpitations, volume depletion
EENT: Blurred vision
ELECT: Hypokalemia, hypercalcemia, hyponatremia, hypochloremia, hypophosphatemia, hypomagnesemia
GI: Nausea, vomiting, anorexia, constipation, diarrhea, cramps, pancreatitis, GI irritation, **hepatitis**
GU: Frequency, polyuria, **uremia,** glucosuria
*HEMA: **Aplastic anemia, hemolytic anemia, leukopenia, agranulocytosis, thrombocytopenia, neutropenia***
INTEG: Rash, urticaria, purpura, photosensitivity, fever

---

italics = common side effects   ***bold italic*** = life threatening reactions

META: Hyperglycemia, *hyperuricemia,* hypomagnesemia, increased creatinine, BUN

Contraindications: Hypersensitivity to thiazides or sulfonamides, anuria, renal decompensation, pregnancy (D), lactation

Precautions: Hypokalemia, renal disease, hepatic disease, gout, COPD, lupus erythematosus, diabetes mellitus, elderly

Pharmacokinetics: Not well absorbed PO

PO: Onset 2 hr, peak 4 hr, duration 6-12 hr; crosses placenta, excreted in breast milk, excreted unchanged by the kidneys; half-life 2 hr

Interactions/incompatibilities:

• Incompatible in sol with amikacin, chlorpromazine, codeine, hydralazine, insulin, ionosol sol, levarterenol, levorphanol, methadone, morphine, polymyxin B, procaine, prochlorperazine, promazine, promethazine, streptomycin, tetracycline, triflupromazine, vancomycin, Vit C, Vit B with C, warfarin

• Increased toxicity: lithium, nondepolarizing skeletal muscle relaxants, digitalis

• Increased hypotension: other antihypertensives, alcohol

• Decreased effects of: antidiabetics, sulfonylureas

• Decreased absorption of thiazides: cholestyramine, colestipol

• Decreased hypotensive response: indomethacin

• Hypokalemia: ticarcillin, glucocorticoids, amphotericin, mezlocillin, piperacillin

• Hyperglycemia, hyperuricemia, hypotension: diazoxide

Lab test interferences:

False negative: Phentolamine and tyramine tests

Interference: Urine steroid tests

Increase: BSP retention, Ca, amylase, parathyroid test

Decrease: PBI, PSP

NURSING CONSIDERATIONS

Assess:

• Weight, I&O daily to determine fluid loss; effect of drug may be decreased if used qd

• Rate, depth, rhythm of respirations; effect of exertion

• B/P lying, standing; postural hypotension may occur, especially in elderly

• Electrolytes: K, Na, Cl; include BUN, blood glucose, CBC, serum creatinine, blood pH, ABGs, uric acid, Ca, Mg

• Glucose in urine if patient is diabetic

• Improvement in CVP q8h

• Signs of metabolic alkalosis: drowsiness, restlessness

• Rashes, temperature elevation qd

• Confusion, especially in elderly; take safety precautions if needed

Administer:

• IV after diluting 0.5 g/18 ml or more of sterile water for inj; may be diluted further with Ringer's, LR, 0.45% NaCl, 0.9% NaCl, D_5W, $D_{10}W$, check for extravasation; give over 5 min (0.5g/5m)

• In AM to avoid interference with sleep if using drug as a diuretic

• K replacement if K is less than 3.0

• With food if nausea occurs; absorption may be decreased slightly; tablets may be crushed

• After shaking suspension

Evaluate:

• Therapeutic response: improvement in edema of feet, legs, sacral area daily if medication is being used CHF

Teach patient/family:

• To rise slowly from lying or sit-

ting position; orthostatic hypotension may occur
• To notify physician of muscle weakness, cramps, nausea, dizziness
• That drug may be taken with food or milk; to take at same time each day; not to double doses; dehydration may occur
• That blood sugar may be increased in diabetics
• To take early in day to avoid nocturia
• To use sunscreen (avoid sunscreen with PABA); use protective clothing against sun to prevent photosensitivity
• To weigh weekly and notify physician of change of >3 lb
• To eat diet high in Vit K
• Not to take OTC medications without consulting physician
Treatment of overdose: Lavage if taken orally; monitor electrolytes; administer dextrose in saline; monitor hydration, CV, renal status

---

chlorotrianisene
(klor-oh-trye-an'i-seen)
TACE
Func. class.: Estrogen
Chem. class.: Nonsteroidal synthetic estrogen

Action: Needed for adequate functioning of female reproductive system, it affects release of pituitary gonadotropins, inhibits ovulation, adequate calcium use in bone structures
Uses: Prostatic cancer, menopause, female hypogonadism, atrophic vaginitis, kraurosis vulvae
Dosage and routes:
Prostatic cancer
• *Adult:* PO 12-25 mg qd
Menopause

• *Adult:* PO 12-25 mg qd × 30 days or 3 wk on 1 wk off
Female hypogonadism
• *Adult:* PO 12-25 mg × 21 days, then progesterone 100 mg IM or 5 days of progesterone PO given with last 5 days of medroxyprogesterone 5-10 mg
Vaginitis
• *Adult:* PO 12-25 mg qd × 30-60 days
Available forms: Caps 12, 25, 72 mg
Side effects/adverse reactions:
CNS: Dizziness, headache, migraines, depression
CV: Hypotension, ***thrombophlebitis***, edema, ***thromboembolism, stroke, pulmonary embolism, myocardial infarction***
GI: Nausea, vomiting, diarrhea, anorexia, pancreatitis, cramps, constipation, increased appetite, increased weight, ***cholestatic jaundice***
EENT: Contact lens intolerance, increased myopia, astigmatism
GU: Amenorrhea, cervical erosion, breakthrough bleeding, dysmenorrhea, vaginal candidiasis, breast changes, *gynecomastia, testicular atrophy,* impotence
INTEG: Rash, urticaria, acne, hirsutism, alopecia, oily skin, seborrhea, purpura, melasma
META: Folic acid deficiency, hypercalcemia, hyperglycemia
Contraindications: Breast cancer, thromboembolic disorders, reproductive cancer, genital bleeding (abnormal, undiagnosed), pregnancy (X)
Precautions: Hypertension, asthma, blood dyscrasias, gallbladder disease, CHF, diabetes mellitus, bone disease, depression, migraine headache, convulsive disorders, hepatic disease, renal

italics = common side effects   ***bold italic*** = life threatening reactions

disease, family history of cancer of the breast or reproductive tract

Pharmacokinetics:

PO: Degraded in liver; excreted in urine; crosses placenta; excreted in breast milk

Interactions/incompatibilities:

• Decreased action of: anticoagulants, oral hypoglycemics

• Toxicity: tricyclic antidepressants

• Decreased action of chlorotrianisene: anticonvulsants, barbiturates, phenylbutazone, rifampin

• Increased action of: corticosteroids

Lab test interferences:

Increase: BSP retention test, PBI, T_4, serum sodium, platelet aggressability, thyroxine-binding globulin (TBG), prothrombin, factors VII, VIII, IX, X, triglycerides

Decrease: Serum folate, serum triglyceride, T_3 resin uptake test, glucose tolerance test, antithrombin III, pregnanediol, metyrapone test

False positive: LE prep, antinuclear antibodies

NURSING CONSIDERATIONS

Assess:

• Urine glucose in patient with diabetes; increased urine glucose may occur

• Weight daily; notify physician if weekly weight gain is >5 lb; if increase, diuretic may be ordered

• B/P q4h; watch for increase caused by water and Na retention

• I&O ratio; be alert for decreasing urinary output and increasing edema

• Liver function studies, including AST, ALT, bilirubin, alk phosphatase

• Edema, hypertension, cardiac symptoms, jaundice

• Mental status: affect, mood, behavioral changes, aggression

• Hypercalcemia

Administer:

• Titrated dose, use lowest effective dose

• In one dose in AM, for prostatic cancer, vaginitis, hypogonadism

• With food or milk to decrease GI symptoms

Evaluate:

• Therapeutic response: reversal of menopause or decrease in tumor size in prostatic cancer

Teach patient/family:

• To weigh weekly, report gain >5 lb

• To report breast lumps, vaginal bleeding, edema, jaundice, dark urine, clay-colored stools, dyspnea, headache, blurred vision, abdominal pain, numbness, stiffness, or pain in legs, chest pain; male to report impotence or gynecomastia

• To check with physician before using OTC drugs

---

chlorphenesin carbamate

(klor-fen'e-sin)

Maolate, Mycil*

Func. class.: Skeletal muscle relaxant, central acting

Chem. class.: Carbamate

Action: Unknown; may be related to sedative properties; does not directly relax muscle or depress nerve conduction

Uses: Adjunct for relieving pain in acute, painful musculoskeletal conditions

Dosage and routes:

• *Adult:* PO 800 mg tid, maintenance 400 mg qid, not to exceed 8 wk

Available forms: Tabs 400 mg

Side effects/adverse reactions:

CNS: Dizziness, weakness, drows-

---

* Available in Canada only

iness, headache, tremor, depression, insomnia, confusion
EENT: Diplopia, temporary loss of vision
HEMA: **Blood dyscrasias**
CV: Postural hypotension, tachycardia
GI: Nausea, vomiting, hiccups
INTEG: Rash, pruritus, fever, facial flushing
SYST: Anaphylaxis
Contraindications: Hypersensitivity, child <12 yr, intermittent porphyria
Precautions: Renal disease, hepatic disease, addictive personality, pregnancy (C), elderly
Pharmacokinetics:
PO: Onset ½ hr, peak 1-2 hr, duration 4-6 hr; metabolized by liver; excreted in urine; crosses placenta; excreted in breast milk (large amounts); half-life 4 hr
Interactions/incompatibilities:
• Increased CNS depression: alcohol, tricyclic antidepressants, narcotics, barbiturates, sedatives, hypnotics

NURSING CONSIDERATIONS
Assess:
• Blood studies: CBC, WBC, differential; blood dyscrasias may occur
• Liver function studies: AST, ALT, alk phosphatase; hepatitis may occur
• Kidney function studies
• ECG in epileptic patients; poor seizure control has occurred with patients taking this drug
• B/P lying and standing; postural hypotension may occur
• Allergic reactions: rash, fever, respiratory distress
• Severe weakness, numbness in extremities
• Psychologic dependency: increased need for medication, more

frequent requests for medication, increased pain
• CNS depression: dizziness, drowsiness, psychiatric symptoms
Administer:
• With meals for GI symptoms
Perform/provide:
• Storage in tight container at room temperature
• Assistance with ambulation if dizziness/drowsiness occurs, especially elderly
Evaluate:
• Therapeutic response: decreased pain, spasticity
Teach patient/family:
• Not to discontinue medication quickly: insomnia, nausea, headache, spasticity, tachycardia will occur; drug should be tapered off over 1-2 wk
• Not to take with alcohol, other CNS depressants
• To avoid altering activities while taking this drug
• To avoid hazardous activities if drowsiness/dizziness occurs
• To avoid using OTC medication: cough preparations, antihistamines, unless directed by physician
Treatment of overdose: Give physostigmine IV; monitor cardiac function

---

italics = common side effects   ***bold italic*** = life threatening reactions

chlorpheniramine maleate

(klor-fen-eer'a-meen)
Aller-Chlor, Allergy, Chlo-Amine, Chlor-100, Chlor-Pro, Chlorate, Chlorpheniramine Maleate, Chlor-Pro 10, Chlorspan-12, Chlortab-B, Chlortab-4, Chlor-Trimeton, Chlor-Trimeton Repetabs, Pedia Care Allergy Formula, Pfeiffer's Allergy, Phenetron, Telachlor, Teldrin

Func. class.: Antihistamine
Chem. class.: Alkylamine, H_1-receptor antagonist

Action: Acts on blood vessels, GI system, respiratory system, by competing with histamine for H_1-receptor site; decreases allergic response by blocking histamine

Uses: Allergy symptoms, rhinitis

Dosage and routes:
• *Adult:* PO 2-4 mg tid-qid, not to exceed 36 mg/day; TIME-REL 8-12 mg bid-tid, not to exceed 36 mg/day; IM/IV/SC 5-40 mg/day
• *Child 6-12 yr:* PO 2 mg q4-6h, not to exceed 12 mg/day; SUS REL 8 mg hs or qd, SUS REL not recommended for child <6 yr
• *Child 2-5 yr:* PO 1 mg q4-6h, not to exceed 4 mg/day

Available forms: Tabs, chewable 2 mg; tabs 4 mg; tabs, time-rel 8, 12 mg, caps, time-rel 8, 12 mg; syr 2 mg/5 ml; inj IM, SC, IV 10, 100 mg/ml

Side effects/adverse reactions:
CNS: Dizziness, drowsiness, poor coordination, fatigue, anxiety, euphoria, confusion, paresthesia, neuritis
RESP: Increased thick secretions, wheezing, chest tightness

HEMA: **Thrombocytopenia, agranulocytosis, hemolytic anemia**
GI: Dry mouth, nausea, anorexia, diarrhea
INTEG: Photosensitivity
GU: Retention, dysuria, frequency
EENT: Blurred vision, dilated pupils, tinnitus, nasal stuffiness, dry nose, throat, mouth

Contraindications: Hypersensitivity to H_1-receptor antagonists, acute asthma attack, lower respiratory tract disease

Precautions: Increased intraocular pressure, renal disease, cardiac disease, hypertension, bronchial asthma, seizure disorder, stenosed peptic ulcers, hyperthyroidism, prostatic hypertrophy, bladder neck obstruction, pregnancy (B), elderly

Pharmacokinetics:
PO: Onset 20-60 min, duration 8-12 hr; detoxified in liver; excreted by kidneys; (metabolites/free drug); half-life 20-24 hr

Interactions/incompatibilities:
• Incompatible with calcium chloride, kanamycin, levarterenol, pentobarbital
• Increased CNS depression: barbiturates, narcotics, hypnotics, tricyclic antidepressants, alcohol
• Decreased effect of: oral anticoagulants, heparin
• Increased effect of chlorpheniramine: MAOIs

Lab test interferences:
False negative: Skin allergy tests

NURSING CONSIDERATIONS

Assess:
• I&O ratio; be alert for urinary retention, frequency, dysuria; drug should be discontinued if these occur
• CBC during long-term therapy
• Blood dyscrasias: thrombocytopenia, agranulocytosis (rare)
• Respiratory status: rate, rhythm,

increase in bronchial secretions, wheezing, chest tightness

Administer:
• IV undiluted at a rate of 10 mg/ 1 min or longer
• With meals if GI symptoms occur; absorption may slightly decrease

Perform/provide:
• Hard candy, gum, frequent rinsing of mouth for dryness
• Storage in tight container at room temperature

Evaluate:
• Therapeutic response: absence of running or congested nose or rashes

Teach patient/family:
• Not to chew or crush sustained-release forms
• All aspects of drug use; to notify physician if confusion/sedation/ hypotension occurs
• That this drug decreases anticoagulant (oral) effect
• To avoid driving or other hazardous activity if drowsiness occurs, especially elderly
• To avoid concurrent use of alcohol or other CNS depressants

Treatment of overdose: Administer ipecac syrup or lavage, diazepam, vasopressors, barbiturates (short-acting)

---

chlorpromazine HCl
(klor-proe′ma-zeen)
Chlorpromazine HCl, Chlorpromanyl,* Ormazine, Thorazine, Thorazine Spansules
Func. class.: Antipsychotic/ neuroleptic
Chem. class.: Phenothiazine-aliphatic

Action: Depresses cerebral cortex, hypothalamus, limbic system, which control activity aggression; blocks neurotransmission produced by dopamine at synapse; exhibits a strong α-adrenergic, anticholinergic blocking action; mechanism for antipsychotic effects is unclear

Uses: Psychotic disorders, mania, schizophrenia, anxiety, intractable hiccups, nausea, vomiting; preoperatively for relaxation; acute intermittent porphyria, behavioral problems in children

Dosage and routes:
Psychiatry
• *Adult:* PO 10-50 mg q1-4h initially, then increase up to 2 g/day if necessary
• *Adult:* IM 10-50 mg q1-4h
• *Child:* PO 0.25 mg/lb q4-6h or 0.5 mg/kg
• *Child:* IM 0.25 mg/lb q6-8h or 0.5 mg/kg
• *Child:* REC 0.5 mg/lb q6-8h or 1 mg/kg

Nausea and vomiting
• *Adult:* PO 10-25 mg q4-6h prn; IM 25-50 mg q3h prn; REC 50-100 mg q6-8h prn, not to exceed 400 mg/day
• *Child:* PO 0.25 mg/lb q4-6h prn, IM 0.25 mg/lb q6-8h prn not to exceed 40 mg/day (<5 yr) or 75 mg/day (5-12 yr); REC 0.5 mg/lb: q6-8h prn
• *Adult:* IV 25-50 mg qd-qid
• *Child:* IV 0.55 mg/kg q6-8h

Intractable hiccups
• *Adult:* PO 25-50 mg tid-qid; IM 25-50 mg (used only if PO dose does not work); IV 25-50 mg in 500-1000 ml saline (only for severe hiccups)

Available forms: Tabs 10, 25, 50, 100, 200 mg; time-rel caps 30, 75, 150, 200, 300 mg; syr 10 mg/5ml; conc 30, 100 mg/ml; supp 25, 100 mg; inj IM, IV 25 mg/ml

Side effects/adverse reactions:
CV: Orthostatic hypotension, hy-

---

italics = common side effects   ***bold italic*** = life threatening reactions

pertension, *cardiac arrest,* ECG changes, *tachycardia*

EENT: Blurred vision, glaucoma, dry eyes

GI: Dry mouth, nausea, vomiting, anorexia, constipation, diarrhea, jaundice, weight gain

GU: Urinary retention, urinary frequency, enuresis, impotence, amenorrhea, gynecomastia, breast engorgement

HEMA: Anemia, *leukopenia, leukocytosis, agranulocytosis*

INTEG: Rash, photosensitivity, dermatitis

RESP: Laryngospasm, dyspnea, *respiratory depression*

CNS: Extrapyramidal symptoms: pseudoparkinsonism, akathisia, dystonia, tardive dyskinesia, seizures, *headache*

Contraindications: Hypersensitivity, circulatory collapse, liver damage, cerebral arteriosclerosis, coronary disease, severe hypertension/hypotension, coma, blood dyscrasias, child <2 years, brain damage, bone marrow depression, alcohol and barbiturate withdrawal

Precautions: Pregnancy (C), lactation, seizure disorders, hypertension, hepatic disease, cardiac disease, elderly

Pharmacokinetics:

PO: Absorption variable, widely distributed; onset erratic 30-60 min, duration 4-6 hours

IM: Well absorbed; peak 15-20 min, duration 4 to 8 hours

IV: Onset 5 min, peak 10 min, duration unknown

PO-ER: Onset 30-60 minutes, peak unknown, duration 10-12 hours

REC: Onset erratic, duration 3 hr; metabolized by liver, excreted in urine (metabolites), crosses placenta, enters breast milk; 95%

bound to plasma proteins; elimination half-life 10-30 hr

Interactions/incompatibilities:

• Incompatible with aminophylline, amphotericin B, ampicillin, atropine, caffeine and sodium benzoate, cephalothin, chloramphenicol, chlorothiazide, dimenhydrinate, epinephrine, folic acid, hydrocortisone, kanamycin, magnesium sulfate, methicillin, methohexital, methylprednisolone, paraldehyde, penicillin G, pentobarbital, phenobarbital, ranitidine, secobarbital, $NaCo_3$, tetracycline, thiopental in sol or syringe

• Oversedation: other CNS depressants, alcohol, barbiturate anesthetics, antihistamines, sedatives/hypnotics, antidepressants

• Toxicity: epinephrine

• Decreased absorption: aluminum hydroxide, magnesium hydroxide antacids

• Decreased antiparkinson activity: levodopa, bromocriptine

• Decreased serum chlorpromazine: lithium

• Increased effects of both drugs: β-adrenergic blockers, alcohol

• Increased anticholinergic effects: anticholinergics

• Agranulocystosis: antithyroid agents

Lab test interferences:

Increase: Liver function tests, cardiac enzymes, cholesterol, blood glucose, prolactin, bilirubin, PBI, cholinesterase, ^{131}I, alk phosphatase, leukocytes, granulocytes, platelets

Decrease: Hormones (blood and urine)

False positive: Pregnancy tests, PKU

False negative: Urinary steroids, 17-OHCS

---

* Available in Canada only

NURSING CONSIDERATIONS
Assess:
• Mental status: orientation, mood, behavior, presence of hallucinations and type before initial administration and monthly
• Swallowing of PO medication; check for hoarding or giving of medication to other patients
• I&O ratio; palpate bladder if low urinary output occurs, especially in elderly
• Bilirubin, CBC, liver function studies monthly
• Urinalysis recommended before, during prolonged therapy
• Affect, orientation, LOC, reflexes, gait, coordination, sleep pattern disturbances
• B/P sitting, standing and lying; take pulse and respirations q4h during initial treatment; establish baseline before starting treatment; report drops of 30 mm Hg; obtain baseline ECG, Q-wave and T-wave changes
• Dizziness, faintness, palpitations, tachycardia on rising
• For neuroleptic malignant syndrome: hyperpyrexia, muscle rigidity, increased CPK, altered mental status
• Extrapyramidal symptoms including akathisia (inability to sit still, no pattern to movements), tardive dyskinesia (bizarre movements of the jaw, mouth, tongue, extremities), pseudoparkinsonism (rigidity, tremors, pill rolling, shuffling gait)
• Skin turgor daily
• Constipation, urinary retention daily; if these occur, increase bulk, water in diet

Administer:
• IM, inject in deep muscle mass, do not give SC
• IV after diluting 1 mg/1 ml with NS, give 1 mg or less/2 min or more; may be further diluted in 500-1000 ml of NS
• Antiparkinsonian agent to be used if extrapyramidal symptoms occur
• Rectal after placing in refrigerator or ½ hour if too soft to insert
• Drug in liquid form mixed in glass of juice or cola if hoarding is suspected
• Decreased dose in elderly
• PO with full glass of water, milk; or give with food to decrease GI upset

Perform/provide:
• Decreased stimuli by dimming lights, avoiding loud noises
• Supervised ambulation until stabilized on medication; do not involve in strenuous exercise program because fainting is possible; patient should not stand still for long periods
• Increased fluids to prevent constipation
• Sips of water, candy, gum for dry mouth
• Storage in tight, light-resistant container, oral sol in amber bottle

Evaluate:
• Therapeutic response: decrease in emotional excitement, hallucinations, delusions, paranoia, reorganization of patterns of thought, speech

Teach patient/family:
• To use good oral hygiene; frequent rinsing of mouth, sugarless gum for dry mouth
• To avoid hazardous activities until drug response is determined
• That orthostatic hypotension occurs often and to rise from sitting or lying position gradually
• To remain lying down after IM injection for at least 30 min
• To avoid hot tubs, hot showers,

---

italics = common side effects   ***bold italic*** = life threatening reactions

tub baths, since hypotension may occur

• To avoid abrupt withdrawal of this drug, or extrapyramidal symptoms may result; drug should be withdrawn slowly

• To avoid OTC preparations (cough, hay fever, cold) unless approved by physician, since serious drug interactions may occur; avoid use with alcohol, CNS depressants; increased drowsiness may occur

• To use a sunscreen and sunglasses during exposure to prevent burns

• About extrapyramidal symptoms and necessity of meticulous oral hygiene, since oral candidiasis may occur

• To take antacids 2 hours before or after this drug

• To report sore throat, malaise, fever, bleeding, mouth sores; if these occur, CBC should be drawn and drug discontinued

• That in hot weather, heat stroke may occur; take extra precautions to stay cool

• That urine may turn pink or red

Treatment of overdose: Lavage if orally ingested; provide airway; *do not induce vomiting or use epinephrine*

---

chlorpropamide

(klor-proe′pa-mide)
Chloronase,* Chlorpropamide, Diabinese, Novopropamide*
Func. class.: Antidiabetic
Chem. class.: Sulfonylurea (1st generation)

Action: Causes functioning β-cells in pancreas to release insulin, leading to drop in blood glucose levels; may improve insulin binding to insulin receptors or increase the number of insulin receptors with prolonged administration. May also reduce basal hepatic glucose secretion; not effective if patient lacks functioning β-cells

Uses: Stable adult-onset diabetes mellitus (type II) NIDDM

Dosage and routes:

• *Adult:* PO 100-250 mg qd, initially, then 100-500 mg maintenance according to response; not to exceed 750 mg/day

Available forms: Tabs 100, 250 mg scored

Side effects/adverse reactions:

CNS: Headache, weakness, dizziness, drowsiness, tinnitus, fatigue, vertigo

GI: Hepatotoxicity, cholestatic jaundice, nausea, vomiting, diarrhea, heartburn

HEMA: Leukopenia, thrombocytopenia, agranulocytosis, aplastic anemia, pancytopenia, hemolytic anemia

INTEG: Rash, allergic reactions, pruritus, urticaria, eczema, photosensitivity, erythema

ENDO: Hypoglycemia, hyponatremia

Contraindications: Hypersensitivity to sulfonylureas, juvenile or brittle diabetes, pregnancy (D), renal failure

Precautions: Elderly, cardiac disease, thyroid disease, renal disease, hepatic disease, severe hypoglycemic reactions

Pharmacokinetics:

PO: Completely absorbed by GI route, onset 1 hr, peak 3-6 hr, duration 60 hr, half-life 36 hr; metabolized in liver; excreted in urine (metabolites and unchanged drug), breast milk; 90%-95% is plasma protein bound

Interactions/incompatibilities:

• Increased hypoglycemic effects:

oral anticoagulants, salicylates, sulfonamides, nonsteroidal antiinflammatories, chloramphenicol, cimetidine, MAOIs, insulin, guanethidine, methyldopa, probenecid, ranitidine
• Increased effects of chlorpropamide: insulin, MAOIs
• Decreased digoxin levels: digoxin
• Decreased effect of both drugs; diazoxide
• Disulfiram-like reaction: alcohol
• Decreased action of chlorpropamide: calcium channel blockers, corticosteroids, oral contraceptives, thiazide diuretics, thyroid preparations, estrogens, phenobarbital, phenytoin, rifampin, sympathomimetics

NURSING CONSIDERATIONS
Assess:
• Hypoglycemic/hyperglycemic reaction that can occur soon after meals
Administer:
• Drug 30 min before meals
Perform/provide:
• Storage in tight container in cool environment
Evaluate:
• Therapeutic response: decrease in polyuria, polydipsia, polyphagia, clear sensorium, absence of dizziness, stable gait
Teach patient/family:
• To check for symptoms of cholestatic jaundice: dark urine, pruritus, yellow sclera; if these occur, physician should be notified
• To use capillary blood glucose test or Chemstrip 3 × /day
• Symptoms of hypo/hyperglycemia, what to do about each
• That this drug must be continued on daily basis; explain consequence of discontinuing drug abruptly
• To take drug in morning to prevent hypoglycemic reactions at night; have glucagon emergency kit available
• To avoid OTC medications unless prescribed by physician
• That diabetes is lifelong illness; drug will not cure disease
• That all food included in diet plan must be eaten to prevent hypoglycemia
• To carry Medic-Alert ID for emergency purposes
• Not to drink alcohol
Treatment of overdose: glucose 25 g IV, via dextrose 50% solution, 50cc or 1 mg glucogon

---

chlortetracycline HCl (topical)
(klor-te-tra-sye'kleen)
Aureomycin
Func. class.: Local antiinfective
Chem. class.: Antibacterial

Action: Interferes with bacterial protein cell synthesis
Uses: Pyogenic skin infections
Dosage and routes:
• *Adult and child:* TOP rub into affected area bid-qid
Available forms: Oint 3%
Side effects/adverse reactions:
INTEG: Rash, urticaria, stinging, burning, dry skin, photosensitivity
Contraindications: Hypersensitivity to this drug or wool
Precautions: Pregnancy (D), lactation
NURSING CONSIDERATIONS
Assess:
• Allergic reaction: burning, stinging, swelling, redness
Administer:
• Enough medication to cover lesions completely
• After cleansing with soap, water before each application; dry well

---

Perform/provide:
• Storage at room temperature in dry place in light-resistant container

Evaluate:
• Therapeutic response: decrease in size, number of lesions

Teach patient/family:
• To watch for superimposed infections
• To use medical asepsis (hand washing) before, after each application
• To apply with glove to prevent further infection
• To avoid use of OTC creams, ointments, lotions unless directed by physician
• To avoid squeezing or poking lesions, or spreading may occur
• To notify physician if condition worsens or rash, irritation, or swelling occurs
• To avoid sunlight or ultraviolet light
• That skin may be stained

---

chlorthalidone
(klor-thal′i-done)
Chlorthalidone, Hygroton, Hylidone, Novothalidone,* Thalitone
Func. class.: Diuretic
Chem. class.: Thiazide-like;
phthalimidine derivative

Action: Acts on distal tubule by increasing excretion of water, sodium, chloride, potassium, magnesium, bicarbonate

Uses: Edema, hypertension, diuresis, CHF, nephrotic syndrome

Dosage and routes:
• *Adult:* PO 25-100 mg/day or 100 mg every other day
• *Child:* PO 2 mg/kg 3 × /wk

Available forms: Tabs 25, 50, 100 mg

Side effects/adverse reactions:
GU: Frequency, polyuria, **uremia,** glucosuria, impotence
CNS: Drowsiness, paresthesia, anxiety, depression, headache, *dizziness, fatigue, weakness*
GI: Nausea, vomiting, anorexia, constipation, diarrhea, cramps, pancreatitis, GI irritation, *hepatitis*
EENT: Blurred vision
INTEG: Rash, urticaria, purpura, photosensitivity, fever
META: Hyperglycemia, hyperuremia, increased creatinine, BUN, gout
HEMA: **Aplastic anemia, hemolytic anemia, leukopenia, agranulocytosis, thrombocytopenia, neutropenia**
CV: Irregular pulse, orthostatic hypotension, palpitations, volume depletion
ELECT: Hypokalemia, hypomagnesemia, hypercalcemia, hyponatremia, hypochloremia

Contraindications: Hypersensitivity to thiazides or sulfonamides, anuria, renal decompensation, lactation

Precautions: Hypokalemia, renal disease, pregnancy (C), hepatic disease, gout, diabetes mellitus, elderly

Pharmacokinetics:
PO: Onset 2 hr, peak 6 hr, duration 24-72 hr; excreted unchanged by kidneys; crosses placenta; enters breast milk; half-life 40 hr

Interactions/incompatibilities:
• Increased toxicity: lithium, nondepolarizing skeletal muscle relaxants
• Decreased effects of: antidiabetics
• Decreased absorption of thiazides: cholestyramine, colestipol

• Decreased hypotensive response: indomethacin, NSAIDs
• Hyperglycemia, hyperuricemia, hypotension: diazoxide

Lab test interferences:

Increase: BSP retention, Ca, cholesterol, triglycerides, amylase

Decrease: PBI, PSP, parathyroid test

NURSING CONSIDERATIONS

Assess:

• Weight, I&O daily to determine fluid loss; effect of drug may be decreased if used qd
• Rate, depth, rhythm of respiration, effect of exertion
• B/P lying, standing; postural hypotension may occur
• Electrolytes: K, Mg, Na, Cl; include BUN, blood sugar, CBC, serum creatinine, blood pH, ABGs, uric acid, Ca
• Glucose in urine if patient is diabetic
• Signs of metabolic alkalosis: drowsiness, restlessness
• Signs of hypokalemia: postural hypotension, malaise, fatigue, tachycardia, leg cramps, weakness
• Rashes, temperature elevation qd
• Confusion, especially in elderly; take safety precautions if needed

Administer:

• In AM to avoid interference with sleep if using drug as a diuretic
• K replacement if K is less than 3.0
• With food if nausea occurs; absorption may be decreased slightly

Evaluate:

• Therapeutic response: improvement in edema of feet, legs, sacral area daily if medication is being used in CHF

Teach patient/family:

• To increase fluid intake to 2-3 L/day unless contraindicated, to rise slowly from lying or sitting position

• To notify physician of muscle weakness, cramps, nausea, dizziness
• That drug may be taken with food or milk
• That blood sugar may be increased in diabetics
• To use sunscreen to protect against photosensitivity
• To take early in day to avoid nocturia

Treatment of overdose: Lavage if taken orally, monitor electrolytes, administer dextrose in saline, monitor hydration, CV, renal status

---

chlorzoxazone

(klor-zox′a-zone)
Chlorzoxazone, Paraflex, Parafon Forte DSC, Remular-S

Func. class.: Skeletal muscle relaxant

Chem. class.: Benzoxazole derivative

Action: Inhibits multisynaptic reflex arcs

Uses: Relieving pain, spasm in musculoskeletal conditions

Dosage and routes:

• *Adult:* PO 250-750 mg tid-qid
• *Child:* PO 20 mg/kg/day in divided doses bid-tid

Available forms: Tabs 250 mg

Side effects/adverse reactions:

GU: Urine discoloration

HEMA: **Granulocytopenia, anemia**

CNS: Dizziness, drowsiness, headache, insomnia, stimulation, malaise

GI: Nausea, vomiting, anorexia, diarrhea, constipation, **hepatotoxicity, jaundice**

INTEG: Rash, pruritus, petechiae, ecchymoses, **angioedema**

SYST: **Anaphylaxis**

---

italics = common side effects   ***bold italic*** = life threatening reactions

Contraindications: Hypersensitivity, impaired hepatic function
Precautions: Pregnancy (C), lactation, hepatic disease, elderly
Pharmacokinetics:
PO: Onset 1 hr, peak 3-4 hr, duration 6 hr, half-life 1 hr; metabolized in liver; excreted in urine (metabolites)
Interactions/incompatibilities:
• Increased CNS depression: alcohol, tricyclic antidepressants, narcotics, barbiturates, sedatives, hypnotics
NURSING CONSIDERATIONS
Assess:
• Blood studies: CBC, WBC, differential; blood dyscrasias may occur
• Liver function studies: AST, ALT, alk phosphatase; hepatitis may occur; hold dose and notify physician if signs of hepatotoxicity occur
• EEG in epileptic patients; poor seizure control has occurred with patients taking this drug
• Allergic reactions: rash, fever, respiratory distress
• Severe weakness, numbness in extremities
• Psychologic dependency: increased need for medication, more frequent requests for medication, increased pain
• CNS depression: dizziness, drowsiness, psychiatric symptoms
Administer:
• With meals for GI symptoms
Perform/provide:
• Storage in tight container at room temperature
• Assistance with ambulation if dizziness or drowsiness occurs, especially elderly
Evaluate:
• Therapeutic response: decreased pain, spasticity

Teach patient/family:
• Not to discontinue the medication quickly; insomnia, nausea, headache, spasticity, tachycardia will occur; drug should be tapered off over 1-2 wk
• Not to take with alcohol, other CNS depressants
• To avoid altering activities while taking this drug
• To avoid hazardous activities if drowsiness, dizziness occurs
• To avoid using OTC medication: cough preparations, antihistamines, unless directed by physician
• That urine may be orange or purple
Treatment of overdose: Gastric lavage or induce emesis, then administer activated charcoal; use other supportive treatment as necessary; monitor cardiac function

---

cholestyramine
(koe-less-tir′a-meen)
Cholybar, Questran, Questran Light
Func. class.: Antilipemic
Chem. class.: Bile acid sequestrant

Action: Absorbs, combines with bile acids to form insoluble complex that is excreted through feces; loss of bile acids lowers cholesterol levels
Uses: Primary hypercholesterolemia, pruritus associated with biliary obstruction, diarrhea caused by excess bile acid, digitalis toxicity, xanthomas
Dosage and routes:
• *Adult:* PO 4 g ac, and hs, not to exceed 32 g/day
• *Child:* PO 240 mg/kg/day in 3 divided doses; administer with food or drink

Available forms: Powder 9 g/4 g cholestyramine

Side effects/adverse reactions:

CNS: Headache, dizziness, drowsiness, vertigo, tinnitus

MS: Muscle, joint pain

GI: Constipation, abdominal pain, nausea, fecal impaction, hemorrhoids, flatulence, vomiting, steatorrhea, peptic ulcer

INTEG: Rash, irritation of perianal area, tongue, skin

HEMA: Decreased Vit A, D, K, red cell folate content, *hyperchloremic acidosis, bleeding,* decreased protime

Contraindications: Hypersensitivity, biliary obstruction

Precautions: Pregnancy (C), lactation, children

Pharmacokinetics:

PO: Excreted in feces, maximum effect in 2 wk

Interactions/incompatibilities:

• Decreased absorption of: phenylbutazone, warfarin, thiazides, digitalis, penicillin G, tetracyclines, cephalexin, phenobarbital, folic acid, corticosteroids, iron, thyroid, clindamycin, trimethoprim, chenodiol, fat-soluble vitamins

Lab test interferences:

Increase: Liver function studies, Cl, PO_4

NURSING CONSIDERATIONS

Assess:

• Cardiac glycoside level, if both drugs are being administered

• For signs of Vit A, D, K deficiency

• Serum cholesterol, triglyceride levels, electrolytes if on extended therapy

• Bowel pattern daily; increase bulk, water in diet if constipation develops

Administer:

• Drug ac, hs; give all other medications 1 hr before cholestyramine or 4 hr after cholestyramine to avoid poor absorption

• Drug mixed/applesauce or stirred into beverage (2-6 oz), do not take dry, let stand for 2 min

• Supplemental doses of Vit A, D, K, if levels are low

Evaluate:

• Therapeutic response: decreased cholesterol level (hyperlipidemia); diarrhea, pruritus (excess bile acids)

Teach patient/family:

• Symptoms of hypoprothrombinemia: bleeding mucous membranes, dark tarry stools, hematuria, petechiae; report immediately

• Importance of compliance, since toxicity may result if doses are missed

• That risk factors should be decreased: high-fat diet, smoking, alcohol consumption, absence of exercise

• Not to discontinue suddenly

---

choline salicylate

(koe'leen)

Arthropan, Teejel*

Func. class.: Nonnarcotic analgesic

Chem. class.: Salicylate

Action: Blocks pain impulses in CNS that occur in response to inhibition of prostaglandin synthesis; antipyretic action results from inhibition of hypothalamic heat-regulating center to produce vasodilation to allow heat dissipation

Uses: Mild to moderate pain or fever including arthritis, juvenile rheumatoid arthritis

italics = common side effects   ***bold italic*** = life threatening reactions

Dosage and routes:
Arthritis
• *Adult and Child >12 yrs:* PO 870-1740 mg qid; max 6 × /day
Pain/fever
• *Adult:* PO 870 mg q3-4h prn
• *Child 3-6 yr:* PO 105-210 mg q4h prn
Available forms: Liq 870 mg/5 ml
Side effects/adverse reactions:
*HEMA: **Thrombocytopenia, agranulocytosis, leukopenia, neutropenia, hemolytic anemia,** increased pro-time*
CNS: Stimulation, drowsiness, dizziness, confusion, ***convulsion,*** headache, flushing, hallucinations, ***coma***
*GI: Nausea, vomiting, GI bleeding, diarrhea, heartburn, anorexia, **hepatitis***
INTEG: Rash, urticaria, bruising
EENT: Tinnitus, hearing loss
CV: Rapid pulse, pulmonary edema
RESP: Wheezing, hyperpnea
ENDO: Hypoglycemia, hyponatremia, hypokalemia
Contraindications: Hypersensitivity to salicylates, GI bleeding, bleeding disorders, children < 3 yr, Vit K deficiency, children with flu-like symptoms
Precautions: Anemia, hepatic disease, renal disease, Hodgkin's disease, pregnancy (C), lactation
Pharmacokinetics:
PO: Onset 15-30 min; metabolized by liver; excreted by kidneys; crosses placenta; excreted in breast milk
Interactions/incompatibilities:
• Decreased effects of choline: antacids, steroids, urinary alkalizers
• Increased blood loss: alcohol, heparin
• Increased effects of: anticoagulants, insulin, methotrexate
• Decreased effects of: probenecid,

spironolactone, sulfinpyrazone, sulfonylamides
• Toxic effects: PABA, furosemide, carbonic anhydrase inhibitors
• Decreased blood sugar levels: salicylates
• GI bleeding: steroids, antiinflammatories
Lab test interferences:
Increase: Coagulation studies, liver function studies, serum uric acid, amylase, CO_2, urinary protein
Decrease: Serum potassium, PBI, cholesterol
Interference: Urine catecholamines, pregnancy test
NURSING CONSIDERATIONS
Assess:
• Liver function studies: AST, ALT, bilirubin, creatinine if patient is on long-term therapy
• Renal function studies: BUN, urine creatinine if patient is on long-term therapy
• Blood studies: CBC, Hct, Hgb, pro-time if patient is on long-term therapy
• I&O ratio; decreasing output may indicate renal failure (long-term therapy)
• Hepatotoxicity: dark urine; clay-colored stools; yellowing of skin, sclera; itching; abdominal pain; fever; diarrhea if patient is on long-term therapy
• Allergic reactions: rash, urticaria; if these occur, drug may have to be discontinued
• Renal dysfunction: decreased urine output
• Ototoxicity: tinnitus, ringing, roaring in ears; audiometric testing needed before, after long-term therapy
• Visual changes: blurring, halos, corneal, retinal damage
• Edema in feet, ankles, legs

• Prior drug history; there are many drug interactions

Administer:

• Mixed with fruit juice, carbonated beverage, water

Evaluate:

• Therapeutic response: decreased pain, fever, stiffness of joints

Teach patient/family:

• To report any symptoms of hepatotoxicity, renal toxicity, visual changes, ototoxicity, allergic reactions, bleeding (long-term therapy)

• Not to exceed recommended dosage; acute poisoning may result

• To read label on other OTC drugs; many contain aspirin

• That therapeutic response takes 2 wk (arthritis)

• To avoid alcohol ingestion; GI bleeding may occur

• That if anticoagulants are given with this drug, this drug should be decreased 2 wk before surgery

Treatment of overdose: Lavage, activated charcoal, monitor electrolytes, VS

---

chorionic gonadotropin, human

(go-nad′oh-troe-pin)

APL, Chorex-5, Chorex-10, Chorigon, Choron 10, Follutein, Gonic, Glukor, Pregnyl, Profasi HP

Func. class.: Human chorionic gonadotropin

Chem. class.: Polypeptide hormone

Action: Stimulates production of gonadal steroids, androgens; stimulates corpus luteum to produce progesterone

Uses: Infertility, anovulation, hypogonadism, nonobstructive cryptorchidism

Dosage and routes:

Infertility/anovulation

• *Adult:* IM 10,000 U 1 day after last dose of menotropins

Hypogonadism

• *Adult:* IM 500-1000 U 3 × wk × 3 wk, then 2 × wk × 3 wk, or 4000 U 3 × wk × 6-9 mo, then 2000 U 3 × wk × 3 mo

Cryptorchidism

• *Child (boy 4-9 yr):* IM 5000 U qod × 4 doses

Available forms: Powder for inj 200, 1000, 2000 U/ml

Side effects/adverse reactions:

CNS: Headache, depression, fatigue, anxiety, irritability

GU: Gynecomastia, early puberty, edema, ***ectopic pregnancy***

INTEG: Pain at injection site

Contraindications: Hypersensitivity, pituitary hypertrophy/tumor, early puberty, prostatic CA

Precautions: Asthma, migraine headache, convulsive disorders, cardiac disease, renal disease

Pharmacokinetics:

IM: Peak 6 hr, half-life 11-24 hr, excreted by kidneys

NURSING CONSIDERATIONS

Assess:

• Weight weekly; notify physician if weekly weight gain is >5 lb

• B/P before, during treatment

• Be alert for decreasing urinary output, increasing edema

• Edema, hypertension

Administer:

• Only after clomiphene citrate has been tried on anovulatory client

• After reconstitution with diluent enclosed in package

Perform/provide:

• Refrigeration for up to 2 mo

Evaluate:

• Therapeutic response: ovulation, fertility

---

italics = common side effects   ***bold italic*** = life threatening reactions

Teach patient/family:
• To report facial, axillary, pubic hair, change in voice, penile enlargement, acne in male, abdominal pain, distention, vaginal bleeding in women
• To report symptoms of ectopic pregnancy: dizziness, pain on one side, shoulder, pallor, weak thready pulse, hemorrhage; shock may proceed rapidly

---

chymopapain
(kye'moe-pa-pane)
Chymodiactin
Func. class.: Enzyme
Chem. class.: Proteolytic

Action: Hydrolyzes noncollagenous polypeptides that maintain structure of chondromucoprotein; this activity decreases pressure on disk

Uses: Herniated lumbar intervertebral disk

Dosage and routes:
• *Adult:* Inj 2-4 mKat U/disk injected intradiskally, not to exceed 10 mKat U in a multiple herniation
Available forms: Powder for inj 4, 10 mKat U/vial

Side effects/adverse reactions:
*CNS: **Paraplegia, cerebral hemorrhage**,* headache, dizziness, paresthesia, numbness of extremities
INTEG: Rash, urticaria, itching
GI: Nausea, paralytic ileus
MS: Back pain, stiffness, spasm, acute transverse myelitis, weakness, leg pain
*SYSTEM: **Anaphylaxis***
GU: Urinary retention

Contraindications: Hypersensitivity to this drug, papaya, meat tenderizer; severe spondylolisthesis; severe progressing paralysis; spinal cord tumor; cauda equina lesion, previous use

Precautions: Pregnancy (C), children

Pharmacokinetics: Onset 30 min, duration 24 hr

Interactions/incompatibilities:
• Dysrhythmias: halothane anesthetics plus epinephrine

NURSING CONSIDERATIONS
Assess:
• RBCs, ESR before treatment
• Respiratory rate, rhythm, depth; notify physician of abnormalities
• Anaphylaxis for several days after injection
• Neuro status after surgery; elimination status, since paralytic ileus can occur
• For allergies: iodine, papaya, meat tenderizer; if allergies are identified, drug should not be used
Administer:
• Only with epinephrine available for anaphylaxis
• Only in lumbar spine by physician
• After diluting with sterile water for injection, use within 60 min
• After completing allergy test (ChymoFAST)
Evaluate:
• Therapeutic response: absence of back pain, increased mobility
Teach patient/family:
• To report allergic reactions that have occurred up to 2 wk after injection
• To be aware of possible infection; redness, swelling, pain

---

ciclopirox olamine (topical)
(sye-kloe-peer'ox)
Loprox
Func. class.: Local antiinfective
Chem. class.: Antifungal

Action: Interferes with fungal cell

---

membrane, which increases permeability, leaking of cell nutrients

Uses: Tinea cruris, tinea corporis, tinea pedis, tinea versicolor, cutaneous candidiasis

Dosage and routes:
• *Adult and child >10 yr:* TOP rub into affected area bid

Available forms: Cream 1%

Side effects/adverse reactions:
INTEG: Rash, urticaria, stinging, burning, pruritus, pain

Contraindications: Hypersensitivity

Precautions: Pregnancy (B), lactation, child <10 yr

NURSING CONSIDERATIONS

Assess:
• Allergic reaction: burning, stinging, swelling, redness

Administer:
• Enough medication to cover lesions completely
• After cleansing with soap, water before each application; dry well

Perform/provide:
• Storage at room temperature in dry place

Evaluate:
• Therapeutic response: decrease in size, number of lesions

Teach patient/family:
• To apply with glove to prevent further infection
• To avoid use of OTC creams, ointments, lotions unless directed by physician
• To continue even though condition improves
• To use medical asepsis (hand washing) before, after each application
• Not to cover with occlusive dressing
• To change shoes and socks once a day during treatment of tinea pedis

• To report blisters, burning, oozing, swelling

---

cimetidine

(sye-met'i-deen)
Tagamet, Peptol*, Novocimetine*

Func. class.: H$_2$ Histamine receptor antagonist

Chem. class.: Imidazole derivative

Action: Inhibits histamine at H$_2$ receptor site in the gastric parietal cells, which inhibits gastric acid secretion

Uses: Short-term treatment of duodenal and gastric ulcers and maintenance

Dosage and routes:
• *Adult and child:* PO 300 mg qid with meals, hs × 8 wk or 400 mg bid, 800 mg hs; after 8 wk give hs dose only; IV BOL 300 mg/20 ml 0.9% NaCl over 1-2 min q6h; IV INF 300 mg/50 ml D$_5$W over 15-20 min; IM 300 mg q6h, not to exceed 2400 mg

Prophylaxis of duodenal ulcer
• *Adult and child >16 yr:* 400 mg hs

Available forms: Tabs 200, 300, 400, 800 mg; liq 300 mg/5 ml; inj IV 300 mg/2 ml, 300 mg/50 ml 0.9% NaCl

Side effects/adverse reactions:
CNS: Confusion, headache, depression, dizziness, anxiety, weakness, psychosis, tremors, **convulsions**
CV: Bradycardia, tachycardia
GI: Diarrhea, abdominal cramps, **paralytic ileus, jaundice**
GU: Gynecomastia, galactorrhea, impotence, increase in BUN, creatinine
HEMA: Agranulocytosis, thrombocytopenia, neutropenia, aplas-

---

tic anemia, increase in pro-time
INTEG: Urticaria, rash, alopecia, sweating, flushing, *exfoliative dermatitis*

Contraindications: Hypersensitivity

Precautions: Pregnancy (B), lactation, child <16 yr, organic brain syndrome, hepatic disease, renal disease, elderly

Pharmacokinetics: Well absorbed (PO, IM)

IM/IV: Onset 10 min, peak ½ hour, duration 4-5 hours

PO: Peak 1-1½ hr, half-life 1½-2 hrs; 30-40% metabolized by liver, excreted in urine (unchanged), crosses placenta, enters breast milk

Interactions/incompatibilities:

• Incompatible in solution with aminophylline, amphotericin B, barbiturates, cefamandole, cefazolin, cephalothin

• Increased toxicity: oral anticoagulants, benzodiazepines, metoprolol, propranolol, phenytoins, quinidine, theophyllines, tricyclic antidepressants, lidocaine, procainamide

• Decreased absorption of cimetidine: antacids

• Decrease effectiveness: smoking

• Decreased absorption: ketoconazole, iron salts, tetracyclines, lindomethacin

• Decreased absorption of: tocainide

Lab test interferences:

Increase: Alk phosphatase, AST, creatinine

False positive: Gastric bleeding test

NURSING CONSIDERATIONS
Assess:

• Gastric pH (5 should be maintained), also epigastric pain and duration, intensity; aggravating, ameliorating factors

• I&O ratio, BUN, creatinine, CBC with differential monthly

Administer:

• IV after diluting 300 mg/20 ml of normal saline for inj; give over 2 min or more; may be diluted 300 mg/50 ml of D$_5$W; run over 15-20 min; or total daily dose (900 mg) diluted in 100-1000 ml D$_5$W given over 24 hr

• With meals for prolonged drug effect; antacids 1 hr before or 1 hr after cimetidine

Perform/provide:

• Storage of diluted sol at room temperature up to 48 hr

Evaluate:

• Therapeutic response: decreased pain in abdomen; healing of ulcers, absence of gastroesophageal reflex

Teach patient/family:

• That gynecomastia, impotence may occur, are reversible

• To avoid driving, other hazardous activities until patient is stabilized on this medication; drowsiness or dizziness may occur

• To avoid black pepper, caffeine, alcohol, harsh spices, extremes in temperature of food

• To avoid OTC preparations: aspirin, cough, cold preparations; condition may worsen

• That smoking decreases the effectiveness of the drug

• That drug must be continued for prescribed time to be effective and taken exactly as prescribed; doses are not to be doubled

• To report bruising, fatigue, malaise; blood dyscrasias may occur

• To report to physician diarrhea, black tarry stools, sore throat, rash

C

cinoxacin

(sin-ox'a-sin)
Cinobac, Cinoxacin
Func. class.: Urinary tract anti-
bacterial

Action: Interferes with conversion
of intermediate DNA fragments
into high-molecular-weight DNA
in bacteria; DNA gynase inhibitor
Uses: Urinary tract infections
caused by *E. coli, Klebsiella, Enterobacter, P. mirabilis, P. vulgaris, P. morgani, Serratia, Citrobacter*
Dosage and routes:
• *Adult and child >12 yr:* PO 1 g/
day in 2-4 divided doses × 1-2 wk
Available forms: Caps 250, 500 mg
Side effects/adverse reactions:
INTEG: Pruritus, rash, urticaria,
photosensitivity, edema
CNS: Dizziness, headache, agitation, insomnia, confusion
*GI: Nausea, vomiting, anorexia,
abdominal cramps,* diarrhea
EENT: Sensitivity to light, visual
disturbances, blurred vision, tinni-
tus
Contraindications: Hypersensitiv-
ity to this drug, anuria, CNS dam-
age
Precautions: Renal disease, he-
patic disease, pregnancy (B), nurs-
ing mothers
Pharmacokinetics:
PO: Duration 6-8 hr, half-life 1½
hr; excreted in urine (unchanged/
inactive metabolites)
Interactions/incompatibilities:
• Increased levels of cinoxacin:
probenecid
NURSING CONSIDERATIONS
Assess:
• Kidney, liver function studies:
BUN, creatinine, AST, ALT
• I&O ratio, urine pH; <5.5 is ideal

• CNS symptoms: insomnia, vertigo, headache, agitation, confusion
• Allergic reactions: fever, flushing, rash, urticaria, pruritus
Administer:
• After clean-catch urine is obtained for C&S
• Two daily doses if urine output is
high or if patient has diabetes
Perform/provide:
• Limited intake of alkaline foods,
drugs: milk, dairy products, peanuts, vegetables, alkaline antacids,
sodium bicarbonate
Evaluate:
• Therapeutic response: decreased
pain, frequency, urgency, C&S ab-
sence of infection
Teach patient/family:
• That photophobic reactions oc-
cur; that patient should avoid sun-
light or use sunglasses, sunscreen
• That fluids must be increased to 3
L/day to avoid crystallization in
kidneys
• That if dizziness occurs, ambu-
late/activities with assistance
• To complete full course of drug
therapy
• To contact physician if adverse
reactions occur
• To take with food/milk to de-
crease GI irritation
Lab test interferences:
Increase: AST/ALT, BUN, creat-
inine, alk phosphatase

ciprofloxacin

(sip-ro-floks'a-sin)
Cipro, Cipro IV
Func. class.: Urinary antiinfec-
tive
Chem. class.: Fluoroquinolone
antibacterial

Action: Interferes with conversion

---

of intermediate DNA fragments into high-molecular-weight DNA in bacteria; DNA gyrase inhibitor

Uses: Adult urinary tract infections (including complicated) caused by *E. coli, E. cloacae, P. mirabilis, K. pneumoniae, P. vulgans, C. freusdil,* group D strep; respiratory, bone, joint infections

Dosage and routes:

Uncomplicated urinary tract infections

• *Adult:* PO 250 mg q12h; IV 200 mg q12h

Complicated/severe urinary tract infections

• *Adult:* PO 500 mg q12h; IV 400 mg q12h

Respiratory, bone, skin, joint infections

• *Adult:* PO 500-750 mg q12h

Available forms: Tabs 250, 500, 750 mg; IV 200 mg/100 ml D₅, 400 mg/200 ml D₅; 200, 400 mg vial

Side effects/adverse reactions:

CNS: Headache, dizziness, fatigue, insomnia, depression, restlessness

GI: Nausea, constipation, increased ALT, AST, flatulence, insomnia, heartburn, vomiting, diarrhea, oral candidiasis, dysphagia

INTEG: Rash, pruritus, urticaria, photosensitivity, flushing, fever, chills

MS: Blurred vision, tinnitus

Contraindications: Hypersensitivity to quinolones

Precautions: Pregnancy (C), lactation, children, renal disease

Pharmacokinetics:

PO: Peak 1 hr, half-life 3-4 hr; steady state 2 days; excreted in urine as active drug, metabolites

Interactions/incompatibilities:

• Considered incompatible with all drugs in syringe or sol

• Decreased absorption: magne-sium antacids, aluminum hydrox-ide, zinc, iron, sucralfate

• Increased serum levels of cipro-floxacin: probenecid

• Increased theophylline levels when used with ciprofloxacin

Lab test interferences:

Increase: AST, ALT, BUN, creat-inine, alk phosphatase

NURSING CONSIDERATIONS

Assess:

• CNS symptoms: headache, diz-ziness, fatigue, insomnia, depres-sion

• Kidney, liver function studies: BUN, creatinine, AST, ALT

• I&O ratio, urine pH <5.5 is ideal

• Allergic reactions: fever, flush-ing, rash, urticaria, pruritus

Administer:

• IV over 1 hr as an INF, comes in premixed plastic INF container or diluted 20 or 40 ml vial to a final conc of 0.5-2 mg/ml of NS or D₅W. Give through Y-tube or 3-way stopcock

• After clean-catch urine is ob-tained for C&S

• Two daily doses if urine output is high or if patient has diabetes

Perform/provide:

• Limited intake of alkaline foods, drugs: milk, dairy products, pea-nuts, vegetables, alkaline antacids, sodium bicarbonate

Evaluate:

• Therapeutic response: decreased pain, frequency, urgency, C&S—absence of infection

Teach patient/family:

• Not to take antacids containing magnesium or aluminum with this drug or within 2 hr of drug

• That photosensitivity may occur; patient should avoid sunlight or use sunscreen to prevent burns

• That fluids must be increased to

---

3 L/day to avoid crystallization in kidneys
• If dizziness occurs, to ambulate, perform activities with assistance
• To complete full course of drug therapy
• To contact physician if adverse reaction occurs
• To take with food, milk to decrease GI irritation

cisapride
(sis'-a-pride)
Propulsid
Func. class.: Cholinergic

Action: Enhances response to acetylcholine at the myenteric plexus
Uses: Treatment of heartburn
Dosage and routes:
• *Adult:* PO 10 mg qid at least 15 min ac and hs; may increase to 20 mg; elderly may need higher dosage
Available forms: Tabs 10 mg
Side effects/adverse reactions:
CNS: Headache, sleeplessness, anxiety, nervousness, pain, fever
GI: Constipation, nausea, anorexia, abdominal pain, flatulence, dyspepsia
GU: UTI, frequency
INTEG: Pruritus, rash
Contraindications: Hypersensitivity; GI hemorrhage, obstruction, perforation
Precautions: Pregnancy (C), lactation, children, elderly
Pharmacokinetics: Rapidly absorbed PO; peak 1-1½ hr
PO: Onset ½-1 hr
Extensively metabolized by liver, excreted in urine, (metabolite); 98% bound to plasma proteins; terminal half-life 6-12 hr
Interactions/incompatibilities:
• Decreased action of cisapride: anticholinergics

• Increased peak plasma levels: cimetidine, H_2 antagonists
• Increased coagulation time: anticoagulants
NURSING CONSIDERATIONS
Assess:
• GI complaints: nausea, vomiting, anorexia, constipation
Administer:
• ½-1 hr before meals for better absorption
Evaluate:
• Therapeutic response: absence of heartburn
Teach patient/family:
• To avoid alcohol, other CNS depressants that will enhance sedating properties of this drug

cisplatin
(sis'pla-tin)
Platinol, Platinol-AQ
Func. class.: Antineoplastic alkylating agent
Chem. class.: Inorganic heavy metal

Action: Alkylates DNA, RNA; inhibits enzymes that allow synthesis of amino acids in proteins; activity is not cell cycle phase specific
Uses: Advanced bladder cancer, adjunctive in metastatic testicular cancer, adjunctive in metastatic ovarian cancer, head, neck cancer, esophagus, prostate, lung and cervical cancer, lymphoma
Dosage and routes:
Testicular cancer
• *Adult:* IV 20 mg/m² qd × 5 days, repeat q3wk for 3 cycles or more, depending on response
Bladder cancer
• *Adult:* IV 50-70 mg/m² q3-4wk
Ovarian cancer
• *Adult:* IV 100 mg/m² q4wk or 50 mg/m² q3wk with doxorubicin

therapy; mix with 2 L of NaCl and 37.5 g mannitol over 6 hr

Available forms: Inj IV 10, 50 mg

Side effects/adverse reactions:

EENT: Tinnitus, hearing loss, vestibular toxicity

HEMA: **Thrombocytopenia, leukopenia, pancytopenia**

CV: Cardiac abnormalities

GI: Severe nausea, vomiting, diarrhea, weight loss

GU: **Renal tubular damage,** renal insufficiency, impotence, sterility, amenorrhea, gynecomastia, hyperuremia

INTEG: Alopecia, dermatitis

CNS: **Convulsions,** peripheral neuropathy

RESP: **Fibrosis**

META: Hypomagnesemia, hypocalcemia, hypokalemia, hypophosphatemia

SYST: **Hypersensitivity reaction**

Contraindications: Radiation therapy within 1 mo, chemotherapy within 1 mo, thrombocytopenia, smallpox vaccination

Precautions: Pneumococcus vaccination, pregnancy (D)

Pharmacokinetics: Well absorbed orally, metabolized in liver, excreted in urine; half-life 2 hr

Interactions/incompatibilities:

• Increased nephrotoxicity: aminoglycosides

• Decreased effects of: phenytoin

• Incompatible with metoclopramide; considered incompatible in syringe or sol with all other drugs except mannitol

NURSING CONSIDERATIONS

Assess:

• CBC, differential, platelet count weekly; withhold drug if WBC is <4000 or platelet count is <75,000; notify physician of results

• Renal function studies: BUN, creatinine, serum uric acid, urine CrCl before, electrolytes during therapy

• I&O ratio; report fall in urine output of 30 ml/hr

• Monitor temperature q4h (may indicate beginning infection)

• Liver function tests before, during therapy (bilirubin, AST, ALT, LDH) as needed or monthly

• Bleeding: hematuria, guaiac, bruising or petechiae, mucosa or orifices q8h, obtain prescription for viscous lidocaine (Xylocaine)

• Dyspnea, rales, unproductive cough, chest pain, tachypnea

• Food preferences; list likes, dislikes

• Effects of alopecia on body image; discuss feelings about body changes

• Yellowing of skin, sclera; dark urine; clay-colored stools; itchy skin; abdominal pain; fever; diarrhea

• Edema in feet, joint pain, stomach pain, shaking

• Inflammation of mucosa, breaks in skin

Administer:

• IV after diluting 10 mg/10 ml or 50 mg/50 ml sterile H_2O for inj; withdraw prescribed dose, dilute ½ dose with 1000 ml D_5 O.2 NaCl or D_5 O.45 NaCl with 37.5 g mannitol; IV INF is given over 3-4 hr; use a 0.45 μm filter; total dose 2000 ml over 6-8 hr; check site for irritation; phlebitis; do not use equipment containing aluminum

• Hydrate patient with 1-2 L of fluids over 8-12 hr before treatment

• Epinephrine for hypersensitivity reaction

• Antiemetic 30-60 min before giving drug to prevent vomiting, and PRN

• Allopurinol or sodium bicarbon-

ate to maintain uric acid levels, alkalinization of urine
• Antibiotics for prophylaxis of infection
• Diuretic (furosemide 40 mg IV) or mannitol after infusion

Perform/provide:
• Strict medical asepsis, protective isolation if WBC levels are low
• Comprehensive oral hygiene
• Storage protected from light in refrigerator (dry powder)
• Deep breathing exercises with patient tid-qid; place in semi-Fowler's position
• Increase fluid intake to 2-3 L/day to prevent urate deposits, calculi formation, elimination of drug
• Diet low in purines: organ meats (kidney, liver), dried beans, peas to maintain alkaline urine

Evaluate:
• Therapeutic response: decreased tumor size, spread of malignancy

Teach patient/family:
• To report signs of infection: increased temperature, sore throat, flu symptoms
• To report signs of anemia: fatigue, headache, faintness, shortness of breath, irritability
• To report bleeding: avoid use of razors or commercial mouthwash
• To avoid use of aspirin or ibuprofen
• About protective isolation precautions
• To report any complaints or side effects to nurse or physician
• That impotence or amenorrhea can occur; reversible after discontinuing treatment
• To report any changes in breathing or coughing
• That hair may be lost during treatment; a wig or hairpiece may make patient feel better; new hair may be different in color, texture

cladribine (CdA)

(clay-dry-bine)
Leustatin
Func. class.: Antineoplastic antibiotic
Chem. class.: Purine nucleoside analog

Action: Phosphylated while passively crossing the cell membrane, causing cell death by not properly repairing single-strand DNA

Uses: Treatment of active hairy cell leukemia; may be useful in chronic lymphocytic leukemia, non-Hodgkin's lymphomas, acute myeloid leukemia, autoimmune hemolytic anemia

Dosage and routes:
Single daily dose
• *Adult:* IV 1 day × 0.09 mg/kg diluted with 0.9% NaCl 500 ml; give over 24 hr × 7 days
Seven-day infusion
• *Adult:* IV 7 days × 0.09 mg/kg diluted with 0.9% NaCl qs to 100 ml; pass through 0.22 microfilter
Available forms: Sol 1 mg/ml

Side effects/adverse reactions:
CNS: Headache, dizziness, insomnia
CV: Edema, tachycardia
GI: Nausea, vomiting, anorexia, diarrhea, constipation, abdominal pain
HEMA: **Neutropenia, anemia, thrombocytopenia, bone marrow hypocellularity,** purpura, epistaxis, petechia
INTEG: Rash, inj site reactions pruritus
MS: Myalgia, arthralgia
RESP: Cough, upper respiratory infection, dyspnea, shortness of breath, abnormal chest sounds, pneumonia

---

italics = common side effects   ***bold italic*** = life threatening reactions

SYST: Fever, infection, fatigue, pain, allergic reaction, chills, ***death, sepsis***

Contraindications: Hypersensitivity

Precautions: Renal disease, pregnancy (D), lactation, children, bone marrow depression, hepatic disease, neurologic disease

Pharmacokinetics:

IV: Terminal half-life 5.4 hr

NURSING CONSIDERATIONS
Assess:

• CBC, differential, platelet count weekly; withhold drug if WBC <4000/mm³ or platelet count <75,000/mm³; notify physician

• Renal function studies: BUN, serum uric acid, urine CrCl, electrolytes before, during therapy

• I&O ratio; report urine output <30 ml/hr

• Monitor temperature q4h; fever may indicate beginning infection

• Liver function tests before, during therapy: bilirubin, AST, ALT, alk phosphatase, as needed or monthly

• Local irritation, pain, burning at injection site

• Symptoms indicating severe allergic reaction: rash, pruritus, urticaria, purpuric skin lesions, itching, flushing

• GI symptoms: frequency of stools, cramping

Administer:

• Antiemetic 30-60 min before giving drug to prevent vomiting

• Use gloves and gown to mix IV sol

• Use bacteriostatic (0.9% NaCl, 0.9% benzyl alcohol preserved) to prepare 7-day inf; pass both cladribine and diluent through sterile 0.22-micron hydrophilic syringe filter as each sol is introduced into inf reservoir; add dose of cladribine to inf reservoir using filter, then bacteriostatic 0.9% NaCl to bring sol total to 100 ml; after preparation, clamp line, disconnect filter, and discard; aspirate air bubbles (reservoir) using syringe and dry filter or sterile vat filter assembly; reclamp line, discard filter and syringe; infuse continuously × 7 days

• Add dose for single daily dose to inf bag (500 ml 0.9% NaCl); infuse continuously over 24 hr; repeat daily dose × 7 days

• Do not admix with other IV drugs or sol

Perform/provide:

• Hydrocortisone, sodium thiosulfate to infiltration area, ice compress after stopping inf

• Strict hand-washing technique, gloves, protective covering

• Liquid diet: carbonated beverages; gelatin may be added if patient is not nauseated or vomiting

• Storage in refrigerator; protect from light; reconstituted or diluted sol may be stored at room temperature no longer than 8 hr; discard single-use vials of unused sol

Evaluate:

• Therapeutic response: decrease in symptoms of hairy cell leukemia

Teach patient/family:

• To report any complaints, side effects to nurse or physician

• To avoid crowds and sources of infection when granulocyte count is low

---

clarithromycin
(clare-i-thro-mye'sin)
Biaxin

Func. class.: Antibacterial
Chem. class.: Macrolide antibiotic

Action: Binds to 50S ribosomal

subunits of susceptible bacteria and suppresses protein synthesis

Uses: Mild to moderate infections of the upper respiratory tract, lower respiratory tract, uncomplicated skin and skin structure infections caused by *S. pneumoniae, M. pneumoniae, C. diphtheriae, B. pertussis, L. monocytogenes, H. influenzae, S. pyogenes, S. aureus*

Dosage and routes:
• *Adult:* PO 250-500 mg bid for 7-14 days

Available forms: Tabs 250, 500 mg

Side effects/adverse reactions:
INTEG: Rash, urticaria, pruritus
GI: Nausea, vomiting, diarrhea, **hepatotoxicity**, abdominal pain, stomatitis, heartburn, anorexia, abnormal taste
GU: Vaginitis, moniliasis
MISC: Headache

Contraindications: Hypersensitivity

Precautions: Pregnancy (C), lactation, hepatic, renal disease, elderly

Pharmacokinetics: Peak 2 hr, duration 12 hr, half-life 4-6 hr; metabolized by the liver; excreted in bile, feces

Interactions/incompatibilities:
• Arrhythmias: terfenadine, astemizole
• Increased effects of oral anticoagulants, digoxin, theophylline, methylprednisolone, cyclosporine, bromocriptine, disopyramide
• Decreased action: clindamycin
• Toxicity: carbamazepine
• Increased or decreased action: penicillins

Lab test interferences:
False increase: 17-OHCS/17-KS, AST, ALT
Decrease: Folate assay

NURSING CONSIDERATIONS
Assess:
• I&O ratio; report hematuria, oliguria in renal disease
• Liver studies: AST, ALT
• Renal studies: urinalysis, protein, blood
• C&S before drug therapy; drug may be taken as soon as culture is taken; C&S may be repeated after treatment
• Bowel pattern before, during treatment
• Skin eruptions, itching
• Respiratory status: rate, character, wheezing, tightness in chest; discontinue drug if these occur
• Allergies before treatment, reaction of each medication; place allergies on chart, notify all people giving drugs

Administer:
• Adequate intake of fluids (2 L) during diarrhea episodes

Perform/provide:
• Storage at room temperature

Evaluate:
• Therapeutic response: C&S negative for infection

Teach patient/family:
• To take with a full glass of water; may give with food if GI symptoms occur
• Do not take with fruit juices
• To report sore throat, fever, fatigue; may indicate superimposed infection
• To notify nurse of diarrhea stools, dark urine, pale stools, yellow discoloration of eyes or skin, severe abdominal pain
• To take at evenly spaced intervals; complete dosage regimen

Treatment of overdose: Withdraw drug, maintain airway, administer epinephrine, aminophylline, O$_2$, IV corticosteroids

italics = common side effects   ***bold italic*** = life threatening reactions

clemastine fumarate

(klem'as-teen)

Tavist, Tavist-1

Func. class.: Antihistamine

Chem. class.: Ethanolamine derivative, H_1-receptor antagonist

Action: Acts on blood vessels, GI, respiratory system by competing with histamine for H_1-receptor site; decreases allergic response by blocking histamine

Uses: Allergy symptoms, rhinitis, angioedema, urticaria

Dosage and routes:

• *Adult and child >12 yr:* PO 1.34-2.68 mg bid-tid, not to exceed 8.04 mg/day

Available forms: Tabs 1.34, 2.68 mg; syr 0.67 mg/ml

Side effects/adverse reactions:

CNS: Dizziness, drowsiness, poor coordination, fatigue, anxiety, euphoria, confusion, paresthesia, neuritis

CV: Hypotension, palpitations, tachycardia

RESP: Increased thick secretions, wheezing, chest tightness

HEMA: Thrombocytopenia, agranulocytosis, hemolytic anemia

GI: Constipation, dry mouth, nausea, vomiting, anorexia, diarrhea

INTEG: Rash, urticaria, photosensitivity

GU: Retention, dysuria, frequency

EENT: Blurred vision, dilated pupils, tinnitus, nasal stuffiness, dry nose, throat, mouth

Contraindications: Hypersensitivity to H_1-receptor antagonists, acute asthma attack, lower respiratory tract disease

Precautions: Increased intraocular pressure, renal disease, cardiac disease, hypertension, bronchial asthma, seizure disorder, stenosed peptic ulcers, hyperthyroidism, prostatic hypertrophy, bladder neck obstruction, pregnancy (B), elderly

Pharmacokinetics:

PO: Peak 5-7 hr, duration 10-12 hr or more; metabolized in liver, excreted by kidneys

Interactions/incompatibilities:

• Increased CNS depression: barbiturates, narcotics, hypnotics, tricyclic antidepressants, alcohol

• Decreased effect of: oral anticoagulants, heparin

• Increased effect of clemastine: MAOIs

Lab test interferences:

False negative: Skin allergy tests

NURSING CONSIDERATIONS

Assess:

• I&O ratio; be alert for urinary retention, frequency, dysuria; drug should be discontinued if these occur

• CBC during long-term therapy

• Blood dyscrasias: thrombocytopenia, agranulocytosis (rare)

• Respiratory status: rate, rhythm, increase in bronchial secretions, wheezing, chest tightness

• Cardiac status: palpitations, increased pulse, hypotension

Administer:

• With meals if GI symptoms occur; absorption may slightly decrease

Perform/provide:

• Hard candy, gum, frequent rinsing of mouth for dryness

• Storage in tight container at room temperature

Evaluate:

• Therapeutic response: absence of running or congested nose or rashes

Teach patient/family:

• All aspects of drug use; to notify

physician if confusion, sedation, hypotension occurs
• To avoid driving or other hazardous activity if drowsiness occurs
• To avoid concurrent use of alcohol or other CNS depressants
• That drug decreases anticoagulant (oral) effect
• To change position slowly, as drug may cause dizziness, hypotension (elderly)

Treatment of overdose: Administer ipecac syrup or lavage, diazepam, vasopressors, barbiturates (short-acting)

---

clidinium bromide

(kli′di-nee-um)
Quarzan
Func. class.: GI anticholinergic
Chem. class.: Synthetic quaternary ammonium antimuscarinic

Action: Inhibits muscarinic actions of acetylcholine at postganglionic parasympathetic neuroeffector sites
Uses: Treatment of peptic ulcer disease in combination with other drugs

Dosage and routes:
• *Adult:* PO 2.5-5 mg tid-qid ac, hs
• *Elderly:* PO 2.5 mg tid ac
Available forms: Caps 2.5, 5 mg

Side effects/adverse reactions:
CNS: Confusion, stimulation in elderly, headache, insomnia, dizziness, drowsiness, anxiety, weakness, hallucination
*GI: Dry mouth, constipation, **paralytic ileus,*** heartburn, nausea, vomiting, dysphagia, absence of taste
GU: Hesitancy, retention, impotence
CV: Palpitations, tachycardia
EENT: Blurred vision, photophobia, mydriasis, cycloplegia, increased ocular tension
INTEG: Urticaria, rash, pruritus, anhidrosis, fever, allergic reactions
Contraindications: Hypersensitivity to anticholinergics, narrow-angle glaucoma, GI obstruction, myasthenia gravis, paralytic ileus, GI atony, toxic megacolon
Precautions: Hyperthyroidism, coronary artery disease, dysrhythmias, CHF, ulcerative colitis, hypertension, hiatal hernia, hepatic disease, renal disease, pregnancy (C), urinary retention, prostatic hypertrophy, elderly

Pharmacokinetics:
PO: Onset 1 hr, duration 3 hr; ionized, excreted in urine

Interactions/incompatibilities:
• Increased anticholinergic effect: amantadine, tricyclic antidepressants, MAOIs
• Decreased effect of: phenothiazines, levodopa, ketoconazole

NURSING CONSIDERATIONS
Assess:
• VS, cardiac status: checking for dysrhythmias, increased rate, palpitations
• I&O ratio; check for urinary retention or hesitancy, especially elderly
• GI complaints: pain, bleeding (frank or occult), nausea, vomiting, anorexia

Administer:
• ½-1 hr ac for better absorption
• Decreased dose to elderly patients, since their metabolism may be slowed
• Gum, hard candy, frequent rinsing of mouth for dryness of oral cavity

Perform/provide:
• Storage in tight container protected from light
• Increased fluids, bulk, exercise to

---

italics = common side effects   ***bold italic*** = life threatening reactions

patient's life-style to decrease constipation

Evaluate:

• Therapeutic response: absence of epigastric pain, bleeding, nausea, vomiting

Teach patient/family:

• To avoid driving or other hazardous activities until stabilized on medication

• To avoid alcohol or other CNS depressants; will enhance sedating properties of this drug

• To avoid hot environments; stroke may occur, drug suppresses perspiration

• To use sunglasses when outside to prevent photophobia, may cause blurred vision

• To drink plenty of fluids

• To report dysphagia

---

clindamycin HCl/ clinda- mycin palmitate HCl/ clindamycin phosphate

(klin-da-mye'sin)

Cleocin HCl, Clindamycin HCl, Dalacin C*/Cleocin Pediatric/ Cleocin Phosphate, Clindamycin Phosphate

Func. class.: Antibacterial macrolide

Chem. class.: Lincomycin derivative

Action: Binds to 50S subunit of bacterial ribosomes, suppresses protein synthesis

Uses: Infections caused by staphylococci, streptococci, pneumococci, *Rickettsia, Fusobacterium, Actinomyces, Peptococcus, Clostridium*

Dosage and routes:

• *Adults:* PO 150-450 mg q6h; IM/ IV 300 mg q6-12h, not to exceed 4800 mg/day

• *Child >1 mo:* PO 8-25 mg/kg/ day in divided doses q6-8h; IM/IV 15-40 mg/kg/day in divided doses q6-8h 3-4 equal doses

• *PID:* Adult IV 600 mg qid plus gentamicin

Available forms: Inj 150-300 mg/ ml; caps 75, 150-300 mg; oral sol 75 mg/ml

Side effects/adverse reactions:

HEMA: **Leukopenia, eosinophilia, agranulocytosis, thrombocytopenia, polyarthritis**

GI: Nausea, vomiting, abdominal pain, diarrhea, **pseudomembranous colitis,** anorexia, weight loss

GU: Increased AST, ALT, bilirubin, alk phosphatase, jaundice, *vaginitis,* urinary frequency

EENT: Rash, urticaria, pruritus, erythema, pain, abscess at injection site

Contraindications: Hypersensitivity to this drug or lincomycin, ulcerative colitis/enteritis, infants <1 mo

Precautions: Renal disease, liver disease, GI disease, elderly, pregnancy (B), lactation, tartrazine sensitivity

Pharmacokinetics:

PO: Peak 45 min, duration 6 hr

IM: Peak 3 hr, duration 8-12 hr

Half-life 2½ hr; metabolized in liver; excreted in urine, bile, feces as active/inactive metabolites; crosses placenta; excreted in breast milk

Interactions/incompatibilities:

• Increased neuromuscular blockage: nondepolarizing muscle relaxants

• Decreased action of: chloramphenicol, erythromycin

• Incompatible with aminophylline, ampicillin, all barbiturates,

---

calcium gluconate, magnesium SO₄, phenytoin, ranitidine, tobramycin, Ringer's sol

Lab test interferences:
Increase: Alk phosphatase, bilirubin, CPK, AST, ALT

NURSING CONSIDERATIONS
Assess:
• Any patient with compromised renal system; drug is excreted slowly in poor renal system function; toxicity may occur rapidly
• Liver studies: AST, ALT
• Blood studies: WBC, RBC, Hct, Hgb, platelets, serum iron, reticulocytes; drug should be discontinued if bone marrow depression occurs
• Renal studies: urinalysis, protein, blood, BUN, creatinine
• C&S before drug therapy; drug may be taken as soon as culture is taken
• Drug level in impaired hepatic, renal systems
• B/P, pulse in patient receiving drug parenterally
• Bowel pattern before, during treatment
• Skin eruptions, itching, dermatitis after administration
• Respiratory status: rate, character, wheezing, tightness in chest
• Allergies before treatment, reaction of each medication; place allergies on chart, Kardex in bright red letters; notify all people giving drugs

Administer:
• IV by infusion only; do not administer bolus dose; dilute 300 mg or less/50 ml or more of D₅W, NS; may be further diluted in greater amounts of D₅W, NS and given as a cont inf in acute pelvic inflammatory disease (PID); give first dose 10 mg/min over ½ hr, then 0.75 mg/min; increased rates may

be used to keep serum blood levels higher; run over >10 min; no more than 1200 mg in a single 1-hr inf
• IM deep injection; rotate sites
• Orally with at least 8 oz water

Perform/provide:
• Storage at room temperature (capsules) and up to 2 wk (reconstituted solution)
• Adrenalin, suction, tracheostomy set, endotracheal intubation equipment on unit
• Adequate intake of fluids (2 L) during diarrhea episodes

Evaluate:
• Therapeutic response: decreased temperature, negative C&S

Teach patient/family:
• To take oral drug with full glass of water; may give with food if GI symptoms occur; antiperistaltic drugs may worsen diarrhea
• Aspects of drug therapy: need to complete entire course of medication to ensure organism death (10-14 days); culture may be taken after completed medication course
• To report sore throat, fever, fatigue; may indicate superimposed infection
• That drug must be taken in equal intervals around clock to maintain blood levels
• To notify nurse of diarrhea

Treatment of hypersensitivity: Withdraw drug; maintain airway; administer epinephrine, aminophylline, O₂, IV corticosteroids

---

clioquinol (iodochlorhydroxyquin)
(klee-oh-kwee'nole)
Vioform
Func. class.: Local antiinfective
Chem. class.: Halogenated hydroxyquinoline

Action: Increases cell membrane

italics = common side effects   ***bold italic*** = life threatening reactions

permeability in susceptible organisms by binding sterols; decreases potassium, sodium, and nutrients in cell

Uses: Cutaneous infections: athlete's foot, eczema, and other fungal infections

Dosage and routes:

TOP: apply to affected area bid or tid ×7 days only

Available forms: cream, oint 3%

Side effects/adverse reactions:

INTEG: Rash, urticaria, stinging, burning, dry skin, pruritus, contact dermatitis, erythema, redness, staining of hair and skin

Contraindications: Hypersensitivity to iodine, chloroxine

Precautions: Pregnancy (C), varicella, viral skin conditions, deep or puncture wounds, serious burns

Pharmacokinetics: Some absorbed through the skin, excreted in urine (conjugated form), the rest excreted slowly

Lab test interference:

Interference: Thyroid function tests

NURSING CONSIDERATIONS

Assess:

• Allergic reaction: burning, stinging, swelling, redness

Administer:

• Enough medication to cover lesions completely

• After cleansing with soap and water before each application; dry well

Perform/provide:

• Storage at room temperature in dry place

Evaluate:

• Therapeutic response: decrease in size, number of lesions

Teach patient/family:

• To avoid use of OTC creams, ointments, lotions unless directed by physician

• To use medical asepsis (hand washing) before, after each application to prevent further infection

• Not to cover with occlusive dressing

• To continue even if condition improves

• That drug may stain clothing, skin, hair

---

clobetasol propionate
(klo-bet'-a-sol)
Temovate
Func. class.: Topical corticosteroid
Chem. class.: Synthetic fluorinated agent, group I potency

Action: Antipruritic, antiinflammatory

Uses: Psoriasis, eczema, contact dermatitis, pruritus; usually reserved for severe dermatoses that have not responded to less potent formulation

Dosage and routes:

• *Adult and child:* Apply to affected area bid

Available forms: Oint 0.05%; cream 0.05%

Side effects/adverse reactions:

INTEG: Burning, dryness, itching, irritation, acne, folliculitis, hypertrichosis, perioral dermatitis, hypopigmentation, atrophy, striae, miliaria, allergic contact dermatitis, secondary infection

Contraindications: Hypersensitivity to corticosteroids, fungal infections

Precautions: Pregnancy (C), lactation, viral infections, bacterial infections

NURSING CONSIDERATIONS

Assess:

• Temperature; if fever develops, drug should be discontinued

• For systemic absorption: increased temperature, inflammation, irritation

Administer:
• Only to affected areas; do not get in eyes
• Leaving uncovered or lightly covered; occlusive dressing is not recommended; systemic absorption may occur
• Only to dermatoses; do not use on weeping, denuded, or infected area

Perform/provide:
• Cleansing before application of drug
• Treatment for a few days after area has cleared
• Storage at room temperature

Evaluate:
• Therapeutic response: absence of severe itching, patches on skin, flaking

Teach patient/family:
• To avoid sunlight on affected area; burns may occur
• To limit treatment to 14 days using <50 g/wk

---

clocortolone pivalate
(klo-kort'-o-lone)
Cloderm
Func. class.: Topical corticosteroid
Chem. class.: Synthetic fluorinated agent, group IV potency

Action: Antipruritic, antiinflammatory
Uses: Psoriasis, eczema, contact dermatitis, pruritus
Dosage and routes:
• *Adult and child:* Apply to affected area tid or qid
Available forms: Cream 0.1%
Side effects/adverse reactions:
INTEG: Burning, dryness, itching, irritation, acne, folliculitis, hypertrichosis, perioral dermatitis, hy-

popigmentation, atrophy, striae, miliaria, allergic contact dermatitis, secondary infection

Contraindications: Hypersensitivity to corticosteroids, fungal infections
Precautions: Pregnancy (C), lactation, viral infections, bacterial infections

NURSING CONSIDERATIONS
Assess:
• Temperature; if fever develops, drug should be discontinued
• For systemic absorption: increased temperature, inflammation, irritation

Administer:
• Only to affected areas; do not get in eyes
• Medication, then cover with occlusive dressing (only if prescribed), seal to normal skin, change q12h; systemic absorption may occur
• Only to dermatoses; do not use on weeping, denuded, or infected area

Perform/provide:
• Cleansing before application of drug
• Treatment for a few days after area has cleared
• Storage at room temperature

Evaluate:
• Therapeutic response: absence of severe itching, patches on skin, flaking

Teach patient/family:
• To avoid sunlight on affected area; burns may occur

---

clofazimine
(kloe-faz'-i-meen)
Lamprene
Func. class.: Leprostatic

Action: Inhibits mycobacterial growth, binds to mycobacterial

---

DNA; exerts antiinflammatory properties in controlling leprosy reactions

Uses: Lepromatous leprosy, dapsone-resistant leprosy, lepromatous leprosy complicated by erythema nodosum leprosum

Dosage and routes:

Erythema nodosum leprosum
• *Adult:* PO: 100-200 mg qd × 3 mo, then taper dosage to 100 mg when disease is controlled; do not exceed 200 mg/day

Dapsone-resistant leprosy
• *Adult:* PO: 100 mg/day in combination with at least one other antileprosy drug × 3 yr, then 100 mg qd clofazimine (only)

Available forms: Caps 50, 100 mg

Side effects/adverse reactions:

GI: Diarrhea, nausea, vomiting, abdominal pain, intolerance, GI bleeding, obstruction, anorexia, constipation, *hepatitis,* jaundice

EENT: Pigmentation of cornea, conjunctive, drying, burning, itching, irritation

INTEG: Pink or brown discoloration, dryness, pruritus, rash, photosensitivity, acne, monilial cheilosis

CNS: Dizziness, headache, fatigue, drowsiness

MISC: Discolored urine, feces, sputum, sweat

Precautions: Pregnancy (C), lactation, children, abdominal pain, diarrhea, depression

Pharmacokinetics: Deposited in fatty tissue, reticuloendothelial system; half-life 70 days; small amount excreted in feces, sputum, sweat

Lab test interferences:

Increase: Albumin, bilirubin, AST, eosinophilia, hypokalemia

NURSING CONSIDERATIONS
Assess:

• Liver studies qwk: ALT, AST, bilirubin
• Renal studies: BUN, creatinine, I&O, sp gr, urinalysis before; qmo
• Blood level of drug
• Mental status often: affect, mood, behavioral changes; psychosis may occur
• Hepatic status: decreased appetite, jaundice, dark urine, fatigue

Administer:

• With meals to decrease GI symptoms
• Antiemetic if vomiting occurs
• After C&S is completed; qmo to detect resistance

Perform/provide:

• Infants to be kept with mother infected with leprosy; breastfeeding during drug therapy is encouraged

Evaluate:

• Therapeutic response: decreased symptoms of infection

Teach patient/family:

• That therapeutic effects may occur after 3-6 mo of drug therapy
• That compliance with dosage schedule, length is necessary
• That scheduled appointments must be kept or relapse may occur
• That drug must be taken with meals
• Skin, sweat, sputum, urine, feces discoloration, although reversible, may take several months or years to disappear

---

clofibrate

(kloe-fye′brate)

Atromid-S, Claripen,* Claripex*, Clofibrate

Func. class.: Antilipemic
Chem. class.: Aryloxisobutyric acid derivative

Action: Inhibits biosynthesis of VLDL, LDL, which are responsible for triglyceride development, mobilizes triglycerides from tissue, increases excretion of neutral sterols

Uses: Hyperlipidemia; xanthoma tuberosum; types III, IV, V hyperlipidemia

Dosage and routes:
• *Adult:* PO 2 g/day in 4 divided doses
Available forms: Caps 500 mg

Side effects/adverse reactions:
GI: Nausea, vomiting, dyspepsia, increased liver enzymes, stomatitis, flatulence, hepatomegaly, gastritis, increased cholelithiasis, weight gain
INTEG: Rash, urticaria, pruritus, dry hair and skin, alopecia
*HEMA: **Leukopenia,** anemia, **eosinophilia,** bleeding*
CNS: Fatigue, weakness, drowsiness, dizziness
GU: Decreased libido, impotence, dysuria, proteinuria, oliguria, *hematuria*
MS: Myalgias, arthralgias
CV: Angina, dysrhythmias, thrombophlebitis, ***pulmonary emboli***
MISC: Polyphagia, weight gain

Contraindications: Severe hepatic disease, severe renal disease, primary biliary cirrhosis
Precautions: Peptic ulcer, pregnancy (C), lactation
Pharmacokinetics:
PO: Peak 2-6 hr, plasma protein binding >90%; half-life 6-25 hr, excreted in urine, metabolized in liver

Interactions/incompatibilities:
• Increased effects of: sulfonylureas, insulin
• Increased toxicity of clofibrate: probenecid
• Increased anticoagulant effects: oral anticoagulants

• Decreased effects of clofibrate: rifampin
Lab test interferences:
Increase: Liver function studies, CPK, BSP, thymol turbidity

NURSING CONSIDERATIONS
Assess:
• Renal and hepatic levels if patient is on long-term therapy
• Bowel pattern daily; increase bulk, water in diet if constipation develops
Administer:
• Drug with meals if GI symptoms occur
Evaluate:
• Therapeutic response: decreased triglycerides, diarrhea, pruritus (excess bile acids)
Teach patient/family:
• That patient compliance is needed since toxicity may result if doses are missed
• That risk factors should be decreased: high-fat diet, smoking, alcohol consumption, absence of exercise
• That birth control should be practiced while on this drug
• To report GU symptoms: decreased libido, impotence, dysuria, proteinuria, oliguria, hematuria

clomiphene citrate
(kloe'mi-feen)
Clomid, Clomiphene Citrate, Milophene, Serophene
Func. class.: Ovulation stimulant
Chem. class.: Nonsteroidal antiestrogenic

Action: Increases LH, FSH release from the pituitary, which increase maturation of ovarian follicle, ovulation, development of corpus luteum

Uses: Female infertility (ovulatory failure)

Dosage and routes:
• *Adult:* PO 50-100 mg qd × 5 days or 50-100 mg qd beginning on day 5 of cycle; may be repeated until conception occurs or 3 cycles of therapy have been completed

Available forms: Tabs 50 mg

Side effects/adverse reactions:
CV: Vasomotor flushing, phlebitis, deep-vein thrombosis

EENT: Blurred vision, diplopia, photophobia

CNS: Headache, depression, restlessness, anxiety, nervousness, fatigue, insomnia, dizziness, flushing

GI: Nausea, vomiting, constipation, abdominal pain, bloating

INTEG: Rash, dermatitis, urticaria, alopecia

GU: Polyuria, frequency, birth defects, spontaneous abortions, multiple ovulation, breast pain, oliguria, abnormal uterine bleeding

Contraindications: Hypersensitivity, pregnancy (X), hepatic disease, undiagnosed vaginal bleeding

Precautions: Hypertension, depression, convulsions, diabetes mellitus

Pharmacokinetics: Metabolized in liver, excreted in feces

Lab test interferences:
Increase: FSH/LH, BSP, thyroxine, TBG

NURSING CONSIDERATIONS
Administer:
• After discontinuing estrogen therapy
• At same time qd to maintain drug level

Evaluate:
• Therapeutic response: fertility

Teach patient/family:
• That multiple births are common after drug is taken

• To notify physician if low abdominal pain occurs; may indicate ovarian cyst, cyst rupture
• If dose is missed, double at next time; if more than one dose is missed, call physician
• That response usually occurs 4-10 days after last day of treatment
• Method for taking, recording basal body temperature to determine whether ovulation has occurred
• If ovulation can be determined (there is a slight decrease in temperature, then a sharp increase for ovulation), to attempt coitus 3 days before and qod until after ovulation
• If pregnancy is suspected, to notify physician immediately

---

clomipramine
(klom-ip′ra-meen)
Anafranil
Func. class.: Tricyclic antidepressant
Chem. class.: Tertiary amine

Action: Not known. Potent inhibitor of serotonin uptake; also increases dopamine metabolism

Uses: Depression, dysphoria, phobias, anxiety, agoraphobia, obsessive-compulsive disorder

Dosage and routes:
Obsessive-compulsive disorder
• *Adult:* PO 25 mg hs and increase gradually over 4 wk to a dose of 75-300 mg/day in divided doses
• *Child (10-18 yr):* PO 25-50 mg/day gradually increased; not to exceed 200 mg/day

Depression
• *Adult:* PO 50-150 mg/day in a single or divided dose

Anxiety/agoraphobia
• *Adult:* PO 25-75 mg/day

Available forms: Caps 25, 50, 75 mg

Side effects/adverse reactions:

HEMA: **Agranulocytosis, neutropenia, pancytopenia**

CV: Hypotension, tachycardia, **cardiac arrest**

CNS: Dizziness, tremors, mania, seizures, aggressiveness

ENDO: Galactorrhea, hyperprolactinemia

META: Hyponatremia

GI: Constipation, dry mouth, nausea, dyspepsia

GU: Delayed ejaculation, anorgasmy, retention

INTEG: Diaphoresis

Contraindications: Hypersensitivity

Precautions: Seizures, suicidal patients, elderly, pregnancy (C)

Pharmacokinetics: Extensively bound to tissue and plasma proteins; demethylated in liver; active metabolites excreted in urine; half-life: 21 hr parent compound, 36 hr metabolite

Interactions/incompatibilities:

• Hypotensive antagonism: bethanidine

• Toxicity: phenothiazines, cimetidine

• Ethanol reaction: disulfiram, guanadrel increased or decreased effects

• Increased or decreased effects of clomipramine: estrogens

• Delirium: ethchlorvynol

• Hypertensive crisis, convulsions, hypertensive episode: MAOIs

• Decreased seizure threshold: phenytoin, phenobarbital

Lab test interferences:

Increase: Prolactin, TBG

Decrease: Serum thryoid hormone

NURSING CONSIDERATIONS

Assess:

• B/P (lying, standing), pulse q4h; if systolic B/P drops 20 mm Hg, withhold drug, notify physician;

take vital signs q4h in patients with cardiovascular disease

• Blood studies: CBC, leukocytes, differential, cardiac enzymes if patient is receiving long-term therapy

• Hepatic studies: AST, ALT, bilirubin

• Mental status: mood, sensorium, affect, suicidal tendencies; increase in psychiatric symptoms: depression, panic

• Urinary retention, constipation; constipation is more likely to occur in children

• Withdrawal symptoms: headache, nausea, vomiting, muscle pain, weakness; do not usually occur unless drug is discontinued abruptly

• Alcohol consumption; if alcohol is consumed, withhold dose until morning

Administer:

• Increased fluids, bulk in diet if constipation occurs, especially elderly

• With food or milk for GI symptoms

• Gum, hard candy, or frequent sips of water for dry mouth

Perform/provide:

• Storage in tight container at room temperature; do not freeze

• Assistance with ambulation during beginning therapy, since drowsiness/dizziness occurs

• Safety measures, including side rails, primarily in elderly

• Checking to see PO medication swallowed

Evaluate:

• Therapeutic response: decreased anxiety, depression

Teach patient/family:

• That the effects may take 2-3 wk

• To use caution in driving or other activities requiring alertness be-

cause of drowsiness, dizziness, blurred vision
• To avoid alcohol ingestion, other CNS depressants
• Not to discontinue medication quickly after long-term use; may cause nausea, headache, malaise
Treatment of overdose: ECG monitoring; induce emesis; lavage, activated charcoal; administer anticonvulsant

---

clonazepam

(kloe-na'zi-pam)
Klonopin
Func. class.: Anticonvulsant
Chem. class.: Benzodiazepine derivative

Controlled Substance Schedule IV
Action: Inhibits spike, wave formation in absence seizures (petit mal), decreases amplitude, frequency, duration, spread of discharge in minor motor seizures
Uses: Absence, atypical absence, akinetic, myoclonic seizures
Dosage and routes:
• *Adult:* PO Not to exceed 1.5 mg/day in 3 divided doses; may be increased 0.5-1 mg q3 days until desired response, not to exceed 20 mg/day
• *Child <10 yr or 30 kg:* PO 0.01-0.03 mg/kg/day in divided doses q8h, not to exceed 0.05 mg/kg/day; may be increased 0.25-0.5 mg q3 days until desired response, not to exceed 0.1-0.2 mg/kg/day
Available forms: Tabs 0.5, 1, 2 mg
Side effects/adverse reactions:
HEMA: Thrombocytopenia, leukocytosis, eosinophilia
CNS: Drowsiness, dizziness, confusion, behavioral changes, trem-

ors, insomnia, headache, suicidal tendencies, slurred speech
GI: Nausea, constipation, polyphagia, anorexia, xerostomia, diarrhea, gastritis, sore gums
INTEG: Rash, alopecia, hirsutism
EENT: Increased salivation, nystagmus, diplopia, abnormal eye movements
*RESP: **Respiratory depression,** dyspnea, congestion
CV: Palpitations, bradycardia
GU: Dysuria, enuresis, nocturia, retention
Contraindications: Hypersensitivity to benzodiazepines, acute narrow-angle glaucoma
Precautions: Open-angle glaucoma, chronic respiratory disease, pregnancy (C), renal, hepatic disease, elderly
Pharmacokinetics:
PO: Peak 1-2 hr; metabolized by liver; excreted in urine; half-life 18-50 hr
Interactions/incompatibilities:
• Increased CNS depression: alcohol, barbiturates, narcotics, antidepressants, other anticonvulsants, general anesthetics, hypnotics, sedatives
• Decreased effect of carbamazepine
• Seizures: valproic acid
Lab test interferences:
Increase: AST, alk phosphatase
NURSING CONSIDERATIONS
Assess:
• Renal studies: urinalysis, BUN, urine creatinine
• Blood studies: RBC, Hct, Hgb, reticulocyte counts qwk for 4 wk then qmo
• Hepatic studies: ALT, AST, bilirubin, creatinine
• Drug levels during initial treatment
• Signs of physical withdrawal if

---

*Available in Canada only

medication suddenly discontinued
• Mental status: mood, sensorium, affect, oversedation, behavioral changes; if mental status changes, notify physician
• Eye problems: need for ophthalmic examinations before, during, after treatment (slit lamp, fundoscopy, tonometry)
• Allergic reaction: red raised rash; if this occurs, drug should be discontinued
• Blood dyscrasias: fever, sore throat, bruising, rash, jaundice
• Toxicity: bone marrow depression, nausea, vomiting, ataxia, diplopia, cardiovascular collapse

Administer:
• With food, milk to decrease GI symptoms

Perform/provide:
• Storage at room temperature
• Hard candy, frequent rinsing of mouth, gum for dry mouth
• Assistance with ambulation during early part of treatment; dizziness occurs, especially elderly

Evaluate:
• Therapeutic response: decreased seizure activity, document on patient's chart

Teach patient/family:
• To carry ID card or Medic Alert bracelet stating patient's name, drugs taken, condition, physician's name, phone number
• To avoid driving, other activities that require alertness
• To avoid alcohol ingestion or CNS depressants; increased sedation may occur
• Not to discontinue medication quickly after long-term use; taper off over several weeks

Treatment of overdose: Lavage, activated charcoal, monitor electrolytes, VS, administer vasopressors

italics = common side effects

clonidine HCl
(klon'i-deen)
Catapres, Clonidine HCl, Dixarit*

Func. class.: Antihypertensive
Chem. class.: Central α-adrenergic agonist

Action: Inhibits sympathetic vasomotor center in CNS, which reduces impulses in sympathetic nervous system; blood pressure, pulse rate, cardiac output decrease

Uses: Mild to moderate hypertension, used alone or in combination

Dosage and routes:
Hypertension
• *Adult:* PO/TRANS 0.1 mg bid, then increase by 0.1 mg/day or 0.2 mg/day until desired response; range 0.2-0.8 mg/day in divided doses

Available forms: Tabs 0.1, 0.2, 0.3 mg; trans sys 2.5, 5, 7.5 mg delivering 0.1, 0.2, 0.3 mg/24 hr, respectively

Side effects/adverse reactions:
CNS: Drowsiness, sedation, headache, fatigue, nightmares, insomnia, mental changes, anxiety, depression, hallucinations, delirium
*CV: Orthostatic hypotension, palpitations, **CHF;*** ECG abnormalities
EENT: Taste change, parotid pain
ENDO: Hyperglycemia
GI: Nausea, vomiting, malaise, constipation, dry mouth
GU: Impotence, dysuria, *nocturia,* gynecomastia
INTEG: Rash, alopecia, facial pallor, pruritus, hives, edema, burning papules, excoriation (transdermal patches)
MS: Muscle, joint pain; leg cramps

bold italic = life threatening reactions

Contraindications: Hypersensitivity

Precautions: MI (recent), diabetes mellitus, chronic renal failure, Raynaud's disease, thyroid disease, depression, COPD, child <12 (patches), asthma, pregnancy (C), lactation, elderly

Pharmacokinetics: Absorbed well
PO: Onset ½ to 1 hour, peak 2-4 hours, duration 8 hours; half-life 12-16 hr
TOP: Onset 3 days, duration 1 week; metabolized by liver (metabolites), excreted in urine (30% unchanged, inactive metabolites, feces), crosses blood-brain barrier, excreted in breast milk

Interactions/incompatibilities:

• Increased CNS depression: narcotics, sedatives, hypnotics, anesthetics, alcohol

• Decreased hypotensive effects: tricyclic antidepressants, MAOIs, appetite suppressants, amphetamines

• Increased hypotensive effects: diuretics, other antihypertensive nitrates

• Increased bradycardia: β-blockers, cardiac glycosides

Lab test interferences:

Increase: Blood glucose

Decrease: VMA, catecholamines aldosterone

NURSING CONSIDERATIONS
Assess:

• Blood studies: neutrophils, decreased platelets

• Renal studies: protein, BUN, creatinine; watch for increased levels that may indicate nephrotic syndrome

• Baselines in renal, liver function tests before therapy begins; K levels, although hyperkalemia rarely occurs

• Dipstick of urine for protein qd in first morning specimen; if protein is increased, a 24-hr urinary protein should be collected

• B/P, pulse if the drug is being used for hypertension

• For narcotic withdrawal including fever, diarrhea, nausea, vomiting, cramps, insomnia, shivering, dilated pupils

• Edema in feet, legs daily; monitor I&O; check for decreasing output

• Allergic reaction: rash, fever, pruritus, urticaria; drug should be discontinued if antihistamines fail to help

• Allergic reaction from patches: rash, urticaria, angioedema; should not continue to use

• Symptoms of CHF: edema, dyspnea, wet rales, B/P

• Renal symptoms: polyuria, oliguria, frequency

• For retinal degeneration: periodic eye exam

Administer:

• IV infusion of 0.9% NaCl (as ordered) to expand fluid volume if severe hypotension occurs

• SL if patient is unable to swallow

• PO: give last dose at hs

• Topical patch q/wk; apply to site without hair; best absorption over chest or upper arm; rotate sides with each application; clean site before application; apply firmly, especially around edges

Perform/provide:

• Storage of patches in cool environment, tablets in tight container

Evaluate:

• Therapeutic response: decrease in B/P in hypertension, decrease in withdrawal symptoms (narcotic)

Teach patient/family:

• To avoid hazardous activities, since drug may cause drowsiness

• To administer 1 hr before meals

- Not to discontinue drug abruptly, or withdrawal symptoms may occur: anxiety, increased B/P, headache, insomnia, increased pulse, tremors, nausea, sweating
- Not to use OTC (cough, cold, or allergy) products unless directed by physician
- To avoid sunlight or wear sunscreen if in sunlight; photosensitivity may occur
- To comply with dosage schedule even if feeling better
- To rise slowly to sitting or standing position to minimize orthostatic hypotension, especially elderly
- To notify physician of mouth sores, sore throat, fever, swelling of hands or feet, irregular heartbeat, chest pain, signs of angioedema
- About excessive perspiration, dehydration, vomiting; diarrhea may lead to fall in blood pressure; consult physician if these occur
- That drug may cause dizziness, fainting; light-headedness may occur during 1st few days of therapy
- That drug may cause dry mouth; use hard candy, saliva product, or frequent rinsing of mouth
- That compliance is necessary; not to skip or stop drug unless directed by physician
- That drug may cause skin rash or impaired perspiration
- That response may take 2-3 days if drug is given transdermally; instruct on administration of patch

Treatment of overdose: Supportive treatment; administer tolazdine, atropine, dopamine prn

clorazepate dipotassium

(klor-az'e-pate)
Clorazepate Dipotassium, Gen-Xene, Tranxene, Tranxene-SD, Tranxene-SD Half Strength
Func. class.: Antianxiety
Chem. class.: Benzodiazepine

Controlled Substance Schedule IV

Action: Potentiates the actions of GABA, especially in limbic system, reticular formation

Uses: Anxiety, acute alcohol withdrawal, adjunct in seizure disorders

Dosage and routes:

Anxiety
- *Adult:* PO 15-60 mg/day

Alcohol withdrawal
- *Adult:* PO 30 mg then 30-60 mg in divided doses; day 2, 45-90 mg in divided doses; day 3, 22.5-45 mg in divided doses; day 4, 15-30 mg in divided doses; then reduce daily dose to 7.5-15 mg

Seizure disorders
- *Adult and child >12 yr:* PO 7.5 mg tid; may increase by 7.5 mg/wk or less, not to exceed 90 mg/day
- *Child 9-12 yr:* PO 7.5 mg bid; may increase by 7.5 mg/wk or less, not to exceed 60 mg/day

Available forms: Caps 3.75, 7.5, 15 mg; tabs 3.75, 7.5, 15 mg, single-dose tab 11.25, 22.5 mg

Side effects/adverse reactions:

CNS: Dizziness, drowsiness, confusion, headache, anxiety, tremors, stimulation, fatigue, depression, insomnia, hallucinations, lethargy
GI: Constipation, dry mouth, nausea, vomiting, anorexia, diarrhea
INTEG: Rash, dermatitis, itching
CV: Orthostatic hypotension, **ECG**

italics = common side effects   ***bold italic*** = life threatening reactions

changes, tachycardia, hypotension
EENT: Blurred vision, tinnitus, my-driasis
Contraindications: Hypersensitivity to benzodiazepines, narrow-angle glaucoma, psychosis, pregnancy (D), child <18 yr
Precautions: Elderly, debilitated, hepatic disease, renal disease
Pharmacokinetics:
PO: Onset 15 min, peak 1-2 hr, duration 4-6 hr; metabolized by liver, excreted by kidneys; crosses placenta, breast milk; half-life 30-100 hr
Interactions/incompatibilities:
• Decreased effects of clorazepate: valproic acid
• Increased effects of clorazepate: CNS depressants, alcohol, disulfiram, oral contraceptives, antidepressants, MAOIs, cimetidine
Lab test interferences:
Increase: AST/ALT, serum bilirubin
Decrease: RAIU
False increase: 17-OHCS
NURSING CONSIDERATIONS
Assess:
• B/P (lying, standing), pulse; if systolic B/P drops 20 mm Hg, hold drug, notify physician
• Blood studies: CBC during long-term therapy; blood dyscrasias have occurred rarely
• Hepatic studies: AST, ALT, bilirubin, creatinine, LDH, alk phosphatase
• I&O; may indicate renal dysfunction
• Mental status: mood, sensorium, affect, sleeping pattern, drowsiness, dizziness
• Physical dependency, withdrawal symptoms: headache, nausea, vomiting, muscle pain, weakness after long-term use
• Suicidal tendencies

Administer:
• With food or milk for GI symptoms
• Crushed if patient is unable to swallow medication whole
• Sugarless gum, hard candy, frequent sips of water for dry mouth
Perform/provide:
• Assistance with ambulation during beginning therapy, since drowsiness/dizziness occurs, especially elderly
• Safety measures, including side rails
• Check to see PO medication has been swallowed
Evaluate:
• Therapeutic response: decreased anxiety, restlessness, insomnia
Teach patient/family:
• That drug may be taken with food
• Not to be used for everyday stress or used longer than 4 mo, unless directed by physician; not to take more than prescribed amount; may be habit forming
• To avoid OTC preparations unless approved by physician
• To avoid driving, activities that require alertness; drowsiness may occur, especially elderly
• To avoid alcohol ingestion or other psychotropic medications, unless prescribed by physician
• Not to discontinue medication abruptly after long-term use
• To rise slowly or fainting may occur
• That drowsiness may worsen at beginning of treatment
Treatment of overdose: Lavage, VS, supportive care, flumazenil

---

*Available in Canada only

clotrimazole

(kloe-trim'a-zole)

Mycelex Troches, Lotrimin, Lotrimin AF, Mycelex, Mycelex OTC, Canesten*, FemCare, Gyne-Lotrimin, Mycelex-G, Mycelex-7, Mycelex Twin Pack

Func. class.: Local antiinfective
Chem. class.: Imidazole derivative

Action: Interferes with fungal DNA replication; binds sterols in fungal cell membrane, which increases permeability, leaking of cell nutrients; fungicidal

Uses: Tinea pedis, tinea cruris, tinea corporis, tinea versicolor, *C. albicans* infection of the vagina, vulva, throat, mouth

Dosage and routes:
• *Adult and child:* TOP rub into affected area bid × 1-8 wk; LOZ dissolve in mouth 5×/day × 2 wk; INTRA VAG 1 applicator/1 tab × 1-2 wk hs, oral troches 10 mg 5×/day ×14 days

Available forms: Cream, sol, lotion 1%; vag tabs 100, 500 mg; vag cream 1%, troches 10 mg

Side effects/adverse reactions:
INTEG: Rash, urticaria, stinging, burning, peeling, blistering, skin fissures
OTHER: Abdominal cramps, bloating, urinary frequency, dyspareunia

Contraindications: Hypersensitivity

Precautions: Pregnancy (B), lactation

NURSING CONSIDERATIONS
Assess:
• Allergic reaction: burning, stinging, swelling, redness
Administer:
• 1 applicator or 1 tablet intravaginally each night

• Enough medication to cover lesions completely
• After cleansing with soap, water before each application; dry well
Perform/provide:
• Storage at room temperature in dry place
Evaluate:
• Therapeutic response: decrease in size, number of lesions, decrease in itching or white patches around vulva
Teach patient/family:
• To apply with glove to prevent further infection
• To avoid use of OTC creams, ointments, lotions unless directed by physician
• To use medical asepsis (hand washing) before, after each application
• To abstain from sexual intercourse during vaginal/vulvular treatment
• To use continuously even during menstrual period
• To report to physician if infection persists or returns in 2 mo; pregnancy or a serious medical condition may be the cause

cloxacillin sodium

(klox-a-sill'in)

Apo Cloxi,* Bactopen,* Cloxacillin Sodium, Cloxapen, Novocloxin,* Orbenin,* Tegopen

Func. class.: Broad-spectrum antibiotic
Chem. class.: Penicillinase-resistant penicillin

Action: Interferes with cell wall replication of susceptible organisms; the cell wall, rendered osmotically unstable, swells, bursts from osmotic pressure

Uses: Effective for gram-positive

italics = common side effects   ***bold italic*** = life threatening reactions

cocci *(S. aureus, S. pyogenes, E. pyogenes, S. pneumoniae), penicillinase-producing staphylococci*

Dosage and routes:
• *Adult:* PO 1-4 g/day in divided doses q6h
• *Child:* PO 50-100 mg/kg in divided doses q6h
Available forms: Caps 250, 500 mg; powder for oral susp 125 mg/ 5 ml

Side effects/adverse reactions:
HEMA: Anemia, increased bleeding time, **bone marrow depression, granulocytopenia**
GI: Nausea, vomiting, diarrhea, increased AST, ALT, abdominal pain, glossitis, colitis
GU: Oliguria, proteinuria, hematuria, *vaginitis, moniliasis,* **glomerulonephritis**
CNS: Lethargy, hallucinations, anxiety, depression, twitching, **coma, convulsions**

Contraindications: Hypersensitivity to penicillins; neonates
Precautions: Pregnancy (B), hypersensitivity to cephalosporins

Pharmacokinetics:
PO: Peak 1 hr, duration 6 hr; half-life 30-60 min; metabolized in liver; excreted in urine, bile, breast milk; crosses placenta

Interactions/incompatibilities:
• Decreased antimicrobial effectiveness of cloxacillin: tetracyclines, erythromycins
• Increased cloxacillin concentrations: aspirin, probenecid

Lab test interferences:
False positive: Urine glucose, urine protein
Decreased: Uric acid

NURSING CONSIDERATIONS
Assess:
• I&O ratio; report hematuria, oli-

guria, since penicillin in high doses is nephrotoxic
• Any patient with compromised renal system, since drug is excreted slowly in poor renal system function; toxicity may occur rapidly
• Liver studies: AST, ALT
• Blood studies: WBC, RBC, H&H, bleeding time
• Renal studies: urinalysis, protein, blood
• Culture, sensitivity before drug therapy; drug may be taken as soon as culture is taken
• Bowel pattern before, during treatment
• Skin eruptions after administration of penicillin to 1 wk after discontinuing drug
• Respiratory status: rate, character, wheezing, tightness in chest
• Allergies before initiation of treatment; reaction of each medication; place allergies on chart, Kardex in bright red

Administer:
• After C&S completed

Perform/provide:
• Adrenaline, suction, tracheostomy set, endotracheal intubation equipment on unit
• Adequate intake of fluids (2 L) during diarrhea episodes
• Scratch test to assess allergy after securing order from physician; usually done when penicillin is only drug of choice
• Storage in tight container; after reconstituting, store in refrigerator for 2 wk, room temperature 1 wk

Evaluate:
• Therapeutic response: absence of temperature, draining wounds

Teach patient/family:
• Aspects of drug therapy including need to complete entire course of medication to ensure organism death (10-14 days); culture may be

---

*Available in Canada only

taken after completed course of medication
• To report sore throat, fever, fatigue (may indicate superimposed infection)
• To wear or carry a Medic Alert ID if allergic to penicillins
• To notify nurse of diarrhea
• To take on an empty stomach with a full glass of water
Treatment of overdose: Withdraw drug; maintain airway; administer epinephrine, aminophylline, O_2, IV corticosteroids for anaphylaxis

clozapine
(kloz-a'pin)
Clozaril
Func. class.: Antipsychotic
Chem. class.: Tricyclic dibenzodiazepine derivative

Action: Interferes with dopamine receptor binding with lack of extrapyramidal symptoms; also acts as an adrenergic, cholinergic, histaminergic, serotonergic antagonist
Uses: Management of psychotic symptoms in schizophrenic patients for whom other antipsychotics have failed
Dosage and routes:
• *Adult:* PO 25 mg qd or bid; may increase by 25-50 mg/day; normal range 300-450 mg/day after 2 wk; do not increase dose more than 2 ×/wk; do not exceed 900 mg/day; use lowest dose to control symptoms
Available forms: Tabs 25, 100 mg
Side effects/adverse reactions:
*CNS: Sedation, salivation, dizziness, headache, tremors, sleep problems, akinesia, fever, **seizures,** sweating, akathisia, confusion, fatigue, insomnia,* depression, slurred speech, anxiety

GI: Drooling or excessive salivation, constipation, nausea, abdominal discomfort, vomiting, diarrhea, anorexia
MS: Weakness; pain in back, neck, legs; spasm
CV: Tachycardia, hypotension, hypertension, chest pain, ECG changes
GU: Urinary abnormalities, incontinence, ejaculation dysfunction, frequency, urgency, retention
RESP: Dyspnea, nasal congestion, throat discomfort
*HEMA: **Leukopenia, neutropenia, agranulocytosis, eosinophilia***
Contraindications: Hypersensitivity, myeloproliferative disorders, severe granulocytopenia, CNS depression, coma, narrow-angle glaucoma
Precautions: Pregnancy (B); lactation; children <16; hepatic, renal, cardiac disease; seizures; prostatic enlargement; elderly
Pharmacokinetics:
Steady state 2.5 hr; 95% protein bound; completely metabolized by the liver; excreted in urine and feces (metabolites); half-life 8-12 hr
Interactions/incompatibilities:
• Increased anticholinergic effects: anticholinergics
• Increased hypotension: antihypertensives
• Increased CNS depression: CNS drugs
• Increased bone marrow suppression: antineoplastics, other drugs suppressing bone marrow
• Increased plasma concentrations: warfarin, digoxin, other highly protein-bound drugs
Lab test interferences:
Increase: Liver function tests, cardiac enzymes, cholesterol, blood glucose, bilirubin, PBI, cholinesterase, [131]I

---

italics = common side effects   ***bold italic*** = life threatening reactions

False positive: Pregnancy tests, PKU

False negative: Urinary steroids, 17-OHCS

NURSING CONSIDERATIONS

Assess:

• Swallowing of PO medication; check for hoarding or giving of medication to other patients

• I&O ratio; obtain baseline before treatment begins; palpate bladder if low urinary output occurs

• Bilirubin, CBC, liver function studies monthly

• Urinalysis is recommended before, during prolonged therapy

• Affect, orientation, LOC, reflexes, gait, coordination, sleep pattern disturbances

• B/P standing and lying; take pulse and respirations q4h during initial treatment; establish baseline before starting treatment; report drops of 30 mm Hg

• Dizziness, faintness, palpitations, tachycardia on rising

• EPS including akathisia (inability to sit still, no pattern to movements), tardive dyskinesia (bizarre movements of the jaw, mouth, tongue, extremities), pseudoparkinsonism (rigidity, tremors, pill rolling, shuffling gait)

• Skin turgor daily

• Constipation, urinary retention daily; if these occur, increase bulk, water in diet, especially elderly

Adminster:

• Antiparkinsonian agent, to be used if extrapyramidal symptoms occur

Perform/provide:

• Decreased noise input by dimming lights, avoiding loud noises

• Supervised ambulation until stabilized on medication; do not involve in strenuous exercise program because fainting is possible; patient should not stand still for long periods

• Increased fluids to prevent constipation

• Storage in tight, light-resistant container

Evaluate:

• Therapeutic response: decrease in emotional excitement, hallucinations, delusions, paranoia, reorganization of patterns of thought, speech

Teach patient/family:

• That orthostatic hypotension occurs often, and to rise from sitting or lying position gradually

• To avoid hot tubs, hot showers, or tub baths; since hypotension may occur

• To avoid abrupt withdrawal of this drug, or EPS may result; drug should be withdrawn slowly

• To avoid OTC preparations (cough, hay fever, cold) unless approved by physician, since serious drug interactions may occur; avoid use with alcohol or CNS depressants; increased drowsiness may occur

• Regarding compliance with drug regimen

• About EPS and necessity for meticulous oral hygiene, since oral candidiasis may occur

• To report sore throat, malaise, fever, bleeding, mouth sores; if these occur, CBC should be drawn and drug discontinued

• In hot weather, heat stroke may occur; take extra precautions to stay cool

• To avoid driving or other hazardous activities; seizures may occur

• To notify physician if pregnant or if pregnancy is intended

Treatment of overdose: Lavage, activated charcoal; provide an airway; do not induce vomiting

---

* Available in Canada only

codeine sulfate/codeine phosphate
(koe'deen)

Func. class.: Narcotic analgesics
Chem. class.: Opiate, phenanthrene derivative

Controlled Substance Schedule II
Action: Depresses pain impulse transmission at the spinal cord level by interacting with opioid receptors
Uses: Moderate to severe pain, nonproductive cough
Dosage and routes:
Pain
• *Adult:* PO 15-60 mg q4h prn; IM/SC 15-60 mg q4h prn
• *Child:* PO 3 mg/kg/day in divided doses q4h prn
Cough
• *Adult:* PO 10-20 mg q4-6h, not to exceed 120 mg/day
• *Child:* PO 1-1.5 mg/kg/day in 4 divided doses, not to exceed 60 mg/day
Available forms: Inj IM, SC 15, 30, 60 mg/ml; tabs 15, 30, 60 mg
Side effects/adverse reactions:
CNS: Drowsiness, sedation, dizziness, agitation, dependency, lethargy, restlessness
GI: Nausea, vomiting, anorexia, constipation
RESP: **Respiratory depression, respiratory paralysis**
CV: Bradycardia, palpitations, orthostatic hypotension, tachycardia
GU: Urinary retention
INTEG: Flushing, rash, urticaria
Contraindications: Hypersensitivity to opiates, respiratory depression, increased intracranial pressure, seizure disorders, severe respiratory disorders
Precautions: Elderly, cardiac dysrhythmias, pregnancy (C)

Pharmacokinetics: Onset 15-30 min, peak 1-2 hr, duration 4-6 hr; metabolized by liver; excreted by kidneys; crosses placenta; excreted in breast milk; half-life 2½-4 hr
Interactions/incompatibilities:
• Effects may be increased with other CNS depressants: alcohol, narcotics, sedative/hypnotics, antipsychotics, skeletal muscle relaxants

NURSING CONSIDERATIONS
Assess:
• I&O ratio; check for decreasing output; may indicate urinary retention, especially elderly
• By using pain-scoring method
• For productive cough
• Cough: type, duration, ability to raise secretion
• CNS changes, dizziness, drowsiness, hallucinations, euphoria, LOC, pupil reaction
• Allergic reactions: rash, urticaria
• Respiratory dysfunction: respiratory depression, character, rate rhythm; notify physician if respirations are <10/min, shallow
• Need for pain medication, physical dependence
Administer:
• With antiemetic if nausea, vomiting occur
• When pain is beginning to return; determine dosage interval by patient response
Perform/provide:
• Storage in light-resistant container at room temperature
• Assistance with ambulation
• Safety measures: top side rails, night-light, call bell
Evaluate:
• Therapeutic response: decrease in pain, absence of grimacing or decreased cough
Teach patient/family:
• To report any symptoms of CNS changes, allergic reactions

---

italics = common side effects   ***bold italic*** = life threatening reactions

• That physical dependency may result when used for extended periods
• To change position slowly; orthostatic hypotension may occur
• To avoid hazardous activities if drowsiness or dizziness occurs
• To avoid alcohol, other CNS depressants unless directed by physician

---

colchicine
(kol′chi-seen)

Func. class.: Antigout agent
Chem. class.: Colchicum autumnale alkaloid

Action: Inhibits microtubule formation of lactic acid in leukocytes, which decreases phagocytosis and inflammation in joints

Uses: Gout, gouty arthritis (prevention, treatment); to arrest progression of neurologic disability in multiple sclerosis

Dosage and routes:
Prevention
• *Adult:* PO 0.5-1.8 mg qd depending on severity; IV 0.5-1 mg 1-2 × day
Treatment
• *Adult:* PO 0.5-1.2 mg, then 0.5-1.2 mg q1h, until pain decreases or side effects occur; IV 2 mg, 0.5 mg q6h, not to exceed 4 mg/24 hr
Available forms: Tabs 0.5, 0.6 mg; inj IV 1 mg/2 ml

Side effects/adverse reactions:
MISC: Myopathy, alopecia, reversible azoospermia, peripheral neuritis
GU: Hematuria, oliguria, renal damage
HEMA: **Agranulocytosis, thrombocytopenia, aplastic anemia, pancytopenia**
GI: Nausea, vomiting, anorexia,

malaise, metallic taste, cramps, peptic ulcer, diarrhea
INTEG: Chills, dermatitis, pruritus, purpura, erythema

Contraindications: Hypersensitivity; serious GI, renal, hepatic, cardiac disorders; blood dyscrasias
Precautions: Severe renal disease, blood dyscrasias, pregnancy (C), hepatic disease, elderly, lactation, children

Pharmacokinetics:
PO: Peak ½-2 hr, half-life 20 min; deacetylates in liver; excreted in feces (metabolites/active drug)

Interactions/incompatibilities:
• Decreased action of colchicine: acidifying agents
• Decreased action of: vitamin B$_{12}$
• Increased action of: CNS depressants, sympathomimetics
• Increased action of colchicine: alkalinizers
• Considered incompatible in syringe with other drugs

Lab test interferences:
Increase: Alk phosphatase, AST/ALT
False positive: RBC, Hgb

NURSING CONSIDERATIONS
Assess:
• I&O ratio; observe for decrease in urinary output
• CBC, platelets, reticulocytes before, during therapy (q3mo)
• Coombs' test to determine Coombs' negative hemolytic anemia

Administer:
• IV undiluted or diluted 1 mg/10-20 ml normal saline or sterile H$_2$O for inj; give over 2-5 min
• Oral: on empty stomach only, to facilitate absorption

Evaluate:
• Therapeutic response: decreased stone formation on x-ray, decreased

---

* Available in Canada only

pain in kidney region, absence of hematuria, decreased pain in joints
Teach patient/family:
• To increase fluids to 3-4 L/day
• To avoid alcohol, OTC preparations that contain alcohol; skin rashes have occurred
• To report any pain, redness, or hard area, usually in legs
• Importance of complying with medical regimen; bone marrow depression may occur

colestipol HCl
(koe-les'ti-pole)
Colestid
Func. class.: Antilipemic
Chem. class.: Bile sequestrant, resin exchange agent

Action: Absorbs, combines with bile acids to form insoluble complex that is excreted through feces; loss of bile acids lowers cholesterol levels
Uses: Primary hypercholesterolemia, xanthomas, digitalis toxicity, pruritus due to biliary obstruction, diarrhea due to bile acids
Dosage and routes:
• *Adult:* PO 15-30 g/day in 2-4 divided doses
Available forms: Granules
Side effects/adverse reactions:
GI: Constipation, abdominal pain, nausea, fecal impaction, hemorrhoids, flatulence, vomiting, steatorrhea, peptic ulcer
INTEG: Rash, irritation of perianal area, tongue, skin
HEMA: Decreased Vit A, D, K, red folate content **hyperchloremic acidosis,** bleeding, decreased protime
Contraindications: Hypersensitivity, biliary obstruction
Precautions: Pregnancy (B), lactation, children, bleeding disorders

Pharmacokinetics:
PO: Excreted in feces
Interactions/incompatibilities:
• May reduce action of: thiazide, digitalis, warfarin, penicillin G, folic acid, phenylbutazone, tetracycline, corticosteroids, iron, thyroid agents, clindamycin, trimethoprim, chenodiol, fat-soluble vitamins, cephalexin, phenobarbital
Lab test interferences:
Increase: Liver function studies, chloride, PO_4
NURSING CONSIDERATIONS
Assess:
• Cardiac glycoside levels, if both drugs are being administered
• For signs of Vit A, D, K deficiency
• Serum cholesterol, triglyceride levels, electrolytes if on extended therapy
• Bowel pattern daily; increase bulk, water in diet if constipation develops
Administer:
• Drug ac, hs; give all other medications 1 hr before colestipol or 4 hr after colestipol to avoid poor absorption
• Drug mixed in applesauce or stirred into beverage (2-6 oz); do not take dry; let stand for 2 min
• Supplemental doses of Vit A, D, K if levels are low
Evaluate:
• Therapeutic response: decreased triglycerides, diarrhea, pruritus (excess bile acids)
Teach patient/family:
• Symptoms of hypoprothrombinemia: bleeding mucous membranes, dark tarry stools, hematuria, petechiae; report immediately
• That patient compliance is needed, since toxicity may result if doses are missed
• That risk factors should be de-

italics = common side effects   ***bold italic*** = life threatening reactions

creased: high-fat diet, smoking, alcohol consumption, absence of exercise

---

colfosceril palmitate
(kohl-foss'sir-ill)
Exosurf Neonatal
Func. class.: Synthetic lung surfactant
Chem. class.: dipalmitoylphosphatidylcholine (DPPC)

Action: Surfactant maintains lung inflation and prevents collapse by lowering surface tension

Uses: Treatment of respiratory distress syndrome (RDS) in premature infants

Dosage and routes:
Prophylactic treatment
Endotracheally: 5 ml/kg as soon as possible after birth and repeat doses 12 and 24 hr later to infants remaining on mechanical ventilation
Rescue treatment
Endotracheally: administer in two 5 ml/kg doses; give initial dose after treatment of RDS, then second dose in 12 hr
Available forms: 10 ml/vial with sterile H_2O for inj and 5 endotracheal tube adapters

Side effects/adverse reactions:
RESP: Apnea, pulmonary hemorrhage, pulmonary air leak, congenital pneumonia
SYST: Nonpulmonary fatal infections

Precautions: Congenital anomalies, prophylactic treatment

Pharmacokinetics: Distributed to all lobes, alveolar spaces, distal airways; alveolar half-life 12 hr; 90% of alveolar phospholipids are recycled

NURSING CONSIDERATIONS
Assess:
• Respiratory rate, rhythm, char-

acter, chest expansion, color, transcutaneous saturation, ABGs
• Endotracheal tube placement before dosing
• For apnea after endotracheal administration
• Reflux of drug into the endotracheal tube during administration; stop drug administration if this occurs, and, if needed, increase peak inspiratory pressure on the ventilator by 4-5 cm H_2O until tube is cleared

Administer:
• Infants should be suctioned before administration
• After selecting an adapter size that corresponds to the diameter of the endotracheal tube, insert the adapter into the tube by twisting, connect the breathing circuit to the adapter, remove the cap from the adapter sideport, and attach the syringe to the sideport; after dose is completed, remove the syringe and recap the sideport
• After reconstituting each vial with 8 ml preservative-free sterile water for injection, fill a 10-12 ml syringe with 8 ml preservative-free sterile water for injection, using an 18-19 gauge needle; allow the vacuum in the vial to draw the liquid into the vial; aspirate the 8 ml out of the vial into the syringe while maintaining the vacuum and then release the syringe plunger; repeat the aspiration and release until adequately mixed; draw the dose required into the syringe from below the froth in the vial; do not use if large particles are present
• By endotracheal administration only by persons trained in neonatal intubation and ventilation

Perform/provide:
• Reduction in peak ventilator in-

spiratory pressures immediately if chest expansion improves substantially after dose

• Reduction in Fio$_2$ in small, repeated steps when infant becomes pink and transcutaneous oxygen saturation is in excess of 95%; oxygen saturation should remain between 90% and 95%

• Suctioning of all infants before administration to prevent mucus plugging; if endotracheal tube obstruction is suspected, remove the obstruction and replace tube immediately

• Storage at room temperature in dry place

Evaluate:

• Therapeutic response: decreased respiratory distress

---

corticotropin (ACTH)

(kor-ti-koe-troe′pin)
ACTH, Acthar, Corticotropin, ACTH-40, ACTH-80, Duracton*, H.P. Acthar Gel

Func. class.: Pituitary hormone
Chem. class.: Adrenocorticotropic hormone

Action: Stimulates adrenal cortex to produce, secrete corticosterone, cortisol

Uses: Testing adrenocortical function, treatment of adrenal insufficiency caused by administration of corticosteroids (long term), multiple sclerosis

Dosage and routes:

Testing of adrenocortical function

• *Adult:* IM/SC up to 80 U in divided doses; IV 10-25 U in 500 ml D$_5$W given over 8 hr

Inflammation

• *Adult:* SC/IM 40 U in 4 divided doses (aqueous) or 40 U q12-24h (gel/repository form)

Available forms: Inj IM, IV, SC 25, 40 U/vial, repository inj IM, SC 40, 80/ml

Side effects/adverse reactions:

INTEG: Impaired wound healing, rash, urticaria, hirsutism, petechiae, ecchymoses, sweating, acne, hyperpigmentation

CNS: **Convulsions,** dizziness, euphoria, insomnia, headache, mood swings, behavioral changes, depression, psychosis

GI: Nausea, vomiting, ***peptic ulcer perforation,*** pancreatitis, distention, ulcerative esophagitis

GU: Water, sodium retention, hypokalemia

EENT: Cataracts, glaucoma

MS: Weakness, osteoporosis, compression fractures, muscle atrophy, steroid myopathy, myalgia, arthralgia

ENDO: Cushingoid symptoms, diabetes mellitus, antibody formation, growth retardation in children, menstrual irregularities

Contraindications: Hypersensitivity, scleroderma, osteoporosis, CHF, peptic ulcer disease, hypertension, systemic fungal infections, smallpox vaccination, recent surgery, ocular herpes simplex, primary adrenocortical insufficiency/ hyperfunction

Precautions: Pregnancy (C), lactation, latent TB, hepatic disease, hypothyroiditis, childbearing-age women, psychiatric diagnosis, myasthenia gravis, acute gouty arthritis

Pharmacokinetics:

IV/IM/SC: Onset <6 hr, duration 2-4 hr, repository duration up to 3 days, half-life <20 min, excreted in urine

Interactions/incompatibilities:

• Possible ulceration: salicylates, alcohol, corticosteroids

---

italics = common side effects   ***bold italic*** = life threatening reactions

• Hypokalemia: diuretics (K-depleting), amphotericin B
• Hyperglycemia: insulin, or oral hypoglycemic agents
• Incompatible with aminophylline, $NaCO_3$ in sol or syringe

NURSING CONSIDERATIONS
Assess:
• Baseline ECG, B/P, chest x-ray, GTT
• Pulse, B/P
• I&O ratio; weight qwk, report gain over 5 lb/wk
• 2 hr postprandial, chest x-ray, serum K, 17 KS, 17-OHCS, cortisol, during long-term treatment
• Dependent edema, moon face, pulmonary edema, cerebral edema
• Infection; drug may mask infections
• Increased stress in patient's life that may require increased corticosteroids
• Mental status: affect, mood, increased aggressiveness, irritability; a change in mental status may require decreased steroids
• Growth rate of child
• Hypoadrenalism in neonates if drug was given during pregnancy
• Allergic reaction: rash, urticaria, fever, nausea, vomiting, dyspnea; drug should be discontinued immediately, administer epinephrine 1:1000

Administer:
• Test for hypersensitivity for individuals allergic to pork products
• Decreased Na, increase K for dependent edema
• Increase protein diet for N loss
• Gel at room temperature, give deep IM using 21G needle
• May be used to treat edema
• IV; give over 2 min; dilute 25 U/1 ml sterile H_2O or normal saline or 40 U/2 ml; may dilute 10-25 U/500 ml compatible sol; give over 8 hr

Perform/provide:
• Storage in refrigerator of unused portion; use within 24 hr

Evaluate:
• Therapeutic response: absence of inflammation, pain, increased muscle strength in myasthenia gravis

Teach patient/family:
• To avoid vaccinations during drug treatment
• To maintain adequate hydration up to 2 L/day unless contraindicated
• To avoid OTC products: salicylates, products with alcohol
• Not to discontinue medication abruptly; adrenal crisis may occur; drug should be tapered off over several wk
• To wear Medic Alert ID specifying steroid therapy
• That drug does not cure condition, only decreases symptoms
• To notify physician of infection: increased temperature, sore throat, muscular pain
• To tell patient to notify anyone involved in medical or dental care that this drug is being taken

---

cortisone acetate
(kor'-ti-sone)
Cortone
Func. class.: Corticosteroid, synthetic
Chem. class.: Glucocorticoid, short-acting

Action: Decreases inflammation by suppression of migration of polymorphonuclear leukocytes, fibroblasts, reversal of increased capillary permeability and lysosomal stabilization

Uses: Inflammation, severe allergy,

adrenal insufficiency, collagen disorders, respiratory, dermatologic disorders

Dosage and routes:
• *Adult:* PO 25-300 mg qd or q2 days, titrated to patient response
Available forms: Tabs 5, 10, 25 mg

Side effects/adverse reactions:
INTEG: Acne, poor wound healing, ecchymosis, bruising, petechiae
CNS: Depression, flushing, sweating, headache, mood changes
*CV: Hypertension, **circulatory collapse, thrombophlebitis, embolism,** tachycardia, **necrotizing angiitis, CHF,** edema*
*HEMA: **Thrombocytopenia***
MS: Fractures, osteoporosis, weakness
*GI: Diarrhea, nausea, abdominal distention, **GI hemorrhage,** increased appetite, pancreatitis*
EENT: Fungal infections, increased intraocular pressure, blurred vision

Contraindications: Psychosis, hypersensitivity, idiopathic thrombocytopenia, acute glomerulonephritis, amebiasis, fungal infections, nonasthmatic bronchial disease, child <2 yr, AIDS, TB

Precautions: Pregnancy (C), diabetes mellitus, glaucoma, osteoporosis, seizure disorders, ulcerative colitis, CHF, myasthenia gravis, renal disease, esophagitis, peptic ulcer

Pharmacokinetics:
PO: Peak 2 hr, duration 1½ days
IM: Peak 20-48 hr, duration 1½ days

Interactions/incompatibilities:
• Decreased action of cortisone: cholestyramine, colestipol, barbiturates, rifampin, ephedrine, phenytoin, theophylline
• Decreased effects of: anticoagulants, anticonvulsants, antidiabetics, ambenonium, neostigmine,

isoniazid, toxoids, vaccines, anticholinesterases, salicylates, somatrem
• Increased side effects: alcohol, salicylates, indomethacin, amphotericin B, digitalis, cyclosporine, diuretics
• Increased action of cortisone: salicylates, estrogens, indomethacin, oral contraceptives, ketoconazole, macrolide antibiotics

Lab test interferences:
Increase: Cholesterol, Na, blood glucose, uric acid, Ca, urine glucose
Decrease: Ca, K, T_4, T_3, thyroid ^{131}I uptake test, urine 17-OHCS, 17-KS, PBI
False negative: Skin allergy tests

NURSING CONSIDERATIONS
Assess:
• K, blood sugar, urine glucose while on long-term therapy; hypokalemia and hyperglycemia
• Weight daily; notify physician of weekly gain >5 lb
• B/P q4h, pulse; notify physician if chest pain occurs
• I&O ratio; be alert for decreasing urinary output and increasing edema
• Plasma cortisol levels during long-term therapy (normal level: 138-635 nmol/L SI units if drawn at 8 AM)
• Infection: increased temperature, WBC even after withdrawal of medication; drug masks symptoms of infection
• K depletion: paresthesias, fatigue, nausea, vomiting, depression, polyuria, dysrhythmias, weakness
• Edema, hypertension, cardiac symptoms
• Mental status: affect, mood, behavioral changes, aggression

Administer:
• After shaking suspension (parenteral)
• Titrated dose; use lowest effective dose
• IM inj deeply in large mass; rotate sites; avoid deltoid; use a 21G needle
• In one dose in AM to prevent adrenal suppression; avoid SC administration; damage may be done to tissue
• With food or milk to decrease GI symptoms

Perform/provide:
• Assistance with ambulation in patient with bone tissue disease to prevent fractures

Evaluate:
• Therapeutic response: ease of respirations, decreased inflammation

Teach patient/family:
• That ID as steroid user should be carried at all times
• To notify physician if therapeutic response decreases; dosage adjustment may be needed
• Not to discontinue this medication abruptly or adrenal crisis can result
• To avoid OTC products: salicylates, alcohol in cough products, cold preparations unless directed by physician
• All aspects of drug usage, including cushingoid symptoms
• Symptoms of adrenal insufficiency: nausea, anorexia, fatigue, dizziness, dyspnea, weakness, joint pain

---

cosyntropin
(koe-sin-troe′pin)
Cortrosyn
Func. class.: Pituitary hormone
Chem. class.: Synthetic polypeptide

Action: Stimulates adrenal cortex

to produce, secrete corticosterone, cortisol

Uses: Testing adrenocortical function

Dosage and routes:
• *Adult and child >2 yr:* IM/IV 0.25-1 mg between blood sampling
• *Child <2 yr:* IM/IV 0.125 mg
Available forms: Inj IM, IV 0.25 mg/vial

Side effects/adverse reactions:
INTEG: Rash urticaria, pruritus, flushing

Contraindications: Hypersensitivity

Precautions: Pregnancy (C)

Pharmacokinetics:
IV/IM: Onset 5 min, peak 1 hr, duration 2-4 hr

Interactions/incompatibilities:
• Considered incompatible with any drug in syringe or sol
• Incompatible with blood, blood products

NURSING CONSIDERATIONS
Assess:
• Plasma cortisol levels at ½-1 hr after drug administered (>5 µg/dl is normal), at end of 1 hr, levels should have doubled
• Dependent edema, moon face, pulmonary edema, cerebral edema
• Infection; drug may mask infections
• Increased stress in patient's life that may require increased corticosteroids
• Mental status: affect, mood, increased aggressiveness, irritability; a change in mental status may require decreased steroids
• Growth rate of child
• Hypoadrenalism in neonates if drug was given during pregnancy
• Allergic reaction: rash, urticaria, fever, nausea, vomiting, dyspnea; drug should be discontinued im-

mediately; administer epinephrine
1 : 1000

Administer:

• After reconstitution with 1 ml
0.9% NaCl/0.25 mg by direct IV
over 2 min; may be further diluted
in D$_5$ or normal saline; run 40 mg/
hr over 4-8 hr as an inf

Perform/provide:

• Storage at room temperature for
24 hr or refrigerated for 3 wk

Evaluate:

• Therapeutic response: absence of
inflammation, pain, increased muscle strength in myasthenia gravis

Teach patient/family:

• To avoid vaccinations during
drug treatment

• To maintain adequate hydration
up to 2 L/day unless contraindicated

• To avoid OTC products: salicylates, products with alcohol

• Not to discontinue medication
abruptly; thyroid crisis may occur;
drug should be tapered off over several wk

• To wear Medic Alert ID specifying steroid therapy

• That drug does not cure condition, only decreases symptoms

• To notify physician of infection:
increased temperature, sore throat,
muscular pain

• To tell patient to notify anyone
involved in medical or dental care
that this drug is being taken

co-trimoxazole (sulfa-methoxazole and tri-methoprim)

(koe-trye-mox′a-zole)
Apo-Sulfatrim,* Bactrim, Co-
trim, Comoxol, Septra, Sulfa-
trim, Bethaprim

Func. class.: Antibiotic
Chem. class.: Miscellaneous
sulfonamide

Action: Sulfamethoxazole (SMZ)
interferes with bacterial biosynthesis of proteins by competitive
antagonism of PABA when adequate levels are maintained; trimethoprim (TMP) blocks synthesis
of tetrahydrofolic acid; combination blocks 2 consecutive steps in
bacterial synthesis of essential nucleic acids, protein

Uses: Urinary tract infections, otitis media, acute and chronic prostatitis, shigellosis, *P. carinii* pneumonitis, chronic bronchitis, chancroid, traveler's diarrhea

Dosage and routes:

Urinary tract infections

• *Adult:* PO 160 mg TMP/800 mg
SMZ q12h × 10-14 days

• *Child:* PO 8 mg/kg TMP/40 mg/
kg SMZ qd in 2 divided doses q12h

Otitis media

• *Child:* PO 8 mg/kg TMP/40 mg/
kg SMZ qd in 2 divided doses q12h
× 10 days

Chronic bronchitis

• *Adult:* PO 160 mg TMP/800
mg SMZ q12h × 14 days

Pneumocystis carinii pneumonitis

• *Adult and child:* PO 20 mg/kg
TMP/100 mg/kg SMZ qd in 4 divided doses q6h × 14 days; IV 15-
20 mg/kg/day (based on TMP) in
3-4 divided doses for up to 14 days

• Dosage reduction necessary in

moderate to severe renal impairment (CrCL 30 ml/min)

Available forms: Tabs 80 mg trimethoprim (TMP)/400 mg sulfamethoxazole (SMZ), 160 mg trimethoprim/800 mg sulfamethoxazole; susp 40 mg/200 mg/5 ml; IV inj 16 mg/80 mg/ml

Side effects/adverse reactions:

CNS: Headache, insomnia, hallucinations, depression, vertigo, fatigue, anxiety, convulsions, drug fever, chills, aseptic meningitis

CV: Allergic myocarditis

GI: Nausea, vomiting, abdominal pain, stomatitis, *hepatitis,* glossitis, pancreatitis, diarrhea, *enterocolitis,* anorexia

GU: Renal failure, toxic nephrosis; increased BUN, creatinine, crystalluria

HEMA: Leukopenia, neutropenia, thrombocytopenia, agranulocytosis, hemolytic anemia, hypoprothrombinemia, Henoch-Schönlein purpura, methemoglobinemia, eosinophilia I

INTEG: Rash, dermatitis, urticaria, *Stevens-Johnson syndrome,* erythema, photosensitivity, pain, inflammation at injection site

RESP: Cough, shortness of breath

SYST: Anaphylaxis, SLE

Contraindications: Hypersensitivity to trimethoprim or sulfonamides, pregnancy at term, megaloblastic anemia, infants <2 mo, CrCl <15 ml/min, lactation

Precautions: Pregnancy (C), renal disease, elderly, G-6-PD deficiency, impaired hepatic function, possible folate deficiency, severe allergy, bronchial asthma

Pharmacokinetics:

PO: Rapidly absorbed, peak 1-4 hr; half-life 8-13 hr, excreted in urine (metabolites and unchanged), breast milk; crosses placenta; highly bound to plasma proteins; TMP achieves high levels in prostatic tissue and fluid

Interactions/incompatibilities:

• Increased hypoglycemic response: sulfonylurea agents

• Increased anticoagulant effects: oral anticoagulants

• Decreased hepatic clearance of: phenytoin

• Increased nephrotoxicity: cyclosporine

• Increased bone marrow depressant effects: methotrexate

• Thrombocytopenia: thiazide diuretics

Lab test interferences:

Increase: Alk phosphatase, creatinine, bilirubin

False positive: Urinary glucose test

NURSING CONSIDERATIONS

Assess:

• Allergic reactions: rash, fever (AIDS patients are more susceptible)

• I&O ratio; note color, character, pH of urine if drug administered for urinary tract infections; output should be 800 ml less than intake; if urine is highly acidic, alkalization may be needed

• Kidney function studies: BUN, creatinine, urinalysis if on long-term therapy

• Type of infection; obtain C&S before starting therapy

• Blood dyscrasias, skin rash, fever, sore throat, bruising, bleeding, fatigue, joint pain

• Allergic reaction: rash, dermatitis, urticaria, pruritus, dyspnea, bronchospasm

Administer:

• With full glass of water to maintain adequate hydration; increase fluids to 2 L/day to decrease crystallization in kidneys

• Medication after C&S; repeat

C&S after full course of medication completed
• After diluting 5 ml of drug/125 ml D$_5$W, run over 1-1½ hr
• With resuscitative equipment and epinephrine available; severe allergic reactions may occur
Perform/provide:
• Storage in tight, light-resistant container at room temperature
Evaluate:
• Therapeutic response: absence of pain, fever, C&S negative
Teach patient/family:
• To take each oral dose with full glass of water to prevent crystalluria; drink 8-10 glasses of water/day
• To complete course of full treatment to prevent superimposed infection
• To avoid sunlight or use sunscreen to prevent burns
• To avoid OTC medications (aspirin, Vit C) unless directed by physician
• If diabetic, to use Clinistix or Tes-Tape
• To use alternative contraceptive measures; decreased effectiveness of oral contraceptives may result
• To notify physician if skin rash, sore throat, fever, mouth sores, unusual bruising, bleeding occur

---

cromolyn sodium (disodium cromoglycate)
(kroe'moe-lin)
Intal, Intal p,* Nasalcrom, Rynacrom,* Gastrocrom
Func. class.: Antiasthmatic
Chem. class.: Mast cell stabilizer

Action: Stabilizes the membrane of the sensitized mast cell, preventing release of chemical mediators after an antigen-IgE interaction

Uses: Allergic rhinitis, severe perennial bronchial asthma, exercise-induced bronchospasm (prevention), prevention of acute bronchospasm induced by environmental pollutants, mastocytosis
Dosage and routes:
Allergic rhinitis
• *Adult and child >6 yr:* nasal sol 1 spray in each nostril tid-qid, not to exceed 6 doses/day
Bronchospasm
• *Adult and child >5 yr:* INH 20 mg <1 hr before exercise
Bronchial asthma
• *Adult and child >5 yr:* INH 20 mg qid; NEB 20 mg qid by nebulization
Available forms: Sol 40 mg/ml; inh, caps for inh, 20 mg; oral caps 100 mg, neb sol 20 mg, aerosol 800 µg/actuation
Side effects/adverse reactions:
EENT: Throat irritation, cough, nasal congestion, burning eyes
CNS: Headache, dizziness, neuritis
GU: Frequency, dysuria
GI: Nausea, vomiting, anorexia, dry mouth, bitter taste
INTEG: Rash, urticaria, angioedema
MS: Joint pain/swelling
Contraindications: Hypersensitivity to this drug or lactose, status asthmaticus
Precautions: Pregnancy (B), lactation, renal disease, hepatic disease, child <5 yr
Pharmacokinetics:
INH: Peak 15 min, duration 4-6 hr; excreted unchanged in feces; half-life 80 min
NURSING CONSIDERATIONS
Assess:
• Eosinophil count during treatment
• Respiratory status: respiratory

---

italics = common side effects   ***bold italic*** = life threatening reactions

rate, rhythm, characteristics, cough, wheezing, dyspnea
Administer:
• By inhalation/nebulizer only
• Gargle, sip of water to decrease irritation in throat
Evaluate:
• Therapeutic response: decrease in asthmatic symptoms, congested, runny nose
Teach patient/family:
• To clear mucus before using
• Proper inhalation technique: exhale; using inhaler, inhale deeply with head tipped back to open airway; remove; hold breath; exhale; repeat until all of drug is inhaled
• That therapeutic effect may take up to 4 wk
• Not to swallow capsule
• That drug is preventive only, not restorative

---

crotamiton
(kroe-tam′i-ton)
Eurax
Func. class.: Scabicide
Chem. class.: Synthetic chloroformate salt

Action: Unknown; toxic to *Sarcoptes scabiei*
Uses: Scabies, pruritus
Dosage and routes:
Scabies
• *Adult and child:* CREAM wash area with soap, water; remove visible crusts, apply cream, apply another coat in 24 hr, remove with soap, water in 48 hr
Pruritus
Massage into affected area, repeat as necessary
Available forms: Cream 10%; lotion 10%
Side effects/adverse reactions:
INTEG: Itching, rash, irritation, contact dermatitis

Contraindications: Hypersensitivity, inflammation of skin, abrasions, or breaks in skin, mucous membranes
Precautions: Children, pregnancy (C)

NURSING CONSIDERATIONS
Assess:
• Area of body involved, including crusts, brownish trails on skin, itching papules in skin folds
Administer:
• After patient bathes with soap, water; remove all crusts
• From chin down; do not apply to face, lips, mouth, eyes, any mucous membrane, anus, or meatus
• Topical corticosteroids as ordered to decrease contact dermatitis; antihistamines for pruritus
• Lotions of menthol or phenol to control itching
• Topical antibiotics for infection
Perform/provide:
• Storage in tight, light-resistant container
• Isolation until areas on skin, scalp have cleared; treatment is complete
Evaluate:
• Therapeutic response: decreased itching after several wk, decreased redness
Teach patient/family:
• To change clothing and bed linen the morning after treatment
• To shake well before using
• To wash all inhabitants' clothing, using hot water, dried in hot dryers for >20 min; preventive treatment may be required of all persons living in same house to decrease spread of infection
• That itching may continue for 4-6 wk
• That drug must be reapplied if accidentally washed off, or treatment will be ineffective

---

- To avoid contact with eyes, face, meatus or mucous membranes, or irritation may occur
- To discontinue use and notify physician if irritation or sensitization occurs

---

cyanocobalamin (vitamin B₁₂)/hydroxocobalamin (vitamin B₁₂a)

(sye-an-oh-koe-bal′a-min)

Bedoz*, B₁₂ Resin, Cobex, Crystamine, Crysti-12, Cyanabin*, Cyanoject, Cyomin, Ener-B, Pernavite, Redisol, Rubesol-1000, Rubion*, Rubramin PC, Sytobex, Vitamin B₁₂

Func. class.: Vit B₁₂, water-soluble vitamin

Action: Needed for adequate nerve functioning, protein and carbohydrate metabolism, normal growth, RBC development and cell reproduction

Uses: Vit B₁₂ deficiency, pernicious anemia, Vit B₁₂ malabsorption syndrome, Schilling test, increased requirements with pregnancy, thyrotoxicosis, hemolytic anemia, hemorrhage, renal and hepatic disease

Dosage and routes:
- *Adult:* PO 25 μg qd × 5-10 days, maintenance 100-200 mg IM qmo; IM/SC 30-100 μg qd × 5-10 days, maintenance 100-200 μg IM qmo
- *Child:* PO 1 μg qd × 5-10 days, maintenance 60 μg IM qmo or more; IM/SC 1-30 μg qd × 5-10 days, maintenance 60 μg IM qmo or more

Pernicious anemia/malabsorption syndrome
- *Adult:* IM 100-1000 μg qd × 2 wk, then 100-1000 μg IM qmo

- *Child:* IM 100-500 μg over 2 wk or more given in 100-500 μg doses, then 60 μg IM/SC monthly

Schilling test
- *Adult and child:* IM 1000 μg in one dose

Available forms: Tabs 25, 50, 100, 250, 500, 1000 μg; inj IM 100, 120, 1000 μg/ml

Side effects/adverse reactions:
CNS: Flushing, optic nerve atrophy
GI: Diarrhea
CV: **CHF,** peripheral vascular thrombosis, *pulmonary edema*
INTEG: Itching, rash, pain at site
META: Hypokalemia
SUST: Anaphylactic shock

Contraindications: Hypersensitivity, optic nerve atrophy

Precautions: Pregnancy (A), lactation, children

Pharmacokinetics: Stored in liver, kidneys, stomach; 50%-90% excreted in urine; crosses placenta, breast milk

Interactions/incompatibilities:
- Decreased absorption: aminoglycosides, anticonvulsants, colchicine, chloramphenicol, aminosalicylic acid, K preparation, cimetidine
- Increased absorption: prednisone

Lab test interferences:
False positive: Intrinsic factor

NURSING CONSIDERATIONS
Assess:
- GI function: diarrhea, constipation
- K levels during beginning treatment
- CBC for increase in reticulocyte count during 1st week of therapy, then increase in RBC and hemoglobin
- Nutritional status: egg yolks, fish, organ meats, dairy products, clams, oysters, which are good sources for Vit B₁₂

---

italics = common side effects   ***bold italic*** = life threatening reactions

• For pulmonary edema, or worsening of CHF in cardiac patients
Administer:
• With fruit juice to disguise taste; administer immediately after mixing
• With meals if possible for better absorption
• By IM injection for pernicious anemia for life unless contraindicated
• IV route not recommended but may be admixed in TPN solution
Perform/provide:
• Protection from light and heat
Evaluate:
• Therapeutic response: decreased anorexia, dyspnea on exertion, palpitations, paresthesias, psychosis, visual disturbances
Teach patient/family
• That treatment must continue for life if diagnosed as having pernicious anemia
• To eat well-balanced diet
• To avoid contact with persons with infection, since infections are more common
Treatment of overdose: Discontinue drug

---

cyclandelate
(sye-klan'da-late)
Cyclan, Cyclandelate, Cyclospasmol
Func. class.: Peripheral vasodilator
Chem. class.: Nonnitrate

Action: Relaxes vascular smooth muscle, dilates peripheral vascular smooth muscle by direct action
Uses: Intermittent claudication, thrombophlebitis, Raynaud's phenomenon, ischemic cerebrovascular disease, arteriosclerosis obliterans, nocturnal leg cramps

Dosage and routes:
• *Adult:* PO 200 mg qid, not to exceed 400 mg qid; maintenance dose is 400-800 mg/day in 2-4 divided doses
Available forms: Tabs 200, 400 mg; caps 200, 400 mg
Side effects/adverse reactions:
HEMA: Increased bleeding time (rare)
CV: Tachycardia
CNS: Headache, paresthesias, dizziness, weakness
GI: Heartburn, eructation, nausea, pyrosis
INTEG: Sweating, flushing
Contraindications: Hypersensitivity
Precautions: Glaucoma, pregnancy (C), lactation, recent MI, hypertension, severe obliterative coronary artery or cerebrovascular disease
Pharmacokinetics:
PO: Onset 15 min, peak 1½ hr, duration 4 hr
NURSING CONSIDERATIONS
Assess:
• Bleeding time in individuals with bleeding disorders
• Cardiac status: B/P, pulse, rate, rhythm, character; watch for increasing pulse
Administer:
• With meals to reduce GI symptoms
Perform/provide:
• Storage in tight container at room temperature
Evaluate:
• Therapeutic response: ability to walk without pain, increased temperature in extremities, increased pulse volume
Teach patient/family:
• That medication is not cure; may have to be taken continuously
• That it is necessary to quit smok-

ing to prevent excessive vasoconstriction

• That improvement may be sudden but usually occurs gradually over several weeks

• To report headache, weakness, increased pulse, as drug may have to be decreased or discontinued

• To avoid hazardous activities until stabilized on medication; dizziness may occur

cyclizine HCl/ cyclizine lactate

(sye'kli-zeen)
Marezine

Func. class.: Antiemetic, antihistamine, anticholinergic
Chem. class.: H₂-receptor antagonist, piperazine derivative

Action: Acts centrally by blocking chemoreceptor trigger zone, which in turn acts on vomiting center
Uses: Motion sickness, prevention of postoperative vomiting
Dosage and routes:
Vomiting
• *Adult:* IM 50 mg ½ hr before termination of surgery, then q4-6h prn (lactate)
• *Child:* IM 3 mg/kg divided in 3 equal doses
Motion sickness
• *Adult:* PO 50 mg then q4-6h prn, not to exceed 200 mg/day (HCl)
• *Child:* PO 25 mg q4-6h prn
Available forms: Tabs 50 mg; inj 50 mg/ml
Side effects/adverse reactions:
CNS: Drowsiness, dizziness, vertigo, fatigue, restlessness, headache, insomnia, hallucinations (auditory/visual), hallucinations and *convulsions* in children
GI: Nausea, anorexia

EENT: Dry mouth, blurred vision, tinnitus
Contraindications: Hypersensitivity to cyclizines, shock
Precautions: Children, narrow-angle glaucoma, urinary retention, lactation, prostatic hypertrophy, elderly, pregnancy (B)
Pharmacokinetics:
PO: Duration 4-6 hr; other pharmacokinetics not known
Interactions/incompatibilities:
• May increase effect: alcohol, tranquilizers, narcotics
Lab test interferences:
False negative: Allergy skin testing
NURSING CONSIDERATIONS
Assess:
• VS, B/P
• Signs of toxicity of other drugs or masking of symptoms of disease: brain tumor, intestinal obstruction
• Observe for drowsiness, dizziness
Administer:
• IM injection in large muscle mass; aspirate to avoid IV administration
• Tablets may be swallowed whole, chewed, or allowed to dissolve
Evaluate:
• Therapeutic response: absence of motion sickness, vomiting
Teach patient/family:
• That a false-negative result may occur with skin testing; skin testing procedures should not be scheduled for 4 days after discontinuing use
• To avoid hazardous activities or activities requiring alertness; dizziness may occur; instruct patient to request assistance with ambulation
• To avoid alcohol, other depressants

italics = common side effects   ***bold italic*** = life threatening reactions

cyclobenzaprine HCl
(sye-kloe-ben′za-preen)
Cyclobenzaprine HCl, Flexeril
Func. class.: Skeletal muscle relaxant, central acting
Chem. class.: Tricyclic amine salt

Action: Unknown; may be related to antidepressant effects
Uses: Adjunct for relief of muscle spasm and pain in musculoskeletal conditions
Dosage and routes:
• *Adult:* PO 10 mg tid × 1 wk, not to exceed 60 mg/day × 3 wk
Available forms: Tabs 10 mg
Side effects/adverse reactions:
CNS: Dizziness, weakness, drowsiness, headache, tremor, depression, insomnia, confusion, paresthesia
EENT: Diplopia, temporary loss of vision
CV: Postural hypotension, tachycardia, dysrhythmias
GI: Nausea, vomiting, hiccups, dry mouth
INTEG: Rash, pruritus, fever, facial flushing, sweating
GU: Urinary retention, frequency, change in libido
Contraindications: Acute recovery phase of myocardial infarction, dysrhythmias, heart block, CHF, hypersensitivity, child <12 yr, intermittent porphyria, thyroid disease
Precautions: Renal disease, hepatic disease, addictive personality, pregnancy (B), elderly
Pharmacokinetics:
PO: Onset 1 hr, peak 3-8 hr, duration 12-24 hr, half-life 1-3 days; metabolized by liver; excreted in urine; crosses placenta; excreted in breast milk

Interactions/incompatibilities:
• Decreased effects of: guanethidine
• Increased CNS depression: alcohol, tricyclic antidepressants, narcotics, barbiturates, sedatives, hypnotics
• Do not use within 14 days of MAOI
NURSING CONSIDERATIONS
Assess:
• Blood studies: CBC, WBC, differential; blood dyscrasias may occur
• Liver function studies: AST, ALT, alk phosphatase; hepatitis may occur
• ECG in epileptic patients; poor seizure control has occurred with patients taking this drug
• Allergic reactions: rash, fever, respiratory distress
• Severe weakness, numbness in extremities
• Psychologic dependency: increased need for medication, more frequent requests for medication, increased pain
• CNS depression: dizziness, drowsiness, psychiatric symptoms
Administer:
• With meals for GI symptoms
Perform/provide:
• Storage in tight container at room temperature
• Assistance with ambulation if dizziness, drowsiness occur, especially elderly
Evaluate:
• Therapeutic response: decreased pain, spasticity; muscle spasms of acute, painful musculoskeletal conditions are generally short term; long-term therapy is seldom warranted
Teach patient/family:
• Not to discontinue medication quickly; insomnia, nausea, head-

ache, spasticity, tachycardia will occur; drug should be tapered off over 1-2 wk
• Not to take with alcohol, other CNS depressants
• To avoid altering activities while taking this drug
• To avoid hazardous activities if drowsiness/dizziness occurs
• To avoid using OTC medication: cough preparations, antihistamines, unless directed by physician
• To use gum, frequent sips of water for dry mouth

Treatment of overdose: Empty stomach with emesis, gastric lavage, then administer activated charcoal; use anticonvulsants if indicated; monitor cardiac function

---

cyclopentolate HCl (optic)

(sye-kloe-pen'toe-late)
AK-Pentolate, Cyclogyl, Cyclopentolate
Func. class.: Mydriatic, cycloplegic, anticholinergic

Action: Blocks response of iris sphincter muscle, muscle of accommodation of ciliary body to cholinergic stimulation, resulting in dilation, paralysis of accommodation

Uses: Cycloplegic refraction, mydriasis

Dosage and routes:
• *Adult:* INSTILL SOL 1 gtt of a 1-2% sol, then 1 gtt in 5 min
• *Child >6 yr:* INSTILL SOL 1 gtt of a 0.5%-2% sol, then 1 gtt in 5 min of a 0.5%-1% sol
Available forms: Sol 0.5%, 1%, 2%

Side effects/adverse reactions:
SYST: Tachycardia, confusion, fever, flushing, dry skin, dry mouth, abdominal discomfort (infants: bladder distention, irregular pulse, ***respiratory depression***)
EENT: Blurred vision, temporary burning sensation on instillation, eye dryness, photophobia, conjunctivitis, increased intraocular pressure
CNS: Psychotic reaction, behavior disturbances, ataxia, restlessness, hallucinations, somnolence, disorientation, failure to recognize people, ***grand mal seizures,*** irritability
GI: Abdominal distention, vomiting

Contraindications: Hypersensitivity, infants <3 mo, open or narrow glaucoma, conjunctivitis

Precautions: Pregnancy (C), elderly, lactation, children, Down syndrome

Pharmacokinetics:
INSTILL: Peak 30-60 min (mydriasis), 25-74 min (cycloplegia), duration ¼-1 day

NURSING CONSIDERATIONS
Administer:
• After shaking vial to mix drug to clear solution, push stopper to mix sterile water with powder
• After cleaning stopper with alcohol (rubbing)
• Immediately after reconstituting, discard unused portion

Evaluate:
• Therapeutic response: mydriasis

Teach patient/family:
• To report change in vision, blurring, or loss of sight, trouble breathing, sweating, flushing
• Method of instillation: pressure on lacrimal sac for 1 min; do not touch dropper to eye
• That blurred vision will decrease with repeated use of drug
• That drug will burn when instilled

---

italics = common side effects   ***bold italic*** = life threatening reactions

• To wear dark sunglasses for photophobia
• Not to do hazardous activities until able to see

---

cyclophosphamide

(sye-kloe-foss'fa-mide)
Cytoxan, Neosar, Procytox*
Func. class.: Antineoplastic alkylating agent
Chem. class.: Nitrogen mustard

Action: Alkylates DNA, RNA; inhibits enzymes that allow synthesis of amino acids in proteins; is also responsible for cross-linking DNA strands, breast neuroblastoma; activity is not cell cycle phase specific
Uses: Hodgkin's disease; lymphomas; leukemia; cancer of female reproductive tract, lung, prostate; multiple myeloma; neuroblastoma; retinoblastoma; Ewing's sarcoma
Dosage and routes:
• *Adult:* PO initially 1-5 mg/kg over 2-5 days, maintenance is 1-5 mg/kg; IV initially 40-50 mg/kg in divided doses over 2-5 days, maintenance 10-15 mg/kg q7-10 days, or 3-5 mg/kg q3 days
• *Child:* PO/IV 2-8 mg/kg or 60-250 mg/m^2 in divided doses for 6 or more days; maintenance 10-15 mg/kg q7-10 days or 30 mg/kg q3-4 wk; dose should be reduced by half when bone marrow depression occurs
Available forms: Powder for inj IV 100, 200, 500 mg, 1, 2 g; tabs 25, 50 mg
Side effects/adverse reactions:
CV: Cardiotoxicity (high doses)
HEMA: Thrombocytopenia, leukopenia, pancytopenia; myelosuppression
GI: Nausea, vomiting, diarrhea, weight loss, colitis, *hepatotoxicity*

GU: Hemorrhagic cystitis, hematuria, neoplasms, amenorrhea, azoospermia, sterility, ovarian fibrosis
INTEG: Alopecia, dermatitis
RESP: Fibrosis
ENDO: Syndrome of inappropriate antidiuretic hormone (SIADH)
CNS: Headache, dizziness
Contraindications: Lactation, pregnancy (D)
Precautions: Radiation therapy
Pharmacokinetics:
Metabolized by liver; excreted in urine; half-life 4-6½ hr; 50% bound to plasma proteins
Interactions/incompatibilities:
• Increased toxicity: aminoglycosides
• Increased metabolism of cyclophosphamide: phenobarbital
• Potentiation of cyclophosphamide: succinylcholine
• Increased bone marrow depression: allopurinol, thiazides
• Decreased digoxin levels: digoxin
• Incompatibility information unknown, give separately
Lab test interferences:
Increase: Uric acid
False positive: Pap test
False negative: PPD, mumps trichophytin, *Candida*
Decrease: Pseudocholinesterase
NURSING CONSIDERATIONS
Assess:
• CBC, differential, platelet count weekly; withhold drug if WBC is <4000 or platelet count is <75,000; notify physician of results
• Pulmonary function tests, chest x-ray films before, during therapy; chest film should be obtained q2 wk during treatment
• Renal function studies: BUN, se-

---

rum uric acid, urine CrCl before, during therapy

• I&O ratio; report fall in urine output of 30 ml/hr

• Monitor temperature q4h (may indicate beginning infection)

• Liver function tests before, during therapy (bilirubin, AST, ALT, LDH) as needed or monthly

• Bleeding: hematuria, guaiac, bruising or petechiae, mucosa or orifices q8h

• Dyspnea, rales, unproductive cough, chest pain, tachypnea

• Food preferences; list likes, dislikes

• Effects of alopecia on body image, discuss feelings about body changes

• Yellowing of skin, sclera; dark urine; clay-colored stools; itchy skin; abdominal pain; fever; diarrhea

• Edema in feet, joint pain, stomach pain, shaking

• Inflammation of mucosa, breaks in skin

• Buccal cavity q8h for dryness, sores or ulceration, white patches, oral pain, bleeding, dysphagia; obtain prescription for viscous lidocaine (Xylocaine)

• Symptoms indicating severe allergic reaction: rash, pruritus, urticaria, purpuric skin lesions, itching, flushing

• Tachypnea, ECG changes, dyspnea, edema, fatigue

Administer:

• Fluids IV or PO before chemotherapy to hydrate patient

• Antacid before oral agent, give drug after evening meal, before bedtime

• Antiemetic 30-60 min before giving drug to prevent vomiting, and prn

• Allopurinol or sodium bicarbon-ate to maintain uric acid levels, alkalinization of urine

• Prevent hyperuricemia

• Antibiotics for prophylaxis of infection

• IV after diluting 100 mg/5 ml of sterile H_2O or bacteriostatic H_2O; shake; let stand until clear; may be further diluted in up to 250 ml D_5 or NS; give 100 mg or less/min through 3-way stopcock of glucose or saline inf

• Using 21-, 23-, 25-gauge needle; check site for irritation, phlebitis

• Topical or systemic analgesics for pain

• Local or systemic drugs for infection

• In AM so drug can be eliminated before hs

Perform/provide:

• Storage in tight container at room temperature

• Strict medical asepsis, protective isolation if WBC levels are low

• Special skin care

• Deep-breathing exercises with patient tid-qid; place in semi-Fowler's position

• Increase fluid intake to 2-3 L/day to prevent urate deposits, calculi formation, reduce incidence of hemorrhagic cystitis

• Diet low in purines: organ meats (kidney, liver), dried beans, peas to maintain alkaline urine

• Rinsing of mouth tid-qid with water, club soda; brushing of teeth bid-tid with soft brush or cotton-tipped applicators for stomatitis; use unwaxed dental floss

• Warm compresses at injection site for inflammation

Evaluate:

• Therapeutic response: decreased tumor size, spread of malignancy

Teach patient/family:

• Of protective isolation precautions

---

italics = common side effects   ***bold italic*** = life threatening reactions

• That amenorrhea can occur; reversible after discontinuing treatment
• To report any changes in breathing or coughing
• That hair may be lost during treatment; a wig or hairpiece may make patient feel better; new hair may be different in color, texture
• To avoid foods with citric acid, hot or rough texture
• To report any bleeding, white spots, ulcerations in mouth to physician; tell patient to examine mouth qd
• To report signs of infection: increased temperature, sore throat, flu symptoms
• To report signs of anemia: fatigue, headache, faintness, shortness of breath, irritability
• To report bleeding: avoid use of razors, or commercial mouthwash
• To avoid use of aspirin products or ibuprofen

---

cycloserine

(sye-kloe-ser′een)
Seromycin Pulvules
Func. class.: Antitubercular
Chem. class.: S. orchidaceus,
antibiotic

Action: Inhibits cell wall synthesis, analog of D-alanine
Uses: Pulmonary tuberculosis, extrapulmonary as adjunctive
Dosage and routes:
• *Adult:* PO 250 mg q12h × 14 days, then 250 mg q8h × 2 wk if there are no signs of toxicity, then 250 mg q6h if there are no signs of toxicity, not to exceed 1 g/day
• *Child:* PO 10-20 mg/kg/day (max 0.75-1 g) individual doses
Available forms: Caps 250 mg

Side effects/adverse reactions:
INTEG: Dermatitis, photosensitivity
CV: **CHF**
CNS: Headache, anxiety, drowsiness, tremors, **convulsions,** lethargy, depression, confusion, psychosis, aggression
HEMA: **Megaloblastic anemia,** Vit B$_{12}$, folic acid deficiency, leukocytosis
Contraindications: Hypersensitivity, seizure disorders, renal disease, alcoholism (chronic), depression, severe anxiety, lactation, anemia
Precautions: Pregnancy (C), children
Pharmacokinetics:
PO: Peak 3-8 hr; excreted unchanged in urine; crosses placenta; excreted in breast milk
Interactions/incompatibilities:
• Seizures: alcohol
• May increase CNS toxicity: isoniazid, ethionamide
Lab test interferences:
Increase: AST/ALT
NURSING CONSIDERATIONS
Assess:
• Liver studies qwk: ALT, AST, bilirubin
• Blood levels of drug; keep at <30 μg/ml or toxicity may occur
• Mental status often: affect, mood, behavioral changes, psychosis may occur
Administer:
• Using pipette provided; use glass container to prevent adherence to sides
• After C&S is completed, qmo to detect resistance
• Pyridoxine (200-300 mg/day) if ordered to prevent neurotoxicity
Perform/provide:
• Storage in tight container at room temperature
Evaluate:
• Therapeutic response: decreased symptoms of TB

Teach patient/family:
• To avoid alcohol while taking drug
• That compliance with dosage schedule, length is necessary
• To report neurotoxicity: confusion, headache, drowsiness, tremors, paresthesias, mental changes
• To avoid hazardous activities if drowsiness or dizziness occurs
Treatment of overdose: Administer Vit B₆, anticonvulsants, lavage, O₂, assisted respiration

cyclosporine
(sye'kloe-spor-een)
Sandimmune
Func. class.: Immunosuppressant
Chem. class.: Fungus-derived peptide

Action: Produces immunosuppression by inhibiting lymphocytes (T)
Uses: Organ transplants to prevent rejection
Dosage and routes:
• *Adult and child:* PO 15 mg/kg several hours before surgery, daily for 2 wk, reduce dosage by 2.5 mg/kg/wk to 5-10 mg/kg/day; IV 5-6 mg/kg several hours before surgery, daily, switch to PO form as soon as possible
Available forms: Oral sol 100 mg/ml; inj IV 50 mg/ml
Side effects/adverse reactions:
GI: Nausea, vomiting, diarrhea, *oral Candida, gum hyperplasia, hepatotoxicity,* pancreatitis
INTEG: Rash, acne, *hirsutism*
CNS: Tremors, headache
GU: **Albuminuria, hematuria, proteinuria, renal failure**
Contraindications: Hypersensitivity
Precautions: Severe renal disease,

severe hepatic disease, pregnancy (C)
Pharmacokinetics: Peak 4 hr, highly protein bound, half-life (biphasic) 1.2 hr, 25 hr; metabolized in liver; excreted in feces; crosses placenta; excreted in breast milk
Interactions/incompatibilities:
• Increased action of cyclosporine: amphotericin B, cimetidine, ketoconazole
• Decreased action of cyclosporine: phenytoin, rifampin
• Compatibility information unknown; give separately
NURSING CONSIDERATIONS
Assess:
• Renal studies: BUN, creatinine at least monthly during treatment, 3 mo after treatment
• Liver function studies: alk phosphatase, AST, ALT, bilirubin
• Drug blood levels during treatment
• Hepatotoxicity: dark urine, jaundice, itching, light-colored stools; drug should be discontinued
Administer:
• IV after diluting each 50 mg/20-100 ml of normal saline or D₅W; run over 2-6 hr; use an infusion pump, glass inf bottles only
• For several days before transplant surgery
• With corticosteroids
• With meals for GI upset or drug placed in chocolate milk
• With oral antifungal for *Candida* infections
Evaluate:
• Therapeutic response: absence of rejection
Teach patient/family:
• To report fever, chills, sore throat, fatigue, since serious infections may occur
• To use contraceptive measures

italics = common side effects   ***bold italic*** = life threatening reactions

during treatment, for 12 wk after ending therapy

---

cyproheptadine HCl
(si-proe-hep'-ta-deen)
Cyproheptadine HCl, Periactin, Vimicon*

Func. class.: Antihistamine, H₁-receptor antagonist

Chem. class.: Piperidine

Action: Acts on blood vessels, GI, respiratory system by competing with histamine for H₁-receptor site; decreases allergic response by blocking histamine

Uses: Allergy symptoms, rhinitis, pruritus, cold urticaria

Dosage and routes:
• *Adult:* PO 4 mg tid-qid, not to exceed 0.5 mg/kg/day
• *Child 7-14 yr:* PO 4 mg bid-tid, not to exceed 16 mg/day
• *Child 2-6 yr:* PO 2 mg bid-tid, not to exceed 12 mg/day

Available forms: Tabs 4 mg; syr 2 mg/5 ml

Side effects/adverse reactions:

CNS: Dizziness, drowsiness, poor coordination, fatigue, anxiety, euphoria, confusion, paresthesia, neuritis

CV: Hypotension, palpitations, tachycardia

RESP: Increased thick secretions, wheezing, chest tightness

GI: Constipation, dry mouth, nausea, vomiting, anorexia, diarrhea, weight gain

INTEG: Rash, urticaria, photosensitivity

GU: Retention, dysuria, frequency, increased appetite

EENT: Blurred vision, dilated pupils; tinnitus; nasal stuffiness; dry nose, throat, mouth

Contraindications: Hypersensitivity to H₁-receptor antagonist, acute asthma attack, lower respiratory tract disease

Precautions: Increased intraocular pressure, renal disease, cardiac disease, hypertension, bronchial asthma, seizure disorder, stenosed peptic ulcers, hyperthyroidism, prostatic hypertrophy, bladder neck obstruction, pregnancy (B), elderly

Pharmacokinetics:
PO: Duration 4-6 hr; metabolized in liver; excreted by kidneys; excreted in breast milk

Interactions/incompatibilities:
• Increased CNS depression: barbiturates, narcotics, hypnotics, tricyclic antidepressants, alcohol
• Decreased effect of: oral anticoagulants, heparin
• Increased effect of cyproheptadine: MAOIs

Lab test interferences:
False negative: Skin allergy tests

NURSING CONSIDERATIONS

Assess:
• I&O ratio; be alert for urinary retention, frequency, dysuria; drug should be discontinued if these occur
• CBC during long-term therapy
• Respiratory status: rate, rhythm, increase in bronchial secretions, wheezing, chest tightness
• Cardiac status: palpitations, increased pulse, hypotension

Administer:
• With meals if GI symptoms occur; absorption may slightly decrease

Perform/provide:
• Hard candy, gum, frequent rinsing of mouth for dryness
• Storage in tight container at room temperature

Evaluate:
• Therapeutic response: absence of running or congested nose or rashes

---

*Available in Canada only

Teach patient/family:
- All aspects of drug use; to notify physician if confusion, sedation, hypotension occurs
- That this drug decreases anticoagulant (oral) effect
- To avoid driving or other hazardous activity if drowsiness occurs, especially elderly
- To avoid concurrent use of alcohol or other CNS depressants

Treatment of overdose: Administer ipecac syrup or lavage, diazepam, vasopressors, barbiturates (short-acting)

---

cytarabine (ARA-C, cytosine arabinoside)

(sye-tare′a-been)
Cytarabine, Cytosar-U, Tarabine PFS

Func. class.: Antineoplastic, antimetabolite
Chem. class.: Pyrimidine nucleoside

Action: Competes with physiologic substrate of DNA synthesis, thus interfering with cell replication in the S phase of the cell cycle (before mitosis)

Uses: Acute myelocytic leukemia, acute lymphocytic leukemia, chronic myelocytic leukemia, and in combination for non-Hodgkin's lymphomas in children

Dosage and routes:
Acute myelocytic leukemia
- *Adult:* IV INF 200 mg/m^2/day × 5 days; INTRATHECAL 5-50 mg/m^2/day × 3 days/wk or 30 mg/m^2/day q4d
In combination
- *Child:* IV INF 100 mg/m^2/day × 5-10 days

Available forms: Inj IV, intrathecal 100, 500 mg, 1, 2 g

Side effects/adverse reactions:
HEMA: Thrombophlebitis, bleeding, **thrombocytopenia, leukopenia, myelosuppression, anemia**
GI: Nausea, vomiting, anorexia, diarrhea, stomatitis, **hepatotoxicity,** abdominal pain, hematemesis, **GI hemorrhage**
EENT: Sore throat, conjunctivitis
GU: Urinary retention, **renal failure, hyperuricemia**
INTEG: Rash, fever, freckling, cellulitis
RESP: **Pneumonia,** dyspnea
CV: Chest pain, **cardiopathy**
CNS: Neuritis, dizziness, headache, personality changes, ataxia, mechanical dysphasia, **coma**
CYTARABINE SYNDROME: Fever, myalgia, bone pain, chest pain, rash, conjunctivitis, malaise (6-12 hr after administration)

Contraindications: Hypersensitivity, infants, pregnancy (1st trimester)

Precautions: Renal disease, hepatic disease, pregnancy (C)

Pharmacokinetics:
INTRATHECAL: Half-life 2 hr; metabolized in liver; excreted in urine (primarily inactive metabolite); crosses blood-brain barrier, placenta
IV: Distribution half-life 10 min, elimination half-life 1-3 hr

Interactions/incompatibilities:
- Increased toxicity: radiation or other antineoplastics
- Decreased effects of: oral digoxin
- Incompatible with methylprednisolone sodium succinate, fluorouracil

NURSING CONSIDERATIONS
Assess:
- CBC (RBC, Hct, Hgb), differential, platelet count weekly; withhold drug if WBC is <4000/mm,^{3} platelet count is <75,000/mm,^{3} or

---

italics = common side effects   ***bold italic*** = life threatening reactions

RBC, Hct, Hgb are low; notify physician of these results
• Renal function studies: BUN, serum uric acid, urine creatinine clearance, electrolytes before and during therapy
• I&O ratio; report fall in urine output to <30 ml/hr
• Monitor temperature q4h; fever may indicate beginning infection; no rectal temperatures
• Liver function tests before and during therapy: bilirubin, ALT, AST, alk phosphatase, as needed or monthly
• Blood uric acid levels during therapy
• Cytarabine syndrome: fever, myalgia, bone pain, chest pain, rash, conjunctivitis, malaise; corticosteroids may be ordered
• Bleeding: hematuria, guaiac, bruising or petechiae, mucosa or orifices q8h
• Dyspnea, rales, unproductive cough, chest pain, tachypnea, fatigue, increased pulse, pallor, lethargy, personality changes, with high doses
• Food preferences; list likes, dislikes
• Edema in feet, joint pain, stomach pain, shaking
• Inflammation of mucosa, breaks in skin
• Yellowing of skin, sclera; dark urine; clay-colored stools; itchy skin; abdominal pain; fever; diarrhea
• Buccal cavity q8h for dryness, sores or ulceration, white patches, oral pain, bleeding, dysphagia
• Local irritation, pain, burning, discoloration at injection site
• GI symptoms: frequency of stools, cramping
• Acidosis, signs of dehydration: rapid respirations, poor skin turgor, decreased urine output, dry skin, restlessness, weakness

Administer:
• IV after diluting 100 mg/5 ml of sterile H_2O for inj; given by direct IV over 1-3 min through free-flowing tubing (IV); may be further diluted in 50-100 ml normal saline or D_5W and given over 30 min to 24° depending on dose
• Antiemetic 30-60 min before giving drug to prevent vomiting, and prn
• Allopurinol or sodium bicarbonate to maintain uric acid levels and alkalinization of the urine
• Prevent hyperuricemia
• Topical or systemic analgesics for pain
• Transfusion for anemia
• Antispasmodic for GI symptoms

Perform/provide:
• Strict medical asepsis and protective isolation if WBC levels are low
• Increase fluid intake to 2-3 L/day to prevent urate deposits and calculi formation, unless contraindicated
• Diet low in purines: absence of organ meats (kidney, liver), dried beans, peas to prevent increased urate deposits
• Rinsing of mouth tid-qid with water, club soda; brushing of teeth bid-tid with soft brush or cotton-tipped applicators for stomatitis; use unwaxed dental floss
• HOB increased to facilitate breathing if dyspnea or pneumonia occurs

Evaluate:
• Therapeutic response: decreased tumor size, spread of malignancy

Teach patient/family:
• Why protective isolation precautions are necessary
• To report any coughing, chest pain, or changes in breathing,

which may indicate beginning pneumonia
• To avoid foods with citric acid, hot or rough texture if stomatitis is present
• To report stomatitis: any bleeding, white spots, ulcerations in mouth; tell patient to examine mouth qd, report any symptoms
• To report signs of infection: increased temperature, sore throat, flu symptoms
• To report signs of anemia: fatigue, headache, faintness, shortness of breath, irritability
• To report bleeding; avoid use of razors or commercial mouthwash
• To avoid use of aspirin products or ibuprofen

dacarbazine (DTIC)
(da-kar′ba-zeen)
DTIC-Dome
Func. class.: Antineoplastic alkylating agent
Chem. class.: Cytotoxic triazine

Action: Alkylates DNA, RNA; inhibits enzymes that allow synthesis of amino acids in proteins; also responsible for cross-linking DNA strands; activity is not cell cycle phase specific
Uses: Hodgkin's disease, sarcomas, neuroblastoma, malignant melanoma
Dosage and routes:
• *Adult:* IV 2-4.5 mg/kg or 70-160 mg/m^2 qd × 10 days; repeat q4wk depending on response or 250 mg/m^2 qd × 5 days; repeat q3wk
Available forms: Inj IV 100, 200 mg
Side effects/adverse reactions:
*HEMA: **Thrombocytopenia, leukopenia,** anemia*

*GI: Nausea, anorexia, vomiting, **hepatotoxicity***
CNS: Facial paresthesia, flushing, fever, malaise
INTEG: Alopecia, dermatitis, pain at injection site
Contraindications: Lactation
Precautions: Radiation therapy, pregnancy (1st trimester) (C)
Pharmacokinetics:
Metabolized by liver; excreted in urine; half-life 35 min, terminal 5 hr, 5% protein bound
Interactions/incompatibilities:
• Decreased effectiveness of dacarbazine: phenytoin, phenobarbital
• Incompatible heparin, hydrocortisone, lidocaine
• Considered incompatible in sol or syringe with any drug
NURSING CONSIDERATIONS
Assess:
• CBC, differential, platelet count weekly; withhold drug if WBC is <4000 or platelet count is <75,000; notify physician of results
• Monitor temperature q4h (may indicate beginning infection)
• Liver function tests before, during therapy (bilirubin, AST, ALT, LDH) as needed or monthly
• Bleeding: hematuria, guaiac, bruising or petechiae, mucosa or orifices q8h
• Food preferences; list likes, dislikes
• Effects of alopecia on body image, discuss feelings about body changes
• Yellowing of skin, sclera; dark urine; clay-colored stools; itchy skin; abdominal pain; fever; diarrhea
• Inflammation of mucosa, breaks in skin

italics = common side effects   ***bold italic*** = life threatening reactions

Administer:

• Antiemetic 30-60 min before giving drug to prevent vomiting

• Antibiotics for prophylaxis of infection

• After diluting 100 mg/9.9 ml of sterile H₂O for inj (10 mg/ml), give by direct IV over 1 min through Y-tube or 3-way stopcock; may be further diluted in 50-250 ml of D₅W or normal saline for inj and given as an inf over ½ hr

• Watch for extravasation; give Na thiosulfate 10% 4 ml plus sterile H₂O 5 ml 3-5 ml SC if needed

Perform/provide:

• Storage in light-resistant container, dry area

• Strict medical asepsis, protective isolation if WBC levels are low

• Increase fluid intake to 2-3 L/day to prevent urate deposits, calculi formation

• Warm compresses at injection site for inflammation

Evaluate:

• Therapeutic response: decreased tumor size, spread of malignancy

Teach patient/family:

• Of protective isolation precautions

• Advise patient to avoid prolonged exposure to sun

• That hair may be lost during treatment; a wig or hairpiece may make the patient feel better; new hair may be different in color, texture

• To report signs of infection: increased temperature, sore throat, flu symptoms

• To report signs of anemia: fatigue, headache, faintness, shortness of breath, irritability

• To report bleeding; avoid use of razors or commercial mouthwash

• To avoid use of aspirin products or ibuprofen

dactinomycin (actinomycin D)

(dak-ti-noe-mye'sin)
Cosmegen
Func. class.: Antineoplastic, antibiotic

Action: Inhibits DNA, RNA, protein synthesis; derived from *S. parrullus;* replication is decreased by binding to DNA, which causes strand splitting; cell cycle nonspecific; a vesicant

Uses: Sarcomas, melanomas, trophoblastic tumors in women, testicular cancer, Wilms' tumor, rhabdomyosarcoma

Dosage and routes:

• *Adult:* IV 500 μg/m²/day × 5 days; stop drug for 2-4 wk; then repeat cycle

• *Child:* IV 15 μg/kg/day × 5 days, not to exceed 500 μg/day; stop drug until bone marrow recovery, then repeat cycle

Available forms: Inj IV 0.5 mg/vial

Side effects/adverse reactions:

*HEMA: **Thrombocytopenia, leukopenia, aplastic anemia***

*GI: Nausea, vomiting, anorexia, stomatitis, **hepatotoxicity,** abdominal pain, diarrhea*

*INTEG: Rash, alopecia, pain at injection site, folliculitis, acne, desquamation, **extravasation***

EENT: Chelitis, dysphagia, esophagitis

CNS: Malaise, fatigue, lethargy, fever

MS: Myalgia

Contraindications: Hypersensitivity, herpes infections, child <6 months

Precautions: Renal disease, hepatic disease, pregnancy (C), lac-

tation, bone marrow depression
Pharmacokinetics: Half-life 36 hr
IV: onset 2-5 min; concentrates in
kidneys, liver, spleen; does not
cross blood-brain barrier; excreted
in feces and urine
Interactions/incompatibilities:
• Increased toxicity: other antineo-
plastics or radiation
• Considered incompatible in sol or
syringe with any drug
Lab test interferences:
Increase: Uric acid

NURSING CONSIDERATIONS
Assess:
• CBC, differential, platelet count
weekly; withhold drug if WBC is
<4000/mm^3 or platelet count is
<75,000/mm^3; notify physician of
these results
• Renal function studies: BUN, serum uric acid, urine CrCl, electrolytes before, during therapy
• I&O ratio; report fall in urine output to <30 ml/hr
• Monitor temperature q4h; fever
may indicate beginning infection
• Liver function tests before, during therapy: bilirubin, AST, ALT,
alk phosphatase, as needed or
monthly
• Bleeding: hematuria, guaiac
stools, bruising, petechiae, mucosa
or orifices q8h
• Food preferences; list likes, dislikes
• Effects of alopecia on body image; discuss feelings about body
changes
• Inflammation of mucosa, breaks
in skin
• Yellowing of skin, sclera; dark
urine; clay-colored stools; itchy
skin; abdominal pain; fever; diarrhea
• Buccal cavity q8h for dryness,
sores, ulceration, white patches,
oral pain, bleeding, dysphagia

• Local irritation, pain, burning at
injection site
• Symptoms indicating severe allergic reaction: rash, pruritus, urticaria, purpuric skin lesions, itching, flushing
• GI symptoms: frequency of
stools, cramping
• Acidosis, signs of dehydration:
rapid respirations, poor skin turgor,
decreased urine output, dry skin,
restlessness, weakness
Administer:
• After diluting 0.5 mg/1.1 ml of
sterile H$_2$O for inj without preservative; use 2.2 ml (0.25 mg/ml),
give by direct IV at 0.5 mg or less/
min through Y-tube or 3-way stopcock of inf in progress; may be further diluted in 50 ml D$_5$W or normal
saline for infusion; run over 10-15
min
• Antiemetic 30-60 min before giving drug to prevent vomiting
• Check for extravasation
• Topical or systemic analgesics for
pain
• Local or systemic drugs for infection
• Hydrocortisone, sodium thiosulfate to infiltration area, and ice
compress after stopping infusion
• Antispasmodic for GI symptoms
Perform/provide:
• Strict hand-washing technique,
gloves and protective covering
• Liquid diet: carbonated beverages; gelatin may be added if patient is not nauseated or vomiting
• Rinsing of mouth tid-qid with
water, club soda; brushing of teeth
bid-qid with soft brush or cotton-
tipped applicators for stomatitis;
use unwaxed dental floss
• Storage in darkness in cool environment
Evaluate:
• Therapeutic response: decreased
tumor size, spread of malignancy

Teach patient/family:
• To report any complaints, side effects to nurse or physician
• That hair may be lost during treatment and wig or hairpiece may make patient feel better; tell patient that new hair may be different in color, texture
• To avoid foods with citric acid, hot or rough texture
• To report any bleeding, white spots, ulcerations in mouth to physician; tell patient to examine mouth qd
• To avoid crowds and sources of infection when granulocyte count is low

---

danazol

(da′na-zole)
Cyclomen,* Danazol, Danocrine
Func. class.: Androgen
Chem. class.: α-Ethinyl testosterone derivative

Action: Atrophy of endometrial tissue; decreases FSH, LH, which are controlled by pituitary; this leads to amenorrhea/anovulation
Uses: Endometriosis, prevention of hereditary angioedema, fibrocystic breast disease
Dosage and routes:
Endometriosis
• *Adult:* PO initial dose 500 mg bid, then decreased to 400 mg bid × 3-9 mo
Fibrocystic breast disease
• *Adult:* PO 100-400 mg qd in 2 divided doses × 2-6 mo
Hereditary angioedema
• *Adult:* PO 200 mg bid-tid until desired response, then decrease dose to 100 mg at 1-3 mo intervals
Available forms: Caps 50, 100, 200 mg

Side effects/adverse reactions:
INTEG: Rash, acneiform lesions, oily hair, skin, flushing, sweating, acne vulgaris, alopecia, hirsutism
CNS: Dizziness, headache, fatigue, tremors, paresthesias, flushing, sweating, anxiety, lability, insomnia, carpal tunnel syndrome
MS: Cramps, spasms
CV: Increased B/P
GU: Hematuria, amenorrhea, atrophic vaginitis, decreased libido, decreased breast size, clitoral hypertrophy, testicular atrophy
GI: Nausea, vomiting, constipation, weight gain, *cholestatic jaundice*
EENT: Conjunctional edema, nasal congestion
ENDO: Abnormal GTT
Contraindications: Severe renal disease, severe cardiac disease, severe hepatic disease, hypersensitivity, genital bleeding (abnormal)
Precautions: Migraine headaches, seizure disorders, pregnancy (C)
Interactions/incompatibilities:
• Increased effects of: oral antidiabetics, oxyphenbutazone
• Increased prothrombin time: anticoagulants
• Edema: ACTH, adrenal steroids
• Decreased effects of: insulin
Lab test interferences:
Increase: Cholesterol
Decrease: Cholesterol, T_4, T_3, thyroid ^{131}I uptake test, 17-KS, PBI
Interferences: GTT
NURSING CONSIDERATIONS
Assess:
• K, blood sugar, urine glucose while on long-term therapy
• Weight daily; notify physician if weekly weight gain is >5 lb
• I&O ratio; be alert for decreasing urinary output, increasing edema
• Edema, hypertension, cardiac symptoms, jaundice

• Mental status: affect, mood, behavioral changes, aggression, sleep disorders, depression
• Signs of virilization: deepening of voice, decreased libido, facial hair (may not be reversible)
• Hypercalcemia: GI symptoms, polydipsia, polyuria, increased calcium levels, decrease in muscle tone

Administer:
• With food or milk to decrease GI symptoms

Perform/provide:
• Storage in tight container at room temperature
• ROM exercise for patients who are immobile

Evaluate:
• Therapeutic response: decreased pain in endometriosis; decreased size, pain in fibrocystic breast disease

Teach patient/family:
• To notify physician if therapeutic response decreases
• Not to discontinue medication abruptly but to taper over several weeks
• To report menstrual irregularities; that amenorrhea usually occurs but menstruation resumes 2-3 mo after termination of therapy
• About routine breast self-exam, report any increase in nodule size
• That drug should induce anovulation; reversible within 60-90 days after drug is discontinued
• That endometriosis tends to recur after drug is discontinued

---

dantrolene sodium
(dan'troe-leen)
Dantrium, Dantrium Intravenous
Func. class.: Skeletal muscle relaxant, direct acting
Chem. class.: Hydantoin

D

Action: Interferes with intracellular release of calcium necessary to initiate contraction

Uses: Spasticity in multiple sclerosis, stroke, spinal cord injury, cerebral palsy, malignant hyperthermia

Dosage and routes:
Spasticity
• *Adult:* PO 25 mg/day; may increase by 25-100 mg bid-qid, not to exceed 400 mg/day × 1 wk
• *Child:* PO 1 mg/kg/day given in divided doses bid-tid; may increase gradually, not to exceed 100 mg qid
Malignant hyperthermia
• *Adult and child:* IV 1 mg/kg, may repeat to total dose of 10 mg/kg; PO 4-8 mg/kg/day in 4 divided doses × 3 days to prevent further hyperthermia

Available forms: Caps 25, 50, 100 mg; powder for inj IV 20 mg/vial

Side effects/adverse reactions:
CNS: Dizziness, weakness, fatigue, drowsiness, headache, disorientation, insomnia, paresthesias, tremors
EENT: Nasal congestion, blurred vision, mydriasis
*HEMA: **Eosinophilia***
CV: Hypotension, chest pain, palpitations
GI: Nausea, constipation, vomiting, increased AST, alk phosphatase, abdominal pain, dry mouth, anorexia, hepatitis
GU: Urinary frequency, nocturia, impotence, crystalluria

---

italics = common side effects   ***bold italic*** = life threatening reactions

INTEG: Rash, pruritus, photosensitivity

Contraindications: Hypersensitivity, compromised pulmonary function, active hepatic disease, impaired myocardial function

Precautions: Peptic ulcer disease, renal disease, hepatic disease, stroke, seizure disorder, diabetes mellitus, pregnancy (C), elderly

Pharmacokinetics:

PO: Peak 5 hr; highly protein bound; half-life 8 hr; metabolized in liver; excreted in urine (metabolites)

Interactions/incompatibilities:

• Increased CNS depression: alcohol, tricyclic antidepressants, narcotics, barbiturates, sedatives, hypnotics

• Considered incompatible in sol or syringe; compatibility information unknown

NURSING CONSIDERATIONS

Assess:

• For increased seizure activity in epilepsy patient

• I&O ratio; check for urinary retention, frequency, hesitancy, especially elderly

• ECG in epileptic patients; poor seizure control has occurred with patients taking this drug

• Hepatic function by frequent determination of AST, ALT, renal function studies, CBC

• Allergic reactions: rash, fever, respiratory distress

• Severe weakness, numbness in extremities

• Psychologic dependency: increased need for medication, more frequent requests for medication, increased pain

• CNS depression: dizziness, drowsiness, psychiatric symptoms

• Signs of hepatitis: jaundice, yellow sclera, pain in abdomen, nausea, fever

Administer:

• With meals for GI symptoms

• IV after diluting 20 mg/60 ml sterile H_2O for inj without bacteriostatic agent; shake until clear; give by rapid IV push through Y-tube or 3-way stopcock; follow by prescribed doses immediately

Perform/provide:

• Storage in tight container at room temperature

• Gum, frequent sips of water for dry mouth

• Assistance with ambulation if dizziness/drowsiness occurs

Evaluate:

• Therapeutic response: decreased pain, spasticity

Teach patient/family:

• Not to discontinue medication quickly; hallucinations, spasticity, tachycardia will occur; drug should be tapered off over 1-2 wk; notify physician of abdominal pain, jaundiced sclera, clay-colored stools, change in color of urine

• Not to take with alcohol, other CNS depressants

• That if improvement does not occur within 6 wk, physician may discontinue

• To avoid altering activities while taking this drug

• To avoid hazardous activities if drowsiness, dizziness occurs

• To avoid using OTC medication: cough preparations, antihistamines, unless directed by physician

Treatment of overdose: Induce emesis of conscious patient; lavage, dialysis

---

dapiprazole HCl
Rev-Eyes

Func. class.: Ophthalmic α-adrenergic blocking agents

Action: Blocks α-adrenergic receptors in smooth muscle in the eye; miosis occurs through effect on the iris dilator muscle

Uses: Iatrogenically induces mydriasis produced by adrenergic or parasympatholytic agents

Dosage and routes:
• *Adult:* Instill 2 gtts, then 2 gtts 5 min later applied to the conjunctiva; do not use more than once a week

Available forms: Pwd for lyophilized 25 mg (0.5% sol reconstituted)

Side effects/adverse reactions:
EENT: Burning, ptosis, lid erythema, lid edema, itching, keratitis, corneal edema; browache, photophobia, headaches, eye dryness, tearing, blurring vision

Contraindications: Hypersensitivity, acute iritis

Precautions: Pregnancy (B), lactation, children, severe cardiovascular disease

NURSING CONSIDERATIONS
Assess:
• Cardiac status; watch for bradycardia, palpitations, especially in cardiac disease (including hypertension)

Administer:
• By instillation after tearing off aluminum seals; remove and discard rubber plugs from drugs and diluent; remove dropper and attach to vial; shake

Perform/provide:
• Storage at room temperature after reconstituting × 21 days

Teach patient/family:
• That drug may cause burning, itching, blurring dryness of eye

---

dapsone (DDS)
(dap′sone)
Avlosulfon*, Dapsone
Func. class.: Leprostatic
Chem. class.: Sulfone

Action: Bactericidal and bacteriostatic against *M. leprae*

Uses: Hansen's disease

Dosage and routes:
• *Adult:* PO 100 mg qd with rifampin 600 mg qd × 6 mo

Available forms: Tabs 25, 100 mg

Side effects/adverse reactions:
INTEG: **Exfoliative dermatitis,** photosensitivity

CNS: Peripheral neuropathy, headache, anxiety, drowsiness, tremors, **convulsions,** lethargy, depression, confusion, psychosis, aggression

GI: Nausea, vomiting, abdominal pain, anorexia

GU: Proteinuria, nephrotic syndrome, renal papillary necrosis

EENT: Blurred vision, optic neuritis, photophobia

HEMA: **Megaloblastic anemia**

Contraindications: Hypersensitivity to sulfones, severe anemia

Precautions: Renal disease, hepatic disease, G-6-PD deficiency, pregnancy (A), lactation

Pharmacokinetics:
Rapid complete absorption; half-life 25-31 hr; highly bound to plasma protein; metabolized in liver; excreted in urine

Interactions/incompatibilities:
• Increased side effects: hemolytic agents
• Increased action of dapsone: probenecid, folic acid antagonists
• Decreased blood levels of dapsone: rifampin
• Decreased bactericidal action: PABA

---

italics = common side effects   ***bold italic*** = life threatening reactions

• Decreased GI absorption of dapsone: activated charcoal

NURSING CONSIDERATIONS
Assess:
• Temperature, if <101° F (38.3° C), drug should be reduced
• Liver studies qwk: ALT, AST, bilirubin
• Renal status: BUN, creatinine, output, sp gr, urinalysis before; qmo
• Blood levels of drug
• For anemia: Hct, Hgb, fatigue; for peripheral neuritis; or exfoliative dermatitis
• Mental status often: affect, mood, behavioral changes; psychosis may occur
• Hepatic status: decreased appetite, jaundice, dark urine, fatigue
Administer:
• With meals to decrease GI symptoms
• Antiemetic if vomiting occurs
• After C&S is completed; qmo to detect resistance
Perform/provide:
• Infants to be kept with mothers infected with leprosy; breastfeeding during drug therapy is encouraged
Evaluate:
• Therapeutic response: decreased symptoms of Hansen's disease
Teach patient/family:
• That therapeutic effects may occur after 3-6 mo of drug therapy
• That compliance with dosage schedule, duration is necessary
• To avoid hazardous machinery if drowsiness occurs

---

daunorubicin HCl
(daw-noe-roo'bi-sin)
Cerubidine
Func. class.: Antineoplastic, antibiotic
Chem. class.: Anthracycline glycoside

Action: Inhibits DNA synthesis, primarily; derived from *S. verticillus;* replication is decreased by binding to DNA, which causes strand splitting; cell cycle specific (S phase); a vesicant

Uses: Myelogenous, monocytic leukemia, acute nonlymphocytic leukemia, Ewing's sarcoma, Wilms' tumor, neuroblastoma, rhabdomyosarcoma

Dosage and routes:
Single agent
• *Adult:* IV 60 mg/m²/day × 3-5 day q4wk
In combination
• *Adult:* IV 45 mg/m²/day × 3 days, then 2 days of subsequent courses with cytosine arabinoside
Available forms: Inj IV 20 mg powder/vial

Side effects/adverse reactions:
*HEMA: **Thrombocytopenia, leukopenia, anemia***
*GI: Nausea, vomiting, anorexia, mucositis, **hepatotoxicity***
GU: Impotence, sterility, amenorrhea, gynecomastia, hyperuricemia
*INTEG: Rash, **extravasation,** dermatitis, reversible alopecia, cellulitis, thrombophlebitis at injection site
*CV: **Dysrhythmias, CHF, pericarditis, myocarditis,** peripheral edema
CNS: Fever, chills
Contraindications: Hypersensitivity, pregnancy (1st trimester) (D),

---

lactation, systemic infections, cardiac disease

Precautions: Renal, hepatic disease; gout; bone marrow depression

Pharmacokinetics: Half-life 18½ hr; metabolized by liver; crosses placenta; appears in breast milk; excreted in urine, bile

Interactions/incompatibilities:

• Increased toxicity: other antineoplastics or radiation

• Incompatible with dexamethasone, heparin

• Considered incompatible with any drug in sol or syringe

Lab test interferences:

Increase: Uric acid

NURSING CONSIDERATIONS
Assess:

• CBC, differential, platelet count weekly; withhold drug if WBC is <4000/mm³ or platelet count is <75,000/mm³; notify physician of these results

• Blood, urine uric acid levels

• Renal function studies: BUN, serum uric acid, urine CrCl, electrolytes before, during therapy

• I&O ratio; report fall in urine output to <30 ml/hr

• Monitor temperature q4h; fever may indicate beginning infection

• Liver function tests before, during therapy: bilirubin, AST, ALT, alk phosphatase as needed or monthly

• ECG; watch for ST-T wave changes, low QRS and T, possible dysrhythmias (sinus tachycardia, heart block, PVCs)

• Bleeding: hematuria, guaiac stools, bruising or petechiae, mucosa or orifices q8h

• Food preferences; list likes, dislikes

• Effects of alopecia on body image; discuss feelings about body changes

• Inflammation of mucosa, breaks in skin

• Yellowing of skin, sclera; dark urine; clay-colored stools; itchy skin; abdominal pain; fever; diarrhea

• Buccal cavity q8h for dryness, sores or ulceration, white patches, oral pain, bleeding, dysphagia

• Local irritation, pain, burning at injection site

• GI symptoms: frequency of stools, cramping

• Acidosis, signs of dehydration: rapid respirations, poor skin turgor, decreased urine output, dry skin, restlessness, weakness

• Cardiac status: B/P, pulse, character, rhythm, rate

Administer:

• IV after diluting 20 mg/4 ml sterile H₂O for inj (5 mg/ml), rotate, further dilute in 10-15 ml normal saline; give over 3-5 min by direct IV through Y-tube or 3-way stopcock of inf of D₅ or NS

• Antiemetic 30-60 min before giving drug and 6-10 hr after treatment to prevent vomiting

• Allopurinol or sodium bicarbonate to reduce uric acid levels, alkalinization of urine

• Transfusion for anemia

• Antispasmodic for GI symptoms

• Hydrocortisone for extravasation; apply ice compress after stopping infusion

Perform/provide:

• Strict hand-washing technique, gloves, protective clothing

• Liquid diet: carbonated beverages, gelatin may be added if patient is not nauseated or vomiting

• Increased fluid intake to 2-3 L/day to prevent urate and calculi formation

• Diet low in purines: absence of organ meats (kidney, liver), dried

---

italics = common side effects   ***bold italic*** = life threatening reactions

beans, peas to reduce uric acid level
• Rinsing of mouth tid-qid with water, club soda; brushing of teeth bid-qid with soft brush or cotton-tipped applicators for stomatitis; use unwaxed dental floss
• Storage at room temperature for 24 hr after reconstituting or 48 hr refrigerated

Evaluate:
• Therapeutic response: decreased tumor size, spread of malignancy

Teach patient/family:
• To report any complaints, side effects to nurse or physician
• That hair may be lost during treatment and wig or hairpiece may make patient feel better; tell patient that new hair may be different in color, texture
• To avoid foods with citric acid, hot or rough texture
• To report any bleeding, white spots, ulcerations in mouth; tell patient to examine mouth qd
• That urine and other body fluids may be red-orange for 48 hr

---

deferoxamine mesylate

(de-fer-ox′a-meen)
Desferal Mesylate
Func. class.: Heavy metal antagonist
Chem. class.: Chelating agent

Action: Binds iron ions (ferric ions) to form water-soluble complex that is removed by kidneys
Uses: Acute, chronic iron intoxication, hemochromatosis, hemosiderosis

Dosage and routes:
Acute
• *Adult and child:* IM/IV 1 g, then 500 mg q4h × 2 doses, then 500 mg q4-12h × 2 doses, not to exceed 15 mg/kg/hr or 6 g/24 hr

Chronic
• *Adult and child:* IM 500 mg-1 g/day plus IV INF 2 g given by separate line with each blood transfusion, not to exceed 15 mg/kg/hr or 6 g/24 hr; SC 1-2 g over 8-24 hr by SC infusion pump

Available forms: Powder for inj IV, IM, SC 500 mg/vial

Side effects/adverse reactions:
INTEG: Urticaria, erythema, pruritus, pain at injection site, fever
CV: Hypotension, tachycardia
GI: Diarrhea, abdominal cramps
EENT: Blurred vision, cataracts, decreased healing, *ototoxicity*
MS: Leg cramps
GU: Dysuria, pyelonephritis
*SYST: **Anaphylaxis***

Contraindications: Hypersensitivity, anuria, severe renal disease, child <3 yr
Precautions: Pregnancy (C), lactation

Pharmacokinetics:
Primarily forms a complex, which is then excreted by kidneys as complex, unchanged drug

Interactions/incompatibilities:
• Incompatible with other drugs in sol or syringe

NURSING CONSIDERATIONS
Assess:
• Inj site for redness, inflammation, pain
• For blood in stools
• Vision and hearing periodically
• VS
• I&O, kidney function studies: BUN, creatinine, CrCl, serum iron levels
• Allergic reactions: rash, urticaria; if these occur, drug should be discontinued

Administer:
• IV (used for shock) after diluting 500 mg/2 ml H₂O for inj; when

---

dissolved, must be further diluted with D₅W or LR or NS; run at <15 mg/kg/hr; 2g/1000 ml usually given over 24 hr; to be used only for short time; IM is preferred route
• IM after diluting with 2 ml sterile water for injection per 500 mg of drug; rotate injection sites
• Only when epinephrine 1:1000 is on unit for anaphylaxis
Evaluate:
• Therapeutic response: decreased symptoms of heavy metal intoxication
Teach patient/family:
• That urine may turn red

---

demeclocycline HCl
(dem-e-kloe-sye′kleen)
Declomycin
Func. class.: Broad-spectrum antibiotic/antiinfective
Chem. class.: Tetracycline

Action: Inhibits protein synthesis, phosphorylation in microorganisms by binding to 30S ribosomal subunits, reversibly binding to 50S ribosomal subunits; bacteriostatic
Uses: Uncommon gram-positive/gram-negative bacteria, protozoa, *Rickettsia, Mycoplasma*
Dosage and routes:
• *Adult:* PO 150 mg q6h or 300 mg q12h
• *Child >8 yr:* PO 6-12 mg/kg/day in divided doses q6-12h
Gonorrhea
• *Adult:* PO 600 mg, then 300 mg q12h × 4 days, total 3 g
SIADH
• *Adult:* PO 600-1200 mg/day in divided doses
Available forms: Tabs 150, 300 mg; caps 150 mg
Side effects/adverse reactions:
CNS: Fever, headache, paresthesia

*HEMA: **Eosinophilia, neutropenia, thrombocytopenia, leukocytosis, hemolytic anemia***
EENT: Dysphagia, glossitis, decreased calcification of deciduous teeth, abdominal pain, oral candidiasis
GI: Nausea, vomiting, diarrhea, anorexia, enterocolitis, **hepatotoxicity,** flatulence, abdominal cramps, epigastric burning, stomatitis, **psuedomembranous colitis**
CV: Pericarditis
GU: Increased BUN, polyuria, polydipsia, **renal failure, nephrotoxicity**
INTEG: Rash, urticaria, photosensitivity, increased pigmentation, **exfoliative dermatitis,** pruritus, angioedema
Contraindications: Hypersensitivity to tetracyclines, children <8 yr, pregnancy (D)
Precautions: Renal disease, hepatic disease, lactation, nephrogenic diabetes insipidus
Pharmacokinetics:
PO: Peak 3-6 hr, duration 48-72 hr, half-life 10-17 hr; excreted in urine; crosses placenta; excreted in breast milk; 36%-91% bound to serum protein
Interactions/incompatibilities:
• Decreased effect of demeclocycline: antacids, NaHCO₃, dairy, alkali products, iron, kaolin, pectin, cimetidine
• Increased effect: anticoagulants
• Decreased effect: penicillins, oral contraceptives
• Nephrotoxicity: methoxyflurane
Lab test interferences:
False negative: Urine glucose with Clinistix or Tes-Tape
False increase: Urinary catecholamines, AST, ALT, BUN

---

italics = common side effects   ***bold italic*** = life threatening reactions

NURSING CONSIDERATIONS
Assess:
• I&O ratio
• Blood studies: PT, CBC, AST, ALT, BUN, creatinine
• Urine sp gr, sodium
• Signs of infection
• Allergic reactions: rash, itching, pruritus, angioedema
• Nausea, vomiting, diarrhea; administer antiemetic, antacids as ordered
• Overgrowth of infection: increased temperature, malaise, redness, pain, swelling, drainage, perineal itching, diarrhea, changes in cough, sputum

Administer:
• On empty stomach 1 hr ac or 2 hr pc with 8 oz of water
• After C&S obtained
• 2 hr before or after laxative or ferrous products; 3 hr after antacid or kaolin-pectin products

Perform/provide:
• Storage in tight, light-resistant container at room temperature

Evaluate:
• Therapeutic response: decreased temperature, absence of lesions, negative C&S

Teach patient/family:
• To avoid sun exposure, since burns may occur; sunscreen does not seem to decrease photosensitivity
• If diabetic, to avoid use of Clinistix, Diastix, or Tes-Tape for urine glucose testing
• That all prescribed medication must be taken to prevent superimposed infection
• To avoid milk products; take with full glass of water

---

desipramine HCl
(dess-ip′ra-meen)
Desipramine HCl, Norpramin, Pertofrane
Func. class.: Antidepressant—tricyclic
Chem. class.: Dibenzazepine, secondary amine

Action: Blocks reuptake of norepinephrine, serotonin into nerve endings, increasing action of norepinephrine, serotonin in nerve cells

Uses: Depression

Dosage and routes:
• *Adult:* PO 75-150 mg/day in divided doses; may increase to 300 mg/day or may give daily dose hs
• *Adolescent/geriatric:* PO 25-50 mg/day, may increase to 100 mg/day

Available forms: Tabs 10, 25, 50, 75, 100, 150 mg; caps 25, 50 mg

Side effects/adverse reactions:
HEMA: Agranulocytosis, thrombocytopenia, eosinophilia, leukopenia
CNS: Dizziness, drowsiness, confusion, headache, anxiety, tremors, stimulation, weakness, insomnia, nightmares, EPS (elderly), increased psychiatric symptoms, paresthesia
GI: Diarrhea, dry mouth, nausea, vomiting, *paralytic ileus,* increased appetite, cramps, epigastric distress, jaundice, *hepatitis,* stomatitis, constipation
GU: Retention, acute renal failure
INTEG: Rash, urticaria, sweating, pruritus, photosensitivity
CV: Orthostatic hypotension, ECG changes, tachycardia, hypertension, palpitations
EENT: Blurred vision, tinnitus, mydriasis, ophthalmoplegia

Contraindications: Hypersensitivity to tricyclic antidepressants, recovery phase of myocardial infarction, narrow-angle glaucoma, convulsive disorders, prostatic hypertrophy, child <12 yr

Precautions: Suicidal patients, severe depression, increased intraocular pressure, elderly, pregnancy (C)

Pharmacokinetics:

PO: Steady state 2-11 days; metabolized by liver; excreted by kidneys; crosses placenta; half-life 14-62 hr

Interactions/incompatibilities:

• Decreased effects of: guanethidine, clonidine, indirect acting sympathomimetics (ephedrine)

• Increased effects of: direct-acting sympathomimetics (epinephrine) alcohol, barbiturates, benzodiazepines, CNS depressants

• Hyperpyretic crisis, convulsions, hypertensive episode: MAOI (pargyline [Eutonyl])

Lab test interferences:

Increase: Serum bilirubin, blood glucose, alk phosphatase

False increase: Urinary catecholamines

Decrease: VMA, 5-HIAA

NURSING CONSIDERATIONS

Assess:

• B/P (lying, standing), pulse q4h; if systolic B/P drops 20 mm Hg, hold drug, notify physician; take vital signs q4h in patients with cardiovascular disease

• Blood studies: CBC, leukocytes, differential, cardiac enzymes if patient is receiving long-term therapy

• Hepatic studies: AST, ALT, bilirubin

• Weight qwk, appetite may increase with drug

• ECG for flattening of T wave, bundle branch block, AV block, dysrhythmias in cardiac patients

• EPS primarily in elderly: rigidity, dystonia, akathisia

• Mental status: mood, sensorium, affect, suicidal tendencies, an increase in psychiatric symptoms: depression, panic

• Urinary retention, constipation; constipation is more likely to occur in children

• Withdrawal symptoms: headache, nausea, vomiting, muscle pain, weakness; do not usually occur unless drug was discontinued abruptly

• Alcohol consumption; if alcohol is consumed, hold dose until morning

Administer:

• Increased fluids, bulk in diet if constipation occurs, especially in elderly

• With food or milk for GI symptoms

• Crushed if patient is unable to swallow medication whole

• Dosage hs if oversedation occurs during day; may take entire dose hs; elderly may not tolerate once/day dosing

• Gum, hard candy, or frequent sips of water for dry mouth

Perform/provide:

• Storage at room temperature

• Assistance with ambulation during beginning therapy, since drowsiness/dizziness occurs

• Safety measures, including side rails, primarily in elderly

• Checking to see PO medication swallowed

Evaluate:

• Therapeutic response: decreased depression

Teach patient/family:

• That therapeutic effects may take 2-3 wk

• To use caution in driving or other

activities requiring alertness because of drowsiness, dizziness, blurred vision

• To avoid alcohol ingestion, other CNS depressants

• Not to discontinue medication quickly after long-term use; may cause nausea, headache, malaise

• To wear sunscreen or large hat, since photosensitivity occurs

Treatment of overdose: ECG monitoring; induce emesis; lavage, activated charcoal; administer anticonvulsant

---

desmopressin acetate
(des-moe-press'in)
Concentraid, DDAVP
Func. class.: Pituitary hormone
Chem. class.: Synthetic antidiuretic hormone

Action: Promotes reabsorption of water by action on renal tubular epithelium; causes smooth muscle constriction, increase in plasma factor VIII levels, which increases platelet aggregation resulting in vasopressor effect

Uses: Hemophilia A, von Willebrand's disease type 1, non-nephrogenic diabetes insipidus, symptoms of polyuria/polydipsia caused by pituitary dysfunction, nocturnal enuresis

Dosage and routes:
Diabetes insipidus
• *Adult:* INTRANASAL 0.1-0.4 ml qd in divided doses (1-4 sprays with pump) IV/SC 0.5-1 ml qd in divided doses
• *Child 3 mo to 12 yr:* INTRANASAL 0.05-0.3 ml qd in divided doses

Hemophilia/von Willebrand's disease
• *Adult and child:* IV 0.3 μg/kg in

NaCl over 15-30 min; may repeat if needed

Available forms: INTRANASAL 0.01 mg/ml, inj IV, SC 4 μg/ml

Side effects/adverse reactions:
EENT: Nasal irritation, congestion, rhinitis
CNS: Drowsiness, headache, lethargy, flushing
GU: Vulval pain
GI: Nausea, heartburn, cramps
CV: Increased B/P

Contraindications: Hypersensitivity, nephrogenic diabetes insipidus
Precautions: Pregnancy (B), CAD, lactation, hypertension

Pharmacokinetics:
NASAL: Onset 1 hr, peak 1-2 hr, duration 8-20 hr, half-life 8 min, 76 min (terminal)

Interactions/incompatibilities:
• Increased response: carbamazepine, chlorpropamide, clofibrate
• Decreased response: lithium, alcohol, demeclocyclines, heparin or large doses of epinephrine
• Compatibility not known

NURSING CONSIDERATIONS
Assess:
• Pulse, B/P when giving drug IV or SC
• I&O ratio, weight daily; check for edema in extremities; if water retention is severe, diuretic may be prescribed
• Water intoxication: lethargy, behavioral changes, disorientation, neuromuscular excitability
• Intranasal use: nausea, congestion, cramps, headache; usually decreased with decreased dose

Administer:
• Undiluted over 1 min in diabetes insipidus
• Diluted, one single dose/50 ml of NS (Adult & Child >10 kg), a single dose/10 ml as an IV inf over

---

15-30 min in von Willebrand's disease or hemophilia A

Perform/provide:

• Storage in refrigerator or cool environment

Evaluate:

• Therapeutic response: absence of severe thirst, decreased urine output, osmolality

Teach patient/family:

• Technique for nasal instillation: to insert tube into nasal cavity to instill drug

• To avoid OTC products: cough, hay fever products, since these preparations may contain epinephrine, decrease drug response; do not use with alcohol

• To wear Medic Alert ID specifying therapy

---

desonide

(dess'oh-nide)

DesOwen, Tridesilon

Func. class.: Topical corticosteroid

Chem. class.: Synthetic non-fluorinated agent, group IV potency

Action: Antipruritic, antiinflammatory

Uses: Psoriasis, eczema, contact dermatitis, pruritus

Dosage and routes:

• *Adult and child:* Apply to affected area bid-tid

Available forms: Cream 0.05%; oint 0.05%

Side effects/adverse reactions:

INTEG: Burning, dryness, itching, irritation, acne, folliculitis, hypertrichosis, perioral dermatitis, hypopigmentation, atrophy, striae, miliaria, allergic contact dermatitis, secondary infection

Contraindications: Hypersensitivity to corticosteroids, fungal infections

Precautions: Pregnancy (C), lactation, viral infections, bacterial infections

NURSING CONSIDERATIONS

Assess:

• Temperature; if fever develops, drug should be discontinued

• For systemic absorption: increased temperature, inflammation, irritation

Administer:

• Only to affected areas; do not get in eyes

• Medication; then cover with occlusive dressing (only if prescribed); seal to normal skin; change q12h; systemic absorption may occur

• Only to dermatoses; do not use on weeping, denuded, or infected area

Perform/provide:

• Cleansing before application of drug

• Treatment for a few days after area has cleared

• Storage at room temperature

Evaluate:

• Therapeutic response: absence of severe itching, patches on skin, flaking

Teach patient/family:

• To avoid sunlight on affected area; burns may occur

---

desoximetasone

(des-ox-i-met'a-sone)

Desoximetasone, Topicort, Topicort LP

Func. class.: Topical corticosteroid

Chem. class.: Synthetic fluorinated agent, group II potency (0.25%), group III potency (0.05%)

Action: Antipruritic, antiinflammatory

Uses: Psoriasis, eczema, contact dermatitis, pruritus

Dosage and routes:

• *Adult and child:* TOP apply to affected area bid-tid

Available forms: Cream 0.05% (LP), 0.25%; oint 0.25%; gel 0.05%

Side effects/adverse reactions:

INTEG: Burning, dryness, itching, irritation, acne, folliculitis, hypertrichosis, perioral dermatitis, hypopigmentation, atrophy, striae, miliaria, allergic contact dermatitis, secondary infection

Contraindications: Hypersensitivity to corticosteroids, fungal infections

Precautions: Pregnancy (C), lactation, viral infections, bacterial infections

NURSING CONSIDERATIONS

Assess:

• Temperature; if fever develops, drug should be discontinued

• For systemic absorption: increased temperature, inflammation, irritation

Administer:

• Only to affected areas; do not get in eyes

• Medication; then cover with occlusive dressing (only if prescribed); seal to normal skin; change q12h; use occlusive dressing with extreme caution (group II potency); systemic absorption may occur

• Only to dermatoses; do not use on weeping, denuded, or infected area

Perform/provide:

• Cleansing before application of drug

• Treatment for a few days after area has cleared

• Storage at room temperature

Evaluate:

• Therapeutic response: absence of severe itching, patches on skin, flaking

Teach patient/family:

• To avoid sunlight on affected area; burns may occur

dexamethasone

(dex-a-meth'a-sone)

Aeroseb-Dex, Decaderm, Decaspray

Func. class.: Topical corticosteroid

Chem. class.: Synthetic fluorinated agent

Action: Possesses antipruritic, antiinflammatory actions

Uses: Corticosteroid-responsive dermatoses

Dosage and routes:

• *Adult and child:* TOP apply to affected area bid-qid

Available forms: Gel 0.1%; aerosol 0.01%, 0.04%

Side effects/adverse reactions:

INTEG: Burning, dryness, itching, irritation, acne, folliculitis, hypertrichosis, perioral dermatitis, hypopigmentation, atrophy of the epidermis, striae, miliaria, allergic contact dermatitis, secondary infection

Contraindications: Hypersensitivity to corticosteroids, fungal infections, viral infections

Precautions: Pregnancy (C), lactation, viral infections, bacterial infections

NURSING CONSIDERATIONS

Assess:

• Temperature; if fever develops, drug should be discontinued

• Systemic absorption: fever, infection, irritation

Administer:

• Only to affected areas; do not get in eyes

• Then cover with occlusive dressing if ordered; seal to normal skin; change q12h; systemic absorption may occur

• Only to dermatoses; do not use on weeping, denuded, or infected area

Perform/provide:

• Cleansing before application of drug

• Treatment for a few days after area has cleared

• Storage at room temperature

Evaluate:

• Therapeutic response: absence of severe itching, patches on skin, flaking

Teach patient/family:

• To avoid sunlight on affected area; burns may occur

---

dexamethasone/ dexamethasone acetate/dexamethasone sodium phosphate
(dex-a-meth′a-sone)
Aeroseb-Dex, Decaderm, Decaspray, Dalalone D.P., Dalalone L.A., Decadron-LA, Decaject-L.A., Dexacen LA-8, Dexamethasone Acetate, Dexasone L.A., Dexone LA, Solurex LA, Dalalone, Decadron Phosphate, Decaject, Dexacen-4, Dexamethasone Sodium Phosphate, Dexasone, Dexone, Hexadrol Phosphate, Solurex, Decadron Phosphate Respihaler

Func. class.: Corticosteroid
Chem. class.: Glucocorticoid, long-acting

Action: Decreases inflammation by suppression of migration of polymorphonuclear leukocytes, fibroblasts, reversal of increased capillary permeability and lysosomal stabilization

Uses: Inflammation, allergies, neoplasms, cerebral edema, septic shock, collagen disorders

Dosage and routes:

Inflammation

• *Adult:* PO 0.25-4 mg bid-qid IM 4-16 mg q1-3 wk (acetate)

Shock

• *Adult:* IV 1-6 mg/kg or 40 mg q2-6h (phosphate)

Cerebral edema

• *Adult:* IV 10 mg, then 4-6 mg IM q6h × 2-4 days, then taper over 1 wk

• *Child:* PO 0.2 mg/kg/day in divided doses

Available forms: Tabs 0.25, 0.5, 0.75, 1, 1.5, 3, 4, 6 mg; inj IM acetate 8, 16 mg/ml; inj IV phosphate 4, 10 mg/ml; elix 0.5 mg/5 ml; oral sol 0.5 mg/5 ml, 0.5 mg/1 ml

Side effects/adverse reactions:

INTEG: Acne, poor wound healing, ecchymosis, petechiae

CNS: Depression, flushing, sweating, headache, mood changes

CV: Hypertension, **circulatory collapse, thrombophlebitis, embolism,** tachycardia, edema

HEMA: **Thrombocytopenia**

MS: Fractures, osteoporosis, weakness

GI: Diarrhea, nausea, abdominal distention, **GI hemorrhage,** *increased appetite,* **pancreatitis**

EENT: Fungal infections, increased intraocular pressure, blurred vision

Contraindications: Psychosis, hypersensitivity, idiopathic thrombocytopenia, acute glomerulonephritis, amebiasis, fungal infections,

---

italics = common side effects   ***bold italic*** = life threatening reactions

nonasthmatic bronchial disease, child <2 yr, AIDS, TB

Precautions: Pregnancy (C), diabetes mellitus, glaucoma, osteoporosis, seizure disorders, ulcerative colitis, CHF, myasthenia gravis, renal disease, peptic ulcer, esophagitis

Pharmacokinetics:

PO: Peak 1-2 h, duration 2⅓ days
IM: Peak 8 h, duration 6 days
Half-life 3-4½ hr

Interactions/incompatibilities:

• Decreased action of dexamethasone: cholestyramine, colestipol, barbiturates, rifampin, ephedrine, phenytoin, theophylline, antacids
• Decreased effects of: anticoagulants, anticonvulsants, antidiabetics, ambenonium, neostigmine, isoniazid, toxoids, vaccines, anticholinesterases, salicylates, somatrem
• Increased side effects: alcohol, salicylates, indomethacin, amphotericin B, digitalis, cyclosporine, diuretics
• Increased action of dexamethasone: salicylates, estrogens, indomethacin, oral contraceptives, ketoconazole, macrolide antibiotics
• Incompatible with amikacin, daunorubicin, doxorubicin, metaraminol, prochlorperazine, vancomycin

Lab test interferences:

Increase: Cholesterol, Na, blood glucose, uric acid, Ca, urine glucose
Decrease: Ca, K, T_4, T_3, thyroid ^{131}I uptake test, urine 17-OHCS, 17-KS, PBI
False negative: Skin allergy tests

NURSING CONSIDERATIONS

Assess:

• K, blood sugar, urine glucose while on long-term therapy; hypokalemia and hyperglycemia

• Weight daily; notify physician of weekly gain >5 lb
• B/P q4h, pulse; notify physician if chest pain occurs
• I&O ratio; be alert for decreasing urinary output and increasing edema
• Plasma cortisol levels during long-term therapy (normal level: 138-635 nmol/L SI units when drawn at 8 AM)
• Infection: increased temperature, WBC even after withdrawal of medication; drug masks symptoms of infection
• Potassium depletion: paresthesias, fatigue, nausea, vomiting, depression, polyuria, dysrhythmias, weakness
• Edema, hypertension, cardiac symptoms
• Mental status: affect, mood, behavioral changes, aggression

Administer:

• IV undiluted direct over 1 min or less or diluted with normal saline or D_5W and give as an IV inf as prescribed rate
• After shaking suspension (parenteral); do not give suspension IV
• Titrated dose; use lowest effective dose
• IM inj deeply in large mass; rotate sites; avoid deltoid; use 21G needle
• In one dose in AM to prevent adrenal suppression; avoid SC administration; damage may be done to tissue
• With food or milk to decrease GI symptoms

Perform/provide:

• Assistance with ambulation in patient with bone tissue disease to prevent fractures

Evaluate:

• Therapeutic response: ease of respirations, decreased inflammation

Teach patient/family:

• That ID as steroid user should be carried

• To notify physician if therapeutic response decreases; dosage adjustment may be needed

• Not to discontinue this medication abruptly or adrenal crisis can result

• To avoid OTC products: salicylates, alcohol in cough products, cold preparations unless directed by physician

• To teach patient all aspects of drug usage, including cushingoid symptoms

• Symptoms of adrenal insufficiency: nausea, anorexia, fatigue, dizziness, dyspnea, weakness, joint pain

---

**dexamethasone/
dexamethasone sodium phosphate**

(dex-a-meth'a-sone)

AK-Dex Ophthalmic, Dexamethasone Ophthalmic Suspension, Decadron Phosphate, Maxidex

Func. class.: Ophthalmic antiinflammatory

Action: Results in decreased inflammation, resulting in decreased pain, photophobia, hyperemia, cellular infiltration

Uses: Inflammation of eye, lids, conjunctiva, cornea; uveitis; iridocyclitis; allergic condition; burns; foreign bodies

Dosage and routes:

• *Adult and child:* Instill 1-2 gtts into conjunctival sac q1-4h depending on condition

Available forms: Oint 0.05%; ophthalmic sol 0.1%

italics = common side effects

Side effects/adverse reactions:

EENT: ***Increased intraocular pressure****, poor corneal wound healing, increased possibility of corneal infection, glaucoma exacerbation, **optic nerve damage,** decreased acuity, visual field, cataracts

Contraindications: Hypersensitivity, acute superficial herpes simplex, fungal/viral diseases of the eye or conjunctiva, active diabetes mellitus, ocular TB, infections of the eye

Precautions: Corneal abrasions, glaucoma, pregnancy (C)

NURSING CONSIDERATIONS

Perform/provide:

• Storage in light-resistant container

Evaluate:

• Therapeutic response: absence of swelling, redness, exudate

Teach patient/family:

• Instillation method: pressure on lacrimal duct for 1 min

• Not to share eye medications with others

• Not to use if purulent drainage is present

• To shake before using

• Not to discontinue abruptly; taper over 1-2 wk

---

dexamethasone sodium phosphate

(dex-a-meth'a-sone)

Decadron Phosphate

Func. class.: Topical corticosteroid

Chem. class.: Synthetic fluorinated agent, group VI potency

Action: Possesses antipruritic, antiinflammatory actions

Uses: Psoriasis, eczema, contact dermatitis, pruritus

bold italic = life threatening reactions

Dosage and routes:
• *Adult and child:* Apply to affected area tid-qid
Available forms: Cream 0.1%
Side effects/adverse reactions:
INTEG: Burning, dryness, itching, irritation, acne, folliculitis, hypertrichosis, perioral dermatitis, hypopigmentation, atrophy, striae, miliaria, allergic contact dermatitis, secondary infection
Contraindications: Hypersensitivity to corticosteroids, fungal infections
Precautions: Pregnancy (C), lactation, viral infections, bacterial infections
• For systemic absorption: increased temperature, inflammation, irritation
NURSING CONSIDERATIONS
Assess:
• Temperature; if fever develops, drug should be discontinued
Administer:
• Only to affected areas; do not get in eyes
• Medication; then cover with occlusive dressing (only if prescribed); seal to normal skin; change q12h; systemic absorption may occur
• Only to dermatoses; do not use on weeping, denuded, or infected area
Perform/provide:
• Cleansing before application of drug
• Treatment for a few days after area has cleared
• Storage at room temperature
Evaluate:
• Therapeutic response: absence of severe itching, patches on skin, flaking
Teach patient/family:
• To avoid sunlight on affected area; burns may occur

dexamethasone sodium phosphate (nasal)

(dex-a-meth'a-sone)
Decadron Phosphate Turbinaire
Func. class.: Steroid, intranasal
Chem. class.: Glucocorticoid

Action: Long-acting synthetic adrenocorticoid with antiinflammatory activity, minimal mineralocorticoid properties
Uses: Inflammation (not within sinuses), nasal polyps, allergic conditions of nose
Dosage and routes:
• *Adult:* SPRAY 1-2 sprays bid-tid, not to exceed 12/day
• *Child 6-12 yr:* SPRAY 1-2 sprays bid, not to exceed 8/day
Available forms: 84 μg/metered spray
Side effects/adverse reactions:
EENT: Nasal irritation, dryness, rebound congestion, epistaxis, sneezing, *infarction of nasal mucosa*
INTEG: Urticaria
CNS: Headache, dizziness
SYSTEMIC: CHF, convulsions, increased Na, hypertension
Contraindications: Hypersensitivity, child <12 yr, localized infection of nose, acute status asthmaticus
Precautions: Lactation, nasal trauma, pregnancy (C)
NURSING CONSIDERATIONS
Assess:
• Adrenal suppression: 17-KS, plasma cortisol for decreased levels
• Nasal passages during long-term treatment for changes in mucus
• For edema, increased B/P, increase in K^+ during treatment, which indicates systemic absorption

Administer:
• After cleaning spray container daily with warm water; dry thoroughly

Perform/provide:
• Storage in cool environment; do not puncture or incinerate container

Evaluate:
• Therapeutic response: decreased inflammation, redness

Teach patient/family:
• To clear nasal passages if sneezing attack occurs, repeat dose
• To continue using product even if mild nasal bleeding occurs; is usually transient
• Method of instillation after providing written instructions from manufacturer
• To clear nasal passages before administration; use decongestant if needed; shake inhaler; invert; tilt head backward; insert nozzle into nostril away from septum; hold other nostril closed; depress activator; inhale through nose; exhale through mouth
• To decrease gradually if drug has been used consistently
• That only 1 person should use a single-container drug
• If irritation, dryness, epistaxis occur, that drug may have to be discontinued
• That benefit requires regular use, will not occur until after several days

dexchlorpheniramine maleate
(dex-klor-fen-eer′a-meen)
Dexchlor, Dexchlorpheniramine Maleate, Poladex, Polaramine

Func. class.: Antihistamine
Chem. class.: Alkylamine derivative, H_1-receptor antagonist

Action: Acts on blood vessels, GI, respiratory system by competing with histamine for H_1-receptor site; decreases allergic response by blocking histamine

Uses: Allergy symptoms, rhinitis, pruritus, contact dermatitis

Dosage and routes:
• *Adult:* PO 1-2 mg tid-qid; REPEAT ACTION 4-6 mg bid-tid
• *Child 6-11 yr:* PO 1 mg q4-6h, or TIME REL 4 mg hs
• *Child 2-5 yr:* PO 0.5 mg q4-6h; do not use repeat action form

Available forms: Tabs 2 mg; repeat-action tab 4, 6 mg; syr 2 mg/5 ml

Side effects/adverse reactions:
CNS: Dizziness, drowsiness, poor coordination, fatigue, anxiety, euphoria, confusion, paresthesia, neuritis
CV: Hypotension, palpitations, tachycardia
RESP: Increased thick secretions, wheezing, chest tightness
GI: Constipation, dry mouth, nausea, vomiting, anorexia, diarrhea
INTEG: Rash, urticaria, photosensitivity
GU: Retention, dysuria, frequency
EENT: Blurred vision, dilated pupils, tinnitus, nasal stuffiness, dry nose, throat, mouth

Contraindications: Hypersensitivity to H_1-receptor antagonist; acute asthma attack, lower respiratory tract disease

---

italics = common side effects   ***bold italic*** = life threatening reactions

Precautions: Increased intraocular pressure, renal disease, cardiac disease, hypertension, bronchial asthma, seizure disorder, stenosed peptic ulcers, hyperthyroidism, prostatic hypertrophy, bladder neck obstruction, pregnancy (B), elderly

Pharmacokinetics:
PO: Onset 15 min, peak 3 hr, duration 3-6 hr; metabolized in liver; excreted by kidneys (inactive metabolites); excreted in breast milk (small amounts)

Interactions/incompatibilities:
• Increased CNS depression: barbiturates, narcotics, hypnotics, tricyclic antidepressants, alcohol
• Decreased effect: oral anticoagulants, heparin
• Increased effect of dexchlorpheniramine: MAOIs

Lab test interferences:
False negative: Skin allergy tests

NURSING CONSIDERATIONS
Assess:
• I&O ratio; be alert for urinary retention, frequency, dysuria; drug should be discontinued if these occur
• CBC during long-term therapy
• Respiratory status: rate, rhythm, increase in bronchial secretions, wheezing, chest tightness
• Cardiac status: palpitations, increased pulse, hypotension

Administer:
• With meals if GI symptoms occur; absorption may slightly decrease

Perform/provide:
• Hard candy, gum, frequent rinsing of mouth for dryness
• Storage in tight container at room temperature

Evaluate:
• Therapeutic response: absence of running or congested nose or rashes

Teach patient/family:
• All aspects of drug use; to notify physician if confusion/sedation/hypotension occurs
• To avoid driving or other hazardous activity if drowsiness occurs, especially elderly
• That this drug decreases anticoagulant (oral) effect
• To avoid concurrent use of alcohol or other CNS depressants

Treatment of overdose: Administer ipecac syrup or lavage, diazepam, vasopressors, barbiturates (short-acting)

---

dextran 40

Dextran 40, Gentran 40, LMD 10%, Rheomacrodex

Func. class.: Plasma volume expander
Chem. class.: Low molecular weight polysaccharide

Action: Similar to human albumin, which expands plasma volume by drawing fluid from interstitial space to intravascular space

Uses: Expand plasma volume, prophylaxis of embolism, thrombosis

Dosage and routes:
Shock
• *Adult:* IV INF 500 ml over 15-30 min, total dose in 24 hr not to exceed 20 ml/kg; then subsequent doses given slowly; if given >24 hr, not to exceed 10 ml/kg/day; not to exceed therapy >5 days

Thrombosis/embolism
• *Adult:* IV INF 500-1000 ml, then 500 ml/day × 3 days, then 500 ml q2-3 days × 2 wk if needed

Available forms: 10% dextran 40/5% dextrose, 10% dextran 40/0.9% sodium chloride

Side effects/adverse reactions:
HEMA: Decreased hematocrit,

platelet function, increased bleeding/coagulation times

INTEG: Rash, urticaria, pruritus, angioedema, chills, fever, flushing
RESP: Wheezing, dyspnea, ***bronchospasm, pulmonary edema***
CV: Hypotension, ***cardiac arrest***
*GU: **Osmotic nephrosis, renal failure, stasis,*** hyponatremia
GI: Nausea, vomiting, increased AST, ALT
*SYST: **Anaphylaxis***

Contraindications: Hypersensitivity, renal failure, CHF (severe), extreme dehydration

Precautions: Active hemorrhage, pregnancy (C)

Pharmacokinetics:
IV: Expands blood volume 1-2 × amount infused; excreted in urine and feces

Interactions/incompatibilities
• Incompatible with chlortetracycline, phytonadione, promethazine
• Incompatible with any drug in dextran sol

Lab test interferences:
False increase: Blood glucose, urinary protein, bilirubin, total protein
Interference: Rh test, blood typing/crossmatching

NURSING CONSIDERATIONS
Assess:
• VS q5min × 30 min
• CVP during infusion (5-10 cm H₂O—normal range)
• Urine output q1h; watch for increase in urinary output, which is common; if output does not increase, infusion should be decreased or discontinued
• I&O ratio and specific gravity, urine osmolarity; if specific gravity is very low, renal clearance is low; drug should be discontinued
• Allergy: rash, urticaria, pruritus, wheezing, dyspnea, broncho-

spasm, drug should be discontinued immediately
• Circulatory overload: increased pulse, respirations, SOB, wheezing, chest tightness, chest pain
• Dehydration after infusion: decreased output, decreased sp. gravity of urine, increased temperature, poor skin turgor, increased specific gravity, dry skin

Administer:
• After prescribed dilution; may give inital 500 mg at 15-30 min; distribute remainder of daily dose over 8-24 hr
• After crossmatch is drawn, if blood is to be given also
• Dextran 1 (Promit) to prevent anaphylaxis if ordered

Perform/provide:
• Storage at constant temperature 15° C (59° F) to 30° C (86° F); discard unused portions, protect from freezing

Evaluate:
• Therapeutic response: increased plasma volume

---

dextran 70/75
Dextran 70, Dextran 75, Gentran 75, Macrodex
Func. class.: Plasma volume expander
Chem. class.: High molecular weight polysaccharide

Action: Similar to human albumin, which expands plasma volume by drawing fluid from interstitial spaces to intravascular space
Uses: Expand plasma volume in hypovolemic shock or impending shock
Dosage and routes:
• *Adult:* IV INF 500-1000 ml not to exceed 20-40 ml/min, not to ex-

ceed 10 ml/kg/24 hr if therapy >24 hr

Available forms: 70/75 dextran in 0.9% NaCl, D₅%

Side effects/adverse reactions:

HEMA: Decreased hematocrit, platelet function; increased bleeding/coagulation times

INTEG: Rash, urticaria, pruritus, angioedema, chills, fever, flushing

RESP: Wheezing, dyspnea, ***bronchospasm, pulmonary edema***

CV: Hypotension, ***cardiac arrest***

GU: ***Osmotic nephrosis, renal failure, stasis,*** hypernatremia

GI: Nausea, vomiting, increased AST, ALT

SYST: ***Anaphylaxis***

Contraindications: Hypersensitivity, renal failure, CHF (severe), extreme dehydration

Precautions: Active hemorrhage, pregnancy (C)

Pharmacokinetics:

IV: Expands blood volume 1-2 × amount infused; excreted in urine and feces

Lab test interferences:

False increase: Blood glucose, urinary protein, bilirubin, total protein

Interferences: Rh test, blood typing/crossmatching

NURSING CONSIDERATIONS

Assess:

• VS q5min × 30 min

• CVP during infusion (5-10 cm H₂O—normal range)

• Urine output q1h; watch for increase in urinary output, which is common; if output does not increase, infusion should be decreased or discontinued

• I&O ratio and specific gravity, urine osmolarity; if specific gravity is very low, renal clearance is low; drug should be discontinued

• Allergy: rash, urticaria, pruritus, wheezing, dyspnea, broncho-

spasm; drug should be discontinued immediately

• Circulatory overload: increased pulse, respirations, SOB, wheezing, chest tightness, chest pain

• Dehydration after infusion: decreased output, increased temperature, poor skin turgor, increased specific gravity, dry skin

Administer:

• After prescribed dilution, may give inital 500 mg at 20-40 ml/min, then reduce flow to lowest rate

• After crossmatch is drawn, if blood is to be given also

• Dextran 1 (Promit) to prevent anaphylaxis

Perform/provide:

• Storage at constant temperature <25° C (77° F); discard unused portions; do not use unless clear

Evaluate:

• Therapeutic response: increased plasma volume

---

dextroamphetamine sulfate

(dex-troe-am-fet'a-meen)

Dexedrine, Dexedrine Spansules, Dextroamphetamine Sulfate, Oxydess II, Spancap #1

Func. class.: Cerebral stimulant

Chem. class.: Amphetamine

Controlled Substance Schedule II

Action: Increases release of norepinephrine, dopamine in cerebral cortex to reticular activating system

Uses: Narcolepsy, exogenous obesity, attention deficit disorder with hyperactivity

Dosage and routes:

Narcolepsy

• *Adult:* PO 5-60 mg qd in divided doses
• *Child >12 yr:* PO 10 mg qd increasing by 10 mg/day at weekly intervals
• *Child 6-12 yr:* PO 5 mg qd increasing by 5 mg/wk (max 60 mg/day)

Attention deficit disorder
• *Child >6 yr:* PO 5 mg qd-bid increasing by 5 mg/day at weekly intervals
• *Child 3-6 yr:* PO 2.5 mg qd increasing by 2.5 mg/day at weekly intervals

Obesity
• *Adult:* PO 10-15 mg/day (sus rel) in AM or 5-10 mg qd 30-60 min before meals

Available forms: Tabs 5, 10 mg; caps sus rel 5, 10, 15 mg; elix 5 mg/5 ml

Side effects/adverse reactions:
CNS: Hyperactivity, insomnia, restlessness, talkativeness, dizziness, headache, chills, stimulation, dysphoria, irritability, aggressiveness, tremor, dependence, addiction
GI: Anorexia, dry mouth, diarrhea, constipation, weight loss, metallic taste
GU: Impotence, change in libido
CV: Palpitations, tachycardia, hypertension, decrease in heart rate, dysrhythmias
INTEG: Urticaria

Contraindications: Hypersensitivity to sympathomimetic amines, hyperthyroidism, hypertension, glaucoma, severe arteriosclerosis, drug abuse, cardiovascular disease, anxiety

Precautions: Gilles de la Tourette's disorder, pregnancy (C), lactation, child <3 yr

Pharmacokinetics:
PO: Onset 30 min, peak 1-3 hr, duration 4-20 hr; metabolized by liver; urine excretion pH dependent; crosses placenta, breast milk; half-life 10-30 hr

Interactions/incompatibilities:
• Hypertensive crisis: MAOIs or within 14 days of MAOIs, furazolidine
• Increased effect of dextroamphetamine: acetazolamide, antacids, sodium bicarbonate, phenothiazines, haloperidol
• Decreased effect of dextroamphetamine: barbiturates, ascorbic acid, ammonium chloride, tricyclics
• Decreased effect: guanethidine

NURSING CONSIDERATIONS
Assess:
• VS, B/P; since this drug may reverse antihypertensives, check patients with cardiac disease more often
• CBC, urinalysis; in diabetes: blood sugar, urine sugar; insulin changes may be required, since eating will decrease
• Height, growth rate in children; growth rate may be decreased
• Mental status: mood, sensorium, affect, stimulation, insomnia, irritability
• Tolerance or dependency: an increased amount may be used to get same effect; will develop after long-term use
• Overdose: pain, fever, dehydration, insomnia, hyperactivity

Administer:
• At least 6 hr before hs to avoid sleeplessness
• For obesity only if the patient is on a weight-reduction program including dietary changes and exercise; patient will develop tolerance, and weight loss won't occur without additional methods; give 30-60 min before meals

---

italics = common side effects   ***bold italic*** = life threatening reactions

• Gum, hard candy, frequent sips of water for dry mouth

Evaluate:
• Therapeutic response: increased CNS stimulation, decreased drowsiness

Teach patient/family:
• Not to crush or chew sus rel forms
• To decrease caffeine consumption (coffee, tea, cola, chocolate), which may increase irritability, stimulation
• To avoid OTC preparations unless approved by the physician
• To taper off drug over several weeks or depression, increased sleeping, lethargy
• To avoid alcohol ingestion
• To avoid hazardous activities until patient is stabilized on medication
• To get needed rest; patient will feel more tired at end of day

Treatment of overdose: Administer fluids, hemodialysis or peritoneal dialysis; antihypertensive for increased B/P, ammonium Cl for increased excretion

---

dextromethorphan hydrobromide
(dex-troe-meth-or'fan)
Benylin DM, Children's Hold, Delsym, Dextromethorphan, Hold DM, Pertussin, Pertussin ES, Robitussin Cough Calmers, Robitussin Pediatric, St. Joseph Cough Suppressant, Sucrets Cough Control, Suppress, Trocal, Vicks Formula 44
Func. class.: Antitussive, non-narcotic
Chem. class.: Levorphanol derivative

Action: Depresses cough center in medulla
Uses: Nonproductive cough

Dosage and routes:
• *Adult:* PO 10-20 mg q4h, or 30 mg q6-8h, not to exceed 120 mg/day; CON-REL LIQ 60 mg bid, not to exceed 120 mg/day
• *Child 6-12 yr:* PO 5-10 mg q4h; CON-REL LIQ 30 mg bid, not to exceed 60 mg/day
• *Child 2-6 yr:* PO 2.5-5 mg q4h, or 7.5 mg q6-8h, not to exceed 30 mg/day

Available forms: Loz 5 mg; sol 5, 7.5, 10, 15 mg/5 ml

Side effects/adverse reactions:
CNS: Dizziness
GI: Nausea

Contraindications: Hypersensitivity, asthma/emphysema, productive cough

Precautions: Nausea/vomiting, increased temperature, persistent headache, pregnancy (C)

Pharmacokinetics:
PO: Onset 15-30 min, duration 3-6 hr

Interactions/incompatibilities:
• Do not give with MAOIs or within 2 wk of MAOIs, penicillins, salicylates, tetracyclines, phenobarbital, iodines (high doses)

NURSING CONSIDERATIONS
Assess:
• Cough: type, frequency, character including sputum

Administer:
• Decreased dose to elderly patients; their metabolism may be slowed

Perform/provide:
• Increased fluids to liquefy secretions
• Humidification of patient's room

Evaluate:
• Therapeutic response: absence of cough

Teach patient/family:
• To avoid driving or other hazard-

ous activities until patient is stabilized on this medication
• To avoid smoking, smoke-filled rooms, perfumes, dust, environmental pollutants, cleaners that increase cough

---

dextrose (*D*-glucose)
Func. class.: Caloric

Action: Needed for adequate utilization of amino acids; decreases protein, nitrogen loss; prevents ketosis
Uses: Increases intake of calories; increases fluids in patients unable to take adequate fluids, calories orally
Dosage and routes:
• *Adult and child:* IV depends on individual requirements
Available forms: Inj IV 2.5%, 5%, 10%, 20%, 40%, 50%
Side effects/adverse reactions:
CNS: Confusion, *loss of consciousness,* dizziness
CV: Hypertension, ***CHF, pulmonary edema***
GU: Glycosuria, osmotic diuresis
ENDO: Hyperglycemia, rebound hypoglycemia, hyperosmolar syndrome, hyperglycemic nonketotic syndrome
INTEG: Chills, flushing, warm feeling, rash, urticaria, extravasation necrosis
Contraindications: Hyperglycemia, delirium tremens, hemorrhage (cranial/spinal), CHF
Precautions: Renal, liver, cardiac disease, diabetes mellitus
NURSING CONSIDERATIONS
Assess:
• Electrolytes (K, Na, Ca, Cl, Mg), blood glucose, ammonia, phosphate
• Renal, liver function studies:

BUN, creatinine, ALT, AST, bilirubin
• Injection site for extravasation: redness along vein, edema at site, necrosis, pain, hard tender area; site should be changed immediately
• Monitor respiratory function q4h: auscultate lung fields bilaterally for crackles, respirations, quality, rate, rhythm
• Monitor temperature q4h for increased fever, indicating infection; if infection suspected, infusion is discontinued, tubing, bottle, catheter tip cultured
• Urine glucose q6h using Chemstrips, which are not affected by infusion substances
• Nutritional status: calorie count by dietitian
Administer:
• Only (4%) protein and dextrose (up to 12.5%) via peripheral vein; stronger solutions require central IV administration
• May be given undiluted via prepared sol give 10% sol, 5 ml/15 sec, 10% sol, 1000 ml/3 hr or more 20% sol, 500 ml/½-1 hr 50% sol, 10 ml/min
• After changing IV catheter, dressing q24h with aseptic technique
Evaluate:
• Therapeutic response: increased weight
Teach patient/family
• Reason for dextrose infusion

---

dextrothyroxine sodium
(dex-troe-thye-rox'een)
Choloxin
Func. class.: Antilipemic
Chem. class.: Hormone isomer

Action: Stimulates hepatic catab-

---

olism, excretion of cholesterol; increases bile products into feces

Uses: Hyperlipidemia in euthyroid patients with no evidence of organic heart disease

Dosage and routes:
• *Adult:* PO 1-2 mg/day, may increase 1-2 mg/day qmo, not to exceed 8 mg/day
• *Child:* PO 0.05 mg/kg/day, may increase 0.05 mg/kg/day qmo, not to exceed 4 mg/day

Available forms: Tabs 1, 2, 4, 6 mg

Side effects/adverse reactions:
GI: Nausea, vomiting, diarrhea, constipation, anorexia, weight loss, jaundice, gallstones
INTEG: Flushing, alopecia, sweating, hyperthermia
CV: Palpitations, dysrhythmias, **myocardial infarction, ischemic myocardial changes,** angina
EENT: Visual disturbances, ptosis, retinopathy, lid lag
GU: Menstrual irregularities, change in libido
CNS: Insomnia, tremors, headache, dizziness, paresthesia, decreased sensorium

Contraindications: Severe hepatic disease, severe renal disease, organic heart disease, Hx of myocardial infarction, cardiac dysrhythmias, rheumatic heart disease, CHF, hypertension, iodism, angina, obesity

Precautions: Hepatic disease, renal disease, pregnancy (C), lactation, surgery, elderly

Interactions/incompatibilities:
• Decreased effects of dextrothyroxine: cholestyramine, colestipol
• Increased effects of: digitalis, oral anticoagulants, sympathomimetics
• Increased CNS stimulation: tricyclic antidepressants

• Increased blood sugar levels in patients with diabetes
• Decreased effects of: β-blockers
• May increase blood sugar levels: assess for loss of diabetic control

NURSING CONSIDERATIONS
Assess:
• Renal and hepatic function tests if patient is on long-term therapy
• CV status: rate, rhythm, character, chest pain
• Bowel pattern daily; increase bulk, water in diet if constipation develops

Evaluate:
• Therapeutic response: decreased cholesterol levels, (hyperlipidemia); diarrhea, pruritus (excess bile acids)

Teach patient/family:
• That compliance is needed, since toxicity may result if doses are missed
• That risk factors should be decreased: high-fat diet, smoking, alcohol consumption, absence of exercise
• That birth control should be practiced while on this drug
• That if anticoagulants are given with this drug, this drug should be discontinued 2 wk before surgery

---

dezocine
Dalgan
Func. class.: Narcotic agonist-antagonist analgesic
Chem. class.: Opioid, synthetic

Action: Depresses pain impulse transmission at the spinal cord level by interacting with opioid receptors
Uses: Severe pain
Dosage and routes:
Adult: IM 5-20 mg q3-6h, not to exceed 120 mg/day; IV 2.5-10 mg q2-4h

Available forms: IM, IV inj 5, 10, 15 mg single-dose vials, multiple dose 10 mg/ml

Side effects/adverse reactions:

CV: Hypotension, pulse irregularity, hypertension, chest pain, pallor, edema, thrombophlebitis

CNS: Drowsiness, dizziness, confusion, sedation, anxiety, headache, depression, delirium, sleep disturbances, dependency

GI: Nausea, vomiting, anorexia, constipation, cramps, abdominal pain, dry mouth, diarrhea

INTEG: Injection site reactions, pruritus, rash, sweating, chills

*RESP: **Respiratory depression,** hiccups*

GU: Urinary frequency, hesitancy, retention

EENT: Blurred vision, slurred speech, diplopia

Contraindications: Hypersensitivity

Precautions: Addictive personality, pregnancy (C), lactation, increased intracranial pressure, respiratory depression, hepatic disease, renal disease, child <18 yr, elderly, biliary surgery, COPD, sulfite sensitivity

Pharmacokinetics: IM: Onset 30 min, peak 50-90 min, duration 2-4 hr; IV: Onset 10 min, peak 30 min, duration 2-4 hr; metabolized by liver; excreted by kidneys; may cross placenta

Interactions/incompatibilities:

• Incompatibility: information not known

• Increased CNS depression: alcohol, narcotics, sedative/hypnotics, antipsychotics, skeletal muscle relaxants, general anesthetics, tranquilizers

NURSING CONSIDERATIONS

Assess:

• I&O ratio; check for decreasing output; may indicate urinary retention

• CNS changes: dizziness, drowsiness, hallucinations, euphoria, LOC, pupil reaction

• Allergic reactions: rash, urticaria

• Respiratory dysfunction: respiratory depression, character, rate, rhythm of respirations; notify physician if respirations are <10/min, shallow

• Need for pain medication, physical dependence

Administer:

• Undiluted 5 mg or less over 2-3 min

• With antiemetic if nausea, vomiting occur

• When pain is beginning to return; determine dosage interval by patient response

Perform/provide:

• Storage in light-resistant area at room temperature

• Assistance with ambulation

• Safety measures: top side rails, night-light, call bell within easy reach

Evaluate:

• Therapeutic response: decrease in pain

Teach patient/family:

• To report any symptoms of CNS changes, allergic reactions

• That physical dependency may result when used for extended periods of time

• That withdrawal symptoms may occur: nausea, vomiting, cramps, fever, faintness, anorexia

Treatment of overdose: Naloxone 0.2-0.8 IV, O$_2$, IV fluids, vasopressors

---

italics = common side effects   ***bold italic*** = life threatening reactions

diazepam

(dye-az'-e-pam)
Diazepam, Diazepam Intensol, D-Tran,* E-Pam,* Meval,* Novodipam,* Stress-Pam,* Valium, Valrelease, Vivol,* Vazepam, Zetran
Func. class.: Antianxiety
Chem. class.: Benzodiazepine

Controlled Substance Schedule IV

Action: Potentiates the actions of GABA, especially in limbic system, reticular formation; enhances presympathetic inhibition, inhibits spinal polysynaptic afferent paths

Uses: Anxiety, acute alcohol withdrawal, adjunct in seizure disorders; preoperatively, skeletal muscle relaxation

Dosage and routes:

Anxiety/convulsive disorders
• *Adult:* PO 2-10 mg tid-qid; EXT REL 15-30 mg qd
• *Child >6 mo:* PO 1-2.5 mg tid-qid

Tetanic muscle spasms
• *Child <5 yr:* IM/IV 5-10 mg q3-4 hr prn
• *Infants >30 days:* IM/IV 1-2 mg q3-4 hr prn

Status epilepticus
• *Adult:* IV BOL 5-20 mg, 2 mg/min, may repeat q5-10 min, not to exceed 60 mg; may repeat in 30 min if seizures reappear
• *Child:* IV BOL 0.1-0.3 mg/kg (1 mg/min over 3 min); may repeat q15 min × 2 doses

Available forms: Tabs 2, 5, 10 mg; caps ext rel 15 mg, IM/IV inj

Side effects/adverse reactions:

CNS: Dizziness, drowsiness, confusion, headache, anxiety, tremors, stimulation, fatigue, depression, insomnia, hallucinations

CV: Orthostatic hypotension, *ECG changes, tachycardia,* hypotension

EENT: Blurred vision, tinnitus, mydriasis

GI: Constipation, dry mouth, nausea, vomiting, anorexia, diarrhea

INTEG: Rash, dermatitis, itching

Contraindications: Hypersensitivity to benzodiazepines, narrow-angle glaucoma, psychosis, pregnancy (D)

Precautions: Elderly, debilitated, hepatic disease, renal disease

Pharmacokinetics:

PO: Rapidly absorbed; onset ½ hr, duration 2-3 hr

IM: Onset 15-30 min, duration 1-1½ hr; absorption slow and erratic

IV: Onset 1-5 min, duration 15 min Metabolized by liver, excreted by kidneys, crosses placenta, excreted in breast milk, crosses the blood-brain barrier; half-life 20-50 hr, more effective by mouth

Interactions/incompatibilities:

• Decreased effects of diazepam: oral contraceptives, rifampin, valproic acid, cimetidine, disulfiram, narcotic analgesics
• Increased CNS depression: CNS depressants, alcohol
• Incompatible with all drugs in sol or syringe

Lab test interferences:

Increase: AST/ALT, serum bilirubin

False increase: 17-OHCS

Decrease: RAIU

NURSING CONSIDERATIONS

Assess:

• B/P (lying, standing), pulse; respiratory rate; if systolic B/P drops 20 mm Hg, hold drug, notify physician; respirations q5-15 min if given IV
• Blood studies: CBC during long-

D

term therapy; blood dyscrasias have occurred (rarely)

• Degree of anxiety; what precipitates anxiety and whether drug controls symptoms

• For alcohol withdrawal symptoms, including hallucinations (visual, auditory, delirium, irritability, agitation, fine to coarse tremors

• For seizure control and type, duration, intensity of convulsions

• Hepatic studies: AST, ALT, bilirubin, creatinine, LDM, alk phosphatase

• IV site for thrombosis or phlebitis, which may occur rapidly

• Mental status: mood, sensorium, affect, sleeping pattern, drowsiness, dizziness

• Physical dependency, withdrawal symptoms: headache, nausea, vomiting, muscle pain, weakness after long-term use

• Suicidal tendencies

Administer:

• IV into large vein; do not dilute or mix with any other drug; give IV 5 mg or less/1 min or total dose over 3 min or more (children, infants); continuous infusion is not recommended

• With food or milk for GI symptoms; crushed if patient is unable to swallow medication whole; do not crush ext rel capsules

• Sugarless gum, hard candy, frequent sips of water for dry mouth

• Reduced narcotic dose by ⅓ if given concomitantly with diazepam

Perform/provide:

• Assistance with ambulation during beginning therapy, for drowsiness, dizziness

• Safety measures, including side rails

• Check to see PO medication has been swallowed

Evaluate:

• Therapeutic response: decreased anxiety, restlessness, insomnia

Teach patient/family:

• That drug may be taken with food

• Not to be used for everyday stress or used longer than 4 mo unless directed by physician; no more than prescribed amount; may be habit forming

• To avoid OTC preparations unless approved by physician

• To avoid driving, activities that require alertness; drowsiness may occur

• To avoid alcohol, other psychotropic medications unless prescribed by physician

• Not to discontinue medication abruptly after long-term use

• To rise slowly or fainting may occur, especially in elderly

• That drowsiness may worsen at beginning of treatment

Treatment of overdose: Lavage, VS, supportive care

---

diazoxide
(dye-az-ox′ide)
Diazoxide Injection, Hyperstat
Func. class.: Antihypertensive
Chem. class.: Vasodilator

Action: Vasodilates arteriolar smooth muscle by direct relaxation; a reduction in blood pressure with concomitant increases in heart rate, cardiac output

Uses: Hypertensive crisis when urgent decrease of diastolic pressure required; increase blood glucose levels in hyperinsulinism

Dosage and routes:

• *Adult:* IV BOL 1-3 mg/kg rapidly up to a max of 150 mg in a single injection; dose may be repeated at 5-15 min intervals until

---

italics = common side effects   ***bold italic*** = life threatening reactions

desired response is achieved; give IV in 30 sec or less
• *Child:* IV BOL 1-2 mg/kg rapidly; administration same as adult, not to exceed 150 mg
Available forms: Inj IV 15 mg/ml
Side effects/adverse reactions:
CV: **Hypotension,** T-wave changes, angina pectoris, palpitations, *supraventricular tachycardia, edema,* rebound hypertension
CNS: Headache, sleepiness, euphoria, anxiety, extrapyramidal symptoms, confusion, tinnitus, blurred vision, dizziness, weakness
GI: Nausea, vomiting, dry mouth
INTEG: Rash
HEMA: Decreased hemoglobin, hematocrit, *thrombocytopenia*
GU: Breast tenderness; increased BUN, fluid, electrolyte imbalances; Na, water retention
ENDO: Hyperglycemia in diabetics, transient hyperglycemia in nondiabetics
Contraindications: Hypersensitivity to thiazides, sulfonamides, hypertension associated with aortic coarctation or AV shunt, pheochromocytoma, dissecting aortic aneurysm
Precautions: Tachycardia, fluid, electrolyte imbalances, pregnancy (B), lactation, impaired cerebral or cardiac circulation, children
Pharmacokinetics:
IV: Onset 1-2 min, peak 5 min, duration 3-12 hr
Half-life 20-36 hr, excreted slowly in urine, crosses blood-brain barrier, placenta
Interactions/incompatibilities:
• Increased effects: thiazide diuretics, antihypertensives, coumadin, guanethidine, sympathomimetics
• Do not mix with any drug in syringe or solution

• Increased effects of: warfarin, other coumarins
• Hyperglycemia/hyperuricemia: thiazides, diuretics
• Decreased pharmacologic effects of both: sulfonylureas
NURSING CONSIDERATIONS
Assess:
• B/P q5min × 2 hr, then q1h × 2 hr, then q4h
• Pulse, jugular venous distention q4h
• Electrolytes, blood studies: K, Na, Cl, CO_2, CBC, serum glucose
• Weight daily, I&O
• Edema in feet, legs daily
• Skin turgor, dryness of mucous membranes for hydration status
• Rales, dyspnea, orthopnea
• IV site for extravasation, rate
• Signs of CHF: dyspnea, edema, wet rales
• Postural hypotension, take B/P sitting, standing
Administer:
• Undiluted; give over ½ min or less
• To patient in recumbent position; keep in that position for 1 hr after administration
Perform/provide:
• Protection from light
Evaluate:
• Therapeutic response: decreased B/P, primarily diastolic pressure
Treatment of overdose: Administer levarterenol, dopamine, or norepinephrine for hypotension, dialysis

---

diazoxide (oral)
(dye-az-ox'ide)
Proglycem
Func. class.: Hyperglycemic
Chem. class.: Benzothiadiazine

Action: Decreases release of insulin from β-cells in pancreas, resulting in an increase in blood glucose

Uses: Hypoglycemia caused by hyperinsulinism

Dosage and routes:
• *Adult and child:* PO 3-8 mg/kg/day in 2-3 divided doses q8-12h
• *Infants and neonates:* PO 8-15 mg/kg/day in 2-3 divided doses 8-12h

Available forms: Caps 50 mg; oral susp 50 mg/ml

Side effects/adverse reactions:
GU: Reversible nephrotic syndrome, decreased urinary output, hematuria
CNS: Headache, weakness, malaise, anxiety, dizziness, insomnia, paresthesia
EENT: Diplopia, cataracts, ring scotoma, subconjunctival hemorrhage, lacrimation
HEMA: **Thrombocytopenia, leukopenia,** eosinophilia, decreased hemoglobulin, hematocrit
INTEG: Increased hair growth or loss of scalp hair, rash, dermatitis, herpes
GI: Nausea, vomiting, anorexia, abdominal pain, transient loss of taste, diarrhea
CV: Tachycardia, palpitations, hypotension, transient hypertension
META: Hyperuricemia, Na/fluid retention, ketoacidosis, hyperglycemia, azotemia

Contraindications: Hypersensitivity to this drug or thiazides, functional hypoglycemia

Precautions: Pregnancy (C), lactation, renal disease, diabetes mellitus, CV disease, gout

Pharmacokinetics:
PO: Onset 1 hr, duration 8 hr, half-life 28 hrs; excreted unchanged by kidneys; crosses blood-brain barrier, placenta

Interactions/incompatibilities:
• Increased effects of diazoxide: phenothiazines, thiazide diuretics
• Decreased effects of: phenytoin
• Increased effects of: antihypertensives, oral anticoagulants
• Decreased effects of diazoxide: α-adrenergic blockers, sulfonylureas, insulin

Lab test interferences:
Increase: Bilirubin, uric acid, blood glucose
Decrease: Creatinine, Hgb, Hct, plasma-free fatty acids

NURSING CONSIDERATIONS
Assess:
• I&O ratio, weight weekly
• Electrolytes (K, Na, Cl), glucose, Hct, Hgb, platelets, differential
• Urine for glucose, ketones qd
Administer:
• Shake susp before using
Perform/provide:
• Susp storage: protect from light
Evaluate:
• Therapeutic response: adequate blood, urine glucose, absence of ketones in urine
Teach patient/family:
• That if drug is not effective within 2-3 wk, drug may be discontinued
• That if hirsutism occurs, it is reversible after discontinuing treatment

---

dibucaine HCl (topical)

(dye'byoo-kane)
Dibucaine, Nupercainal
Func. class.: Topical anesthetic
Chem. class.: Amide

Action: Inhibits nerve impulses from sensory nerves, which produces anesthesia

---

italics = common side effects   ***bold italic*** = life threatening reactions

Uses: Pruritus, sunburn, toothache, sore throat, cold sores, oral pain, rectal pain and irritation

Dosage and routes:
• *Adult and child:* TOP apply qid as needed; REC insert tid and after each BM

Available forms: Cream 0.5%; rec or top oint 1%

Side effects/adverse reactions:
INTEG: Rash, irritation, sensitization

Contraindications: Hypersensitivity, infants <1 yr, application to large areas

Precautions: Child <6 yr, sepsis, pregnancy (C), denuded skin

NURSING CONSIDERATIONS
Assess:
• Allergy: rash, irritation, reddening, swelling
• Infection: if affected area is infected, do not apply

Administer:
• After cleansing and drying of affected area

Evaluate:
• Therapeutic response: absence of pain, itching of affected area

Teach patient/family:
• To report rash, irritation, redness, swelling
• How to apply cream, ointment

---

diclofenac

(dye-kloe'-fen-ac)

Voltaren

Func. class.: Nonsteroidal antiinflammatory

Chem. class.: Phenylacetic acid

Action: Inhibits prostaglandin synthesis by decreasing enzyme needed for biosynthesis; analgesic, antiinflammatory, antipyretic properties

Uses: Acute, chronic rheumatoid arthritis, osteoarthritis, ankylosing spondylitis

Dosage and routes:
Osteoarthritis
• *Adult:* PO 100-150 mg/day in divided doses

Rheumatoid arthritis
• *Adult:* PO 150-200 mg/day in divided doses

Ankylosing spondylitis
• *Adult:* PO 100-125 mg/day; give 25 mg qid and 25 mg hs if needed

Available forms: Tabs enteric coated 25, 50, 75 mg

Side effects/adverse reactions:
GI: Nausea, anorexia, vomiting, diarrhea, *jaundice, cholestatic hepatitis,* constipation, flatulence, cramps, dry mouth, peptic ulcer, GI bleeding

CNS: Dizziness, drowsiness, fatigue, tremors, confusion, insomnia, anxiety, depression, nervousness, paresthesia, muscle weakness

CV: **CHF,** tachycardia, peripheral edema, palpitations, *dysrhythmias,* hypotension, hypertension, fluid retention

INTEG: Purpura, rash, pruritus, sweating, erythema, petechiae, photosensitivity, alopecia

GU: **Nephrotoxicity: dysuria, hematuria, oliguria, azotemia, cystitis, UTI**

HEMA: **Blood dyscrasias,** epistaxis, bruising

EENT: Tinnitus, hearing loss, blurred vision

RESP: Dyspnea, hemoptysis, pharyngitis, *bronchospasm, laryngeal edema,* rhinitis, shortness of breath

Contraindications: Hypersensitivity to aspirin, iodides, other nonsteroidal antiinflammatory agents, asthma

Precautions: Pregnancy (B) 1st, 2nd trimester, lactation, children, bleeding disorders, GI disorders,

---

cardiac disorders, hypersensitivity to other antiinflammatory agents

Pharmacokinetics:

PO: Peak 2-3 hr, elimination half-life 1-2 hr, 90% bound to plasma proteins, metabolized in liver to metabolite, excreted in urine

Interactions/incompatibilities:

• Decreased antihypertensive effect: β-blockers, diuretics

• Increased anticoagulant effect: coumarin

• Increased toxicity: phenytoin, sulfonamides, sulfonylurea, digoxin, lithium

• Increased plasma levels of diclofenac: probenecid, K-sparing diuretics

NURSING CONSIDERATIONS

Assess:

• Blood counts during therapy; watch for decreasing platelets; if low, therapy may need to be discontinued, restarted after hematologic recovery

• Blood dyscrasias (thrombocytopenia): bruising, fatigue, bleeding, poor healing

Evaluate:

• Therapeutic response: decreased inflammation in joints

Teach patient/family:

• That drug must be continued for prescribed time to be effective

• To report bleeding, bruising, fatigue, malaise since blood dyscrasias do occur

• To avoid aspirin, alcoholic beverages

• To take with food, milk, or antacids to avoid GI upset, to swallow whole

• To use caution when driving; drowsiness, dizziness may occur

• To take with a full glass of water to enhance absorption; do not crush, break, or chew

---

dicloxacillin sodium

(dye-klox-a-sill'-in)

Dicloxacillin sodium, Dycill, Dynapen, Pathocil

Func. class.: Broad-spectrum antibiotic

Chem. class.: Penicillinase-resistant penicillin

Action: Interferes with cell wall replication of susceptible organisms; osmotically unstable cell wall swells, bursts from osmotic pressure

Uses: Effective for gram-positive cocci *(S. aureus, S. pyogenes, S. viridans, S. faecalis, S. bovis, S. pneumoniae)*, infections caused by penicillinase-producing *Staphylococcus*

Dosage and routes:

• *Adult:* PO 0.5-4 g/day in divided doses q6h

• *Child:* PO 12.5-25 mg/kg in divided doses q6h, max 4 g/d

Available forms: Caps 125, 250, 500 mg; powder for oral susp 62.5 mg/5 ml

Side effects/adverse reactions:

HEMA: Anemia, increased bleeding time, ***bone marrow depression, granulocytopenia***

GI: Nausea, vomiting, diarrhea, increased AST, ALT, abdominal pain, glossitis, colitis

GU: ***Oliguria, proteinuria, hematuria,*** vaginitis, moniliasis, ***glomerulonephritis***

CNS: Lethargy, hallucinations, anxiety, depression, twitching, ***coma, convulsions***

Contraindications: Hypersensitivity to penicillins; neonates

Precautions: Hypersensitivity to cephalosporins, pregnancy (B)

Pharmacokinetics:

PO: Peak 1 hr, duration 4-6 hr, half-

---

italics = common side effects   ***bold italic*** = life threatening reactions

life 30-60 min; metabolized in liver; excreted in urine, bile, breast milk; crosses placenta

Interactions/incompatibilities:
• Decreased antimicrobial effectiveness of dicloxacillin: tetracyclines, erythromycins
• Increased dicloxacillin concentrations: aspirin, probenecid

Lab test interferences:
False positive: Urine glucose, urine protein

NURSING CONSIDERATIONS
Assess:
• I&O ratio; report hematuria, oliguria, since penicillin in high doses is nephrotoxic
• Any patient with compromised renal system, since drug is excreted slowly in poor renal system function; toxicity may occur rapidly
• Liver studies: AST, ALT
• Blood studies: WBC, RBC, H&H, bleeding time
• Renal studies: urinalysis, protein, blood
• C&S before drug therapy; drug may be given as soon as culture is taken
• WBC and diff., ALT, AST, BUN, creatine for patients on long-term therapy
• Bowel pattern before, during treatment
• Skin eruptions after administration of penicillin to 1 wk after discontinuing drug
• Respiratory status: rate, character, wheezing, tightness in chest
• Allergies before initiation of treatment, reaction of each medication; highlight allergies on chart, Kardex

Administer:
• Drug after C&S has been completed
• On an empty stomach with a full glass of water

Perform/provide:
• Adrenalin, suction, tracheostomy set, endotracheal intubation equipment
• Adequate fluid intake (2 L) during diarrhea episodes
• Scratch test to assess allergy after securing order from physician; usually done when penicillin is only drug of choice
• Storage in tight container; after reconstituting, store in refrigerator up to 2 wk

Evaluate:
• Therapeutic response: absence of fever, draining wounds

Teach patient/family:
• Aspects of drug therapy, including need to complete course of medication to ensure organism death (10-14 days); culture may be taken after completed course
• To report sore throat, fever, fatigue (could indicate superimposed infection)
• To wear or carry Medic Alert ID if allergic to penicillins
• To notify nurse of diarrhea

Treatment of overdose: Withdraw drug; maintain airway; administer epinephrine, aminophylline, O_2, IV corticosteroids for anaphylaxis

---

dicyclomine HCl
(dye-sye'kloe-meen)
Antispas, Bentyl, Bentylol,* Byclomine, Dibent, Dicyclomine HCL, Di-Spaz, Formulex,* Neoquess, OR-Tyl, Spasmoject, Viserol

Func. class.: Gastrointestinal anticholinergic
Chem. class.: Synthetic tertiary amine

Action: Inhibits muscarinic actions of acetylcholine at postganglionic

---

parasympathetic neuroeffector sites

Uses: Treatment of peptic ulcer disease in combination with other drugs; infant colic

Dosage and routes:
• *Adult:* PO 10-20 mg tid-qid; IM 20 mg q4-6h
• *Child >2 yr:* PO 10 mg tid-qid
• *Child 6 mo-2 yr:* PO 5 mg tid-qid

Available forms: Caps 10, 20 mg; tabs 20 mg; syr 10 mg/5 ml; inj IM 10 mg/ml

Side effects/adverse reactions:

CNS: Confusion, stimulation in elderly, headache, insomnia, dizziness, drowsiness, anxiety, weakness, hallucination; *seizures, coma* (child <3 mo)

GI: Dry mouth, constipation, paralytic ileus, heartburn, nausea, vomiting, dysphagia, absence of taste

GU: Hesitancy, rentention, impotence

CV: Palpitations, tachycardia

EENT: Blurred vision, photophobia, mydriasis, cycloplegia, increased ocular tension

INTEG: Urticaria, rash, pruritus, anhidrosis, fever, allergic reactions

Contraindications: Hypersensitivity to anticholinergics, narrow-angle glaucoma, GI obstruction, myasthenia gravis, paralytic ileus, GI atony, toxic megacolon

Precautions: Hyperthyroidism, coronary artery disease, dysrhythmias, CHF, ulcerative colitis, hypertension, hiatal hernia, hepatic disease, renal disease, pregnancy (B), urinary retention, prostatic hypertrophy

Pharmacokinetics:

PO: Onset 1-2 hr, duration 3-4 hr; metabolized by liver; excreted in urine

Interactions/incompatibilities:
• Increased anticholinergic effect: amantadine, tricylic antidepressants, MAOIs, H₁ antihistamines
• Decreased effect of: phenothiazines, levodopa, ketoconazole

NURSING CONSIDERATIONS

Assess:
• VS, cardiac status: checking for dysrhythmias, increased rate, palpitations
• I&O ratio; check for urinary retention or hesitancy
• GI complaints: pain, bleeding (frank or occult), nausea, vomiting, anorexia

Administer:
• ½-1 hr ac for better absorption
• Decreased dose to elderly patients; their metabolism may be slowed
• Gum, hard candy, frequent rinsing of mouth for dryness of oral cavity

Perform/provide:
• Storage in tight container protected from light
• Increased fluids, bulk, exercise to patient's lifestyle to decrease constipation

Evaluate:
• Therapeutic response: absence of epigastric pain, bleeding, nausea, vomiting

Teach patient/family:
• To avoid driving or other hazardous activities until stabilized on medication; may cause blurred vision
• To avoid alcohol or other CNS depressants; will enhance sedating properties of this drug
• To avoid hot environments; stroke may occur; drug suppresses perspiration
• To use sunglasses when outside to prevent photophobia

---

italics = common side effects   ***bold italic*** = life threatening reactions

- To drink plenty of fluids
- To report dysphagia

---

didanosine (ddI, dideoxyinosine)

(dye-dan′-o-seen)

Videx, ddI, Dideoxyinosine

Func. class.: Antiviral

Chem. class.: Synthetic purine nucleoside of deoxyadenosine

Action: Nucleoside analog incorporating into cellular DNA by viral reverse transcriptase, thereby terminating the cellular DNA chain

Uses: Advanced HIV infections in adults and children who have been unable to use zidovudine or who have not responded to treatment

Dosage and routes:

- *Adult:* PO >75 kg, 300 mg bid tabs, or 375 mg bid buffered powder

50-74 kg, 200 mg bid tabs, or 250 mg bid buffered powder

35-49 kg, 125 mg bid tabs, or 167 mg bid buffered powder

- *Child:* PO 1.1-1.4 m², 100 mg bid tabs, or 125 mg bid pedi powder

0.8-1 m², 75 mg bid tabs, or 94 mg bid pedi powder

0.5-0.7 m², 50 mg bid tabs, or 62 mg bid pedi powder

< 0.4 m², 25 mg bid tabs, or 31 mg bid pedi powder

Available forms: Tabs, buffered, chewable/dispersible 25, 50, 100, 150 mg; powder for oral sol, buffered 100, 167, 250, 375 mg; powder for oral sol, pedi 2, 4 g

Side effects/adverse reactions:

GI: **Pancreatitis,** diarrhea, nausea, vomiting, abdominal pain, constipation, stomatitis, dyspepsia, liver abnormalities, flatulence, taste perversion, dry mouth, oral thrush, melena, increased ALT, AST, Alk phosphatase, amylase

GU: Increased bilirubin, uric acid

CNS: **Peripheral neuropathy, seizures,** confusion, anxiety, hypertonia, abnormal thinking, asthenia, insomnia, **CNS depression,** pain, dizziness, chills, fever

RESP: Cough, pneumonia, dyspnea, asthma, epistaxis, hypoventilation, sinusitis

INTEG: Rash, pruritus, alopecia, ecchymosis, hemorrhage, petechiae, sweating

MS: Myalgia, arthritis, myopathy, muscular atrophy

CV: Hypertension, vasodilation, dysrhythmia, syncope, CHF, palpitation

EENT: Ear pain, otitis, photophobia, visual impairment

HEMA: **Leukopenia, granulocytopenia, thrombocytopenia, anemia**

Contraindications: Hypersensitivity

Precautions: Renal, hepatic disease, pregnancy (B), lactation, children, Na-restricted diets, elevated amylase, preexistant peripheral neuropathy

Pharmacokinetics:

PO: Elimination half-life 1.62 hr, extensive metabolism is thought to occur; administration within 5 min of food will decrease absorption

Interactions/incompatibilities:

- Decreased absorption: ketoconazole, dapsone, food
- Do not administer with tetracyclines
- Decreased concentrations of: fluoroquinolone antibiotics

NURSING CONSIDERATIONS

Assess:

- Neuropathy: tingling or pain in hands and feet, distal numbness
- Pancreatitis: Abdominal pain, nausea, vomiting, elevated liver en-

---

zymes; drug should be discontinued, since condition can be fatal
• Children by dilated retinal examination q6mo to rule out retinal depigmentation
• CBC, differential, platelet count qmo; withhold drug if WBC is <4000 or platelet count is <75,000; notify physician of results; monitor amylase
• Renal function studies: BUN, serum uric acid, urine CrCl before, during therapy
• Temperature q4h, may indicate beginning infection
• Liver function tests before, during therapy (bilirubin, AST, ALT) as needed or qmo

Administer:
• Antibiotics for prophylaxis of infection

Perform/provide:
• Strict medical asepsis, protective isolation if WBC levels are low
• Clean-up of powdered products; use wet mop or damp sponge

Evaluate:
• Therapeutic response: absence of infection; symptoms of HIV

Teach patient/family:
• To take on an empty stomach; not to take dapsone at same time as ddi
• To report signs of infection: increased temperature, sore throat, flu symptoms
• To report signs of anemia: fatigue, headache, faintness, shortness of breath, irritability
• To report bleeding; avoid use of razors or commercial mouthwash
• That hair may be lost during therapy; a wig or hairpiece may make patient feel better (rare)

dienestrol
(dye-en-ess'trole)
DV, Ortho Dienestrol
Func. class.: Estrogen
Chem. class.: Nonsteroidal synthetic estrogen

Action: Needed for adequate functioning of female reproductive system, it affects release of pituitary gonadotropins, inhibits ovulation, adequate calcium use in bone structures

Uses: Atrophic vaginitis, kraurosis vulvae

Dosage and routes:
• *Adult:* VAG CREAM 1-2 applications qd × 2 wk, then ½ dose × 2 wk, then 1 application

Available forms: Vag cream 0.01%

Side effects/adverse reactions:
CNS: Dizziness, headache, migraines, depression
CV: Hypotension, thrombophlebitis, edema, *thromboembolism, stroke, pulmonary embolism, myocardial infarction*
GI: Nausea, vomiting, diarrhea, anorexia, pancreatitis, cramps, constipation, increased appetite, increased weight, *cholestatic jaundice*
EENT: Contact lens intolerance, increased myopia, astigmatism
GU: Amenorrhea, cervical erosion, breakthrough bleeding, dysmenorrhea, vaginal candidiasis, breast changes, gynecomastia, testicular atrophy, impotence
INTEG: Rash, urticaria, acne, hirsutism, alopecia, oily skin, seborrhea, purpura, melasma
META: Folic acid deficiency, hypercalcemia, hyperglycemia

Contraindications: Breast cancer, thromboembolic disorders, repro-

---

italics = common side effects   ***bold italic*** = life threatening reactions

ductive cancer, genital bleeding (abnormal, undiagnosed), pregnancy (X)

Precautions: Hypertension, asthma, blood dyscrasias, gallbladder disease, CHF, diabetes mellitus, bone disease, depression, migraine headache, convulsive disorders, hepatic disease, renal disease, family history of cancer of the breast or reproductive tract

Pharmacokinetics:

TOP: Degraded in liver; excreted in urine; crosses placenta; excreted in breast milk

Interactions/incompatibilities:

• Decreased action of: anticoagulants, oral hypoglycemics

• Toxicity: tricyclic antidepressants

• Decreased action of dienestrol: anticonvulsants, barbiturates, phenylbutazone, rifampin

• Increased action of: corticosteroids

NURSING CONSIDERATIONS

Assess:

• Weight daily; notify physician of weekly weight gain >5 lb

• B/P q4h

• I&O ratio; be alert for decreasing urinary output and increasing edema

• Liver function studies including ALT, AST, bilirubin

• Edema, hypertension, cardiac symptoms, jaundice

• Mental status: affect, mood, behavioral changes, aggression

• Hypercalcemia

Administer:

• At hs for better absorption

• Titrated dose; use lowest effective dose to prevent adverse reactions

• Dosage reduction should continue at 3-6 month intervals

Perform/provide:

• Storage in tight, light-resistant container in refrigerator

Evaluate:

• Therapeutic response: decreased symptoms of vaginitis, kraurosis

Teach patient/family:

• How to fill applicator and insert cream

• To check with physician before using any OTC drugs

• To report breast lumps, vaginal bleeding, edema, jaundice, dark urine, clay-colored stools, dyspnea, headache, blurred vision, abdominal pain, numbness or stiffness in legs, chest pain

---

diethylpropion HCl

Dospan, Diethylpropion HCl, Tenuate, Tenuate Dospan, Tepanil, Tepanil Ten-Tab

Func. class.: Andrexiant
Chem. class.: Amphetamine-like analog

Controlled Substance Schedule IV

Action: Direct stimulation of partial adrenergic pathways to suppress appetite

Uses: Exogenous obesity

Dosage and routes:

• *Adult:* PO 25 mg tid 1 hr ac, or 75 mg controlled release qd mid-morning

Available forms: Tabs 25 mg, tabs sus rel 75 mg

Side effects/adverse reactions:

MISC: Hair loss, ecchymosis, muscle/chest pain, excessive sweating, chills, flushing, fever

EENT: mydriosis, blurred vision, eye irritation

HEMA: **Bone marrow depression,** leukopenia, agranulocytosis

CNS: Hyperactivity, restlessness,

---

anxiety, insomnia, dizziness, dysphoria, depression, tremors, headache, incoordination, fatigue, malaise, euphoria, depression, tremor, confusion

GI: Nausea, vomiting, anorexia, unpleasant taste, pain, dry mouth, diarrhea, constipation

GU: Impotence, change in libido, menstrual irregularities, dysuria, polyuria, urinary frequency

CV: Palpitations, tachycardia, hypertension, dysrhythmias, pulmonary hypertension, ECG changes

INTEG: Urticaria, rash, erythema

Contraindications: Hypersensitivity, hyperthyroidism, hypertension, glaucoma, angina pectoris, drug abuse, cardiovascular disease, children <12 yr, severe arteriosclerosis, agitated states

Precautions: Convulsive disorders, pregnancy (B), lactation

Pharmacokinetics:

PO: Duration 4 hr

CONT REL: Duration 10-14 hr; metabolized by liver; excreted by kidneys; crosses placenta, breast milk; half-life 1-3½ hr

Interactions/incompatibilities:

• Hypertensive crisis: MAOIs or within 14 days of MAOIs

• Decreased effects of: diethylpropion, tricyclics

• Decreased effects of: guanethidine

NURSING CONSIDERATIONS

Assess:

• VS, B/P since this drug may reverse antihypertensives; check patients with cardiac disease more often

• CBC, urinalysis, in diabetes: blood sugar, urine sugar; insulin changes may be required since eating will decrease

• Height, growth rate in children; growth rate may be decreased

• Mental status: mood, sensorium, affect, stimulation, insomnia, aggressiveness

• Physical dependency: should not be used for extended time; dose should be discontinued gradually; drug tolerance occurs after long-term use

• Withdrawal symptoms: headache, nausea, vomiting, muscle pain, weakness

Administer:

• At least 6 hr before hs to avoid sleeplessness

• For obesity only if patient is on weight reduction program, including dietary changes, exercise; patient will develop tolerance, and weight loss won't occur without additional methods; give 1 hour before meals

• Gum, hard candy, frequent sips of water for dry mouth

Evaluate:

• Therapeutic response: decreased weight

Teach patient/family:

• To take on empty stomach; do not take more than amount prescribed

• Not to crush or chew sus rel preps; not to take more frequently than prescribed

• To decrease caffeine consumption (coffee, tea, cola, chocolate); may increase irritability, stimulation

• To avoid OTC preparations unless approved by physician

• To taper off drug over several weeks, or depression, increased sleeping, lethargy will occur

• To avoid alcohol ingestion

• To avoid hazardous activities until patient is stabilized on medication

• To get needed rest; patient will feel more tired at end of day

Treatment of overdose: Admin-

---

italics = common side effects   ***bold italic*** = life threatening reactions

ister fluids, hemodialysis for peritoneal dialysis; antihypertensive for increased B/P; ammonium Cl for increased excretion

---

diethylstilbestrol/diethylstilbestrol diphosphate

(dye-eth-il-stil-bess'trole)
DES, Diethylstilbestrol, Honvol*, Stilboestrol*, Stilphostrol

Func. class.: Estrogen
Chem. class.: Nonsteroidal synthetic estrogen

Action: Needed for adequate functioning of female reproductive system, it affects release of pituitary gonadotropins, inhibits ovulation, adequate calcium use in bone structures

Uses: Atrophic vaginitis, kraurosis vulvae, menopause, postcoital contraception, hypogonadism, castration, primary ovarian failure, breast engorgement, breast cancer, prostatic cancer

Dosage and routes:
Atrophic vaginitis/kraurosis vulvae
• *Adult:* VAG SUPP 0.1-1 mg qd × 10-14 days with oral therapy or up to 5 mg qwk
Menopause
• *Adult:* PO 0.1-2 mg qd 3wk on, 1 wk off
Contraception
• *Adult:* PO 25 mg bid × 5 days, within 72 hr of intercourse
Hypogonadism/castration/ovarian failure
• *Adult:* PO 0.2-0.5 mg qd
Breast engorgement
• *Adult:* PO 5 mg qd-tid, not to exceed 30 mg
Prostatic cancer
• *Adult:* PO 1-3 mg qd, then 1

mg qd; PO 50-200 mg tid (diphosphate); IM 5 mg 2×/wk, then 4 mg 2×/wk; IV 0.25-1 g qd × 5 days, then 1-2×/wk
Breast cancer
• *Adult:* PO 15 mg qd
Available forms: Tabs 1, 5 mg; tabs enteric coated 0.1, 0.25, 0.5, 1, 5 mg; vag supp 0.1, 0.5 mg, IV
Side effects/adverse reactions:
CNS: Dizziness, headache, migraines, depression
CV: Hypotension, thrombophlebitis, edema, *thromboembolism, stroke, pulmonary embolism, myocardial infarction*
GI: Nausea, vomiting, diarrhea, anorexia, pancreatitis, cramps, constipation, increased appetite, increased weight, *cholestatic jaundice*
EENT: Contact lens intolerance, increased myopia, astigmatism
GU: Amenorrhea, cervical erosion, breakthrough bleeding, dysmenorrhea, vaginal candidiasis, breast changes, *gynecomastia, testicular atrophy, impotence*
INTEG: Rash, urticaria, acne, hirsutism, alopecia, oily skin, seborrhea, purpura, melasma
META: Folic acid deficiency, hypercalcemia, hyperglycemia
Contraindications: Breast cancer, thromboembolic disorders, reproductive cancer, genital bleeding (abnormal, undiagnosed), pregnancy (X)
Precautions: Hypertension, asthma, blood dyscrasias, gallbladder disease, CHF, diabetes mellitus, bone disease blocking agents
Interactions/incompatibilities:
• Decreased action of: anticoagulants, oral hypoglycemics
• Toxicity: tricyclic antidepressants

---

* Available in Canada only

• Decreased action of diethylstilbestrol: anticonvulsants, barbiturates, phenylbutazone, rifampin
• Increased action of: corticosteroids
• Incompatibility: not known

Lab test interferences:

Increase: BSP retention test, PBI, T₄, serum Na, platelet aggressability, thyroxine-binding globulin (TBG), prothrombin, factors VII, VIII, IX, X, triglycerides

Decrease: Serum folate, serum triglyceride, T₃ resin uptake test, glucose tolerance test, antithrombin III, pregnanediol, metyraponetest

False positive: LE prep, antinuclear antibodies

NURSING CONSIDERATIONS
Assess:
• Urine glucose in patient with diabetes; increased urine glucose may occur
• Weight daily, notify physician of weekly weight gain >5 lb; if increase, diuretic may be ordered
• B/P q4h, watch for increase caused by H₂O and Na retention
• I&O ratio; be alert for decreasing urinary output and increasing edema
• Liver function studies, including AST, ALT, bilirubin, alk phosphatase
• Edema, hypertension, cardiac symptoms, jaundice
• Mental status: affect, mood, behavioral changes, aggression
• Hypercalcemia

Administer:
• IV after diluting in 300 ml of dextrose or saline sol; give at a rate of 1-2 ml/min × 15 min; may increase rate to complete infusion 1 hr after starting
• Titrated dose; use lowest effective dose

• IM injection deeply in large muscular mass
• In one dose in AM for prostatic cancer, vaginitis, hypogonadism
• With food or milk to decrease GI symptoms

Evaluate:
• Therapeutic response: absence of breast engorgement, reversal of menopause or decrease in tumor size in prostatic cancer

Teach patient/family:
• To weigh weekly, report gain >5 lb
• To report breast lumps, vaginal bleeding, edema, jaundice, dark urine, clay-colored stools, dyspnea, headache, blurred vision, abdominal pain, numbness or stiffness in legs, chest pain; male to report impotence or gynecomastia
• To check with physician before taking any OTC drugs

---

difenoxin HCl with atropine sulfate
(dye-fen-ox' -in)
Motofen
Func. class.: Antidiarrheal
Chem. class.: Phenylpiperidine derivative, opiate agonist

Controlled Substance Schedule IV
Action: Inhibits gastric motility by acting on mucosal receptors responsible for peristalsis
Uses: Acute nonspecific and acute exacerbations of chronic functional diarrhea

Dosage and routes:
• *Adult:* PO 2 mg, then 1 mg after each loose stool or 1 mg q3-4h as needed, not to exceed 8 mg/24 hr
Available forms: Tab 1 mg difenoxin HCl, 0.025 mg atropine sulfate

---

italics = common side effects   ***bold italic*** = life threatening reactions

Side effects/adverse reactions:
CNS: Dizziness, drowsiness, light-headedness, headache, fatigue, nervousness, insomnia, confusion
GI: Nausea, vomiting, dry mouth, epigastric distress, constipation
EENT: Burning eyes, blurred vision
Contraindications: Hypersensitivity, pseudomembranous enterocolitis, jaundice, glaucoma, child <2 yr, severe electrolyte imbalances, diarrhea associated with organisms that penetrate intestinal mucosa
Precautions: Hepatic disease, renal disease, ulcerative colitis, pregnancy (C), lactation, severe liver disease
Pharmacokinetics:
PO: Onset 40-60 min, peak 2 hrs, duration 3-4 hr, terminal half-life 12-14 hr; metabolized in liver to inactive metabolite; excreted in urine, feces
Interactions/incompatibilities:
• Do not use with MAOIs; hypertensive crisis may occur
• Increased action of: alcohol, narcotics, barbituates, other CNS depressants, anticholinergics
NURSING CONSIDERATIONS
Assess:
• Electrolytes (K, Na, Cl) if on long-term therapy
• Bowel pattern before; for rebound constipation after termination of medication
• Response after 48 hr; if no response, drug should be discontinued
• Abdominal distention, toxic megacolon, which may occur in ulcerative colitis
Administer:
• For 48 hr only
Evaluate:
• Therapeutic response: decreased diarrhea

Teach patient/family:
• To avoid OTC products unless directed by physician; may contain alcohol
• Not to exceed recommended dose
• That drug may be habit forming

---

diflorasone diacetate
(die-floor'-a-sone)
Florone, Florone E, Maxiflor, Psorcon
Func. class.: Topical corticosteroid
Chem. class.: Synthetic fluorinated agent, group II potency

Action: Antipruritic, antiinflammatory
Uses: Psoriasis, eczema, contact dermatitis, pruritus
Dosage and routes:
• *Adult and child:* Apply to affected area qd-tid
Available forms: Cream 0.05%; oint 0.05%
Side effects/adverse reactions:
INTEG: Burning, dryness, itching, irritation, acne, folliculitis, hypertrichosis, perioral dermatitis, hypopigmentation, atrophy, striae, miliaria, allergic contact dermatitis, secondary infection
Contraindications: Hypersensitivity to corticosteroids, fungal infections
Precautions: Pregnancy (C), lactation, viral infections, bacterial infections
NURSING CONSIDERATIONS
Assess:
• Temperature; if fever develops, drug should be discontinued
• For systemic absorption: increased temperature, inflammation, irritation
Administer:
• Only to affected areas; do not get in eyes

---

*Available in Canada only

• Medication; then cover with occlusive dressing (only if prescribed); seal to normal skin; change q12h; use occlusive dressing with extreme caution; systemic absorption may occur

• Only to dermatoses; do not use on weeping, denuded, or infected area

Perform/provide:

• Cleansing before application of drug

• Treatment for a few days after area has cleared

• Storage at room temperature

Evaluate:

• Therapeutic response: absence of severe itching, patches on skin, flaking

Teach patient/family:

• To avoid sunlight on affected area; burns may occur

---

diflunisal

(dye-floo′ni-sal)

Diflunisal, Dolobid

Func. class.: Nonsteroidal antiinflammatory

Chem. class.: Salicylate derivative

Action: May block pain impulses in CNS that occur in response to inhibition of prostaglandin synthesis; antipyretic action results from inhibition of hypothalamic heat-regulating center to produce vasodilation to allow heat dissipation

Uses: Mild to moderate pain or fever including arthritis; 3-4 times more potent than aspirin

Dosage and routes:

Pain/fever

• *Adult:* PO loading dose 1 g; then 500-1000 mg/day in 2 divided doses, q12h, not to exceed 1500 mg/day

Available forms: Tabs 250, 500 mg

Side effects/adverse reactions:

*HEMA: **Thrombocytopenia, agranulocytosis, leukopenia, neutropenia, hemolytic anemia,** in-creased pro-time*

CNS: Stimulation, drowsiness, dizziness, confusion, ***convulsions,*** headache, flushing, hallucinations, coma

GI: Nausea, vomiting, GI bleeding, diarrhea, heartburn, anorexia, **hepatitis**

INTEG: Rash, urticaria, bruising

EENT: Blurred vision, decreased acuity, corneal deposits

CV: Rapid pulse, ***pulmonary edema***

RESP: Wheezing, hyperpnea

ENDO: Hypoglycemia, hyponatremia, hypokalemia

Contraindications: Hypersensitivity to salicylates, GI bleeding, bleeding disorders, children <12 yr, Vit K deficiency

Precautions: Anemia, hepatic disease, renal disease, Hodgkin's disease, pregnancy (C), lactation

Pharmacokinetics:

PO: Onset 15-30 min, peak 2-3 hr, half-life 10-12 hr; metabolized by liver; excreted by kidneys; crosses placenta; 99% protein bound; excreted in breast milk

Interactions/incompatibilities:

• Decreased effects of diflunisal: antacids, steroids, urinary alkalizers

• Increased blood loss: alcohol, heparin

• Increased effects of: anticoagulants, insulin, methotrexate, hydrochlorothiazide, acetaminophen

• Decreased effects of: probenecid, spironolactone, sulfinpyrazone, sulfonylmides

• Toxic effects: PABA

• Decreased blood sugar levels: salicylates

---

italics = common side effects   ***bold italic*** = life threatening reactions

Lab test interferences:
Increase: Coagulation studies, liver function studies, serum uric acid, amylase, CO_2, urinary protein
Decrease: Serum K, PBI, cholesterol
Interfere: Urine catecholamines, pregnancy test

NURSING CONSIDERATIONS
Assess:
• Liver function studies: AST, ALT, bilirubin, creatinine if patient is on long-term therapy
• Renal function studies: BUN, urine creatinine if patient is on long-term therapy
• Blood studies: CBC, Hct, Hgb, pro-time if patient is on long-term therapy
• I&O ratio; decreasing output may indicate renal failure (long-term therapy)
• Hepatotoxicity: dark urine; clay-colored stools; yellowing of skin, sclera; itching; abdominal pain; fever; diarrhea if patient is on long-term therapy
• Allergic reactions: rash, urticaria; if these occur, drug may need to be discontinued
• Renal dysfunction: decreased urine output
• Ototoxicity: tinnitus, ringing, roaring in ears; audiometric testing is needed before, after long-term therapy
• Visual changes: blurring, halos, corneal, retinal damage
• Edema in feet, ankles, legs
• Prior drug history; there are many drug interactions
Administer:
• To patient whole
• With food or milk to decrease gastric symptoms
Evaluate:
• Therapeutic response: decreased pain, stiffness of joints

Teach patient/family:
• To report any symptoms of hepatotoxicity, renal toxicity, visual changes, ototoxicity, allergic reactions (long-term therapy)
• Not to exceed recommended dosage; acute poisoning may result
• To read label on other OTC drugs; many contain aspirin
• That therapeutic response takes 2 wk (arthritis)
• To avoid alcohol ingestion; GI bleeding may occur
Treatment of overdose: Lavage, activated charcoal, monitor electrolytes, VS

digitoxin
(di-ji-tox'in)
Digitaline*, Digitoxin
Func. class.: Antidysrhythmic, cardiac glycoside cardiotonic
Chem. class.: Digitalis preparation

Action: Acts by increased influx of calcium ions from extracellular to intracellular cytoplasm, increasing force of contraction and cardiac output; decreases conduction velocity through AV node; prolongs effective refractory period
Uses: CHF, atrial fibrillation, atrial flutter, atrial tachycardia, rapid digitalization in these disorders
Dosage and routes:
• *Adult and child >12 yr:* 1.2-1.6 initially; give in divided doses over 24 hr; 150 μg qd
• *Neonates:* 22 μg/kg; 2 wk-1 yr: 45 μg/kg; 1-2 yr: 40 μg/kg; 2-12 yr: 30 μg/kg
Maintenance dose: 10% initial dose
Available forms: Powder, tabs 50, 100, 150, 200 μg
Side effects/adverse reactions:
CNS: Headache, drowsiness, apa-

thy, confusion, disorientation, fatigue, depression, hallucinations
*CV: **Dysrhythmias**, hypotension, bradycardia, AV block*
GI: Nausea, vomiting, anorexia, abdominal pain, diarrhea
EENT: Blurred vision, yellow-green halos, photophobia, diplopia
MS: Muscular weakness
Contraindications: Hypersensitivity to digitalis, ventricular fibrillation, ventricular tachycardia, carotid sinus syndrome, 2nd or 3rd degree heart block

Precautions: Hepatic disease, acute MI, AV block, hypokalemia, hypomagnesemia, sinus node disease, lactation, severe respiratory disease, hypothyroidism, elderly, pregnancy (C)

Pharmacokinetics:
PO: Onset ½-2 hr, peak 4-12 hr; duration 2-3 wk, half-life 4-20 days; metabolized in liver; excreted in urine

Interactions/incompatibilities:
• Hypokalemia: thiazides
• Increased blood levels: spironolactone
• Decreased effects: hydantoins, aminoglutethimide, rifampin, phenylbutazone, barbiturates, cholestyramine, colestipol
• Toxicity: adrenergics, diuretics, succinylcholine, quinidine, thioamines
• Decreased level of digitoxin: thyroid agents

Lab test interferences:
Increase: CPK

NURSING CONSIDERATIONS
Assess:
• Apical pulse for 1 min before giving drug; if pulse <60, take again in 1 hr; if <60, call physician
• Electrolytes: K, Na, Cl, Ca renal function studies: BUN, creatinine; blood studies: ALT, AST, bilirubin

• Monitor drug levels (therapeutic level 25-35 ng/ml)
• Cardiac status: apical pulse, character, rate, rhythm

Administer:
• K supplements if ordered for K levels <3.0

Evaluate:
• Therapeutic response: decreased weight, edema, pulse, respiration and increased urine output

Teach patient/family:
• Not to stop drug abruptly; teach all aspects of drug, digitalis toxicity
• To avoid OTC medications, since many adverse drug interactions may occur

Treatment of overdose: Discontinue drug, administer K, digoxin immune FAB, monitor ECG

---

digoxin
(di-jox'in)
Digoxin, Lanoxicaps, Lanoxin
Func. class.: Antidysrhythmic, cardiac glycoside
Chem. class.: Digitalis preparation

Action: Inhibits the sodium-potassium ATPase, which makes more calcium available for contractile proteins, resulting in increased cardiac output

Uses: CHF, atrial fibrillation, atrial flutter, atrial tachycardia, rapid digitalization in these disorders

Dosage and routes:
• *Adult:* IV 0.5 mg given over >5 min, then PO 0.125-0.5 mg qd in divided doses q4-6hr as needed
• *Elderly:* PO 0.125 mg qd maintenance
• *Child >2 yr:* PO 0.02-0.04 mg/kg divided q8h over 24 hr; maintenance 0.006-0.012 mg/kg qd in divided doses q12hr; IV loading

---

italics = common side effects   ***bold italic*** = life threatening reactions

dose 0.015-0.035 mg/kg over >5 min

• *Child 1 mo-2 yr:* IV 0.03-0.05 mg/kg in divided doses over >5 min q48h; change to PO as soon as possible; PO 0.035-0.060 mg/kg divided in 3 doses over 24 hr; maintenance 0.01-0.02 mg/kg in divided doses q12h

• *Neonates:* IV loading dose 0.02-0.03 mg/kg over >5 min in divided doses q4-8h; change to PO as soon as possible; PO loading dose 0.035 mg/kg divided q8h over 24hr; maintenance 0.01 mg/kg in divided doses q12hr

• *Premature infants:* IV 0.015-0.025 mg/kg divided in 3 doses over 24 hr, given over >5 min; maintenance 0.003-0.009 mg/kg in divided doses q12h

Available forms: Caps 50, 100, 200 µg; elix 50 µg/ml; tabs 125, 250, 500 µg; inj 100, 250 µg/ml

Side effects/adverse reactions:
CNS: Headache, drowsiness, apathy, confusion, disorientation, fatigue, depression, hallucinations
CV: **Dysrhythmias,** *hypotension,* bradycardia, **AV block**
EENT: Blurred vision, yellow-green halos, photophobia, diplopia
GI: Nausea, vomiting, anorexia, abdominal pain, diarrhea

Contraindications: Hypersensitivity to digitalis, ventricular fibrillation, ventricular tachycardia, carotid sinus syndrome, 2nd or 3rd degree heart block

Precautions: Renal disease, acute MI, AV block, severe respiratory disease, hypothyroidism, elderly, pregnancy (C), sinus nodal disease, lactation, hypokalemia

Pharmacokinetics:
PO: Onset ½-2 hr, peak 6-8 hrs, duration 3-4 days
IV: Onset 5-30 min, peak 1-5 hr, duration variable, half-life 1.5 days excreted in urine

Interactions/incompatibilities:
• Hypokalemia: diuretics, amphotericin B, carbenicillin, ticarcillin, corticosteroids, piperacillin
• Decreased digoxin level: thyroid agents
• Increased blood levels: propantheline bromide, spironolactone quinidine, verapamil, aminoglycosides PO, amiodarone, anticholinergics, quinine
• Increased bradycardia: β-adrenergic blockers, antidysrhythmics
• Toxicity: adrenergics, amphotericin, corticosteroids, diuretics, glucose, insulin, reserpine, succinylcholine, quinidine, thioamines
• Incompatible with acids, alkalies, Ca salts

Lab test interferences:
Increase: CPK

NURSING CONSIDERATIONS
Assess:
• Apical pulse for 1 min before giving drug; if pulse <60 in adult or <90 in an infant, take again in 1 hr; if <60 in adult, call physician; note rate, rhythm, character
• Electrolytes: K, Na, Cl, Mg, Ca; renal function studies: BUN, creatinine; blood studies: ALT, AST, bilirubin, Hct, Hgb before initiating treatment and periodically thereafter
• I&O ratio, daily weights; monitor turgor, lung sounds, edema
• Monitor drug levels (therapeutic level 0.5-2 ng/ml)
• Cardiac status: apical pulse, character, rate, rhythm

Administer:
• PO with or without food; may crush tabs
• K supplements if ordered for K levels <3, or foods high in K: bananas, orange juice

---

* Available in Canada only

• IV undiluted or 1 ml of drug/4 ml sterile H$_2$O, D$_5$, or NS; give over >5 min through Y-tube or 3-way stopcock; during digitalization close monitoring is necessary

Perform/provide:

• Storage protected from light

Evaluate:

Therapeutic response: decreased weight, edema, pulse, respiration, rales; increased urine output; serum digoxin level (0.5-2 ng/ml)

Teach patient/family:

• Not to stop drug abruptly; teach all aspects of drug, to take exactly as ordered

• To avoid OTC medications, since many adverse drug interactions may occur; do not take antacid at same time

• To notify physician of any loss of appetite, lower stomach pain, diarrhea, weakness, drowsiness, headache, blurred or yellow vision, rash, depression, toxicity

• Toxic symptoms of this drug and when to notify physician

• To maintain a sodium-restricted diet as ordered

• To report shortness of breath, difficulty breathing, weight gain, edema, persistent cough

Treatment of overdose: Discontinue drug; administer K; monitor ECG, administer an adrenergic blocking agent, digoxin immune FAB

---

digoxin immune FAB (ovine)
Digibind

Func. class.: Antidote—digoxin specific

Action: Antibody fragments bind to free digoxin to reverse digoxin toxicity by not allowing digoxin to bind to sites of action

Uses: Life-threatening digoxin or digitoxin toxicity

Dosage and routes:

Digoxin toxicity

• *Adult:* IV dose (mg) =
Dose ingested (mg) × 0.8 × 66.7; if ingested amount is unknown, give 800 mg IV

If digoxin liquid caps or digitoxin used, do not multiply ingested dose by 0.8

Available forms: Inj 40 mg/vial (binds 0.6 mg digoxin or digitoxin)

Side effects/adverse reactions:

CV: **CHF,** ventricular rate increase, **atrial fibrillation,** low cardiac output

RESP: **Impaired respiratory function, rapid respiratory rate**

META: Hypokalemia

INTEG: **Hypersensitivity,** allergic reactions

Contraindications: Mild digoxin toxicity

Precautions: Children, lactation, cardiac disease, renal disease, pregnancy (C)

Pharmacokinetics:

IV: Peaks after completion of infusion, onset 30 min (variable); not known if crosses placenta, breast milk; half-life biphasic—14-20 hr; prolonged in renal disease; excreted by kidneys

Interactions/incompatibilities

• Considered incompatible with all drugs in syringe or sol

Lab test interferences:

Interfere: Immunoassay digoxin

NURSING CONSIDERATIONS

Assess:

• K levels may decrease rapidly

Administer:

• After diluting 40 mg/4 ml of sterile H$_2$O for inj 10 mg/ml mix; may

---

italics = common side effects   ***bold italic*** = life threatening reactions

be further diluted with normal saline
• By bolus if cardiac arrest is eminent or IV over 30 min using a 0.22 μm filter

Perform/provide:
• Storage of reconstituted solution for up to 4 hr in refrigerator

Evaluate:
• Therapeutic response: correction of digoxin toxicity; check digoxin levels

---

dihydroergotamine mesylate

(dye-hye-droe-er-got'a-meen)
D.H.E. 45

Func. class.: α-Adrenergic blocker
Chem. class.: Ergot alkaloid (dihydrogenated)

Action: Constricts smooth muscle in periphery, cranial blood vessels; inhibits norepinephrine uptake

Uses: Vascular headache (migraine or histamine)

Dosage and routes:
• *Adult:* IM/IV 1 mg; may repeat q1-2h if needed, not to exceed 3 mg/day or 6 mg/wk
Available forms: Inj 1 mg/ml

Side effects/adverse reactions:
CNS: Numbness in fingers, toes, weakness
CV: Transient tachycardia, chest pain, bradycardia, increase or decrease in B/P, *gangrene*
GI: Nausea, vomiting
MS: Muscle pain

Contraindications: Hypersensitivity to ergot preparations, occlusion (peripheral, vascular), CAD, hepatic disease, pregnancy (X), renal disease, peptic ulcer, hypertension, lactation, children, uremia

Pharmacokinetics:
IM: Onset 15-30 min, peak 2 hr, duration 3-4 hr
IV: Onset 5 min, peak 45 min, duration 3-4 hr
Half-life 1.3-4 hr

Interactions/incompatibilities:
• Increased effects: troleandomycin
• Increased vasoconstriction: β-blockers
• Incompatible with any drug in syringe or sol

NURSING CONSIDERATIONS
Assess:
• Weight daily, check for peripheral edema in feet, legs
• For stress level, activity, recreation, coping mechanisms of patient
• Neurologic status: LOC, blurring vision, nausea, vomiting, tingling in extremities that occur preceding the headache
• Ingestion of tyramine foods (pickled products, beer, wine, aged cheese), food additives, preservatives, colorings, artificial sweeteners, chocolate, caffeine, which may precipitate these types of headaches

Administer:
• IV undiluted; give 1 mg or less/min
• IM dose, which takes 20 min for effect, or use IV for immediate effect
• At beginning of headache; dose must be titrated to patient response
• Only to women who are not pregnant; harm to fetus may occur

Perform/provide:
• Storage in dark area; do not use discolored solutions
• Quiet, calm environment with decreased stimulation for noise, bright light, excessive talking

---

*Available in Canada only

Evaluate:
• Therapeutic response: decrease in frequency, severity of headache
Teach patient/family:
• Not to use OTC medications; serious drug interactions may occur
• To report side effects: increased vasoconstriction starting with cold extremities, then paresthesia, weakness
• That an increase in headaches may occur when this drug is discontinued after long-term use
• To keep drug out of reach of children; death may occur

---

dihydrotachysterol
(dye-hye-droe-tak-iss'ter-ole)
DHT Intensol, DHT, Hytakerol
Func. class.: Parathyroid agent (calcium regulator)
Chem. class.: Vitamin D analog

Action: Increases intestinal absorption of calcium for bones, increases renal tubular absorption of phosphate
Uses: Renal osteodystrophy, hypoparathyroidism, pseudohypoparathyroidism, familial hypophosphatemia, postoperative tetany
Dosage and routes:
Hypophosphatemia
• *Adult and child:* PO 0.5-2 mg qd, maintenance 0.3-1.5 mg qd
Hypoparathyroidism/pseudohypoparathyroidism
• *Adult:* PO 0.8-2.4 mg qd × 1 wk, maintenance 0.2-2 mg qd regulated by serum Ca levels
• *Child:* PO 1-5 mg qd × 1 wk, maintenance 0.2-1 mg qd regulated by serum Ca levels
Renal osteodystrophy
• *Adult:* PO 0.1-0.6 mg qd
Available forms: Tabs 0.125, 0.2, 0.4 mg; caps 0.125, 0.2, 0.25 mg/5 ml

Side effects/adverse reac...
EENT: Tinnitus
CNS: Drowsiness, headache, vertigo, fever, lethargy
GI: Nausea, diarrhea, vomiting, jaundice, anorexia, dry mouth, constipation, cramps, metallic taste
MS: Myalgia, arthralgia, decreased bone development
GU: Polyuria, hypercalciuria, hyperphosphatemia, *hematuria*
Contraindications: Hypersensitivity, renal disease, hyperphosphatemia, hypercalcemia
Precautions: Pregnancy (C), renal calculi, lactation, CV disease
Pharmacokinetics:
PO: Onset 2 wk; metabolized by liver, excreted in feces (active/inactive)
Interactions/incompatibilities:
• Decreased absorption of dihydrotachysterol: cholestyramine, colestipol, HCl, mineral oil
• Hypercalcemia: thiazide diuretics, Ca supplements
• Cardiac dysrhythmias: cardiac glycosides, verapamil
• Decreased effect of dihydrotachysterol: corticosteroids, phenytoin, barbiturates
Lab test interferences:
False increase: Cholesterol
NURSING CONSIDERATIONS
Assess:
• BUN, urinary Ca, AST, ALT, cholesterol, creatinine, uric acid, Cl, Mg, electrolytes, urine pH, phosphate; may increase Ca, should be kept at 9-10 mg/dl, Vit D 50-135 IU/dl, phosphate 70 mg/dl
• Alk phosphatase; may be decreased
• For increased blood level, since toxic reactions may occur rapidly

---

italics = common side effects   *bold italic* = life threatening reactions

: taste,
e weak-
tinnitus,
ır pulse,
respira-
vomiting,
stipation;
emia

• Renal status, ~~~~eased urinary output (oliguria, anuria), edema in extremities, weight gain >5 lb, periorbital edema
• Nutritional status, diet for sources of Vit D (milk, some seafood), Ca (dairy products, dark green vegetables), phosphates (dairy products) must be avoided

Administer:
• PO, may be increased q4wk depending on blood level

Perform/provide:
• Storage in tight, light-resistant containers at room temperature
• Restriction of Na, K if required
• Restriction of fluids if required for chronic renal failure

Evaluate:
• Therapeutic response: prevention of bone deficiencies

Teach patient/family:
• Symptoms of hypercalcemia
• About foods rich in calcium

Available forms: Chewable tab 334 mg
Side effects/adverse reactions:
GI: Constipation, obstruction
Contraindications: Hypersensitivity to aluminum products
Precautions: Elderly, Na/fluid restriction, decreased GI motility, GI obstruction, dehydration, severe renal disease, CHF, pregnancy (C)
Pharmacokinetics:
PO: Onset 20-40 min, excreted in feces
Interactions/incompatibilities:
• Decreased effectiveness of: tetracyclines, ketoconazole, isoniazid, phenothiazines, iron salts, digitalis
• Constipation; increase bulk in the diet if needed

NURSING CONSIDERATIONS
Administer:
• Laxatives or stool softeners if constipation occurs
Evaluate:
• Therapeutic response: absence of pain, decreased acidity
Teach patient/family:
• To increase fluids to 2 L/day unless contraindicated
• To avoid long-term use; high sodium content

---

dihydroxyaluminum sodium carbonate

(dye-hye-drox'-ee-a-loom-aa-nim)
Rolaids Antacid
Func. class.: Antacid
Chem. class.: Aluminum product

Action: Neutralizes gastric acidity, reduces pepsin
Uses: Antacid
Dosage and routes:
• *Adult:* PO 1-2 as needed; may give up to 2-4 tabs

---

diltiazem HCl

(dil-tye'a-zem)
Cardizem, Cardizem SR, Cardizem CD, Diltiazem, Dilacor-XR
Func. class.: Calcium channel blocker
Chem. class.: Benzothiazepine

Action: Inhibits calcium ion influx across cell membrane during cardiac depolarization; produces relaxation of coronary vascular smooth muscle, dilates coronary arª

---

*Available in Canada only

teries, slows SA/AV node conduction times, dilates peripheral arteries

Uses: Oral: angina pectoris due to coronary insufficiency, hypertension. Parenteral: atrial fibrillation, flutter, paroxysmal supraventricular tachycardia

Dosage and routes:
• *Adult:* PO 30 mg qid, increasing dose gradually to 180-360 mg/day in divided doses or 60-120 mg bid; may increase to 240-360 mg/day
• *Adult IV:* 0.25 mg/kg over BOL 2 min initially, then 0.35 mg/kg may be given after 15 min; if no response, may give Cont Inf 5-15 mg/hr for up to 24 hrs
• *Adult:* PO (Cardizem CD) qd
Available forms: Tabs 30, 60, 90, 120 mg, sus rel 60, 90, 120, 150 mg; Inj (IV) 5 mg/ml (5, 10 ml)

Side effects/adverse reactions:
CV: Dysrhythmia, edema, **CHF,** bradycardia, hypotension, palpitations, heart block, peripheral edema, angina
GI: Nausea, vomiting, diarrhea, gastric upset, constipation, increased liver function studies
GU: Nocturia, polyuria, **acute renal failure**
INTEG: Rash, pruritus, flushing, photosensitivity
CNS: Headache, fatigue, drowsiness, dizziness, depression, weakness, insomnia, tremor, paresthesia

Contraindications: Sick sinus syndrome, 2nd or 3rd degree heart block, hypotension less than 90 mm Hg systolic, acute MI, pulmonary congestion

Precautions: CHF, hypotension, hepatic injury, pregnancy (C), lactation, children, renal disease

Pharmacokinetics: Onset 30-60 min, peak 2-3 hr, immediate rel, 6-11 sus rel, half-life 3½-9 hr; metabolized by liver; excreted in urine (96% as metabolites)

Interactions/incompatibilities:
• Increased effects of: β-blockers, digitalis, lithium, carbamazepine, cyclosporine
• Increased effects of diltiazem: cimetidine

NURSING CONSIDERATIONS
Assess:
• Blood levels (therapeutic levels: 0.025-0.1 µg/ml)
• Cardiac status: B/P, pulse, respiration, ECG and intervals PR, QRS, QT

Administer:
• Before meals, hs

Perform/provide:
• Storage in tight container at room temperature

Evaluate:
• Therapeutic response: decreased anginal pain, decreased B/P

Teach patient/family:
• How to take pulse before taking drug; record or graph should be kept
• To avoid hazardous activities until stabilized on drug, dizziness is no longer a problem
• To limit caffeine consumption
• To avoid OTC drugs unless directed by a physician
• Importance of complying with all areas of medical regimen: diet, exercise, stress reduction, drug therapy; sit on side of bed for 5-10 min. prior to OOB; do not lift heavy items
• Not to crush SR capsules
• To report dizziness, shortness of breath, palpitations
• Not to discontinue abruptly
• To take with a full glass of water

Treatment of overdose: Defibrillation, atropine for AV block, vasopressor for hypotension

dimenhydrinate

(dye-men-hye'dri-nate)

Calm-X, Dimenhydrinate, Dinate, Dommanate, Dramamine, Dramanate, Dramocen, Dramoject, Dymenate, Gravol*, Hydrate, Marmine, Nauseal*, Nauseatol*, Nico-Vert, Novodimenate*, Travamine*, Triptone Caplets, Vertab

Func. class.: Antiemetic, antihistamine, anticholinergic

Chem. class.: H₁-receptor antagonist, ethanolamine derivative

Action: Acts centrally by blocking chemoreceptor trigger zone, which in turn acts on vomiting center

Uses: Motion sickness, nausea, vomiting

Dosage and routes:
• *Adult:* PO 50-100 mg q4h; REC 100 mg qd or bid; IM/IV 50 mg as needed
• *Child:* IM/PO 5 mg/kg divided in 4 equal doses

Available forms: Tabs 50 mg; inj 500 mg/ml; liq 12.5 mg/4 ml; supp 50, 100 mg

Side effects/adverse reactions:
CNS: Drowsiness, restlessness, headache, dizziness, insomnia, confusion, nervousness, tingling, vertigo; hallucinations and *convulsions* in young children
GI: Nausea, anorexia, diarrhea, vomiting, constipation
CV: Hypertension, hypotension, palpitation
INTEG: Rash, urticaria, fever, chills, flushing
EENT: Dry mouth, blurred vision, diplopia, nasal congestion, photosensitivity

Contraindications: Hypersensitivity to narcotics, shock

Precautions: Children, cardiac dysrhythmias, elderly, asthma, pregnancy (B), prostatic hypertrophy, bladder-neck obstruction, narrow-angle glaucoma, stenosing peptic ulcer, pyloroduodenal obstruction

Pharmacokinetics:
IM/PO: Duration 4-6 hr

Interactions/incompatibilities:
• Incompatible with aminophylline, ammonium chloride, amobarbital, butorphanol, chlordiazepoxide, chlorpromazine, diphenhydramine, glycopyrrolate, heparin, hydrocortisone, hydroxyzine, midazolam, pentobarbital, phenobarbital, phenytoin, prednisolone, prochlorperazine, promazine, promethazine, tetracyclines, trifluoperzine, thiopental
• Increased effect: alcohol, other CNS depressants
• May mask ototoxic symptoms associated with aminoglycosides

Lab test interferences:
False negative: Allergy skin testing

NURSING CONSIDERATIONS

Assess:
• VS, B/P; check patients with cardiac disease more often
• Signs of toxicity of other drugs or masking of symptoms of disease: brain tumor, intestinal obstruction
• Observe for drowsiness, dizziness

Administer:
• IV after diluting 50 mg/10 ml of NaCl inj; give 50 mg or less over 2 min
• IM injection in large muscle mass; aspirate to avoid IV administration
• Tablets may be swallowed whole, chewed, or allowed to dissolve

Evaluate:
• Therapeutic response: absence of nausea, vomiting

*Available in Canada only

Teach patient/family:
• That a false-negative result may occur with skin testing; these procedures should not be scheduled for 4 days after discontinuing use
• To avoid hazardous activities, activities requiring alertness; dizziness may occur; instruct patient to request assistance with ambulation
• To avoid alcohol, other depressants

---

dimercaprol

(dye-mer-kap'role)
BAL in Oil, British Anti-Lewis-ite*
Func. class.: Heavy metal antagonist
Chem. class.: Chelating agent (dithiol compound)

Action: Binds ions from arsenic, gold, mercury, lead, copper to form water-soluble complex removed by kidneys

Uses: Arsenic, gold, mercury, lead poisoning

Dosage and routes:
Severe gold/arsenic poisoning
• *Adult:* IM 3 mg/kg q4h × 2d then qid × 1d, then bid × 10d
Mild gold/arsenic poisoning
• *Adult:* IM 2.5 mg/kg qid × 2d, then bid × 1d, then qd × 10d
Acute lead poisoning
• *Adult:* IM 4 mg/kg, then q4h with edetate Ca disodium 12.5 mg/kg IM, not to exceed 5 mg/kg/dose
Mercury poisoning
• *Adult:* IM 5 mg/kg, then 2.5 mg/kg/day or bid × 10 days
Available forms: Inj IM 100 mg/ml

Side effects/adverse reactions:
CNS: Headache, paresthesia, anxiety, tremors, ***convulsions, shock***

INTEG: Urticaria, erythema, pruritus, pain at injection site, fever, burning of lips, mouth, throat
CV: Hypertension, tachycardia
GI: Nausea, vomiting, salivation
EENT: Rhinorrhea, throat pain or constriction, lacrimation
GU: Burning sensation in penis, ***nephrotoxicity***
SYST: ***Anaphylaxis,*** metabolic acidosis
Contraindications: Hypersensitivity, anuria, hepatic insufficiency, poisoning of other metals, severe renal disease, child <3 yr, pregnancy (D)
Precautions: Hypertension, lactation G-6-PD deficiency
Pharmacokinetics:
Metabolized by plasma enzymes, excreted by kidneys as complex, unchanged drug within 4 hr
Interactions/incompatibilities:
• Increased toxicity: iron, selenium, uranium, cadmium
Lab test interferences:
Decrease: RAIU test
NURSING CONSIDERATIONS
Assess:
• B/P, increasing B/P or tachycardia, respirations, pulse
• Monitor I&O, kidney function studies: BUN, creatinine, CrCl; report decreases in output
• Urine: pH, albumin, casts, blood
• Metal levels daily, temperature
• Allergic reactions (rash, urticaria); if these occur, drug should be discontinued
Administer:
• IM in deep muscle mass; rotate injection sites; if giving EDTA also, give in separate site; observe for sterile abscesses
• Only when epinephrine 1:1000 is on unit for anaphylaxis
• Being careful not to allow drug

---

italics = common side effects   ***bold italic*** = life threatening reactions

to touch skin; contact dermatitis can occur
• Acetazolamide or sodium citrate to decrease pH of urine, which decreases renal damage

Evaluate:
• Therapeutic response: decreasing level of metal exposed to in the blood

Teach patient/family:
• That breath may be odorous

---

dinoprostone
(dye-noe-prost'one)
Prepidil Gel, Prostin E$_2$
Func. class.: Oxytocic
Chem. class.: Prostaglandin E$_2$

Action: Stimulates uterine contractions, causing abortion; acts within 30 hr for complete abortion

Uses: Abortion during 2nd trimester, benign hydatidiform mole, expulsion of uterine contents in fetal deaths to 28 wk, missed abortion

Dosage and routes:
• *Adult:* VAG SUPP 20 mg, repeat q3-5h until abortion occurs, max dose is 240 mg

Available forms: Vag supp 20 mg, gel

Side effects/adverse reactions:
CNS: Headache, dizziness, chills, fever
CV: Hypotension
GI: Nausea, vomiting, diarrhea
GU: Vaginitis, vaginal pain, vulvitis, vaginismus
INTEG: Rash, skin color changes
MS: Leg cramps, joint swelling, weakness
EENT: Blurred vision

Contraindications: Hypersensitivity, uterine fibrosis, cervical stenosis, pelvic surgery, pelvic inflammatory disease (PID), respiratory disease

Precautions: Hepatic disease, renal disease, cardiac disease, asthma, anemia, jaundice, diabetes mellitus, convulsive disorders, hypertension, hypotension

Pharmacokinetics:
SUPP: Onset 10 min, duration 2-3 hr; metabolized in spleen, kidney, lungs; excreted in urine

NURSING CONSIDERATIONS
Assess:
• Respiratory rate, rhythm, depth; notify physician of abnormalities, pulse, B/P, temperature
• Vaginal discharge: check for itching, irritation; indicates vaginal infection
• For length, duration of contraction; notify physician of contractions lasting over 1 min or absence of contractions
• For fever, chills: increase fluids or give tepid sponge bath or blanket

Administer:
• Antiemetic/antidiarrheal before administration of this drug
• High in vagina
• After warming suppository by running warm water over package

Evaluate:
• Therapeutic response: expulsion of fetus

Teach patient/family:
• To remain supine for 10-15 min after insertion
• To report excessive cramping, bleeding, chills, fever
• Methods of pain, comfort control

D

diphenhydramine HCl
(dye-fen-hye′dra-meen)
Allermax, Banophen, Belix,
Bena-D 10, Bena-D 50, Bena-
dryl, Benadryl 25, Benadryl
Kapseals, Benahist 10, Benahist
50, Ben-Allergin-50, Benoject,
Benoject-10, Benoject-50, Ben-
ylin Cough, Bydramine, Com-
pōz, Dermamycin, Diahist, Di-
phenacen-50, Diphen Cough,
Diphenhist, Diphenhydramine
HCl, Dormarex 2, Dormin, Dy-
rexin, Genahist, Hydramine,
Hydramyn, Hyrexin-50,
Nidryl, Nordryl, Nordryl Cough,
Nytol, Phendry, Scot-Tussin Al-
lergy, Silphen Cough, Sleep-
Eze 3, Sleepinal, Sominex 2,
Sominex Caplets, Tusstat, Twil-
ite, Uni-Bent Cough, Wehdryl
Func. class.: Antihistamine
Chem. class.: Ethanolamine
derivative, H$_1$-receptor antago-
nist

Action: Acts on blood vessels, GI,
respiratory system by competing
with histamine for H$_1$-receptor site;
decreases allergic response by
blocking histamine
Uses: Allergy symptoms, rhinitis,
motion sickness, antiparkinsonism,
nighttime sedation, infant colic,
nonproductive cough
Dosage and routes:
• *Adult:* PO 25-50 mg q4-6h, not
to exceed 400 mg/day; IM/IV 10-
50 mg, not to exceed 400 mg/day
• *Child >12 kg:* PO/IM/IV 5 mg/
kg/day in 4 divided doses, not to
exceed 300 mg/day
Available forms: Caps 25, 50 mg;
tabs 50 mg; elix 12.5 mg/5 ml; syr
12.5 mg/5 ml; inj IM, IV 10, 50
mg/ml

Side effects/adverse reactions:
CNS: Dizziness, drowsiness, poor
coordination, fatigue, anxiety, euphoria, confusion, paresthesia,
neuritis
RESP: Increased thick secretions,
wheezing, chest tightness
HEMA: ***Thrombocytopenia, agranulocytosis, hemolytic anemia***
GI: Dry mouth, nausea, anorexia,
diarrhea
INTEG: Photosensitivity
GU: Retention, dysuria, frequency
EENT: Blurred vision, dilated pupils, tinnitus, nasal stuffiness, dry
nose, throat, mouth
Contraindications: Hypersensitivity to H$_1$-receptor antagonist, acute
asthma attack, lower respiratory
tract disease
Precautions: Increased intraocular
pressure, renal disease, cardiac
disease, hypertension, bronchial
asthma, seizure disorder, stenosed
peptic ulcers, hyperthyroidism,
prostatic hypertrophy, bladder neck
obstruction, pregnancy (C)
Pharmacokinetics:
PO: Peak 1-3 hr, duration 4-7 hr;
IM: Onset ½ hr, peak 1-4 hr, duration 4-7 hr; *IV:* Onset immediate,
duration 4-7 hr; metabolized in
liver, excreted by kidneys; crosses
placenta, excreted in breast milk;
half-life 2-7 hr
Interactions/incompatibilities:
• Incompatible with: amobarbital,
amphotericin B, cephalothin, dexamethasone, furosemide, methylprednisolone, pentobarbital, phenytoin, secobarbital
• Increased CNS depression: barbiturates, narcotics, hypnotics, tricyclic antidepressants, alcohol
• Decreased effect of: oral anticoagulants, heparin
• Increased effect of: diphenhydramine: MAOIs

---

italics = common side effects   ***bold italic*** = life threatening reactions

Lab test interferences:
False negative: Skin allergy tests

NURSING CONSIDERATIONS
Assess:
• I&O ratio; be alert for urinary retention, frequency, dysuria; drug should be discontinued if these occur
• CBC during long-term therapy; blood dyscrasias
• Respiratory status: rate, rhythm, increase in bronchial secretions, wheezing, chest tightness

Administer:
• With meals if GI symptoms occur, absorption may slightly decrease
• IV undiluted; give 25 mg/1 min
• Deep IM in large muscle; rotate site
• Hs only if using for sleep aid

Perform/provide:
• Hard candy, gum, frequent rinsing of mouth for dryness
• Storage in tight container at room temperature

Evaluate:
• Therapeutic response: absence of running or congested nose or rashes, improved sleep

Teach patient/family:
• All aspects of drug use; to notify physician of confusion, sedation, hypotension
• To avoid driving or other hazardous activity if drowsiness occurs
• That this drug may decrease anticoagulant (oral)
• To avoid concurrent use of alcohol or other CNS depressants

Treatment of overdose: Administer ipecac syrup or lavage, diazepam, vasopressors, barbiturates (short-acting)

diphenidol
(dye-fen'-i-dole)
Vontrol
Func. class.: Antiemetic
Chem. class.: Trihexyphenidyl derivative

Action: May act as dopamine antagonist at chemoreceptor trigger zone to inhibit vomiting
Uses: Nausea, vomiting, peripheral dizziness

Dosage and routes:
• *Adult:* PO 25-50 mg q4h
• *Children >23 kg:* PO 25 mg q4h prn; do not exceed 5.5 mg/kg/24 hr
Available forms: Tabs 25 mg

Side effects/adverse reactions:
CNS: Drowsiness, fatigue, restlessness, tremor, headache, stimulation, dizziness, insomnia, twitching, disorientation, confusion, sleep disturbance, auditory, visual hallucination, depression
GI: Nausea, indigestion
CV: Hypotension
INTEG: Rash
EENT: Dry mouth, blurred vision
Contraindications: Hypersensitivity, psychosis, anuria
Precautions: Children, prostatic hypertrophy, glaucoma, pyloric and duodenal stenosis, elderly, pregnancy (C), lactation

Pharmacokinetics:
PO: Onset 30-45 min, duration 3-6 hr, metabolized by liver, excreted by kidneys

NURSING CONSIDERATIONS
Assess:
• VS, B/P; check patients with cardiac disease more often
• Observe for CNS adverse effects: confusion, hallucination
• Monitor I&O (90% excreted in urine)

• Signs of toxicity of other drugs or masking of symptoms of disease: brain tumor, intestinal obstruction
• Drowsiness, dizziness

Administer:
• Tabs may be swallowed whole, chewed, or allowed to dissolve

Evaluate:
• Therapeutic response: absence of nausea, vomiting

Teach patient/family:
• To avoid alcohol, other depressants
• That drug should be used only under close supervision

---

diphenoxylate HCl with atropine sulfate

(dye-fen-ox'i-late)
Diphenatol, Lofene, Lomotil, Lo-Trol

Func. class.: Antidiarrheal
Chem. class.: Phenylipeperidine derivative, opiate agonist

Controlled Substance Schedule V
Action: Inhibits gastric motility by acting on mucosal receptors responsible for peristalsis
Uses: Diarrhea (cause undetermined)

Dosage and routes:
• *Adult:* PO 2.5-5 mg qid, titrated to patient response
• *Child 2-12 yr:* PO 0.3-0.4 mg/kg/day in divided doses
Available forms: Tabs 2.5 mg

Side effects/adverse reactions:
CNS: Drowsiness, headache, sedation, depression, weakness, lethargy, flushing, hyperthermia
GI: Nausea, vomiting, abdominal pain, glossitis, colitis, *paralytic ileus, toxic megacolon,* dry mucous membranes
EENT: Blurred vision, nystagmus, mydriasis

INTEG: Rash, urticaria, pruritus, *angioneurotic edema*
CV: Tachycardia
GU: Urine retention
Contraindications: Hypersensitivity, severe liver disease, pseudomembranous enterocolitis, glaucoma, child <2 yr, electrolyte imbalances
Precautions: Hepatic disease, renal disease, ulcerative colitis, pregnancy (C), lactation, elderly

Pharmacokinetics:
PO: Onset 45-60 min, peak 2 hr, duration 3-4 hr, half-life 2½ hr; metabolized in liver to active, terminal half-life 12-14 hr; excreted in urine, feces, breast milk

Interactions/incompatibilities:
• Do not use with MAOIs; hypertensive crisis may occur
• Increased action of: alcohol, narcotics, barbiturates, other CNS depressants, anticholinergics

NURSING CONSIDERATIONS
Assess:
• Electrolytes (K, Na, Cl) if on long-term therapy
• Bowel pattern before; for rebound constipation after termination of medication
• Response after 48 hr; if no response, drug should be discontinued
• Dehydration in children
• Abdominal distention, toxic megacolon, which may occur in ulcerative colitis

Administer:
• For 48 hr only

Evaluate:
• Therapeutic response: decreased diarrhea

Teach patient/family:
• To avoid OTC products unless directed by physician; may contain alcohol
• Not to exceed recommended dose

---

italics = common side effects   ***bold italic*** = life threatening reactions

• That drug may be habit forming
• May give with food to prevent GI irritation
• May cause drowsiness; avoid hazardous activities
• Interventions for relieving dry mouth
• To avoid alcohol and CNS depressants

---

diphtheria and tetanus toxoids and pertussis vaccine (DPT)
Diphtheria and Tetanus Toxoids and Pertussis Vaccine, Tri-Immunol
Func. class.: Vaccine/toxoid

Action: Provide immunity to diphtheria, tetanus, pertussis by stimulating antibody/antitoxin production

Uses: Prevention of diphtheria, tetanus, pertussis

Dosage and routes:
• *Child >6 wk-6 yr:* IM 0.5 ml at 2, 4, 6 mos, 1½ yr; booster needed 0.5 ml at age 6

Available forms: Inj IM diphtheria 12.5 LfU, tetanus 5 LfU, pertussis 4 U/0.5 ml

Side effects/adverse reactions:
GI: Nausea, vomiting, anorexia
INTEG: Skin abscess, urticaria, itching, swelling, erythema, edema at site
CV: Tachycardia, hypotension
SYST: Lymphadenitis, ***anaphylaxis***, fever, chills, malaise
CNS: Crying, fretfulness, fever, drowsiness, *seizures*
MS: Osteomyelitis

Contraindications: Hypersensitivity, active infection, poliomyelitis outbreak, immunosuppression, febrile illness

Precautions: Pregnancy

Interactions/incompatibilities:
• Decreased response to toxoid: immunosuppressive agents: antineoplastics, corticosteroids, radiation therapy; alkylating agents

NURSING CONSIDERATIONS
Assess:
• For skin reactions: swelling, rash, urticaria
• For anaphylaxis: inability to breathe, bronchospasm

Administer:
• At least 4 wk apart × 3 doses
• Only with epinephrine 1:1000 on unit to treat laryngospasm
• IM only; not to be given SC (vastus lateralis in infants)

Perform/provide:
• Storage in refrigerator, do not freeze
• Written record of immunization

Evaluate:
• For history of allergies, skin conditions (eczema, psoriasis, dermatitis), reactions to vaccinations

Teach patient/family:
• That doses are given at least 4 wk apart × 3 doses; booster needed at 10 yr intervals, diphtheria/tetanus

---

dipivefrin HCl
(dye-pi′ve-frin)
Propine
Func. class.: Adrenergic agonist
Chem. class.: Diesterified epinephrine

Action: Converted to epinephrine, which decreases aqueous production and increases outflow

Uses: Open-angle glaucoma

Dosage and routes:
• *Adult:* INSTILL 1 gtt q12h

Available forms: Sol 0.1%

Side effects/adverse reactions:
CV: Hypertension, tachycardia, dysrhythmias

---

*Available in Canada only

EENT: Burning, stinging, mydriasis, photophobia

Contraindications: Hypersensitivity, narrow-angle glaucoma

Precautions: Pregnancy (B), lactation, children, aphakia

Pharmacokinetics:

INSTILL: Onset 30 min, peak 1 hr, duration 12 hr

NURSING CONSIDERATIONS

Perform/provide:

• Storage at room temperature

Evaluate:

• Therapeutic response: decrease in aqueous humor of eye

Teach patient/family:

• To report stinging, burning, itching, lacrimation, puffiness

• Method of instillation, including pressure on lacrimal sac for 1 min and not to touch dropper to eye

---

dipyridamole

(dye-peer-id'a-mole)

Dipyridamole, Persantine, Persantine IV, Pyridamole

Func. class.: Coronary vasodilator, antiplatelet

Chem. class.: Nonnitrate

Action: Increases oxygen saturation in coronary tissues, coronary blood flow; acts on small resistance vessels with little effect on vascular resistance; may increase development of collateral circulation

Uses: Prevention of transient ischemic attacks, inhibition of platelet adhesion to prevent myocardial reinfarction, thromboembolism, with warfarin in prosthetic heart valves, prevention of coronary bypass graft occlusion with aspirin; possibly effective for long-term therapy of chronic angina pectoris

Dosage and routes:

TIA

• *Adult:* PO 50 mg tid, 1 hr ac, not to exceed 400 mg qd

Inhibition of platelet adhesion

• *Adult:* PO 50-75 mg qid in combination with aspirin or warfarin

Available forms: Tabs 25, 50, 75 mg, IV

Side effects/adverse reactions:

CV: Postural hypotension

CNS: Headache, dizziness, weakness, fainting, syncope

GI: Nausea, vomiting, anorexia, diarrhea

INTEG: Rash, flushing

Contraindications: Hypersensitivity, hypotension

Precautions: Pregnancy (C)

Pharmacokinetics:

PO: Peak 2-2½ hr, duration 6 hr; therapeutic response may take several months; metabolized in liver; excreted in bile; undergoes enterohepatic recirculation

Interactions/incompatibilities:

• Incompatibility not known

• Additive antiplatelet effects: ASA, NSAID

• Increased bleeding: Coumadin

NURSING CONSIDERATIONS

Assess:

• B/P, pulse during treatment until stable; take B/P lying, standing; orthostatic hypotension is common

• Cardiac status: chest pain, what aggravates or ameliorates condition

Administer:

• IV after diluting each 5 mg/2 ml or more D₅W, 0.45% NS, or NS to a total vol of 20-50 ml; give over 4 min; do not give undiluted

• On an empty stomach: 1 hr before meals or 2 hr after

Perform/provide:

• Storage at room temperature

Evaluate:

• Therapeutic response: decreased

---

italics = common side effects   ***bold italic*** = life threatening reactions

chest pain (angina), decreased platelet adhesion

Teach patient/family:

• That medication is not cure; may have to be taken continuously

• That it is necessary to quit smoking to prevent excessive vasoconstriction

• To avoid hazardous activities until stabilized on medication; dizziness may occur

Treatment of overdose: Administer IV phenylephrine

---

disopyramide

(dye-soe-peer'a-mide)

Disopyramide, Norpace, Norpace CR

Func. class.: Antidysrhythmic (Class IA)

Chem. class.: Nonnitrate

Action: Prolongs action, potential duration, and effective refractory period; reduces disparity in refractory between normal and infarcted myocardium

Uses: PVCs, ventricular tachycardia, supraventricular tachycardia, atrial flutter, fibrillation

Dosage and routes:

• *Adult:* PO 100-200 mg q6h, in renal dysfunction 100 mg q6h; SUS REL CAPS 200 mg q12h

• *Child 12-18 yr:* PO 6-15 mg/kg/day, in divided doses q6h

• *Child 4-12 yr:* PO 10-15 mg/kg/day in divided doses q6h

• *Child 1-4 yr:* PO 10-20 mg/kg/day in divided doses q6h

• *Child <1 yr:* PO 10-30 mg/kg/day, in divided doses q6h

Available forms: Caps 100, 150 mg (as phosphate), caps, sus rel 100, 150 mg

Side effects/adverse reactions:

GU: Retention, hesitancy, impotence, urinary frequency, urgency

CNS: Headache, dizziness, psychosis, fatigue, depression, paresthesias, anxiety, insomnia

GI: Dry mouth, constipation, nausea, anorexia, flatulence, diarrhea, vomiting

CV: Hypotension, bradycardia, angina, PVCs, tachycardia, increases QRS, QT segments, *cardiac arrest,* edema, weight gain, AV block, *CHF,* syncope, chest pain

META: Hypoglycemia

INTEG: Rash, pruritus, urticaria

MS: Weakness, pain in extremities

EENT: Blurred vision, dry nose, throat, eyes, narrow-angle glaucoma

HEMA: Thrombocytopenia, agranulocytosis, anemia (rare), decreased hemoglobin, hematocrit

Contraindications: Hypersensitivity, 2nd or 3rd degree block, cardiogenic shock, CHF (uncompensated), sick sinus syndrome, QT prolongation

Precautions: Pregnancy (C), lactation, diabetes mellitus, renal disease, children, hepatic disease, myasthenia gravis, narrow-angle glaucoma, cardiomyopathy, conduction abnormalities

Pharmacokinetics:

PO: Peak 30 min-3 hr, duration 6-12 hr; half-life 4-10 hr; metabolized in liver; excreted in feces, urine, breast milk; crosses placenta

Interactions/incompatibilities:

• Increased effects of disopyramide: quinidine, procainamide, propranolol, lidocaine, atenolol, other antidysrhythmics

• Do not administer within 48 hr of verapamil

• Increased side effects of disopyramide: anticholinergics

• Decreased effects of disopyramide: phenytoin, rifampin

Lab test interferences:
Increase: Liver enzymes, lipids, BUN, creatinine
Decrease: Hgb/Hct, blood glucose
NURSING CONSIDERATIONS
Assess:
• Apical pulse for 1 min; if less than 60, check again in 1 hr; if still less than 60, notify physician
• ECG; check for increased QT, widening QRS; drug should be discontinued
• Blood level during treatment (therapeutic level 2-8 μg/ml)
• Weight daily; a rapid weight gain should be reported
• For dehydration or hypovolemia, I&O ratio, electrolytes (Na, K, Cl)
• Liver, kidney function studies (AST, ALT, bilirubin, BUN, creatinine) during treatment
• Diabetics for signs of hypoglycemia
• B/P continuously for hypotension, hypertension
• Increase in QRS, QT; drug should be discontinued
• For rebound hypertension after 1-2 hr
• Constipation: increased bulk in diet, water, stool softeners, or laxatives needed
• Cardiac rate, respiration: rate, rhythm, character
• Urinary hesitancy, frequency or a change in I&O ratio; check for edema daily; check for toxicity
Administer:
• Sugar-free gum, frequent sips of water for dry mouth
• Reduced dosage slowly with ECG monitoring
Evaluate:
• Therapeutic response: decreased dysrhythmias
Teach patient/family:
• To take drug exactly as prescribed

• To avoid alcohol, or severe hypotension may occur; to avoid OTC drugs, or serious drug interactions may occur
• To make position change slowly during early therapy to prevent fainting
• To avoid hazardous activities if dizziness or blurred vision occurs
• Importance of complying with drug regimen; tell patient that this drug does not cure condition
Treatment of overdose: O₂, artificial ventilation, ECG, administer dopamine for circulatory depression, administer diazepam or thiopental for convulsions, gastric lavage

disulfiram
(dye-sul'fi-ram)
Antabuse, Disulfiram
Func. class.: Alcohol deterrent
Chem. class.: Aldehyde dehydrogenase inhibitor

Action: Blocks oxidation of alcohol at acetaldehyde stage; accumulation of acetaldehyde produces the disulfiram-alcohol reaction
Uses: Chronic alcoholism (as adjunct)
Dosage and routes:
• *Adult:* PO 250-500 mg qd × 1-2 wk, then 125-500 mg qd until fully socially recovered
Available forms: Tabs 250, 500 mg
Side effects/adverse reactions:
CNS: Headache, drowsiness, restlessness, dizziness, fatigue, tremors, psychosis, neuritis, sweating, *convulsions, death,* peripheral neuropathy
GI: Nausea, vomiting, anorexia, severe thirst, *hepatotoxicity,* metallic, garliclike aftertaste
INTEG: Rash, dermatitis, urticaria

italics = common side effects   ***bold italic*** = life threatening reactions

Disulfiram Reaction: Alcohol reaction: flushing, throbbing, headache, respiratory difficulty, nausea, vomiting, sweating, thirst, chest pain, palpitations, dyspnea, hyperventilation, tachycardia, confusion, CV collapse, MI, CHF, convulsions, death

Contraindications: Hypersensitivity, alcohol intoxication, psychoses, CV disease, pregnancy (X)

Precautions: Hypothyroidism, hepatic disease, diabetes mellitus, seizure disorders, nephritis, cerebral damage

Pharmacokinetics:
PO: Onset 12 hr; oxidized by liver; excreted unchanged in feces

Interactions/incompatibilities:
• Increased effects of: tricyclic antidepressants, diazepam, oral anticoagulants, paraldehyde, phenytoin, chlordiazepoxide, isoniazid, caffeine
• Disulfiram reaction: alcohol
• Psychosis: metronidazole

Lab test interferences:
Increase: Cholesterol
Decrease: ^{131}I uptake, PBI, VMA

NURSING CONSIDERATIONS
Assess:
• Liver function studies q2wk during therapy: AST, ALT
• CBC, SMA q3-6 mo to detect any abnormality, including increased cholesterol
• Mental status: affect, mood, drug history, ability to follow treatment, abstain from alcohol
• For signs of hepatotoxicity: jaundice, dark urine, clay-colored stools, abdominal pain

Administer:
• Only with patient's knowledge; do not give to intoxicated individuals
• Once per day in the AM or hs if drowsiness occurs

• Only after patient has not been drinking for >12 hr

Evaluate:
• Therapeutic response: prevention of alcohol intake

Teach patient/family:
• Effect of this drug if alcohol is taken; written consent for disulfiram therapy should be obtained
• That shaving lotions, creams, lotions, cough preparations, skin products must be checked for alcohol content; even in small amount, alcohol can produce a reaction
• That tolerance will not develop if treatment is prolonged
• That reaction may occur for 2 wk after last dose
• That tablets can be crushed, mixed with beverage
• To carry ID listing disulfiram therapy
• To avoid driving or hazardous tasks if drowsiness occurs
• That disulfiram reaction can be fatal; occurs 15 min after drinking and may last several hours

Treatment of overdose: IV Vit C, ephedrine sulfate, antihistamines, O_2

DNase (recombinant human deoxyribonuclease I)
Pulmozyme
Func. class.: Cystic fibrosis agent (orphan drug)

Action: May break down molecules in large amounts of infected sputum; improves air flow, and lessens chances of bacterial infection

Uses: Management of cystic fibrosis

Dosage and routes:
Child 5-20 yr: INH 2.5 mg qd
Available forms: Neb 2.5 mg
Side effects/adverse reactions:
RESP: Possibly laryngitis, hoarseness, hemoptysis, transient decrease in pulmonary function
Contraindications: Hypersensitivity

NURSING CONSIDERATIONS
Assess:
• Resp. function: B/P, pulse, lung sounds
Administer:
• By nebulization only
Evaluate:
• Therapeutic response: decreased thick tenacious secretions, ease of respirations
Teach patient/family:
• To rinse mouth after use
• About all aspects of drug; avoid smoking, smoke-filled rooms, persons with respiratory infections

---

dobutamine HCl
(doe-byoo'ta-meen)
Dubutrex
Func. class.: Adrenergic direct-acting β_1-agonist
Chem. class.: Catecholamine

Action: Causes increased contractility, increased coronary blood flow and heart rate by acting on β-1 receptors in heart
Uses: Cardiac surgery, refractory heart failure
Dosage and routes:
• *Adult:* IV INF 2.5-10 μg/kg/min; may increase to 40 μg/kg/min if needed
Available forms: Inj 250 mg vial IV
Side effects/adverse reactions:
CNS: Anxiety, headache, dizziness

CV: Palpitations, tachycardia, hypertension, PVCs, angina
GI: Heartburn, nausea, vomiting
MS: Muscle cramps (leg)
Contraindications: Hypersensitivity, idiopathic hypertrophic subaortic stenosis
Precautions: Pregnancy (C), lactation, children, hypertension
Pharmacokinetics:
IV: Onset 1-5 min, peak 10 min, half-life 2 min; metabolized in liver (inactive metabolites); excreted in urine
Interactions/incompatibilities:
• Dysrhythmias: general anesthetics
• Decreased action of dobutamine: other β-blockers
• Increased B/P: oxytocics
• Increased pressor effect and dysrhythmias: tricyclic antidepressant, MAOIs
• Incompatible with $NaHCO_3$, acyclovir, aminophylline, bretylium, bumetamide, Ca Cl, calcium gluconate, cefamandole, cefazolin, cephalothin, diazepam, digoxin, furosemide, heparin, hydrocortisone, insulins, Mg SO_4, penicillin, phenytoin, potassium phosphate, sodium ethacrynate
NURSING CONSIDERATIONS
Assess:
• I&O ratio
• ECG during administration continuously; if B/P increases, drug is decreased
• B/P and pulse q5min after parenteral route
• CVP or PWP during infusion if possible
Administer:
• IV diluting each 250 mg/10 ml of sterile H_2O or D_5 for inj; may be further diluted to 50 ml or more given at prescribed rate; should be gradually increased to desired rate

---

italics = common side effects   ***bold italic*** = life threatening reactions

• Plasma expanders for hypovolemia

• Parenteral (IV) dose slowly, after reconstituting, then diluting with at least 50 ml of D_5W, 0.9% NS, or Na lactate

Perform/provide:

• Storage of reconstituted solution if refrigerated for <24 hr

Evaluate:

• Therapeutic response: increased B/P with stabilization

Teach patient/family:

• Reason for drug administration

Treatment of overdose: Administer a β_1 adrenergic blocker

---

docusate calcium/docusate potassium/docusate sodium

(dok'yoo-sate)

DC Softgels, Docusate Calcium, Pro-Cal-Sof, Sulfalax Calcium, Surfak/Dialose, Diocto-K, Kasof/Colace, Correctol Extra Gentle, Diocto, Dioeze, Disonate, Docusate Sodium, DOK, DOS Softgel, Doxinate, D-S-S, Modane Soft, Regulex SS, Regutol,

Func. class.: Laxative, emollient

Chem. class.: Anionic surfactant

Action: Increases water, fat penetration in intestine; allows for easier passage of stool

Uses: To soften stools

Dosage and routes:

• *Adult:* PO 50-300 mg qd (Na) or 240 mg (Ca or K) prn; ENEMA 5 ml (sodium)

• *Child >12 yr:* ENEMA 2 ml (sodium)

• *Child 6-12 yr:* PO 40-120 mg qd (sodium)

• *Child 3-6 yr:* PO 20-60 mg qd (sodium)

• *Child <3 yr:* PO 10-40 mg qd (sodium)

Available forms: Caps 50, 100, 240, 250, 300 mg; tabs 50, 100 mg; oral sol 10, 50 mg/ml, 16.7, 20 mg/5 ml, enema conc 18 g/100 ml

Side effects/adverse reactions:

GI: Nausea, anorexia, cramps, diarrhea

INTEG: Rash

EENT: Bitter taste, throat irritation

Contraindications: Hypersensitivity, obstruction, fecal impaction, nausea/vomiting

Precautions: Pregnancy (C)

Pharmacokinetics: Onset 24-72 hrs

NURSING CONSIDERATIONS

Assess:

• Blood, urine electrolytes if drug is used often by patient

• I&O ratio to identify fluid loss

• Cause of constipation; identify whether fluids, bulk, or exercise is missing from life-style

• Cramping, rectal bleeding, nausea, vomiting; if these symptoms occur, drug should be discontinued

Administer:

• Alone with 8 oz H_2O only for better absorption; do not take within 1 hr of other drugs or within 1 hr of antacids, milk, or H_2 blockers

• In morning or evening (oral dose)

Perform/provide:

• Storage in cool environment; do not freeze

Evaluate:

• Therapeutic response: decrease in constipation

Teach patient/family:

• To swallow tabs whole; do not chew

• That normal bowel movements do not always occur daily

• Do not use in presence of abdominal pain, nausea, vomiting
• To notify physician if constipation unrelieved or if symptoms of electrolyte imbalance occur: muscle cramps, pain, weakness, dizziness, excessive thirst
• To keep out of children's reach

---

dopamine HCl
(doe'pa-meen)
Dopamine HCl, Intropin, Revimine*

Func. class.: Agonist
Chem. class.: Catecholamine

Action: Causes increased cardiac output; acts on α-receptors, causing vasoconstriction in blood vessels; when low doses are administered, causes renal and mesenteric vasodilation

Uses: Shock; increase perfusion; hypotension

Dosage and routes:
• *Adult:* IV INF 2-5 μg/kg/min, not to exceed 50 μg/kg/min, titrate to patient's response

Available forms: Inj 0.8, 1.6, 40, 80, 160 mg/ml

Side effects/adverse reactions:
CNS: Headache
CV: Palpitations, tachycardia, hypertension, ectopic beats, angina, wide QRS complex, peripheral vasoconstriction
GI: Nausea, vomiting, diarrhea
INTEG: Necrosis, tissue sloughing with extravasation, **gangrene**
RESP: Dyspnea

Contraindications: Hypersensitivity, ventricular fibrillation, tachydysrhythmias, pheochromocytoma
Precautions: Pregnancy (C), lactation, arterial embolism, peripheral vascular disease

Pharmacokinetics:
IV: Onset 5 min, duration <10 min; metabolized in liver; excreted in urine (metabolites)

Interactions/incompatibilities:
• Incompatible with acyclovir, amphotericin B, cephalothin, gentamicin, sodium bicarbonate, alkaline sol
• Do not use within 2 wk of MAOIs, phenytoin, barbiturates, or hypertensive crisis may result
• Dysrhythmias: general anesthetics
• Decreased action of dopamine: other β-blockers
• Increased B/P: oxytocics
• Increased pressor effect: tricyclic antidepressant, MAOIs
• Additive effect: diuretics

NURSING CONSIDERATIONS
Assess:
• I&O ratio
• ECG during administration continuously; if B/P increases, drug is decreased
• B/P and pulse q5min after parenteral route
• CVP or PWP during infusion if possible
• Paresthesias and coldness of extremities; peripheral blood flow may decrease
• Injection site: tissue sloughing; if this occurs, administer phentolamine mixed with NS

Administer:
• Plasma expanders for hypovolemia
• IV after diluting 200 mg/250-500 ml of NS, D₅W, D₅ 0.45% NaCl, D₅ 0.9% NaCl, D₅LR, LR
• Parenteral IV dose slowly; after reconstituting, use infusion pump; flush line before infusing; infuse as secondary IV line

Perform/provide:
• Storage of reconstituted solution

---

italics = common side effects   **bold italic** = life threatening reactions

if refrigerated for no longer than 24 hr
• Do not use discolored solutions
Evaluate:
• Therapeutic response: increased B/P with stabilization
Teach patient/family:
• Reason for drug administration
Treatment of overdose: Administer a β₁ adrenergic blocker

---

doxacurium chloride
(dox′a-cure-ee-um)
Nuromax
Func. class.: Neuromuscular blocker (nondepolarizing)

Action: Inhibits transmission of nerve impulses by binding with cholinergic receptor sites, antagonizing action of acetylcholine
Uses: Facilitation of endotracheal intubation, skeletal muscle relaxation during mechanical ventilation, surgery, or general anesthesia
Dosage and routes:
• *Adult:* IV 0.05 mg/kg; 0.08 mg/kg is used for prolonged neuromuscular blockade; maintenance 0.025 mg/kg
Available forms: Inj 1 mg/ml
Side effects/adverse reactions:
CV: Decreased B/P, ventricular fibrillation, myocardial infarction, cardiovascular accident
RESP: Prolonged apnea, bronchospasm, wheezing, respiratory depression
EENT: Diplopia
MS: Weakness, prolonged skeletal muscle relaxation, *paralysis*
INTEG: Rash, urticaria
Contraindications: Hypersensitivity
Precautions: Pregnancy (C), renal, hepatic disease, lactation, children <3 mo, fluid and electrolyte

imbalances, neuromuscular disease, respiratory disease, obesity, elderly, severe burns
Pharmacokinetics: Not metabolized; excretion of unchanged drug in urine and bile
Interactions/incompatibilities:
• Increased neuromuscular blockade: Aminoglycosides, quinidine, local anesthetics, polymyxin antibiotics, enflurane, isoflurane, tetracyclines, halothane, Mg, colistin, procainamide, bacitracin, lincomycin, clindamycin, lithium
• Longer onset and shorter duration of doxacurium: phenytoin, carbamazepine
NURSING CONSIDERATIONS
Assess:
• For electrolyte imblances (K, Mg); may lead to increased action of this drug
• Vital signs (B/P, pulse, respirations, airway) until fully recovered; rate, depth, pattern of respirations, strength of hand grip
• I&O ratio; check for urinary retention, frequency, hesitancy
• Recovery: decreased paralysis of face, diaphragm, leg, arm, rest of body
• Allergic reactions: rash, fever, respiratory distress, pruritus; drug should be discontinued
Administer:
• Using nerve stimulator by anesthesiologist to determine neuromuscular blockade
• After succinylcholine effects subside
• Anticholinesterase to reverse neuromuscular blockade
• By slow IV over 1-2 min (only by qualified persons, usually an anesthesiologist)
• Only fresh solution
Perform/provide:
• Storage at room temperature; do not freeze

• Reassurance if communication is difficult during recovery from neuromuscular blockade
• Use reconstituted solution within 24 hr
• Frequent (q2h) instillation of artificial tears and covering eyes to prevent drying of cornea

Evaluate:
• Therapeutic response: paralysis of jaw, eyelid, head, neck, rest of body

Treatment of overdose: Neostigmine; monitor VS; may require mechanical ventilation

---

doxapram HCl
(dox'a-pram)
Dopram
Func. class.: Analeptic

Action: Respiratory stimulation through activation of peripheral carotid chemoreceptor; with higher doses medullary respiratory centers are stimulated

Uses: Chronic obstructive pulmonary disease (COPD), postanesthesia respiratory stimulation, acute hypercapnia, drug-induced CNS depression

Dosage and routes:
Postanesthesia
• *Adult:* IV inj 0.5-1 mg/kg, not to exceed 1.5 mg/kg total as a single injection; IV inf 250 mg in 250 ml sol, not to exceed 4 mg/kg; run at 1-3 mg/min

Drug-induced CNS depression
Priming IV dose of 2 mg/kg, repeated in 5 min; repeat q1-2 h till patient awakes; IV inf priming dose 2 mg/kg at 1-3 mg/min, not to exceed 3 g/d

COPD
• *Adult:* IV inf 1-2 mg/min, not to exceed 3 mg/min for no longer than 2 hr

Available forms: Inj IV 20 mg/ml

Side effects/adverse reactions:
CNS: **Convulsions,** (clonus/generalized), *headache,* restlessness, dizziness, confusion, paresthesias, flushing, sweating, bilateral Babinski's sign, rigidity, depression
GI: Nausea, vomiting, diarrhea, hiccups
GU: Retention, incontinence
CV: Chest pain, hypertension, change in heart rate, lowered T waves, tachycardia, arrhythmias
INTEG: Pruritus, irritation at injection site
EENT: Pupil dilation, sneezing
RESP: **Laryngospasm, bronchospasm,** rebound hypoventilation, dyspnea, cough, tachypnea, hiccoughs

Contraindications: Hypersensitivity, seizure disorders, severe hypertension, severe bronchial asthma, severe dyspnea, severe cardiac disorders, pneumothorax, pulmonary embolism, severe respiratory disease, newborns

Precautions: Bronchial asthma, pheochromocytoma, severe tachycardia, dysrhythmias, pregnancy (B), hypertension, lactation, children

Pharmacokinetics:
IV: Onset 20-40 sec, peak 1-2 min, duration 5-10 min; metabolized by liver; excreted by kidneys (metabolites); half-life 2.5-4 hr

Interactions/incompatibilities:
• Synergistic pressor effect: MAOIs, sympathomimetics
• Cardiac dysrhythmias: halothane, cyclopropane, enflurane
• Incompatible with aminophylline, carbenicillin, cefaperazone cefotaxime, cefetetan, cefuroxime, dexamethasone, diazepam, di-

---

goxin, dobutamine, furosemide, hydrocortisone, ketamine, methylprednisolone, minocycline, pentobarbital, phenobarbital, secobarbital, thiopental, ticarcillin

NURSING CONSIDERATIONS
Assess:
• BP, HR, deep tendon reflexes, ABGs before administration, q30min
• PO_2, PCO_2, O_2 saturation during treatment
• Hypertension, dysrhythmias, tachycardia, dyspnea, skeletal muscle hyperactivity; may indicate overdosage; discontinue if these occur
• Respiratory stimulation: increased respiratory rate, abnormal rhythm
• Extravasation; change IV site q48h

Administer:
• IV undiluted or diluted with equal parts of sterile H_2O for inj; may be diluted 250 mg/250 ml of D_5W, $D_{10}W$ and run as infusion
• IV undiluted over 5 min; IV inf at 1-3 mg/min; adjust for desired respiratory response, using infusion pump IV; if an inf is used after initial dose, start at 1-3 mg/min depending on patient response; D/C after 2 hr; wait 1-2 hr and repeat
• Only after adequate airway is established
• After O_2, IV barbiturates, resuscitative equipment available

Perform/provide:
• Placing patient in Sims' position to prevent aspiration of vomitus
• Discontinue infusion if side effects occur; narrow margin of safety

Evaluate:
• Therapeutic response: increased breathing capacity

Treatment of overdose: Lavage, activated charcoal; monitor electrolytes, vital signs

doxazosin mesylate
Cardura
Func. class.: Peripheral α_1-adrenergic blocker
Chem. class.: Quinozoline

Action: Peripheral blood vessels are dilated, peripheral resistance lowered; reduction in blood pressure results from α-adrenergic receptors being blocked
Uses: Hypertension
Dosage and routes:
*Adult: PO 1 mg qd, increasing up to 16 mg qd if required; usual range 4-16 mg/day
Available forms: Tabs 1, 2, 4, 8 mg
Side effects/adverse reactions:
CV: Palpitations, orthostatic hypotension, tachycardia, edema, dysrhythmias, chest pain
CNS: Dizziness, headache, drowsiness, anxiety, depression, vertigo, weakness, fatigue, asthenia
GI: Nausea, vomiting, diarrhea, constipation, abdominal pain
GU: Incontinence, polyuria
EENT: Epistaxis, tinnitus, dry mouth, red sclera, pharyngitis, rhinitis
Contraindications: Hypersensitivity to quinazolines
Precautions: Pregnancy (C), children, lactation, hepatic disease
Pharmacokinetics:
PO: Onset 2 hr, peak 2-6 hr, duration 6-12 hr; half-life 22 hr; metabolized in liver; excreted via bile/feces (<63%) and in urine (9%); extensively protein bound (98%)
Interaction/incompatibilities:
• Increased hypotensive effects: β-blockers, verapamil

---

* Available in Canada only

• Decreased hypotensive effects: indomethacin

NURSING CONSIDERATIONS
Assess:
• B/P 2-6 hr after each dose and with each increase; postural effects may occur
• Pulse, jugular venous distention q4h
• BUN, uric acid if on long-term therapy
• I&O, weight daily
• Edema in feet, legs daily
• Skin turgor, dryness of mucous membranes for hydration status
• Rales, dyspnea, orthopnea q30min
Administer:
• Whole; do not chew or crush tablets
Perform/provide:
• Storage in tight container in cool environment
Evaluate:
• Therapeutic response: decreased B/P
Teach patient/family:
• That fainting occasionally occurs after 1st dose; do not drive or operate machinery for 4 hr after 1st dose or after dosage increase or take 1st dose hs
Treatment of overdose: Administer volume expanders or vasopressors; discontinue drug; place in supine position

---

doxepin HCl
(dox′e-pin)
Adapin, Doxepin HCl, Sinequan, Sinequan Concentrate, Triadapin*
Func. class.: Antidepressant, tricyclic
Chem. class.: Dibenzoxepin, tertiary amine

Action: Blocks reuptake of nor-

epinephrine, serotonin into nerve endings, increasing action of norepinephrine, serotonin in nerve cells
Uses: Major depression, anxiety
Dosage and routes:
• *Adult:* PO 50-75 mg/day in divided doses; may increase to 300 mg/day or may give daily dose hs
Available forms: Caps 10, 25, 50, 75, 100, 150 mg; oral conc 10 mg/ml
Side effects/adverse reactions:
HEMA: Agranulocytosis, thrombocytopenia, eosinophilia, leukopenia
CNS: Dizziness, drowsiness, confusion, headache, anxiety, tremors, stimulation, weakness, insomnia, nightmares, EPS (elderly), increased psychiatric symptoms, paresthesia
GI: Diarrhea, dry mouth, nausea, vomiting, *paralytic ileus,* increased appetite, cramps, epigastric distress, jaundice, *hepatitis,* stomatitis, constipation
GU: Retention, acute renal failure
INTEG: Rash, urticaria, sweating, pruritus, photosensitivity
CV: Orthostatic hypotension, ECG changes, tachycardia, hypertension, palpitations
EENT: Blurred vision, tinnitus, mydriasis, ophthalmoplegia, glossitis
Contraindications: Hypersensitivity to tricyclic antidepressants, urinary retention, narrow-angle glaucoma, prostatic hypertrophy
Precautions: Suicidal patients, elderly, pregnancy (C)
Pharmacokinetics:
PO: Steady state 2-8 days; metabolized by liver; excreted by kidneys; crosses placenta; excreted in breast milk; half-life 8-24 hr
Interactions/incompatibilities:
• Decreased effects of: guanethi-

dine, clonidine, indirect-acting sympathomimetics (ephedrine)
• Increased effects of: direct-acting sympathomimetics (epinephrine), alcohol, barbiturates, benzodiazepines, CNS depressants
• Hyperpyretic crisis, convulsions, hypertensive episode: MAOI (pargyline [Eutonyl])

Lab test interferences:
Increase: Serum bilirubin, blood glucose, alk phosphatase
False increase: Urinary catecholamines
Decrease: VMA, 5-HIAA

NURSING CONSIDERATIONS
Assess:
• B/P (lying, standing), pulse q4h; if systolic B/P drops 20 mm Hg, hold drug, notify physician; take vital signs q4h in patients with cardiovascular disease
• Blood studies: CBC, leukocytes, differential, cardiac enzymes if patient is receiving long-term therapy
• Hepatic studies: AST, ALT, bilirubin
• Weight qwk; appetite may increase with drug
• ECG for flattening of T wave, bundle branch block, AV block, dysrhythmias in cardiac patients
• EPS primarily in elderly: rigidity, dystonia, akathisia
• Mental status: mood, sensorium, affect, suicidal tendencies, an increase in psychiatric symptoms: depression, panic
• Urinary retention, constipation; constipation is more likely to occur in children
• Withdrawal symptoms: headache, nausea, vomiting, muscle pain, weakness; do not usually occur unless drug is discontinued abruptly
• Alcohol consumption; if alcohol is consumed, hold dose until morning

Administer:
• Increased fluids, bulk in diet if constipation, urinary retention occur
• With food or milk for GI symptoms
• Dosage hs if oversedation occurs during day; may take entire dose hs; elderly may not tolerate qd dosing
• Gum, hard candy, or frequent sips of water for dry mouth
• Concentrate with fruit juice, water, or milk to disguise taste

Perform/provide:
• Storage in tight container protected from direct sunlight
• Assistance with ambulation during beginning therapy, since drowsiness/dizziness occurs
• Safety measures, including side rails, primarily for elderly
• Checking to see PO medication swallowed

Evaluate:
• Therapeutic response: decreased anxiety, depression

Teach patient/family:
• That therapeutic effects may take 2-3 wk
• To use caution in driving, other activities requiring alertness, because of drowsiness, dizziness, blurred vision
• To avoid alcohol ingestion, other CNS depressants
• Not to discontinue medication quickly after long-term use; may cause nausea, headache, malaise
• To wear sunscreen or large hat, since photosensitivity occurs

Treatment of overdose: ECG monitoring; induce emesis; lavage, activated charcoal; administer anticonvulsant

---

* Available in Canada only

doxorubicin HCl
(dox-oh-roo'bi-sin)
Adriamycin, Adriamycin PFS, Adriamycin RDF, Doxorubicin HCl, Rubex
Func. class.: Antineoplastic, antibiotic
Chem. class.: Anthracycline glycoside

Action: Inhibits DNA synthesis primarily; derived from *Streptomyces peucetius;* replication is decreased by binding to DNA, which causes strand splitting; active throughout entire cell cycle; a vesicant

Uses: Wilms' tumor; bladder, breast, cervical, head, neck, liver, lung, ovarian, prostatic, stomach, testicular, thyroid cancer; Hodgkin's disease; acute lymphoblastic leukemia; myeloblastic leukemia; neuroblastomas; lymphomas; sarcomas

Dosage and routes:
• *Adult:* 60-75 mg/m² q3 wk, or 30 mg/m² on days 1-3 of 4-wk cycle, not to exceed 550 mg/m² cumulative dose
Available forms: Inj IV 10, 20, 50 mg

Side effects/adverse reactions:
*HEMA: **Thrombocytopenia, leukopenia, anemia***
GI: Nausea, vomiting, anorexia, mucositis, ***hepatotoxicity***
GU: Impotence, sterility, amenorrhea, gynecomastia, hyperuricemia
INTEG: Rash, *necrosis at injection site,* dermatitis, <u>reversible alopecia</u>, cellulitis, thrombophlebitis at injection site
CV: Increased B/P, ***sinus tachycardia, PVCs,*** chest pain, ***bradycardia, extra systoles***

Contraindications: Hypersensitivity, pregnancy (1st trimester) (D), lactation, systemic infections

Precautions: Renal, hepatic, cardiac disease, gout, bone marrow depression (severe)

Pharmacokinetics: Triphasic pattern of elimination; half-life 12 min, 3⅓ hr, 29⅔ hr; metabolized by liver; crosses placenta; appears in breast milk; excreted in urine, bile

Interactions/incompatibilities:
• Increased toxicity: other antineoplastics or radiation
• Decreased serum digoxin levels: digoxin
• Incompatible with aminophyline, cephalothin, dexamethasone, diazepam, fluorouracil, heparin, hydrocortisone, methotrexate; considered incompatible with all other drugs

Lab test interferences:
Increase: Uric acid

NURSING CONSIDERATIONS
Assess:
• CBC, differential, platelet count weekly; withhold drug if WBC is <4000/mm³ or platelet count is <75,000/mm³; notify physician of these results
• Blood, urine uric acid levels
• Renal function studies: BUN, serum uric acid, urine CrCl, electrolytes before, during therapy
• I&O ratio; report fall in urine output to <30 ml/hr
• Monitor temperature q4h; fever may indicate beginning infection
• Liver function tests before, during therapy: bilirubin, AST, ALT, alk phosphatase as needed or monthly
• ECG; watch for ST-T wave changes, low QRS and T, possible dysrhythmias (sinus tachycardia, heart block, PVCs)

---

italics = common side effects   ***bold italic*** = life threatening reactions

- Bleeding: hematuria, guaiac, bruising or petechiae, mucosa or orifices q8h
- Food preferences; list likes, dislikes
- Effects of alopecia on body image; discuss feelings about body changes
- Inflammation of mucosa, breaks in skin
- Yellowing of skin and sclera, dark urine, clay-colored stools, itchy skin, abdominal pain, fever, diarrhea
- Buccal cavity q8h for dryness, sores, ulceration, white patches, oral pain, bleeding, dysphagia
- Alkalosis if severe vomiting is present
- Local irritation, pain, burning at injection site
- GI symptoms: frequency of stools, cramping
- Acidosis, signs of dehydration: rapid respirations, poor skin turgor, decreased urine output, dry skin, restlessness, weakness
- Cardiac status: B/P, pulse, character, rhythm, rate, ABGs, ECG

Administer:
- Hydrocortisone, dexamethasone or sodium bicarbonate (1 mEq/1 ml) for extravasation; apply ice compresses
- Antiemetic 30-60 min before giving drug to prevent vomiting
- Allopurinol or sodium bicarbonate to maintain uric acid levels, alkalinization of urine
- IV after diluting 10 mg/5 ml of NaCl for inj; another 5 ml of diluent/10 mg is recommended shake; give over 3-5 min; give through Y-tube or 3-way stopcock through free-flowing 5% dextrose inf or NS
- Topical or systemic analgesics for pain

- Transfusion for anemia
- Antispasmodic for GI symptoms

Perform/provide:
- Strict hand-washing technique, gloves, protective clothing
- Liquid diet: carbonated beverages, Jell-O may be added if patient is not nauseated or vomiting
- Increased fluid intake to 2-3 L/day to prevent urate, calculi formation
- Diet low in purines: absence of organ meats (kidney, liver), dried beans, peas to maintain alkaline urine
- Rinsing of mouth tid-qid with water, club soda; brushing of teeth bid-tid with soft brush or cotton-tipped applicators for stomatitis; use unwaxed dental floss
- Storage at room temperature for 24 hr after reconstituting or 48 hr refrigerated

Evaluate:
- Therapeutic response: decreased tumor size, spread of malignancy

Teach patient/family:
- To report any complaints, side effects to nurse or physician
- That hair may be lost during treatment and wig or hairpiece may make the patient feel better; tell patient that new hair may be different in color, texture
- To avoid foods with citric acid, hot or rough texture
- To report any bleeding, white spots, ulcerations in mouth to physician; tell patient to examine mouth qd
- That urine and other body fluids may be red-orange for 48 hr
- To avoid crowds and persons with infections when granulocyte count is low

* Available in Canada only

D

doxycycline hyclate
(dox-i-sye'kleen)
Bio-Tab, Doryx, Doxy 100,
Doxy 200, Doxy-Caps, Doxy-
chel Hyclate, Doxycin,* Doxy-
cycline, Monodox, Vibramycin,
Vibramycin IV, Vibra-Tabs
Func. class.: Broad-spectrum
antibiotic/antiinfective
Chem. class.: Tetracycline

Action: Inhibits protein synthesis,
prosphorylation in microorganisms
by binding to 30S ribosomal subunits, reversibly binding to 50S ribosomal subunits; bacteriostatic
Uses: Syphilis, *C. trachomatis,*
gonorrhea, lymphogranuloma venereum, uncommon gram-nega-
tive/positive organisms, malaria
prophylaxis
Dosage and routes:
• *Adult:* PO 100 mg q12h on day
1, then 100 mg/d; IV 200 mg in 1-
2 inf on day 1, then 100-200 mg/d
• *Child >8 yr:* PO/IV 4.4 mg/kg/
d in divided doses q12h on day 1,
then 2.2-4.4 mg/kg/d
Gonorrhea (uncomplicated)
• *Adult:* PO 200 mg, then 100 mg
hs and 100 mg bid × 3d or 300
mg, then 300 mg in 1 hr
• Disseminated; 100 mg PO bid ×
at least 7d
Malaria prophylaxis
• *Adult:* 100 mg qd 1-2d prior to
travel and daily during travel
C. trachomatis
• *Adult:* PO 100 mg bid × 7d
Syphilis
• *Adult:* PO 300 mg/day in divided
doses × 10d
Available forms: Tabs 50, 100 mg;
caps 50, 100 mg; syr 50 mg/ml;
powder for inj IV 100, 200 mg,
powder for oral susp 25 mg/5 ml

Side effects/adverse reactions:
CNS: Fever
*HEMA: **Eosinophilia, neutropenia,
thrombocytopenia, hemolytic anemia***
EENT: Dysphagia, glossitis, decreased calcification of deciduous
teeth, oral candidiasis
*GI: Nausea, abdominal pain, vom-
iting, diarrhea, anorexia, enterocolitis, **hepatotoxicity,** flatulence, abdominal cramps, gastric
burning, stomatitis*
CV: Pericarditis
GU: Increased BUN
*INTEG: Rash, urticaria, photosen-
sitivity, increased pigmentation,
exfoliative dermatitis, pruritus, **angioedema***
Contraindications: Hypersensitivity to tetracyclines, children <8 yr,
pregnancy (D)
Precautions: Hepatic disease, lactation
Pharmacokinetics:
PO: Peak 1½-4 hr, half-life 15-22
hr; excreted in bile, 25%-93% protein bound
Interactions/incompatibilities:
• Decreased effects of doxycy-
line: antacids, NaHCO₃, dairy
products, alkali products, iron, ka-
olin/pectin, barbiturates, carbem-
azine, phenytoin, cimetidine
• Increased effect: anticoagulants
• Decreased effects: penicillins,
oral contraceptives
• Incompatible with cephalothin;
do not mix with D₅LR, LR
Lab test interferences:
False negative: Urine glucose with
Clinistix or Tes-Tape
False increase: Urinary catechol-
amines; ALT, AST
NURSING CONSIDERATIONS
Assess:
• I&O ratio

---

italics = common side effects   ***bold italic*** = life threatening reactions

• Blood studies: PT, CBC, AST, ALT, BUN, creatinine
• Signs of infection
• Allergic reactions: rash, itching, pruritus, angioedema
• Nausea, vomiting, diarrhea; administer antiemetic, antacids as ordered
• Overgrowth of infection: increased temperature, malaise, redness, pain, swelling, drainage, perineal itching, diarrhea, changes in cough or sputum
• IV site for phlebitis/thrombosis; drug is highly irritating

Administer:
• IV after diluting 100 mg or less/10 ml of sterile H_2O or normal saline for inj; further dilute with 100-1000 ml of NaCl, D_5, Ringer's 10% invert sugar in water, LR D_5LR, Normosol-M, Normosol-R in D_5W; run 100 mg or less over 1-4 hr; do not give IM/SC; inf must be completed in 6 hr, when diluted in LR sol, or 12 hr in other sol
• After C&S obtained
• 2 hr before or after laxative or ferrous products; 3 hr after antacid or kaolin-pectin products

Perform/provide:
• Storage in tight, light-resistant container at room temperature

Evaluate:
• Therapeutic response: decreased temperature, absence of lesions, negative C&S

Teach patient/family:
• To avoid sun exposure, since burns may occur; sunscreen does not seem to decrease photosensitivity
• If diabetic to avoid use of Clinistix, Diastix, or Tes-Tape for urine glucose testing
• That all prescribed medication must be taken to prevent superimposed infection

• To take with a full glass of water; may take with food or milk

---

D-penicillamine
(pen-i-sill'a-meen)
Cuprimine, Depen
Func. class.: Heavy metal antagonist
Chem. class.: Chelating agent (thiol compound)

Action: Binds with ions of lead, mercury, copper, iron, zinc to form a water-soluble complex excreted by kidneys

Uses: Wilson's disease, rheumatoid arthritis, cystinuria, lead poisoning

Dosage and routes:
Cystinuria
• *Adult:* PO 250 mg qid ac, not to exceed 5 g/day
• *Child:* PO 30 mg/kg/day in divided doses qid ac
Wilson's disease
• *Adult:* PO 250 mg qid ac
• *Child:* PO 20 mg/kg/day in divided doses ac
Rheumatoid arthritis
• *Adult:* PO 125-250 mg/day, then increased 250 mg q2-3 mo if needed, not to exceed 1 g/day
Available forms: Caps 125, 250 mg; tabs 250 mg

Side effects/adverse reactions:
*HEMA: **Thrombocytopenia, granulocytopenia, leukopenia, hemolytic anemia, aplastic anemia, eosinophilia,** Lupus syndrome,* increased sedimentation rate
INTEG: Urticaria, erythema, pruritus, fever, ecchymosis, alopecia
CV: Hypotension, tachycardia
*GI: Diarrhea, abdominal cramping, nausea, vomiting, **hepatotoxicity,** anorexia, pain, peptic ulcer
EENT: Tinnitus, optic neuritis

MS: *Arthralgia*
GU: **Proteinuria, nephrotic syndrome, glomerulonephritis**
SYST: **Anaphylaxis**
RESP: *Pneumonitis,* **asthma, pulmonary fibrosis**
Contraindications: Hypersensitivity to penicillins, anuria, agranulocytosis, severe renal disease, pregnancy (D), lactation
Pharmacokinetics:
PO: Peak 1 hr, metabolized in liver, excreted in urine
Interactions/incompatibilities:
• Increased side effects: oxyphenbutazone, phenylbutazone, gold salts, antimalarials, cytotoxics
• Decreased absorption of D-penicillamine: oral iron, antacids, food
NURSING CONSIDERATIONS
Assess:
• Monitor hepatic, renal studies: AST/ALT, alk phosphatase, BUN, creatinine
• Monitor I&O, temperature
• Monitor platelet, neutropenia, WBC, H&H; if WBC <3500/mm³ or if platelets <100,000/mm³, drug should be discontinued
• Allergic reactions (rash, urticaria); if these occur, drug should be discontinued
Administer:
• On an empty stomach, ½-1 hr before meals or at least 2 hr after meals
• Vit B$_6$ daily, depleted when this drug is used
• Only when epinephrine 1:1000 is on unit for anaphylaxis
• Fluids to 3 L/day to prevent renal failure
Evaluate:
• Therapeutic response: absence of pain, rigidity in joints (rheumatoid arthritis)
Teach patient/family:
• That urine may be red in color

• That therapeutic effect may take 1-3 mo
• To report sore throat, easy bruising, bleeding from mucous membranes; may indicate bone marrow depression

---

D

droperidol
(droe-per′i-dole)
Droperidol, Inapsine
Func. class.: Neuroleptic
Chem. class.: Butyrophenone derivative

Action: Acts on CNS at subcortical levels, produces tranquilization, sleep; antiemetic
Uses: Premedication for surgery; induction, maintenance in general anesthesia
Dosage and routes:
Induction
• *Adult:* IV 2.5 mg/20-25 lb given with analgesic or general anesthetic
• *Child 2-12 yr:* IV 1-1.5 mg/20-25 lb, titrated to response needed
Premedication
• *Adult:* IM 2.5-10 mg ½-1 hr before surgery
• *Child 2-12 yr:* IM 1-1.5 mg/20-25 lb
Maintaining general anesthesia
• *Adult:* IV 1.25-2.5 mg
Available forms: Inj IM, IV 2.5 mg/ml
Side effects/adverse reactions:
RESP: **Laryngospasm, bronchospasm**
CNS: *Dystonia, akathisia, flexion of arms, fine tremors, dizziness, anxiety, drowsiness, restlessness, hallucination, depression*
CV: Tachycardia, hypotension
EENT: Upward rotation of eyes, oculogyric crisis
INTEG: *Chills, facial sweating, shivering*

---

italics = common side effects   ***bold italic*** = life threatening reactions

Contraindications: Hypersensitivity, child <2 yr, pregnancy (C)
Precautions: Elderly, cardiovascular disease (hypotension, bradydysrhythmias), renal disease, liver disease, Parkinson's disease
Pharmacokinetics:
IM/IV: Onset 3-10 min, peak ½ hr, duration 3-6 hr; metabolized in liver; excreted in urine as metabolites; crosses placenta
Interactions/incompatibilities:
• Increased CNS depression: alcohol, narcotics, barbiturates, antipsychotics or other CNS depressants
• Decreased effects of: amphetamines, anticonvulsants, anticoagulants, when given with this drug
• Increased intraocular pressure: anticholinergics, antiparkinson drugs
• Increased side effects of: lithium
• Incompatible with barbiturates, epinephrine
NURSING CONSIDERATIONS
Assess:
• VS q10 min during IV administration, q30 min after IM dose
• Extrapyramidal reactions: dystonia, akathisia
• For increasing heart rate or decreasing B/P, notify physician at once; do not place patient in Trendelenburg position, or sympathetic blockade may occur, causing respiratory arrest
Administer:
• IV undiluted; give through Y-tube or 3-way stopcock at 10 mg or less/ min; titrate to patient response; may be given as an infusion by adding dose to 250 ml LR, D₅W, 0.9% NaCl
• Anticholinergics (benztropine, diphenhydramine) for extrapyramidal reaction

• Only with crash cart, resuscitative equipment nearby
Perform/provide:
• Slow movement of patient to avoid orthostatic hypotension
Evaluate:
• Therapeutic response: decreased anxiety, absence of vomiting during and after surgery

---

dyphylline
(dye′fi-lin)
Dilor, Dyflex-200, Dyflex-400, Dylline, Dyphylline, Lufyllin, Lufyllin-400, Neothylline, Protophylline*
Func. class.: Spasmolytic
Chem. class.: Xanthine, ethylenediamide

Action: Relaxes smooth muscle of respiratory system by blocking phosphodiesterase, which increases cyclic AMP
Uses: Bronchial asthma, bronchospasm in chronic bronchitis, COPD
Dosage and routes:
• *Adult:* PO 200-800 mg q6h; IM 250-500 mg q6h injected slowly
• *Child >6 yr:* PO 4-7 mg/kg/day in 4 divided doses
Available forms: Tabs 200, 400 mg; elix 100, 160 mg/15 ml; inj IM 250 mg/ml
Side effects/adverse reactions:
CNS: Anxiety, restlessness, insomnia, dizziness, convulsions, headache, light-headedness, muscle twitching
CV: Palpitations, sinus tachycardia, hypotension, flushing, dysrhythmias
GI: Nausea, vomiting, anorexia, dyspepsia, epigastric pain
INTEG: Flushing, urticaria
RESP: Tachypnea

---

* Available in Canada only

Other: Fever, dehydration, ***albuminuria,*** hyperglycemia

Contraindications: Hypersensitivity to xanthines, tachydysrhythmias

Precautions: Elderly, CHF, cor pulmonale, hepatic disease, active peptic ulcer disease, diabetes mellitus, hyperthyroidism, hypertension, children, renal disease, pregnancy (C), glaucoma

Pharmacokinetics: Peak 1 hr, half-life 2 hr, excreted in urine unchanged

Interactions/incompatibilities:

• Do not mix in syringe with other drugs
• Increased action of dyphylline: cimetidine, propranolol, erythromycin, troleandomycin
• May increase effects of: anticoagulants
• Cardiotoxicity: β-blockers
• Increased metabolism: barbiturates, phenytoin
• Decreased elimination of dyphylline: uricosurics

NURSING CONSIDERATIONS

Assess:

• Dyphylline blood levels; toxicity may occur with small increase above 20 µg/ml
• Monitor I&O; diuresis occurs; dehydration may result in elderly or children
• Whether theophylline was given recently
• Auscultate lung fields bilaterally; notify physician of abnormalities
• Allergic reactions: rash, urticaria; if these occur, drug should be discontinued

Administer:

• PO after meals to decrease GI symptoms; absorption may be affected
• Avoid IM injection; pain occurs

Perform/provide

• Storage protected from light, at room temperature

Evaluate:

• Therapeutic response: decreased dyspnea, respiratory rate, rhythm

Teach patient/family

• To check OTC medications, current prescription medications for ephedrine; will increase stimulation; not to drink alcohol or caffeine
• To avoid hazardous activities; dizziness, drowsiness, blurred vision may occur
• If GI upset occurs, to take drug with 8 oz of water; avoid food, since absorption may be decreased

---

echothiophate iodide
(ek-oh-thye′oh-fate)
Phospholine Iodide
Func. class.: Miotic
Chem. class.: Cholinesterase inhibitor, irreversible

Action: Prevents breakdown of neurotransmitter acetylcholine, which then accumulates, causing enhancement, prolongation of its physiologic effects

Uses: Glaucoma (open-angle), accommodative esotropia, treatment of obstructed aqueous outflow; extremely effective in control of chronic wide-angle glaucoma, aphakic glaucoma, congenital glaucoma

Dosage and routes:

• *Adult and child:* INSTILL 1 gtt of 0.03%, or 0.125% sol qd in conjunctival sac, not to exceed 1 gtt bid

Available forms: Powder for reconstitution, 1.5 mg (0.03%), 3 mg (0.06%), 6.25 mg (0.125%), 12.5 mg (0.25%) with 5 ml diluent

Side effects/adverse reactions:

GU: Frequency
CV: Hypotension, bradycardia, ***cardiac arrest***

---

italics = common side effects   ***bold italic*** = life threatening reactions

INTEG: Sweating, pallor, cyanosis
RESP: **Bronchospasm**
GI: Nausea, vomiting, abdominal cramps, diarrhea
EENT: Blurred vision; stinging; burning; lacrimation; lid muscle twitching; conjunctival, ciliary redness; browache; headache; induced myopia; iris cysts; hyperemia; hyphema

Contraindications: Hypersensitivity, ureitis

Precautions: Asthma, bradycardia, parkinsonism, peptic ulcer, pregnancy (C)

Interactions/incompatibilities:
• Decreased effect of echothiophate: pilocarpine
• Increased effect of both drugs: ambenonium, edrophonium, neostigmine, physostigmine, pyridostigmine
• Increased effects of: general anesthetics

NURSING CONSIDERATIONS
Assess:
• Specific condition being treated
• History of patient's previous/current conditions (e.g., asthma, cardiac), possible sensitivity, contraindications, drug interactions

Administer:
• After checking vial for concentration
• Immediately after reconstituting; discard unused portion
• After reconstituting powder with diluent provided

Evaluate:
• Therapeutic response: decreased aqueous humor in eye

Teach patient/family:
• Why patient is receiving medication; patient, family should have a clear regimen as well as name of medication
• To report change in vision, blur-

ring or loss of sight, trouble breathing, sweating, flushing
• Method of instillation, including pressure on lacrimal sac for 1 min, not to touch dropper to eye
• That long-term therapy may be required
• That blurred vision will decrease with repeated use of drug
• That patient may experience stinging sensation, dull ache or tearing, which should subside in a few minutes; if it persists, contact physician
• That patient may experience decreased visual ability at night; instruct not to drive
• To use drops at night to eliminate hazardous, transient blurring

---

econazole nitrate (topical)

(e-kone'a-zole)
Spectazole

Func. class.: Local antiinfective
Chem. class.: Imidazole derivative, antifungal

Action: Interferes with fungal cell membrane, which increases permeability, leaking of cell nutrients

Uses: Tinea pedis, tinea cruris, tinea corporis, tinea versicolor, cutaneous candidiasis

Dosage and routes:
• *Adult and child:* TOP apply to affected area bid-qid depending on condition

Available forms: Cream 1%

Side effects/adverse reactions:
INTEG: Rash, urticaria, stinging, burning, pruritus

Contraindications: Hypersensitivity

Precautions: Pregnancy (C), lactation

NURSING CONSIDERATIONS
Assess:
• Allergic reaction: burning, sting-ing, swelling, redness
Administer:
• Enough medication to cover le-sions completely
• After cleansing with soap, water before each application, dry well
• For 2 wk in tinea cruris, tinea cor-poris, *Candida* infections; 1 month tinea pedis
Perform/provide:
• Storage at room temperature in dry place
Evaluate:
• Therapeutic response: decrease in size, number of lesions
Teach patient/family:
• To use medical asepsis (hand washing) before, after each applica-tion
• To apply with glove to prevent further infection
• To avoid use of OTC creams, ointments, lotions unless directed by physician
• Not to cover with occlusive dressing
• To continue even though condi-tion improves
• To notify physician if condition worsens

---

edetate calcium disodium
(ed'e-tate)
Calcium Disodium Versenate
Func. class.: Heavy metal an-tagonist
Chem. class.: Chelating agent

Action: Binds ions of lead to form a water-soluble complex that is re-moved by kidneys
Uses: Lead poisoning, acute lead encephalopathy

Dosage and routes:
Acute lead encephalopathy
• *Adult and child:* 1.5 g/m^2/day × 3-5 days, with dimerca-prol, may be given again after 4 days off drug
Lead poisoning
• *Adult:* IV 1 g/250-500 ml D$_5$W or 0.9% NaCl over 1-2 hr or q12h × 3-5 days; may repeat after 2 days; not to exceed 50 mg/kg/day; may be given as a continuous infusion over 8-24 hr
• *Adult:* IM 35 mg/kg bid
• *Child:* IM 35 mg/kg/day in di-vided doses q8-12h, not to exceed 50 mg/kg/day; may give for 3-5 days, off 4 days before next course
Available forms: Inj IM, IV 200 mg/ml
Side effects/adverse reactions:
CNS: Headache, paresthesia, numbness
INTEG: Urticaria, erythema, pruri-tus, pain at injection site, fever, cheilosis
CV: Hypotension, dysrhythmias, thrombophlebitis
GI: Vomiting, *diarrhea, abdominal cramps, anorexia,* cheilosis, his-tamine-like reaction with GI dis-tress
EENT: Nasal congestion, sneezing
MS: Leg cramps, myalgia, arthral-gia, weakness
GU: Hematuria, renal tubular ne-crosis, proteinuria
Contraindications: Hypersensitiv-ity, anuria, poisoning of other met-als, severe renal disease, child <3 yr
Precautions: Hypertension, preg-nancy (C), lactation, gout, active TB
Pharmacokinetics:
Not metabolized; excreted in urine; half-life 20-60 min (IV), 90 min (IM)

---

italics = common side effects   ***bold italic*** = life threatening reactions

Lab test interferences:

Decrease: Cholesterol/triglycerides, K

NURSING CONSIDERATIONS
Assess:

• VS, B/P, pulse, respirations, weigh daily

• Monitor I&O, kidney function studies: BUN, creatinine, CrCl; watch for decreasing urine output

• Neuro status: Watch for paresthesias, beginning convulsions

• Urine: pH, albumin, casts, blood, coproporphyrins, calcium

• For febrile reactions that may occur 4-8 hr following drug therapy

• Cardiac abnormalities: dysrhythmias, hypotension, tachycardia

• Allergic reactions (rash, urticaria); if these occur; drug should be discontinued

Administer:

• EDTA, BAL separately

• IV slowly; IM is preferred route

• IM in large muscle mass; rotate injection sites; procaine HCl should be added to IM injection (1 ml of procaine 1% to each ml of concentrated drug) to minimize pain at injection site

• Only when epinephrine 1:1000 is on unit for anaphylaxis

• IV fluids to ensure adequate hydration before administration of drug

Evaluate:

• Therapeutic response: decreased symptoms of lead poisoning

---

edetate disodium

(ed'e-tate)

Chealamide, Disodium EDTA, Disotate, Endrate

Func. class.: Metal antagonist
Chem. class.: Chelating agent

Action: Binds with ions of calcium, zinc, magnesium to form a water-soluble complex excreted from kidneys

Uses: Hypercalcemic crisis, control of ventricular arrhythmias associated with digitalis toxicity

Dosage and routes:

• *Adult and child:* IV INF 15-50 mg/kg/day, diluted in 500 ml of D_5W or 0.9% NaCl, given over 3-4 hr, not to exceed 3 g/day (adult) or 70 mg/kg/day (child); allow 5 days between courses (child), 2 days (adult)

Available forms: Inj conc 150 mg/ml

Side effects/adverse reactions:

CNS: Headache, paresthesia, numbness

INTEG: Urticaria, erythema, pain at injection site

CV: Hypotension, *exfoliative dermatitis*, thrombophlebitis

GI: Nausea, vomiting, diarrhea

GU: Dysuria, pyelonephritis, *nephrotoxicity*, hyperuricemia, hypomagnesemia, polyuria, *proteinuria, renal tubular necrosis, hypocalcemia*

Contraindications: Hypersensitivity, anuria, hepatic insufficiency, poisoning of other metals, severe renal disease, child <3 yr, seizure disorders, active/inactive TB

Precautions: Hypertension, pregnancy (C), lactation

Pharmacokinetics:

Excreted in urine as Ca chelate

Interactions/incompatibilities:

• Incompatible in 5% alcohol

Lab test interferences:

False decrease: Ca

Decrease: Mg, alk phosphatase

NURSING CONSIDERATIONS
Assess:

• VS, B/P, pulse; if hypotension occurs, drug should be discontinued

---

• Monitor I&O, kidney function studies: BUN, creatinine, CrCl, Ca (must be done following each administration)
• Hypocalcemia: numbness of feet, hands, tongue, lips; positive Chvostek's, Trousseau's signs; convulsions; stupor
• Cardiac abnormalities: dysrhythmias, hypotension, tachycardia
• Allergic reactions (rash, urticaria); if these occur, drug should be discontinued
Administer:
• IV inf after diluting in 500 ml dextrose, or isotonic saline sol, not to exceed 15 mg of actual medication/min, total dose is usually given over 3-4 hr
• Only when IV Ca preparation is on unit for emergency use
• EDTA, BAL separately
• IV use infusion pump, rotate infusion sites, observe site for redness, inflammation
• IV fluids to ensure adequate hydration before administration of drug
Perform/provide:
• Assistance with ambulation
Evaluate:
• Therapeutic response: Ca levels 9-10 mg/dl; absence of hypercalcemic symptoms
Teach patient/family:
• To remain recumbent for ½ hr to prevent postural hypotension
• To make position changes slowly to prevent fainting
• That dosage schedule must be followed
• That breath may be odorous

edrophonium chloride
(ed-roe-foe′nee-um)
Enlon, Reversol, Tensilon
Func. class.: Cholinergics, anticholinesterase
Chem. class.: Quaternary ammonium compound

E

Action: Inhibits destruction of acetylcholine, which increases concentration at sites where acetylcholine is released; this facilitates transmission of impulses across myoneural junction
Uses: To diagnose myasthenia gravis; curare antagonist; differentiation of myasthenic crisis from cholinergic crisis
Dosage and routes:
Tensilon test
• *Adult:* IV 1-2 mg over 15-30 sec, then 8 mg if no response; IM: 10 mg; if cholinergic reaction occurs, retest after ½ hr with 2 mg IM
• *Child >34 kg:* IV 2 mg; if no response in 45 sec, then 1 mg q45 sec, not to exceed 10 mg
• *Child <34 kg:* IV 1 mg; if no response in 45 sec, then 1 mg q45 sec, not to exceed 5 mg
• *Infant:* IV 0.5 mg
Curare antagonist
• *Adult:* IV 10 mg over 30-45 sec, may repeat, not to exceed 40 mg
Differentiation of myasthenic crisis from cholinergic crisis
• *Adult:* IV 1 mg, if no response in 1 min, may repeat
Available forms: Inj IV 10 mg/ml
Side effects/adverse reactions:
INTEG: Rash, urticaria
CNS: Dizziness, headache, sweating, weakness, *convulsions,* incoordination, *paralysis,* drowsiness, *loss of consciousness*
GI: Nausea, diarrhea, vomiting,

cramps, increased salivary and gastric secretions, dysphagia, increased peristalsis
CV: Tachycardia, dysrhythmias, bradycardia, hypotension, AV block, ECG changes, ***cardiac arrest***, syncope
GU: Frequency, incontinence, urgency
*RESP: **Respiratory depression, bronchospasm, constriction, laryngospasm, respiratory arrest***, dyspnea
EENT: Miosis, blurred vision, lacrimation, visual changes
Contraindications: Obstruction of intestine, renal system, hypersensitivity
Precautions: Seizure disorders, bronchial asthma, coronary occlusion, hyperthyroidism, dysrhythmias, peptic ulcer, megacolon, poor GI motility, pregnancy (C), bradycardia, hypotension
Pharmacokinetics:
IV: Onset 30-60 sec, duration 6-24 min
IM: Onset 2-10 min, duration 12-45 min
Interactions/incompatibilities:
• Decreased action of edrophonium: procainamide, quinidine, aminoglycosides, anesthetics, mecamylamine, polymyxin, Mg, corticosteroids, antidysrhythmics
• Bradycardia: digitalis
• Considered incompatible with any drug in syringe or sol
NURSING CONSIDERATIONS
Assess:
• VS, respiration during test
• Diabetic patient carefully, since this drug lowers blood glucose
Administer:
• IV undiluted 2 mg or less over 15-30 sec; as a curare antagonist, over 30-45 sec; or given as continuous infusion in myasthenia crisis

• Only with atropine sulfate available for cholinergic crisis
• Only after all other cholinergics have been discontinued
Perform/provide:
• Storage at room temperature
Evaluate:
• Therapeutic response: increased muscle strength, hand grasp; improved gait; absence of labored breathing (if severe)
Teach patient/family:
• To wear Medic Alert ID specifying myasthenia gravis, drugs taken
Treatment of overdose:
Respiratory support, atropine 1-4 mg (IV)

---

enalapril maleate/ enalaprilat
(en-al-a′prel)
Vasotec, Vasotec IV
Func. class.: Antihypertensive
Chem. class.: Angiotensin-converting enzyme inhibitor

Action: Selectively suppresses renin-angiotensin-aldosterone system; inhibits ACE; prevents conversion of angiotensin I to angiotensin II, dilation of arterial, venous vessels
Uses: Hypertension, CHF
Dosage and routes:
• *Adult:* PO 5 mg/day, may increase or decrease to desired response range 10-40 mg/day
Hypertension
• *Adult:* IV 1.25 mg q6h over 5 min
Patients on diuretics
• *Adult:* IV 0.625 mg over 5 min, may give additional doses of 1.25 mg q6h
Renal impairment
• *Adult:* IV 1.25 mg q6h with CrCl

<3 mg/dl or 0.625 mg if CrCl >3 mg/dl

Available forms: Tabs 2.5, 5, 10, 20 mg, inj 1.25 mg/ml

Side effects/adverse reactions:

CV: Hypotension, chest pain, tachycardia, dysrhythmias

CNS: Insomnia, dizziness, paresthesias, headache, fatigue, anxiety

GI: Nausea, vomiting, colitis, cramps, diarrhea, constipation, flatulence, dry mouth, loss of taste

INTEG: Rash, purpura, alopecia, hyperhidrosis

*HEMA: **Agranulocytosis, neutropenia***

EENT: Tinnitus, visual changes, sore throat, double vision, dry burning eyes

*GU: **Proteinuria, renal failure,*** increased frequency of polyuria or oliguria

RESP: Dyspnea, cough, rales, angioedema

META: Hyperkalemia

Contraindications: Pregnancy (C), lactation

Precautions: Renal disease, hyperkalemia

Pharmacokinetics:

PO: Peak 4-6 hr; half-life 1½ hr; metabolized by liver to active metabolite, excreted in urine

IV: Onset 5-15 min, peak up to 4 hr

Interactions/incompatibilities:

• Hypersensitivity: allopurinol

• Severe hypotension: diuretics, other antihypertensives

• Decreased effects of enalapril: aspirin, antacids

• Increased K levels: salt substitutes, K-sparing diuretics, K supplements

• May increase effects of: ergots, neuromuscular blocking agents, antihypertensives, hypoglycemics, barbiturates, reserpine, levodopa

• Effects may be increased by phenothiazines, diuretics, phenytoin, quinidine, nifedipine

Lab test interferences:

Interference: Glucose/insulin tolerance tests

NURSING CONSIDERATIONS

Assess:

• B/P, pulse q4h; note rate, rhythm, quality

• Electrolytes: K, Na, Cl

• Baselines in renal, liver function tests before therapy begins

• Edema in feet, legs daily

• Skin turgor, dryness of mucous membranes for hydration status

• Symptoms of CHF: edema, dyspnea, wet rales

Administer:

• IV, undiluted over 5 min, use diluent provided or 50 ml of D$_5$W, 0.9% NaCl, 0.9% NaCl in D$_5$W or LR, Isolyte E, give through Y-tube of free-flowing inf of NS, D$_5$W, LR, Isolyte E

Evaluate:

• Therapeutic response: decreased B/P

Teach patient/family:

• Not to use OTC (cough, cold, or allergy) products unless directed by physician

• To avoid sunlight or wear sunscreen if in sunlight; photosensitivity may occur

• To comply with dosage schedule, even if feeling better

• To notify physician of mouth sores, sore throat, fever, swelling of hands or feet, irregular heartbeat, chest pain, signs of angioedema

• Excessive perspiration, dehydration, vomiting, diarrhea; may lead to fall in blood pressure—consult physician if these occur

• That drug may cause dizziness, fainting; light-headedness may oc-

---

italics = common side effects   ***bold italic*** = life threatening reactions

cur during 1st few days of therapy
• That drug may cause skin rash or impaired perspiration
• Not to discontinue drug abruptly
• Not to use OTC products unless directed by physician
• To rise slowly to sitting or standing position to minimize orthostatic hypotension

Treatment of overdose: Lavage, IV atropine for bradycardia, IV theophylline for bronchospasm, digitalis, O_2, diuretic for cardiac failure, hemodialysis

---

enoxacin
(en-ox′aa-sin)
Penetrex
Func. class.: Antiinfective
Chem. class.: Fluoroquinolone

Action: Inhibits the enzyme that repairs bacterial DNA, thereby preventing bacterial replication
Uses: Uncomplicated urethral or cervical gonorrhea, uncomplicated and complicated urinary tract infections (UTI)
Dosage and routes:
Gonorrhea
• *Adult:* PO 400 mg as a single dose
Uncomplicated UTI
• *Adult:* PO 200 mg bid × 7 days
Complicated UTI
• *Adult:* PO 400 mg bid × 14 days
Available forms: Tabs 200, 400 mg
Side effects/adverse reactions:
CNS: Dizziness, headache, fatigue, somnolence, depression, insomnia, anxiety
GI: Diarrhea, nausea, vomiting, anorexia, flatulence, heartburn, abdominal pain, dry mouth, increased AST, ALT
INTEG: Rash, pruritus, photosensitivity

EENT: Visual disturbances, dizziness
Contraindications: Hypersensitivity to quinolones
Precautions: Pregnancy (C), lactation, children, elderly, renal disease, seizure disorders
Pharmacokinetics:
PO: Peak 1 hr, half-life 3-6 hr, steady state 2 days; excreted in urine as unchanged drug, metabolites
Interactions/incompatibilities:
• Decreased effects of enoxacin: antacids, nitrofurantoin, iron salts, sucralfate, antineoplastics
• Increased enoxacin levels: probenecid, cimetidine
• Increased toxicity: theophylline, cyclosporin, caffeine
NURSING CONSIDERATIONS
Assess:
• Kidney, liver function studies: BUN, creatinine, AST, ALT
• I&O ratio, urine pH; <5.5 is ideal
• CNS symptoms: insomnia, vertigo, headache, agitation, confusion
• Allergic reactions: rash, flushing, urticaria, pruritus
Administer:
• After clean-catch urine is obtained for C&S
Perform/provide:
• Limited intake of alkaline foods, drugs; milk, dairy products, peanuts, vegetables, alkaline actacids, sodium bicarbonate
Evaluate:
• Therapeutic response: negative C&S
Teach patient/family:
• Fluids must be increased to 3L/ day to avoid crystallization in kidneys
• If dizziness occurs, to ambulate, perform activities with assistance

---

* Available in Canada only

• To complete full course of drug therapy, take 1 hr ac or 2 hr pc
• To contact physician if adverse reactions occur

E

enoxaparin sodium
(in-ox'a-par-in)
Lovenox
Func. class.: Anticoagulant
Chem. class.: Unfractionated porcine heparin

Action: Prevents conversion of fibrinogen to fibrin and prothrombin to thrombin by enhancing inhibitory effects of antithrombin III; produces higher ratio of anti-factor Xa to anti-factor IIa

Uses: Prevention of deep vein thrombosis, pulmonary emboli in hip and knee replacement

Dosage and routes:
• *Adult:* SC 30 mg bid immediately after surgery; continue to administer until deep vein thrombosis no longer a threat (7-14 days)

Available forms: Inj 30 mg/0.3 ml

Side effects/adverse reactions:
CNS: Fever, confusion
GI: Nausea
GU: Edema, peripheral edema
HEMA: Hypochromic anemia
INTEG: Ecchymosis

Contraindications: Hypersensitivity to this drug, heparin, or pork; hemophilia, leukemia with bleeding, peptic ulcer disease, thrombocytopenic purpura

Precautions: Alcoholism, elderly, pregnancy (C), hepatic disease (severe), renal disease (severe), blood dyscrasias, severe hypertension, subacute bacterial endocarditis, acute nephritis, lactation, children

Pharmacokinetics:
SC: Maximum antithrombin activity (3-5 hr)
Elimination half-life 4½ hr

Interactions/incompatibilities:
• Increased action of enoxaprin: oral anticoagulants, salicylates
• Do not mix with other drugs or infusion fluids

NURSING CONSIDERATIONS
Assess:
• Blood studies (Hct, platelets, occult blood in stools); thrombocytopenia may occur
• Bleeding gums, petecchiae, ecchymosis, black tarry stools, hematuria

Administer:
• Only after screening patient for bleeding disorders
• SC only; do not give IM
• To recumbent patient; give deep SC; rotate inj sites (left/right anterolateral, left/right posterolateral abdominal wall)
• Insert whole length of needle into skin fold held with thumb and forefinger
• Only this drug when ordered; not interchangeable with heparin
• At same time each day to maintain steady blood levels
• Do not massage area or aspirate when giving SC injection
• Avoiding all IM injections that may cause bleeding

Perform/provide:
• Storage at 77° F (25° C); do not freeze

Evaluate:
• Therapeutic response: prevention of deep vein thrombosis

Teach patient/family:
• To use soft-bristle toothbrush to avoid bleeding gums, to use electric razor
• To report any signs of bleeding: gums, under skin, urine, stools

Treatment of overdose:
Protamine SO_4 10% sol; dose should equal dose of enoxaprin

---

italics = common side effects   ***bold italic*** = life threatening reactions

ephedrine sulfate (nasal)

(e-fed'rin)

Vatronol Nose Drops

Func. class.: Nasal decongestant

Chem. class.: Indirect/direct sympathomimetic amine

Action: Relaxes bronchial smooth muscle, increases diameter of nasal passage by action on β_2-adrenergic receptors

Uses: Nasal congestion associated with colds, hay fever, sinusitis, other allergic conditions, adjunct in middle ear infections

Dosage and routes:

• *Adult and child:* Instill 3-4 gtts, q4h or small amount of gel in each nostril q4h

Available forms: Sol 0.5% sulfate, gel 0.6% HCl

Side effects/adverse reactions:

GI: Nausea, vomiting, anorexia

EENT: Irritation, burning, sneezing, stinging, dryness, rebound congestion

INTEG: Contact dermatitis

CNS: Anxiety, restlessness, tremors, weakness, insomnia, dizziness, fever, headache

Contraindications: Hypersensitivity to sympathomimetic amines

Precautions: Child <6 yr, elderly, diabetes, cardiovascular disease, hypertension, hyperthyroidism, increased ICP, prostatic hypertrophy, pregnancy (C)

Interactions/incompatibilities:

• Hypertension: MAOIs, β-adrenergic blockers

• Hypotension: methyldopa, mecamylamine, reserpine

NURSING CONSIDERATIONS

Assess:

• Redness, swelling, pain in nasal passages

Administer:

• No more than q4h

• For <4 consecutive days

Perform/provide:

• Environmental humidification to decrease nasal congestion, dryness

• Storage in light-resistant containers; do not expose to high temperatures

Evaluate:

• Therapeutic response: decreased congestion, runny nose

Teach patient/family:

• That stinging may occur for a few applications; drying of mucosa may be decreased by environmental humidification

• To notify physician if irregular pulse, insomnia, dizziness, or tremors occur

• Proper administration to avoid systemic absorption

ephedrine sulfate

(e-fed'rin)

Ephedrine, Ephedrine sulfate, Neorespin

Func. class.: Adrenergic, mixed direct and indirect effects

Chem. class.: Phenylisopropylamine

Action: Causes increased contractility and heart rate by acting on β-receptors in the heart; also acts on α-receptors, causing vasoconstriction in blood vessels

Uses: Shock; increased perfusion; hypotension, bronchodilation

Dosage and routes:

• *Adult:* IM/SC 25-50 mg, not to exceed 150 mg/24 hr

IV 10-25 mg, not to exceed 150 mg/24 hr

• *Child:* SC/IV 3 mg/kg/day in divided doses q4-6h

---

* Available in Canada only

Bronchodilator
• *Adult:* PO 12.5-50 mg bid-qid, not to exceed 400 mg/day
• *Child:* PO 2-3 mg/kg/day in 4-6 divided doses
Available forms: Inj 25, 50 mg/ml, IM, SC, IV; caps 25, 50 mg; syr 11, 20 mg/5 ml
Side effects/adverse reactions:
CNS: Tremors, anxiety, insomnia, headache, dizziness, confusion, hallucinations, ***convulsions, CNS depression***
GU: Dysuria, urinary retention
CV: Palpitations, tachycardia, hypertension, chest pain, ***dysrhythmias***
GI: Anorexia, nausea, vomiting
*RESP: **Dyspnea***
Contraindications: Hypersensitivity to sympathomimetics, narrow-angle glaucoma
Precautions: Pregnancy (C), cardiac disorders, hyperthyroidism, diabetes mellitus, prostatic hypertrophy
Pharmacokinetics:
PO: Onset 15-60 min, duration 2-4 hr
IV: Onset 5 min, duration 2 hr
Metabolized in liver; excreted in urine (unchanged); crosses blood-brain barrier, placenta, breast milk
Interactions/incompatibilities:
• Do not use with MAOIs or tricyclic antidepressants; hypertensive crisis may occur
• Decreased effect of ephedrine: methyldopa, urinary acidifiers, rauwolfia alkaloids
• Increased effect of this drug: urinary alkalizers
• Dysrhythmia: halothane, anesthetics, digitalis
• Decreased effect of: guanethidine
• Incompatible with alkaline sol,

hydrocortisone, pentobarital, phenobarbital, secobarbital, thiopental
NURSING CONSIDERATIONS
Assess:
• I&O ratio
• ECG during administration continuously; if B/P increases, drug is decreased
• B/P and pulse q5min after parenteral route
• CVP or PWP during infusion if possible
• For paresthesias and coldness of extremities; peripheral blood flow may decrease
• Injection site: tissue sloughing; if this occurs, administer phentolamine mixed with NS
Administer:
• IV undiluted given through Y-tube or 3-way stopcock; give 10 mg or less over 1 min
• Plasma expanders for hypovolemia
Perform/provide:
• Storage of reconstituted solution if refrigerated for no longer than 24 hr
• Do not use discolored solutions
Evaluate:
• Therapeutic response: increased B/P with stabilization
Teach patient/family:
• Reason for drug administration
Treatment of overdose: Administer phentolamine for hypertension, diazepam for convulsions

---

italics = common side effects   ***bold italic*** = life threatening reactions

---

epinephrine/epi-nephrine bitartrate/epinephrine HCl
(ep-i-nef'rin)

Adrenalin Chloride, Adrenalin Chloride Solution, Asthma Haler, Asthma Nefrin, Bronitin Mist, Bronkaid Mist, Epinephrine, Epinephrine HCl, Epinephrine Pediatric, Medihaler-Epi, Micro-Nefrin, Nephron Inhalant, Primatene Mist, S-2 Inhalant, Sus-Phrine, Vaponefrin

Func. class.: Adrenergic
Chem. class.: Catecholamine

Action: β₁- and β₂-agonist causing increased levels of cyclic AMP producing bronchodilation, cardiac, and CNS stimulation; large doses cause vasoconstriction; small doses can cause vasodilation via β₂-vascular receptors

Uses: Acute asthmatic attacks, hemostasis, bronchospasm, anaphylaxis, allergic reactions, cardiac arrest

Dosage and routes:
• *Adult:* IM/SC 0.1-0.5 ml of 1:1000 sol, may repeat q10-15 min IV 0.1-0.25 ml of 1:1000 sol
• *Child:* SC 0.01 ml of 1:1000/kg, may repeat q20min to 4 hr; INH 0.005 ml/kg of 1:200 solution, may repeat q8-12h

Asthma
• *Adult and child:* INH 1-2 puffs of 1:100 or 2.25% racemic q1-5min

Hemostasis
• *Adult:* TOP 1:50,000-1:1000 applied as needed to stop bleeding

Cardiac arrest
• *Adult:* IC, IV, endotracheal 0.1-1 mg repeat q5min PRN
• *Child:* IC, IV, endotracheal 5-10

μg q5min, may use 0.1 μ/kg/min IV inf after inital dose

Available forms: Aerosol 0.16 mg/spray, 0.2 mg/spray, 0.25 mg/spray, inj 1:1000 (1 mg/ml), 1:200 (5 mg/ml), 0.01 mg/ml (1:100,000), 0.1 mg/ml (1:10,000), 0.5 mg/ml (1:2,000); IM, IV, SC; sol for nebulization 1:100, 1.25% 2.25% (base)

Side effects/adverse reactions:
GU: Urinary retention
CNS: Tremors, anxiety, insomnia, headache, dizziness, confusion, hallucinations, *cerebral hemorrhage*
CV: Palpitations, tachycardia, hypertension, *dysrhythmias,* increased T wave
GI: Anorexia, nausea, vomiting
RESP: Dyspnea

Contraindications: Hypersensitivity to sympathomimetics, narrow-angle glaucoma

Precautions: Pregnancy (C), cardiac disorders, hyperthyroidism, diabetes mellitus, prostatic hypertrophy

Pharmacokinetics:
SC: Onset 3-5 min, duration 20 min
PO, INH: Onset 1 min

Interactions/incompatibilities:
• Do not use with MAOIs or tricyclic antidepressants; hypertensive crisis may occur
• Decreased effect of epinephrine: methyldopa, urinary acidifiers, rauwolfia alkaloids and β-blockers
• Increased effect of epinephrine: urinary alkalizers
• Incompatible with any other drug in syringe; unstable in sol with aminophylline, cephapirin, mephentermine, NaCO₃, warfarin

NURSING CONSIDERATIONS
Assess:
• ECG during administration con-

tinuously; if B/P increases, drug is decreased
• B/P and pulse q5min after parenteral route
• CVP or PCWP during infusion if possible
• Injection site: tissue sloughing; if this occurs, administer phentolamine mixed with NS

Administer:
• Parenteral IV dose slowly, after reconstituting 1 mg (1:1000 sol)/10 ml or more normal saline; to prepare a 1:10,000 sol for maintenance, may be further diluted in 500 ml D₅W; give 1 mg or less over 1 min or more through Y-tube or 3-way stopcock; 1 mg = 1 ml of 1:1,000 or 10 ml of 1:10,000

Perform/provide:
• Storage of reconstituted sol if refrigerated for no longer than 24 hr
• Do not use discolored solutions

Evaluate:
• Therapeutic response: increased B/P with stabilization or ease of breathing

Teach patient/family:
• Reason for drug administration
• To rinse mouth after use to prevent dryness after inhalation
• Not to take OTC preparations

Treatment of overdose: Administer an α-blocker and a β-blocker

---

epinephrine bitartrate/epinephrine HCl/epinephryl borate (optic)
(ep-i-nef′rin)
Epitrate, Mytrate/Epifrin, Glaucon/Epinal, Eppy*
Func. class.: Mydriatic
Chem. class.: Sympathomimetic amine

Action: Blocks response of iris sphincter muscle, muscle of accommodation of ciliary body to cholinergic stimulation, resulting in dilation, paralysis of accommodation

Uses: During ocular surgery, open-angle glaucoma

Dosage and routes:
• *Adult and child:* INTRAOCULAR INJ 0.1-0.2 ml of a 0.01 or 0.1% sol (HCl); INSTILL SOL 1-2 gtts of a 1%-2% sol, determined by tonometric reading (bitartrate); 1 gtt of a 0.5%-2% sol (HCl) or 0.5%-1% (Borate)

During surgery
• *Adult and child:* INSTILL SOL 1 or more gtts of a 0.1% sol (HCl) up to 3 × /day

Available forms: Sol 0.1%, 0.25%, 0.5%, 1.2% (HCl), borate 0.5%, 1, 2%

Side effects/adverse reactions:
CV: Palpitations, tachycardia, headache, hypertension, faintness, trembling
EENT: Blurred vision, eye pain, ocular irritation, and tearing

Contraindications: Hypersensitivity to sympathomimetic amines, narrow-angle glaucoma, dysrhythmias, cardiogenic shock, cerebral arteriosclerosis

Precautions: Elderly, prostatic hypertrophy, diabetes mellitus, hypertension, TB, Parkinson's disease, pregnancy (C), asthma, lactation, children

Pharmacokinetics:
INSTILL: Onset 1 hr, peak 4-8 hr, duration 12-24 hr

Interactions/incompatibilities:
• Dysrhythmias: cyclopropane, halogenated hydrocarbons
• Increased pressor effects: tricyclic antidepressants, antihistamines, β-blockers, MAOIs

NURSING CONSIDERATIONS
Assess:
• Allergic reaction: itching, edema of eyelids, eye discharge; drug should be discontinued
• Tonometer readings during long-term treatment
• B/P, pulse, respirations
Evaluate:
• Therapeutic response: mydriasis
Teach patient/family:
• To report change in vision, blurring or loss of sight, trouble breathing, sweating, pallor
• Method of instillation: pressure on lacrimal sac for 1 min; do not touch dropper to eye
• That long-term therapy may be required if using for glaucoma
• To check OTC drugs for other sympathetic nervous system stimulants (e.g., phenylephrine)
• Not to use solution if brown or contains a precipitate
• Not to use while wearing soft contact lenses

---

epinephrine HCl (nasal)
(ep-i-nef'rin)
Adrenalin Chloride
Func. class.: Nasal decongestant
Chem. class.: Sympathomimetic amine

Action: Relaxes bronchial smooth muscle, increases diameter of nasal passage by action on β-adrenergics
Uses: Nasal congestion, superficial bleeding
Dosage and routes:
• *Adult and child >6 yr old:* TOP apply to affected area with sterile swab
Available forms: Sol 0.1%

Side effects/adverse reactions:
GI: Nausea, vomiting, anorexia
EENT: Irritation, burning, sneezing, stinging, dryness, rebound congestion
INTEG: Contact dermatitis
CNS: Anxiety, restlessness, tremors, weakness, insomnia, dizziness, fever, headache
Contraindications: Hypersensitivity to sympathomimetic amines
Precautions: Child <6 yr, elderly, diabetes, cardiovascular disease, hypertension, hyperthyroidism, increased ICP, prostatic hypertrophy, pregnancy (C)
Interactions/incompatibilities:
• Hypertension: MAOIs, β-adrenergic blockers
• Hypotension: methyldopa, mecamylamine, reserpine
NURSING CONSIDERATIONS
Assess:
• For redness, swelling, pain in nasal passages
Administer:
• No more than q4h
• For <4 consecutive days
Perform/provide:
• Environmental humidification to decrease nasal congestion, dryness
• Storage in light-resistant containers; do not expose to high temperatures
Evaluate:
• Therapeutic response: decreased congestion, bleeding
Teach patient/family:
• That stinging may occur for a few applications; drying of mucosa may be decreased by environmental humidification
• To notify physician of irregular pulse, insomnia, dizziness, or tremors
• Proper administration to avoid systemic absorption

ergoloid mesylate

(er'goe-loid mess'i-late)
Ergoloid Mesylates, Gerimal, Hydergine, Hydergine LC
Func. class.: Migraine agent
Chem. class.: Ergot alkaloid–amino acid

Action: May increase cerebral metabolism and blood flow

Uses: Senile dementia, Alzheimer's dementia, multiinfarct dementia, primary progressive dementia

Dosage and routes:
• *Adult:* PO/SL 1 mg tid, may increase to 4.5-12 mg/day

Available forms: Tabs SL 0.5, 1 mg, tabs 1 mg, cap 1 mg, liquid 1 mg/ml

Side effects/adverse reactions:
GI: Nausea, vomiting, sublingual irritation

Contraindications: Hypersensitivity to ergot preparations; psychosis

Precautions: Acute intermittent porphyria, pregnancy (C)

Pharmacokinetics:
PO: Peak 1 hr; metabolized in liver; excreted as metabolites in feces; crosses blood-brain barrier; half-life 3½ hr

NURSING CONSIDERATIONS
Assess:
• Weight daily; check for peripheral edema in feet, legs
• B/P and pulse, check regularly
• Neurologic status: LOC, blurring vision, nausea, vomiting, tingling in extremities that occur preceding the headache
• Toxicity: dyspnea; hypotension or hypertension; rapid, weak pulse; delirium; nausea; vomiting; bradycardia

Administer:
• With meals or after meals to avoid GI symptoms; do not crush or chew SL tab

Perform/provide:
• Storage in well-closed container at room temperature

Evaluate:
• Therapeutic response: decreased forgetfulness, increased mental alertness and ability for self-care

Teach family/patient:
• To change positions slowly and to move extremities before walking
• To maintain dosage at approved level; not to increase drug
• To report side effects, including increased vasoconstriction starting with cold extremities, then paresthesia, weakness
• That 6 months of treatment may be required; some improvement occurs in 1 month
• To keep drug out of reach of children; death may occur

Treatment of overdose: Induce emesis if orally ingested, or gastric lavage; administer saline cathartic, keep warm

ergonovine maleate

(er-goe-noe'veen)
Ergotrate Maleate, Ergonovine Maleate
Func. class.: Oxytocic
Chem. class.: Ergot alkaloid

Action: Stimulates uterine contractions, decreases bleeding

Uses: Treatment of hemorrhage associated with postpartum or postabortion

Dosage and routes:
• *Adult:* IM 0.2 mg q2-4h, not to exceed 5 doses; IV 0.2 mg given over 1 min; PO 0.2-0.4 mg q6-12h × 2-7 days after initial IM or IV dose

---

italics = common side effects   ***bold italic*** = life threatening reactions

Available forms: Inj IM, IV 0.2 mg/ml; tabs 0.2 mg

Side effects/adverse reactions:
CNS: Headache, dizziness, fainting
CV: Hypertension, chest pain
GI: Nausea, vomiting
INTEG: Sweating
RESP: Dyspnea
EENT: Tinnitus
GU: Cramping

Contraindications: Hypersensitivity to ergot medication, augmentation of labor, before delivery of placenta, spontaneous abortion (threatened), pelvic inflammatory disease (PID)

Precautions: Hepatic disease, renal disease, cardiac disease, asthma, anemia, convulsive disorders, hypertension, glaucoma, obliterative vascular disease

Pharmacokinetics:
PO: Onset 5-25 min, duration 3 hr
IM: Onset 2-5 min, duration 3 hr
IV: Onset immediate, duration 45 min
Metabolized in liver, excreted in urine

Interactions/incompatibilities:
• Hypertension: sympathomimetics, ergots

NURSING CONSIDERATIONS
Assess:
• B/P, pulse; watch for change that may indicate hemorrhage
• Respiratory rate, rhythm, depth; notify physician of abnormalities
• Fundal tone, nonphasic contractions; check for relaxation

Administer:
• IV undiluted through Y-tube or 3-way stopcock
• IM in deep muscle mass; rotate injection sites if additional doses are given
• With crash cart available on unit

Evaluate:
• Therapeutic response: decreased blood loss, severe cramping

Teach patient/family:
• To report increased blood loss, increased temperature or foul-smelling lochia; that cramping is normal

ergotamine tartrate
(er-got'a-meen)
Ergostat
Func. class.: α-Adrenergic blocker
Chem. class.: Ergot alkaloid-amino acid

Action: Constricts smooth muscle in peripheral, cranial blood vessels, relaxes uterine muscle

Uses: Vascular headache (migraine or histamine)

Dosage and routes:
• *Adult:* 2 mg, then 1-2 mg qh or q½ hr for SL, not to exceed 6 mg/day or 10 mg/wk; INH 1 puff, may repeat in 5 min, not to exceed 6/24 hr

Available forms: SL tabs 2 mg; tabs 1 mg; oral inh 360 μg/dose

Side effects/adverse reactions:
CNS: Numbness in fingers, toes, headache, weakness
CV: Transient tachycardia, chest pain, bradycardia, edema, claudication, increase or decrease in B/P
GI: Nausea, vomiting
MS: Muscle pain

Contraindications: Hypersensitivity to ergot preparations, occlusion (peripheral, vascular), CAD, hepatic disease, renal disease, peptic ulcer, hypertension, pregnancy (X)

Precautions: Lactation, children, anemia

Pharmacokinetics:
PO: Peak 30 min-3 hr; metabolized in liver; excreted as metabolites in feces; crosses blood-brain barrier; excreted in breast milk

Interactions/incompatibilities:
• Increased effects: troleandomycin
• Increased vasoconstriction: β-blockers
NURSING CONSIDERATIONS
Assess:
• Weight daily, check for peripheral edema in feet, legs
• Check for coldness of extremities and tingling of fingers; drug should be discontinued
• For stress level, activity, recreation, coping mechanisms
• Neurologic status: LOC, blurring vision, nausea, vomiting, tingling in extremities that occur preceding the headache
• Ingestion of tyramine foods (pickled products, beer, wine, aged cheese), food additives, preservatives, colorings, artificial sweeteners, chocolate, caffeine, which may precipitate these types of headaches
• Toxicity: dyspnea, hypotension or hypertension, rapid, weak pulse, delirium, nausea, vomiting
Administer:
• At beginning of headache; dose must be titrated to patient response
• By SL route if possible for better, faster absorption
• With meals or after meals to avoid GI symptoms
• Only to women who are not pregnant; harm to fetus may occur
Perform/provide:
• Quiet, calm environment with decreased stimulation for noise, or bright light or excessive talking
Evaluate:
• Therapeutic response: decrease in frequency, severity of headache
Teach patient/family:
• Not to use OTC medications; serious drug interactions may occur
• To maintain dose at approved level; not to increase even if drug does not relieve headache
• To report side effects including increased vasoconstriction starting with cold extremities, then paresthesia, weakness
• That an increase in headaches may occur when this drug is discontinued after long-term use
• To keep drug out of reach of children; death may occur
• How to use inhaler
Treatment of overdose: Induce emesis if orally ingested; orgastric lavage; administer saline cathartic; keep warm

erythrityl tetranitrate
(e-ri'thri-till)
Cardilate
Func. class.: Vasodilator, coronary
Chem. class.: Nitrate

Action: Decreases preload, afterload, which is responsible for decreasing left ventricular end diastolic pressure, systemic vascular resistance; improves exercise tolerance
Uses: Chronic stable angina pectoris, prophylaxis of angina pain, pulmonary arteriolar dilation
Dosage and routes:
• *Adult:* PO 10-30 mg tid; SL 5-15 mg before stressful activity
Available forms: Chew tabs 10 mg; tabs PO, SL 5, 10 mg
Side effects/adverse reactions:
CV: Postural hypotension, tachycardia, ***collapse,*** syncope, edema
GI: Nausea, vomiting
INTEG: Pallor, sweating, rash
*CNS: Headache, flushing, dizziness **weakness, fainting***
MISC: Twitching, hemolytic anemia, ***methemoglobinemia***

italics = common side effects   ***bold italic*** = life threatening reactions

Contraindications: Hypersensitivity to this drug or nitrites, severe anemia, increased intracranial pressure, cerebral hemorrhage, acute MI, head trauma

Precautions: Postural hypotension, pregnancy (C), lactation, children, hypertropic cardiomyopathy, glaucoma

Pharmacokinetics:
PO: Onset 30 min, peak 1-1½ hr, duration 6 hr
SL: Onset 5-10 min, peak 30-45 min, duration 3 hr; metabolized by liver, excreted in urine

Interactions/incompatibilities:
• Increased effects: β-blockers, diuretics, antihypertensives, alcohol products

Lab test interferences:
Decrease: Cholesterol

NURSING CONSIDERATIONS
Assess:
• For orthostatic B/P, pulse during beginning therapy
• Pain: duration, time started, activity being performed, character
• Tolerance if taken over long period
• Headache, light-headedness, decreased B/P; may indicate a need for decreased dosage

Administer:
• With 8 oz of water on empty stomach (oral tablet)
• After checking expiration date

Evaluate:
• Therapeutic response: decrease or prevention of anginal pain

Teach patient/family:
• To keep tabs in original container
• If 3 SL tabs do not relieve pain, activate EMS
• To avoid alcohol products
• That drug may cause headache; tolerance occurs over time
• That drug may be taken before stressful activity: exercise, sexual activity
• Not to chew or swallow SL tablets
• That SL may sting when drug comes in contact with mucous membranes
• To avoid hazardous activities if dizziness occurs
• Importance of complying with complete medical regimen
• To make position changes slowly to prevent fainting

erythromycin (ophthalmic)
(er-ith-roe-mye'sin)
AK-Mycin, Erythromycin, Ilotycin
Func. class.: Antiinfective

Action: Inhibits bacterial protein synthesis

Uses: Infection of external eye, prophylaxis of ophthalmia neonatorium due to N. gonorrhoeae, C. trachomatis

Dosage and routes:
• *Adult and child:* Apply oint qd-qid as needed
Ophthalmia neonatorum
• *Neonates:* Apply oint to conjunctival sacs immediately after delivery
Available forms: Oint 0.5%

Side effects/adverse reactions:
EENT: Poor corneal wound healing, temporary visual haze, overgrowth of nonsusceptible organisms

Contraindications: Hypersensitivity, epitheleal herpes, varicella, mycobacterial, fungal infections, simplex keratitis

Precautions: Antibiotic hypersensitivity

NURSING CONSIDERATIONS
Assess:
• Allergy: itching, lacrimation, redness, swelling

Administer:
• After washing hands, cleanse crusts or discharge from eye before application

Perform/provide:
• Storage at room temperature, in tight container

Evaluate:
• Therapeutic response: absence of redness, inflammation, tearing

Teach patient/family:
• To use drug exactly as prescribed
• Not to use eye makeup, towels, washcloths, eye medication of others; reinfection may occur
• That drug container tip should not be touched to eye
• To report itching, increased redness, burning, stinging, swelling; drug should be discontinued
• That drug may cause blurred vision when ointment is applied

---

erythromycin (topical)

(er-ith-roe-mye'sin)
A/T/S, Akne-Mycin, C-Solve 2, Erycette, Eryderm, Erygel, Erymax, Erythromycin, E-Solve 2, ETS-2%, Staticin, Theramycin Z, T-Stat

Func. class.: Local antiinfective

Chem. class.: Macrolide antibacterial

Action: Interferes with bacterial protein synthesis

Uses: Pyoderma, acne vulgaris

Dosage and routes:
• Adult and child: TOP apply to affected area tid-qid

Available forms: Top sol, ointment 1.5%, 2%, gel 2%

Side effects/adverse reactions:
INTEG: Rash, urticaria, stinging, burning, pruritus, dry, scaly, oily skin

Contraindications: Hypersensitivity

Precautions: Pregnancy (C), lactation, child <12 yr

Interactions/incompatibilities:
Avoid use with clindamycin, abrasive agents, acids, alkaline media

NURSING CONSIDERATIONS

Assess:
• Allergic reaction: burning, stinging, swelling, redness

Administer:
• Enough medication to cover lesions completely
• After cleansing with soap, water before each application; dry well

Perform/provide:
• Storage at room temperature in dry place; after reconstitution, store in refrigerator

Evaluate:
• Therapeutic response: decrease in size, number of lesions

Teach patient/family:
• To use medical asepsis (hand washing) before, after each application
• To apply with glove to prevent further infection
• To avoid use of OTC creams, ointments, lotions unless directed by physician
• To avoid use near eyes, nose, mouth
• To monitor for superimposed infection
• To report skin irritation to physician

---

italics = common side effects   **bold italic** = life threatening reactions

---

**erythromycin base,
erythromycin esto-
late, erythromycin
ethylsuccinate, eryth-
romycin gluceptate,
erythromycin lacto-
bionate, erythromy-
cin stearate**

(er-ith-roe-mye'sin)

E-Base, E-Mycin, Eryc, Ery-Tab,
Erythromycin, Erythromycin
Base, Erthromycin Filmtabs,
Novorythro,* PCE Dispertab,
Robimycin Robitabs/Ery-
thromid,* Erythromycin Esto-
late, Ilosone, Ilosone Pulvules/
E.E.S. 200, E.E.S. 400,
Eryped, Ery Ped Drops, Eryped
200, Eryped 400, Erythromycin
Ethylsuccinate/Erythromycin
Lactobionate, Ilotycin Glucep-
tate

Func. class.: Antibacterial
Chem. class.: Macrolide antibiotic

Action: Binds to 50S ribosomal
subunits of susceptible bacteria and
suppresses protein synthesis

Uses: Infections caused by *N. gonorrhoeae;* mild to moderate respiratory tract, skin, soft tissue infections caused by *D. pneumoniae, M.
pneumoniae, C. diphtheriae, B.
pertussis, B. burgdorferi, L. monocytogenes;* syphilis; Legionnaire's
disease; *C. trachomatis; H. influenzae*

Dosage and routes:
Soft tissue infections
• *Adult:* PO 250-500 mg q6h (base,
estolate, stearate); PO 400-800 mg
q6h (ethylsuccinate); IV INF 15-20
mg/kg/day (lactobionate)
• *Child:* PO 30-50 mg/kg/day in
divided doses q6h (salts); IV 15-20

mg/kg/day in divided doses q4-6h
(lactobionate)
N. gonorrhoeae/PID
• *Adult:* IV 500 mg q6h × 3 days
(gluceptate, lactobionate), then PO
250 mg (base, estolate, stearate)
or 400 mg (ethylsuccinate) q6h ×
1 wk
Syphilis
Adult: PO 20 g in divided doses
over 15 days (base, estolate, stearate)
Chlamydia
• *Adult:* PO 500 mg q6h × 1 wk
or 250 mg qid × 2 wk
• *Infant:* PO 50 mg/kg/day in 4
divided doses × 3 wk or more
• *Newborn:* PO 50 mg/kg/day in
4 divided doses × 2 wk or more
Intestinal amebiasis
• *Adult:* PO 250 mg q6h × 10-14
days (base, estolate, stearate)
• *Child:* PO 30-50 mg/kg/day in
divided doses q6h × 10-14 days
(base, estolate, stearate)
Available forms: Base: tabs, enteric-coated 250, 333, 500 mg; tabs
film-coated 250, 500 mg; caps, enteric-coated 125, 250 mg; estolate:
tabs chewable 125, 250 mg; tabs
500 mg; caps 125, 250 mg; drops
100 mg/ml; susp 125, 250 mg/
5ml; stearate: tabs, film-coated
250, 500 mg; ethylsuccinate: tabs,
chewable 200, 400 mg; 100 mg/
2.5 ml, 200, 400 mg/5 ml; susp
200, 400 mg powder for suspension
100 mg/2.5 ml, 200 and 400 mg/
5 ml powder for inj; 500 mg and 1
g (lactobionate); 250 mg, 500 mg,
1 g (as gluceptate)
Side effects/adverse reactions:
INTEG: Rash, urticaria, pruritus,
thrombophlebitis (IV site)
GI: Nausea, vomiting, diarrhea,
hepatotoxicity, abdominal pain,
stomatitis, heartburn, anorexia,
pruritus ani

---

*Available in Canada only

GU: Vaginitis, moniliasis
EENT: Hearing loss, tinnitus
Contraindications: Hypersensitivity, preexisting liver disease (estolate)
Precautions: Pregnancy (C), hepatic disease, lactation
Pharmacokinetics: Peak 4 hr, duration 6 hr, half-life 1-3 hr; metabolized in liver; excreted in bile, feces
Interactions/incompatabilities:
• Arrhythmias: astemizole, terfenadine
• Increased action of: oral anticoagulants, digitalis, theophylline, methylprednisolone, cyclosporine, bromocriptine, disopyramide, ergots, triazolam
• Decreased action of: clindamycin, penicillins
• Serious CV effects: astemizole, terfenadine
• Toxicity: carbamazepine
• Incompatible with: amikacin, aminophylline, Vit C, carbenicillin, cephalothin, cephapirin, chloramphenicol, colistimethate, heparin, lincomycin, metaraminol, metoclopramide, pentobarbital, phenobarbital, phenytoin, prochlorperazine, secobarbital, Na salts, tetracycline, thiopental, vancomycin, Vit B complex with C, warfarin in sol or syringe
Lab test interferences:
False increase: 17-OHCS/17-KS, AST/ALT
Decrease: Folate assay
NURSING CONSIDERATIONS
Assess:
• I&O ratio; report hematuria, oliguria in renal disease
• Liver studies: AST, ALT
• Renal studies: urinalysis, protein, blood
• C&S before drug therapy; drug may be given as soon as culture is taken; C&S may be repeated after treatment
• Bowel pattern before, during treatment
• Skin eruptions, itching
• Respiratory status: rate, character, wheezing, tightness in chest; discontinue drug if these occur
• Allergies before treatment, reaction of each medication; place allergies on chart, Kardex in bright red letters; notify all people giving drugs
Administer:
• IV after diluting 500 mg or less/ 10 ml sterile H_2O without preservatives; dilute further in 80-250 ml of NS, LR, Normosol-R; may be further diluted to 1 mg/ml and given as continuous infusion; run 1 g or less/100 ml over ½-1 hr; continuous infusion over 6 hr, may require buffers to neutralize pH if dilution is < 250 ml, use infusion pump
• Enteric-coated tablets may be given with food
Perform/provide:
• Storage at room temperature
• Adequate intake of fluids (2 L) during diarrhea episodes
Evaluate:
• Therapeutic response: decreased symptoms of infection
Teach patient/family:
• To take oral drug with full glass of water; give with food if GI symptoms occur
• Do not take with fruit juice
• To report sore throat, fever, fatigue; could indicate superimposed infection
• To notify nurse of diarrhea stools, dark urine, pale stools, yellow discoloration of eyes or skin, and severe abdominal pain
• To take at evenly spaced intervals; complete dosage regimen

italics = common side effects   ***bold italic*** = life threatening reactions

Treatment of overdose: Withdraw drug; maintain airway; administer epinephrine, aminophylline, O_2, IV corticosteroids

---

erythropoietin recombinant

(er-ith-row-poe'-ee-tin)
rHU-EPO, eprex*
Func. class.: Hormone
Chem. class.: Amino acid polypeptide

Action: Erythropoietin is one factor controlling rate of red cell production; drug is developed by recombinant DNA technology
Uses: Anemia caused by reduced endogenous erythropoietin production, primarily end-stage renal disease; to correct hemostatic defect in uremia
Dosage and routes:
• *Adult:* IV 5-500 U/kg 3 × /wk
Side effects/adverse reactions:
CV: Hypertension, **hypertensive encephalopathy**
CNS: Seizures, coldness, sweating
MS: Bone pain
Contraindications: Hypersensitivity
Pharmacokinetics:
IV: Metabolized in body; extent of metabolism unknown; onset of increased reticulocyte count 1-2 wk
NURSING CONSIDERATIONS
Assess:
• Renal studies: urinalysis, protein, blood, BUN, creatinine
• Blood studies: reticulocyte count weekly
• I&O; report drop in output to <50 ml/hr
• CNS symptoms: coldness, sweating
• CV status: B/P; hypertension

may occur rapidly leading to hypertension encephalopathy
Evaluate:
• Therapeutic response: increase in reticulocyte count in 1-2 wk, increased appetite, enhanced sense of well-being

---

esmolol HCl

(ess'moe-lol)
Brevibloc
Func. class.: β-Adrenergic blocker

Action: Competitively blocks stimulation of β_1-adrenergic receptors in the myocardium; produces negative chronotropic, inotropic activity (decreases rate of SA node discharge, increases recovery time), slows conduction of AV node, decreases heart rate, decreases O_2 consumption in myocardium; also decreases renin-aldosterone-angiotensin system at high doses; inhibits β_2-receptors in bronchial system slightly
Uses: Supraventricular tachycardia, noncompensatory tachycardia, hypertensive crisis
Dosage and routes:
• *Adult:* IV loading dose—500 μg/kg/min over 1 min; maintenance—50 μg/kg/min for 4 min; may repeat q5min, increasing maintenance inf by 50 μg/kg/min (max of 200 μg/kg/min), titrate to patient response
Available forms: Inj IV 10 mg, conc 250 mg/ml
Side effects/adverse reactions:
INTEG: Induration, inflammation at site, discoloration, edema, erythema, burning pallor, flushing, rash, pruritus, dry skin, alopecia
CNS: Confusion, light-headedness, paresthesia, somnolence, fever,

dizziness, fatigue, headache, depression, anxiety

GI: Nausea, vomiting, anorexia, gastric pain, flatulence, constipation, heartburn, bloating

CV: Hypotension, bradycardia, chest pain, peripheral ischemia, shortness of breath, CHF, conduction disturbances

GU: Urinary retention, impotence, dysuria

*RESP: **Bronchospasm,*** dyspnea, cough, wheeziness, nasal stuffiness

Contraindications: 2nd or 3rd degree heart block, cardiogenic shock, CHF, cardiac failure, hypersensitivity

Precautions: Hypotension, pregnancy (C), peripheral vascular disease, diabetes, hypoglycemia, thyrotoxicosis, renal disease, lactation

Pharmacokinetics: Onset very rapid, duration short, half-life 9 min; metabolized by hydrolysis of the ester linkage; excreted via kidneys

Interactions/incompatibilities:
• Increased digoxin levels: digoxin
• Increased esmolol levels: morphine
• Reversal of esmolol effects: isoproterenol, norepinephrine, dopamine, dobutamine
• Increased effects of both drugs: disopyramide
• Increased effects of: lidocaine
• Incompatible with $NaCO_3$, furosemide; do not mix with any drug before full dilution

Lab test interferences:
Interference: Glucose/insulin tolerance test

NURSING CONSIDERATIONS
Assess:
• I&O ratio, weight daily
• B/P, pulse q4h; note rate, rhythm, quality; rapid changes can cause shock; if systolic <100 or

diastolic <60, notify physician before giving drug
• Apical/radial pulse before administration; notify physician if less than 60 bpm
• Baselines in renal, liver function tests before therapy begins
• Breath sounds and respiratory pattern
• Respiratory pattern: wheezing from bronchospasm
• Edema in feet, legs daily
• Skin turgor, dryness of mucous membranes for hydration status

Administer:
• Reduced dosage in cool environment
• IV diluted 5 g/20 ml of D_5W, D_5R, D_5 0.9% NaCl, 0.45% NaCl, LR D_5 0.45% NaCl 0.9% NaCl further dilute in the remaining 480 ml (10 mg/ml) and give as infusion

Perform/provide:
• Storage protected from light, moisture; place in cool environment

Evaluate:
• Therapeutic response: decreased B/P immediately, decreased heart rate

Treatment of overdose: Discontinue drug

---

essential crystalline amino acid solution
Aminosyn-RF, Nephramine, Ren-Amine 6.5
Func. class.: Nitrogen product

Action: Needed for anabolism to maintain structure, decrease catabolism, promote healing

Uses: Renal decompensation

Dosage and routes:
• *Adult:* CENT IV 0.3-0.5 g/kg, 250 ml of amino acid/500 ml D70, given at rate of 20-30 ml/hr, in-

creased by 10 ml/hr q24h, not to exceed 100 ml/hr
• *Child:* CENT IV 1 g/kg/day or less, depending on patient's needs
Available forms: Inj central line only, many types

Side effects/adverse reactions:
CNS: Dizziness, headache, confusion, *loss of consciousness*
CV: Hypertension, *CHF, pulmonary edema*
GI: Nausea, vomiting, liver fat deposits, abdominal pain
GU: Glycosuria, osmotic diuresis
ENDO: Hyperglycemia, rebound hypoglycemia, electrolyte imbalances, hyperosmolar syndrome, hyperosmolar hyperglycemic nonketotic syndrome, alkalosis, acidosis, hypophosphatemia, hyperammonemia, dehydration, hypocalcemia
INTEG: Chills, flushing, warm feeling, rash, urticaria, extravasation necrosis, phlebitis at injection site
Contraindications: Hypersensitivity, severe electrolyte imbalances, anuria, severe liver damage, maple syrup urine disease, PKU
Precautions: Renal disease, pregnancy (C), children, diabetes mellitus, CHF

NURSING CONSIDERATIONS
Assess:
• Electrolytes (K, Na, Ca, Cl, Mg), blood glucose, ammonia, phosphate
• Renal, liver function studies: BUN, creatinine, ALT, AST, bilirubin
• Injection site for extravasation: redness along vein, edema at site, necrosis, pain, hard tender area; site should be changed immediately
• Monitor respiratory function q4h: auscultate lung fields bilaterally for crackles, respirations, quality, rate, rhythm

• Monitor temperature q4h for increased fever, indicating infection; if infection suspected, infusion is discontinued; tubing, bottle, catheter tip cultured
• Urine glucose q6h using Tes-Tape, Clinistix, Keto-Diastix, which are not affected by infusion substances
• Hyperammonemia: nausea, vomiting, malaise, tremors, anorexia, convulsions

Administer:
• TPN must be used only mixed with dextrose to promote protein synthesis
• Immediately after mixing in pharmacy under strict aseptic technique using laminar flowhood; use infusion pump, in-line filter
• Using careful monitoring technique; do not speed up infusion; pulmonary edema, glucose overload will result

Perform/provide:
• Storage depends on type of solution; consult manufacturer
• Changing dressing, IV tubing to prevent infection q24-48h

Evaluate:
• Therapeutic response: weight gain, decreased jaundice in liver disorders, increased serum albumin

Teach patient/family:
• Reason for use of TPN
• To report chills, sweating at once

---

estazolam
ProSom
Func. class.: Sedative-hypnotic
Chem. class.: Benzodiazepine derivative

Controlled Substance Schedule IV (US)
Action: Produces CNS depression at the limbic, thalamic, hypotha-

lamic levels of the CNS; may be mediated by neurotransmitter γ-aminobutyric acid (GABA); results are sedation, hypnosis, skeletal muscle relaxation, anticonvulsant activity, anxiolytic action

Uses: Insomnia

Dosage and routes:

Adult: PO 1-2 mg hs

Available forms: Tabs 1, 2 mg

Side effects/adverse reactions:

INTEG: Dermatitis, allergy, sweating, flushing, pruritus

*HEMA: **Leukopenia, granulocytopenia (rare)***

CNS: Lethargy, drowsiness, daytime sedation, dizziness, confusion, light-headedness, headache, anxiety, irritability, weakness, tremors, depression, lack of coordination

GI: Nausea, vomiting, diarrhea, heartburn, abdominal pain, constipation, anorexia, taste alteration

CV: Chest pain, pulse changes, palpitations, tachycardia

MISC: Joint pain, congestion

Contraindications: Hypersensitivity to benzodiazepines, pregnancy (X), sleep apnea

Precautions: Hepatic disease, renal disease, suicidal individuals, drug abuse, elderly, psychosis, child <18, lactation, depression, *pulmonary insufficiency*

Pharmacokinetics: Onset 15-45 min, peaks 1½-2 hr, duration 7-8 hr; metabolized by liver; excreted by kidneys (inactive/active metabolites); crosses placenta; excreted in breast milk

Interactions/incompatibilities:

• Increased effects of estazolam: cimetidine, disulfiram, isoniazid, probenecid, oral contraceptives

• Increased CNS depression: alcohol, CNS depressants

• Decreased effect of estazolam: theophylline, rifampin, smoking, caffeine

NURSING CONSIDERATIONS

Assess:

• Blood studies: Hct, Hgb, RBCs (if on long-term therapy)

• For REM rebound if abruptly discontinued after 3 wks of use

• Hepatic studies: AST, ALT, bilirubin

• Mental status: mood, sensorium, affect, memory (long, short)

• Blood dyscrasias: fever, sore throat, bruising, rash, jaundice, epistaxis (rare)

• Type of sleep problem: falling asleep, staying asleep

Administer:

• After removal of cigarettes to prevent fire

• After trying conservative measures for insomnia

• ½-1 hr before hs for sleeplessness

• On empty stomach for fast onset, but may be taken with food if GI symptoms occur

Perform/provide:

• Assistance with ambulation after receiving dose

• Safety measures: side rails, nightlight, call bell within easy reach

• Checking to see PO medication has been swallowed

• Storage in tight container in cool environment

Evaluate:

• Therapeutic response: ability to sleep at night, decreased amount of early morning awakenings

Teach patient/family:

• To avoid driving or other activities requiring alertness until drug is stabilized

E

---

italics = common side effects   ***bold italic*** = life threatening reactions

esterified estrogens

Climestrone,* Estratab, Menest, Neo-Estrone*

Func. class.: Estrogen
Chem. class.: Nonsteroidal synthetic estrogen

Action: Needed for adequate functioning of female reproductive system; affects release of pituitary gonadotropins, inhibits ovulation, adequate calcium use in bone structures

Uses: Menopause, breast cancer, prostatic cancer hypogonadism, castration, primary ovarian failure

Dosage and routes:
Menopause
• *Adult:* PO 0.3-3.75 mg qd 3wk on, 1 wk off
Hypogonadism/castration/ovarian failure
• *Adult:* PO 2.5 mg qd-tid 3wk on, 1 wk off
Prostatic cancer
• *Adult:* PO 1.25-2.5 mg tid
Breast cancer
• *Adult:* PO 10 mg tid × 3 months or longer
Available forms: Tabs 0.3, 0.625, 1.25, 2.5 mg

Side effects/adverse reactions:
CNS: Dizziness, headache, migraines, depression
CV: Hypotension, thrombophlebitis, edema, *thromboembolism, stroke, pulmonary embolism, myocardial infarction*
GI:Nausea, vomiting, diarrhea, anorexia, pancreatitis, cramps, constipation, increased appetite, increased weight, *cholestatic jaundice*
EENT: Contact lens intolerance, increased myopia, astigmatism
GU: Amenorrhea, cervical erosion, breakthrough bleeding, dysmenorrhea, vaginal candidiasis, breast changes, *gynecomastia, testicular atrophy, impotence*
INTEG: Rash, urticaria, acne, hirsutism, alopecia, oily skin, seborrhea, purpura, melasma
META: Folic acid deficiency, hypercalcemia, hyperglycemia

Contraindications: Breast cancer, thromboembolic disorders, reproductive cancer, genital bleeding (abnormal, undiagnosed), pregnancy (X)

Precautions: Hypertension, asthma, blood dyscrasias, gallbladder disease, CHF, diabetes mellitus, bone disease, depression, migraine headache, convulsive disorders, hepatic disease, renal disease, family history of cancer of breast or reproductive tract

Pharmacokinetics:
PO: Degraded in liver; excreted in urine; crosses placenta; excreted in breast milk

Interactions/incompatibilities:
• Decreased action of: anticoagulants, oral hypoglycemics
• Toxicity: tricyclic antidepressants
• Decreased action of estrogens: anticonvulsants barbiturates, phenylbutazone, rifampin
• Increased action of: corticosteroids

NURSING CONSIDERATIONS
Assess:
• Blood glucose in patient with diabetes
• Weight daily; notify physician of weekly weight gain >5 lb; if increase, diuretic may be ordered
• B/P q4h; watch for increase caused by H_2O and Na retention
• I&O ratio; be alert for decreasing urinary output and increasing edema
• Liver function studies, including

AST, ALT, bilirubin, alk phosphatase

• Edema, hypertension, cardiac symptoms, jaundice

• Mental status: affect, mood, behavioral changes, aggression

• Hypercalcemia

Administer:

• Titrated dose; use lowest effective dose

• With food or milk to decrease GI symptoms

Evaluate:

• Therapeutic response: reversal of menopause or decrease in tumor size in prostatic cancer

Teach patient/family:

• To weigh weekly, report gain >5 lb

• To check with physician before using OTC drugs

• To report breast lumps, vaginal bleeding, edema, jaundice, dark urine, clay-colored stools, dyspnea, headache, blurred vision, abdominal pain, numbness or stiffness in legs, chest pain; male to report impotence or gynecomastia

estradiol/estradiol cypionate/estradiol valerate

(ess-tra-dye'ole)

Cypionate, depGynogen, Depo Estadiol, Depogen, Dura-Estrin, Estra-D, Estradiol Cypionate, Estro-Cyp, Estroject-LA, Estronol-LA/Estrace, Estraderm/Deladiol-40, Delestrogen, Dioval 40, Dioval XX, Duragen-10, Duragen-20, Duragen-40, Estradiol Valerate, Estra-L 20, Estra-L 40, Gynogen L.A. "10", Gynogen L.A. "20", Gynogen L.A. "40", L.A.E. 20, Valergen 10, Valergen 20, Valergen 40

Func. class.: Estrogen

Chem. class.: Nonsteroidal synthetic estrogen

Action: Needed for adequate functioning of female reproductive system; affects release of pituitary gonadotropins, inhibits ovulation, adequate calcium use in bone structures

Uses: Menopause, breast cancer, prostatic cancer, atrophic vaginitis, kraurosis vulvae, hypogonadism, castration, primary ovarian failure, prevention of osteoporosis

Dosage and routes:

Menopause/hypogonadism/castration/ovarian failure

• *Adult:* PO 1-2 mg qd 3wk on, 1 wk off or 5 days on, 2 days off; IM 0.2-1 mg qwk

Prostatic cancer

• *Adult:* IM 30 mg q1-2wk (valerate); PO 1-2 mg tid (oral estradiol)

Breast cancer

• *Adult:* PO 10 mg tid × 3 mo or longer

---

italics = common side effects   ***bold italic*** = life threatening reactions

Atropic vaginitis
• *Adult:* VAG CREAM 2-4 g qd × 1-2 wk, then 1 g 1-3 × /wk
Kraurosis vulvae
• *Adult:* IM 1-1.5 mg 1-2 × /wk
Available forms: Estradiol tabs 1, 2 mg; cypionate injection IM 1, 5 mg/ml; valerate injection IM 10, 20, 40 mg/ml

Side effects/adverse reactions:
CNS: Dizziness, headache, migraines, depression
CV: Hypotension, thrombophlebitis, edema, *thromboembolism, stroke, pulmonary embolism, myocardial infarction*
GI:Nausea, vomiting, diarrhea, anorexia, pancreatitis, cramps, constipation, increased appetite, increased weight, *cholestatic jaundice*
EENT: Contact lens intolerance, increased myopia, astigmatism
GU: Amenorrhea, cervical erosion, breakthrough bleeding, dysmenorrhea, vaginal candidiasis, breast changes, *gynecomastia, testicular atrophy, impotence*
INTEG: Rash, urticaria, acne, hirsutism, alopecia, oily skin, seborrhea, purpura, melasma
META: Folic acid deficiency, hypercalcemia, hyperglycemia

Contraindications: Breast cancer, thromboembolic disorders, reproductive cancer, genital bleeding (abnormal, undiagnosed), pregnancy (X)

Precautions: Hypertension, asthma, blood dyscrasias, gallbladder disease, CHF, diabetes mellitus, bone disease, depression, migraine headache, convulsive disorders, hepatic disease, renal disease, family history of cancer of breast or reproductive tract

Pharmacokinetics:
PO/IH/TOP: Degraded in liver; excreted in urine; crosses placenta; excreted in breast milk

Interactions/incompatibilities:
• Decreased action of: anticoagulants, oral hypoglycemics
• Toxicity: tricyclic antidepressants
• Decreased action of estradiol: anticonvulsants, barbiturates, phenylbutazone, rifampin, milk products, Ca
• Increased action of: corticosteroids

Lab test interferences:
Increase: BSP retention test, PBI, T_4, serum sodium, platelet aggregation, thyroxine-binding globulin (TBG), prothrombin, factors VII, VIII, IX, X, triglycerides
Decrease: Serum folate, serum triglyceride, T_3 resin uptake test, glucose tolerance test, antithrombin III, pregnanediol, metyrapone test
False positive: LE prep, antinuclear antibodies

NURSING CONSIDERATIONS
Assess:
• Blood glucose in patient with diabetes
• Weight daily, notify physician of weekly weight gain >5 lb; if increase, diuretic may be ordered
• B/P q4h, watch for increase caused by H_2O and Na retention
• I&O ratio; be alert for decreasing urinary output and increasing edema
• Liver function studies, including AST, ALT, bilirubin, alk phosphatase
• Hypertension, cardiac symptoms, jaundice, hypercalcemia
• Mental status: affect, mood, behavioral changes, aggression

Administer:
• Titrated dose; use lowest effective dose
• IM injection deeply in large muscle mass
• With food or milk to decrease GI symptoms (oral)

Evaluate:
• Therapeutic response: reversal of menopause or decrease in tumor size in prostatic cancer

Teach patient/family:
• To weigh weekly, report gain >5 lb
• To report breast lumps, vaginal bleeding, edema, jaundice, dark urine, clay-colored stools, dyspnea, headache, blurred vision, abdominal pain, numbness or stiffness in legs, chest pain; male to report impotence or gynecomastia

---

estramustine phosphate sodium
(ess-tra-muss'teen)
Emcyt
Func. class.: Antineoplastic
Chem. class.: Hormone: estrogen

Action: Combination drug consisting of nitrogen mustard/estrogen; estrogen is a carrier for the nitrogen mustard into estrogen-dependent tissue; acts like a weak alkylating agent

Uses: Metastatic prostate cancer

Dosage and routes:
• *Adult:* PO 10-16 mg/kg in 3-4 divided doses/day; treatment may continue for ≥ 3 mo
Available forms: Caps 140 mg (12.5 mg Na/cap)

Side effects/adverse reactions:
GI: Nausea, vomiting, anorexia, **hepatotoxicity**

GU: **Renal failure,** impotence, gynecomastia
INTEG: Rash, urticaria, pruritus, flushing, alopecia
RESP: Dyspnea, **emboli,** hoarseness
CV: **Myocardial infarction,** hypertension, **CHF, CVA**
CNS: Headache, anxiety, seizures, insomnia, mood swings

Contraindications: Hypersensitivity to estradiol, thromboembolic disorders, pregnancy (D)

Precautions: Edema, hepatic disease, CVA, MI, seizures, hypertension, diabetes mellitus

Pharmacokinetics:
PO: Peak 1-2 hr, executed via biliary tract; excreted in bile; half-life 20 hr (terminal)

NURSING CONSIDERATIONS
Assess:
• Renal function studies: BUN, serum uric acid, urine CrCl, electrolytes before, during therapy
• I&O ratio; report fall in urine output of 30 ml/hr
• Liver function tests before, during therapy (bilirubin, AST, ALT, LDH) as needed or monthly
• Dyspnea, chest pain, tachypnea, fatigue, increased pulse, pallor, lethargy
• Food preferences; list likes, dislikes
• Edema in feet, joint, stomach pain, shaking
• Inflammation of mucosa, breaks in skin
• Yellowing of skin and sclera, dark urine, clay-colored stools, itchy skin, abdominal pain, fever, diarrhea
• Symptoms indicating severe allergic reaction: rash, pruritus, urticaria, purpuric skin lesions, itching, flushing
• Tachycardia, ECG changes, dys-

---

italics = common side effects   ***bold italic*** = life threatening reactions

pnea, edema, fatigue, leg cramps; may indicate cardiac toxicity

Administer:
• In divided doses over 1-3 mo; give antiemetic if nausea, vomiting or anorexia become severe

Evaluate:
• Therapeutic response: decreased tumor size, spread of malignancy

Teach patient/family:
• To report any complaints, side effects to nurse or physician
• That gynecomastia, impotence can occur and are reversible after discontinuing treatment
• To report any changes in breathing, coughing
• Importance of immediately reporting GI bleeding
• To use contraception during use; positive mutagenic effects

---

estrogenic substances, conjugated

C.E.S.,* Conjugated Estrogens, Premarin, Premarin Intravenous

Func. class.: Estrogen
Chem. class.: Nonsteroidal synthetic estrogen

Action: Needed for adequate functioning of female reproductive system; it affects release of pituitary gonadotropins, inhibits ovulation, adequate calcium use in bone structures

Uses: Menopause, breast cancer, prostatic cancer, abnormal uterine bleeding, hypogonadism, castration, primary ovarian failure, osteoporosis

Dosage and routes:
Menopause
• *Adult:* PO 0.3-1.25 mg qd 3wk on, 1 wk off

Prostatic cancer
• *Adult:* PO 1.25-2.5 mg tid
Breast cancer
• *Adult:* PO 10 mg tid × 3 mo or longer
Abnormal uterine bleeding
• *Adult:* IV/IM 25 mg, repeat in 6-12 hr
Castration/primary ovarian failure/osteoporosis
• *Adult:* PO 1.25 mg qd 3wk on, 1 wk off
Hypogonadism
• *Adult:* PO 2.5 mg bid-tid × 20 days/mo

Available forms: Tabs 0.3, 0.625, 0.9, 1.25, 2.5 mg

Side effects/adverse reactions:
CNS: Dizziness, headache, migraine, depression
CV: Hypotension, thrombophlebitis, edema, ***thromboembolism, stroke, pulmonary embolism, myocardial infarction***
GI: Nausea, vomiting, diarrhea, anorexia, pancreatitis, cramps, constipation, increased appetite, increased weight, ***cholestatic jaundice***
EENT: Contact lens intolerance, increased myopia, astigmatism
GU: Amenorrhea, cervical erosion, breakthrough bleeding, dysmenorrhea, vaginal candidiasis, breast changes, *gynecomastia, testicular atrophy, impotence*
INTEG: Rash, urticaria, acne, hirsutism, alopecia, oily skin, seborrhea, purpura, melasma
META: Folic acid deficiency, hypercalcemia, hyperglycemia

Contraindications: Breast cancer, thromboembolic disorders, reproductive cancer, genital bleeding (abnormal, undiagnosed), pregnancy (X), lactation

Precautions: Hypertension, asthma, blood dyscrasias, gallbladder disease, CHF, diabetes melli-

---

*Available in Canada only

tus, bone disease, depression, migraine headache, convulsive disorders, hepatic disease, renal disease, family history of cancer of breast or reproductive tract

Pharmacokinetics:
PO/IV/IM: Degraded in liver, excreted in urine, crosses placenta, excreted in breast milk

Interactions/incompatibilities:
• Decreased action of: anticoagulants, oral hypoglycemics
• Toxicity: tricyclic antidepressants
• Decreased action of estrogens: anticonvulsants, barbiturates, phenylbutazone, rifampin
• Increased action of: corticosteroids

NURSING CONSIDERATIONS
Assess:
• Blood glucose in patient with diabetes
• Weight daily; notify physician of weekly weight gain >5 lb; if increase, diuretic may be ordered
• B/P q4h; watch for increase caused by H_2O and Na retention
• I&O ratio; be alert for decreasing urinary output and increasing edema
• Liver function studies, including AST, ALT, bilirubin, alk phosphatase
• Hypertension, cardiac symptoms, jaundice, hypercalcemia
• Mental status: affect, mood, behavioral changes, aggression

Administer:
• Titrated dose, use lowest effective dose
• IM injection deeply in large muscle mass
• With food or milk to decrease GI symptoms PO

Evaluate:
• Therapeutic response: absence of breast engorgement, reversal of

menopause, or decrease in tumor size in prostatic cancer

Teach patient/family:
• To avoid breastfeeding, since drug is secreted in breast milk
• To weigh weekly, report gain >5 lb
• To report breast lumps, vaginal bleeding, edema, jaundice, dark urine, clay-colored stools, dyspnea, headache, blurred vision, abdominal pain, numbness or stiffness in legs, chest pain; male to report impotence or gynecomastia
• To avoid sunlight or wear sunscreen; burns may occur

---

estrone
(ess'trone)
Aquest, Estrone Aqueous, Estrone-5, Estronol, Femogen Forte,* Kestrone-5, Theelin Aqueous
Func. class.: Estrogen
Chem. class.: Nonsteroidal synthetic estrogen

Action: Needed for adequate functioning of female reproductive system; affects release of pituitary gonadotropins, inhibits ovulation, promotes adequate calcium use in bone structures

Uses: Menopause, prostatic cancer, atrophic vaginitis, hypogonadism, primary ovarian failure

Dosage and routes:
Menopause/atrophic vaginitis
• *Adult:* IM 0.1-0.5 mg 2-3 × /wk
Prostatic cancer
• *Adult:* IM 2-4 mg 2-3 × /wk
Female hypogonadism/primary ovarian failure
• *Adult:* IM 0.1-1 mg qwk in one dose or divided doses
Available forms: Inj IM 2, 5 mg/ml

Side effects/adverse reactions:

CNS: Dizziness, headache, migraine, depression

CV: Hypotension, thrombophlebitis, edema, *thromboembolism, stroke, pulmonary embolism, myocardial infarction*

GI:Nausea, vomiting, diarrhea, anorexia, pancreatitis, cramps, constipation, increased appetite, increased weight, *cholestatic jaundice*

EENT: Contact lens intolerance, increased myopia, astigmatism

GU: Amenorrhea, cervical erosion, breakthrough bleeding, dysmenorrhea, vaginal candidiasis, breast changes, *gynecomastia, testicular atrophy, impotence*

INTEG: Rash, urticaria, acne, hirsutism, alopecia, oily skin, seborrhea, purpura, melasma

META: Folic acid deficiency, hypercalcemia, hyperglycemia

Contraindications: Breast cancer, thromboembolic disorders, reproductive cancer, genital bleeding (abnormal, undiagnosed), pregnancy (X)

Precautions: Hypertension, asthma, blood dyscrasias, gallbladder disease, CHF, diabetes mellitus, bone disease, depression, migraine headache, convulsive disorders, hepatic disease, renal disease, family history of cancer of the breast or reproductive tract

Pharmacokinetics:

IM: Degraded in liver; excreted in urine; crosses placenta; excreted in breast milk

Interactions/incompatibilities:

• Decreased action of: anticoagulants, oral hypoglycemics

• Toxicity: tricyclic antidepressants

• Decreased action of estrone: anticonvulsants, barbiturates, phenylbutazone, rifampin

• Increased action of: corticosteroids

NURSING CONSIDERATIONS

Assess:

• Blood glucose in patient with diabetes

• Weight daily, notify physician of weekly weight gain >5 lb; if increase, diuretic may be ordered

• B/P q4h, watch for increase caused by H_2O, Na retention

• I&O ratio; be alert for decreasing urinary output and increasing edema

• Liver function studies, including AST, ALT, bilirubin, alk phosphatase

• Hypertension, cardiac symptoms, jaundice, hypercalcemia

• Mental status: affect, mood, behavioral changes, aggression

Administer:

• Titrated dose; use lowest effective dose

• IM injection deeply in large muscle mass

Evaluate:

• Therapeutic response: absence of breast engorgement, reversal of menopause, or decrease in tumor size in prostatic cancer

Teach patient/family:

• To weigh weekly, report gain >5 lb

• To report breast lumps, vaginal bleeding, edema, jaundice, dark urine, clay-colored stools, dyspnea, headache, blurred vision, abdominal pain, numbness or stiffness in legs, chest pain; male to report impotence or gynecomastia

• To avoid sunlight or wear sunscreen, burns may occur

---

*Available in Canada only

ethacrynate sodium/ethacrynic acid
(eth-a-kri'nate)
Edecrin, Edecrin Sodium
Func. class.: Loop diuretic
Chem. class.: Ketone derivative

Action: Acts on loop of Henle by increasing excretion of chloride, sodium

Uses: Pulmonary edema, edema in CHF, liver disease, nephrotic syndrome, ascites

Dosage and routes:
• *Adult:* PO 50-200 mg/day; may give up to 200 mg bid
• *Child:* PO 25 mg, increased by 25 mg/day until desired effect occurs

Pulmonary edema
• *Adult:* IV 50 mg given over several minutes or 0.5-1 mg/kg
Available forms: Tabs 25, 50 mg; powder for inj 50 mg

Side effects/adverse reactions:
GU: Polyuria, **renal failure,** *glycosuria*
ELECT: Hypokalemia, hypochloremic alkalosis, hypomagnesemia, hyperuricemia, hypocalcemia, hyponatremia, decreased glucose tolerance
CNS: Headache, fatigue, weakness, vertigo
GI: Nausea, *severe diarrhea,* dry mouth, vomiting, anorexia, cramps, upset stomach, abdominal pain, *acute pancreatitis,* jaundice, *GI bleeding*; abdominal distention
EENT: Loss of hearing, ear pain, tinnitus, blurred vision
INTEG: Rash, pruritus, purpura, ***Stevens-Johnson syndrome,*** sweating, photosensitivity
MS: Cramps, arthritis, stiffness

ENDO: Hyperglycemia
HEMA: ***Thrombocytopenia, agranulocytosis, leukopenia, neutropenia***
CV: **Chest pain,** hypotension, ***circulatory collapse,*** ECG changes
Contraindications: Hypersensitivity to sulfonamides, anuria, hypovolemia, lactation, electrolyte depletion, infants
Precautions: Dehydration, ascites, severe renal disease, pregnancy (D), hypoproteinemia
Pharmacokinetics:
PO: Onset ½ hr, peak 2 hr, duration 6-8 hr
IV: Onset 5 min, peak 15-30 min, duration 2 hr
Excreted by kidneys; crosses placenta; half-life 30-70 min
Interactions/incompatibilities:
• Increased hypotension: antihypertensives
• Decreased diuretic effect: indomethacin, NSAIDs
• Increased ototoxicity: cisplatin, aminoglycosides, rancomycin
• Increased toxicity: lithium, nondepolarizing skeletal muscle relaxants, digitalis
• Increased anticoagulant activity: warfarin
• Incompatible with hydralazine, procainamide, reserpine, tolazine, triflupromazine, blood, blood products

NURSING CONSIDERATIONS
Assess:
• Weight, I&O daily to determine fluid loss; effect of drug may be decreased if used qd
• Rate, depth, rhythm of respiration, effect of exertion
• B/P lying, standing; postural hypotension may occur
• Electrolytes: K, Na, Cl; include BUN, blood sugar, CBC, serum

---

italics = common side effects   ***bold italic*** = life threatening reactions

creatinine, blood pH, ABGs, uric acid, Ca, Mg
• Glucose in urine if patient is diabetic
• Hearing when giving high IV doses
• Improvement in CVP q8h
• Signs of metabolic alkalosis: drowsiness, restlessness
• Signs of hypokalemia: postural hypotension, malaise, fatigue, tachycardia, leg cramps, weakness
• Rashes, temperature elevation qd
• Confusion, especially in elderly; take safety precautions if needed
Administer:
• IV after diluting with 50 ml NaCl inj; give through Y-tube or 3-way stopcock or heplock; give 10 mg or less over 1 min or run infusion over ½ hr; do not add to IV sol
• In AM to avoid interference with sleep if using drug as a diuretic
• K replacement if K is less than 3.0
• With food if nausea occurs; absorption may be decreased slightly
• PO, IV only; do not give IM/SC
Evaluate:
• Therapeutic response: improvement in edema of feet, legs, sacral area daily if medication is being used in CHF
Teach patient/family:
• To increase fluid intake to 2-3 L/day unless contraindicated; to rise slowly from lying or sitting position
• About adverse reactions: muscle cramps, weakness, nausea, dizziness
• To take with food or milk for GI symptoms
• To take early in day to prevent nocturia
• To use sunscreen for photosensitivity
Treatment of overdose: Lavage if taken orally; monitor electrolytes; administer dextrose in saline; monitor hydration, CV, renal status

---

ethambutol HCl
(e-tham'byoo-tole)
Etibi,* Myambutol
Func. class.: Antitubercular
Chem. class.: Diisopropylethylene diamide derivative

Action: Inhibits RNA synthesis, decreases tubercle bacilli replication
Uses: Pulmonary tuberculosis, as an adjunct
Dosage and routes:
• *Adult and child >13 yr:* PO 15 mg/kg/day as a single dose
Retreatment
• *Adult and child >13 yr:* PO 25 mg/kg/day as single dose × 2 mo with at least 1 other drug, then decrease to 15 mg/kg/day as single dose
Available forms: Tabs 100, 400 mg
Side effects/adverse reactions:
GI: Abdominal distress, anorexia, nausea, vomiting
INTEG: Dermatitis, pruritis
CNS: Headache, confusion, fever, malaise, dizziness, disorientation, hallucinations
EENT: Blurred vision, optic neuritis, photophobia, decreased visual acuity
META: Elevated uric acid, acute gout, liver function impairment
MISC: Thrombocytopenia, joint pain, bloody sputum
Contraindications: Hypersensitivity, optic neuritis, child <13 yr
Precautions: Pregnancy (D), renal disease, diabetic retinopathy, cataracts, ocular defects, hepatic and hematopoietic disorders

Pharmacokinetics:
PO: Peak 2-4 hr, half-life 3 hr; metabolized in liver; excreted in urine (unchanged drug/inactive metabolites, unchanged drug in feces)

Interactions/incompatibilities:
• Increased renal toxicity: aminoglycosides, cisplatin
• Delayed absorption of ethambutol: aluminum salts

NURSING CONSIDERATIONS
Assess:
• Liver studies qwk: ALT, AST, bilirubin
• Signs of anemia: Hct, Hgb, fatigue
• Mental status often: affect, mood, behavioral changes; psychosis may occur
• Hepatic status: decreased appetite, jaundice, dark urine, fatigue

Administer:
• With meals or antacids to decrease GI symptoms
• Antiemetic if vomiting occurs
• After C&S is completed; qmo to detect resistance

Evaluate:
• Therapeutic response: decreased symptoms of TB

Teach patient/family:
• To avoid alcohol products
• That compliance with dosage schedule, duration is necessary
• That scheduled appointments must be kept or relapse may occur

---

ethchlorvynol
(eth-klor-vi′nole)
Placidyl
Func. class.: Sedative-hypnotic
Chem. class.: Tertiary acetylenic alcohol

Controlled Substance Schedule IV (USA), Schedule F (Canada)
Action: Produces cerebral depression; exact action is unknown
Uses: Sedation, insomnia

Dosage and routes:
Sedation
• *Adult:* PO 100-200 mg bid or tid
Insomnia
• *Adult:* PO 500 mg-1g ½ hr before hs; may repeat 100-200 mg if needed
Medication for EEG
• *Child:* PO 25 mg/kg in one dose not to exceed 1 g
Available forms: Caps 100, 200, 500, 750 mg

Side effects/adverse reactions:
*HEMA: **Thrombocytopenia***
CNS: Fatigue, drowsiness, dizziness, sedation, ataxia, nightmares, hangover, giddiness, weakness, hysteria
GI: Nausea, vomiting
INTEG: Rash, urticaria
EENT: Blurred vision, bitter aftertaste
CV: Hypotension

Contraindications: Hypersensitivity to this drug, severe pain, porphyria, pregnancy (C)
Precautions: Depression, hepatic disease, renal disease, suicidal individual, pregnancy (3rd trimester) (C), elderly

Pharmacokinetics:
PO: Onset 15-30 min, peak 1-1½ hr, duration 5 hr; metabolized by liver; excreted by kidneys; half-life 10-20 hr, 21-100 hr terminal

Interactions/incompatibilities:
• Decreased hypoprothrombinemic effect: dicumarol, warfarin
• Increased CNS effects of ETOH, barbiturates, other CNS depressants, MAOIs

Lab test interferences:
Interferences: Clinitest

NURSING CONSIDERATIONS
Assess:
• Blood studies: Hct, Hgb, RBCs

before and after treatment if blood dyscrasias are suspected
• Hepatic studies: AST, ALT, bilirubin if hepatic disease is present
• Mental status: mood, sensorium, affect, memory (long, short)
• Physical dependency: more frequent requests for medication, shakes, anxiety
• Toxicity: hypotension, hypothermia, weakness, poor muscle coordination, visual problems; drug should be discontinued
• Respiratory dysfunction: respiratory depression, character, rate, rhythm; hold drug if respirations are <10/min or if pupils are dilated (rare)
• Blood dyscrasias: fever, sore throat, bruising, rash, jaundice, epistaxis (rare)
• Allergy to tartrazine: this drug contains tartrazine and should not be used in patients allergic to this dye

Administer:
• After removal of cigarettes to prevent fires
• After trying conservative measures for insomnia
• ½-1 hr before hs for sleeplessness
• With food or meals to decrease dizziness, giddiness
• For only 1 wk; not intended for long-term treatment

Perform/provide:
• Assistance with ambulation after receiving dose, especially elderly
• Safety measures: side rails, nightlight, call bell within easy reach
• Checking to see PO medication swallowed
• Storage in tight, light-resistant container in cool environment

Evaluate:
• Therapeutic response: ability to sleep at night, decreased amount of early morning awakening if taking drug for insomnia

Teach patient/family:
• To avoid driving or other activities requiring alertness
• To avoid alcohol ingestion or CNS depressants; serious CNS depression may result
• That effects may take 2 nights for benefits to be noticed
• Alternate measures to improve sleep: reading, exercise several hours before hs, warm bath, warm milk, TV, self-hypnosis, deep breathing

Treatment of overdose: Lavage, activated charcoal; monitor electrolytes, vital signs

---

ethinyl estradiol
(eth'in-il ess-tra-dye'ole)
Estinyl, Feminone
Func. class.: Estrogen
Chem. class.: Nonsteroidal synthetic estrogen

Action: Needed for adequate functioning of female reproductive system; affects release of pituitary gonadotropins, inhibits ovulation, promotes adequate calcium use in bone structures

Uses: Menopause, prostatic cancer, breast cancer, breast engorgement, hypogonadism

Dosage and routes:
Menopause
• *Adult:* PO 0.02-0.5 mg qd 3wk on, 1 wk off
Prostatic cancer
• *Adult:* PO 0.15-2 mg qd
Hypogonadism
• *Adult:* PO 0.05 mg qd-tid × 2 wk/mo, then 2 wk progesterone, then 3-6 mo cycles, then 2 mo off
Breast cancer
• *Adult:* PO 1 mg tid

Breast engorgement
• *Adult:* PO 0.5-1 mg qd × 3 days, then tapered off over 7 days
Available forms: Tabs 0.02, 0.05, 0.5 mg
Side effects/adverse reactions:
CNS: Dizziness, headache, migraine, depression
CV: Hypotension, thrombophlebitis, edema, ***thromboembolism, stroke, pulmonary embolism, myocardial infarction***
GI: Nausea, vomiting, diarrhea, anorexia, pancreatitis, cramps, constipation, increased appetite, increased weight, ***cholestatic jaundice***
EENT: Contact lens intolerance, increased myopia, astigmatism
GU: Amenorrhea, cervical erosion, breakthrough bleeding, dysmenorrhea, vaginal candidiasis, breast changes, *gynecomastia, testicular atrophy, impotence*
INTEG: Rash, urticaria, acne, hirsutism, alopecia, oily skin, seborrhea, purpura, melasma
META: Folic acid deficiency, hypercalcemia, hyperglycemia
Contraindications: Breast cancer, thromboembolic disorders, reproductive cancer, genital bleeding (abnormal, undiagnosed), pregnancy (X)
Precautions: Hypertension, asthma, blood dyscrasias, gallbladder disease, CHF, diabetes mellitus, bone disease, depression, migraine headache, convulsive disorders, hepatic disease, renal disease, family history of cancer of breast or reproductive tract
Pharmacokinetics:
PO: Degraded in liver; excreted in urine; crosses placenta; excreted in breast milk
Interactions/incompatibilities:
• Decreased action of: anticoagulants, oral hypoglycemics

• Toxicity: tricyclic antidepressants
• Decreased action of estradiol: anticonvulsants, barbiturates, phenylbutazone, rifampin
• Increased action of: corticosteroids

NURSING CONSIDERATIONS
Assess:
• Blood glucose in patient with diabetes
• Weight daily, notify physician of weekly weight gain >5 lb; if increase, diuretic may be ordered
• B/P q4h; watch for increase caused by H_2O, Na retention
• I&O ratio; be alert for decreasing urinary output and increasing edema
• Liver function studies: AST, ALT, bilirubin, alk phosphatase
• Hypertension, cardiac symptoms, jaundice, hypercalcemia
• Mental status: affect, mood, behavioral changes, aggression
Administer:
• Titrated dose; use lowest effective dose
• IM injection deeply in large muscle mass
• With food or milk to decrease GI symptoms
Evaluate:
• Therapeutic response: absence of breast engorgement, reversal of menopause, or decrease in tumor size in prostatic cancer
Teach patient/family:
• To weigh weekly, report gain >5 lb
• To report breast lumps, vaginal bleeding, edema, jaundice, dark urine, clay-colored stools, dyspnea, headache, blurred vision, abdominal pain, numbness or stiffness in legs, chest pain; male to report impotence or gynecomastia

---

italics = common side effects   ***bold italic*** = life threatening reactions

ethionamide

(e-thye-on-am-ide)

Trecator-SC

Func. class.: Antitubercular

Chem. class.: Thiomine derivative

Action: Bacteriostatic against *M. tuberculosis*

Uses: Pulmonary, extrapulmonary TB when other antitubercular drugs have failed

Dosage and routes:

• *Adult:* PO 500 mg-1 g qd in divided doses, with another antitubercular drug and pyridoxine

• *Child:* PO 15-20 mg/kg/day in 3-4 doses, not to exceed 1g

Available forms: Tabs 250 mg

Side effects/adverse reactions:

INTEG: Dermatitis, alopecia, acne

CV: Severe postural hypotension

CNS: Headache, drowsiness, tremors, *convulsions,* depression, psychosis, dizziness, peripheral neuritis

GI: Anorexia, nausea, vomiting, diarrhea, metallic taste

EENT: Blurred vision, optic neuritis

HEMA: Thrombocytopenia, purpura

MISC: Gynecomastia, impotence, menorrhagia, difficulty managing diabetes mellitus

Contraindications: Hypersensitivity, severe hepatic disease

Precautions: Pregnancy (D), renal disease, diabetic retinopathy, cataracts, ocular defects, child <13 yr

Pharmacokinetics:

PO: Peak 3 hr, duration 9 hr, half-life 3 hr; metabolized in liver; excreted in urine (unchanged drug/inactive); crosses placenta

Interactions/incompatibilities:

• Increased neurotoxicity: cycloserine, ethyl alcohol

• Increased adverse reactions: TB test agents, anti-TB drugs

NURSING CONSIDERATIONS

Assess:

• Signs of anemia: Hgb, Hct, fatigue

• Liver studies qwk: ALT, AST, bilirubin

• Mental status often: affect, mood, behavioral changes; psychosis may occur

• Hepatic status: decreased appetite, jaundice, dark urine, fatigue

Administer:

• With meals or antacids to decrease GI symptoms

• Antiemetic if vomiting occurs

• After C&S is completed, qmo to detect resistance

• Pyridoxine to prevent neuritis

Evaluate:

• Therapeutic response: decreased symptoms of TB

Teach patient/family:

• That compliance with dosage schedule, duration are necessary

• To avoid alcohol while taking this drug

• To notify physician of depression, mood changes, which are symptoms of toxicity

ethosuximide

(eth-oh-sux'i-mide)

Zarontin

Func. class.: Anticonvulsant

Chem. class.: Succinimide

Action: Inhibits spike, wave formation in absence seizures (petit mal), decreases amplitude, frequency, duration, spread of discharge in minor motor seizures

Uses: Absence seizures, partial seizures, tonic-clonic seizures

Dosage and routes:

• *Adult and child >6 yr:* PO 250

mg bid initially; may increase by 250 mg q4-7d, not to exceed 1.5 g/day
• *Child 3-6 yr:* PO 250 mg/day or 125 mg bid; may increase by 250 mg q4-7d, not to exceed 1.5 g/day
Available forms: Caps 250 mg, syr 250 mg/5 ml

Side effects/adverse reactions:
*HEMA: **Agranulocytosis, aplastic anemia, thrombocytopenia, leukocytosis, eosinophilia, pancytopenia***
CNS: Drowsiness, dizziness, fatigue, euphoria, lethargy, anxiety, aggressiveness, irritability, depression, insomnia, headache
GI: Nausea, vomiting, heartburn, anorexia, diarrhea, abdominal pain, cramps, constipation, hiccups, weight loss, gum hypertrophy, tongue swelling
GU: Vaginal bleeding, ***hematuria, renal damage***
INTEG: Urticaria, pruritic erythema, hirsutism, ***Stevens-Johnson syndrome***
EENT: Myopia, blurred vision
Contraindications: Hypersensitivity to succinimide derivatives
Precautions: Lactation, pregnancy (C), hepatic disease, renal disease
Pharmacokinetics:
PO: Peak 1-7 hr, steady state 4-7 days; metabolized by liver; excreted in urine, bile, feces; half-life 24-60 hr
Interactions/incompatibilities:
• Antagonist effect: tricyclic antidepressants (imipramine, doxepin)
• Decreased effects of: estrogens, oral contraceptives
Lab test interferences:
False positive: Direct Coombs' test
NURSING CONSIDERATIONS
Assess:
• Renal studies: urinalysis, BUN, urine creatinine

• Blood studies: CBC, Hᵴ reticulocyte counts qwk for ·, then qmo
• Hepatic studies: AST, ALT, bilirubin
• Drug levels during initial treatment, therapeutic range (40-100 μg/ml
• Mental status: mood, sensorium, affect, behavioral changes; if mental status changes, notify physician
• Eye problems: need for ophthalmic examinations before, during, after treatment (slit lamp, fundoscopy, tonometry)
• Allergic reaction: red raised rash, exfoliative dermatitis; if these occur, drug should be discontinued
• Blood dyscrasias: fever, sore throat, bruising, rash, jaundice
• Toxicity: bone marrow depression, nausea, vomiting, ataxia, diplopia, cardiovascular collapse, Stevens-Johnson syndrome
Administer:
• With food, milk to decrease GI symptoms
Perform/provide:
• Hard candy, frequent rinsing of mouth, gum for dry mouth
• Assistance with ambulation during early part of treatment; dizziness occurs
Evaluate:
• Therapeutic response: decreased seizure activity; document on patient's chart
Teach patient/family:
• To carry ID card or Medic Alert bracelet stating patient's name, drugs taken, condition, physician's name, phone number
• To avoid driving, other activities that require alertness
• To avoid alcohol ingestion, CNS depressants; increased sedation may occur
• Not to discontinue medication

E

---

italics = common side effects   ***bold italic*** = life threatening reactions

Hgb,
wk,

455

rm use; ab-
:cur
)se: Lavage,
monitor electro-

ethotoin

(eth'oh-toyin)
Peganone
Func. class.: Anticonvulsant
Chem. class.: Hydantoin deriv-
ative

Action: Inhibits nerve in impulses
in the motor cortex by decreasing
sodium ion influx, limiting tetanic
stimulation

Uses: Generalized tonic-clonic or
complex-partial seizures

Dosage and routes:
• *Adult:* PO 250 mg qid initially;
may increase over several days to
3 g/day in divided doses
• *Child:* PO 250 mg bid; may increase by 250 mg qid
Available forms: Tabs 250, 500 mg

Side effects/adverse reactions:
*HEMA: Agranulocytosis, throm-
bocytopenia, leukopenia, pancy-
topenia, megaloblastic anemia,*
lymphadenopathy
*CNS: Fatigue, insomnia, numbness,
fever, headache, dizziness*
GI: Nausea, vomiting, diarrhea,
gingival hypertrophy
INTEG: Rash
EENT: Nystagmus, diplopia
CV: Chest pain

Contraindications: Hypersensitivity to hydantoins, blood dyscrasias,
hematologic disease, hepatic disease, pregnancy (D)

Pharmacokinetics: Metabolized
by liver; excreted in urine; half-life
3-9 hr

Interactions/incompatibilities:
• Decreased effects of: rifampin,

chronic alcohol, barbiturates, antihistamines, antacids, other anticonvulsants antineoplastics, Ca products, folic acid, oxacillin
• Increased effects of: benzodiazepines, cimetidine, salicylates, sulfonamide, pyrazolones, phenothiazines, estrogens, disulfiram,
chloramphenicol, anticoagulants
• Seizures: valproic acid
• Paranoia: Phenacemide
• Myocardial depressions: lidocaine, propranolol, sympathomimetics

Lab test interferences:
Increase: Serum glucose, urine
glucose, BSP, alk phosphatase
Decrease: Urinary steroids, PBI,
dexamethasone/metyrapone tests

NURSING CONSIDERATIONS
Assess:
• Renal studies: urinalysis, BUN,
urine creatinine
• Blood studies: RBC, Hct, Hgb,
reticulocyte counts qwk for 4 wk
then qmo
• Hepatic studies: AST, ALT, bilirubin, creatinine periodically
• For signs, symptoms of infection:
sore throat, fever, bruising, petechiae
• Drug levels during initial treatment, therapeutic level (15-50 µg/
ml)
• Mental status: mood, sensorium,
affect, behavioral changes; if mental status changes, notify physician
• Eye problems: need for ophthalmic examinations before, during,
after treatment (slit lamp, fundoscopy, tonometry)
• Allergic reaction: red raised rash;
if this occurs, drug should be discontinued
• Blood dyscrasias: fever, sore
throat, bruising, rash, jaundice
• Toxicity: bone marrow depression, nausea, vomiting, ataxia, dip-

lopia, cardiovascular collapse, Stevens-Johnson syndrome, lupuslike syndrome

Administer:
• With food, milk to decrease GI symptoms
• After meals

Perform/provide:
• Hard candy, frequent rinsing of mouth, gum for dry mouth
• Assistance with ambulation during early part of treatment; dizziness occurs

Evaluate:
• Therapeutic response: decreased seizure activity, document on patient's chart

Teach patient/family:
• To carry ID card or Medic Alert bracelet stating patient's name, drugs taken, condition, physician's name, phone number
• To avoid driving, other activities that require alertness
• To avoid alcohol ingestion, CNS depressants; increased sedation may occur
• Notify dentist; use good oral hygiene; monitor gums
• Not to discontinue medication quickly after long-term use; taper off over several weeks

Treatment of overdose: Lavage, activated charcoal; monitor electrolytes, VS

---

ethylestrenol
(eth-il-ess′tre-nole)
Maxibolin
Func. class.: Androgenic anabolic steroid
Chem. class.: Hydantoin derivative

Action: Increases weight by building body tissue, increases potassium, phosphorus, chloride, and ni-

trogen levels, increases bone development

Uses: To increase weight, combat tissue depletion, osteoporosis, immobility, refractory anemias, catabolic effects of corticosteroid therapy

Dosage and routes:
• *Adult:* PO 4-8 mg qd, decreased at beginning clinical response
• *Child:* PO 1-3 mg qd, not to exceed treatment of 6 wk, lupuslike syndrome

Available forms: Tabs 2 mg; elix 2 mg/5 ml

Side effects/adverse reactions:
INTEG: Rash, acneiform lesions, oily hair, skin, flushing, sweating, acne vulgaris, alopecia, hirsutism
CNS: Dizziness, headache, fatigue, tremors, paresthesias, flushing, sweating, anxiety, lability, insomnia, carpal tunnel syndrome
MS: Cramps, spasms
CV: Increased B/P
GU: **Hematuria,** amenorrhea, vaginitis, decreased libido, decreased breast size, clitoral hypertrophy, testicular atrophy
GI: Nausea, vomiting, constipation, weight gain, **cholestatic jaundice**
EENT: Conjunctival edema, nasal congestion
ENDO: Abnormal GTT

Contraindications: Severe renal disease, severe cardiac disease, severe hepatic disease, hypersensitivity, pregnancy (C), lactation, genital bleeding (abnormal)

Precautions: Migraine headaches, seizure disorders

Pharmacokinetics:
PO: Metabolized in liver; excreted in urine; crosses placenta; excreted in breast milk

Interactions/incompatibilities:
• May increase effects of: oral an-

---

italics = common side effects   ***bold italic*** = life threatening reactions

ticoagulants, antidiabetics, oxyphenbutazone, phenylbutazone

• May decrease effect of ethylestrenol: barbiturates

Lab test interferences:

Increase: Cholesterol

Decrease: Cholesterol, T_4, T_3, thyroid ^{131}I uptake test, 17-KS, PBI

Interferes: GTT

NURSING CONSIDERATIONS

Assess:

• Weight daily, notify physician if weekly weight gain is >5 lb

• B/P q4h

• I&O ratio; be alert for decreasing urinary output, increasing edema

• Growth rate in children, since growth rate may be uneven (linear/bone growth), used for extended periods of time; periodic x-ray films to assure changes in bone growth

• Electrolytes: K, Na, Cl; cholesterol

• Liver function studies; ALT, AST, bilirubin

• Blood sugar in diabetes (may become hypoglycemic)

• Hypertension, cardiac symptoms, jaundice

• Mental status: affect, mood, behavioral changes, aggression

• Signs of masculinization in female: increased libido, deepening of voice, increased breast tissue, enlarged clitoris, menstrual irregularities;

male: gynecomastia, impotence, testicular atrophy

• Hypercalcemia: lethargy, polyuria, polydipsia, nausea, vomiting, constipation, drug may need to be decreased

• Hypoglycemia in diabetics, since oral antidiabetic action is increased

Administer:

• Increased Ca, Vit D in diet for osteoporosis, decrease in high-P

foods (bread, soft drinks, phosphate-based preservatives)

• Titrated dose; use lowest effective dose

• With food or milk to decrease GI symptoms

Perform/provide:

• Diet with increased calories, protein; decrease Na if edema occurs

Evaluate:

• Therapeutic response: increased appetite, increased stamina

Teach patient/family:

• Drug must be combined with complete health plan: diet, rest, exercise

• To notify physician if therapeutic response decreases

• Not to discontinue medication abruptly

• About change in sex characteristics

---

ethylnorepinephrine HCl

(eth-il-nor-ep-i-nef′rin)

Bronkephrine

Func. class.: Adrenergic

Chem. class.: Catecholamine

Action: α-Stimulation with vasoconstriction, pressor response, nasal decongestion and $β_2$-stimulation with vasodilation and bronchial dilation

Uses: Bronchospasm

Dosage and routes:

• *Adult:* IM/SC 0.5-1 ml

• *Child:* IM/SC 0.1-0.5 ml

Available forms: Inj 2 mg/ml IM, SC

Side effects/adverse reactions:

CNS: Tremors, anxiety, insomnia, headache, dizziness, confusion,

CV: Palpitations, tachycardia, hypertension, chest pain, ***dysrhythmias***

GI: Anorexia, nausea, vomiting
Contraindications: Hypersensitivity to sympathomimetics, narrow-angle glaucoma
Precautions: Pregnancy (C), cardiac disorders, hyperthyroidism, diabetes mellitus, prostatic hypertrophy
Pharmacokinetics:
IM/SC: Onset 6-12 min, duration 1-2 hr
Interactions/incompatibilities:
• Do not use with MAOIs or tricyclic antidepressants; hypertensive crisis may occur
• Decreased effect of ethylnorepinephrine when used with methyldopa, urinary acidifiers, rauwolfia alkaloids
• Increased effect of ethylnorepinephrine when used with urinary alkalizers
NURSING CONSIDERATIONS
Assess:
• B/P and pulse q5min after parenteral route
Perform/provide:
• Storage of reconstituted solution if refrigerated for no longer than 24 hr
• Do not use discolored solutions
Evaluate:
• Therapeutic response: ease of breathing after several min
Teach patient/family:
• The reason for drug administration

---

etidocaine HCl
(et-ee′-doe-kane)
Duranest HCl
Func. class.: Local anesthetic
Chem. class.: Amide

Action: Competes with calcium for sites in nerve membrane that control sodium transport across cell membrane; decreases rise of depolarization phase of action potential
Uses: Peripheral nerve block, caudal anesthesia, central neural block, vaginal block
Dosage and routes:
Varies with route of anesthesia
Available forms: Inj 1%, 1.5%
Side effects/adverse reactions:
CNS: Anxiety, restlessness, ***convulsions, loss of consciousness,*** drowsiness, disorientation, tremors, shivering
*CV: **Myocardial depression, cardiac arrest, dysrhythmias,*** bradycardia, hypotension, hypertension, ***fetal bradycardia***
GI: Nausea, vomiting
EENT: Blurred vision, tinnitus, pupil constriction
INTEG: Rash, urticaria, allergic reactions, edema, burning, skin discoloration at injection site, tissue necrosis
*RESP: **Status asthmaticus, respiratory arrest, anaphylaxis***
Contraindications: Hypersensitivity, child <12 yr, elderly, severe liver disease
Precautions: Severe drug allergies, pregnancy (B)
Pharmacokinetics: Onset 2-8 min, duration 3-6 hr; metabolized by liver, excreted in urine (metabolites)
Interactions/incompatibilities:
• Dysrhythmias: epinephrine, halothane, enflurane
• Hypertension: MAOIs, tricyclic antidepressants, phenothiazines
• Decreased action of etidocaine: chloroprocaine
NURSING CONSIDERATIONS
Assess:
• B/P, pulse, respiration during treatment

---

italics = common side effects   ***bold italic*** = life threatening reactions

• Fetal heart tones if drug is used during labor
• Allergic reactions: rash, urticaria, itching
• Cardiac status: ECG for dysrhythmias, pulse, B/P during anesthesia

Administer:
• Only with crash cart, resuscitative equipment nearby
• Only drugs without preservatives for epidural or caudal anesthesia

Perform/provide:
• Use of new solution; discard unused portions

Evaluate:
• Therapeutic response: anesthesia necessary for procedure

Treatment of overdose: Airway, O_2, vasopressor, IV fluids, anticonvulsants for seizures

---

etidronate disodium
(e-ti-droe′nate)
Didronel, Didronel IV
Func. class.: Parathyroid agent (calcium regulator)
Chem. class.: Diphosphate

Action: Decreases bone resorption and new bone development (accretion)

Uses: Paget's disease, heterotopic ossification, hypercalcemia of malignancy

Dosage and routes:
Paget's disease
• *Adult:* PO 5-10 mg/kg/day 2 hr ac with H_2O, not to exceed 20 mg/kg/day, max 6 mo

Heterotropic ossification
• *Adult:* PO 20 mg/kg qd × 2 wk, then 10 mg/kg/day for 10 wk, total 12 wk

Available forms: Tabs 200, 400 mg

Side effects/adverse reactions:
GI: Nausea, diarrhea

MS: Bone pain, hypocalcemia, decreased mineralization of nonaffected bones

Contraindications: Pathologic fractures, children, colitis, severe renal disease with creatinine >5 mg/dl

Precautions: Pregnancy (B), renal disease, lactation, restricted Vit D/Ca

Pharmacokinetics: Not metabolized excreted in urine/feces therapeutic response: 1-3 mo

NURSING CONSIDERATIONS
Assess:
• I&O ratio; check for decreased output in renal patients
• BUN, creatinine, uric acid, phosphate chloride, electrolytes, pH, urine Ca, Mg, alk phosphatase, urinalysis; Ca should be kept at 9-10 mg/dl, Vit D 50-135 IU/dl
• Muscle spasm, laryngospasm, paresthesias, facial twitching, colic; may indicate hypocalcemia
• Nutritional status, diet for sources of Vit D (milk, some seafood), Ca (dairy products, dark green vegetables), phosphates—adequate intake is necessary
• Persistent nausea or diarrhea

Administer:
• On empty stomach with H_2O 2 hr ac
• Drug therapy should not last longer than 6 mo
• IV after diluting in 250 ml or more of normal saline; give over 2 hr or longer
• Food, especially high in Ca and vitamins with mineral supplements or antacids high in metals should not be given within 2 hr of dose

Evaluate:
• Therapeutic response: prevention of bone deficiencies

Teach patient/family:
• To avoid OTC products

---

* Available in Canada only

• That therapeutic response may take 1-3 mo; effects persist for months after drug is discontinued
• That adequate intake of Ca$^+$, Vit D is necessary

---

etodolac
(e-toe-doe'lack)
Lodine
Func. class.: Nonsteroidal antiinflammatory

Action: Inhibits prostaglandin synthesis by decreasing an enzyme needed for biosynthesis; analgesic, antiinflammatory, antipyretic

Uses: Mild to moderate pain, osteoarthritis

Dosage and routes:
Osteoarthritis
• *Adult:* PO 800-1200 mg/day in divided doses initially, then adjust dose to 600-1200 mg/day in divided doses; do not exceed 1200 mg/day; patients <60 kg not to exceed 20 mg/kg

Analgesia
• *Adult:* PO 200-400 mg q6-8h prn for acute pain; do not exceed 1200 mg/day; patients 60 kg, not to exceed 20 mg/kg
• *Available forms:* Caps 200, 300 mg

Side effects/adverse reactions:
CV: Tachycardia, peripheral edema, fluid retention, palpitations, dysrhythmias, CHF
GU: Nephrotoxicity: dysuria, hematuria, oliguria, azotemia, cystitis, urinary tract infection
HEMA: Blood dyscrasias
INTEG: Erythema, urticaria, purpura, rash, pruritus, sweating
GI: Nausea, anorexia, vomiting, diarrhea, jaundice, *cholestatic hepatitis,* constipation, flatulence,

cramps, dry mouth, peptic ulcer, dyspepsia, *GI bleeding*
CNS: Dizziness, headache, drowsiness, fatigue, tremors, confusion, insomnia, anxiety, depression, light-headedness, vertigo
EENT: Tinnitus, hearing loss, blurred vision

Contraindications: Hypersensitivity; patients in whom aspirin, iodides, or other nonsteroidal antiinflammatories have produced asthma, rhinitis, urticaria, nasal polyps, angioedema, bronchospasm

Precautions: Pregnancy (C); lactation; children; bleeding; GI, cardiac disorders; elderly; renal, hepatic disorders

Pharmacokinetics:
PO: Peak 1-2 hr, serum protein binding >90%, half-life 7 hr; metabolized by liver (metabolites excreted in urine)

Interactions/incompatibilities:
• Increased action of: coumarin, phenytoin, cyclosporin, lithium
• Decreased antihypertensive effects: β-blockers
• Decreased plasma concentration of etodolac: salicylates
• Increased concentration and toxicity of etodolac: probenecid

NURSING CONSIDERATIONS
Assess:
• Blood, renal, liver studies: BUN, creatinine, AST, ALT, Hgb, before treatment, periodically thereafter
• Audiometric, ophthalmic examination before, during, after treatment
• For eye, ear problems: blurred vision, tinnitus; may indicate toxicity
Administer:
• With food to decrease GI symptoms, since extent of absorption is not affected by food

---

italics = common side effects   ***bold italic*** = life threatening reactions

Perform/provide:
• Storage at room temperature
Evaluate:
• Therapeutic response: decreased pain, stiffness, swelling in joints, ability to move more easily
Teach patient/family:
• To report blurred vision or ringing, roaring in ears; may indicate toxicity
• To avoid driving or other hazardous activities if dizziness or drowsiness occurs
• To report change in urine pattern, weight increase, edema, pain increase in joints, fever, blood in urine; indicates nephrotoxicity
• That therapeutic effects may take up to 1 mo
• To avoid aspirin, alcoholic beverages while taking this medication

---

etomidate
(e-tom′i-date)
Amidate
Func. class.: General anesthetic
Chem. class.: Nonbarbiturate hypnotic

Action: Acts at level of reticular-activating system to produce anesthesia
Uses: Induction of general anesthesia
Dosage and routes:
• *Adult and child >10 yr:* IV 0.2-0.6 mg/kg over ½-1 min
Available forms: Inj IV 2 mg/ml
Side effects/adverse reactions:
GI: Nausea, vomiting (postoperatively)
CNS: Tonic movements, myoclonic movements, averting movements
CV: Tachycardia, hypotension, hypertension, bradycardia

ENDO: Decreases steroid production
*RESP: **Laryngospasm***
INTEG: Pain on administration
Contraindications: Hypersensitivity, labor/delivery
Precautions: Pregnancy (C), child <10 yr, lactation, liver disease
Pharmacokinetics:
IV: Onset 20 sec, peak 1 min, duration 3-5 min; half-life 75 min; metabolized in liver; excreted in urine
NURSING CONSIDERATIONS
Assess:
• I&O ratio for increasing urine output
• VS q10min during IV administration
• Plasma cortisol levels if administered over several hours (5-20 μg/100 ml normal level of cortisol)
• Increasing or decreasing heart rate or dysrhythmias shown on ECG
Administer:
• Corticosteroids for severe hypotension
• Only with crash cart, resuscitative equipment nearby
• IV slowly only; muscular twitching is reduced with fentanyl before anesthesia induction
Evaluate:
• Therapeutic response: induction of anesthesia

---

etoposide (VP-16)
(e-toe-poe′side)
VePesid
Func. class.: Antineoplastic
Chem. class.: Semisynthetic podophyllotoxin

Action: Inhibits mitotic activity through metaphase to mitosis; also inhibits cells from entering mitosis,

---

depresses DNA, RNA synthesis
Uses: Leukemias, lung, testicular cancer, lymphomas, neuroblastoma, melanoma, ovarian cancer

Dosage and routes:
• *Adult:* IV 45-75 mg/m^2/day × 3-5 days given q3-5wk or 200-250 mg/m^2/wk, or 125-140 mg/m^2/day 3 × wk, q5wk

Available forms: Inj IV 20 mg/ml, caps 50 mg

Side effects/adverse reactions:
*HEMA: **Thrombocytopenia, leukopenia, myelosuppression, anemia***
*GI: Nausea, vomiting, anorexia, **hepatotoxicity***
INTEG: Rash, alopecia, phlebitis at IV site
*RESP: **Bronchospasm***
CV: Hypotension
CNS: Headache, fever
*GU: **Nephrotoxicity***

Contraindications: Hypersensitivity, bone marrow depression, severe hepatic disease, severe renal disease, bacterial infection, pregnancy (D)

Precautions: Renal disease, hepatic disease, lactation, children, gout

Pharmacokinetics: Half-life 3 hr, terminal 15 hr; metabolized in liver; excreted in urine; crosses placental barrier

Interactions/incompatibilities:
• Do not use with radiation
• Incompatible with any drug in sol or syringe; incompatible with any sol except NS or dextrose in H$_2$O
• Increased pro-time: warfarin

NURSING CONSIDERATIONS
Assess:
• CBC, differential, platelet count weekly; withhold drug if WBC is <4000 or platelet count is <75,000; notify physician of results
• Renal function studies: BUN, serum uric acid, urine CrCl, electrolytes before, during therapy
• I&O ratio; report fall in urine output of 30 ml/hr; check blood pressure BID and report any significant decrease
• Monitor temperature q4h; may indicate beginning infection
• Liver function tests before, during therapy (bilirubin, AST, ALT, LDH) as needed or monthly
• RBC, Hct, Hgb, since these may be decreased
• Bleeding: hematuria, guaiac stools, bruising or petechiae, mucosa or orifices q8h
• Food preferences; list likes, dislikes
• Effects of alopecia on body image; discuss feelings about body changes
• Yellowing of skin and sclera, dark urine, clay-colored stools, itchy skin, abdominal pain, fever, diarrhea
• Buccal cavity q8h for dryness, sores or ulceration, white patches, oral pain, bleeding, dysphagia
• Local irritation, pain, burning, discoloration at injection site
• Symptoms indicating severe allergic reaction: rash, pruritus, urticaria, purpuric skin lesions, itching, flushing
• Symptoms of anaphylaxis: flushing, restlessness, coughing, difficulty breathing
• Frequency of stools, characteristics: cramping, acidosis; signs of dehydration: rapid respirations, poor skin turgor, decreased urine output, dry skin, restlessness, weakness

Administer:
• After diluting 100 mg/250 ml or more D$_5$W or NaCl to a concentration of 0.2-0.4 mg/ml, infuse over 30-60 min

italics = common side effects   ***bold italic*** = life threatening reactions

• Antiemetic 30-60 min before giving drug and prn to prevent vomiting
• Allopurinol or sodium bicarbonate to maintain uric acid levels, alkalinization of urine
• Hyaluronidase 150 U/ml to 1 ml NaCl to infiltration area, ice compress for treatment of vesicant activity
• Transfusion for anemia
• Antispasmodic

Perform/provide:
• Liquid diet: cola, Jell-O; dry toast or crackers may be added if patient is not nauseated or vomiting
• Increase fluid intake to 2-3 L/day to prevent urate deposits, calculi formation
• Diet low in purines: organ meats (kidney, liver), dried beans, peas to maintain alkaline urine
• Nutritious diet with iron, vitamin supplements
• HOB raised to facilitate breathing

Evaluate:
• Therapeutic response: decreased tumor size, spread of malignancy

Teach patient/family:
• To report any complaints or side effects to nurse or physician
• To report any changes in breathing or coughing
• That hair may be lost during treatment; a wig or hairpiece may make patient feel better; tell patient that new hair may be different in color, texture
• To make position changes slowly to prevent fainting

---

etretinate
(e-tret′-in-ate)
Tegison
Func. class.: Systemic antipsoriatic
Chem. class.: Retinol derivative

Action: Unknown; drug is related to retinol

Uses: Severe recalcitrant psoriasis, including erythrodermic and generalized pustular types

Dosage and routes:
• *Adult:* PO 0.75-1 mg/kg/day in divided doses, not to exceed 1.5 mg/kg/day; maintenance dose 0.5-0.75 mg/kg/day generally beginning after 8-16 wk of therapy

Available forms: Caps 10, 25 mg

Side effects/adverse reactions:
INTEG: Alopecia; peeling of palms, soles, fingertips; itching; rash; dryness; red scaling face; bruising; sunburn; pyogenic granuloma; paronychia; onycholysis; perspiration change; nail changes

CNS: Fatigue, headache, dizziness, fever, pain, anxiety, amnesia, depression

EENT: Eye irritation, pain, double vision, change in lacrimation, earache, otitis externa, dry nose, eyes, mouth, nosebleed, cheilitis, sore tongue

*GI: Anorexia, abdominal pain, nausea, **hepatitis,*** constipation, diarrhea, flatulence, weight loss

*CV: Edema, **CV obstruction, atrial fibrillation,*** chest pain, coagulation disorders

RESP: Dyspnea, cough

*GU: WBC in urine, **proteinuria,*** glycosuria, *increased BUN, creatinine, **hematuria,*** casts, ***acetonuria, hemoglobinuria, dysuria***

META: Increase or decrease K, Ca, P, Na, Cl

MS: Hyperostosis, bone pain, cramps, myalgia, gout, hypertonia

Contraindications: Pregnancy (X)

Precautions: Lactation, children, hepatic disease, diabetes, obesity

Pharmacokinetics: 99% plasma protein binding; excreted in bile, urine; terminal half-life 120 days; stored in fatty tissue

Interactions/incompatibilities:
• Increased absorption of etretinate: milk

NURSING CONSIDERATIONS
Assess:
• For pseudotumor cerebri: headache, nausea, vomiting, visual problems, papilledema
• Hepatic studies: AST, ALT, LDH, since hepatotoxicity may occur
• Visual problems: blurring, decreased night vision, poor visual acuity; drug should be discontinued and ophthalmologist consulted
• Lipids before, q1-2wk during treatment; after discontinuing treatment, lipids will return to normal

Evaluate:
• Therapeutic response: decrease in scaling, itching, amount of psoriasis

Teach patient/family:
• To take with food
• Not to use during pregnancy; contraception must be used for 1 mo before or after therapy
• Not to take Vit A supplements
• That contact lens intolerance is common

---

factor IX complex (human)

Alphanine, Konyne HT, Proplex T, Proplex SX-T, Profilnine Heat-Treated

Func. class.: Hemostatic
Chem. class.: Factors II, VII, IX, X

Action: Causes an increase in blood levels of clotting factors II, VII, IX, X

Uses: Hemophilia B (Christmas disease), factor IX deficiency, anticoagulant reversal, control of bleeding in patients with factor VIII inhibitors

Dosage and routes:
• *Adult and child:* IV 1 U/kg × desired % increase

Available forms: Inj IV (number of units noted on label)

Side effects/adverse reactions:
GI: Nausea, vomiting, abdominal cramps, jaundice, *viral hepatitis*
INTEG: Rash, flushing, *urticaria*
CNS: Headache, dizziness, malaise, paresthesia, *lethargy, chills, fever, flushing*
HEMA: **Thrombosis, hemolysis, AIDS, DIC**
CV: Hypotension, tachycardia, *MI,* **venous thrombosis, pulmonary embolism**
RESP: **Bronchospasm**

Contraindications: Hypersensitivity, hepatic disease, DIC, elective surgery, mild factor IX deficiency

Precautions: Neonates/infants, pregnancy (C)

Pharmacokinetics:
IV: Half-life factor VII—3-6 hr, factor IX—24-36 hr; rapidly cleared from plasma

Interactions/incompatiblilities:
• Incompatible with protein products

---

italics = common side effects   ***bold italic*** = life threatening reactions

• Increased risk of thrombosis: aminocaproic acid; do not administer

NURSING CONSIDERATIONS
Assess:
• Blood studies (coagulation factors assays by % normal: 5% prevents spontaneous hemorrhage, 30%-50% for surgery, 80%-100% for severe hemorrhage)
• Increased B/P, pulse
• For bleeding q15-30min, immobilize and apply ice to affected joints
• I&O; if urine becomes orange or red, notify physician
• Allergic or pyrogenic reaction: fever, chills, rash, itching, slow infusion rate if not severe
• DIC: bleeding, ecchymosis, hypersensitivity, changes in coagulation tests

Administer:
• IV after warming to room temperature 3 ml/min or less, with plastic syringe only; do not admix
• After dilution with provided diluent, 50 U/ml or 25 U/ml; give not to exceed 10 ml/min; decrease rate if fever, headache, flushing, tingling occur
• After crossmatch is completed if patient has blood type A, B, AB, to determine incompatibility with factor

Perform/provide:
• Storage of reconstituted solution for 3 hr at room temp or up to 2 yr refrigeration (powder); check expiration date

Evaluate:
• Therapeutic response: prevention of hemorrhage

Teach patient/family:
• To report any signs of bleeding: gums, under skin, urine, stools, emesis
• Risk of viral hepatitis, AIDS

• That immunization for hepatitis B may be given first
• To be tested q2-3mo for HIV
• To carry ID identifying disease; avoid salicylates, to inform other health professionals about condition

---

famotodine
(fam-oo'-te-dine)
Pepcid, Pepcid IV
Func. class.: H₂ histamine receptor antagonist

Action: Competitively inhibits histamine at histamine H_2 receptor site, decreasing gastric secretion while pepsin remains at stable level
Uses: Short-term treatment of active duodenal ulcer, maintenance therapy for duodenal ulcer, Zollinger-Ellison syndrome, multiple endocrine adenomas, gastric ulcers
Dosage and routes:
Duodenal ulcer
• *Adult:* PO 40 mg qd hs × 4-8 wk, then 20 mg qd hs if needed (maintenance); IV 20 mg q12h if unable to take PO
Hypersecretory conditions
• *Adult:* PO 20 mg q6h; may give 160 mg q6h if needed; IV 20 mg q12h if unable to take PO
Available forms: Tabs 20, 40 mg; powder for oral susp 40 mg/5 ml; inj IV 10 mg/ml
Side effects/adverse reactions:
*HEMA: **Thrombocytopenia***
CNS: Headache, dizziness, paresthesia, *seizure,* depression, anxiety, somnolence, insomnia, fever
EENT: Taste change, tinnitus, orbital edema
GI: Constipation, nausea, vomiting, anorexia, cramps, abnormal liver enzymes
INTEG: Rash

MS: Myalgia, arthralgia
RESP: Bronchospasm
Contraindications: Hypersensitivity
Precautions: Pregnancy (B), lactation, children, severe renal disease, severe hepatic function, elderly
Pharmacokinetics: Absorption 50% (PO)
PO: Onset 30-60 minutes, duration 6-12 hours, peak 1-3 hr
IV: Onset immediate, peak 30-60 minutes, duration 6-12 hours, plasma protein-binding 15%-20%; metabolized in liver 30% (active metabolites), 70% excreted by kidneys, half-life 2½-3½ hr
Interactions/incompatibilities:
• Decreased absorption: ketoconazole
• Decreased absorption of famotidine: antacids
NURSING CONSIDERATIONS
Assess:
• Blood counts during therapy; watch for decreasing platelets; if low, therapy may have to be discontinued and restarted after hematologic recovery
• For bleeding, hematuria, hematuresis, occult blood in stools
• Blood dyscrasias (thrombocytopenia): bruising, fatigue, bleeding, poor healing
Administer:
• Antacids 1 hr before or 2 hr after famotidine; may be given with foods or liquids
• After shaking oral suspension
• IV direct after diluting 20 mg of drug in (0.9% NaCl) to total volume of 5-10 ml; inject over 2 min to prevent hypotension
• IV infusion after diluting 20 mg of drug in 100 ml of LR, 0.9% NaCl, D₅W, D₁₀W; run over 15-30 min

Perform/provide:
• Storage in cool environment (oral); IV solution is stable for 48 hr at room temperature; do not use discolored sol; discard unused oral solution after 1 mo
Evaluate:
• Therapeutic response: decreased abdominal pain
Teach patient/family:
• That drug must be continued for prescribed time in prescribed method to be effective; do not double dose
• To report bleeding, bruising, fatigue, malaise, since blood dyscrasias occur
• About possibility of decreased libido, reversible after discontinuing therapy
• To avoid irritating foods, alcohol, aspirin and extreme temperatures of foods that may irritate the GI system
• That smoking should be avoided, since it diminishes the effectiveness of this drug
• To avoid tasks requiring alertness; dizziness, drowsiness may occur
• To increase bulk and fluids in the diet to prevent constipation

fat emulsions
Intralipid 10%, Intralipid 20%, Liposyn II 10%, Liposyn II 20%, Liposyn III 10%, Liposyn III 20%, Soyacal 20%
Func. class.: Caloric
Chem. class.: Fatty acid, long chain

Action: Needed for energy, heat production; consist of neutral triglycerides, primarily unsaturated fatty acids

italics = common side effects   ***bold italic*** = life threatening reactions

Uses: Increase calorie intake, fatty acid deficiency, prevention

Dosage and routes:

Deficiency

• *Adult and child:* IV 8%-10% of required calorie intake (intralipid)

Adjunct to TPN

• *Adult:* IV 1 ml/min over 15-30 min (10%) or 0.5 ml/min over 15-30 min (20%); may increase to 500 ml over 4-8 hr if no adverse reactions occur; not to exceed 2.5 g/kg

• *Child:* IV 0.1 ml/min over 10-15 min (10%) or 0.05 ml/min over 10-15 min (20%); may increase to 1 g/kg over 4 hr if no adverse reactions occur; not to exceed 4 g/kg

Prevention of deficiency

• *Adult:* IV 500 ml 2 × / wk (10%), given 1 ml/min for 30 min, not to exceed 500 ml over 6 hr

• *Child:* IV 5-10 ml/kg/day (10%), given 0.1 ml/min for 30 min, not to exceed 100 ml/hr

Available forms: Inj IV many types

Side effects/adverse reactions:

CNS: Dizziness, headache, drowsiness, focal seizures

CV: Shock

GI: Nausea, vomiting, *hepatomegaly*

RESP: Dyspnea, *fat in lung tissue*

HEMA: Hyperlipemia, hypercoagulation, thrombocytopenia, leukopenia, leukocytosis

Contraindications: Hypersensitivity, hyperlipemia, lipid necrosis, acute pancreatitis accompanied by hyperlipemia, hyperbilirubinemia of the newborn

Precautions: Severe liver disease, diabetes mellitus, thrombocytopenia, gastric ulcers, premature, term newborns, pregnancy (C), sepsis

Interactions/incompatibilities:

• Do not mix with any drug, electrolytes, solutions, vitamin, unless added to TPN

NURSING CONSIDERATIONS

Assess:

• Triglycerides, free fatty acid levels, platelet counts daily to prevent fat overload, thrombocytopenia

• Liver function studies: AST, ALT

• Nutritional status: calorie count by dietician

Administer:

• After changing IV tubing at each infusion: infection may occur with old tubing

• With infusion pump at prescribed rate; do not use in-line filter sized for lipid emulsion; clogging will occur

Perform/provide:

• Use of mixed solutions that are not separated or oily looking

Evaluate:

• Therapeutic response: increased weight

Teach patient/family

• Reason for use of lipids

---

felbamate

(fell-ba′mate)

Felbatol

Func. class.: Anticonvulsant

Chem. class.: Carbamate derivative

Action: Mechanism of action unknown; may increase seizure threshold; has weak inhibitory effects on GABA-receptor and benzodiazinepine-receptor binding

Uses: Partial seizures, with or without generalization in adults; partial and generalized seizures in children with Lennox-Gastaut syndrome

Dosage and routes:

Adjunctive therapy

• *Adult:* PO add 1.2 g/day in 3-4

---

divided doses; reduce other anticonvulsants (valproic acid, phenytoin, carbamazepine and derivatives) by 20% to control plasma
concentrations; may increase felbamate 1.2 g/day increments qwk,
up to 3.6 g/day

Monotherapy

Adult: PO 1.2 g/day in 3-4 divided
doses; titrate with close supervision; increase dose by 600-mg increments q2wk to 3.6 g/day if
needed

Lennox-Gastaut syndrome
Adjunctive therapy

Child (2-14 yr): PO add 15 mg/kg/
day in 3-4 divided doses; reduce
other anticonvulsants (valproic
acid, phenytoin, carbamazepine
and derivatives) by 20% to control
plasma concentrations; may increase felbamate 15 mg/kg/day
qwk up to 45 mg/day

Available forms: Tabs 400, 600
mg; susp 600 mg/5 ml

Side effects/adverse reactions:

CNS: Dizziness, fatigue, headache,
insomnia, anxiety, tremor, unsteady gait, depression, paresthesia

CV: Chest pain

EENT: Dry mouth, blurred vision,
diplopia

GI: Nausea, constipation, diarrhea,
anorexia, vomiting, abdominal
pain, increased liver enzymes, hiccups

GU: Urinary incontinence, intra-
menstrual bleeding, *UTI*

HEMA: Purpura, **leukopenia**

INTEG: Rash, acne

RESP: Upper respiratory tract infection, rhinitis, sinusitis, pharyngitis, coughing

Contraindications: Hypersensitivity to this drug, other carbamates

Precautions: Hepatic disease, renal disease, cardiac disease, psy-

chosis, pregnancy (C), lactation,
child <6 yr, elderly

Pharmacokinetics:

PO: well absorbed, metabolized by
liver, excreted in urine (40%-50%
unchanged); crosses placenta, excreted in breast milk, terminal half-
life 20-23 hr; protein binding (22%-
25% to albumin)

Interactions/incompatibilities:

• Increased levels of: phenytoin,
valproic acid

• Decreased levels: carbamazepine

NURSING CONSIDERATIONS

Assess:

• Renal studies: urinalysis, BUN,
urine creatinine q3mo

• Hepatic studies: ALT, AST, bilirubin

• Description of seizures

• Mental status: mood, sensorium,
affect, behavioral changes; if mental status changes, notify physician

• Eye problems: need for ophthalmic examinations before, during,
after treatment (slit lamp, fundoscopy, tonometry)

• Allergic reaction: purpura, red
raised rash; if these occur, drug
should be discontinued

Administer:

• With food, milk to decrease GI
symptoms

• Shake susp well

Perform/provide:

• Storage at room temperature,
away from heat and light

• Hard candy, frequent rinsing of
mouth, gum for dry mouth

• Assistance with ambulation during early part of treatment; dizziness occurs

Evaluate:

• Therapeutic response: decreased
seizure activity; document on patient's chart

Teach patient/family:

• To carry Medic Alert ID stating

patient's name, drugs taken, condition, physician's name, phone number
• To avoid driving, other activities that require alertness
• Not to discontinue medication quickly after long-term use
Treatment of overdose:
Lavage, VS

---

felodipine
(fell-od'a-pine)
Plendil
Func. class.: Calcium-channel blocker
Chem. class.: Dihydropyridine

Action: Inhibits calcium ion influx across cell membrane, resulting in dilation of peripheral arteries
Uses: Essential hypertension, alone or with other antihypertensives
Dosage and routes:
• *Adult:* PO 5 mg qd initially, usual range 5-10 mg qd; do not exceed 20 mg qd; do not adjust dosage at intervals of <2 wk
Available forms: Ext rel tabs 5, 10 mg
Side effects/adverse reactions:
CV: Dysrhythmia, edema, CHF, hypotension, palpitations, *MI, pulmonary edema,* tachycardia, syncope, AV block, angina
GI: Nausea, vomiting, diarrhea, gastric upset, constipation, increased liver function studies, dry mouth
GU: Nocturia, polyuria
INTEG: Rash, pruritus
MISC: Flushing, sexual difficulties, cough, nasal congestion, shortness of breath, wheezing, epistaxis, respiratory infection, chest pain
CNS: Headache, fatigue, drowsiness, dizziness, anxiety, depression, nervousness, insomnia, light-headedness, paresthesia, tinnitus, psychosis, somnolence
HEMA: Anemia
Contraindications: Hypersensitivity, sick sinus syndrome, 2nd or 3rd degree heart block
Precautions: CHF, hypotension <90 mm Hg systolic, hepatic injury, pregnancy (C), lactation, children, renal disease, elderly
Pharmacokinetics: Peak plasma levels 2.5-5 hr; highly protein bound, >99% metabolized in liver, 0.5% excreted unchanged in urine; elimination half-life 11-16 hr
Interactions/incompatibilities:
• Increased effects of: β-blockers, antihypertensives, digitalis
• Increased felodipine level: cimetidine, ranitidine
NURSING CONSIDERATIONS
Assess:
• Cardiac status: B/P, pulse, respiration, ECG
Administer:
• Once daily as whole tablet
Evaluate:
• Therapeutic response: decreased B/P
Teach patient/family:
• To swallow whole; do not crush or chew
• To avoid hazardous activities until stabilized on drug, dizziness is no longer a problem
• To limit caffeine consumption
• To avoid OTC drugs unless directed by a physician
• Importance of complying with all areas of medical regimen: diet, exercise, stress reduction, drug therapy
Treatment of overdose: Defibrillation, atropine for AV block, vasopressor for hypotension

---

fenfluramine HCl
(fen-fluer′a-meen)
Pondimin
Func. class.: Anorexiant
Chem. class.: Amphetamine derivative

Controlled Substance Schedule IV

Action: Influences serotonin pathways in CNS; may also increase glucose utilization

Uses: Exogenous obesity

Dosage and routes:
• *Adult:* PO 20 mg tid ac, not to exceed 40 mg tid; total not to exceed 120 mg/day

Available forms: Tabs 20, 40 mg

Side effects/adverse reactions:
HEMA: Bone marrow depression, leukopenia, agranulocytosis
MISC: Hair loss, flushing, fever
EENT: Mydriasis, blurred vision, eye irritation
CNS: Insomnia, talkativeness, dizziness, drowsiness, headache, irritability, confusion, mood changes, anxiety, weakness, vivid dreams, uncoordination, depression, fatigue, malaise, euphoria, tremor, confusion
GI: Nausea, vomiting, anorexia, *dry mouth, diarrhea,* constipation, abdominal pain
GU: Impotence, change in libido, dysuria, urinary frequency
CV: Palpitations, tachycardia, hypertension, hypotension, dysrythmias, pulmonary hypertension
INTEG: Urticaria, rash, burning, sweating, chills, fever, erythma

Contraindications: Hypersensitivity to sympathomimetic amine, glaucoma, drug abuse, cardiovascular disease, alcoholism, children <12 yr, hypertension, hyperthy-roidism, severe arteriosclerosis, agitated states

Precautions: Diabetes mellitus, hypertension, depression, pregnancy (C), lactation

Pharmacokinetics:
PO: Onset 1-2 min, duration 4-6 hr; metabolized by liver; excreted by kidneys; half-life 20 hr; elimination rate by kidneys is dependent on pH of urine

Interactions/incompatibilities:
• Hypertensive crisis: MAOIs or within 14 days of MAOIs furazolidone
• Increased effect of fenfluramine: acetazolamide, antacids, sodium bicarbonate
• Increased hypoglycemic effects: insulin, sulfonylureas
• Decreased effects of fenfluramine: tricyclics, ascorbic acid, ammonium chloride
• Decreased effects of: guanethidine

NURSING CONSIDERATIONS
Assess:
• VS, B/P, since this drug may reverse antihypertensives; check patients with cardiac disease more often
• CBC, urinalysis, in diabetes: blood sugar, urine sugar; insulin changes may have to be made, since eating will decrease
• Height, growth rate in children; growth rate may be decreased
• Mental status: mood, sensorium, affect, stimulation, insomnia, aggressiveness may occur
• Physical dependency: should not be used for extended time; dose should be discontinued gradually; drug tolerance will occur after long-term use
• Withdrawal symptoms: headache, nausea, vomiting, muscle pain, weakness

---

italics = common side effects   ***bold italic*** = life threatening reactions

Administer:
• At least 6 hr before hs to avoid sleeplessness
• For obesity only if patient is on weight reduction program, including dietary changes, exercise; patient will develop tolerance and weight loss won't occur without additional methods; give 1 hr before meals
• Gum, hard candy, frequent sips of water for dry mouth

Perform/provide:
• Check to see PO medication has been swallowed

Evaluate:
• Therapeutic response: decreased weight

Teach patient/family:
• Not to take more frequently than prescribed
• To decrease caffeine consumption (coffee, tea, cola, chocolate); may increase irritability, stimulation
• Avoid OTC preparations unless approved by physician
• To taper off drug over several weeks, or depression, increased sleeping, lethargy may ensue
• To avoid alcohol ingestion
• To avoid hazardous activities until patient is stabilized on medication
• To get needed rest; patients will feel more tired at end of day

Treatment of overdose: Administer fluids, gastric lavage, hemodialysis or peritoneal dialysis; antihypertensive for increased B/P; ammonium Cl for increased excretion

---

fenoprofen calcium
(fen-oh-proe'fen)
Fenoprofen, Nalfon
Func. class.: Nonsteroidal antiinflammatory
Chem. class.: Propionic acid derivative

Action: May inhibit prostaglandin synthesis by decreasing enzyme needed for biosynthesis; analgesic, antiinflammatory, antipyretic

Uses: Mild to moderate pain, osteoarthritis, rheumatoid arthritis, acute gout, arthritis, ankylosing spondylitis, inflammation, dysmenorrhea

Dosage and routes:
Pain
• *Adult:* PO 200 mg q4-6h as needed
Arthritis
• *Adult:* PO 300-600 mg qid, not to exceed 3.2 g/day

Available forms: Caps 200, 300 mg; tabs 600 mg

Side effects/adverse reactions:
GI: Nausea, anorexia, vomiting, diarrhea, jaundice, ***cholestatic hepatitis,*** constipation, flatulence, cramps, dry mouth, peptic ulcer
CNS: Dizziness, headache, drowsiness, fatigue, tremors, confusion, insomnia, anxiety, depression
CV: Tachycardia, peripheral edema, palpitations, dysrhythmias
INTEG: Purpura, rash, pruritus, sweating
GU: ***Nephrotoxicity: dysuria, hematuria, oliguria, azotemia***
*HEMA: **Blood dyscrasias***
EENT: Tinnitus, hearing loss, blurred vision

Contraindications: Hypersensitivity, asthma, severe renal disease, severe hepatic disease

---

Precautions: Pregnancy, (B) 1st and 2nd trimester, lactation, children, bleeding disorders, GI disorders, cardiac disorders, hypersensitivity to other antiinflammatory agents

Pharmacokinetics:
PO: Peak 2 hr, half-life 3-3½ hr; metabolized in liver; excreted in urine (metabolites), breast milk; 99% plasma protein binding

Interactions/incompatibilities:
• May increase the action of: coumarin, sulfonamides, salicylates
• May decrease effects of fenoprofen: phenobarbital, probenecid

NURSING CONSIDERATIONS
Assess:
• Renal, liver, blood studies: BUN, creatinine, AST, ALT, Hgb, before treatment, periodically thereafter
• Audiometric, ophthalmic examination before, during, after treatment
• For eye, ear problems: blurred vision, tinnitus; may indicate toxicity

Administer:
• With food to decrease GI symptoms; however, best to take on empty stomach to facilitate absorption

Perform/provide:
• Storage at room temperature

Evaluate:
• Therapeutic response: decreased pain, stiffness in joints, decreased swelling in joints, ability to move more easily

Teach patient/family:
• To report blurred vision, ringing, roaring in ears; may indicate toxicity
• To avoid driving, other hazardous activities if dizziness, drowsiness occurs
• To report change in urine pattern, increased weight, edema, increased

pain in joints, fever, blood in urine; indicates nephrotoxicity
• That therapeutic effects may take up to 1 mo
• To take with a full glass of water to enhance absorption
• To avoid concurrent use of alcohol, ASA, acetaminophen or other OTC meds without consulting physician

fentanyl citrate
(fen'ta-nill)
Fentanyl, Sublimaze
Func. class.: Narcotic analgesics
Chem. class.: Opiate, synthetic phenylpiperidine derivative

Controlled Substance Schedule II
Action: Inhibits ascending pain pathways in CNS, increases pain threshold, alters pain perception
Uses: Preoperatively, postoperatively; adjunct to general anesthetic, when combined with droperidol

Dosage and routes:
Anesthetic
• *Adult:* IV 0.05-0.1 mg q2-3min prn
Preoperatively
• *Adult:* IM 0.05-0.1 mg q30-60 min before surgery
Postoperatively
• *Adult:* IM 0.05-0.1 mg ql-2h prn
• *Child:* IM 0.02-0.03 mg/9 kg
Available forms: Inj IM, IV 0.05 mg/ml

Side effects/adverse reactions:
CNS: Dizziness, delirium, euphoria
GI: Nausea, vomiting
MS: Muscle rigidity
EENT: Blurred vision, miosis
CV: **Bradycardia, arrest,** hypotension or hypertension
RESP: **Respiratory depression, arrest, laryngospasm**

---

italics = common side effects   ***bold italic*** = life threatening reactions

474   fentanyl citrate

Contraindications: Hypersensitivity to opiates, myasthenia gravis
Precautions: Elderly, respiratory depression, increased intracranial pressure, seizure disorders, severe respiratory disorders, cardiac dysrhythmias, pregnancy (C)
Pharmacokinetics:
IM: Onset 7-15 min, peak 30 min, duration 1-2 hr
IV: Onset immediate, peak 3-5 min, duration ½-1 hr; metabolized by liver; excreted by kidneys; crosses placenta; excreted in breast milk; half-life 2½-4 hr; 80% bound to plasma proteins
Interactions/incompatibilities:
• Effects may be increased with other CNS depressants: alcohol, narcotics, sedative/hypnotics, antipsychotics, skeletal muscle relaxants
• Incompatible with diazepam, methohexitol pentobarbital, phenytoin, $NaCO_3$, thiopental in sol or syringe
NURSING CONSIDERATIONS
Assess:
• VS after parenteral route; note muscle rigidity, drug history, liver, kidney function test
• CNS changes: dizziness, drowsiness, hallucinations, euphoria, LOC, pupil reaction
• Allergic reactions: rash, urticaria
• Respiratory dysfunction: respiratory depression, character, rate, rhythm; notify physician if respirations are <10/min
Administer:
• By injection (IM, IV); give slowly to prevent rigidity
• Only with resuscitative equipment available
• IV undiluted by anesthesiologist or diluted with 5 ml or more sterile H_2O or NS given through Y-tube or

3-way-stopcock given at 0.1 mg or less/1-2 min
Perform/provide:
• Storage in light-resistant area at room temperature
• Coughing, turning, deep breathing for postoperative patients
• Safety measures: side rails, nightlight, call bell within reach
Evaluate:
• Therapeutic response: induction of anesthesia

---

fentanyl citrate/droperidol combination
(fen'ta-nil) (droe-per'i-dole)
Innovar
Func. class.: General anesthetic/narcotic analgesic
Chem. class.: Phenylpiperone derivative

Controlled Substance Schedule II
Action: Action at subcortical levels to reduce motor activity, produces analgesia
Uses: Premedication, adjunct to general anesthesia, maintenance of anesthesia
Dosage and routes:
Induction
• *Adult:* IV 1 ml/20-25 lb
• *Child:* IV 0.5 ml/20 lb
Premedication
• *Adult:* IM 0.5-2 ml 45-60 min before surgery or procedure
• *Child:* IM 0.25 ml/20 lb 45-60 min before surgery or procedure
Available forms: Inj IM, IV 0.05 mg fentanyl, 2.5 mg droperidol/ml
Side effects/adverse reactions:
RESP: Laryngospasm, bronchospasm, respiratory arrest
CNS: Dystonia, akathisia, flexion of arms, fine tremors, dizziness, anxiety, drowsiness, restlessness, hallucination, depression, muscular

* Available in Canada only

rigidity, extrapyramidal symptoms
CV: Tachycardia, hypotension, circulatory depression
EENT: Upward rotation of eyes, oculogyric crisis, blurred vision
INTEG: Chills, facial sweating, shivering, diaphoresis
GI: Nausea, vomiting

Contraindications: Hypersensitivity, child < 2 yr, myasthenia gravis
Precautions: Elderly, increased intracranial pressure, cardiovascular disease (bradydysrhythmias), renal disease, liver disease, Parkinson's disease, COPD, pregnancy (C)

Pharmacokinetics:
IV: Onset 20 sec, peak 2-10 min, duration ½-2 hr; tranquilizing effect may last up to 12h
IM: Onset 7 min, duration 1-2 hr; metabolized in liver; excreted in urine metabolites (90%)

Interactions/incompatibilities:
• Increased CNS depression: alcohol, narcotics, barbiturates, antipsychotics or other CNS depressants
• Decreased effects of: amphetamines, anticonvulsants, anticoagulants
• Increased intraocular pressure: anticholinergics, antiparkinson drugs
• Increased side effects of: lithium
• Incompatible with diazepam, methohexitol, nafcillin, phenobarbital, phenytoin, $NaCO_3$, thiopental in sol or syringe

NURSING CONSIDERATIONS
Assess:
• VS q10min during IV administration, q30min after IM dose
• Liver functions test and BUN creatinine $PaCO_2$
• Rigidity of skeletal muscles
• Extrapyramidal reactions: dystonia, akathisia
• Increasing heart rate or decreasing B/P by >10% from baseline; notify physician at once; do not place patient in Trendelenburg position or sympathetic blockade may occur, causing respiratory arrest

Administer:
• Anticholinergics (benztropine, diphenhydramine) for extrapyramidal reaction
• Only with crash cart, resuscitative equipment nearby; narcotic antagonist for severe respiratory depression, cardiac monitor
• IV direct undiluted through Y-tube or 3-way stopcock; give each 1 ml of undiluted drug/1min or more; 0.1ml/kg may be diluted in 250 ml D_5W and given as IV inf over 5-10 min; titrate to patient response

Perform/provide:
• Slow movement of patient to avoid orthostatic hypotension

Evaluate:
• Therapeutic response: decreased anxiety, absence of vomiting, maintenance of anesthesia

Teach patient/family:
• To use deep breathing, turning, coughing after surgery to prevent increased secretions in lungs

---

fentanyl transdermal

Duragesic-25, Duragesic-50, Duragesic-75, Duragesic-100

Func. class.: Narcotic analgesic
Chem. class.: Opiate, synthetic phenylpiperidine

Controlled Substance Schedule II

Action: Inhibits ascending pain pathways in CNS, increases pain threshold, alters pain perception
Uses: Management of chronic

---

italics = common side effects   ***bold italic*** = life threatening reactions

pains for those requiring opioid analgesia

Dosage and routes:
Adult: 25 μg/hr; may increase until pain relief occurs; apply patch to flat surface on upper torso and wear for 72 hr; apply new patch on different site for continued relief

Available forms: Patch 2.5, 5, 7.5, 10 mg

Side effects/adverse reactions:
CNS: Dizziness, delirium, euphoria, light-headedness, sedation, dysphoria, agitation, anxiety
GI: Nausea, vomiting, diarrhea, cramps
EENT: Blurred vision, miosis
CV: Bradycardia, *cardiac arrest,* hypotension or hypertension, facial flushing, chills
RESP: Respiratory depression, laryngospasm, bronchospasm; depresses cough; hypoventilation

Contraindications: Hypersensitivity to opiates, myasthenia gravis

Precautions: Elderly, respiratory depression, increased intracranial pressure, seizure disorders, severe respiratory disorders, cardiac dysrhythmias, pregnancy (C), fever

Interactions/incompatibilities:
• Effects may be increased with other CNS depressants: alcohol, narcotics, sedative/hypnotics, antipsychotics, skeletal muscle relaxants

NURSING CONSIDERATIONS
Assess:
• Pain contol; check for duration, site, character of pain, fever; use pain and sedation scoring
• CNS changes: dizziness, drowsiness, hallucinations, euphoria, LOC, pupil reaction
• Allergic reactions: rash, urticaria
• Respiratory dysfunction: respiratory depression, character, rate, rhythm; notify physician if respirations are <10/min

Administer:
• q72h for continuous pain relief
Perform/provide:
• Safety measures: side rails, nightlight, call bell within reach
Evaluate:
• Therapeutic response: decreased pain
Teach patient/family:
• Avoid activities that require alertness

ferrous fumarate/ferrous gluconate/ferrous sulfate

Femiron, Feostat, Ferrets, Ferrous Fumarate, Fumasorb, Fumerin, Hemocyte, Ircon, Nephro-Fer, Span-FF, Fergon, Ferralet, Ferralet S.R., Ferrous Gluconate, Simron, Feosol, Feratab, Fer-In-Sol, Fer-Iron, Fero-Gradumet, Ferospace, Ferralyn, Ferra-TD, Ferrous Sulfate, Mol-Iron, Slow-Fe

Func. class.: Hematinic
Chem. class.: Iron preparation

Action: Replaces iron stores needed for red blood cell development, energy and O_2 transport, utilization; fumarate contains 33% elemental iron; gluconate, 12%; sulfate, 20%; iron, 30%; ferrous sulfate exsiccated

Uses:
Iron deficiency anemia, prophylaxis for iron deficiency in pregnancy

Dosage and routes:
Fumarate
• *Adult:* PO 200 mg tid-qid
• *Child:* 2-12 yr: PO 3 mg/kg/day (elemental iron) tid-qid

• *Child 6 mo-2 yr:* PO up to 6 mg/kg/day (elemental iron) tid-qid
• *Child: 6 mo-2 yr:* 6 mg/kg/day in 3-4 divided doses
• *Infants:* PO 10-25 mg/day (elemental iron) in 3-4 divided doses
Gluconate
• *Adult:* PO 200-600 mg tid
• *Child 6-12 yr:* 300-900 mg qd
• *Child <6 yr:* 100-300 mg qd
Sulfate
• *Adult:* PO 0.750-1.5 g/day in divided doses tid
• *Child 6-12 yr:* 600 mg/day in divided doses
Pregnancy
• *Adult:* PO 300-600 mg/day in divided doses

Available forms:
Fumarate
Tabs 63, 195, 200, 324, 325 mg; tabs chewable 100 mg; tabs controlled-release 300 mg; oral susp 100 mg/5 ml, 45 mg/0.6 ml
Gluconate
Tabs 300, 320, 325 mg; caps 86, 325, 435 mg; tabs film-coated 300 mg; elix 300 mg/5 ml
Sulfate
Tabs, 195, 300, 325 mg; tabs enteric-coated 325 mg; tabs extended-release, time-release caps, 525 mg

Side effects/adverse reactions:
GI: Nausea, constipation, epigastric pain, black and red tarry stools, vomiting, diarrhea
INTEG: Temporarily discolored tooth enamel and eyes

Contraindications: Hypersensitivity, ulcerative colitis/regional enteritis, hemosiderosis/hemochromatosis, peptic ulcer disease, hemolytic anemia, cirrhosis

Precautions: Anemia (long-term), pregnancy (A)

Pharmacokinetics:
PO: Excreted in feces, urine, skin, breast milk; enters bloodstream; bound to transferrin; crosses placenta

Interactions/incompatibilities:
• Decreased absorption of: penicillamine, Levodopa, methyldopa, quinolone, tetracycline
• Decreased absorption of iron preparations: antacids, tetracycline, Vit E
• Increased absorption of iron preparation: ascorbic acid, chloramphenicol

Lab test interferences:
False-positive: Occult blood

NURSING CONSIDERATIONS
Assess:
• Blood studies: Hct, Hgb, reticulocytes, bilirubin before treatment, at least monthly
• Toxicity: nausea, vomiting, diarrhea (green, then tarry stools), hematemesis, pallor, cyanosis, shock, coma
• Elimination; if constipation occurs, increase water, bulk, activity
• Nutrition: amount of iron in diet (meat, dark green leafy vegetables, dried beans, dried fruits, eggs)
• Cause of iron loss or anemia, including salicylates, sulfonamides, antimalarials, quinidine

Administer:
• Only with Vit E supplements to infants or hemolytic anemia may occur
• Between meals for best absorption; may give with juice; do not give with antacids or milk, delay at least 1 hr; if GI symptoms occur, give PC even if absorption is decreased; eggs, milk products, chocolate, caffeine interfere with absorption
• Through plastic straw to avoid discoloration of tooth enamel; dilute thoroughly
• At least 1 hr before hs, since corrosion may occur in stomach
• For <6 months for anemia

---

italics = common side effects   ***bold italic*** = life threatening reactions

Perform/provide:
• Storage in tight, light-resistant container
Evaluate:
• Therapeutic response: improvement in Hct, Hgb, reticulocytes, decreased fatigue, weakness
Teach patient/family:
• That iron will change stools black or dark green
• That iron poisoning may occur if increased beyond recommended level
• Not to crush; swallow tablet whole
• To keep out of reach of children
• Do not substitute one iron salt for another; elemental iron content differs (e.g., 300 mg ferrous fumarate contains about 100 mg elemental iron, whereas 300 mg ferrous gluconate contains only about 30 mg elemental iron)
• To avoid reclining position for 15-30 min after taking drug to avoid esophageal corrosion
• To follow diet high in iron
Treatment of overdose: Induce vomiting; give eggs, milk until lavage can be done

---

fibrinolysin/desoxyribonuclease

(fye-bri-noe-lye′sin)
Elase
Func. class.: Enzyme
Chem. class.: Proteolytic-bovine

Action: Dissolves fibrin in clots, attacks DNA in areas of disintegrating cells
Uses: Debridement of wounds, vaginitis, cervicitis, ulcerative colitis, 2nd, 3rd degree burns; irrigating wounds, topically

Dosage and routes:
Debridement/intravaginally
• *Adult:* OINT 5 g × 5 applications
Irrigating
• *Adult:* IRIG dilution depends on type of wound
Available forms: Fibrinolysin with desoxyribonuclease 666.6 U/g; powder for reconstitution fibrinolysin 25 U/desoxyribonuclease 15,000 U
Side effects/adverse reactions:
INTEG: Hyperemia
Contraindications: Hypersensitivity to bovine or mercury products, hematoma
Precautions: Pregnancy (C)
NURSING CONSIDERATIONS
Assess:
• For signs of irritation and inflammation; drug should be discontinued
• Wound: drainage, color, odor, size, depth
Administer:
• After reconstituting with 10 ml sterile NaCl solution; use only fresh solution
• After removing necrotic debris, dry eschar
• Wet dressing by mixing 1 vial elase/10-50 ml saline solution; saturate gauze with solution; pack area; remove in 6-8 hr; repeat tid-qid
Perform/provide:
• Cleansing of wound using aseptic technique; cover with drug, then dressing; change at least qid
Evaluate:
• Therapeutic response: decrease in wound scarring, tissue necrosis

filgrastim (G-CSF)

(fill-grass'stim)

Neupogen

Func. class.: Biologic modifier
Chem. class.: Granulocyte colony-stimulating factor

Action: Stimulates proliferation and differentiation of neutrophils

Uses: To decrease chance of infection in patients receiving antineoplastics that are myelosuppressive; to increase WBC in patients with drug-induced neutropenia

Dosage and routes:
• *Adult:* IV/SC 5 µg/kg/day in a single dose; may increase by 5 µg/kg in each chemotherapy cycle; give qd for up to 2 wk until the absolute neutrophil count (ANC) has reached 10,000/mm³; response to G-CSF is much greater with SC than IV therapy

Available forms: Inj 300 µg/ml

Side effects/adverse reactions:
CNS: Fever

HEMA: Thrombocytopenia

INTEG: Alopecia, exacerbation of skin conditions

MS: Osteoporosis, skeletal pain

GI: Nausea, vomiting, diarrhea, mucositis, anorexia

Contraindications: Hypersensitivity to proteins of *E. coli*

Precautions: Pregnancy (C), lactation, cardiac conditions

Pharmacokinetics: Metabolism, excretion, distribution not known

Interactions/incompatibilities:
• Do not use this drug concomitantly with antineoplastics

Lab test interferences:
Increase: Uric acid, lactate dehydrogenase, alk, phosphatase

NURSING CONSIDERATIONS

Assess:
• Blood studies: CBC, platelet

count before treatment and twice weekly; neutrophil counts may be increased for 2 days after therapy

Administer:
• 300 µg/ml or 480 µg/1.6 ml; allow to warm to room temperature; give single dose over 1 min or less through Y-tube or medport
• Using single-use vials; after dose is withdrawn, do not reenter vial
• For 2 wk or until ANC is 10,000/mm³ after the expected chemotherapy neutrophil nadir

Perform/provide:
• Storage in refrigerator; do not freeze; may store at room temperature for up to 6 hr
• Avoid shaking

Evaluate:
• Therapeutic response: absence of infection

Teach patient/family:
• Technique for self-administration: dose, side effects, disposal of containers and needles; provide instruction sheet

finasteride

(feen-as'-ter-ide)

Proscar

Func. class.: Androgen hormone inhibitor
Chem. class.: 5-α-reductase inhibitor

Action: Inhibits 5-α-reductase and reduction in DHT; DHT induces androgenic effects by binding to androgen receptors in the cell nuclei of the prostate gland, liver, skin; produces lower levels of 5-α-reductase which prevents development of BHP

Uses: Symptomatic benign prostatic hyperplasia

Dosage and routes:
• *Adult:* PO 5 mg qd × 6-12 mo
Available forms: Tab 5 mg

Side effects/adverse reactions:
GU: Impotence, decreased libido, decreased volume of ejaculate

Contraindications: Hypersensitivity, pregnancy (X), children, women

Precautions: Large residual urinary volume, severely diminished urinary flow, liver function abnormalities

Pharmacokinetics: Bioavailability 63%, plasma protein binding 90%; metabolized in the liver; excreted in urine (metabolites) 39%, feces (57%); crosses blood-brain barrier

Interactions/incompatibilities:
• Increases theophylline clearance

NURSING CONSIDERATIONS
Assess:
• Urinary patterns, residual urinary volume, severely diminished urinary flow
• PSA levels and digital rectal exam prior to initiating therapy and periodically thereafter
• Liver function studies prior to treatment; extensively metabolized in liver

Administer:
• Without regard to meals

Perform/provide:
• Storage at temperatures <86° F (30° C); protect from light; keep container tightly closed

Evaluate:
• Therapeutic response: increased urinary flow, decreased postvoiding dribbling, frequency, nocturia

Teach patient/family:
• Pregnant women should not touch crushed tablets or come into contact with semen of a patient taking this drug; may adversely affect developing male fetus
• That volume of ejaculate may be decreased during treatment; impotence and decreased libido may also occur

---

flavoxate HCl
(fla-vox'ate)
Urispas
Func. class.: Spasmolytic
Chem. class.: Flavone derivative

Action: Relaxes smooth muscles in urinary tract

Uses: Relief of nocturia, incontinence, suprapubic pain, dysuria, frequency associated with urologic conditions (symptomatic only)

Dosage and routes:
• *Adult and child >12 yr:* PO 100-200 mg tid-qid

Available forms: Tabs 100 mg

Side effects/adverse reactions:
*HEMA: **Leukopenia, eosinophilia***
*CNS: Anxiety, restlessness, dizziness, **convulsions,** headache,* drowsiness, confusion, decreased concentration
CV: Palpitations, sinus tachycardia, hypotension
GI: Nausea, vomiting, anorexia, abdominal pain, constipation
GU: Dysuria
INTEG: Urticaria, dermatitis
EENT: Blurred vision, increased intraocular tension, dry mouth, throat

Contraindications: Hypersensitivity, GI obstruction, GI hemorrhage, GU obstruction

Precautions: Pregnancy (B), lactation, suspected glaucoma, children <12 yr

Pharmacokinetics: Excreted in urine

NURSING CONSIDERATIONS
Assess:
• Urinary status: dysuria, frequency, nocturia, incontinence
• Allergic reactions: rash, urticaria; if these occur, drug should be discontinued

---

*Available in Canada only

Evaluate:
• Therapeutic response: decreased dysuria
Teach patient/family
• To avoid hazardous activities; dizziness may occur

---

flecainide acetate
(fle-kay'nide)
Tambocor
Func. class.: Antidysrhythmic (Class IC)

Action: Decreases conduction in all parts of the heart, with greatest effect on His-Purkinje system, which stabilizes cardiac membrane
Uses: Life-threatening ventricular dysrhythmias, sustained ventricular tachycardia
Dosage and routes:
• *Adult:* PO 100 mg q12h; may increase q4d by 50 mg q12h to desired response, not to exceed 400 mg/day
Available forms: Tabs 50, 100, 150 mg
Side effects/adverse reactions:
CNS: Headache, dizziness, involuntary movement, confusion, psychosis, restlessness, irritability, paresthesias, ataxia, flushing, somnolence, depression, anxiety, malaise
EENT: Tinnitus, *blurred vision,* hearing loss
GI: Nausea, vomiting, anorexia, constipation, abdominal pain, flatulence, change in taste
CV: Hypotension, bradycardia, angina, PVCs, *heart block, **cardiovascular collapse, arrest,** dysrhythmias, **CHF, fatal ventricular tachycardia***
RESP: Dyspnea, ***respiratory depression***

INTEG: Rash, urticaria, edema, swelling
HEMA: Leukopenia, thrombocytopenia
GU: Impotence, decreased libido, polyuria, urinary retention
Contraindications: Hypersensitivity, severe heart block, cardiogenic shock, nonsustained ventricular dysrhythmias, frequent PVCs, non-life-threatening dysrhythmias
Precautions: Pregnancy (C), lactation, children, renal disease, liver disease, CHF, respiratory depression, myasthenia gravis
Pharmacokinetics:
PO: Peak 3 hr; half-life 12-27 hr; metabolized by liver; excreted unchanged by kidneys (10%); excreted in breast milk
Interactions/incompatibilities:
• Increased levels of both drugs: propranolol
• Increased level of flecainide: amiodarone, cimetidine
• Increased negative inotropic effects: disopyramide, verapamil
• Increased digoxin level: digoxin
Lab test interferences:
Increase: CPK

NURSING CONSIDERATIONS
Assess:
• For hypokalemia, hyperkalemia before administration; correct electrolytes
• Blood levels: trough (0.2-1 μg/ml)
• B/P, ECG continuously for fluctuations
• Malignant hyperthermia: tachypnea, tachycardia, changes in B/P, increased temperature
• Cardiac rate, respiration: rate, rhythm, character, continuously
• Respiratory status: rate, rhythm, lung fields for rales
• CNS effects: dizziness, confusion, psychosis, paresthesias, con-

---

italics = common side effects   ***bold italic*** = life threatening reactions

vulsions; drug should be discontinued
• Increased respiration, increased pulse; drug should be discontinued
Administer:
• Reduced dosage as soon as dysrhythmia is controlled
Evaluate:
• Therapeutic response: decreased dysrhythmias
Treatment of overdose: O_2, artificial ventilation, ECG, administer dopamine for circulatory depression, administer diazepam or thiopental for convulsions, treat ventricular dysrhythmias

---

floxuridine
(flox-yoor'i-deen)
Floxuridine, FUDR
Func. class.: Antineoplastic, antimetabolite
Chem. class.: Pyrimidine antagonist

Action: Inhibits DNA synthesis; interferes with cell replication by competitively inhibiting thymidylate synthesis S phase of cell cycle
Uses: GI adenocarcinoma metastatic to liver; cancer of breast, head, neck, liver, brain, gallbladder, bile duct
Dosage and routes:
• *Adult:* INTRAARTERIAL by continuous inf 0.1-0.6 mg/kg/day × 1-6 wk; HEPATIC ARTERY INJ 0.4-0.6 mg/kg/day × 1-6 wk
Available forms: Powder for inj (intraarterial, hepatic artery) 500 mg/5 ml vial
Side effects/adverse reactions:
HEMA: Thrombocytopenia, leukopenia, myelosuppression, anemia
GI: Anorexia, diarrhea, nausea, vomiting, *hemorrhage*

GU: Renal failure
EENT: Epistaxis
INTEG: Rash, fever
CNS: Lethargy, malaise, weakness
Contraindications: Hypersensitivity, myelosuppression, pregnancy (D), poor nutritional status, serious infections
Precautions: Renal disease, hepatic disease, bone marrow depression
Pharmacokinetics: Half-life 10-20 min, 20 hr terminal; metabolized in liver; excreted in urine (active metabolite); crosses blood-brain barrier
Interactions/incompatibilities:
• Increased toxicity: radiation or other antineoplastics
Lab test interferences:
Increase: Liver function studies
NURSING CONSIDERATIONS
Assess:
• CBC, differential, platelet count weekly; withhold drug if WBC is <3500/mm³ or platelet count is <100,000/mm³; notify physician of these results; drug should be discontinued
• Renal function studies: BUN, serum uric acid, urine CrCl, electrolytes before, during therapy
• I&O ratio: report fall in urine output to <30 ml/hr
• Monitor temperature q4h; fever may indicate beginning infection
• Liver function tests before, during therapy: bilirubin, alk phosphatase, AST, ALT, LDH; as needed or monthly
• Bleeding: hematuria, guaiac, bruising or petechiae, mucosa or orifices q8h
• Food preferences; list likes, dislikes
• Inflammation of mucosa, breaks in skin
• Buccal cavity q8h for dryness,

sores or ulceration, white patches, oral pain, bleeding, dysphagia
• Symptoms indicating severe allergic reaction: rash, urticaria, itching, flushing
• GI symptoms: frequency of stools, cramping; low-residue diet with elimination of milk products when used in conjunction with 5FUDR/radiation therapy
• Acidosis, signs of dehydration: rapid respirations, poor skin turgor, decreased urine output, dry skin, restlessness, weakness

Administer:
• By intraarterial infusion pump after diluting 5 ml drug/5 ml sterile H₂O for inj, dilute further with D₅W or normal saline to required dilution
• Antiemetic 30-60 min before giving drug to prevent vomiting and prn
• Antibiotics for prophylaxis of infection
• Topical or systemic analgesics for pain
• Transfusion for anemia
• Antispasmodic for diarrhea

Perform/provide:
• Wrapping solution; do not expose to light
• Strict medical asepsis and protective isolation if WBC levels are low
• Increased fluid intake to 2-3 L/day to prevent dehydration unless contraindicated
• Rinsing of mouth tid-qid with water, club soda, brushing of teeth bid-tid with soft brush or cotton-tipped applicators for stomatitis; use unwaxed dental floss
• Nutritious diet with iron, vitamin supplements, low fiber, and no dairy products as ordered

Evaluate:
• Therapeutic response: decreased tumor size, spread of malignancy

Teach patient/family:
• Why protective isolation is necessary
• To report signs of infection: increased temperature, sore throat, flu symptoms
• To report signs of anemia: fatigue, headache, faintness, shortness of breath, irritability
• To report bleeding: avoid use of razors, commercial mouthwash
• To avoid use of aspirin products or ibuprofen
• To report stomatitis: any bleeding, white spots, ulcerations in mouth; tell patient to examine mouth qd, report symptoms

---

fluconazole
(floo-con'-a-zole)
Diflucan
Func. class.: Antifungal

Action: Inhibits ergosterol biosynthesis, causes direct damage to membrane phospholipids

Uses: Oropharyngeal candidiasis in AIDS patients, chronic mucocutaneous candidiasis, urinary candidiasis, cryptococcal meningitis

Dosage and routes:
Vaginal candidiasis
• *Adult:* PO 150 mg as a single dose
Serious fungal infections
• *Adult:* PO/IV 50-400 mg initially, then 200 mg once daily for 4 wk
Oropharyngeal candidiasis in AIDS patients:
• *Adult:* PO 200 mg initially, then 100 mg daily for at least 2 wk
Available forms: Tabs 50, 100, 200 mg, IV inj 200, 400 mg

Side effects/adverse reactions:
GI: Nausea, vomiting, diarrhea,

cramping, flatus, increased AST, ALT

Contraindications: Hypersensitivity

Precautions: Renal disease, pregnancy (B)

Interactions/incompatibilities:
• Potentiation of anticoagulation: warfarin
• Increased renal dysfunction: cyclosporines
• Incompatible with other drugs in sol or syringe

NURSING CONSIDERATIONS
Assess:
• VS q15-30min during first infusion; note changes in pulse, B/P
• I&O ratio; watch for decreasing urinary output, change in sp gr; discontinue drug to prevent renal damage
• Weight weekly; if weight gain >2 lb/wk and edema is present, renal damage should be considered
• Renal toxicity: increasing BUN, serum creatinine; if BUN is >40 mg/dl or if serum creatinine is >3 mg/dl, drug may be discontinued or dosage reduced
• For hepatotoxicity: increasing AST, ALT, alk phosphatase, bilirubin

Administer:
• After diluting according to package directions; run at 200 mg/hr or less; do not use plastic containers in connections
• IV using an in-line filter, using distal veins; check for extravasation and necrosis q2h
• Drug only after C&S confirms organism, drug needed to treat condition

Perform/provide:
• Storage; protected from moisture and light, diluted solution is stable for 24 hr

Evaluate:
• Therapeutic response: decreasing oral candidiasis, fever, malaise, rash; negative C&S for infection organism

Teach patient/family:
• That long-term therapy may be needed to clear infection

---

flucytosine
(floo-sye′toe-seen)
Ancobon, Ancotil*
Func. class.: Antifungal
Chem. class.: Pyrimidine (fluorinated)

Action: Converted to fluorouracil after entering fungi; inhibits DNA synthesis

Uses: *Candida* infections (septicemia, endocarditis, pulmonary, urinary tract infections), *Cryptococcus* (meningitis, pulmonary, urinary tract infections)

Dosage and routes:
• *Adult and child >50 kg:* PO 50-150 mg/kg/day q6h
• *Adult and child <50 kg:* PO 1.5-4.5 g/m²/day in 4 divided doses
Available forms: Caps 250, 500 mg

Side effects/adverse reactions:
INTEG: Rash
CNS: Headache, confusion, dizziness, sedation, vertigo
GI: Nausea, vomiting, anorexia, diarrhea, abdominal distention, cramps, enterocolitis, increased AST, ALT, alk phosphatase, *bowel perforation* (rare)
HEMA: **Thrombocytopenia, agranulocytosis, anemia, leukopenia, pancytopenia**
GU: Increased BUN, creatinine

Contraindications: Hypersensitivity

Precautions: Renal disease, impaired hepatic function, bone marrow depression, blood dyscrasias, radiation/chemotherapy, pregnancy (C)

Pharmacokinetics:

PO: Peak 2½-6 hr, half-life 3-6 hr, excreted in urine (unchanged), well-distributed to CSF, aqueous humor, joints

Interactions/incompatibilities:

• Synergisim: Amphotericin B

Lab test interferences:

False increase: Creatinine

NURSING CONSIDERATIONS

Assess:

• VS q15-30min during first infusion; note changes in pulse and B/P

• Blood studies: CBC, including platelets

• Drug level during treatment (therapeutic level 25-100 μg/ml); if renal impairment is present, level usually kept <100 μg/ml

• For renal toxicity: increasing BUN, serum creatinine; if serum creatinine >1.7 mg/100 dl, dosage may be reduced

• For hepatotoxicity: increasing AST, ALT, alk phosphatase

• For allergic reaction: dermatitis, rash; drug should be discontinued, antihistamines (mild reaction) or epinephrine (severe reaction) administered

• For blood dyscrasias, fatigue, bruising, malaise, dark urine

Administer:

• Drug only after C&S confirms organism, drug needed to treat condition

• Few caps at a time to decrease nausea, vomiting over 15 min

Perform/provide:

• Symptomatic treatment as ordered for adverse reactions: aspirin, antihistamines, antiemetics, antispasmodics

• Storage in tight, light-resistant containers at room temperature

Evaluate:

• Therapeutic response: decreased fever, malaise, rash, negative C&S for infecting organism

Teach patient/family:

• That long-term therapy may be needed to clear infection (1-2 mo depending on type of infection)

• To report symptoms of blood dyscrasias: fatigue, bruising, malaise, dark urine

---

fludarabine phosphate

(floo-dar'a-bine)

Fludara

Func. class.: Antineoplastic, antimetabolite

Chem. class.: Vidarabine derivative

Action: Competes with physiologic substrate that inhibits DNA synthesis

Uses: Chronic lymphocytic leukemia

Dosage and routes:

• *Adult:* IV 25 mg/m² over 30 min qd × 5 days, may repeat q28 days; reconstitute with 2 ml of sterile water for inj; dissolution should occur in <15 sec

Available forms: Lyophilized powder for reconstitution 50 mg

Side effects/adverse reactions:

SYST: Fever, chills, malaise, fatigue

META: Hyperuricemia, hyperphosphatemia, hypocalcemia, metabolic acidosis, hyperkalemia

HEMA: Thrombophlebitis, bleeding, ***thrombocytopenia, leukopenia, myelosuppression, anemia***

GI: Nausea, vomiting, anorexia, diarrhea, stomatitis, ***hepatotoxic-***

---

italics = common side effects   ***bold italic*** = life threatening reactions

ity, abdominal pain, hematemesis, *GI hemorrhage*

EENT: Visual disturbances, sinusitis

GU: Dysuria, infection

INTEG: Rash

RESP: ***Pneumonia,*** dyspnea, cough, interstitial pulmonary infiltrate

CV: Edema

CNS: Weakness, confusion, headache, depression, sleep disorder, impaired mentation, *coma,* peripheral neuropathy

Contraindications: Hypersensitivity, pregnancy (D)

Precautions: Renal disease, hepatic disease, infants

Pharmacokinetics: Rapidly converted to active metabolite; half-life of metabolite 10 hr; mean plasma clearance of metabolite 8.9 L/hr/m^2; 23% excreted in urine as unchanged metabolite

Interactions/incompatibilities:

• Increased toxicity: radiation or other antineoplastics

NURSING CONSIDERATIONS
Assess:

• CBC (RBC, Hct, Hgb), differential, platelet count weekly; withhold drug if CBC <4000/mm^3, platelet count is <75,000/mm^3, or RBC, Hct, Hgb are low; notify physician of these results

• Renal function studies: BUN, uric acid, urine creatinine clearance, electrolytes before and during therapy

• I&O ratio; report fall in urine output to <30 ml/hr

• Temperature q4h; fever may indicate beginning infection; no rectal temperature

• Liver function tests before, during therapy: bilirubin, ALT, AST, alk phosphatase, as needed or monthly

• Blood uric acid levels during therapy

• Bleeding: hematuria, guaiac, bruising or petechiae, mucosa or orifices q8h

• Dyspnea, rales, unproductive cough, chest pain, tachypnea, fatigue, increased pulse, pallor, lethargy, personality changes with high doses

• Food preferences: list likes, dislikes

• Edema in feet, joint pain, stomach pain, shaking

• Inflammation of mucosa, breaks in skin

• Yellowing of skin and sclera, dark urine, clay-colored stools, itchy skin, abdominal pain, fever, diarrhea

• Buccal cavity q8h for dryness, sores or ulceration, white patches, oral pain, bleeding, dysphagia

• Local irritation, pain, burning, discoloration at injection site

• GI symptoms: frequency of stools, cramping

• Acidosis, signs of dehydration: rapid respirations, poor skin turgor, decreased urine output, dry skin, restlessness, weakness

Administer:

• Antiemetic 30 to 60 min before giving drug to prevent vomiting, and PRN

• Allopurinol or sodium bicarbonate to maintain uric acid levels and alkalinization or the urine; prevent hyperuricemia

• Antibiotics for prophylaxis of infection

• Topical or systemic analgesics for pain

• Transfusion for anemia

• Antispasmodic for GI symptoms

Perform/provide:

• Strict medical asepsis and protective isolation if WBC levels are low

• Increase fluid intake to 2-3 L/day to prevent urate deposits and calculi formation, unless contraindicated
• Diet low in purines: absence of organ meats (kidney, liver), dried beans, peas to prevent increased urate deposits
• Rinsing of mouth tid-qid with water, club soda; brushing of teeth bid-tid with soft brush or cotton-tipped applicators for stomatitis; use unwaxed dental floss
• HOB raised to facilitate breathing if dyspnea or pneumonia occurs
• Storage in refrigerator
Evaluate:
• Therapeutic response: decrease in tumor size, spread of malignancy
Teach patient/family:
• Why protective isolation is necessary
• To report any coughing, chest pain, or changes in breathing, which may indicate beginning pneumonia
• To avoid foods with citric acid, hot or rough texture if stomatitis is present
• To report stomatitis: any bleeding, white spots, ulcerations in mouth; tell patient to examine mouth qd, report any symptoms
• To report signs of anemia: fatigue, headache, faintness, shortness of breath, irritability
• To report bleeding; avoid use of razors or commercial mouthwash
• To avoid use of aspirin products or ibuprofen
Overdose treatment: Discontinue drug, use supportive therapy

**fludrocortisone ace-
tate**
(floo-droe-kor'ti-sone)
Florinef Acetate
Func. class.: Corticosteroid
Chem. class.: Mineralocorticoid

Action: Promotes increased reabsorption of sodium and loss of potassium from the renal tubules
Uses: Adrenal insufficiency, salt-losing adrenogenital syndrome
Dosage and routes:
• *Adult:* PO 0.1-0.2 mg qd
Available forms: Tabs 0.1 mg
Side effects/adverse reactions:
CNS: Flushing, sweating, headache
CV: Hypertension, ***circulatory col-
lapse, thrombophlebitis, embo-
lism,*** tachycardia
MS: Fractures, osteoporosis, weakness
Contraindications: Hypersensitivity, acute glomerulonephritis, amebiasis
Precautions: Pregnancy (C), osteoporosis, CHF
Pharmacokinetics:
PO: Half-life 3.5 hr, metabolized by liver, excreted in urine
Interactions/incompatibilities:
• Decreased action of fludrocortisone: cholestyramine, colestipol, barbiturates, rifampin, ephedrine, phenytoin, theophylline
• Decreased effects of: diuretics, K-sparing diuretics, K supplements
• Increased side effects: Na-containing food or medication, digitalis preparations
Lab test interferences:
Increase: K, Na
Decrease: Hematocrit
NURSING CONSIDERATIONS
Assess:
• K, while on long-term therapy; hypokalemia

• Weight daily, notify physician of weekly gain >5 lb
• B/P q4h, pulse; notify physician if chest pain occurs
• I&O ratio; be alert for decreasing urinary output and increasing edema
• K depletion: paresthesias, fatigue, nausea, vomiting, depression, polyuria, dysrhythmias, weakness
• Edema, hypertension, cardiac symptoms

Administer:
• Titrated dose; use lowest effective dose
• With food or milk to decrease GI symptoms

Perform/provide:
• Assistance with ambulation in patient with bone tissue disease to prevent fractures

Evaluate:
• Therapeutic response: correction of adrenal insufficiency

Teach patient/family:
• That ID as steroid user should be carried
• Not to discontinue this medication abruptly

---

flumazenil
(floo-maz'een-ill)
Mazicon, Ronazicon
Func. class.: Benzodiazepine receptor antagonist
Chem. class.: Imidazobenzo-diazepine derivative

Action: Antagonizes the actions of benzodiazepines on the CNS, competitively inhibits the activity at the benzodiazepine recognition site on the GABA/benzodiazepine receptor complex

Uses: Reversal of the sedative effects of benzodiazepines

Dosage and routes:
Reversal of conscious sedation or in general anesthesia
• *Adult:* IV 0.2 mg (2 ml) given over 15 sec; wait 45 sec, then give 0.2 mg (2 ml) if consciousness does not occur; may be repeated at 60-sec intervals as needed, up to 4 additional times (max total dose 1 mg); dose is to be individualized
Management of suspected benzodiazepine overdose
• *Adult:* IV 0.2 mg (2 ml) given over 30 sec; wait 30 sec, then give 0.3 mg (3 ml) over 30 sec if consciousness does not occur; further doses of 0.5 mg (5 ml) can be given over 30 sec at intervals of 1 min up to cumulative dose of 3 mg
Available forms: Inj 0.1 mg/ml

Side effects/adverse reactions:
EENT: Abnormal vision, blurred vision, tinnitus
CV: Hypertension, palpitations, cutaneous vasodilation, dysrhythmias, bradycardia, tachycardia, chest pain
GI: Nausea, vomiting, hiccups
CNS: Dizziness, agitation, emotional lability, confusion, *convulsions,* somnolence
SYST: Headache, injection site pain, increased sweating, fatigue, rigors

Contraindications: Hypersensitivity to this drug or benzodiazepines, serious cyclic antidepressant overdose, patients given benzodiazepine for control of life-threatening condition

Precautions: Pregnancy (C), lactation, children, elderly, renal disease, seizure disorders, head injury, labor and delivery, hepatic disease, hypoventilation, panic disorder, drug and alcohol dependency, ambulatory patients

Pharmacokinetics: Terminal half-life 41-79 min; metabolized in liver

---

*Available in Canada only

Interactions/incompatibilities:
• Toxicity: mixed drug overdosage
• Ingestion of food during IV INF: Increased flumazenil clearance

NURSING CONSIDERATIONS
Assess:
• Cardiac status using continuous monitoring
• For seizures; protect patient from injury
• GI symptoms: nausea, vomiting; place in side-lying position to prevent aspiration
• Allergic reactions: flushing, rash, urticaria, pruritus

Administer:
• Over several minutes; check airway and IV access before administration

Evaluate:
• Therapeutic response: decreased sedation

Teach patient/family:
• That amnesia may continue
• Not to engage in hazardous activities for 18-24 hr after discharge
• Not to take any alcohol or nonprescription drugs for 18-24 hr

---

flunisolide
(floo-niss'oh-lide)
AeroBid
Func. class.: Steroid, intranasal
Chem. class.: Glucocorticoid

Action: Long-acting synthetic adrenocorticoid with antiinflammatory activity, minimal mineralocorticoid properties

Uses: Rhinitis (seasonal or perennial)

Dosage and routes:
• *Adult:* INSTILL 2 sprays in each nostril bid, then increase to tid if needed, not to exceed 8 sprays/day in each nostril
• *Child 6-14 yr:* INSTILL 1 spray

in each nostril tid or 2 sprays bid, not to exceed 4 sprays/day in each nostril

Available forms: Aerosol 25µg/spray

Side effects/adverse reactions:
EENT: Nasal irritation, dryness, rebound congestion, epistaxis, sneezing
INTEG: Urticaria
CNS: Headache, dizziness
SYST: **CHF, convulsions,** increased Na, hypertension

Contraindications: Hypersensitivity, child <12 yr, fungal, bacterial infection of nose

Precautions: Lactation, pregnancy (C)

Pharmacokinetics:
AERO: Half-life 6 min, terminal half-life 1.8 hr; metabolized in liver; excreted in urine

NURSING CONSIDERATIONS
Assess:
• Redness, swelling, pain in nasal passages

Administer:
• No more than q4h

Perform/provide:
• Storage in light-resistant container; discard open container after 3 mo

Evaluate:
• Therapeutic response: decreased congestion, runny nose

Teach patient/family:
• That stinging may occur for several applications; drying of mucosa may be decreased by environmental humidification
• To notify physician if irregular pulse, insomnia, dizziness, or tremors occur
• Proper administration to avoid systemic absorption
• To check with physician before using any other nasal medications

---

italics = common side effects   ***bold italic*** = life threatening reactions

flunisolide

(floo-niss'oh-lide)
AeroBid, Nasalide
Func. class.: Corticosteroid
Chem. class.: Glucocorticoid

Action: Decreases inflammation by suppression of migration of polymorphonuclear leukocytes, fibroblasts, reversal of increased capillary permeability and lysosomal stabilization; does not depress hypothalamus

Uses: Rhinitis, allergies, nasal polyps

Dosage and routes:
• *Adult and child >6 yr:* SPRAY 2 puffs bid, not to exceed 4 puffs bid
Available forms: Nasal sol 25 μg/metered dose (Nasalide), 250 μg/metered dose (AeroBid)

Side effects/adverse reactions:
CNS: Headache, nervousness, restlessness
EENT: Hoarseness, *Candida* infection of oral cavity, sore throat
GI: Nausea, vomiting, dry mouth

Contraindications: Hypersensitivity, child <6 yr

Precautions: Nonasthmatic bronchial disease, bacterial, fungal, viral infections of mouth, throat, lungs, respiratory TB, untreated fungal, bacterial, or viral infections, pregnancy (C), glaucoma

Pharmacokinetics:
INH: Duration 1 hr

NURSING CONSIDERATIONS

Assess:
• Infection: increased temperature, WBC, even after withdrawal of medication; drug masks symptoms of infection

Administer:
• Titrated dose; use lowest effective dose

Evaluate:
• Therapeutic response: ease of respirations, decreased inflammation
Teach patient/family:
• To use gum; rinse mouth after each dose
• That ID as steroid user should be carried
• To notify physician if therapeutic response decreases; dosage adjustment may be needed
• Proper administration technique; shake well before use
• Compliance to therapy
• Teach patient about cushingoid symptoms
• Symptoms of adrenal insufficiency: nausea, anorexia, fatigue, dizziness, dyspnea, weakness, joint pain

fluocinonide

(floo-oh-sin'oh-nide)
Flucinolone, Fluocinolone Acetonide, Fluonid, Flurosyn, Synalar, Synalar-HP, Synemol, Fluocinonide, Lidemol,* Lidex, Lidex-E, Vasoderm, Vasoderm E
Func. class.: Topical corticosteroid
Chem. class.: Synthetic fluorinated agent, group II potency

Action: Possesses antipruritic, antiinflammatory actions
Uses: Psoriasis, eczema, contact dermatitis, pruritus
Dosage and routes:
• *Adult and child:* Apply to affected area tid-qid
Available forms: Oint 0.05%; cream 0.05%; sol 0.05%; gel 0.05%
Side effects/adverse reactions:
INTEG: Burning, dryness, itching, irritation, acne, folliculitis, hyper-

trichosis, perioral dermatitis, hypopigmentation, atrophy, striae, miliaria, allergic contact dermatitis, secondary infection

Contraindications: Hypersensitivity to corticosteroids, fungal infections

Precautions: Pregnancy (C), lactation, viral infections, bacterial infections

NURSING CONSIDERATIONS

Assess:

• Temperature: if fever develops, drug should be discontinued

Administer:

• Only to affected areas; do not get in eyes

• Medication, then cover with occlusive dressing (only if prescribed), seal to normal skin, change q12h; use occlusive dressings with extreme caution

• Only to dermatoses; do not use on weeping, denuded, or infected area

Perform/provide:

• Cleansing before application of drug

• Treatment for a few days after area has cleared

• Storage at room temperature

Evaluate:

• Therapeutic response: absence of severe itching, patches on skin, flaking

Teach patient/family:

• To avoid sunlight on affected area; burns may occur

---

fluorescein sodium

(flure′e-seen)

AK-Fluor, Fluorescein, Fluorescite, Fluorets, Fluor-I-Strip, Fluor-I-Strip-A.T., Ful-Glo, Funduscein-10, Funduscein-25, Fluorets

Func. class.: Diagnostic agent, optic

Chem. class.: Fluorescent dye

Action: Allows breaks in the corneal tissue to absorb dye and show up as bright green under cobalt blue light

Uses: Diagnostic aid in identifying foreign bodies, fitting hard contact lenses, fundus photography, tonometry, identifying corneal abrasions, retinal angiography

Dosage and routes:

• *Adult:* INSTILL 1 gtt of 2% sol; irrigate or wet strip with sterile water and touch conjunctiva or fornix; flush eye with irrigating sol

Retinal angiography

• *Adult:* IV 5 ml 10% sol or 3 ml 25% sol injected in antecubital vein

• *Child:* IV 0.077 ml 10% sol or 0.044 ml 25% sol injected in antecubital vein

Available forms: Inj IV 10%, 25%; sol 2%; strips 0.6, 1, 9 mg

Side effects/adverse reactions:

CNS: Headache, dizziness, paresthesia, *convulsions*

CV: Bradycardia, *shock, cardiac arrest,* hypotension, syncope

RESP: Dyspnea, acute pulmonary edema, bronchospasm

GI: Nausea, vomiting, GI distress

EENT: Stinging, burning, conjunctival redness, urticaria, pruritis

Contraindications: Hypersensitivity; do not use with soft lenses

Precautions: Bronchial asthma, pregnancy (C), lactation, children

---

italics = common side effects   ***bold italic*** = life threatening reactions

NURSING CONSIDERATIONS
Assess:
• Eye color after application: epithelial defects are green; normal precorneal tear film appears bright yellow
• For allergic reaction: rash, urticaria, pruritus, angioedema

Administer:
• Only after soft contact lens are removed
• Solution; have patient close eyes for 1 min
• Only with resuscitative equipment nearby
• Test dose (IV) before angiography
• Epinephrine 1:1000 for IV, IM route; an antihistamine and O_2 should always be available

Perform/provide:
• Storage at room temperature

Evaluate:
• IV site for redness, inflammation, swelling

Teach patient/family:
• To report stinging, burning, itching, lacrimation, puffiness
• That urine will be yellow after IV dose

---

fluorometholone
(flure-oh-meth'oh-lone)
Flarex, Fluor-Op, FML, FML Forte, FML Liquifilm
Func. class.: Ophthalmic antiinflammatory

Action: Decreases inflammation, resulting in decreased pain, photophobia, hyperemia, cellular infiltration

Uses: Inflammation of eye, lids, conjunctiva, cornea, uveitis, iridocyclitis, allergic condition, burns, foreign bodies, postoperatively in cataract

Dosage and routes:
• *Adult and child:* INSTILL 1-2 gtts into conjunctival sac qh × 2 days, if needed, then bid-qid
Available forms: Oint 0.1%; ophthalmic susp 0.1%, 0.25%

Side effects/adverse reactions:
*EENT: **Increased intraocular pressure,*** poor corneal wound healing, increased possibility of corneal infections, glaucoma exacerbation, ***optic nerve damage,*** decreased acuity, visual field, cataracts

Contraindications: Hypersensitivity, acute superficial herpes simplex, fungal/viral diseases of the eye or conjunctiva, active diabetes mellitus, ocular TB, infections of the eye

Precautions: Corneal abrasions, glaucoma, pregnancy (C), lactation, children

NURSING CONSIDERATIONS
Evaluate:
• Therapeutic response: absence of swelling, redness, exudate

Administer:
• After shaking suspension

Perform/provide:
• Storage in tight, light-resistant container

Teach patient/family:
• Instillation method: pressure on lacrimal duct for 1 min
• Not to share eye medications with others
• Not to touch applicator to eye
• Not to use if purulent drainage is present
• Not to discontinue steroids abruptly; they should be tapered over 1-2 wk

fluorouracil
(flure-oh-yoor'a-sil)
Efudex, Fluoroplex
Func. class.: Topical antineoplastic
Chem. class.: Antimetabolite

Action: Inhibits synthesis of DNA, RNA in susceptible cells

Uses: Keratosis (multiple/actinic), basal cell carcinoma

Dosage and routes:
• *Adult and child:* TOP apply to affected area bid

Available forms: Sol 1%, 2%, 5%; cream 1%, 5%

Side effects/adverse reactions:
INTEG: Rash, irritation, pain, burning, contact dermatitis, scaling, swelling, soreness, hyperpigmentation, pruritus

Contraindications: Hypersensitivity, pregnancy (D)

NURSING CONSIDERATIONS
Assess:
• WBC, platelets at least monthly
• Area of body involved for redness, swelling
• Check oral cavity qd for stomatitis; if present discontinue drug
Administer:
• Only 5% sol/cream for basal cell carcinoma
• Using gloves or applicator
• A low-residue diet with no dairy product where radiation is also used
Perform/provide:
• Covering of lesion with porous gauze dressing only
• Washing of hands after application if gloves or applicator is not used
• Storage at room temperature
Evaluate:
• Therapeutic response: decreased size of lesion

Teach patient/family:
• To avoid application on normal skin or getting cream in eyes
• To discontinue use if rash or irritation occurs
• To avoid sunlight or use sunscreen; photosensitivity may occur
• To wash hands after application
• Not to change application; use exactly as prescribed
• That lesion will disappear in 1-2 mo

fluorouracil (5-fluorouracil)
(flure-oh-yoor'a-sil)
Adrucil, 5-FU
Func. class.: Antineoplastic, antimetabolite
Chem. class.: Pyrimidine antagonist

Action: Inhibits DNA synthesis; interferes with cell replication by competitively inhibiting thymidylate synthesis, S phase of cell cycle–specific vesicant

Uses: Cancer of breast, colon, rectum, stomach, pancreas

Dosage and routes:
• *Adult:* IV 12 mg/kg/day × 4 days, not to exceed 800 mg/day; may repeat with 6 mg/kg on day 6, 8, 10, 12; maintenance is 10-15 mg/kg/wk as a single dose, not to exceed 1 g/wk

Available forms: Inj IV 50 mg/ml

Side effects/adverse reactions:
CV: Myocardial ischemia, angina
HEMA: **Thrombocytopenia, leukopenia, myelosuppression, anemia, agranulocytosis**
GI: Anorexia, *stomatitis,* diarrhea, nausea, vomiting, **hemorrhage,** *enteritis glossitis*
GU: **Renal failure**

italics = common side effects   ***bold italic*** = life threatening reactions

EENT: Epistaxsis
INTEG: Rash, fever
CNS: Lethargy, malaise, weakness
Contraindications: Hypersensitivity, myelosuppression, pregnancy (D), poor nutritional status, serious infections
Precautions: Renal disease, hepatic disease, bone marrow depression, angina, lactation, children
Pharmacokinetics: Half-life 10-20 min, 20 hr terminal; metabolized in the liver; excreted in the urine; crosses blood-brain barrier
Interactions/incompatibilities:
• Increased toxicity: radiation or other antineoplastics
• Incompatible with droperidol, cytarabine or other antineoplastics, diazepam in sol or syringe
Lab test interferences:
Increase: Liver function studies, 6-HIAA
Decrease: Albumin

NURSING CONSIDERATIONS
Assess:
• CBC, differential, platelet count weekly; withhold drug if WBC is <3500/mm^3 or platelet count is <100,000/mm^3; notify physician of these results; drug should be discontinued
• Renal function studies: BUN, serum uric acid, urine CrCl, electrolytes before, during therapy
• I&O ratio; report fall in urine output to <30 ml/hr
• Temperature q4h; fever may indicate beginning infection
• Liver function tests before, during therapy: bilirubin, alk phosphatase, AST, ALT, LDH; as needed or monthly
• Bleeding: hematuria, guaiac, bruising or petechiae, mucosa or orifices q8h
• Food preferences; list likes, dislikes
• Inflammation of mucosa, breaks in skin
• Buccal cavity q8h for dryness, sores or ulceration, white patches, oral pain, bleeding, dysphagia
• Symptoms indicating severe allergic reaction: rash, urticaria, itching, flushing
• GI symptoms: frequency of stools, cramping
• Acidosis, signs of dehydration: rapid respirations, poor skin turgor, decreased urine output, dry skin, restlessness, weakness
Administer:
• IV undiluted; may inject through Y-tube or 3-way stopcock; give over 1-3 min; may be diluted in NS, D$_5$W, given over 2-8 hr as an IV inf
• Antiemetic 30-60 min before giving drug to prevent vomiting
• Antibiotics for prophylaxis of infection
• Topical or systemic analgesics for pain
• Transfusion for anemia
• Antispasmodic for diarrhea
Perform/provide:
• Protection from light
• Strict medical asepsis, protective isolation if WBC levels are low
• Increase fluid intake to 2-3 L/day to prevent dehydration, unless contraindicated
• Changing of IV site q48h
• Rinsing of mouth tid-qid with water, club soda; brushing of teeth bid-tid with soft brush or cotton-tipped applicator for stomatitis; use unwaxed dental floss
• Nutritious diet with iron, vitamin supplements, low fiber, few dairy products, especially when combined with radiotherapy as ordered
Evaluate:
• Therapeutic response: decreased tumor size, spread of malignancy

Teach patient/family:
• Why protective isolation is necessary
• To avoid foods with citric acid, hot or rough texture if stomatitis is present; to drink adequate fluids
• To report stomatitis: any bleeding, white spots, ulcerations in mouth; tell patient to examine mouth qd, report symptoms
• To report signs of infection: increased temperature, sore throat, flu symptoms
• To report signs of anemia: fatigue, headache, faintness, shortness of breath, irritability
• To report bleeding: avoid use of razors, commercial mouthwash
• To avoid use of aspirin products or ibuprofen
• To use contraception during therapy (men and women)

---

fluoxetine
(floo-ox'e-teen)
Prozac
Func. class.: Bicyclic antidepressant

Action: Inhibits CNS neuron uptake of serotonin, but not of norepinephrine
Uses: Major depressive disorder
Dosage and routes:
• *Adult:* PO 20 mg qd in AM; after 4 wk if no clinical improvement is noted, dose may be increased to 20 mg bid in AM, afternoon, not to exceed 80 mg/day
Available forms: Pulvules 20 mg, cap 10 mg, liquid 20 mg/5 ml
Side effects/adverse reactions:
*CNS: Headache, nervousness, insomnia, drowsiness, anxiety, tremor, dizziness, fatigue, sedation, poor concentration, abnormal dreams, agitation, **convulsions,***

apathy, euphoria, hallucinations, delusions, psychosis
GI: Nausea, diarrhea, dry mouth, anorexia, dyspepsia, constipation, cramps, vomiting, taste changes, flatulence, decreased appetite
INTEG: Sweating, rash, pruritus, acne, alopecia, urticaria
RESP: Infection, pharyngitis, nasal congestion, sinus headache, sinusitus, cough, dyspnea, bronchitis, asthma, hyperventilation, pneumonia
CV: Hot flashes, palpitations, angina pectoris, **hemorrhage,** hypertension, tachycardia, first-degree AV block, bradycardia, *MI,* thrombophlebitis
MS: Pain, arthritis, twitching
GU: Dysmenorrhea, decreased libido, urinary frequency, urinary tract infection, amenorrhea, cystitis, impotence
EENT: Visual changes, ear/eye pain, photophobia, tinnitus
SYST: Asthenia, viral infection, fever, allergy, chills
Contraindications: Hypersensitivity
Precautions: Pregnancy (B), lactation, children, elderly
Pharmacokinetics:
PO: Peak 6-8 hr; metabolized in liver; excreted in urine; half-life 2-7 days
Interactions/incompatibilities:
• Do not use with MAOIs
• Increased agitation: L-tryptophan
• Increased side effects: highly protein-bound drugs (i.e., fluoxetine)
• Increased half-life of: diazepam
Lab test interferences:
Increase: Serum bilirubin, blood glucose, alk phosphatase
Decrease: VMA, 5-HIAA
False increase: Urinary catecholamines

---

italics = common side effects   ***bold italic*** = life threatening reactions

NURSING CONSIDERATIONS
Assess:
• Mental status: mood, sensorium, affect, suicidal tendencies, increase in psychiatric symptoms, depression, panic
• B/P (lying/standing), pulse q4h; if systolic B/P drops 20 mm Hg, hold drug, notify physician; take vital signs q4h in patients with cardiovascular disease
• Blood studies: CBC, leukocytes, differential, cardiac enzymes if patient is receiving long-term therapy
• Hepatic studies: AST, ALT, bilirubin, creatinine
• Weight qwk; appetite may decrease with drug
• ECG for flattening of T wave, bundle branch, AV block, dysrhythmias in cardiac patients
• EPS primarily in elderly: rigidity, dystonia, akathisia
• Urinary retention, constipation
• Withdrawal symptoms: headache, nausea, vomiting, muscle pain, weakness; do not usually occur unless drug was discontinued abruptly
• Alcohol consumption; if alcohol is consumed, hold dose until morning
Administer:
• Increased fluids, bulk in diet if constipation, urinary retention occur
• With food or milk for GI symptoms
• Crushed if patient is unable to swallow medication whole
• Dosage hs if oversedation occurs during the day; may take entire dose hs; elderly may not tolerate once/day dosing
• Gum, hard candy, frequent sips of water for dry mouth
Perform/provide:
• Storage at room temperature; do not freeze

• Assistance with ambulation during therapy, since drowsiness, dizziness occur
• Safety measures including side rails, primarily in elderly
• Checking to see PO medication swallowed
Evaluate:
• Therapeutic response: decreased depression
Teach patient/family:
• That therapeutic effect may take 2-3 wk
• To use caution in driving or other activities requiring alertness because of drowsiness, dizziness, or blurred vision
• Not to discontinue medication quickly after long-term use; may cause nausea, headache, malaise
• To avoid alcohol ingestion or other CNS depressants
• To notify physician if pregnant or plan to become pregnant or breastfeed

---

fluoxymesterone

(floo-ox-ee-mess'te-rone)
Fluoxymesterone, Halotestin
Func. class.: Androgenic anabolic steroid
Chem. class.: Halogenated testosterone derivative

Action: Increases weight by building body tissue, increases potassium, phosphorus, chloride, nitrogen levels, increases bone development
Uses: Impotence from testicular deficiency, hypogonadism; breast engorgement; palliative treatment of female breast cancer
Dosage and routes:
Hypogonadism/impotence
• *Adult:* PO 2-10 mg qd

Breast engorgement
• *Adult:* PO 2.5 mg qd, then 5-10 mg qd × 5 days
Breast cancer
• *Adult:* PO 15-30 mg qd in divided doses until therapeutic effect occurs, then dosage should be reduced
Available forms: Tabs 2, 5, 10 mg
Side effects/adverse reactions:
INTEG: Rash, acneiform lesions, oily hair, skin, flushing, sweating, acne vulgaris, alopecia, hirsutism
CNS: Dizziness, headache, fatigue, tremors, paresthesias, flushing, sweating, anxiety, lability, insomnia, carpal tunnel syndrome
MS: Cramps, spasms
CV: Increased B/P
GU: **Hematuria,** amenorrhea, vaginitis, decreased libido, decreased breast size, clitoral hypertrophy, testicular atrophy
GI: Nausea, vomiting, constipation, weight gain, ***cholestatic jaundice***
EENT: Conjunctional edema, nasal congestion
ENDO: Abnormal GTT
Contraindications: Severe renal disease, severe cardiac disease, severe hepatic disease, hypersensitivity, pregnancy (X), lactation, genital bleeding (abnormal) children
Precautions: Diabetes mellitus, CV disease, MI
Pharmacokinetics:
PO: Metabolized in liver; excreted in urine; crosses placenta; excreted in breast milk
Interactions/incompatibilities:
• Increased effects of: oral antidiabetics, oxyphenbutazone
• Increased PT: anticoagulants
• Edema: ACTH, adrenal steroids
• Decreased effects of: insulin
Lab test interferences:
Increase: Serum cholesterol, blood glucose, urine glucose

Decrease: Serum Ca, serum K, T_4, T_3, thyroid ^{131}I uptake test, urine 17-OHCS, 17-KS, PBI, BSP
NURSING CONSIDERATIONS
Assess:
• Weight daily; notify physician if weekly weight gain is >5 lb
• B/P q4h
• I&O ratio; be alert for decreasing urinary output, increasing edema
• Growth rate in children, since growth rate may be uneven (linear/bone growth) if used for extended periods
• Electrolytes: K, Na, Cl, cholesterol
• Liver function studies: ALT, AST, bilirubin
• Edema, hypertension, cardiac symptoms, jaundice
• Mental status: affect, mood, behavioral changes, aggression
• Signs of masculinization in female: increased libido, deepening of voice, breast tissue, enlarged clitoris, menstrual irregularities; male: gynecomastia, impotence, testicular atrophy
• Hypercalcemia: lethargy, polyuria, polydipsia, nausea, vomiting, constipation; drug may have to be decreased
• Hypoglycemia in diabetics, since oral antidiabetic action is increased
Administer:
• Titrated dose, use lowest effective dose
• With food or milk to decrease GI symptoms
Perform/provide:
• Diet with increased calories, protein; decrease Na, if edema occurs
Evaluate:
• Therapeutic response: increased appetite, stamina
Teach patient/family:
• That drug must be combined with

---

italics = common side effects   ***bold italic*** = life threatening reactions

complete health plan: diet, rest, exercise
• To notify physician if therapeutic response decreases
• Not to discontinue medication abruptly
• About change in sex characteristics
• Females to report menstrual irregularities
• That 1-3 mo course is necessary for response in breast cancer
• That steroids should not be used for body building

---

fluphenazine decanoate/fluphenazine enanthate/fluphenazine HCl

(floo-fen´-a-zeen)

Permitil, Prolixin, Fluphenazine Decanoate, Prolixin Decanoate, Prolixin Enanthate, Fluphenazine HCl

Func. class.: Antipsychotic/neuroleptic

Chem. class.: Phenothiazine, piperazine

Action: Depresses cerebral cortex, hypothalamus, limbic system, which control activity and aggression; blocks neurotransmission produced by dopamine at synapse; exhibits strong α-adrenergic and anticholinergic blocking action; mechanism for antipsychotic effects is unclear

Uses: Psychotic disorders, schizophrenia

Dosage and routes:

Enanthate, decanoate
• *Adult and child >12 yr:* SC 12.5-25 mg q1-3wk

HCl
• *Adult:* PO 2.5-10 mg, in divided doses q6-8h, not to exceed 20 mg qd; IM initially 1.25 mg then 2.5-10 mg in divided doses q6-8h
• *Child:* PO 0.25-3.5 mg qd in divided doses q 4-6 hrs., max 10 mg/qd

Available forms: HCl tabs 1, 2.5, 5, 10 mg; elix 2.5 mg/5 ml; conc 5 mg/ml; inj IM 10 mg/ml, enanthate, decanoate, inj SC, IM 25 mg/ml

Side effects/adverse reactions:

RESP: **Laryngospasm,** dyspnea, **respiratory depression**

CNS: Extrapyramidal symptoms: pseudoparkinsonism, akathisia, dystonia, tardive dyskinesia, drowsiness, headache, **seizures, neuroleptic malignant syndrome**

HEMA: Anemia, **leukopenia, leukocytosis, agranulocytosis**

INTEG: Rash, photosensitivity, dermatitis

EENT: Blurred vision, glaucoma, dry eyes

GI: Dry mouth, nausea, vomiting, anorexia, constipation, diarrhea, jaundice, weight gain, **paralytic ileus, hepatitis**

GU: Urinary retention, urinary frequency, enuresis, impotence, amenorrhea, gynecomastia

CV: Orthostatic hypotension, hypertension, **cardiac arrest,** ECG changes, **tachycardia**

Contraindications: Hypersensitivity, circulatory collapse, liver damage, cerebral arteriosclerosis, coronary disease, severe hypertension/hypotension, blood dyscrasias, coma, child <12 yr, brain damage, bone marrow depression, alcohol and barbiturate withdrawal

Precautions: Pregnancy (C), lactation, seizure disorders, hypertension, hepatic disease, cardiac disease

Pharmacokinetics:

PO/IM (HCl): Onset 1 hr, peak 2-4 hr, duration 6-8 hr

SC (enanthate): Onset 1-2 days, peak 2-3 days, duration 1-3 wk, half-life 3.5-4 days; decanoate: onset 1-3 days, peak 1-2 days, duration over 4 wk, half-life (single dose) 6.8-9.6 days, (multiple dose) 14.3 days; metabolized by liver; excreted in urine (metabolites); crosses placenta; enters breast milk

Interactions/incompatibilities:

• Oversedation: other CNS depressants, alcohol, barbiturate anesthetics
• Toxicity: epinephrine
• Decreased effects of: levodopa, lithium
• Decreased effects of: fluphenazine: smoking, phenobarbital
• Increased effects of both drugs: β-adrenergic blockers, alcohol
• Increased anticholinergic effects: anticholinergics

Lab test interferences:

Increase: Liver function tests, cardiac enzymes, cholesterol, blood glucose, prolactin, bilirubin, PBI, cholinesterase

Decrease: Hormones (blood and urine)

False positive: Pregnancy tests, PKU

False negative: Urinary steroids, 17-OHCS, pregnancy tests

NURSING CONSIDERATIONS

Assess:

• Swallowing of PO medication; check for hoarding or giving of medication to other patients
• I&O ratio; palpate bladder if low urinary output occurs
• Bilirubin, CBC, liver function studies monthly
• Urinalysis is recommended before and during prolonged therapy
• Affect, orientation, LOC, reflexes, gait, coordination, sleep pattern disturbances
• B/P standing and lying; take pulse and respirations q4h during initial treatment; establish baseline before starting treatment; report drops of 30 mm Hg
• Dizziness, faintness, palpitations, tachycardia on rising
• Extrapyramidal symptoms including akathisia (inability to sit still, no pattern to movements), tardive dyskinesia (bizarre movements of jaw, mouth, tongue, extremities), pseudoparkinsonism (rigidity, tremors, pill rolling, shuffling gait)
• Skin turgor daily
• Constipation, urinary retention daily; if these occur, increase bulk, H_2O in diet

Administer:

• Concentrate with juice, milk, or uncaffeinated drinks
• Antiparkinsonian agent if extrapyramidal symptoms occur
• IM injection into large muscle mass; to minimize postural hypotension, give injection and have patient remain seated or recumbent for ½ hr
• Use dry needle, or solution will become cloudy; use No. 21 G or larger due to viscosity

Perform/provide:

• Decreased noise input by dimming lights, avoiding loud noises
• Supervised ambulation until stabilized on medication; do not involve in strenuous exercise program because fainting is possible; patient should not stand still for long periods
• Increased fluids to prevent constipation
• Sips of water, candy, gum for dry mouth

---

italics = common side effects   ***bold italic*** = life threatening reactions

• Storage in tight, light-resistant container in cool environment

Evaluate:

• Therapeutic response: decrease in emotional excitement, hallucinations, delusions, paranoia, reorganization of patterns of thought, speech

Teach patient/family:

• That orthostatic hypotension occurs often; to rise from sitting or lying position gradually; avoid hazardous activities until stabilized on medication

• To avoid hot tubs, hot showers or tub baths, since hypotension may occur

• To avoid abrupt withdrawal of this drug, or extrapyramidal symptoms may result; drug should be withdrawn slowly

• To avoid OTC preparations (cough, hay fever, cold) unless approved by physician, since serious drug interactions may occur; avoid use with alcohol or CNS depressants; increased drowsiness may occur

• To use a sunscreen during sun exposure to prevent burns

• Regarding compliance with drug regimen

• About extrapyramidal symptoms and necessity for meticulous oral hygiene, since oral candidiasis may occur

• To report sore throat, malaise, fever, bleeding, mouth sores; if these occur, CBC should be drawn and drug discontinued

• That in hot weather, heat stroke may occur; take extra precautions to stay cool

• That urine may turn pink to reddish-brown

Treatment of overdose: Lavage; if orally ingested, provide an airway; *do not induce vomiting*

flurandrenolide

(flure-an-dren'oh-lide)
Cordran, Cordran SP, Cordran Tape, Drenison 1/4,* Drenison Tape*

Func. class.: Topical corticosteroid

Chem. class.: Synthetic fluorinated agent

Action: Antipruritic, antiinflammatory

Uses: Corticosteroid-responsive dermatoses, pruritus

Dosage and routes:

• *Adult and child:* TOP apply to affected area tid-qid; apply tape q12-24h

Available forms: Oint 0.025%, 0.05%; cream 0.025%, 0.05%; lotion 0.05%; tape 4 $\mu g/cm^2$

Side effects/adverse reactions:

INTEG: Burning, dryness, itching, irritation, acne, folliculitis, hypertrichosis, perioral dermatitis, hypopigmentation, atrophy, striae, miliaria, allergic contact dermatitis, secondary infection

Contraindications: Hypersensitivity to corticosteroids, fungal infections, viral infections

Precautions: Pregnancy (C), lactation, viral infections, bacterial infections

NURSING CONSIDERATIONS

Assess:

• Temperature; if fever develops drug should be discontinued

• Systemic absorption: fever, infection, irritation

Administer:

• Only to affected areas; do not get in eyes

• Then cover with occlusive dressing if ordered; seal to normal skin; change q12h; systemic absorption may occur

---

• Only to dermatoses; do not use on weeping, denuded, or infected area
• Tape after cutting with scissors; apply only to clean, dry wounds
Perform/provide:
• Cleansing before application of drug
• Treatment for a few days after area has cleared
• Storage at room temperature
Evaluate:
• Therapeutic response: absence of severe itching, patches on skin, flaking
Teach patient/family:
• To avoid sunlight on affected area; burns may occur

---

flurazepam HCl
(flure-az'e-pam)
Dalmane, Flurazepam, Somnol*

Func. class.: Sedative-hypnotic
Chem. class.: Benzodiazepine derivative

Controlled Substance Schedule IV (USA), Schedule F (Canada)
Action: Produces CNS depression at the limbic, thalamic, hypothalamic levels of CNS; may be mediated by neurotransmitter γ-aminobutyric acid (GABA); results are sedation, hypnosis, skeletal muscle relaxation, anticonvulsant activity, anxiolytic action
Uses: Insomnia
Dosage and routes:
• *Adult:* PO 15-30 mg hs; may repeat dose once if needed
• *Geriatric:* PO 15 mg hs; may increase if needed
Available forms: Caps 15, 30 mg
Side effects/adverse reactions:
HEMA: **Leukopenia, granulocytopenia** (rare)

CNS: *Lethargy, drowsiness, daytime sedation,* dizziness, confusion, light-headedness, headache, anxiety, irritability
GI: Nausea, vomiting, diarrhea, heartburn, abdominal pain, constipation
CV: Chest pain, pulse changes
Contraindications: Hypersensitivity to benzodiazepines, pregnancy, lactation, intermittent porphyria, uncontrolled pain
Precautions: Anemia, hepatic disease, renal disease, suicidal individuals, drug abuse, elderly, psychosis, child <15 yr
Pharmacokinetics:
PO: Onset 15-45 min, duration 7-8 hr; metabolized by liver; excreted by kidneys (inactive/active metabolites); crosses placenta; excreted in breast milk; half-life 47-100 hr, additional 100 hr for active metabolites
Interactions/incompatibilities:
• Increased effects of flurazepam: cimetidine, disulfiram, probenicid, isoniazid
• Increased action of both drugs: alcohol, CNS depressants
• Decreased effect of flurazepam: antacids, theophylline, rifampin, smoking
Lab test interferences:
Increase: AST/ALT, serum bilirubin
False increase: Urinary 17-OHCS
Decrease: RAI uptake
NURSING CONSIDERATIONS
Assess:
• Blood studies: Hct, Hgb, RBC (if on long-term therapy)
• Hepatic studies: AST, ALT, bilirubin
• Mental status: mood, sensorium, affect, memory (long, short)
• Blood dyscrasias: fever, sore

italics = common side effects   ***bold italic*** = life threatening reactions

throat, bruising, rash, jaundice, epistaxis (rare)
• Type of sleep problem: falling asleep, staying asleep
Administer:
• After removal of cigarettes to prevent fires
• After trying conservative measures for insomnia
• ½-1 hr before hs for sleeplessness
• On empty stomach for fast onset, but may be taken with food if GI symptoms occur
Perform/provide:
• Assistance with ambulation after receiving dose
• Safety measure: side rails, night-light, call bell within easy reach
• Checking to see PO medication has been swallowed
• Storage in tight container in cool environment
Evaluate:
• Therapeutic response: ability to sleep at night, decreased amount of early morning awakening if taking drug for insomnia
Teach patient/family:
• To avoid driving or other activities requiring alertness until drug is stabilized
• To avoid alcohol ingestion or CNS depressants; serious CNS depression may result
• That effects may take 2 nights for benefits to be noticed
• Alternate measures to improve sleep: reading, exercise several hours before hs, warm bath, warm milk, TV, self-hypnosis, deep breathing
• That hangover is common in elderly but less common than with barbiturates
Treatment of overdose: Lavage, activated charcoal; monitor electrolytes, vital signs

flurbiprofen sodium
(flure-bi′proe-fen)
Ocufen
Func. class.: Nonsteroidal antiinflammatory ophthalmic
Chem. class.: Phenylalkanoic acid

Action: Inhibits enzyme system necessary for biosynthesis of prostaglandins; inhibits miosis
Uses: Inhibition of intraoperative miosis, corneal edema
Dosage and routes:
• *Adult:* 1 gtt q½h 2 hr before surgery (4 gtt total)
Available forms: Sol 0.03%
Side effects/adverse reactions:
EENT: Burning, stinging in the eye, irritation, bleeding or redness
Contraindications: Hypersensitivity, epithelial herpes simplex keratitis
Precautions: Pregnancy (C), lactation, child, aspirin or nonsteroidal antiinflammatory drug hypersensitivity, allergy, bleeding disorder
Interactions/incompatibilities:
• Ineffective action of: acetylcholine, carbachol
NURSING CONSIDERATIONS
Administer:
• Excess solution must be wiped away promptly to prevent its flow into lacrimal system, producing systemic symptoms
Perform/provide:
• Protect solution from sun
Evaluate:
• Therapeutic response: absence of corneal edema, intraoperative miosis
Teach patient/family:
• To report change in vision, blurring, or loss of sight during miosis

• Not to use for any other condition than prescribed

---

flutamide
(floo'-ta-mide)
Eulexin
Func. class.: Antineoplastic hormone
Chem. class.: Antiandrogen

Action: Interferes with testosterone uptake in the nucleus or testosterone activity in target tissues; arrests tumor growth in androgen-sensitive tissue, i.e., prostate gland; prostatic carcinoma is androgen-sensitive, so tumor growth is arrested
Uses: Metastatic prostatic carcinoma, stage D2 in combination with LHRH agonist analogs (leuprolide)
Dosage and routes:
• *Adult:* PO 250 mg q8h tid, for a daily dosage of 750 mg
Available forms: cap 125 mg
Side effects/adverse reactions:
CNS: Hot flashes, drowsiness, confusion, depression, anxiety
GU: Decreased libido, impotence, gynecomastia
GI: Diarrhea, nausea, vomiting, increased liver function studies, **hepatitis,** anorexia
INTEG: Irritation at site, rash, photosensitivity
MISC: Edema, hematopoietic symptoms, neuromuscular and pulmonary symptoms, hypertension
Contraindications: Hypersensitivity, pregnancy (D)
Pharmacokinetics: Rapidly and completely absorbed; excreted in urine and feces as metabolites; half-life 6 hr, geriatric half-life 8 hr; 94% bound to plasma proteins
NURSING CONSIDERATIONS
Assess:
• Liver function studies: AST,

ALT, alk phosphatase, which may be elevated
• For CNS symptoms: drowsiness, confusion, depression, anxiety
Evaluate:
• Therapeutic response: decrease in prostatic tumor size, decrease in spread of cancer
Teach patient/family:
• To report side effects: decreased libido, impotence, breast enlargement, hot flashes, diarrhea
• That this drug is taken with leuprolide
Treatment of overdose: Induce vomiting, provide supportive care

---

folic acid (vitamin B₉)
Apo-Folic, Folvite, Novofolacid*
Func. class.: Vitamin B complex group

Action: Needed for erythropoiesis; increases RBC, WBC, and platelet formation in megaloblastic anemias
Uses: Megaloblastic or macrocytic anemia caused by folic acid deficiency; liver disease, alcoholism, hemolysis, intestinal obstruction, pregnancy
Dosage and routes:
Supplement
• *Adult:* PO/IM/SC/IV 0.1 mg qd
• *Child:* PO/IM/SC/IV 0.05 mg qd
Megaloblastic/macrocytic anemia
• *Adult and child >4 yr:* PO/SC/IM/IV 1 mg qd × 4-5 days
• *Child <4 yr:* PO/SC/IM/IV 0.3 mg or less qd
• *Pregnancy/lactation:* PO/SC/IM/IV 0.8 mg qd
Prevention of megaloblastic/macrocytic anemia
• *Pregnancy:* PO/SC/IM/IV 1 mg qd

---

italics = common side effects   ***bold italic*** = life threatening reactions

Available forms: Tabs 0.1, 0.4, 0.8, 1 mg; inj SC, IM, IV 5, 10 mg/ml

Side effects/adverse reactions:
RESP: **Bronchospasm**
INTEG: Flushing

Contraindications: Hypersensitivity, anemias other than megaloblastic/macrocytic anemia, Vit B$_{12}$ deficiency anemia, uncorrected pernicious anemia

Precautions: Pregnancy (A)

Pharmacokinetics:
PO: Peak ½-1 hr; bound to plasma proteins; excreted in breast milk; methylated in liver; excreted in urine (small amounts)

Interactions/incompatibilities:
• Decreased folate levels: chloramphenicol
• Increased metabolism of: phenobarbitol, hydantoins
• Do not use with methotrexate unless leucovorin rescue is available
• Incompatible with Ca, chlorpromazine, 40% dextrose or greater concentrations, iron sulfate, Vit B complex with C in sol or syringe

NURSING CONSIDERATIONS
Assess:
• Hgb, Hct and reticulocyte count
• Folate levels: 6-15 μg/ml
• Nutritional status: bran, yeast, dried beans, nuts, fruits, fresh vegetables, asparagus
• Drugs currently taken: alcohol, oral contraceptives, hydantoins, trimethoprim; these drugs may cause increased folic acid use by body and contribute to a deficiency

Administer:
• IV direct undiluted 5 mg or less/1 min or may be added to most IV sol or TPN

Perform/provide:
• Storage in light-resistant container

Evaluate:
• Therapeutic response: increased weight, oriented well-being; absence of fatigue

Teach patient/family:
• To take drug exactly as prescribed
• To notify physician of side effects

---

foscarnet sodium
(foss-car′net)
Foscavir
Func. class.: Antiviral
Chem. class.: Inorganic pyrophosphate organic analog

Action: Antiviral activity is produced by selective inhibition at the pyrophosphate binding site on virus-specific DNA polymerases and reverse transcriptases at concentrations that do not affect cellular DNA polymerases

Uses: Treatment of CMV retinitis, colitis in AIDS

Dosage and routes:
• *Adult:* IV INF 60 mg/kg given over at least 1 hr, q8hr × 2-3 wk initially, then 90-120 mg/kg/day over 2 hr, usually give with at least 750-1000 ml NS qd

In renal abnormalities:
• *Adult:* IV Male:

$$\frac{140 - age}{serum\ creatinine \times 72} = Ccr$$

Female: 0.85 × above value
Dose based on table provided in package insert

Available forms: Inj 24 mg/ml

Side effects/adverse reactions:
CNS: Fever, dizziness, headache, *seizures,* fatigue, neuropathy, tremor, ataxia, dementia, stupor, EEG abnormalities, vertigo, *coma,* abnormal gait, hypertonia, extrapyramidal disorders, hemiparesis,

paralysis, hyperreflexia paraplegia, *tetany,* hyporeflexia, neuralgia, neuritis, cerebral edema, paresthesia, depression, confusion, anxiety, insomnia, somnolence, amnesia, hallucinations, agitation
GI: *Nausea, vomiting,* anorexia, abdominal pain, constipation, dysphagia, rectal hemorrhage, dry mouth, melena, flatulence, ulcerative stomatitis, pancreatitis, enteritis, enterocolitis, glossitis, proctitis, stomatitis, increased amylases, gastroenteritis, *pseudomembranous colitis,* duodenal ulcer, *paralytic ileus, esophageal ulceration,* abnormal A-G ratio, increased AST, ALT, cholecystitis, *hepatitis,* dyspepsia, tenesmus, hepatosplenomegaly, jaundice
INTEG: Rash, sweating, pruritus, skin ulceration, seborrhea, skin discoloration, alopecia, acne, dermatitis, pain/inflammation at injection site, facial edema, dry skin, urticaria
HEMA: Anemia, *granulocytopenia, leukopenia, thrombocytopenia,* platelet abnormalities, *thrombosis, pulmonary embolism, coagulation disorders, decreased prothrombin, hypochromic anemia, pancytopenia, hemolysis, leukocytosis,* lymphadenopathy, epistaxis, lymphopenia
SYST: Hypokalemia, hypocalcemia, hypomagnesemia, increased alk phosphatase, LDH, BUN, acidosis, hypophosphatemia, hyperphosphatemia, dehydration, glycosuria, increased creatine phosphokinase, hypervolemia, infection, *sepsis, death, ascites,* hyponatremia, hypochloremia, hypercalcemia
GU: *Acute renal failure,* decreased Ccr and increased serum creatinine, *glomerulonephritis, toxic ne-*phropathy, *nephrosis, renal tubular disorders, pyelonephritis, uremia, hematuria, albuminuria,* dysuria, polyuria
RESP: Coughing, dyspnea, pneumonia, sinusitis, pharyngitis, *pulmonary infiltration,* stridor, *pneumothorax, hemoptysis, bronchospasm,* bronchitis, *respiratory depression, pleural effusion, pulmonary hemorrhage,* rhinitis
EENT: Visual field defects, vocal cord paralysis, speech disorders, taste perversion, eye pain, conjunctivitis, tinnitus, otitis
CV: Hypertension, palpitations, ECG abnormalities, 1st degree AV block, nonspecific ST-T segment changes, hypotension, cerebrovascular disorder, cardiomyopathy, *cardiac arrest,* bradycardia, dysrhythmias
MS: Arthralgia, myalgia
Contraindications: Hypersensitivity
Precautions: Pregnancy (C), lactation, children, elderly, renal disease, seizure disorders, electrolyte/mineral imbalances, severe anemia
Pharmacokinetics: 14%-17% plasma protein bound, half-life 2-8 hr in normal renal function
Interactions/incompatibilities:
• Nephrotoxicity: aminoglycosides, amphotericin B, IV pentamidine
• Hypocalcemia: pentamidine
• Increased anemia: zidovudine
NURSING CONSIDERATIONS
Assess:
• Kidney, liver function studies: BUN, creatinine, AST, ALT
• I&O ratio, urine pH
• Blood counts q2wk; watch for decreasing granulocytes, Hgb; if low, therapy may have to be discontinued and restarted after hematologic

---

italics = common side effects   ***bold italic*** = life threatening reactions

recovery; blood transfusions may be required

• GI symptoms: severe nausea, vomiting, diarrhea; severe symptoms may necessitate discontinuing drug

• Electrolytes and minerals: Ca, P, Mg, Na, K; watch closely for tetany during first administration

• Blood dyscrasias (anemia, granulocytopenia); bruising, fatigue, bleeding, poor healing

• Allergic reactions: flushing, rash, urticaria, pruritus

Administer:

• Increased fluids before and during drug administration to induce diuresis and minimize renal toxicity

• Using infusion device, at no more than 1 mg/kg/min; do not give by rapid or bolus IV; give by CVP or peripheral vein; standard 24 mg/ml solution may be used without dilution if using by CVP; dilute the 24 mg/ml sol to 12 mg/ml with D_5W or normal saline if using peripheral vein

Perform/provide:

• Regular ophthalmologic exams

• Close monitoring during therapy if tingling, numbness, paresthesias; if these occur, stop infusion, obtain lab sample for electrolytes

Evaluate:

• Therapeutic response: improvement in CMV retinitis

Teach patient/family:

• To call physician if sore throat, swollen lymph nodes, malaise, fever occur, since other infections may occur

• To report perioral tingling, numbness in extremities, and paresthesias

• That serious drug interactions may occur if OTC products are ingested; check first with physician

• That drug is not a cure, but will control symptoms

---

fosinopril
(foss-in-o'pril)
Monopril
Func. class.: Antihypertensive
Chem. class.: Angiotension-converting enzyme (ACE) inhibitor

Action: Selectively suppresses renin-angiotensin-aldosterone system; inhibits ACE; prevents conversion of angiotensin I to angiotensin II; results in dilation of arterial, venous vessels

Uses: Hypertension, alone or in combination with thiazide diuretics

Dosage and routes:

• *Adult:* PO 10 mg qd initially, then 20-40 mg/day divided bid or qd

Available forms: Tabs 10, 20 mg

Side effects/adverse reactions:

CV: Hypotension, chest pain, palpitations, angina, orthostatic hypotension

GU: Proteinuria, Increased BUN, creatinine, decreased libido

HEMA: Decreased Hct, Hgb, *eosinophilia, leukopenia, neutropenia*

INTEG: Angioedema, rash, flushing, sweating, photosensitivity, pruritus

RESP: Cough, sinusitis, dyspnea, *bronchospasm*

META: Hyperkalemia

GI: Nausea, constipation, vomiting, diarrhea

CNS: Insomnia, paresthesia, headache, dizziness, fatigue, memory disturbance, tremor, mood change

MS: Arthralgia, myalgia

Contraindications: Hypersensitivity to ACE inhibitors, pregnancy (D), lactation, children

Precautions: Impaired liver function, hypovolemia, blood dyscrasias, CHF, COPD, asthma, elderly

Pharmacokinetics:

PO: Peak 3 hr; serum protein binding 97%; half-life 12 hr; metabolized by liver (metabolites excreted in urine, feces)

Interactions/incompatibilities:

• Increased hypotension: diuretics, other antihypertensives, ganglionic blockers, adrenergic blockers

• Increased toxicity: vasodilators, hydralazine, prazosin, K-sparing diuretics, sympathomimetics

• Decreased absorption: antacids

• Decreased antihypertensive effect: indomethacin

• Increased serum levels of: digoxin, lithium

• Increased hypersensitivity: allopurinol

Lab test interferences:

False positive: Urine acetone

NURSING CONSIDERATIONS

Assess:

• Blood studies: neutrophils, decreased platelets

• B/P, orthostatic hypotension, syncope

• Renal studies: protein, BUN, creatinine; watch for increased levels that may indicate nephrotic syndrome

• Baselines in renal, liver function tests before therapy begins

• K levels, although hyperkalemia rarely occurs

• Dipstick of urine for protein qd in first morning specimen; if protein is increased, a 24-hr urinary protein should be collected

• Edema in feet, legs daily

• Allergic reactions: rash, fever, pruritus, urticaria; drug should be discontinued if antihistamines fail to help

• Renal symptoms: polyuria, oliguria, frequency, dysuria

Administer:

• IV infusion of 0.9% NaCl (as ordered) to expand fluid volume if severe hypotension occurs

Perform/provide:

• Storage in tight container at 86° F (30° C) or less

• Supine or Trendelenburg position for severe hypotension

Evaluate:

• Therapeutic response: decrease in B/P

Teach patient/family:

• Not to discontinue drug abruptly

• Not to use OTC products (cough, cold, allergy) unless directed by physician; do not use salt substitutes containing potassium without consulting physician

• Importance of complying with dosage schedule, even if feeling better

• To rise slowly to sitting or standing position to minimize orthostatic hypotension

• To notify physician of mouth sores, sore throat, fever, swelling of hands or feet, irregular heart beat, chest pain

• To report excessive perspiration, dehydration, vomiting, diarrhea; may lead to fall in B/P

• That drug may cause dizziness, fainting, light-headedness during 1st few days of therapy

• That drug may cause skin rash or impaired perspiration

• How to take B/P; normal readings for age group

Treatment of overdose: 0.9% NaCl IV INF, hemodialysis

---

italics = common side effects   ***bold italic*** = life threatening reactions

furosemide

(fur-oh'se-mide)
Fumide, Furomide M.D., Furosemide, Lasix, Luramide, Novosemide,* Uritol*
Func. class.: Loop diuretic
Chem. class.: Sulfonamide derivative

Uses: Pulmonary edema; edema in CHF, liver disease, nephrotic syndrome, ascites, hypertension

Dosage and routes:

• *Adult:* PO 20-80 mg/day in AM; may give another dose in 6 hr up to 600 mg/day; IM/IV 20-40 mg, increased by 20 mg q2h until desired response

• *Child:* PO/IM/IV 2 mg/kg; may increase by 1-2 mg/kg/q6-8h up to 6 mg/kg

Pulmonary edema

• *Adult:* IV 40 mg given over several minutes, repeated in 1 hr; increase to 80 mg if needed

Available forms: Tabs 20, 40, 80 mg; oral sol 10 mg/ml; inj IM, IV 10 mg/ml

Side effects/adverse reactions:

CNS: Headache, fatigue, weakness, vertigo, paresthesias

CV: Orthostatic hypotension, chest pain, ECG changes, *circulatory collapse*

EENT: Loss of hearing, ear pain, tinnitus, blurred vision

ELECT: Hypokalemia, hypochloremic alkalosis, hypomagnesemia, hyperuricemia, hypocalcemia, hyponatremia, metabolic alkalosis

ENDO: Hyperglycemia

GI: Nausea, diarrhea, dry mouth, vomiting, anorexia, cramps, oral, gastric irritations, pancreatitis

GU: Polyuria, renal failure, glycosuria

HEMA: Thrombocytopenia, agranulocytosis, leukopenia, neutropenia, anemia

INTEG: Rash, pruritus, purpura, *Stevens-Johnson syndrome,* sweating, photosensitivity, urticaria

MS: Cramps, stiffness

Contraindications: Hypersensitivity to sulfonamides, anuria, hypovolemia, infants, lactation, electrolyte depletion

Precautions: Diabetes mellitus, dehydration, severe renal disease, pregnancy (C)

Pharmacokinetics:

PO: Onset 1 hr, peak 1-2 hr, duration 6-8 hr; absorbed 70%

IV: Onset 5 min, peak ½ hr, duration 2 hr (metabolized by the liver 30%)

Excreted in urine, some as unchanged drug, feces; crosses placenta; excreted in breast milk; half-life ½-1 hour

Interactions/incompatibilities:

• Increased toxicity: lithium, nondepolarizing skeletal muscle relaxants, digitalis

• Increased action of: antihypertensives, oral anticoagulants, nitrates

• Increased ototoxicity: aminoglycosides, cisplatin, vancomycin

• Decreased antihypertensive effect of furosemide: indomethacin, metolazone

• Incompatible in sol with acidic sol, Vit C, corticosteroids, diphenhydramine, dobutamine, esmolol, epinephrine, gentamicin, levarterenol, meperidine, milrione, netilmicin, reserpine, spironolactone, tetracyclines; incompatible with any drug in syringe

Lab test interferences:

Interference: GTT

NURSING CONSIDERATIONS
Assess:
• Signs of metabolic alkalosis: drowsiness, restlessness
• Signs of hypokalemia: postural hypotension, malaise, fatigue, tachycardia, leg cramps, weakness
• Rashes, temperature elevation qd
• Confusion, especially in elderly; take safety precautions if needed
• Hearing, including tinnitus and hearing loss, when giving high doses for extended periods
• Weight, I&O daily to determine fluid loss; effect of drug may be decreased if used qd
• Rate, depth, rhythm of respiration, effect of exertion, lung sounds
• B/P lying, standing; postural hypotension may occur
• Electrolytes: K, Na, Cl; include BUN, blood sugar, CBC, serum creatinine, blood pH, ABGs, uric acid, Ca, Mg
• Skin turgor, edema, condition of mucous membranes in mouth and nose
• Glucose in urine if patient is diabetic
• Allergies to sulfonamides, thiazides

Administer:
• IV undiluted; may be given through Y-tube or 3-way stopcock; give 20 mg or less/min; may be added to NS or D₅W if large doses are required and given as IV INF, not to exceed 4 mg/min; use infusion pump
• In AM to avoid interference with sleep if using drug as a diuretic
• K replacement if K is less than 3
• PO with food if nausea occurs; absorption may be decreased slightly; tablets may be crushed

Evaluate:
• Therapeutic response: improvement in edema of feet, legs, sacral area daily if medication is being used CHF

Teach patient/family:
• To discuss the need for a high-K diet or K replacement with physician
• To increase fluid intake 2-3 L/day unless contraindicated
• To rise slowly from lying or sitting position; orthostatic hypotension may occur
• Adverse reactions that may occur: muscle cramps, weakness, nausea, dizziness
• Regarding entire regimen, including exercise, diet, stress relief for hypertension
• To take with food or milk for GI symptoms
• To use sunscreen or protective clothing to prevent photosensitivity
• To take early in day to prevent sleeplessness
• To avoid OTC medication unless prescribed by physician

Treatment of overdose: Lavage if taken orally; monitor electrolytes; administer dextrose in saline; monitor hydration, CV, renal status

---

gabapentin
(gab'a-pen-tin)
Neurontin
Func. class.: Anticonvulsant

Action: Mechanism unknown; may increase seizure threshold; structurally similar to GABA; gabapentin binding sites in neocortex, hippocampus

Uses: Adjunct treatment of partial seizures, with or without generalization in adults

Dosage and routes:
• *Adult:* PO 900-1800 mg/day in 3 divided doses; may titrate by giving 300 mg on the first day, 300 mg

---

bid on second day, 300 mg tid on third day; may increase to 1800 mg/day by adding 300 mg on subsequent days

Available forms: Caps 100, 300, 400 mg

Side effects/adverse reactions:

CNS: Dizziness, fatigue, anxiety, somnolence, ataxia, amnesia, abnormal thinking, unsteady gait, depression

CV: Vasodilation

EENT: Dry mouth, blurred vision, diplopia

GI: Constipation, increased appetite, dental abnormalities

GU: Impotence, bleeding, *UTI*

HEMA: **Leukopenia,** decreased WBC

INTEG: Pruritus, abrasion

MS: Myalgia

RESP: Rhinitis, pharyngitis, coughing

Contraindications: Hypersensitivity to this drug

Precautions: Hepatic disease, renal disease, pregnancy (C), lactation, child <6 yr, elderly

Pharmacokinetics:
Largely unbound to plasma proteins; not metabolized; excreted in urine (unchanged); elimination half-life 5-7 hr

Interactions/incompatibilities:
• Decreased levels of gabapentin: antacids

NURSING CONSIDERATIONS
Assess:
• Renal studies: urinalysis, BUN, urine creatinine q3mo
• Hepatic studies: ALT, AST, bilirubin
• Description of seizures
• Mental status: mood, sensorium, affect, behavioral changes; if mental status changes, notify physician
• Eye problems, need for ophthalmic examinations before, during, after treatment (slit lamp, fundoscopy, tonometry)
• Allergic reaction: purpura, red raised rash; if these occur, drug should be discontinued

Administer:
• With food, milk to decrease GI symptoms

Perform/provide:
• Storage at room temperature away from heat and light
• Hard candy, frequent rinsing of mouth, gum for dry mouth
• Assistance with ambulation during early part of treatment; dizziness occurs

Evaluate:
• Therapeutic response: decreased seizure activity; document on patient's chart

Teach patient/family:
• To carry Medic Alert ID stating patient's name, drugs taken, condition, physician's name and phone number
• To avoid driving, other activities that require alertness
• Not to discontinue medication quickly after long-term use

Treatment of overdose: Lavage, VS

gallamine triethiodide
(gal'a-meen)
Flaxedil
Func. class.: Neuromuscular blocker (nondepolarizing)

Action: Inhibits transmission of nerve impulses by binding with cholinergic receptor sites, antagonizing action of acetylcholine

Uses: Facilitation of endotracheal intubation, skeletal muscle relaxation during mechanical ventilation, surgery, or general anesthesia

---

*Available in Canada only

Dosage and routes:
• *Adult and child >1 mo:* IV 1 mg/kg, not to exceed 100 mg, then 0.5-1 mg/kg q30-40 min
• *Child <1 mo, >5 kg:* IV 0.25-0.75 mg/kg, then 0.01-0.05 mg/kg q30-40 min
Available forms: Inj IV 20 mg/ml
Side effects/adverse reactions:
CV: Bradycardia, tachycardia, increased, decreased B/P
*RESP: **Prolonged apnea, bronchospasm, cyanosis, respiratory depression***
EENT: Increased secretions
INTEG: Rash, flushing, pruritus, urticaria
*CNS: **Malignant hyperthermia***
GI: Decreased motility
Contraindications: Hypersensitivity to iodides
Precautions: Pregnancy (C), thyroid disease, collagen disease, cardiac disease, lactation, children <2 yr, electrolyte imbalances, dehydration, neuromuscular disease (myasthenia gravis), respiratory disease, renal disease
Pharmacokinetics:
IV: Onset 2 min, duration 20-60 min; half-life 2 min, 29 min (terminal); excreted in urine, feces (metabolites); crosses placenta
Interactions/incompatibilities:
• Increased neuromuscular blockade: aminoglycosides, clindamycin, lincomycin, quinidine, local anesthetics, polymyxin antibiotics, lithium, narcotic analgesics, thiazides, enflurane, isoflurane; used with cyclopropane, may provoke ventricular dysrhythmias
• Dysrhythmias: theophylline
• Incompatible with anesthetics, barbiturates in sol; incompatible with any other drug in syringe
NURSING CONSIDERATIONS
Assess:
• For electrolyte imbalances (K,

Mg); may lead to increased action of this drug
• Vital signs (B/P, pulse, respirations, airway) q15min until fully recovered; rate, depth, pattern of respirations, strength of hand grip
• I&O ratio; check for urinary retention, frequency, hesitancy
• Recovery: decreased paralysis of face, diaphragm, leg, arm, rest of body
• Allergic reactions: rash, fever, respiratory distress, pruritus; drug should be discontinued
Administer:
• Using nerve stimulator by anesthesiologist to determine neuromuscular blockade
• Anticholinesterase to reverse neuromuscular blockade
• IV undiluted over 1-2 min (only by qualified person, usually an anesthesiologist)
• Only slightly discolored solution
Perform/provide:
• Storage in light-resistant, cool area
• Reassurance if communication is difficult during recovery from neuromuscular blockade
Evaluate:
• Therapeutic response: paralysis of jaw, eyelid, head, neck, rest of body
Treatment of overdose: Edrophonium or neostigmine, atropine; monitor VS; may require mechanical ventilation

---

gallium nitrate
(gal'ee-yum)
Ganite
Func. class.: Electrolyte modifier
Chem. class.: Hypocalcemic drug

Action: Lowers serum calcium

---

italics = common side effects   ***bold italic*** = life threatening reactions

levels by inhibiting calcium resorption from bone

Uses: Cancer-related hypercalcemia

Dosage and routes:
• *Adult:* IV 100-200 mg/m² qd × 5 days; infuse over 24 hr

Available forms: 25 mg/ml inj

Side effects/adverse reactions:
HEMA: Anemia, leukopenia
CV: Tachycardia
EENT: Blurred vision, optic neuritis, hearing loss
GU: Nephrotoxicity, increased BUN, creatinine
META: Hypophosphatemia, hypocalcemia, decreased serum bicarbonate

Contraindications: Hypersensitivity, severe renal disease

Precautions: Pregnancy (C), lactation, children, mild renal disease

Pharmacokinetics:
IV: Onset 12-24 hr, peak 5 days, duration 8 days

Interactions/incompatibilities:
• Increased nephrotoxicity: aminoglycosides, amphotericin B

NURSING CONSIDERATIONS
Assess:
• Renal status: BUN, creatinine, urine output
• Monitor Ca, phosphate, bicarbonate, since all levels may be decreased and supplements of phosphate may be needed
• For hypercalcemia: nausea, vomiting, fatigue, weakness, thirst, dehydration, dysrhythmias, change in mental status
• For hypocalcemia: dysrhythmias; paresthesia; twitching; colic; laryngospasm; Trousseau's, Chvostek's sign; tremors

Administer:
• Adequate hydration with IV saline, 2 L/day during treatment
• After dilution of dose/1 L 0.9%

NaCl or D₅W, run over 24 hr, use infusion pump

Perform/provide:
• Storage of solution for 48 hr at room temperature or 1 wk in refrigerator

Evaluate:
• Therapeutic response: decreased serum Ca levels

Teach patient/family:
• To follow dietary guidelines given by physician, including adequate Ca (dairy products, broccoli) and Vit D (fortified milk, grain products, fish oil)

---

ganciclovir (DHPG)
(gan-sy-clo-ver)
Cytovene
Func. class.: Antiviral
Chem. class.: Synthetic nucleoside analog

Action: Inhibits replication of herpesviruses in vitro, in vivo by selective inhibition of the human CMV DNA polymerase and by direct incorporation into viral DNA

Uses: Cytomegalovirus (CMV) retinitis in immunocompromised persons, including those with AIDS, after indirect ophthalmoscopy confirms diagnosis

Dosage and routes:
Induction treatment
• *Adult:* IV 5 mg/kg given over 1 hr, q12h × 2-3 wk
Maintenance treatment
• *Adult:* IV INF 5 mg/kg given over 1 hr, qd × 7 days/wk; or 6 mg/kg qd × 5 days/wk
• Dosage must be reduced in renal impairment

Available forms: powder 500 mg/ vial ganciclovir

Side effects/adverse reactions:
HEMA: Granulocytopenia, throm-

G

bocytopenia, irreversible neutropenia, anemia, eosinophilia
GI: Abnormal LFTs, nausea, vomiting, anorexia, diarrhea, abdominal pain, ***hemorrhage***
INTEG: Rash, alopecia, pruritis, urticaria, pain at site, phlebitis
CNS: Fever, chills, ***coma***, confusion, abnormal thoughts, dizziness, bizarre dreams, headache, psychosis, tremors, somnolence, paresthesia
CV: Dysrhythmia, hypertension/hypotension
RESP: Dyspnea
EENT: Retinal detachment in CMV retinitis
GU: Hematuria, increased creatinine, BUN
Contraindications: Hypersensitivity to acyclovir or ganciclovir
Precautions: Preexisting cytopenias, renal function impairment, pregnancy (C), lactation, children <6 mo, elderly, platelet count <25,000/mm
Pharmacokinetics: Half-life 3-4½ hr; excreted by the kidneys (unchanged drug); crosses blood-brain barrier
Interactions/incompatibilities:
• Decreased renal clearance of ganciclovir: probenecid
• Increased toxicity: dapsone, pentamidine, flucytosine, vincristine, vinblastine, adriamycin, doxorubicin, amphotericin B, trimethoprim-sulfa combinations, or other nucleoside analogs
• Severe granulocytopenia: zidovudine; do not give together
• Increased seizures: imipenemcilastatin
• Incompatible with any other drug in sol or syringe
NURSING CONSIDERATIONS
Assess:
• For leukopenia/neutropenia/

thrombocytopenia: WBCs, platelets q2d during 2 × /d dosing and q1wk thereafter
• For leukopenia with qd WBC count in patients with prior leukopenia with other nucleoside analogs or for whom leukopenia counts are <1,000 cells/mm³ at start of treatment
• Serum creatinine or creatine clearance at least q2wk
Administer:
• IV after diluting 500 mg/10 ml sterile H_2O for injection (50 mg/ml); shake; further dilute in 100 ml D_5W, NS, LR and run over 1 hr; use infusion pump
• Slowly; do not give by bolus IV, IM, SC injection
• Using diluted solution within 24 hr
Evaluate:
• Therapeutic response: decreased symptoms of CMV
Teach patient/family:
• That drug does not cure condition, that regular ophthalmologic examinations are necessary
• That major toxicities may necessitate discontinuing drug
• To use contraception during treatment and that infertility may occur; men should use barrier contraception for 90 days after treatment
Treatment of overdose: Discontinue drug, use hemodialysis, and increase hydration

---

gemfibrozil
(gem-fi′broe-zil)
Lopid
Func. class.: Antilipemic
Chem. class.: Aryloxisobutyric
acid derivative

Action: Inhibits biosynthesis of

VLDL, LDL, which are responsible for cholesterol development
Uses: Type III/IV, V hyperlipidemia
Dosage and routes:
• *Adult:* PO 1200 mg in divided doses bid 30 min before meals
Available forms: Caps 300 mg
Side effects/adverse reactions:
GI: Nausea, vomiting, dyspepsia, diarrhea, abdominal pain
INTEG: Rash, urticaria, pruritus
HEMA: Leukopenia, anemia, eosinophilia
CNS: Dizziness, blurred vision
Contraindications: Severe hepatic disease, preexisting gallbladder disease, severe renal disease, primary biliary cirrhosis, hypersensitivity
Precautions: Monitor hematologic and hepatic function, pregnancy (B), lactation
Pharmacokinetics:
PO: Peak 1-2 hr; plasma protein binding >90%; half-life 1.5 hr; excreted in urine; metabolized in liver
Interactions/incompatibilities:
• May increase anticoagulant properties: oral anticoagulants
• Increased risk of myositis, myalgia: lovastatin
Lab test interferences:
Increase: Liver function studies, CPK, BSP, thymol turbidity, glucose
Decrease: Hgb, Hct, WBC
NURSING CONSIDERATIONS
Assess:
• Renal, hepatic levels if patient is on long-term therapy
• Bowel pattern daily; increase bulk, water in diet if constipation develops, especially elderly
Administer:
• 30 min before morning and evening meals
Evaluate:
• Therapeutic response: decreased cholesterol levels

Teach patient/family:
• That compliance is needed, since toxicity may result if doses are missed
• That risk factors should be decreased: high-fat diet, smoking, alcohol consumption, absence of exercise
• Birth control should be practiced while on this drug

---

gentamicin sulfate
(jen-ta-mye'sin)
Alcomicin,* Apogen, Cidomycin,* Garamycin, Garamycin Intrathecal, Garamycin IV Piggyback, Garamycin Pediatric, Gentamicin Sulfate, Gentamicin Sulfate IV Piggyback, Jenamicin, Pediatric Gentamicin Sulfate
Func. class.: Antibiotic
Chem. class.: Aminoglycoside

Action: Interferes with protein synthesis in bacterial cell by binding to ribosomal subunit, causing misreading of genetic code; inaccurate peptide sequence forms in protein chain, causing bacterial death
Uses: Severe systemic infections of CNS, respiratory, GI, urinary tract, bone, skin, soft tissues caused by susceptible strains of *P. aeruginosa, Proteus, Klebsiella, Serratia, E. coli, Enterobacter, Citrobacter, Staphylococcus, Shigella, Salmonella*
Dosage and routes:
Severe systemic infections
• *Adult:* IV INF 3-5 mg/kg/day in 3 divided doses q8h; dilute in 50-200 ml NS or D₅W given over 30 min-2 hr; IM 3 mg/kg/day in divided doses q8h
• *Adult:* INTRATHECAL 4-8 mg qd

• *Child:* IV/IM 2-2.5 mg/kg q8h
• *Neonates and infants:* IV/IM 2.5 mg/kg q8h
• *Neonates <1 wk:* 2.5 mg/kg q12h
• *Infants and child >3 months:* INTRATHECAL 1-2 mg qd

Dental/respiratory procedures/ GI/GU surgery (prophylaxis endocarditis)
• *Adult:* IM 1.5 mg/kg ½-1 hr before procedure with ampicillin
• *Child:* IM 2.5 mg/kg ½-1 hr before procedure with ampicillin

Available forms: Inj IM, IV 10, 40, 60, 80, 100 mg; intrathecal 2 mg/ml

Side effects/adverse reactions:
*GU: **Oliguria, hematuria, renal damage, azotemia, renal failure, nephrotoxicity***
CNS: Confusion, depression, numbness, tremors, ***convulsions,*** muscle twitching, ***neurotoxicity,*** dizziness, vertigo
*EENT: **Ototoxicity,** deafness,* visual disturbances, tinnitus
*HEMA: **Agranulocytosis, thrombocytopenia, leukopenia, eosinophilia,** anemia*
GI: Nausea, vomiting, anorexia, increased ALT, AST, bilirubin, hepatomegaly, ***hepatic necrosis,*** splenomegaly
CV: Hypotension, hypertension, palpitations
INTEG: Rash, burning, urticaria, dermatitis, alopecia

Contraindications: Severe renal disease, hypersensitivity
Precautions: Neonates, mild renal disease, pregnancy (C), hearing deficits, myasthenia gravis, lactation, elderly, Parkinson's disease
Pharmacokinetics:
IM: Onset rapid, peak 1-2 hr
IV: Onset immediate, peak 1-2 hr
Plasma half-life 1-2 hr; duration 6-8 hr; not metabolized; excreted unchanged in urine; crosses placental barrier

Interactions/incompatibilities:
• Increased ototoxicity, neurotoxicity, nephrotoxicity: other aminoglycosides, amphotericin B, polymyxin, vancomycin, ethacrynic acid, furosemide, mannitol, methoxyflurane, cisplatin, cephalosporins, bacitracin, enflurane
• Increased effects: nondepolarizing neuromuscular blockers
• Incompatible with amphotericin B, ampicillin, cefamandole, cephalothin, cephaprin, dopamine, furosemide, heparin; inactivated by penicillins, cephalosporins; administer separately

NURSING CONSIDERATIONS
Assess:
• Weight before treatment; calculation of dosage is usually based on ideal body weight, but may be calculated on actual body weight
• I&O ratio, urinalysis daily for proteinuria, cells, casts; report sudden change in urine output; toxicity is increased in patients with decreased renal function if high doses are given
• VS during infusion; watch for hypotension, change in pulse
• IV site for thrombophlebitis, including pain, redness, swelling, q30min, change site if needed; apply warm compresses to discontinued site
• Serum peak, drawn at 30-60 min after IV infusion or 60 min after IM injection, and trough level drawn just before next dose; blood level should be 2-4 times bacteriostatic level; peak = 4-10 µg/ml, trough = 1-2 µg/ml
• Urine pH if drug is used for UTI; urine should be kept alkaline
• Renal impairment by securing

---

italics = common side effects   ***bold italic*** = life threatening reactions

urine for CrCl testing, BUN, serum creatinine; lower dosage should be given in renal impairment (CrCl <80 ml/min)

• Deafness by audiometric testing, ringing, roaring in ears, vertigo; assess hearing before, during, after treatment

• Dehydration: high sp gr, decrease in skin turgor, dry mucous membranes, dark urine

• Overgrowth of infection including increased temperature, malaise, redness, pain, swelling, perineal itching, diarrhea, stomatitis, change in cough or sputum

• C&S before starting treatment to identify infecting organism

• Vestibular dysfunction: nausea, vomiting, dizziness, headache; drug should be discontinued if severe

• Injection sites for redness, swelling, abscesses; use warm compresses at site

Administer:

• IV after diluting in 50-200 ml of normal saline or D₅W; sol concentration should be 1 mg/ml or less; decrease vol of diluent in child; maintain 0.1% sol run over ½-1 hr (adults) or up to 2 hr (children); flush IV line with NS or D₅W after administration

• IM injection in large muscle mass; rotate injection sites

• Drug in evenly spaced doses to maintain blood level

• Bicarbonate to alkalinize urine if ordered for UTI, as drug is most active in alkaline environment

Perform/provide:

• Adequate fluids of 2-3 L/day, unless contraindicated, to prevent irritation of tubules

• Supervised ambulation, other safety measures with vestibular dysfunction

Evaluate:

• Therapeutic response: absence of fever, draining wounds, negative C&S after treatment

Teach patient/family:

• To report headache, dizziness, symptoms of overgrowth of infection, renal impairment

• To report loss of hearing, ringing, roaring in ears or feeling of fullness in head

Treatment of overdose: Hemodialysis; monitor serum levels of drug

---

gentamicin sulfate (ophthalmic)

(jen-ta-mye'sin)

Garamycin Ophthalmic, Genoptic Ophthalmic, Genoptic S.O.P., Gentacidin, Gent-AK, Gentamicin, Gentamicin Ophthalmic Liquifilm, Gentak

Func. class.: Antiinfective ophthalmic

Action: Inhibits bacterial protein synthesis

Uses: Infection of external eye

Dosage and routes:

• *Adult and child:* INSTILL 1 or 2 gtt q2-4h; TOP apply oint to conjunctival sac bid-qid

Available forms: Oint, sol 3%

Side effects/adverse reactions:

EENT: Poor corneal wound healing, temporary visual haze, overgrowth of nonsusceptible organisms

Contraindications: Hypersensitivity, vaccina, varicella, mycobacterial, fungal infections of eye, epithelial herpes, simplex keratitis

Precautions: Antibiotic hypersensitivity, pregnancy (C)

NURSING CONSIDERATIONS

Assess:

• Allergy: itching, lacrimation, redness, swelling, photosensitivity

---

* Available in Canada only

Administer:
• After washing hands; cleanse crusts or discharge from eye before application

Perform/provide:
• Storage at room temperature

Evaluate:
• Therapeutic response: absence of redness, inflammation, tearing

Teach patient/family:
• To use drug exactly as prescribed
• Not to use eye makeup, towels, washcloths, eye medication of others; reinfection may occur
• That drug container tip should not be touched to eye
• To report itching, increased redness, burning, stinging, swelling; drug should be discontinued
• That drug may cause blurred vision when ointment is applied

---

gentamicin sulfate (topical)

(jen-ta-mye′sin)

G-Myticin, Garamycin, Gentamicin

Func. class.: Local antiinfective

Chem. class.: Aminoglycoside

Action: Interferes with bacterial protein synthesis

Uses: Superficial skin infections; burns, skin ulcers

Dosage and routes:
• *Adult and child:* TOP rub into affected area tid-qid

Available forms: Cream, oint 0.1%

Side effects/adverse reactions:
INTEG: Rash, urticaria, stinging, burning, photosensitivity, pruritus

Contraindications: Hypersensitivity, impaired renal function

Precautions: Pregnancy (C), lactation

NURSING CONSIDERATIONS

Assess:
• Allergic reaction: burning, stinging, swelling, redness, photosensitivity

Administer:
• Enough medication to cover lesions completely; may cover with gauze dressing
• After cleansing with soap, water before each application; dry well

Perform/provide:
• Storage at room temperature in dry place

Evaluate:
• Therapeutic response: decrease in size, number of lesions

Teach patient/family:
• To use medical asepsis (hand washing) before, after each application
• To apply with glove to prevent further infection
• To avoid use of OTC creams, ointments, lotions unless directed by physician
• To avoid sunlight or wear sunscreen to prevent burns
• Not to use in eyes or external ear if eardrum is perforated
• To notify physician if condition worsens
• That overuse may lead to resistant organisms
• To avoid use on large skin lesions or over wide areas
• In impetigo, to remove crusts before applying

---

glipizide

(glip-i′zide)

Glucotrol

Func. class.: Antidiabetic

Chem. class.: Sulfonylurea (2nd generation)

Action: Causes functioning β-cells

---

italics = common side effects   ***bold italic*** = life threatening reactions

in pancreas to release insulin, leading to drop in blood glucose levels; may improve insulin binding to insulin receptors or increase the number of insulin receptors with prolonged administration; may also reduce basal hepatic glucose secretion; not effective if patient lacks functioning β-cells

Uses: Stable adult-onset diabetes mellitus (type II) NIDDM

Dosage and routes:
• *Adult:* PO 5 mg initially, then increase to desired response; do not exceed 15 mg once a day dose or 40 mg/d in divided doses
• *Elderly hepatic disease:* PO 2.5 mg initially, then increase to desired response; max 40 mg/day in divided doses or 15 mg/dose

Available forms: Tabs 5, 10 mg scored

Side effects/adverse reactions:
CNS: Headache, weakness, dizziness, drowsiness, tinnitus, fatigue, vertigo
GI: Hepatotoxicity, cholestatic jaundice, nausea, vomiting, diarrhea, heartburn
HEMA: Leukopenia, thrombocytopenia, agranulocytosis, aplastic anemia, increased AST, ALT, alk phosphatase, *pancytopenia, hemolytic anemia*
INTEG: Rash, allergic reactions, pruritus, urticaria, eczema, photosensitivity, erythema
ENDO: Hypoglycemia

Contraindications: Hypersensitivity to sulfonylureas, juvenile or brittle diabetes

Precautions: Pregnancy (C), elderly, cardiac disease, severe renal disease, severe hepatic disease, thyroid disease

Pharmacokinetics:
PO: Completely absorbed by GI route, onset 1-1½ hr, duration 10-24 hr, half-life 2-4 hr; metabolized in liver; excreted in urine; 90%-95% is plasma protein bound

Interactions/incompatibilities:
• Increased hypoglycemic effects: insulin, MAOIs, cimetidine, chloramphenicol, guanethidine, methyldopa, nonsteroidal antiinflammatories, salicylates, probenecid
• Decreased action of glipizide: calcium channel blockers, corticosteroids, oral contraceptives, thiazide diuretics, thyroid preparations, estrogens, phenothiazines, phenytoin, rifampin, isoniazide, phenobarbital, sympathomimetics
• Disulfiram-like reaction: alcohol
• Decreased effects of both drugs: diazoxide

NURSING CONSIDERATIONS
Assess:
• Blood, urine glucose levels during treatment to determine diabetes control
• Hypo/hyperglycemic reaction that can occur soon after meals

Administer:
• Drug 30 min before meals

Perform/provide:
• Storage in tight light-resistant containers at room temperature

Evaluate:
• Therapeutic response: decrease in polyuria, polydipsia, polyphagia, clear sensorium, absence of dizziness, stable gait

Teach patient/family:
• Not to drink alcohol; explain disulfiram reaction
• To check for symptoms of cholestatic jaundice: dark urine, pruritus, yellow sclera; if these occur, physician should be notified
• To use a capillary blood glucose test while on this drug
• To test urine glucose levels with Chemstrip 3 ×/day
• The symptoms of hypo/hyper-

---

* Available in Canada only

glycemia, what to do about each; to have glucagon emergency kit available

• That drug must be continued on daily basis; explain consequence of discontinuing drug abruptly

• To take drug in morning to prevent hypoglycemic reactions at night

• To avoid OTC medications unless prescribed by a physician

• That diabetes is a life-long illness; drug will not cure disease

• That all food in diet plan must be eaten to prevent hypoglycemia

• To carry Medic Alert ID for emergency purposes

• To test urine for glucose/ketones tid if this drug is replacing insulin

• To continue weight control, dietary restrictions, exercise, hygiene

Treatment of overdose: Glucose 25g IV via dextrose 50% solution 50 ml or 1 mg glucagon

---

glutethimide
(gloo-teth'i-mide)
Glutethimide
Func. class.: Sedative-hypnotic
Chem. class.: Piperidine derivative

Controlled Substance Schedule II (USA), Schedule F (Canada)

Action: Depresses activity in brain cells primarily in reticular activating system in brain stem, also selectively depresses neurons in posterior hypothalamus, limbic structures; pronounced anticholinergic activity; suppressess REM sleep

Uses: Insomnia, labor (stage 1), preoperatively for relaxation

Dosage and routes:
Insomnia
• *Adult:* PO 250-500 mg hs; may repeat dose >4 hr before usual awakening, not to exceed 1 g
Preoperatively
• *Adult:* PO 500 mg hs the night before surgery, then 500 mg-1 g 1 hr before surgery
Labor
• *Adult:* PO 500 mg given at the onset of labor, may repeat

Available forms: Tabs 250, 500 mg; caps 500 mg

Side effects/adverse reactions:
*HEMA: **Thrombocytopenia, aplastic anemia, leukopenia, megaloblastic anemia***
CNS: Residual sedation, dizziness, ataxia, stimulation, headache, hangover
GI: Nausea, vomiting, hiccups, diarrhea, jaundice
GU: Porphyria
INTEG: Rash, urticaria, purpura, ***exfoliative dermatitis** (rare)*
EENT: Dry mouth, blurred vision

Contraindications: Hypersensitivity to this drug or piperidine derivatives, severe pain, severe renal disease, porphyria

Precautions: Depression, suicidal individuals, drug abuse, cardiac dysrhythmias, narrow-angle glaucoma, prostatic hypertrophy, stenosed peptic ulcer, pyloroduodenal/bladder neck obstruction, pregnancy (C)

Pharmacokinetics:
PO: Onset 30 min, peak 1-2 hr, duration 4-8 hr; metabolized by liver; excreted by kidneys (metabolites); crosses placenta; excreted in breast milk; half-life 4 hr, 10-20 hr terminal

Interactions/incompatibilities:
• Decreased hypoprothrombinemic effect: oral anticoagulants
• Increased CNS depression: alcohol and other CNS depressants

---

italics = common side effects   ***bold italic*** = life threatening reactions

• Increased anticholinergic effect: tricyclic antidepressants

Lab test interferences:
Interferences: 17-OHCS

NURSING CONSIDERATIONS
Assess:
• Blood studies: Hct, Hgb, RBCs (if on long-term therapy)
• Hepatic studies: AST, ALT, bilirubin
• Mental status: mood, sensorium, affect, memory (long, short)
• Blood dyscrasias: fever, sore throat, bruising, rash, jaundice, epistaxis (rare)
• Type of sleep problem: falling asleep, staying asleep

Administer:
• After removal of cigarettes to prevent fires
• After trying conservative measures for insomnia
• ½-1 hr before hs for sleeplessness
• Several hours before patient is to arise (to avoid hangover)

Perform/provide:
• Assistance with ambulation after receiving dose
• Safety measures: side rails, nightlight, call bell within easy reach
• Checking to see PO medication has been swallowed
• Storage in tight container in cool environment

Evaluate:
• Therapeutic response: ability to sleep at night, decreased amount of early morning awakening if taking drug for insomnia

Teach patient/family:
• To avoid driving or other activities requiring alertness until drug is stabilized
• To avoid alcohol ingestion or CNS depressants; serious CNS depression may result
• Not to discontinue medication quickly after long-term use; drug should be tapered over 1-2 wk
• That effects may take 2 nights for benefits to be noticed
• Alternate measures to improve sleep: reading, exercise several hours before hs, warm bath, warm milk, TV, self-hypnosis, deep breathing
• That hangover is common in elderly but less common than with barbiturates
• Symptoms of withdrawal: nausea, vomiting, anxiety, hallucinations, insomnia, tachycardia, fever, cramps, tremors, seizures
• Blood dyscrasias: fever, sore throat, bruising, rash, jaundice (rare)
• Allergic reaction: rash; discontinue drug if rash occurs

Treatment of overdose: Lavage, activated charcoal; monitor electrolytes, vital signs

---

glyburide
(glye'byoor-ide)
DiaBeta,* Glynase Prestab, Micronase
Func. class.: Antidiabetic
Chem. class.: Sulfonylurea (2nd generation)

Action: Causes functioning β-cells in pancreas to release insulin, leading to drop in blood glucose levels; may improve insulin binding to insulin receptors and increase number of insulin receptors with prolonged administration; may also reduce basal hepatic glucose secretion; not effective if patient lacks functioning β-cells

Uses: Stable adult-onset diabetes mellitus (type II) NIDDM

Dosage and routes:
• *Adult:* PO 2.5-5 mg initially, then increased to desired response

---

• *Elderly:* PO 1.25 mg initially, then increased to desired response; max 20 mg/day, maintenance 1.25-20 mg/qd

Available forms: Tabs 1.25, 2.5, 5 mg

Side effects/adverse reactions:

CNS: Headache, weakness, paresthesia, tinnitus, fatigue, vertigo

GI: Nausea, fullness, heartburn, ***hepatotoxicity, cholestatic jaundice,*** vomiting, diarrhea

HEMA: ***Leukopenia, thrombocytopenia, agranulocytosis, aplastic anemia,*** increased AST, ALT, alk phosphatase

INTEG: Rash, allergic reactions, pruritus, urticaria, eczema, photosensitivity, erythema

ENDO: ***Hypoglycemia***

MS: Joint pains

Contraindications: Hypersensitivity to sulfonylureas, juvenile or brittle diabetes

Precautions: Pregnancy (B), elderly, cardiac disease, severe renal disease, severe hepatic disease, thyroid disease, severe hypoglycemic reactions

Pharmacokinetics:

PO: Completely absorbed by GI route; onset 2-4 hr, peak 2-8 hr, duration 24 hr; half-life 10 hr; metabolized in liver; excreted in urine, feces (metabolites); crosses placenta; 90%-95% is plasma protein bound

Interactions/incompatibilities:

• Both drugs' effects may be decreased: diazoxide

• Decreased digoxin level: digoxin

• Increased hypoglycemic effects: insulin, MAOIs, cimetidine, oral anticoagulants, chloramphenicol, guanethidine, methyldopa, nonsteroidal antiinflammatories, salicylates, probenecid

• Decreased action of glyburide:

calcium channel blockers, corticosteroids, oral contraceptives, thiazide diuretics, thyroid preparations, estrogens, phenothiazines, phenytoin, rifampin, isoniazide, phenobarbital, sympathomimetics

• Disulfiram-like reaction: alcohol

NURSING CONSIDERATIONS

Assess:

• Hypo/hyperglycemic reaction that can occur soon after meals

Administer:

• With breakfast

Perform/provide:

• Storage in tight container in cool environment

Evaluate:

• Therapeutic response: decrease in polyuria, polydipsia, polyphagia, clear sensorium, absence of dizziness, stable gait

Teach patient/family:

• Not to drink alcohol; explain disulfiram reaction

• To check for symptoms of cholestatic jaundice: dark urine, pruritus, yellow sclera; if these occur, a physician should be notified

• To use a capillary blood glucose test while on this drug

• The symptoms of hypo/hyperglycemia, what to do about each

• That drug must be continued on daily basis; explain consequence of discontinuing drug abruptly

• To take drug in morning to prevent hypoglycemic reactions at night

• To avoid OTC medications unless prescribed by a physician

• That diabetes is a lifelong illness; drug will not cure disease

• That all food included in diet plan must be eaten to prevent hypoglycemia; to have glucagon emergency kit available

• To carry a Medic Alert ID for emergency purposes

---

italics = common side effects   ***bold italic*** = life threatening reactions

Treatment of overdose: Glucose 25 g IV via dextrose 50% solution, 50 ml or 1 mg glucagon

---

glycerin
(gli'ser-in)
Fleet Babylax, Glycerin USP, Glycerol, Osmoglyn, Sani-Supp
Func. class.: Laxative, hyperosmotic
Chem. class.: Trihydric alcohol

Action: Increases osmotic pressure, draws fluid into colon
Uses: Constipation
Dosage and routes:
• *Adult and child >6 yr:* REC SUPP 3 g; ENEMA 5-15 ml
• *Child <6 yr:* REC SUPP 1-1.5 g; ENEMA 2-5 ml
Available forms: Rec sol 4 ml/applicator; supp
Side effects/adverse reactions:
CNS: Headache, confusion, *convulsions*
GI: Nausea, vomiting, diarrhea
META: Dehydration
Contraindications: Hypersensitivity
Precautions: Pregnancy (C)
NURSING CONSIDERATIONS
Assess:
• Cause of constipation; identify whether fluids, bulk, or exercise is missing from life-style
• Cramping, rectal bleeding, nausea, vomiting; if these symptoms occur, drug should be discontinued
Administer:
• In morning or evening (oral dose)
Perform/provide:
• Storage in cool environment; do not freeze
Evaluate:
• Therapeutic response: decrease in constipation

Teach patient/family:
• Not to use laxatives for long-term therapy; bowel tone will be lost
• That normal bowel movements do not always occur daily
• Not to use in presence of abdominal pain, nausea, vomiting
• To notify physician if constipation unrelieved or if symptoms of electrolyte imbalance occur: muscle cramps, pain, weakness, dizziness, excessive thirst

---

glycerin, anhydrous
(gli'ser-in)
Ophthalgan Ophthalmic
Func. class.: Ophthalmic
Chem. class.: Trihydric alcohol

Action: Reduces corneal edema by osmosis of water through corneal epithelium, which is semipermeable
Uses: Reduce corneal edema
Dosage and routes:
• *Adult:* INSTILL 1-2 gtts after local anesthetic
Available forms: Sol
Side effects/adverse reactions:
EENT: Eye pain
CNS: Headache
Contraindications: Hypersensitivity
Precautions: Pregnancy (C), lactation, children
Pharmacokinetics: Onset 10 min, peak 20 min, duration 6-8 hr
NURSING CONSIDERATIONS
Administer:
• Anesthetic (tetracaine or proparacaine) before instillation to decrease pain
Perform/provide:
• Storage in tight container; discard 6 months after opening
Evaluate:
• Therapeutic response: decreased corneal edema

Teach patient/family:
• Method of instillation, including pressure on lacrimal sac for 1 min, and not to touch dropper to eye

---

glycopyrrolate

(glye-koe-pye′roe-late)
Glycopyrrolate, Robinul, Robinul Forte
Func. class.: Cholinergic blocker
Chem. class.: Quaternary ammonium compound

Action: Inhibits acetylcholine at receptor sites in autonomic nervous system, which controls secretions, free acids in stomach

Uses: Decreased secretions before surgery, reversal of neuromuscular blockade, peptic ulcer disease, irritable bowel syndrome

Dosage and routes:
Preoperatively
• *Adult:* IM 0.002 mg/lb ½-1 hr before surgery
• *Child 2-12 yr:* IM 0.002-0.004 mg/lb
• *Child <2 yr:* IM 0.004 mg/lb
Reversal of neuromuscular blockage
• *Adult:* IV 0.2 mg for each 1 mg of neostigmine or 5 mg IV of pyridostigmine simultaneously
GI disorders
• *Adult:* PO 1-2 mg bid-tid; IM/IV 0.1-0.2 mg tid-qid, titrated to patient response
Available forms: Tabs 1, 2 mg; inj 0.2 mg/ml

Side effects/adverse reactions:
INTEG: Urticaria, allergic reactions
MISC: Suppression of lactation, nasal congestion, decreased sweating
CNS: Confusion, anxiety, restlessness, irritability, delusions, hallucinations, headache, sedation, depression, incoherence, dizziness, lethargy, flushing, weakness
EENT: Blurred vision, photophobia, dilated pupils, difficulty swallowing, increased intraocular pressure, mydriasis, cycloplegia
CV: Palpitations, tachycardia, postural hypotension, paradoxical bradycardia
GI: Dryness of mouth, constipation, nausea, vomiting, abdominal distress, paralytic ileus, altered taste perception
GU: Hesitancy, retention, impotence

Contraindications: Hypersensitivity, narrow-angle glaucoma, myasthenia gravis, GI/GU obstruction, child <3 yr, tachycardia, myocardial ischemia, hepatic disease, ulcerative colitis, toxic megacolon

Precautions: Pregnancy (C), elderly, lactation, prostatic hypertrophy, renal disease, CHF, pulmonary disease, hyperthyroidism

Pharmacokinetics:
PO: Peak 1 hr, duration 6 hr
IM: Peak 30-45 min, duration 7 hr
IV: Peak 10-15 min, duration 4 hr
Excreted in urine, bile, feces (unchanged)

Interactions/incompatibilities:
• Increased anticholinergic effect: alcohol, antihistamines, phenothiazines, amantadine, tricyclics
• Incompatible with alkaline sol, dexamethasone, dimenhydrinate, methohexital, methylprednisolone, pentazocine, phenothiazines, secobarbital, thiopental, diazepam, chloramphenicol, pentobarbital, sodium bicarbonate, in syringe or sol

NURSING CONSIDERATIONS
Assess:
• I&O ratio; retention commonly causes decreased urinary output

---

• Urinary hesitancy, retention: palpate bladder if retention occurs
• Constipation; increase fluids, bulk, exercise if this occurs
• For tolerance over long-term therapy; dose may have to be increased or changed
• Mental status: affect, mood, CNS depression, worsening of mental symptoms during early therapy

Administer:
• IV undiluted, give through a Y-tube or 3-way stopcock; give 0.2 mg or less over 1-2 min
• Parenteral dose with patient recumbent to prevent postural hypotension
• With or after meals to prevent GI upset; may give with fluids other than water
• Parenteral dose slowly; keep in bed for at least 1 hr after dose; monitor vital signs
• After checking dose carefully; even slight overdose may lead to toxicity

Perform/provide:
• Storage at room temperature
• Hard candy, frequent drinks, sugarless gum to relieve dry mouth

Evaluate:
• Therapeutic response: decreased secretions

Teach patient/family:
• Not to discontinue this drug abruptly; to taper off over 1 wk
• To avoid driving or other hazardous activities; drowsiness may occur
• To avoid OTC medication: cough, cold preparations with alcohol, antihistamines unless directed by physician

gonadorelin acetate
(goe-nad-oh-rell'in)
Lutrepulse
Func. class.: Gonadotropin
Chem. class.: Synthetic endogenous gonadotropin-releasing hormone (GnRH)

Action: Induces ovulation in women by release of LH in the anterior pituitary gland

Uses: Primary hypothalamic amenorrhea

Dosage and routes:
• IV Pump: 5 μg/min, × 21 days; after three treatment intervals, it may be necessary to raise the dose in a stepwise program

Available forms: Powder for inj, IV 0.8, 3.2 mg

Side effects/adverse reactions:
INTEG: Inflammation at injection site, phlebitis, hematoma at catheter site
SYST: Anaphylaxis (bronchospasm, tachycardia, flushing, urticaria, induration of injection site)
REPRO: Ovarian hyperstimulation, multiple pregnancy

Contraindications: Hypersensitivity; patients with ovarian cysts or hormonally dependent tumors; causes of anovulation other than those of hypothalamic origin

Precautions: Pregnancy (B)

Pharmacokinetics: Excreted by kidneys, half-life (initial) 2-10 min, (terminal 10-40 min)

Interaction/incompatibilities:
• Ovulation stimulators should not be used with this drug

NURSING CONSIDERATIONS
Assess:
• Effects by ovarian ultrasound: baseline, after 1 wk, after 2 wk,

midluteal phase serum progesterone

Administer:

• Using Lutrepulse pump only; detailed instructions are given with pump

• After reconstituting 8 ml of diluent provided and transferring to plastic reservoir, withdraw 8 ml of diluent and inject into lyophile drug cake; shake, fill reservoir bag with reconstituted solution, and administer IV using pump provider; 8 ml = 1 wk supply

Perform/provide:

• Storage at room temperature; use prepared solution within 24 hr

Evaluate:

• Therapeutic response: absence of amenorrhea with drug use

---

gonadorelin HCl

(goe-nad-oh-rell'in)
Factrel

Func. class.: Gonadotropin
Chem. class.: Synthetic luteinizing hormone–releasing hormone

---

Action: Combination luteinizing hormone (releasing hormone) that acts on anterior pituitary

Uses: Evaluation of response of gonadotropic hormone

Dosage and routes:

• *Women:* SC/IV 100 μg usually given between day 1-7 of menstrual cycle

• *Child:* SC/IV 2 μg/kg

Available forms: Powder for inj SC, IV 100, 500 μg/vial

Side effects/adverse reactions:

CNS: Dizziness, headache, flushing
GI: Nausea
INTEG: Inflammation at injection site

Contraindications: Hypersensitivity

Precautions: Pregnancy (B)

Pharmacokinetics: Excreted by kidneys

Interactions/incompatibilities:

• Increased level of gonadorelin: levodopa, spironolactone

• Decreased level of gonadorelin: digoxin, oral contraceptives, phenothiazines, dopamine antagonists

Lab test interferences:

False results when used with androgens, glucocorticoids, estrogens, progestins

NURSING CONSIDERATIONS
Assess:

• Test result: pituitary/hypothalamus dysfunction (decreased LH); postmenopausal (increased LH)

Administer:

• After reconstituting with sterile diluent (1 ml)/100 μg enclosed in package; give over 30 sec

• Repeated doses may be necessary to elevate pituitary gonadotropin reserve

Perform/provide:

• Storage at room temperature; use prepared solution within 24 hr

---

goserelin acetate

(go'seh-rel-in)
Zoladex

Func. class.: Gonadotropin-releasing hormone
Chem. class.: Synthetic decapeptide analog of LHRH

Action: Inhibitor of pituitary gonadotropin secretion. Initially increases LH and FSH, with increases in testosterone, reduction in sex steroid levels

Uses: Advanced prostate cancer, premenopausal breast cancer

Dosage and routes:
• *Adult:* SC 3.6 mg q28d
Available forms: Depot inj 3.6 mg
Side effects/adverse reactions:
CNS: Headaches, **spinal cord compression,** anxiety, depression
CV: **Dysrhythmia, cerebrovascular accident,** hypertension, **MI,** chest pain
ENDO: Gynecomastia, breast tenderness, hot flashes
GI: Nausea, vomiting, constipation, diarrhea, ulcer
GU: Spotting, breakthrough bleeding, decreased libido, renal insufficiency, urinary obstruction, urinary tract infection
INTEG: Rash, pain on injection
MS: Osteoneuralgia
Contraindications: Hypersensitivity, pregnancy
Pharmacokinetics: Peak serum concentrations in 12-15 days
Lab test interferences:
Increased: Alk phosphatase, estradiol, FSH, LH, testosterone levels
Decreased: Testosterone levels, progesterone
NURSING CONSIDERATIONS
Assess:
• For relief of bone pain
Evaluate:
• Therapeutic response: more normal levels of prostate-specific antigen, acid phosphatase, alk phosphatase; testosterone level of <25 ng/dl
Teach patient/family:
• That gynecomastia and postmenopausal symptoms may occur but will decrease after treatment is discontinued

griseofulvin microsize/ griseofulvin ultramicrosize

(gri-see-oh-ful'vin)
Fulvicin-U/F, Grifulvin V, Grisactin, Grisactin 500, Fulvicin P/G, Grisactin-Ultra, Gris-PEG
Func. class.: Antifungal
Chem. class.: Penicillium griseofulvum derivative

Action: Arrests fungal cell division at metaphase; binds to human keratin, making it resistant to disease
Uses: Mycotic infections: tinea corporis, tinea pedis, tinea cruris, tinea barbae, tinea capitis, tinea unguium if caused by *Epidermophyton, Microsporum, Trichophyton*
Dosage and routes:
• *Adult:* PO 500-1000 mg qd in single or divided doses (microsize), 125-165 mg bid (ultramicrosize) or 250-330 mg qd; may need 500-660 mg in divided doses for severe infections
• *Child:* PO 10 mg/kg/day or 30 mg/m^2/day (microsize) or 5 mg/kg/day (ultramicrosize)
Available forms: Microcaps 125, 250 mg; tabs 250, 500 mg; oral susp 125 mg/ml; ultratabs 125, 165, 250, 330 mg
Side effects/adverse reactions:
INTEG: Rash, urticaria, photosensitivity, lichen planus, angioedema
CNS: Headache, peripheral neuritis, paresthesias, confusion, dizziness, fatigue, insomnia, psychosis
EENT: Blurred vision, oral candidiasis, furry tongue, transient hearing loss
GU: Proteinuria, cylinduria, precipitate porphyria, increased thirst
GI: Nausea, vomiting, anorexia, diarrhea, cramps, dry mouth, flatulence

---

*HEMA: **Leukopenia, granulocytopenia, neutropenia, monocytosis***
Contraindications: Hypersensitiv-
ity, porphyria, hepatic disease, lu-
pus erythematosus
Precautions: Penicillin sensitivity,
pregnancy (C)
Pharmacokinetics:
PO: Peak 4 hr, half-life 9-24 hr, me-
tabolized in liver; excreted in urine
(inactive metabolites), feces, per-
spiration
Interactions/incompatibilities:
• Tachycardia: alcohol
• Decreased action of griseofulvin:
barbiturates
• Decreased action of: warfarin,
anticoagulants (oral)
NURSING CONSIDERATIONS
Assess:
• I&O ratio
• Liver studies qwk (ALT, AST,
bilirubin, alk phosphatase)
• Renal studies: BUN, serum cre-
atinine
• Blood studies: CBC, platelets,
q2wk
• Drug level during treatment
• For history of penicillin allergy;
may be cross-sensitive to this drug
• For renal toxicity: increasing
BUN, serum creatinine, protein-
uria, cylinduria
• For hepatotoxicity: increasing
ALT, AST, bilirubin, alk phospha-
tase
• For blood dyscrasias: fatigue,
malaise, dark urine, bruising
Administer:
• Drug carefully, making sure there
is no confusion with dosage form
(microsize vs ultrasize)
• With meals to decrease GI symp-
toms
• Until 3 separate cultures are neg-
ative for infective organism
Perform/provide:
• Storage in tight, light-resistant
containers at room temperature

Evaluate:
• Therapeutic response: decreased
fever, malaise, rash, negative C&S
for infecting organism
Teach patient/family:
• That long-term therapy may be
needed to clear infection (2 wk-6
mo depending on organism)
• Proper hygiene: hand-washing
technique, nail care, use of concomitant topical agents if prescribed
• Importance of compliance even
after feeling better
• To avoid alcohol, since nausea,
vomiting, hypertension may occur
• To use sunscreen or avoid direct
sunlight to prevent photosensitivity
• To notify physician of sore
throat, fever, skin rash, which may
indicate overgrowth of organisms

---

guaifenesin
(gwye-fen'e-sin)
Amonidrin, Anti-tuss, Balmi-
nil,* Breonesin, Fenesin, Gee-
Gee, Genatuss, GG-Cen,
Glyate, Glycotuss, Glytuss,
Guaifenesin, Guiatuss, Halo-
tussin, Humibid, Humibid L.A.,
Hytuss, Hytuss 2X, Malotuss,
Mytussin, Naldecon Senior EX,
Resyl,* Robitussin, Scot-Tussin
Expectorant, Sinumist-SR, Uni-
Tussin
Func. class.: Expectorant

Action: Acts as an expectorant by
stimulating a gastric mucosal reflex
to increase the production of lung
mucus
Uses: Dry, nonproductive cough
Dosage and routes:
• *Adult:* PO 100-400 mg q4-6h, not
to exceed 1.2 g/day
• *Child:* PO 12 mg/kg/day in 6 divided doses

Available forms: Tabs 100, 200 mg; caps 200 mg; syr 100 mg/5 ml

Side effects/adverse reactions:
CNS: Drowsiness
GI: Nausea, anorexia, vomiting

Contraindications: Hypersensitivity, persistent cough

Precautions: Pregnancy (C)

NURSING CONSIDERATIONS
Assess:
• Cough: type, frequency, character, including sputum

Perform/provide:
• Storage at room temperature
• Increased fluids, room humidification to liquefy secretions

Evaluate:
• Therapeutic response: absence of cough

Teach patient/family:
• To avoid driving, other hazardous activities if drowsiness occurs (rare)
• To avoid smoking, smoke-filled room, perfumes, dust, environmental pollutants, cleansers

---

guanabenz acetate
(gwan'a-benz)
Wytensin

Func. class.: Antihypertensive
Chem. class.: Central α_2-adrenergic agonist

Action: Stimulates central α_2-adrenergic receptors, resulting in decreased sympathetic outflow from brain

Uses: Hypertension

Dosage and routes:
• *Adult:* PO 4 mg bid, increasing in increments of 4-8 mg/day q1-2wk, not to exceed 32 mg bid

Available forms: Tabs 4, 8, 16 mg

Side effects/adverse reactions:
CV: Severe rebound hypertension, chest pain, dysrhythmias, palpitations

CNS: Drowsiness, dizziness, sedation, headache, depression, weakness

EENT: Dry mouth, nasal congestion, blurred vision

GI: Nausea, diarrhea, constipation
GU: Impotence

Contraindications: Hypersensitivity to guanabenz

Precautions: Pregnancy (C), lactation, children <12 yr, severe coronary insufficiency, recent myocardial infarction, cerebrovascular disease, severe hepatic or renal failure

Pharmacokinetics:
PO: Peak 2-4 hr; half-life 6 hr; excreted in urine

Interactions/incompatibilities:
• Increased sedation: CNS depressants

NURSING CONSIDERATIONS
Assess:
• Renal studies: protein, BUN, creatinine; watch for increased levels
• Baselines in renal, liver function tests before therapy begins
• B/P during beginning treatment, periodically thereafter
• Edema in feet and legs daily
• Allergic reaction: rash, fever, pruritus, urticaria; drug should be discontinued if antihistamines fail to help
• Renal symptoms: polyuria, oliguria, frequency

Evaluate:
• Therapeutic response: decrease in B/P

Teach patient/family:
• To avoid hazardous activities; sedation may occur
• Not to discontinue drug abruptly, or withdrawal symptoms may occur: anxiety, increased B/P, head-

ache, insomnia, increased pulse, tremors, nausea, sweating

• Not to use OTC (cough, cold, or allergy) products unless directed by physician

• Importance of complying with dosage schedule even if feeling better

• To notify physician of swelling of hands or feet, irregular heart beat, chest pain

• About excessive perspiration, dehydration, vomiting, diarrhea; may lead to fall in blood pressure; consult physician if these occur

• That drug may cause dizziness, fainting; light-headedness may occur during 1st few days of therapy

• That compliance is necessary; not to skip or stop drug unless directed by physician

• That drug may cause skin rash or impaired perspiration

Treatment of overdose: Administer vasopressor, discontinue drug; supine position

---

guanadrel sulfate
(gwahn'a-drel)
Hylorel

Func. class.: Antihypertensive
Chem. class.: Adrenergic blocker, peripheral guanethidine derivative

Action: Inhibits sympathetic vasoconstriction by inhibiting release of norepinephrine, depletes norepinephrine stores in adrenergic nerve endings

Uses: Hypertension

Dosage and routes:

• *Adult:* PO 5 mg bid, adjusted to desired response; may need 20-75 mg/day in divided doses

Available forms: Tabs 10, 25 mg

Side effects/adverse reactions:

CV: Orthostatic hypotension, bradycardia, **CHF,** *palpitations,* chest pain, tachycardia, dysrhythmias

CNS: Drowsiness, fatigue, weakness, feeling of faintness, insomnia, dizziness, mental changes, memory loss, hallucinations, *depression,* anxiety, *confusion, paresthesias, headache*

GI: Nausea, cramps, diarrhea, constipation, dry mouth, anorexia, indigestion

INTEG: Rash, purpura, alopecia

EENT: Nasal stuffiness, tinnitus, visual changes, sore throat, double vision, dry burning eyes

GU: Ejaculation failure, impotence, dysuria, nocturia, frequency

RESP: **Bronchospasm,** dyspnea, cough, rales, SOB

MS: Leg cramps, aching, pain, inflammation

Contraindications: Hypersensitivity, pregnancy (B), pheochromocytoma, lactation, CHF, child <18 yr

Precautions: Elderly, bronchial asthma, peptic ulcer, electrolyte imbalances, vascular disease

Pharmacokinetics:

PO: Onset 0.5-2 hr, peak 1½-2 hr, duration 4-14 hr; half-life 10-12 hr; excreted in urine (50% unchanged)

Interactions/incompatibilities:

• Increased hypotension: diuretics, other antihypertensives

• Do not use with MAOIs

• Increased orthostatic hypotension: alcohol, opioids

• Decreased hypotensive effect: tricyclic antidepressants, phenothiazines, ephedrine, phenylpropanolamine

NURSING CONSIDERATIONS

Assess:

• Renal function studies in renal impairment (BUN, creatinine)

- Bleeding time; check for ecchymosis, thrombocytopenia, purpura
- I&O in renal disease patient
- Cardiac status: B/P lying and standing, pulse; watch for hypotension
- Edema in feet, legs daily; take weight daily
- Skin turgor, dryness of mucous membranes for hydration status
- Symptoms of CHF: edema, dyspnea, wet rales

Evaluate:
- Therapeutic response: decreased B/P

Teach patient/family:
- To avoid driving, hazardous activities if drowsiness occurs
- Not to discontinue drug abruptly
- Not to use OTC cough, cold preparations unless directed by physician
- To report bradycardia, dizziness, confusion, depression, fever or sore throat
- That impotence, gynecomastia may occur but are reversible
- To rise slowly to sitting or standing position to minimize orthostatic hypotension
- That therapeutic effect may take 2-4 wk

---

guanethidine monosulfate

(gwahn-eth'i-deen)
Guanethidine Sulfate, Ismelin
Func. class.: Antihypertensive
Chem. class.: Antiadrenergic agent, peripheral

Action: Inhibits norepinephrine release, depleting norepinephrine stores in adrenergic nerve endings
Uses: Moderate to severe hypertension

Dosage and routes:
- *Adult:* PO 10 mg qd, increase by 10 mg qwk; may require 25-50 mg qd
- *Adult:* (Hospitalized) 25-50 mg; may increase by 25-50 mg/day or every other day
- *Child:* PO 200 µg/kg/day; increase q7-10d, not to exceed 3000 µg/kg/24 hr

Available forms: Tabs 10, 25 mg
Side effects/adverse reactions:
CV: Orthostatic hypotension, dizziness, weakness, lassitude, bradycardia, CHF, fatigue, angina, heart block, chest paresthesia
CNS: Depression
GI: Nausea, vomiting, *diarrhea,* constipation, dry mouth, weight gain, anorexia
INTEG: Dermatitis, loss of scalp hair
HEMA: Thrombocytopenia, leukopenia
EENT: Nasal congestion, ptosis, blurred vision
GU: Ejaculation failure, impotence, nocturia, edema, retention, increased BUN
RESP: Dyspnea
Contraindications: Hypersensitivity, pheochromocytoma, recent MI, CHF, cardiac failure, sinus bradycardia
Precautions: Pregnancy (B), lactation, peptic ulcer, asthma
Pharmacokinetics:
PO: Therapeutic level: 1-3 wk; half-life 5 days; metabolized by liver; excreted in urine (metabolites), breast milk
Interactions/incompatibilities:
- Increased hypotension: diuretics, other antihypertensives
- Do not use with MAOIs
- Increased orthostatic hypotension: alcohol
- Decreased hypotensive effect: tri-

---

cyclic antidepressants, phenothiazines, ephedrine, phenylpropanolamine, oral contraceptives, thiothixine, doxepin, haloperidol, amphetamines

Lab test interferences:
Increase: BUN
Decrease: Blood glucose, VMA excretion, urinary norepinephrine

NURSING CONSIDERATIONS
Assess:
• Renal function studies in renal impairment (BUN, creatinine)
• Bleeding time; check for ecchymosis, thrombocytopenia, purpura
• I&O in renal disease patient
• Cardiac status: B/P, pulse; watch for hypotension
• Edema in feet, legs daily; take weight daily
• Skin turgor, dryness of mucous membranes for hydration status
• Symptoms of CHF: edema, dyspnea, wet rales

Evaluate:
• Therapeutic response: decreased B/P

Teach patient/family:
• To avoid driving, hazardous activities if drowsiness occurs
• Not to discontinue drug abruptly
• Not to use OTC cough, cold preparations unless directed by physician
• To report bradycardia, dizziness, confusion, depression, fever, sore throat
• That impotence, gynecomastia may occur but are reversible
• To rise slowly to sitting or standing position to minimize orthostatic hypotension; more common in AM, hot weather, during exercise, or when using alcohol
• That therapeutic effect may take 2-4 wk
• Notify physician of severe diarrhea

Treatment of overdose: Lavage, vasopressors given cautiously

guanfacine HCI
(gwahn'fa-seen)
Tenex
Func. class.: Antihypertensive
Chem. class.: α₂ Adrenergic receptor agonist

Action: Stimulates central α-adrenergic receptors, resulting in decreased sympathetic outflow from brain

Uses: Hypertension in individual using a thiazide diuretic

Dosage and routes:
• *Adult:* PO 1 mg/day hs; may increase dose in 2-3 wk to 2-3 mg/day

Available forms: Tabs 1 mg

Side effects/adverse reactions:
GI: Dry mouth, constipation, cramps, nausea, diarrhea
CNS: Somnolence, dizziness, headache, fatigue
GU: Impotence, urinary incontinence
EENT: Taste change, tinnitus, vision change, rhinitis, nasal congestion
MS: Leg cramps
RESP: Dyspnea
INTEG: Dermatitis, pruritus, purpura
CV: Bradycardia, chest pain

Contraindications: Hypersensitivity

Precautions: Pregnancy (B), lactation, children <12 yr, severe coronary insufficiency, recent MI, renal or hepatic disease, CVA

Pharmacokinetics:
Peak 1-4 hr; 70% bound to plasma proteins; half-life 17 hr; eliminated via kidneys unchanged and as metabolites

Interactions/incompatibilities:
• Increased sedation: CNS depressants, other antihypertensives
• Decreased hypotensive effect: tricyclic antidepressants

NURSING CONSIDERATIONS
Assess:
• Blood studies: neutrophils, decrease in platelets
• Baselines in renal, liver function tests before therapy begins
• B/P before, during, after treatment; notify physician of significant changes
• Edema in feet, legs daily
• Allergic reaction: rash, fever, pruritus, urticaria; drug should be discontinued if antihistamines fail to help
• Symptoms of CHF: edema, dyspnea, wet rales, B/P
• Renal symptoms: polyuria, oliguria, frequency

Perform/provide:
• Storage of tablets in tight containers

Evaluate:
• Therapeutic response: decreased B/P in hypertension

Teach patient/family:
• To avoid hazardous activities
• Not to discontinue drug abruptly or withdrawal symptoms may occur: anxiety, increased B/P, headache, insomnia, increased pulse, tremors, nausea, sweating
• Not to use OTC (cough, cold, or allergy) products unless directed by physician
• To avoid sunlight or to wear sunscreen; photosensitivity may occur
• Importance of complying with dosage schedule even if feeling better

---

haemophilus b vaccines (polysaccharide, conjugate)
(hee-moef'ii-lus)
Hib-Imune, HibVAX (polysaccharide), b-Capsa 1, ProHIBIT (conjugate)
Func. class.: Vaccine
Chem. class.: H. influenzae capsular polysaccharide

Action: Stimulates antibody production to *H. influenzae b*
Uses: Polysaccharide immunization of children 2-6 yr against *H. influenzae b*, conjugate immunization of child 1½-5 yr against invasive disease of *H. influenzae b*

Dosage and routes:
• *Child:* SC 0.5 ml (polysaccharide), IM 0.5 mg (conjugate)
Available forms: Polysaccharide powder for injection 25 μg/0.5 ml after reconstituting; conjugate powder for injection 25 μg polysaccharide and 18 μg conjugated diphtheria toxoid/0.5 ml

Side effects/adverse reactions:
INTEG: Redness, soreness at injection site, rash
SYST: Low-grade fever, acute febrile reactions

Contraindications: Hypersensitivity, febrile illness, active infection
Precautions: Pregnancy (C)
Lab test interferences:
Interference: Latex agglutination, countercurrent immunoelectrophoresis

NURSING CONSIDERATIONS
Assess:
• For skin reactions: swelling, rash, urticaria
• For anaphylaxis: inability to breathe, bronchospasm

Administer:
• After diluting with 0.6 ml diluent, which will yield 10 doses of 0.5 ml
• Only with epinephrine 1 : 1000 on unit to treat laryngospasm
• Only by SC or IM route

Perform/provide:
• Storage in refrigerator
• Written record of immunization

Evaluate:
• For history of allergies, skin conditions (eczema, psoriasis, dermatitis), reactions to vaccinations

Teach patient/family:
• That usually one dose is required

---

halazepam

(hal-az′e-pam)
Paxipam
Func. class.: Antianxiety
Chem. class.: Benzodiazepine

Controlled Substance Schedule IV

Action: Depresses subcortical levels of CNS, including limbic system, reticular formation

Uses: Anxiety

Dosage and routes:
• *Adult:* PO 20-40 mg tid-qid
• *Geriatric:* PO 20 mg qd-bid

Available forms: Tabs 20, 40 mg

Side effects/adverse reactions:
CNS: Dizziness, drowsiness, confusion, headache, anxiety, tremors, stimulation, fatigue, depression, insomnia, hallucinations
GI: Constipation, dry mouth, nausea, vomiting, anorexia, diarrhea
INTEG: Rash, dermatitis, itching
*CV: Orthostatic hypotension, **ECG changes, tachycardia,*** hypotension
EENT: Blurred vision, tinnitus, mydriasis

Contraindications: Hypersensitivity to benzodiazepines, narrow-angle glaucoma, psychosis, pregnancy (D), child <18 yr

Precautions: Elderly, debilitated, hepatic disease, renal disease

Pharmacokinetics:
PO: Peak 1-3 hr, duration 3-6 hr; metabolized by liver; excreted by kidneys; crosses placenta, breast milk; half-life 14 hr

Interactions/incompatibilities:
• Decreased effects of halazepam: oral contraceptives, valproic acid
• Increased effects of halazepam: CNS depressants, alcohol, disulfiram, oral contraceptives, cimetidine

Lab test interferences:
Increase: AST/ALT, serum bilirubin
False increase: 17-OHCS
Decrease: RAIU

NURSING CONSIDERATIONS
Assess:
• B/P (lying, standing), pulse; if systolic B/P drops 20 mm Hg, hold drug, notify physician
• Blood studies: CBC during long-term therapy; blood dyscrasias have occurred rarely
• Hepatic studies: AST, ALT, bilirubin, creatinine, LDH, alk phosphatase
• Mental status: mood, sensorium, affect, sleeping pattern, drowsiness, dizziness
• Physical dependency, withdrawal symptoms: headache, nausea, vomiting, muscle pain, weakness after long-term use
• Suicidal tendencies

Administer:
• With food or milk for GI symptoms
• Crushed if patient is unable to swallow medication whole
• Sugarless gum, hard candy, frequent sips of water for dry mouth

---

italics = common side effects   ***bold italic*** = life threatening reactions

Perform/provide:
• Assistance with ambulation during beginning therapy, since drowsiness/dizziness occurs
• Safety measures, including side rails
• Check to see PO medication has been swallowed

Evaluate:
• Therapeutic response: decreased anxiety, restlessness, sleeplessness

Teach patient/family:
• That drug may be taken with food
• Not to be used for everyday stress or used longer than 4 mo unless directed by physician; not to take more than prescribed amount; may be habit forming
• To avoid OTC preparations (hay fever, cough, cold) unless approved by physician
• To avoid driving or other activities that require alertness; drowsiness may occur
• To avoid alcohol ingestion or other psychotropic medications unless prescribed by physician
• Not to discontinue medication abruptly after long-term use
• To rise slowly or fainting may occur
• That drowsiness may worsen at beginning of treatment

Treatment of overdose: Lavage, VS, supportive care, flumazenil

---

halcinonide
(hal-sin'oo-nide)
Halog, Halog-E
Func. class.: Corticosteroid, synthetic
Chem. class.: Fluorinated corticosteroid

Action: Antiinflammatory, antipruritic, vasoconstrictor actions

Uses: Inflammation of corticosteroid-responsive dermatoses

Dosage and routes:
• *Adult:* TOP apply to affected area bid-tid

Available forms: Cream 0.025%, 0.1%; oint 0.1%; sol 0.1%

Side effects/adverse reactions:
INTEG: Acne, atrophy, epidermal thinning, purpura, striae

Contraindications: Hypersensitivity, viral infections, fungal infections

Precautions: Pregnancy (C)

NURSING CONSIDERATIONS
Assess:
• Infection: increased temperature, WBC, even after withdrawal of medication; keep in mind, these may be systemically absorbed

Administer:
• Using an occlusive dressing; systemic absorption may occur
• For 3-5 days after lesions are gone

Perform/provide:
• Washing of skin before application
• Dressing change qd; check area for redness, rash, inflammation, discoloration; do not leave dressing in place over 16 hr

Evaluate:
• Therapeutic response: decreased inflammation

Teach patient/family:
• Not to get drug in eyes or mucous membranes

---

halofantrene
(hal-o-fan'-trine)
Halfan
Func. class.: Antimalarial
Chem. class.: Synthetic 4-aminoquinoline derivative

Action: Inhibits parasite replica-

---

tions, transcription of DNA to RNA by forming complexes with DNA of parasite

Uses: Malaria caused by *P. vivax, P. malariae, P. ovale, P. falciparum* (some strains)

Dosage and routes:
• *Adult:* 500 mg PO every 6 hr × 3 doses
• *Children <40 kg:* 8 mg/kg every 6 hr × 3 doses

Available forms: Tablets

Side effects/adverse reactions:
CV: Hypotension, heart block, asystole with syncope, ECG changes
INTEG: Pruritus, pigmentary changes, skin eruptions, lichen planuslike eruptions, eczema, exfoliative dermatitis, alopecia
CNS: Headache, stimulation, fatigue, irritability, convulsion, bad dreams, dizziness, confusion, psychosis, decreased reflexes
EENT: Blurred vision, corneal changes, retinal changes, difficulty focusing, tinnitus, vertigo, deafness, photophobia, corneal edema
GI: Nausea, vomiting, anorexia, diarrhea, cramps, weight loss, stomatitis
HEMA: Thrombocytopenia, agranulocytosis, hemolytic anemia, leukopenia

Contraindications: Hypersensitivity, retinal field changes, porphyria, children (long-term)

Precautions: Pregnancy (C), children, blood dyscrasias, severe GI disease, neurologic disease, alcoholism, hepatic disease, G-6-PD deficiency, psoriasis, eczema

Pharmacokinetics:
PO: Peak 1-2 hr, half-life 3-5 days; metabolized in the liver; excreted in urine, feces, breast milk; crosses placenta

Interactions/incompatibilities:
• Decreased action of chloroquine: Mg Al compounds, kaolin

NURSING CONSIDERATIONS
Assess:
• Ophthalmic test if long-term treatment or drug dosage 150 mg/day
• Liver studies qwk: AST, ALT, bilirubin
• Blood studies: CBC, since blood dyscrasias occur
• For decreased reflexes: knee, ankle
• ECG during therapy
• Watch for depression of T waves, widening of QRS complex
• Allergic reactions: pruritus, rash, urticaria
• Blood dyscrasias: malaise, fever, bruising, bleeding (rare)
• For ototoxicity (tinnitus, vertigo, change in hearing); audiometric testing should be done before, after treatment
• For toxicity: blurring vision, difficulty focusing, headache, dizziness, knee, ankle reflexes; drug should be discontinued immediately

Administer:
• Before or after meals at same time each day to maintain drug level
• IM after aspirating to avoid injection into blood system, which may cause hypotension, asystole, heart block; rotate injection sites

Perform/provide:
• Storage in tight, light-resistant containers at room temperature; injection should be kept in cool environment

Evaluate:
• Therapeutic response: decreased symptoms of infection

Teach patient/family:
• To use sunglasses in bright sunlight to decrease photophobia

H

---

italics = common side effects   **bold italic** = life threatening reactions

• That urine may turn rust or brown color
• To report hearing, visual problems, fever, fatigue, bruising, bleeding, which may indicate blood dyscrasias

Treatment of overdose: Induce vomiting; gastric lavage; administer barbiturate (ultrashort-acting), vasopressin; tracheostomy may be necessary

---

haloperidol/haloperidol decanoate

(ha-loe-per′idole)
Haldol, Haloperidol, Haloperidol Decanoate 50, Haloperidol 100

Func. class.: Antipsychotic/neuroleptic
Chem. class.: Butyrophenone

Action: Depresses cerebral cortex, hypothalamus, limbic system, which control activity and aggression; blocks neurotransmission produced by dopamine at synapse; exhibits strong α-adrenergic, anticholinergic blocking action; mechanism for antipsychotic effects unclear

Uses: Psychotic disorders, control of tics, vocal utterances in Gilles de la Tourette syndrome, short-term treatment of hyperactive children showing excessive motor activity, prolonged parenteral therapy in chronic schizophrenia

Dosage and routes:
Psychosis
• *Adult:* PO 0.5-5 mg bid or tid initially depending on severity of condition; dose is increased to desired dose, max 100 mg/day; IM 2-5 mg q1-8h
• *Child 3-12 yr:* PO/IM 0.05-0.15 mg/kg/day

• *Decanoate:* Initial dose IM is 10-15 × daily oral dose at 4 wk interval; do not administer IV; not to exceed 100 mg

Chronic schizophrenia
• *Adult:* IM 10-15 times the PO dose q4wk (decanoate)
• *Child 3-12 yr:* PO/IM 0.05-0.15 mg/kg/day

Tics/vocal utterances
• *Adult:* PO 0.5-5 mg bid or tid, increased until desired response occurs
• *Child 3-12 yr:* PO 0.05-0.075 mg/kg/day

Hyperactive children
• *Child 3-12 yr:* PO 0.05-0.075 mg/kg/day

Available forms: Tabs 0.5, 1, 2, 5, 10, 20 mg; conc 2 mg/ml; inj IM 5 mg/ml

Side effects/adverse reactions:
RESP: **Laryngospasm,** dyspnea, **respiratory depression**
CNS: Extrapyramidal symptoms: pseudoparkinsonism, akathisia, dystonia, tardive dyskinesia, drowsiness, headache, seizures neuroleptic malignant syndrome, confusion
INTEG: Rash, photosensitivity, dermatitis
EENT: Blurred vision, glaucoma, dry eyes
GI: Dry mouth, nausea, vomiting, anorexia, constipation, diarrhea, jaundice, weight gain, *ileus, hepatitis*
GU: Urinary retention, urinary frequency, enuresis, impotence, amenorrhea, gynecomastia
CV: Orthostatic hypotension, hypertension, *cardiac arrest,* ECG changes, *tachycardia*

Contraindications: Hypersensitivity, blood dyscrasias, coma, child <3 yr, brain damage, bone marrow depression, alcohol and barbiturate

---

withdrawal states, Parkinson's disease, angina, epilepsy, urinary retention, narrow-angle glaucoma

Precautions: Pregnancy (C), lactation, seizure disorders, hypertension, hepatic disease, cardiac disease

Pharmacokinetics:

PO: Onset erratic, peak 2-6 hr, half-life 24 hr

IM: Onset 15-30 min, peak 15-20 min, half-life 21 hr

IM (Decanoate): Peak 4-11 days, half-life 3 wk

Metabolized by liver; excreted in urine, bile; crosses placenta; enters breast milk

Interactions/incompatibilities:

• Oversedation: other CNS depressants, alcohol, barbiturate anesthetics

• Toxicity: epinephrine

• Toxicity: with lithium, neurotoxicity and brain damage possible

• Decreased effects of: lithium, levodopa

• Increased effects of both drugs: β-adrenergic blockers, alcohol

• Increased anticholinergic effects: anticholinergics

• Decreased effects of: haloperidol; phenobarbital

Lab test interferences:

Increase: Liver function tests, cardiac enzymes, cholesterol, blood glucose, prolactin, bilirubin, PBI, cholinesterase

Decrease: Hormones (blood, urine)

False positive: Pregnancy tests, PKU

False negative: Urinary steroids

NURSING CONSIDERATIONS

Assess:

• Swallowing of PO medication; check for hoarding or giving of medication to other patients

• I&O ratio; palpate bladder if low urinary output occurs

• Bilirubin, CBC, liver function studies monthly

• Urinalysis is recommended before and during prolonged therapy

• For depression in bipolar patients; rapid mood swings may occur with this drug

• Affect, orientation, LOC, reflexes, gait, coordination, sleep pattern disturbances

• B/P standing and lying; take pulse and respirations q4h during initial treatment; establish baseline before starting treatment; report drops of 30 mm Hg

• Dizziness, faintness, palpitations, tachycardia on rising

• Extrapyramidal symptoms including akathisia (inability to sit still, no pattern to movements), tardive dyskinesia (bizarre movements of jaw, mouth, tongue, extremities), pseudoparkinsonism (rigidity, tremors, pill rolling, shuffling gait)

• Skin turgor daily

• For neuroleptic malignant syndrome: hyperthermia, muscle rigidity, altered mental status, increased CPK

• Constipation, urinary retention daily; if these occur, increase bulk, water in diet

Administer:

• Reduced dose to elderly

• Antiparkinsonian agent, to be used if extrapyramidal symptoms occur

• IM injection into large muscle mass, use No. 21 G, 2″ needle; give no more than 3 ml/injection site; patient should remain recumbent for ½ hr

• Oral liquid: use calibrated dropper; do not mix in coffee or tea

• PO with food or milk

---

italics = common side effects   ***bold italic*** = life threatening reactions

Perform/provide:

• Decreased noise input by dimming lights, avoiding loud noises
• Supervised ambulation until stabilized on medication; do not involve in strenuous exercise program because fainting is possible; patient should not stand still for long periods
• Increased fluids to prevent constipation
• Sips of water, candy, gum for dry mouth
• Storage in tight, light-resistant container

Evaluate:

• Therapeutic response: decrease in emotional excitement, hallucinations, delusions, paranoia, reorganization of patterns of thought, speech

Teach patient/family:

• That orthostatic hypotension occurs often and to rise from sitting or lying position gradually to avoid hazardous activities until stabilized on medication
• To remain lying down after IM injection for at least 30 min
• To avoid hot tubs, hot showers, tub baths, since hypotension may occur
• To avoid abrupt withdrawal of this drug, or extrapyramidal symptoms may result; drug should be withdrawn slowly
• To avoid OTC preparations (cough, hay fever, cold) unless approved by physician, since serious drug interactions may occur; avoid use with alcohol or CNS depressants; increased drowsiness may occur
• To use a sunscreen during sun exposure to prevent burns
• Regarding compliance with drug regimen
• About EPS and necessity for meticulous oral hygiene, since oral candidiasis may occur
• To report impaired vision, jaundice, tremors, muscle twitching
• That in hot weather, heat stroke may occur; take extra precautions to stay cool

Treatment of overdose: Activated charcoal lavage if orally ingested; provide an airway; *do not induce vomiting*

---

haloprogin (topical)

(ha-loe-proe'jin)
Halotex

Func. class.: Local antiinfective, antifungal
Chem. class.: Iodinated phenolic ester

Action: Interferes with fungal cell membrane permeability

Uses: Tinea pedis, tinea cruris, tinea corporis, tinea manus, tinea versicolor

Dosage and routes:

• *Adult and child:* TOP apply to affected area bid × 14-21 days
Available forms: Cream, sol 1%

Side effects/adverse reactions:

INTEG: Rash, urticaria, stinging, burning, vesiculation, pruritus, erythema, scaling, folliculitis sensitization

Contraindications: Hypersensitivity

Precautions: Pregnancy (B), lactation, children

NURSING CONSIDERATIONS

Assess:

• Allergic reaction: burning, stinging, swelling, redness, vesiculation, scaling

Administer:

• Enough medication to cover lesions completely
• After cleansing with soap, water

before each application; dry well
Perform/provide:
• Storage at room temperature in dry place
Evaluate:
• Therapeutic response: decrease in size, number of lesions
Teach patient/family:
• To use medical asepsis (hand washing) before, after each application
• To apply with glove to prevent further infection
• To avoid use of OTC creams, ointments, lotions unless directed by physician
• To avoid contact with eyes
• To continue even though condition improves
• To use for full duration even if condition subsides or irritation increases; if condition does not improve after 4 wk, another treatment should be considered

---

heparin calcium/heparin sodium
(hep'a-rin)
Calcilean,* Calciparine, Hepalean,* Heparin Sodium and 0.45% Sodium Chloride, Heparin Sodium and 0.9% Sodium Chloride, Heparin Lock Flush, Heparin Sodium, Hep-Lock, Liquaemin Sodium
Func. class.: Anticoagulant

Action: Prevents conversion of fibrinogen to fibrin and prothrombin to thrombin by enhancing inhibitory effects of antithrombin III
Uses: Deep-vein thrombosis, pulmonary emboli, myocardial infarction, open heart surgery, disseminated intravascular clotting syndrome, atrial fibrillation with embolization, as an anticoagulant in transfusion and dialysis procedures, prevention of DVT/PE

Dosage and routes:
Deep vein thrombosis/MI
• *Adult:* IV PUSH 5000-7000 U q4h then titrated to PTT or ACT level; IV BOL 5000-7500 U, then IV INF; IV INF; after bolus dose, then 1000 U/hr titrated to PTT or ACT level
• *Child:* IV INF 50 U/kg, maintenance 100 U/kg q4h or 20,000 U/m² qd
Pulmonary embolism
• *Adult:* IV PUSH 7500-10,000 q4h then titrated to PTT or ACT level; IV BOL 7500-10,000, then IV INF; IV INF after bolus dose, then 1000 U/hr titrated to PTT or ACT level
• *Child:* IV INF 50 U/kg, maintenance 100 U/kg q4h or 20,000 U/m² qd
Open heart surgery
• *Adult:* IV INF 150-300 U/kg Prophylaxis for DVT/PE
• *Adult SC:* 5,000 units q8-12h
Available forms: Heparin sodium inj 1000, 2500, 5000, 7500, 10,000, 15,000, 20,000, 40,000 U/ml; Heparin calcium inj 5000, 12,500, 20,000 U/dose
Side effects/adverse reactions:
CNS: Fever, chills
GI: Diarrhea, nausea, vomiting, anorexia, stomatitis, abdominal cramps, *hepatitis*
GU: Hematuria
HEMA: Hemorrhage, thrombocytopenia
INTEG: Rash, dermatitis, urticaria, alopecia, pruritus
Contraindications: Hypersensitivity, hemophilia, leukemia with bleeding, peptic ulcer disease, thrombocytopenic purpura, hepatic disease (severe), renal disease (severe), blood dyscrasias, severe

---

italics = common side effects   ***bold italic*** = life threatening reactions

hypertension, subacute bacterial endocarditis, acute nephritis

Precautions: Alcoholism, elderly, pregnancy (C)

Pharmacokinetics: Well absorbed (SC)

IV: Peak 5 min, duration 2-6 hr

SC: Onset 20-60 min, duration 8-12 hr

Half-life 1½ hr, excreted in urine, 95% bound to plasma proteins, does not cross placenta or alter breast milk; removed from the system via the lymph and spleen

Interactions/incompatibilities:

• Decreased action of: corticosteroids

• Increased action of: diazepam

• Decreased action of heparin: digitalis, tetracyclines, antihistamines

• Increased action of heparin: oral anticoagulants, salicylates, dextran, steroids, nonsteroidal antiinflammatories

• Incompatible in sol with amikacin, ampicillin, atropine, cephalothin, chlordiazepoxide, chlorpromazine, chlortetracycline, codeine, dacarbazine, daunorubicin, diazepam, dobutamine, erythromycin, ergonovine, gentamicin hyaluronidase, hydrocortisone, hydroxyzine, insulin, kanamycin, levorphanol, meperidine, metaraminol, methadone, methicillin, morphine, penicillin G, polymyxin B, procainamide, prochlorperazine, promazine, promethazine, streptomycin, tetracycline, tobramycin, vancomycin, vinblastine

Lab test interferences:

Increase: T$_3$ uptake

Decrease: Uric acid

NURSING CONSIDERATIONS

Assess:

• Blood studies (Hct, occult blood in stools) q3mo

• Partial prothrombin time, which

should be 1½-2 × control, PTT; often done qd, APTT, ACT

• B/P, watch for increasing signs of hypertension

• Platelet count q 2-3 days; thrombocytopenia may occur

• Bleeding gums, petecchiae, ecchymosis, black tarry stools, hematuria, epistaxis, decrease in B/P; indicate bleeding and possible hemorrhage

• Fever, skin rash, urticaria

• Needed dosage change q1-2wk

Administer:

• IV undiluted or diluted in 0.9% NaCl, dextrose, Ringer's sol and given by direct, intermittent, or continuous infusion; give 1000 U or less over 1 min; then 5000 U or less over 1 min; infusion may run from 4-24 hr; use infusion pump

• Blood after adding 7,500 U/100 ml NaCl inj, add 6-8ml of this sol/100ml of whole blood

• At same time each day to maintain steady blood levels

• SC deep with at 25 G ⅜-in needle; do not massage area or aspirate when giving SC injection; give in abdomen between pelvic bone, rotate sites; do not pull back on plunger, leave in for 10 sec; apply gentle pressure for 1 min

• Changing needles is not recommended

• Avoiding all IM injections that may cause bleeding

• Do not administer concomitantly with IV nitroglycerin

Perform/provide:

• Storage in tight container

Evaluate:

• Therapeutic response: decrease of deep-vein thrombosis

Teach patient/family:

• To avoid OTC preparations that may cause serious drug interactions unless directed by physician

• That drug may be held during active bleeding (menstruation), depending on condition
• To use soft-bristle toothbrush to avoid bleeding gums, avoid contact sports, use electric razor, avoid IM injection
• To carry a Medic Alert ID identifying drug taken
• To report any signs of bleeding: gums, under skin, urine, stools
Treatment of overdose:
Withdraw drug, protamine SO_4 1:1 solution

---

hepatitis B vaccine
Engerix-B, Recombivax HB
Func. class.: Vaccine

Action: Provides active immunity to hepatitis B
Uses: Prevention of hepatitis B virus
Dosage and routes:
• *Adult and child >10 yr:* IM 1 ml, then 1 ml after 1 mo, then 1 ml 6 mo after initial dose
• *Child 3 mo-10 yr:* IM 0.5 ml, then 0.5 ml after 1 mo, then 0.5 ml 6 mo after initial dose
• *Patients with decreased immunity:* IM 2 ml, then 2 ml after 1 mo, then 2 ml 6 mo after initial dose
Available forms: Inj IM 10 mg/0.5 ml, 20 μg/ml
Side effects/adverse reactions:
INTEG: Soreness at injection site, urticaria, erythema, swelling
SYST: Induration
CNS: Headache, dizziness, fever
GI: Nausea, vomiting
Contraindications: Hypersensitivity
Precautions: Pregnancy, elderly, lactation, children; active infection, compromised cardiac or pulmonary status

NURSING CONSIDERATIONS
Assess:
• For skin reactions: rash, induration, urticaria
• For anaphylaxis: inability to breathe, bronchospasm
Administer:
• After rotating vial; do not shake
• Only with epinephrine 1:1000 on unit to treat laryngospasm
• In deltoid for better protection; give 2 ml dose in two different sites
Perform/provide:
• Written record of immunization
• Comfort measures
Evaluate:
• For history of allergies, skin conditions (eczema, psoriasis, dermatitis), reactions to vaccinations

---

hetastarch
(het′a-starch)
Hespan
Func. class.: Plasma expander
Chem. class.: Synthetic polymer

Action: Similar to human albumin, which expands plasma volume by colloidal osmotic pressure
Uses: Plasma volume expander, leukapheresis
Dosage and routes:
• *Adult:* IV INF 500-1000 ml, total dose not to exceed 1500 ml/day, not to exceed 20 ml/kg/hr (hemorrhagic shock)
Leukapheresis
• *Adult:* IV INF 250-700 ml infused at 1:8 ratio with whole blood, may be repeated 2/wk up to 10 treatments
Available forms: 6% hetastarch/ 0.9% NaCl
Side effects/adverse reactions:
HEMA: Decreased hematocrit, platelet function, increased bleed-

---

italics = common side effects   **bold italic** = life threatening reactions

ing/coagulation times, increased sed rate

INTEG: Rash, urticaria, pruritus, angioedema, chills, fever, flushing, peripheral edema

RESP: Wheezing, dyspnea, ***bronchospasm, pulmonary edema***

GI: Nausea, vomiting

SYST: ***Anaphylaxis***

CNS: Headache

Contraindications: Hypersensitivity, severe bleeding disorders, renal failure, CHF (severe)

Precautions: Pregnancy (C), liver disease, pulmonary edema

Pharmacokinetics:

IV: Expands blood volume 1-2 × amount infused, excreted in urine

Lab test interferences:

False increase: bilirubin

NURSING CONSIDERATIONS

Assess:

• VS q5min × 30 min

• CVP during infusion (5-10 cm H_2O normal range)

• Urine output q1h, watch for increase in urinary output, which is common; if output does not increase, infusion should be decreased or discontinued

• I&O ratio and specific gravity, urine osmolarity; if specific gravity is very low, renal clearance is low; drug should be discontinued

• Allergy: rash, urticaria, pruritus, wheezing, dyspnea, bronchospasm; drug should be discontinued immediately

• For circulatory overload: increased pulse, respirations, SOB, wheezing, chest tightness, chest pain

• For dehydration after infusion: decreased output, increased temperature, poor skin turgor, increased specific gravity, dry skin

Administer:

• IV Inf undiluted, run at 20 ml/kg/hr; reduced rate in septic shock, burns

Perform/provide:

• Storage at room temperature; discard unused portions, do not freeze, do not use if turbid or deep brown or precipitate forms

Evaluate:

• Therapeutic response: increased plasma volume

---

hexamethylmelamine
Hexalen
Func. class.: Antineoplastic, alkylating agent

Action: Responsible for inhibition of cell DNA and RNA synthesis, cell death; rapidly degraded; cell cycle nonspecific

Uses: Resistant or recurrent ovarian cancer; may be used alone or in combination

Dosage and routes:

Adult: PO 260 mg/m²; average dose 400 qd × 14 days, then rest for 14 days; cycle should continue until patient no longer responds

Available forms: Caps 50 mg

Side effects/adverse reactions:

EENT: Tinnitus, hearing loss

HEMA: ***Thrombocytopenia, leukopenia***

GI: Nausea, vomiting, diarrhea, stomatitis, weight loss, colitis, hepatotoxicity, anorexia

CNS: Headache, dizziness, drowsiness, paresthesia, peripheral neuropathy, coma, hyporeflexia, muscle weakness

INTEG: Alopecia, pruritus, herpes zoster

Contraindications: Lactation, pregnancy (first trimester) (D), myelosuppression, acute herpes zoster, hypersensitivity

Precautions: Radiation therapy, leukopenia, thrombocytopenia

Pharmacokinetics: Metabolized in liver, excreted in urine

Interactions/incompatibilities:
• Increased toxicity: antineoplastics, radiation
• Reduced efficiency: influenza vaccine, pneumococcal vaccine

NURSING CONSIDERATIONS

Assess:
• CBC, differential, platelet count weekly; withhold drug if WBC is <4000 or platelet count is 75,000; notify physician of these results
• Renal function studies: BUN, serum uric acid, urine CrCl before, during therapy
• I&O ratio; report fall in urine output to <30 ml/hr
• Monitor temperature q4h; fever may indicate beginning infection; no rectal temperatures
• Liver function tests before, during therapy: (bilirubin, AST, ALT, LDH) as needed or monthly
• Bleeding: hematuria, guaiac, bruising, or petechiae, mucosa or orifices q8h
• Food preferences: list likes, dislikes
• Yellowing of skin and sclera, dark urine, clay-colored stools, itchy skin, abdominal pain, fever, diarrhea
• Effects of alopecia on body image; discuss feelings about body changes
• Inflammation of mucosa, breaks in skin
• Buccal cavity q8h for dryness, sores, or ulceration, white patches, oral pain, bleeding, dysphagia
• Symptoms indicating severe allergic reaction: rash, pruritus, urticaria, purpuric skin lesions, itching, flushing

Administer:
• As divided daily doses 1-2 hr pc and hs
• Antiemetic 30-60 min before giving drug to prevent vomiting and prn
• Topical or systemic analgesics for pain
• Local or systemic drugs for infection

Perform/provide:
• Storage at room temperature in dry form
• Strict medical asepsis, protective isolation if WBC levels are low
• Special skin care
• Increase fluid intake to 2-3 L/day to prevent urate deposits, calculi information
• Diet low in purines: organ meats (kidney, liver), dried beans, peas to maintain alkaline urine
• Rinsing of mouth tid-qid with water, club soda; brushing of teeth bid-tid with soft brush or cotton-tipped applicators for stomatitis; use unwaxed dental floss

Evaluate:
• Therapeutic response: decreased tumor size, decreased spread of malignancy

Teach patient/family:
• About protective isolation precautions
• That sterility, amenorrhea can occur; reversible after discontinuing treatment
• That hair may be lost during treatment; a wig or hairpiece may make patient feel better; new hair may be different in color, texture
• To avoid foods with citric acid, hot or rough texture
• To report any bleeding, white spots, or ulcerations in mouth to

---

physician; tell patient to examine mouth qd

• To report signs of infection: increased temperature, sore throat, flu symptoms

• To report signs of anemia: fatigue, headache, faintness, shortness of breath, irritability

---

hexocyclium methylsulfate

(hex-oh-sye′klee-um)

Tral

Func. class.: GI anticholinergic
Chem. class.: Synthetic quaternary ammonium compound

Action: Inhibits muscarinic actions of acetylcholine at postganglionic parasympathetic neuroeffector sites

Uses: Treatment of peptic ulcer disease in combination with other drugs; other GI disorders

Dosage and routes:

• *Adult:* PO 25 mg qid ac, hs

Available forms: Tabs 25 mg

Side effects/adverse reactions:

CNS: Confusion, stimulation in elderly, headache, insomnia, dizziness, drowsiness, anxiety, weakness, hallucination

GI: Dry mouth, constipation, paralytic ileus, heartburn, nausea, vomiting, dysphagia, absence of taste

GU: Hesitancy, retention, impotence

CV: Palpitations, tachycardia

EENT: Blurred vision, photophobia, mydriasis, cycloplegia, increased ocular tension

INTEG: Urticaria, rash, pruritus, anhidrosis, fever, allergic reactions

Contraindications: Hypersensitivity to anticholinergics, narrow-angle glaucoma, GI obstruction, myasthenia gravis, paralytic ileus, GI atony, toxic megacolon

Precautions: Hyperthyroidism, coronary artery disease, dysrhythmias, CHF, ulcerative colitis, hypertension, hiatal hernia, hepatic disease, renal disease, pregnancy (C), urinary retention, prostatic hypertrophy, elderly

Pharmacokinetics:

PO: Onset 1 hr, duration 3-4 hr; metabolized by liver, excreted in urine

Interactions/incompatibilities:

• Increased anticholinergic effect: amantadine, tricyclic antidepressants, MAOIs

• Decreased effect of: phenothiazines, levodopa, ketoconazole

NURSING CONSIDERATIONS

Assess:

• VS, cardiac status: checking for dysrhythmias, increased rate, palpitations

• I&O ratio; check for urinary retention or hesitancy

• GI complaints: pain, bleeding (frank or occult), nausea, vomiting, anorexia

Administer:

• ½-1 hr ac for better absorption

• Decreased dose to elderly patients; their metabolism may be slowed

• Gum, hard candy, frequent rinsing of mouth for dryness of oral cavity

Perform/provide:

• Storage in tight container protected from light

• Increased fluids, bulk, exercise to patient's life-style to decrease constipation

Evaluate:

• Therapeutic response: absence of epigastric pain, bleeding, nausea, vomiting

---

Teach patient/family:
• To avoid driving or other hazardous activities until stabilized on medication
• To avoid alcohol or other CNS depressants; will enhance sedating properties of drug
• To avoid hot environments; stroke may occur; drug suppresses perspiration
• To use sunglasses when outside to prevent photophobia; may cause blurred vision
• To drink plenty of fluids
• To report dysphagia

**homatropine
hydrobromide (optic)**
(hoe'ma-troe-peen)
AK-Homatropine, Homatropine, Homatropine HBr Ophthalmic, Isopto
Func. class.: Mydriatic
Chem. class.: Synthetic alkaloid

Action: Blocks response of iris sphincter muscle, muscle of accommodation of ciliary body to cholinergic stimulation, resulting in dilation, paralysis of accommodation

Uses: Uveitis, iritis, mydriatic, cycloplegic for refraction

Dosage and routes:
• *Adult and child:* INSTILL 1-2 gtts; repeat in 5-10 min for refraction or q3-4h for uveitis
Use only 2% strength in children
Available forms: Sol 2%, 5%

Side effects/adverse reactions:
CV: Tachycardia
CNS: Confusion, somnolence, flushing, fever, restlessness, seizures, ataxic gait, psychiatric disturbances in children
EENT: Blurred vision, photophobia, increased intraocular pressure, irritation, edema

Contraindications: Hypersensitivity, children <6 yr, narrow-angle glaucoma, increased intraocular pressure, infants

Precautions: Children, elderly, hypertension, hyperthyroidism, diabetes, pregnancy (C)

Pharmacokinetics:
INSTILL: Peak ½-1 hr, duration 1-3 days

NURSING CONSIDERATIONS
Assess:
• Eye pain; discontinue use
Evaluate:
• Therapeutic response: decrease in inflammation or cycloplegic refraction

Teach patient/family:
• To report change in vision, blurring or loss of sight, trouble breathing, sweating, flushing
• Method of instillation: pressure on lacrimal sac for 1 min; do not touch dropper to eye
• That blurred vision will decrease with repeated use of drug
• Not to engage in hazardous activities until able to see
• To wait 5 min to use other drops
• Not to blink more than usual

---

hyaluronidase
(hye-al-yoor-on'i-dase)
Wydase
Func. class.: Enzyme

Action: Hydrolyzes hyaluronic acid within areas filled with exudates

Uses: Hypodermoclysis, subcutaneous urography; adjunct to dispersion of other drugs

Dosage and routes:
Adjunct
• *Adult and child:* INJ 150 U with other drug

---

italics = common side effects   ***bold italic*** = life threatening reactions

Urography
• *Adult and child:* SC 75 U over scapula, then contrast medium injected at same site

Hypodermoclysis
• *Adult and child >3 yr:* SC 150 U/L of clysis sol for 1 L of clysis sol

Available forms: Inj powder 150, 1500 U; inj sol 150 U/ml

Side effects/adverse reactions:
INTEG: Rash, urticaria, itching
OTHER: Overhydration (hyperdermoclysis)

Contraindications: Hypersensitivity to bovine products, CHF, hypoproteinemia, around infected/inflamed or cancerous area

Precautions: Pregnancy (C)

Interactions/incompatibilities:
• Systemic reactions: local anesthetics

NURSING CONSIDERATIONS
Assess:
• Site before administration (hypodermoclysis)
• For overhydration in child <3 yr

Administer:
• After test dose: 0.02 ml of 150 u/ml solution is injected if wheal develops, itching test is positive
• Right after mixing, since solution is unstable
• To child <3 yr, not exceeding 200 ml; in neonates not exceeding 2 ml/min

Evaluate:
• Therapeutic response: absence of swelling, pain after hypodermoclysis

---

hydralazine HCl
(hye'dral'a-zeen)
Alazine, Apresoline, Hydralazine HCl
Func. class.: Antihypertensive, direct-acting peripheral vasodilator
Chem. class.: Phthalazine

Action: Vasodilates arteriolar smooth muscle by direct relaxation; reduction in blood pressure with reflex increases in cardiac function

Uses: Essential hypertension; *parenteral:* severe essential hypertension, CHF

Dosage and routes:
• *Adult:* PO 10 mg qid 2-4 days, then 25 mg for rest of 1st wk, then 50 mg qid individualized to desired response, not to exceed 300 mg qd; IV/IM BOL 20-40 mg q4-6h, administer PO as soon as possible; IM 20-40 mg q4-6h
• *Child:* PO 0.75-3 mg/kg/day in 4 divided doses; max 7.5 mg/kg/24 hr; IV BOL 0.1-0.2 mg/kg q4-6h; IM 0.1-0.2 mg/kg q4-6h

Available forms: Inj IV, IM 20 mg/ml; tabs 10, 25, 50, 100 mg

Side effects/adverse reactions:
MISC: Nasal congestion, muscle cramps, *lupuslike symptoms*
CV: Palpitations, reflex tachycardia, angina, **shock,** edema, rebound hypertension
CNS: Headache, tremors, dizziness, anxiety, peripheral neuritis, depression
GI: Nausea, vomiting, anorexia, diarrhea, constipation
INTEG: Rash, pruritus
HEMA: **Leukopenia, agranulocytosis,** anemia
GU: Impotence, urinary retention, Na, H_2O retention

Contraindications: Hypersensitivity to hydralazines, coronary artery disease, mitral valvular rheumatic heart disease, rheumatic heart disease

Precautions: Pregnancy (C), CVA, advanced renal disease

Pharmacokinetics:

PO: Onset 20-30 min, peak 1 hr, duration 2-4 hr

IM: Onset 5-10 min, peak 1 hr, duration 2-4 hr

IV: Onset 5-20 min, peak 10-80 min, duration 2-6 hr; half-life 2-8 hr; metabolized by liver; less than 10% present in urine

Interactions/incompatibilities:

• Increased tachycardia, angina: sympathomimetics (epinephrine, norepinephrine)

• Increased effects of: β-blockers

• Use MAOIs with caution in patients receiving hydralazine

• Incompatible with aminophylline, ampicillin, calcium disodium edetate, chlorothiazide, ethacrynic acid, hydrocortisone, mephentermine, methohexital, nitroglycerin, phenobarbital, verapamil, 10% fructose, $D_{10}LR$

NURSING CONSIDERATIONS

Assess:

• B/P q5min × 2 hr, then q1h × 2 hr, then q4h

• Pulse, jugular venous distention q4h

• Electrolytes, blood studies: K, Na, Cl, CO_2, CBC, serum glucose

• Weight daily, I&O

• LE prep, ANA titer before starting therapy

• Edema in feet, legs daily

• Skin turgor, dryness of mucous membranes for hydration status

• Rales, dyspnea, orthopnea

• IV site for extravasation, rate

• Fever, joint pain, tachycardia, palpitations, headache, nausea

• Mental status: affect, mood, behavior, anxiety; check for personality changes

Administer:

• IV undiluted; give through Y-tube or 3-way stopcock each 10 mg or less/min

• To patient in recumbent position; keep in that position for 1 hr after administration

Evaluate:

• Therapeutic response: decreased B/P

Teach patient/family:

• To take with food to increase bioavailability

• To avoid OTC preparations unless directed by physician

• To notify physician if chest pain, severe fatigue, fever, muscle or joint pain occurs

Treatment of overdose: Administer vasopressors, volume expanders for shock; if PO, lavage or give activated charcoal, digitalization

hydrochlorothiazide

(hye-droe-klor-oh-thye'a-zide)
Diaqua, Diuchlor H,* Esidrix, Hydro-Chlor, Hydrochlorothiazide, HydroDiuril, Hydromal, Hydro-T, Hydrozide,* Neo-Codema,* Novohydrazide,* Oretic, Thiuretic, Urozide*

Func. class.: Thiazide diuretic
Chem. class.: Sulfonamide derivative

Action: Acts on distal tubule by increasing excretion of water, sodium, chloride, potassium

Uses: Edema, hypertension, diuresis, CHF

Dosage and routes:

• *Adult:* PO 25-100 mg/day

• *Child >6 mo:* PO 2.2 mg/kg/day in divided doses

---

italics = common side effects   ***bold italic*** = life threatening reactions

• *Child <6 mo:* PO up to 3.3 mg/kg/day in divided doses

Available forms: Tabs 25, 50, 100 mg; sol 50 mg/5 ml, 100 mg/ml, 10 mg/ml

Side effects/adverse reactions:

GU: Frequency, polyuria, *uremia, glucosuria*

CNS: Drowsiness, paresthesia, depression, headache, *dizziness, fatigue, weakness*

GI: Nausea, vomiting, anorexia, constipation, diarrhea, cramps, pancreatitis, GI irritation, *hepatitis*

EENT: Blurred vision

INTEG: Rash, urticaria, purpura, photosensitivity, fever

META: Hyperglycemia, hyperuricemia, increased creatinine, BUN

HEMA: Aplastic anemia, hemolytic anemia, leukopenia, agranulocytosis, thrombocytopenia, neutropenia

CV: Irregular pulse, orthostatic hypotension, palpitations, volume depletion

ELECT: Hypokalemia, hypercalcemia, hyponatremia, hypochloremia, hypomagnesemia

Contraindications: Hypersensitivity to thiazides or sulfonamides, anuria, renal decompensation, hypomagnesemia

Precautions: Hypokalemia, renal disease, pregnancy (D), hepatic disease, gout, COPD, lupus erythematosus, diabetes mellitus

Pharmacokinetics:

PO: Onset 2 hr, peak 4 hr, duration 6-12 hr; excreted unchanged by kidneys; crosses placenta; enters breast milk

Interactions/incompatibilities:

• Increased toxicity of: lithium, nondepolarizing skeletal muscle relaxants, digitalis

• Decreased effects of: antidiabetics

• Decreased absorption of thiazides: cholestyramine, colestipol

• Decreased hypotensive response: indomethacin, NSAIDs

• Hyperglycemia, hyperuricemia, hypotension: diazoxide

Lab test interferences:

Increase: BSP retention, amylase, parathyroid test

Decrease: PBI, PSP

NURSING CONSIDERATIONS

Assess:

• Weight, I&O daily to determine fluid loss; effect of drug may be decreased if used qd

• Rate, depth, rhythm of respiration, effect of exertion

• B/P lying, standing; postural hypotension may occur

• Electrolytes: K, Mg, Na, Cl; include BUN, blood sugar, CBC, serum creatinine, blood pH, ABGs, uric acid, Ca

• Glucose in urine if patient is diabetic

• Signs of metabolic alkalosis: drowsiness, restlessness

• Signs of hypokalemia: postural hypotension, malaise, fatigue, tachycardia, leg cramps, weakness, dehydration

• Rashes, temperature elevation qd

• Confusion, especially in elderly; take safety precautions if needed

Administer:

• In AM to avoid interference with sleep if using drug as a diuretic

• K replacement if K is less than 3.0

• With food; if nausea occurs, absorption may be decreased slightly

Evaluate:

• Therapeutic response: improvement in edema of feet, legs, sacral area daily if medication is being used in CHF

Teach patient/family:

• To increase fluid intake to 2-3 L/

day unless contraindicated; to rise slowly from lying or sitting position
• To notify physician of muscle weakness, cramps, nausea, dizziness
• That drug may be taken with food or milk
• Use sunscreen for photosensitivity
• That blood sugar may be increased in diabetics
• To take early in day to avoid nocturia
Treatment of overdose: Lavage if taken orally; monitor electrolytes; administer dextrose in saline; monitor hydration, CV, renal status

---

hydrocodone bitartrate
(hye-droe-koe'done)
Hycodan,* Robidone*
Func. class.: Narcotic analgesic
Chem. class.: Opiate

Controlled Substance Schedule III
Action: Acts directly on cough center in medulla to suppress cough
Uses: Hyperactive and nonproductive cough, mild pain
Dosages and routes:
• *Adults:* PO 5 mg q4h prn or 10 mg q12h (long-acting)
• *Child:* PO, 2-12 mg 1.25-5 mg q4h prn
Available forms: Caps 5 mg, susp 5 mg/ml, tabs 5 mg, 10 mg (long-acting)
Side effects/adverse reactions:
CNS: Drowsiness, dizziness, lightheadedness, confusion, headache, sedation, euphoria, dysphoria, weakness, hallucinations, disorientation, mood changes, dependence, *convulsions*

GI: Nausea, vomiting, anorexia, constipation, cramps, dry mouth
GU: Increased urinary output, dysuria, urinary retention
INTEG: Rash, urticaria, flushing, pruritus
EENT: Tinnitus, blurred vision, miosis, diplopia
CV: Palpitations, tachycardia, bradycardia, change in B/P, *circulatory depression,* syncope
RESP: Respiratory depression
Contraindications: Hypersensitivity, addiction (narcotic)
Precautions: Addictive personality, pregnancy (C), lactation, increased intracranial pressure, MI (acute), severe heart disease, respiratory depression, hepatic disease, renal disease, child <18 yr
Pharmacokinetics: Onset 10-20 min, duration 3-6 hr, half-life 3-4 hr; metabolized in liver; excreted in urine; crosses placenta
Interactions/incompatibilities:
• Increased CNS depression: alcohol, narcotics, sedative/hypnotics, phenothiazines, skeletal muscle relaxants, general anesthetics, tricyclic antidepressants
Lab test interferences:
Increase: Amylase, lipase
Treatment of overdose: Naloxone HCl (Narcan) 0.2-0.8 IV, O_2, IV fluids, vasopressors
NURSING CONSIDERATIONS
Assess:
• I&O ratio; check for decreasing output; may indicate urinary retention
• CNS changes: dizziness, drowsiness, hallucinations, euphoria, LOC, pupil reaction
• Allergic reactions: rash, urticaria
• Respiratory dysfunction: respiratory depression, character, rate, rhythm; notify physician if respirations are <10/min

---

italics = common side effects   ***bold italic*** = life threatening reactions

• Need for pain medication, physical dependence
Administer:
• With antiemetic after meals if nausea or vomiting occurs
Perform/provide:
• Storage in light-resistant area at room temperature
• Assistance with ambulation
• Safety measures: side rails, nightlight, call bell within easy reach
Evaluate:
• Therapeutic response: decrease in pain or cough
Teach patient/family:
• To report any symptoms of CNS changes, allergic reactions
• That physical dependency may result when used for extended periods
• Withdrawal symptoms may occur: nausea, vomiting, cramps, fever, faintness, anorexia

NURSING CONSIDERATIONS
Assess:
• For redness, swelling, fever, pain in ear, which indicates infection
Administer:
• After removing impacted cerumen by irrigation
• After cleaning stopper with alcohol
• After restraining child if necessary
• Warming solution to body temperature
Evaluate:
• Therapeutic response: decreased ear pain, inflammation
Teach patient/family:
• Method of instillation using aseptic technique, including not touching dropper to ear
• That dizziness may occur after instillation

---

hydrocortisone/hydrocortisone acetate
(hye-droe-kor'ti-sone)
Cortamed,* Otall
Func. class.: Otic
Chem. class.: Synthetic steroid

Action: Antiinflammatory, antipruritic
Uses: Ear canal inflammation
Dosage and routes:
• *Adult and child:* INSTILL 3-4 gtt bid-qid
Available forms: Otic sol 0.25%, 0.5%, 1%
Side effects/adverse reactions:
EENT: Itching, irritation in ear
INTEG: Rash, urticaria
Contraindications: Hypersensitivity, perforated eardrum
Precautions: Pregnancy (C)

H

hydrocortisone/hydrocortisone acetate/hydrocortisone valerate

(hye-droe-kor'ti-sone)

Acticort 100, Aeroseb-HC, Ala-Cort, Ala-Scalp, Alphaderm, Bactine Hydrocortisone, Caldecort Anti-Itch, Cetacort, Cortaid, Cortaid Maximum Strength, Cort-Dome, Cortef Feminine Itch, Cortizone-5, Cortizone-10, Cortril, Delacort, Delcort, Dermacort, Dermicort, Dermolate Anti-Itch, Dermtex HC, Hi-Cor 1.0, Hi-Cor 2.5, Hycort, HydroTex, Hytone, Lacticare-HC, Nutracort, Penecort, 1% HC, S-T Cort, Synacort, Tega-Cort, Tega-Cort Forte, Texacort, Westcort

Func. class.: Topical corticosteroid

Chem. class.: Natural nonfluorinated, group IV potency (valerate), group VI potency (acetate and plain)

Action: Antipruritic, antiinflammatory

Uses: Psoriasis, eczema, contact dermatitis, pruritus

Dosage and routes:

• *Adult and child >2 yr:* Apply to affected area qd-qid

Available forms: Hydrocortisone—oint 0.5%, 1%, 2.5%; cream 0.25%, 0.5%, 1%, 2.5%; lotion 0.25%, 0.5%, 1%, 2%, 2.5%; gel 1%; sol 1%; aerosol/pump spray 0.5%; *acetate*—oint 0.5%, 1%, 2.5%; cream 0.5%; lotion 0.05%; aerosol 1%; *valerate*—oint 0.2%; cream 0.2% (many others)

Side effects/adverse reactions:

INTEG: Burning, dryness, itching, irritation, acne, folliculitis, hypertrichosis, perioral dermatitis, hypopigmentation, atrophy, striae, miliaria, allergic contact dermatitis, secondary infection

Contraindications: Hypersensitivity to corticosteroids; fungal infections

Precautions: Pregnancy (C), lactation, viral infections, bacterial infections

NURSING CONSIDERATIONS

Assess:

• Temperature; if fever develops, drug should be discontinued

• For systemic absorption: increased temperature, inflammation, irritation

Administer:

• Only to affected areas; do not get in eyes

• Medication, then cover with occlusive dressing (only if prescribed); seal to intact skin; change q12h; systemic absorption may occur; use gloves

• Only to dermatoses; do not use on weeping, denuded, or infected area

• Apply aerosol from 6 in (15 cm) for 1-2 sec

Perform/provide:

• Cleansing before application of drug

• Treatment for a few days after area has cleared

• Storage at room temperature

Evaluate:

• Therapeutic response: absence of severe itching, patches on skin, flaking

Teach patient/family:

• To avoid sunlight on affected area; burns may occur

• Not to use other OTC products unless approved by physician

italics = common side effects   ***bold italic*** = life threatening reactions

---

hydrocortisone/hydrocortisone acetate/hydrocortisone sodium phosphate/hydrocortisone sodium succinate

(hye-dro-kor'ti-sone)

Cortef, Hydrocortone/Cortef Acetate, Hydrocortone Acetate/Hydrocortone Phosphate/A-Hydrocort, Solu-Cortef, Cortenema

Func. class.: Corticosteroid
Chem. class.: Short-acting glucocorticoid

Action: Decreases inflammation by suppression of migration of polymorphonuclear leukocytes, fibroblasts, reversal of increased capillary permeability and lysosomal stabilization

Uses: Severe inflammation, septic shock, adrenal insufficiency, ulcerative colitis, collagen disorders

Dosage and routes:

Adrenal insufficiency/inflammation

• *Adult:* PO 5-30 mg bid-qid; IM/IV 100-250 mg (succinate), then 50-100 mg IM as needed; IM/IV 15-240 mg q12h (phosphate)

Shock

• *Adult:* 500 mg-2 g q2-6h (succinate)

• *Child:* IM/IV 0.16-1 mg/kg bid-tid (succinate)

Colitis

• *Adult:* ENEMA 100 mg nightly for 21 days

Available forms: Retention enema 100 mg/60 ml; tabs 5, 10, 20 mg; inj 25, 50 mg/ml; inj 50 mg/ml; phosphate inj 100, 250, 500, 1000 mg/vial; succinate inj 25, 50 mg/ml

Side effects/adverse reactions:

CNS: Depression, flushing, sweating, headache, mood changes

*CV: Hypertension, **circulatory collapse, thrombophlebitis, embolism,** tachycardia, edema

EENT: Fungal infections, increased intraocular pressure, blurred vision

GI: Diarrhea, nausea, abdominal distention, **GI hemorrhage**, increased appetite, *pancreatitis*

*HEMA: **Thrombocytopenia***

INTEG: Acne, poor wound healing, ecchymosis, petechiae

MS: Fractures, osteoporosis, weakness

Contraindications: Psychosis, hypersensitivity, idiopathic thrombocytopenia, acute glomerulonephritis, amebiasis, fungal infections, nonasthmatic bronchial disease, child <2 yr, AIDS, TB

Precautions: Pregnancy (C), diabetes mellitus, glaucoma, osteoporosis, seizure disorders, ulcerative colitis, CHF, myasthenia gravis, renal disease, esophagitis, peptic ulcer

Pharmacokinetics:

PO: Onset 1-2 hr, peak 1 hr, duration 1-1½ days

IM/IV: Onset 20 min, peak 4-8 hr, duration 1-1½ days

REC: Onset 3-5 days

Metabolized by liver, excreted in urine (17-OHCS, 17-KS), crosses placenta

Interactions/incompatibilities:

• Decreased action of hydrocortisone: cholestyramine, colestipol, barbiturates, rifampin, ephedrine, phenytoin, theophylline

• Decreased effects of: anticoagulants, anticonvulsants, antidiabetics, ambenonium, neostigmine, isoniazid, toxoids, vaccines, anticholinesterases, salicylates, somatrem

---

*Available in Canada only

• Increased side effects: alcohol, salicylates, indomethacin, amphotericin B, digitalis, cyclosporine, diuretics
• Increased action of hydrocortisone: salicylates, estrogens, indomethacin, oral contraceptives, ketoconazole, macrolide antibiotics

Phosphate
• Incompatible with amobarbital, calcium gluconate, cephalothin, chloramphenicol, erythromycin, diazepam, heparin, kanamycin, metaraminol, methicillin, pentobarbital, phentobarbital, phenytoin, phytonadione, prochlorperazine, promazine, tetracycline, vancomycin, Vit B complex with C, warfarin

Succinate
• Incompatible with aminophylline, amobarbital, ampicillin, bleomycin, chlorpromazine, colistimethate, dimenhydrinate, diphenhydramine, doxorubicin, ephedrine, heparin, hyaluronidase, hydralazine, hydroxyzine, kanamycin, lidocaine, meperidine, metaraminol, methicillin, nafcillin, netilmicin, phentobarbital, phenobarbital, prochlorperazine, promazine, promethazine, secobarbital, tetracycline, tolazoline, vancomycin, diazepam, phenytoin

Lab test interferences:
Increase: Cholesterol, Na, blood glucose, uric acid, Ca, urine glucose
Decrease: Ca, K, T_4, T_3, thyroid ^{131}I uptake test, urine 17-OHCS, 17-KS, PBI
False negative: Skin allergy tests

NURSING CONSIDERATIONS
Assess:
• K, blood sugar, urine glucose while on long-term therapy; hypokalemia and hyperglycemia

• Weight daily, notify physician of weekly gain >5 lb
• B/P q4h, pulse; notify physician of chest pain
• I&O ratio; be alert for decreasing urinary output, increasing edema
• Plasma cortisol levels during long-term therapy (normal level: 138-635 nmol/L SI units when drawn at 8 AM)
• Infection: increased temperature, WBC, even after withdrawal of medication; drug masks symptoms of infection
• K depletion: paresthesias, fatigue, nausea, vomiting, depression, polyuria, dysrhythmias, weakness
• Edema, hypertension, cardiac symptoms
• Mental status: affect, mood, behavioral changes, aggression

Administer:
• Daily dose in AM for better results
• Phosphate: IV undiluted or added to dextrose or saline inj and given by infusion; give 25 mg or less/min
• Succinate: IV in mix-o-vial, or reconstitute 250 mg or less/2 ml bacteriostatic H_2O for inj; mix gently; give direct IV over 1 min or more; may be further diluted in 100, 250, 500 or 1000 ml of D_5W, D_5 0.9%, NaCl 0.9% given over ordered rate
• IM inj deeply in large mass; rotate sites; avoid deltoid; use 21G needle
• In one dose in AM to prevent adrenal suppression; avoid SC administration; may damage tissue
• With food or milk to decrease GI symptoms
• Rectal: telling patient to retain for 20 min if possible

Perform/provide:
• Assistance with ambulation in pa-

H

---

italics = common side effects   ***bold italic*** = life threatening reactions

tient with bone tissue disease to prevent fractures

Evaluate:
• Therapeutic response: ease of respirations, decreased inflammation

Teach patient/family:
• That ID as steroid user should be carried
• To notify physician if therapeutic response decreases; dosage adjustment may be needed
• Not to discontinue this medication abruptly, or adrenal crisis can result; drug should be tapered off
• To avoid OTC products: salicylates, alcohol in cough products, cold preparations unless directed by physician
• About cushingoid symptoms of adrenal insufficiency: nausea, anorexia, fatigue, dizziness, dyspnea, weakness, joint pain

---

hydrogen peroxide
(per-ox′ide)
Func. class.: Disinfectant
Chem. class.: Oxidizing drug

Action: Destroys bacteria (primarily anaerobic) by mechanical action
Uses: Douche, cleansing wounds, mouthwash for Vincent's stomatitis, removal of earwax

Dosage and routes:
• *Adult and child:* SOL Use as needed
Available forms: Top sol 1.5%, 3%

Side effects/adverse reactions:
CV: Oxygen emboli
INTEG: Irritation
EENT: Black hairy tongue, decalcification of tooth enamel

Contraindications: Hypersensitivity to this drug, closed wounds

Precautions: 3rd degree burns, deep wounds

Pharmacokinetics:
TOP: Duration to end of bubbling

NURSING CONSIDERATIONS
Assess:
• Area of body involved: irritation, rash, breaks, dryness, scales

Administer:
• To ear canal to facilitate removal of cerumen
• As mouthwash for Vincent's stomatitis; do not use every day as mouthwash
• After dilution with H_2O or saltwater solution
• Only when O_2 can flow in and out of wound; emboli may result

Evaluate:
• Therapeutic response: cleansing of area

---

hydromorphone HCl
(hye-droe-mor′fone)
Dilaudid, Dilaudid HP, Hydromorphone HCl
Func. class.: Narcotic analgesics
Chem. class.: Opiate, semisynthetic phenanthrene

Controlled Substance Schedule II
Action: Inhibits ascending pain pathways in CNS, increases pain threshold, alters pain perception
Uses: Moderate to severe pain

Dosage and routes:
• *Adult:* PO 1-6 mg q4-6h prn; IM/SC/IV 2-4 mg q4-6h; REC 3 mg hs prn
Available forms: Inj IM, IV 1, 2, 3, 4 mg/ml; tabs 1, 2, 3, 4 mg; rec supp 3 mg

Side effects/adverse reactions:
CNS: Drowsiness, dizziness, confusion, headache, sedation, euphoria
GI: Nausea, vomiting, anorexia, constipation, cramps

GU: Increased urinary output, dysuria, urinary retention

INTEG: Rash, urticaria, bruising, flushing, diaphoresis, pruritus

EENT: Tinnitus, blurred vision, miosis, diplopia

CV: Palpitations, bradycardia, change in B/P

*RESP: **Respiratory depression***

Contraindications: Hypersensitivity, addiction (narcotic)

Precautions: Addictive personality, pregnancy (C), lactation, increased intracranial pressure, MI (acute), severe heart disease, respiratory depression, hepatic disease, renal disease, child <18 yr

Pharmacokinetics:

Onset 15-30 min, peak ½-1½ hr, duration 4-5 hr; metabolized by liver; excreted by kidneys; crosses placenta; excreted in breast milk

Interactions/incompatibilities:

• Effects may be increased with other CNS depressants: alcohol, narcotics, sedative/hypnotics, antipsychotics, skeletal muscle relaxants

• Incompatible with alkalies, bromides, iodides, pentobarbital, prochlorperazine, $NaCO_3$, thiopental

Lab test interferences:

Increase: Amylase

NURSING CONSIDERATIONS

Assess:

• I&O ratio; check for decreasing output; may indicate urinary retention

• CNS changes: dizziness, drowsiness, hallucinations, euphoria, LOC, pupil reaction

• Allergic reactions: rash, urticaria

• Respiratory dysfunction: respiratory depression, character, rate, rhythm; notify physician if respirations are <10/min

• Need for pain medication, physical dependence

• Pain control and sedation by scoring

Administer:

• IV Direct diluted with 5 ml of sterile H_2O or normal saline; give through Y-tube or 3-way stopcock; give 2 mg or less/5 min

• IV INF: Dilute each 0.1-1 mg/ml normal saline (0.1-1 mg/m) deliver by narcotic syringe infusor; may be diluted in D_5W, D_5NaCl, 0.45% NaCl or normal saline for larger amounts and delivery through an infusion pump

• With antiemetic if nausea, vomiting occur

• When pain is beginning to return; determine dosage interval by patient response

Perform/provide:

• Storage in light-resistant area at room temperature

• Assistance with ambulation

• Safety measures: side rails, nightlight, call bell within easy reach

Evaluate:

• Therapeutic response: decrease in pain

Teach patient/family:

• To report any symptoms of CNS changes, allergic reactions

• That physical dependency may result when used for extended periods

• Withdrawal symptoms may occur: nausea, vomiting, cramps, fever, faintness, anorexia

Treatment of overdose: Naloxone HCl (Narcan) 0.2-0.8 IV, O_2, IV fluids, vasopressors

---

italics = common side effects   ***bold italic*** = life threatening reactions

hydromorphone HCl

(hye-droe-mor'fone)
Dilaudid Cough Syrup
Func. class.: Antitussive, narcotic
Chem. class.: Phenanthrene derivative, guaifenesin

Controlled Substance Schedule II

Action: Increases respiratory tract fluid by decreasing surface tension, adhesiveness, which increases removal of mucus; analgesic, antitussive

Uses: Cough

Dosage and routes:
• *Adult:* PO 1 mg q3-4h prn
• *Child 6-12 yr:* PO 0.5 mg q3-4h prn

Available forms: Syr 1 mg/5 ml

Side effects/adverse reactions:

CNS: Dizziness, drowsiness

GI: Nausea, constipation, vomiting, anorexia

CV: Hypotension

INTEG: Urticaria, rash

RESP: Respiratory depression

Contraindications: Hypersensitivity, increased intracranial pressure, status asthmaticus

Precautions: Hypothyroidism, Addison's disease, CNS depression, brain tumor, asthma, hepatic disease, renal disease, COPD, psychosis, alcoholism, convulsive disorders, pregnancy (C)

Pharmacokinetics: Metabolized by liver; half-life 2-4 hr

Interactions/incompatibilities:
• Enhanced CNS depression: barbiturates, narcotics, antipsychotics, antidepressants

NURSING CONSIDERATIONS

Assess:
• VS, cardiac status, including hypotension
• Respiratory rate, depth

• Cough: type, frequency, character, including sputum

Administer:
• Decreased dose to elderly patients; their metabolism may be slowed

Perform/provide:
• Storage at room temperature
• Increased fluids, bulk, exercise to patient's life-style to decrease constipation

Evaluate:
• Therapeutic response: absence of cough

Teach patient/family:
• To avoid driving, other hazardous activities until patient is stabilized on this medication if drowsiness occurs
• To avoid alcohol, other CNS depressants; will enhance sedating properties of this drug

hydroquinone

(hye'droe-kwin-one)
Cocrema Mercolized, Eldopaque, Eldopaque-Forte, Eldoquin, Eldoquin-Forte, Esoterica Facial, Esoterica Fortified, Esoterica Regular, Melanex, Porcelana, Porcelana With Sunscreen, Solaquin, Solaquin Forte
Func. class.: Depigmentating agent
Chem. class.: Enzyme inhibitor

Action: Inhibits production of tyrosine, which is needed in formation of melanin

Uses: Bleaching skin, including age spots, freckles, lentigo, chloasma

Dosage and routes:
• *Adult and child:* TOP apply to affected area qd-bid

Available forms: Top cream 2%, 4%; top lotion 2%; gel 4%; sol 3%

Side effects/adverse reactions:

INTEG: Rash, dryness, fissures, stinging, contact dermatitis, erythema, irritation

Contraindications: Hypersensitivity, inflamed skin, prickly heat, sunburn

Precautions: Pregnancy (C), lactation, child <1 yr

NURSING CONSIDERATIONS

Assess:

• Area of body involved, including time involved; what helps or aggravates condition

Administer:

• Topical corticosteroid for irritation

• Test dose to be applied to area 25 mm in diameter; check site after 24 hr; if itching or excessive inflammation occurs, drug should not be used

Perform/provide:

• Storage at room temperature in tight container

Evaluate:

• Therapeutic response: fading of spots over time

Teach patient/family:

• To avoid application on normal skin or getting cream in eyes

• To use opaque sunscreen during day on exposed areas, or bleaching effect may be reversed

• That minor redness is not a contraindication

• To continue to use sunscreen after bleaching is complete

---

hydroxocobalamin (vitamin B₁₂)

Acti-B₁₂,* Alphamin, Hydrobexan, Hydro-Crysti 12, Hydroxo-12, Hydroxycobalamin, LA-12

Func. class.: Vitamin
Chem. class.: B₁₂—water-soluble vitamin

Action: Needed for adequate nerve functioning, protein and carbohydrate metabolism, normal growth, RBC development

Uses: Vit B₁₂ deficiency, pernicious anemia, Vit B₁₂ malabsorption syndrome, Schilling test

Dosage and routes:

• *Adult:* IM 30-100 μg qd × 5-10 days, maintenance 100-200 mg IM qmo

• *Child:* IM 1-30 μg qd × 5-10 days, maintenance 60 μg IM qmo or more often

Pernicious anemia/malabsorption syndrome

• *Adult:* IM 100-1000 μg qd × 2 wk, then 100-1000 μg IM qmo

• *Child:* IM 1000-5000 μg × 2 wk or more given in 100-500 μg doses, then 60 μg IM/SC mo

Schilling test

• *Adult and child:* IM 1000μg in one dose

Available forms: Inj IM 100, 120, 1000 μg/ml

Side effects/adverse reactions:

CNS: Flushing, optic nerve atrophy
GI: Diarrhea
CV: **CHF,** peripheral vascular thrombosis, *pulmonary edema*
INTEG: Itching, rash

Contraindications: Hypersensitivity, optic nerve atrophy, cardiac disease

Precautions: Pregnancy (A), lactation, children

Pharmacokinetics: Stored in liver, kidneys, stomach; 50%-90% excreted in urine; crosses placenta, breast milk

Interactions/incompatibilities:
• Decreased absorption of hydroxocobalamin: aminoglycosides, anticonvulsants, colchicine, chloramphenicol, antineoplastics, cimetidine, alcohol, Vit C, K preparations
• Increased absorption of this drug: prednisone

Lab test interferences:
False positive: Intrinsic factor

NURSING CONSIDERATIONS
Assess:
• K levels during beginning treatment
• CBC for increased reticulocyte count during 1st week of therapy, followed by increase in RBC and hemoglobin
• Nutritional status: egg yolks, fish, organ meats, dairy products, clams, oysters, which are good sources of Vit B₁₂
• For pulmonary edema or worsening of CHF in cardiac patients

Administer:
• By IM inj for pernicious anemia unless contraindicated

Evaluate:
• Therapeutic response: decreased anorexia, dyspnea on excretion, palpitations, paresthesias, psychosis, visual disturbances

Teach patient/family
• That treatment must continue for life if diagnosed as having pernicious anemia
• Importance of well-balanced diet
• To avoid persons with infections

hydroxychloroquine sulfate

(hye-drox-ee-klor'oh-kwin)
Plaquenil Sulfate
Func. class.: Antimalarial
Chem. class.: 4-aminoquinoline derivative

Action: Inhibits parasite replications, transcription of DNA to RNA by forming complexes with DNA of parasite

Uses: Malaria caused by *P. vivax, P. malariae, P. ovale, P. falciparum* (some strains): lupus erythematosus, rheumatoid arthritis

Dosage and routes:
Malaria
• *Adult and child:* PO 5 mg/kg/wk on same day of week, not to exceed 400 mg; treatment should begin 2 wk before entering endemic area, continue 8 wk after leaving; if treatment begins after exposure, 800 mg for adult, 10 mg/kg for children in 2 divided doses 6 hr apart

Lupus erythematosus
• *Adult:* PO 400 mg qd-bid; length depends on patient response; maintenance 200-400 mg qd

Rheumatoid arthritis
• *Adult:* PO 400-600 mg qd, then 200-300 mg qd after good response

Available forms: Tabs 200 mg

Side effects/adverse reactions:
CV: Hypotension, heart block, **asystole with syncope**
INTEG: Pruritus, pigmentation changes, skin eruptions, lichen planuslike eruptions, eczema, **exfoliative dermatitis,** alopecia
CNS: Headache, stimulation, fatigue, irritability, **convulsion,** bad dreams, dizziness, confusion, psychosis, decreased reflexes
EENT: Blurred vision, corneal

changes, *retinal changes, difficulty focusing,* tinnitus, vertigo, deafness, photophobia, corneal edema
GI: Nausea, vomiting, anorexia, diarrhea, cramps
*HEMA: **Thrombocytopenia, agranulocytosis, hemolytic anemia, leukopenia***

Contraindications: Hypersensitivity, retinal field changes, prophyria, children (long-term)

Precautions: Blood dyscrasias, severe GI disease, neurologic disease, alcoholism, hepatic disease, G-6-PD deficiency, psoriasis, eczema, pregnancy (C)

Pharmacokinetics:
PO: Peak 1-2 hr, half-life 3-5 days; metabolized in liver; excreted in urine, feces, breast milk; crosses placenta

Interactions/incompatibilities:
• Decreased action of hydroxychloroquine: Mg or Al compounds
• Increased levels of: digoxin

NURSING CONSIDERATIONS
Assess:
• Ophthalmic test if long-term treatment or drug dosage >150 mg/day
• Liver studies qwk: AST, ALT, bilirubin
• Blood studies: CBC, since blood dyscrasias occur
• For decreased reflexes: knee, ankle
• ECG during therapy
• Watch for depression of T waves, widening of QRS complex
• Allergic reactions: pruritus, rash, urticaria
• Blood dyscrasias: malaise, fever, bruising, bleeding (rare)
• For ototoxicity (tinnitus, vertigo, change in hearing); audiometric testing should be done before, after treatment
• For toxicity: blurring vision, difficulty focusing, headache, dizziness, knee, ankle reflexes; drug should be discontinued immediately

Administer:
• Before or after meals at same time each day to maintain drug level
• IM after aspirating to avoid injection into blood system, which may cause hypotension, asystole, heart block; rotate injection sites

Perform/provide:
• Storage in tight, light-resistant containers at room temperature; injection should be kept in cool environment

Evaluate:
• Therapeutic response: decreased symptoms of malaria

Teach patient/family:
• To use sunglasses in bright sunlight to decrease photophobia
• That urine may turn rust or brown color
• To report hearing, visual problems, fever, fatigue, bruising, bleeding, which may indicate blood dyscrasias

Treatment of overdose: Induce vomiting; gastric lavage; administer barbiturate (ultrashort-acting), vasopressin, ammonium chloride; tracheostomy may be necessary

---

hydroxyprogesterone caproate

(hye-drox-ee-proe-jess'te-rone)
Duralutin, Gesterol L.A. 250, Hylutin, Hyprogest 250, Pro-Depo
Func. class.: Progestogen, hormone

Action: Inhibits secretion of pituitary gonadotropins, which prevents follicular maturation, ovulation, stimulates growth of mammary tissue, antineoplastic action against endometrial cancer

Uses: Uterine cancer, menstrual disorders

Dosage and routes:
• *Adult:* IM 125-375 mg q4wk; discontinue after 4 cycles

Uterine cancer
• *Adult:* IM 1-5 g/wk

Available forms: Inj IM 125, 250 mg/ml

Side effects/adverse reactions:
CNS: Dizziness, headache, migraines, depression, fatigue
CV: Hypotension, thrombophlebitis, edema, *thromboembolism, stroke, pulmonary embolism, myocardial infarction*
GI: Nausea, vomiting, anorexia, cramps, increased weight, *cholestatic jaundice*
EENT: Diplopia
GU: Amenorrhea, cervical erosion, breakthrough bleeding, dysmenorrhea, vaginal candidiasis, breast changes, *gynecomastia, testicular atrophy, impotence,* endometriosis, *spontaneous abortion*
INTEG: Rash, urticaria, acne, hirsutism, alopecia, oily skin, seborrhea, purpura, melasma, photosensitivity
META: Hyperglycemia

Contraindications: Breast cancer, hypersensitivity, thromboembolic disorders, reproductive cancer, genital bleeding (abnormal, undiagnosed), pregnancy (X)

Precautions: Lactation, hypertension, asthma, blood dyscrasias, gallbladder disease, HF, diabetes mellitus, bone disease, depression, migraine headache, convulsive disorders, hepatic disease, renal disease, family history of breast or reproductive tract cancer

Pharmacokinetics:
IM: Half-life 5 min, duration 24 hr; excreted in urine, feces; metabolized in liver

Lab test interferences:
Increase: Alk phosphatase, N (urine), pregnanediol, amino acids
Decrease: GTT, HDL

NURSING CONSIDERATIONS
Assess:
• Weight daily; notify physician of weekly weight gain >5 lb
• B/P at beginning of treatment and periodically
• I&O ratio; be alert for decreasing urinary output, increasing edema
• Liver function studies: ALT, AST, bilirubin, periodically during long-term therapy
• Edema, hypertension, cardiac symptoms, jaundice
• Mental status: affect, mood, behavioral changes, depression
• Hypercalcemia

Administer:
• Titrated dose; use lowest effective dose
• Oil solution deeply in large muscle mass (IM), rotate sites
• In one dose in AM
• With food or milk to decrease GI symptoms
• After warming to dissolve crystals

Perform/provide:
• Storage in dark area

Evaluate:
• Therapeutic response: decreased abnormal uterine bleeding, absence of amenorrhea

Teach patient/family:
• To avoid sunlight or use sunscreen; photosensitivity can occur
• About cushingoid symptoms
• To report breast lumps, vaginal bleeding, edema, jaundice, dark urine, clay-colored stools, dyspnea, headache, blurred vision, ab-

dominal pain, numbness or stiffness in legs, chest pain; male to report impotence or gynecomastia
• To report suspected pregnancy

---

hydroxyurea
(hye-drox'ee-yoo-ree-ah)
Hydrea
Func. class.: Antineoplastic antimetabolite
Chem. class.: Synthetic urea analog

Action: Acts by inhibiting DNA synthesis without interfering with RNA or protein synthesis; incorporates thymidine into DNA, causing direct damage to DNA strands; S phase of cell cycle specific

Uses: Melanoma, chronic myelocytic leukemia, recurrent or metastatic ovarian cancer, squamous cell carcinoma of the head and neck

Dosage and routes:
Solid tumors
• *Adult:* PO 80 mg/kg as a single dose q3d or 20-30 mg/kg as a single dose qd
In combination with radiation
• *Adult:* PO 80 mg/kg as a single dose q3d; should be started 7 days before irradiation
Resistant chronic myelocytic leukemia
• *Adult:* PO 20-30 mg/kg/day as a single daily dose

Available forms: Caps 500 mg

Side effects/adverse reactions:
*HEMA: **Leukopenia, anemia, thrombocytopenia***
GI: Nausea, vomiting, anorexia, diarrhea, stomatitis, constipation
GU: Increased BUN, uric acid, creatinine, temporary renal function impairment
INTEG: Rash, urticaria, pruritus, dry skin

CV: Angina, ischemia
CNS: Headache, confusion, hallucinations, dizziness, ***convulsions***

Contraindications: Hypersensitivity, leukopenia (<2500/mm³), thrombocytopenia (<100,000/mm³), anemia (severe), pregnancy (D)

Precautions: Renal disease (severe)

Pharmacokinetics: Readily absorbed when taken orally, peak level in 2 hr; degraded in liver; excreted in urine, almost totally eliminated in 24 hr; readily crosses blood-brain barrier

Interactions/incompatibilities:
• Increased toxicity: radiation or other antineoplastics

Lab test interferences:
Increase: Renal function studies

NURSING CONSIDERATIONS
Assess:
• CBC, differential, platelet count weekly; withhold drug if WBC is <3500/mm³ or platelet count is <100,000/mm³; notify physician of these results; drug should be discontinued
• Renal function studies: BUN, serum uric acid, urine CrCl, electrolytes before, during therapy
• I&O ratio; report fall in urine output to <30 ml/hr
• Monitor temperature q4h; fever may indicate beginning infection
• Liver function tests before, during therapy: bilirubin, alk phosphatase, AST, ALT, LDH; as needed or monthly
• B/P q3-4h; check for chest pain; angina, ischemia may occur
• Bleeding: hematuria, guaiac, bruising or petechiae, mucosa or orifices q8h
• Food preferences; list likes, dislikes

H

---

italics = common side effects **bold italic** = life threatening reactions

• Inflammation of mucosa, breaks in skin
• Buccal cavity q8h for dryness, sores or ulceration, white patches, oral pain, bleeding, dysphagia
• Symptoms indicating severe allergic reaction: rash, urticaria, itching, flushing
• Neurotoxicity: headaches, hallucinations, convulsions, dizziness

Administer:
• Allopurinol or NaHCO₃ concurrently to prevent high uric acid levels; extra fluids
• Antiemetic 30-60 min before giving drug to prevent vomiting and prn
• Antibiotics for prophylaxis of infection
• Transfusion for anemia

Perform/provide:
• Rinsing of mouth tid-qid with water, club soda; brushing of teeth bid-tid with soft brush or cotton-tipped applicators for stomatitis; use unwaxed dental floss
• Nutritious diet with iron, vitamin supplements as ordered

Evaluate:
• Therapeutic response: decreased tumor size, spread of malignancy

Teach patient/family:
• To report signs of infection: elevated temperature, sore throat, flu symptoms
• To report signs of anemia: fatigue, headache, faintness, shortness of breath, irritability
• To report bleeding: avoid use of razors, commercial mouthwash
• To avoid use of aspirin products or ibuprofen
• To avoid foods with citric acid, hot or rough texture if stomatitis is present
• To report stomatitis: any bleeding, white spots, ulcerations in the mouth; tell patient to examine mouth qd, report symptoms
• That contraceptive measures are recommended during therapy
• To drink 10-12 (8 oz) glasses of fluid/day
• To notify physician of fever, chills, sore throat, nausea, vomiting, anorexia, diarrhea, bleeding, bruising; may indicate blood dyscrasias

---

hydroxyzine HCl/ hydroxyzine pamoate
(hye-drox'i-zeen)
Anxanil, Atarax, Atarax 100, Atozine, Durel, E-Vista, Hydroxacen, Hydroxyzine HCl, Hydroxyzine Pamoate, Hyzine-50, Quiess, Vamate, Vistacon, Vistaject-25, Vistaject-50, Vistaquel 50, Vistaril, Vistazine 50
Func. class.: Antianxiety
Chem. class.: Piperazine derivative

Action: Depresses subcortical levels of CNS, including limbic system, reticular formation
Uses: Anxiety preoperatively, postoperatively to prevent nausea, vomiting, to potentiate narcotic analgesics; sedation; pruritus

Dosage and routes:
• *Adult:* PO 25-100 mg tid-qid
• *Child >6 yr:* 50-100 mg/day in divided doses
• *Child <6 yr:* 50 mg/day in divided doses

Preoperatively/postoperatively
• *Adult:* IM 25-100 mg q4-6h
• *Child:* IM 1.1 mg/kg q4-6h

Available forms: Tabs 10, 25, 50, 100 mg; caps 25, 50, 100 mg; syrup 10 mg/5 ml; oral susp 25 mg/5 ml; IM inj 25, 50 mg/ml

---

Side effects/adverse reactions:
CNS: Dizziness, drowsiness, confusion, headache, tremors, fatigue, depression, ***convulsions***
GI: Dry mouth
Contraindications: Hypersensitivity, pregnancy (C)
Precautions: Elderly, debilitated, hepatic disease, renal disease
Pharmacokinetics:
PO: Onset 15-30 min, duration 4-6 hr, half-life 3 hr
Interactions/incompatibilities:
• Increased CNS depressant effect: barbiturates, narcotics, analgesics, alcohol
Lab test interferences:
False increase: 17-OHCS
NURSING CONSIDERATIONS
Assess:
• B/P (lying, standing), pulse; if systolic B/P drops 20 mm Hg, hold drug, notify physician
• Blood studies: CBC
• Hepatic studies: AST, ALT, bilirubin, creatinine
• Mental status: mood, sensorium, affect
• Increased sedation
Administer:
• By Z-track injection in large muscle for IM to decrease pain, chance of necrosis
• With food or milk for GI symptoms
• Crushed if patient is unable to swallow medication whole
• Gum, hard candy, frequent sips of water for dry mouth
Perform/provide:
• Assistance with ambulation during beginning therapy, since drowsiness/dizziness occurs
• Safety measures, including side rails
• Checking to see PO medication has been swallowed

Evaluate:
• Therapeutic response: decreased anxiety
Teach patient/family:
• Not to be used for everyday stress or used longer than 4 mo
• Avoid OTC preparations (cold, cough, hay fever) unless approved by physician
• To avoid driving, activities that require alertness
• To avoid alcohol ingestion, other psychotropic medications
• Not to discontinue medication quickly after long-term use
• To rise slowly or fainting may occur
Treatment of overdose: Lavage if orally ingested; VS, supportive care; IV norepinephrine for hypotension

H

---

hyoscyamine sulfate
(hye-oh-sye′a-meen)
Anaspaz, Cystospaz, Cystospaz-M, Gastrosed, Levsin, Levsin Drops, Levsinex Timecaps, Neoquess
Func. class.: GI anticholinergic
Chem. class.: Belladonna alkaloid

Action: Inhibits muscarinic actions of acetylcholine at postganglionic parasympathetic neuroeffector sites
Uses: Treatment of peptic ulcer disease in combination with other drugs; other GI disorders, other spastic disorders
Dosage and routes:
• *Adult:* PO/SL 0.125-0.25 mg tid-qid ac, hs; TIME REL 0.375 q12h; IM/SC/IV 0.25-0.5 mg q6h
• *Child 2-10 yr:* ½ adult dose
• *Child <2 yr:* ¼ adult dose
Available forms: Tabs 0.125, 0.13, 0.15 mg; caps time rel 0.375 mg;

sol 0.125 mg/ml; elix 0.125 mg/5 ml; inj IM, IV, SC 0.5 mg/ml

Side effects/adverse reactions:

CNS: Confusion, stimulation in elderly, headache, insomnia, dizziness, drowsiness, anxiety, weakness, hallucination

GI: Dry mouth, constipation, paralytic ileus, heartburn, nausea, vomiting, dysphagia, absence of taste

GU: Hesitancy, retention, impotence

CV: Palpitations, tachycardia

EENT: Blurred vision, photophobia, mydriasis, cycloplegia, increased ocular tension

INTEG: Urticaria, rash, pruritus, anhidrosis, fever, allergic reactions

Contraindications: Hypersensitivity to anticholinergics, narrow-angle glaucoma, GI obstruction, myasthenia gravis, paralytic ileus, GI atony, toxic megacolon, prostatic hypertrophy

Precautions: Hyperthyroidism, coronary artery disease, dysrhythmias, CHF, ulcerative colitis, hypertension, hiatal hernia, hepatic disease, renal disease, pregnancy (C), urinary retention

Pharmacokinetics:

PO: Duration 4-6 hr; metabolized by liver; excreted in urine; half-life 3.5 hr

Interactions/incompatibilities:

• Decreased effect of hyoscyamine: antacids

• Increased anticholinergic effect: amantadine, tricyclic antidepressants, MAOIs, H_1 antihistamines

• Decreased effect of: phenothiazines, levodopa, ketoconazole

NURSING CONSIDERATIONS

Assess:

• VS, cardiac status: checking for dysrhythmias, increased rate, palpitations

• I&O ratio; check for urinary retention or hesitancy

• GI complaints: pain, bleeding (frank or occult), nausea, vomiting, anorexia

Administer:

• ½ hr ac for better absorption

• Decreased dose to elderly patients; their metabolism may be slowed

• Gum, hard candy, frequent rinsing of mouth for dryness of oral cavity

Perform/provide:

• Storage is tight container protected from light

• Increased fluids, bulk, exercise to patient's life-style to decrease constipation

Evaluate:

• Therapeutic response: absence of epigastric pain, bleeding, nausea, vomiting

Teach patient/family:

• To avoid driving or other hazardous activities until stabilized on medication

• To avoid alcohol or other CNS depressants; will enhance sedating properties of this drug

• To avoid hot environments; stroke may occur; drug suppresses perspiration

• To use sunglasses when outside to prevent photophobia; may cause blurred vision

Ibuprofen

(eye-byoo'proe-fen)

Aches-N-Pain, Advil, Children's Advil, Excedrin IS, Genpril, Haltran, Ibuprin, Ibuprofen, Ibuprohm, IBU-Tab, Medipren, Menadol, Midol-200, Motrin, Motrin IB, Nuprin, Pamprin-IB, PediaProfen, Rufen, Saleto-200, Saleto-400, Saleto-600, Saleto-800, Trendar

Func. class.: Nonsteroidal antiinflammatory
Chem. class.: Propionic acid derivative

Action: Inhibits prostaglandin synthesis by decreasing enzyme needed for biosynthesis; analgesic, antiinflammatory, antipyretic

Uses: Rheumatoid arthritis, osteoarthritis, primary dysmenorrhea, gout, dental pain, musculoskeletal disorders

Dosage and routes:
• *Adult:* PO 200-800 mg qid, not to exceed 3.2 g/day

Available forms: Tabs 200, 300, 400, 600, 800 mg

Side effects/adverse reactions:
CV: Tachycardia, peripheral edema, palpitations, dysrhythmias, hypertension
CNS: Dizziness, drowsiness, fatigue, tremors, confusion, insomnia, anxiety, depression
EENT: Tinnitus, hearing loss, blurred vision
GI: Nausea, anorexia, vomiting, diarrhea, jaundice, *cholestatic hepatitis*, constipation, flatulence, cramps, dry mouth, peptic ulcer
GU: Nephrotoxicity; dysuria, hematuria, oliguria, azotemia
HEMA: Blood dyscrasias
INTEG: Purpura, rash, pruritus, sweating

Contraindications: Hypersensitivity, asthma, severe renal disease, severe hepatic disease

Precautions: Pregnancy (B) 1st and 2nd trimester, lactation, children, bleeding disorders, GI disorders, cardiac disorders, hypersensitivity to other antiinflammatory agents

Pharmacokinetics: Well absorbed (PO)
PO: Onset ½ hour; peak 1-2 hr, half-life 2-4 hr, metabolized in liver (inactive metabolites), excreted in urine (inactive metabolites), 90%-99% plasma protein binding, does not enter breast milk

Interactions/incompatibilities:
• May increase action of: coumarin, phenytoin, sulfonamides
• Decreased action of ibuprofen: salicylates

NURSING CONSIDERATIONS
Assess:
• Renal, liver, blood studies: BUN, creatinine, AST, ALT, Hgb, before treatment, periodically thereafter
• Pain: note type, duration, location and intensity with ROM
• Audiometric, ophthalmic examination before, during, after treatment; for eye, ear problems: blurred vision, tinnitus; may indicate toxicity
• Cardiac status: edema (peripheral), tachycardia, palpitations; monitor B/P, pulse for character, quality, rhythm
• For history of peptic ulcer disorder; asthma, aspirin, hypersensitivity, check closely for allergic reactions and lupus

Administer:
• With food, milk or antacid to decrease GI symptoms; however, best to take on empty stomach to facilitate absorption; if nausea and vom-

---

italics = common side effects   ***bold italic*** = life threatening reactions

iting occur/persist, notify physician

Perform/provide:

• Storage at room temperature

Evaluate:

• Therapeutic response: decreased pain, stiffness in joints; decreased swelling in joints; ability to move more easily; reduction in fever or menstrual cramping

Teach patient/family:

• To report blurred vision, ringing, roaring in ears; may indicate toxicity; eye and hearing tests should be done during long-term therapy

• To avoid driving, other hazardous activities if dizziness or drowsiness occurs

• To report change in urine pattern, increased weight, edema, increased pain in joints, fever, blood in urine; indicate nephrotoxicity

• That therapeutic inflammatory effects may take up to 1 mo

• To avoid alcohol, salicylates; bleeding may occur

• To avoid sun, sunlamp

Idarubicin HCl

(eye-dah-roob'ih-sin)

Idamycin

Func. class.: Antineoplastic, antibiotic

Chem. class.: Anthracycline glycoside

Action: Inhibits DNS synthesis derived from daunorubicin by binding to DNA, which causes strand splitting; cell cycle specific (S phase); a vesicant

Uses: Used in combination with other antineoplastics for acute myelocytic leukemia in adults

Dosage and routes:

Adult: IV 12 mg/m^2/day × 3 days in combination with cytosine arabinoside, or 25 mg/m^2 IV bolus followed by 200 mg/m^2/day × 5 days by continuous INF

Available forms: inj IV 5, 10 mg

Side effects/adverse reactions:

*HEMA: **Thrombocytopenia, leukopenia, anemia***

GI: Nausea, vomiting, abdominal pain, mucositis, diarrhea, ***hepatotoxicity***

INTEG: Rash, extravasation, dermatitis, reversible alopecia, urticaria, thrombophlebitis at injection site

*CV: **Dysrhythmias, CHF, pericarditis, myocarditis,*** peripheral edema

CNS: Fever, chills, headache

Contraindications: Hypersensitivity, pregnancy (D)

Precautions: Renal and hepatic disease, gout, bone marrow depression, children

Pharmacokinetics: Half-life 22 hr; metabolized by liver; crosses placenta; excreted in bile, urine (primarily as metabolites)

Interactions/incompatibilities:

• Increased toxicity: other antineoplastics or radiation

• Incompatible with heparin, but considered incompatible with all other drugs in sol or syringe

Lab test interferences:

Increase: Uric acid

NURSING CONSIDERATIONS

Assess:

• CBC, differential, platelet count weekly; withhold drug if WBC is 4000/mm^3 or platelet count is 75,000/mm^3; notify physician of these results

• Blood, urine, uric acid levels

• Renal function studies: BUN, serum uric acid, urine CrCl, electrolytes before, during therapy

• I&O ratio; report fall in urine output to <30 ml/hr

---

*Available in Canada only

• Monitor temperature q4h; fever may indicate beginning infection
• Liver function tests before, during therapy: bilirubin, AST, ALT, alk phosphatase as needed or monthly
• ECG: watch for ST-T wave changes, low QRS and T, possible dysrhythmias (sinus tachycardia, heart block, PVCs)
• Bleeding: hematuria, guaiac stools, bruising or petechiae, mucosa or orifices q8h
• Food preferences: list likes, dislikes
• Effects of alopecia on body image; discuss feelings about body changes
• Inflammation of mucosa, breaks in skin
• Yellowing of skin and sclera, dark urine, clay-colored stools, itchy skin, abdominal pain, fever, diarrhea
• Buccal cavity q8h for dryness, sores, ulceration, white patches, oral pain, bleeding, dysphagia
• Local irritation, pain, burning at injection site
• GI symptoms: frequency of stools, cramping
• Acidosis, signs of dehydration: rapid respirations, poor skin turgor, decreased urine output, dry skin, restlessness, weakness
• Cardiac status: B/P, pulse, character, rhythm, rate

Administer:
• Antiemetic 30-60 min before giving drug and 6-10 hr after treatment to prevent vomiting
• After reconstituting 5 mg vial with 5 ml 0.9% NaCl (1 mg/1 ml); give over 10-15 min through Y-tube or 3-way stopcock of inf of D$_5$ or normal saline; discard unused portion
• Allopurinol or sodium bicarbonate to reduce uric acid levels, alkalinization, or urine
• Transfusion for anemia
• Hydrocortisone for extravasation; apply ice compress after stopping infusion

Perform/provide:
• Strict hand-washing technique, gloves, protective clothing
• Liquid diet: carbonated beverages, gelatin may be added if patient is not nauseated or vomiting
• Increase fluid intake to 2-3 L/day to prevent urate and calculi formation
• Diet low in purines: absence of organ meats (kidney, liver), dried beans, peas to reduce uric acid level
• Rinsing of mouth tid-qid with water, club soda; brushing of teeth tid-qid with soft brush or cotton-tipped applicators for stomatitis; use unwaxed dental floss
• Storage at room temperature for 3 days after reconstituting or 7 days refrigerated

Evaluate:
• Therapeutic response: decreased tumor size, spread of malignancy

Teach patient/family:
• To report any complaints, side effects to nurse or physician
• That hair may be lost during treatment and wig or hairpiece may make patient feel better; tell patient that new hair may be different in color, texture
• To avoid foods with citric acid, hot or rough texture
• To report any bleeding, white spots, ulcerations in mouth; tell patient to examine mouth qd
• That urine may be red-orange for 48 hr

---

italics = common side effects   ***bold italic*** = life threatening reactions

Idoxuridine-IDU (oph-thalmic)

(eye-dox-your'ih-deen)
Herplex
Func. class.: Antiviral
Chem. class.: Pyrimidine nucleoside

Action: Inhibits viral replication by interfering with viral DNA synthesis

Uses: Herpes simplex keratitis, CMV, varicella zoster alone or with corticosteroids

Dosage and routes:
• *Adult and child:* INSTILL 1 gtt q1h during day and 2 hr during night
Available forms: sol 0.1%

Side effects/adverse reactions:
EENT: Poor corneal wound healing, temporary visual haze, overgrowth of nonsusceptible organisms

Contraindications: Hypersensitivity

Precautions: Antibiotic hypersensitivity, pregnancy (C)

Interactions/incompatibilities:
• Do not use boric acid with this drug

NURSING CONSIDERATIONS
Assess:
• Allergy: itching, lacrimation, redness, swelling

Administer:
• After washing hands; cleanse crusts or discharge from eye before application

Perform/provide:
• Storage in refrigerator in light-resistant container until used

Evaluate:
• Therapeutic response: absence of redness, inflammation, tearing, photophobia

Teach patient/family:
• To use drug exactly as prescribed
• Not to use eye makeup, towels, washcloths, eye medication of others; reinfection may occur
• That drug container tip should not be touched to eye
• To report itching, increased redness, burning, stinging, swelling; drug should be discontinued
• That drug may cause blurred vision when ointment is applied

ifosfamide

(i-foss'fa-mid)
Ifex
Func. class.: Antineoplastic alkylating agent
Chem. class.: Nitrogen mustard

Action: Alkylates DNA, RNA, inhibits enzymes that allow synthesis of amino acids in proteins; also responsible for cross-linking DNA strands; activity is not cell cycle stage specific

Uses: Testicular cancer

Dosage and routes:
• *Adult:* IV 1.2 g/m^2/day × 5 days, repeat course q3wk
Available forms: Inj 1, 3 g

Side effects/adverse reactions:
CNS: Facial paresthesia, fever, malaise, somnolence, confusion, depression, hallucinations, dizziness, disorientation, *seizures, coma*

GI: Nausea, vomiting, anorexia, *hepatotoxicity,* stomatitis, constipation

INTEG: Dermatitis, alopecia, pain at injection site

*GU: **Hematuria, nephrotoxicity, hemorrhagic cystitis,*** dysuria, urinary frequency

*HEMA: **Thrombocytopenia, leukopenia, anemia***

Contraindications: Hypersensitivity, bone marrow suppression

Precautions: Renal disease, pregnancy (D), lactation, children

Pharmacokinetics: Metabolized by liver; saturation occurs at high doses; excreted in urine; half-life 7-15 hr

NURSING CONSIDERATIONS
Assess:

• Liver function studies before, during therapy (bilirubin, AST, ALT, LDH) as needed or monthly

• CBC, differential, platelet count weekly; withhold drug if WBC is <4000 or platelet count is <75,000; notify physician of results

• Monitor temperature q4h (may indicate beginning infection)

• Blood dyscrasias (anemia, granulocytopenia); bruising, fatigue, bleeding, poor healing

• Allergic reactions: dermatitis, exfoliative dermatitis, pruritus, urticaria

• Bleeding: hematuria, guaiac, bruising or petechiae, mucosa or orifices q8h

• Food preferences; list likes, dislikes

• Effects of alopecia on body image, discuss feelings about body changes

• Yellowing of skin and sclera, dark urine, clay-colored stools, itchy skin, abdominal pain, fever, diarrhea

• Inflammation of mucosa, breaks in skin

Administer:

• IV after diluting 1 g/20 ml sterile or bacteriostatic H$_2$O for inj with parabens or benzyl only; shake; may be diluted further with D$_5$W, LR, normal saline, sterile water for inj; 1 gm/20 ml = 50 mg/ml; 1 gm/50ml = 20 mg/ml; 1 gm/200 ml = 5 mg/ml; give over 30 min

• Antiemetic 30-60 min before giving drug to prevent vomiting

• Antibiotics for prophylaxis of infection

• Always give with mesna to prevent ifosfamide-induced hemorrhagic cystitis

Perform/provide:

• Storage of powder at room temperature

• Strict medical asepsis, protective isolation if WBC levels are low

• Increase fluid intake to 2-3 L/day to prevent urate deposits, calculi formation

• Warm compresses at injection site for inflammation

Evaluate:

• Therapeutic response: decrease in size and spread of tumor

Teach patient/family:

• To call physician if sore throat, swollen lymph nodes, malaise, fever occur, since other infections may occur

• About protective isolation precautions

• That hair may be lost during treatment; a wig or hairpiece may make the patient feel better; new hair may be different in color, texture

• To report signs of anemia: fatigue, headache, faintness, shortness of breath, irritability

• To report bleeding; avoid use of razors or commercial mouthwash

• To avoid use of aspirin products or ibuprofen

• To use contraceptive measures during therapy

Imipenem/cilastatin
i-me-pen'em sye-la-stat'in
Primaxin IM, Primaxin IV
Func. class.: Antiinfective-misc penicillin

Action: Interferes with cell wall

---

replication of susceptible organisms; osmotically unstable cell wall swells, bursts from osmotic pressure; addition of cilastatin prevents renal inactivation that occurs with high urinary concentrations of imipenem

Uses: Serious infections caused by gram-positive: *S. pneumoniae*, group A β-hemolytic streptococci, *S. aureus*, enterococcus; gram-negative: *Klebsiella, Proteus, E. coli, Acinetobacter, Serratia, P. aeruginosa; Salmonella, Shigella*

Dosage and routes:
• *Adult:* IV 250-500 mg q6h; severe infections may require 1 g q6h; may give IM (total daily IM dosage >1500 mg not recommended)

Available forms: Inj 250, 500, 750 mg vials

Side effects/adverse reactions:
CNS: Fever, somnolence, *seizures,* dizziness, weakness, myoclonia
GI: Diarrhea, nausea, vomiting, *pseudomembranous colitis, hepatitis,* glossitis
CV: Hypotension, palpitations
HEMA: Eosinophilia, neutropenia, decreased Hgb, Hct
INTEG: Rash, urticaria, pruritus, pain at injection site, phlebitis, erythema at injection site
SYST: Anaphylaxis
RESP: Chest discomfort, dyspnea, hyperventilation

Contraindications: Hypersensitivity, IM hypersensitivity to local anesthetics of the amide type

Precautions: Pregnancy (C), lactation, elderly, hypersensitivity to penicillins, seizure disorders, renal disease, children

Pharmacokinetics:
IV: Onset immediate, peak ½-1 hr, half-life 1 hr

Interactions/incompatibilities:
• Increased imipenem plasma levels: probenecid

• Incompatible with aminoglycosides, ganciclovir in sol or syringe

Lab test interferences:
Increase: AST, ALT, LDH, BUN, alk phosphatase, bilirubin, creatinine
False positive: Direct Coombs' test

NURSING CONSIDERATIONS
Assess:
• Sensitivity to penicillin or other cephalosporins
• Renal disease: lower dose may be required
• Bowel pattern qd; if severe diarrhea occurs, drug should be discontinued; may indicate pseudomembranous colitis
• Allergic reactions: rash, urticaria, pruritus; may occur few days after therapy begins
• Overgrowth of infection: perineal itching, fever, malaise, redness, pain, swelling, drainage, rash, diarrhea, change in cough, sputum

Administer:
• After reconstitution of 250 or 500 mg with 10 ml of diluent and shake; add to at least 100 ml of same inf sol
• 250-500 mg over 20-30 min; 1 g over 40-60 min; give through Y-tube or 3-way stopcock; do not give by IV bolus or give cloudy solutions
• After C&S is taken

Evaluate:
• Therapeutic response: negative C&S

Teach patient/family:
• To report severe diarrhea; may indicate pseudomembranous colitis
• To report sore throat, bruising, bleeding, joint pain; may indicate blood dyscrasias (rare)

Treatment of overdose: Epinephrine, antihistamines; resuscitate if needed (anaphylaxis)

---

* Available in Canada only

Imipramine HCl
(im-ip′ra-meen)
Imipramine HCl, Impril,* Janimine, Novopramine,* Tofranil
Func. class.: Antidepressant—tricyclic
Chem. class.: Dibenzazepine—tertiary amine

Action: Blocks reuptake of norepinephrine, serotonin into nerve endings, increasing action of norepinephrine, serotonin in nerve cells

Uses: Depression, enuresis in children

Dosage and routes:
• *Adult:* PO/IM 75-100 mg/day in divided doses, may increase by 25-50 mg to 200 mg, not to exceed 300 mg/day; may give daily dose hs
• *Child:* PO 25-75 mg/day
Available forms: Tabs 10, 25, 50 mg; inj IM 25 mg/2 ml

Side effects/adverse reactions:
*HEMA: **Agranulocytosis, thrombocytopenia, eosinophilia, leukopenia***
CNS: Dizziness, drowsiness, confusion, headache, anxiety, tremors, stimulation, weakness, insomnia, nightmares, EPS (elderly), increased psychiatric symptoms, paresthesia
GI: Diarrhea, dry mouth, nausea, vomiting, ***paralytic ileus,*** increased appetite, cramps, epigastric distress, jaundice, ***hepatitis,*** stomatitis
*GU: Retention, **acute renal failure***
INTEG: Rash, urticaria, sweating, pruritus, photosensitivity
*CV: Orthostatic hypotension, ECG changes, tachycardia, **hypertension,*** palpitations

EENT: Blurred vision, tinnitus, mydriasis

Contraindications: Hypersensitivity to tricyclic antidepressants, recovery phase of myocardial infarction, convulsive disorders, prostatic hypertrophy

Precautions: Suicidal patients, severe depression, increased intraocular pressure, narrow-angle glaucoma, urinary retention, cardiac disease, hepatic disease, hyperthyroidism, electroshock therapy, elective surgery, elderly, pregnancy (C)

Pharmacokinetics:
PO: Steady state 2-5 days; metabolized by liver; excreted by kidneys, feces; crosses placenta; excreted in breast milk; half-life 6-20 hr

Interactions/incompatibilities:
• Decreased effects of: guanethidine, clonidine, indirect-acting sympathomimetics (ephedrine)
• Increased effects of: direct-acting sympathomimetics (epinephrine), alcohol, barbiturates, benzodiazepines, CNS depressants
• Hyperpyretic crisis, convulsions, hypertensive episode: MAOI (pargyline [Eutonyl])

Lab test interferences:
Increase: Serum bilirubin, alk phosphatase, blood glucose
Decrease: 5-HIAA, VMA, urinary catecholamines

NURSING CONSIDERATIONS
Assess:
• B/P (lying, standing), pulse q4h; if systolic B/P drops 20 mm Hg, hold drug, notify physician; take vital signs q4h in patients with cardiovascular disease
• Blood studies: CBC, leukocytes, differential, cardiac enzymes if patient is receiving long-term therapy

italics = common side effects   ***bold italic*** = life threatening reactions

• Hepatic studies: AST, ALT, bilirubin
• Weight qwk; appetite may increase with drug
• ECG for flattening of T wave, bundle branch block, AV block, dysrhythmias in cardiac patients
• EPS primarily in elderly: rigidity, dystonia, akathisia
• Mental status: mood, sensorium, affect, suicidal tendencies, increase in psychiatric symptoms: depression, panic
• Urinary retention, constipation; constipation is more likely to occur in children, elderly
• Withdrawal symptoms: headache, nausea, vomiting, muscle pain, weakness; do not usually occur unless drug was discontinued abruptly
• Alcohol consumption; if alcohol is consumed, hold dose until morning

Administer:
• Increased fluids, bulk in diet if constipation, urinary retention occur
• With food or milk for GI symptoms
• Dosage hs if oversedation occurs during day; may take entire dose hs; elderly may not tolerate once/day dosing
• Gum, hard candy, or frequent sips of water for dry mouth

Perform/provide:
• Storage in tight container at room temperature; do not freeze
• Assistance with ambulation during beginning therapy, since drowsiness/dizziness occurs
• Safety measures, including side rails, primarily in elderly
• Checking to see PO medication swallowed

Evaluate:
• Therapeutic response: decreased depression, enuresis

Teach patient/family:
• That therapeutic effects may take 2-3 wk
• Dispensed in small amounts because of suicide potential, especially in beginning of therapy
• To use caution in driving or other activities requiring alertness because of drowsiness, dizziness, blurred vision
• To avoid alcohol ingestion, other CNS depressants
• Not to discontinue medication quickly after long-term use; may cause nausea, headache, malaise
• To wear sunscreen or large hat, since photosensitivity occurs

Treatment of overdose: ECG monitoring; induce emesis; lavage, activated charcoal; administer anticonvulsant

---

immune globulin (IGIV, IG, ISG)

Gamimune N, Gammagard, Gammar-IV, Iveegam, Sandoglobulin, Venoglobulin-I, Venoglobulin-S, Gammar, Gamastan, Immune Serum Globulin

Func. class.: Immune serum
Chem. class.: IgG

Action: Provides passive immunity to hepatitis A, measles, varicella, rubella, immune globulin deficiency

Uses: Agammaglobulinemia, hepatitis A exposure, measles exposure, measles vaccine complications, purpura, rubella exposure, chickenpox exposure

Dosage and routes:
• *Adult:* IM 30-50 ml q mo; IV 100 mg/kg qmo, 0.01-0.02 ml/kg/min × ½ hr (Gamimune); IV 200 mg/kg q, 0.05-1 ml/min × 15-30

---

min, then increase to 1.5-2.5 ml/min (Sandoglobulin)

• *Child:* IM 20-40 ml qmo

Hepatitis A exposure

• *Child and adult:* IM 0.02-0.04 ml/kg or 0.1 mg/kg if treatment is delayed

Hepatitis B exposure

• *Adult and child:* IM 0.06 ml/kg within 1 wk, qmo

Measles

• *Child:* IM 0.25 ml/kg within 6 days

Immunoglobulin deficiency

• *Child:* IM 1.3 ml/kg, then 0.66 ml/kg after 2-4 wk and q2-4wk thereafter

Idiopathic thrombocytopenia purpura

• *Adult:* IV 0.4 g/kg × 5 days

Available forms: IV, IM inj 2, 10 ml/vial

Side effects/adverse reactions:

INTEG: Pain at injection site, rash, pruritus, chills, chest pain

MS: Arthralgia

SYST: Lymphadenopathy, ***anaphylaxis***

CNS: Headache, fatigue, malaise

GI: Abdominal pain

Contraindications: Hypersensitivity

Precautions: Pregnancy (C)

Interactions/incompatibilities:

• Do not administer live virus vaccines within 3 mo of this drug

• Incompatible with any other drug in sol or syringe

NURSING CONSIDERATIONS
Administer:

• Gamimune: IV undiluted or dilute with D₅; give 0.01 ml/kg/min; may increase to 0.02-0.04 ml/kg/min

• Sandoglobulin: IV diluted with provided diluent; give 0.5-1 ml/min × 15-30 min; may increase to 1.5-2.5 ml/min

• IM ≤3ml in one site, use large muscle mass

• Only after epinephrine 1:1000, resuscitative equipment are available

• Only within 2 wk of exposure to hepatitis A

Perform/provide:

• Storage at 36°-46° F (2°-8° C)

Teach patient/family:

• That passive immunity is temporary

• Treatment of anaphylaxis: Epinephrine, diphenhydramine, O₂, vasopressors, corticosteroids

---

Indapamide

(in-dap′a-mide)

Lozol, Lozide*

Func. class.: Diuretic—thiazide-like

Chem. class.: Indoline

Action: Acts on proximal section of distal renal tubule by inhibiting reabsorption of sodium; may act by direct vasodilation caused by blocking of calcium channel

Uses: Edema, hypertension, diuresis

Dosage and routes:

• *Adult:* PO 2.5 mg qd in AM; may be increased to 5 mg qd if needed

Available forms: Tabs 2.5 mg

Side effects/adverse reactions:

GU: Polyuria, dysuria, frequency

ELECT: Hypochloremic alkalosis, hypomagnesemia, hyperuricemia, hypercalcemia, hyponatremia, hypokalemia, hyperglycemia

CNS: Headache, dizziness, fatigue, weakness, paresthesias, depression

GI: Nausea, diarrhea, dry mouth, vomiting, anorexia, cramps, constipation, pancreatitis, abdominal pain, jaundice, hepatitis

EENT: Loss of hearing, tinnitus,

---

italics = common side effects   ***bold italic*** = life threatening reactions

blurred vision, nasal congestion, increased intraocular pressure

INTEG: Rash, pruritus, photosensitivity, alopecia, urticaria

MS: Cramps

*HEMA: **Thrombocytopenia, agranulocytosis, leukopenia, neutropenia, anemia***

CV: Orthostatic hypotension, volume depletion, palpitations, dysrhythmias

Contraindications: Hypersensitivity, anuria, lactation

Precautions: Hypokalemia, dehydration, ascites, hepatic disease, severe renal disease, pregnancy (B)

Pharmacokinetics:

PO: Onset 1-2 hr, peak 2 hr, duration up to 36 hr; excreted in urine, feces; half-life 14-18 hr

Interactions/incompatibilities:

• Hyperglycemia, hyperuricemia, hypotension: diazoxide

• Muscle relaxants, steroids, lithium, digitalis

• Decreased K: steroids

• Decreased effects: antidiabetics

• Decreased absorption: cholestyramine, colestipol

• Decreased hypotensive effect: indomethacin, NSAIDs

Lab test interferences:

Increase: Ca, parathyroid test

NURSING CONSIDERATIONS

Assess:

• Weight daily, I&O daily to determine fluid loss; effect of drug may be decreased if used qd

• Rate, depth, rhythm of respiration, effect of exertion

• B/P lying, standing; postural hypotension may occur

• Electrolytes: K, Mg, Na, Cl: include BUN, CBC, serum creatinine, blood pH, ABGs, uric acid, Ca, glucose

• Signs of metabolic alkalosis

• Signs of hypokalemia

• Rashes, temperature elevation qd

• Confusion, especially in elderly; take safety precautions if needed

• Hydration: skin turgor, thirst, dry mucous membranes

Administer:

• In AM to avoid interference with sleep

• With food; if nausea occurs, absorption may be decreased slightly

Evaluate:

• Therapeutic response: improvement in edema of feet, legs, sacral area daily if medication is being used in CHF

Teach patient/family:

• To increase fluid intake to 2-3 L/day unless contraindicated; diet high in K; to rise slowly from lying or sitting position

• Adverse reactions: muscle cramps, weakness, nausea, dizziness

• To take with food or milk for GI symptoms

• To use sunscreen for photosensitivity

• To take early in day to prevent nocturia

Treatment of overdose: Lavage if taken orally; monitor electrolytes, administer IV fluids; monitor hydration, CV, renal status

indecainide HCl

(in-de-kane′ide)

Decabid

Func. class.: Antidysrhythmic, (Class Ic)

Action: Unknown; able to slow conduction, reduce membrane responsiveness; inhibits automaticity, increases ratio of effective refractory period to action potential duration

Uses: Life-threatening dysrhyth-

mias, sustained ventricular tachycardia

Dosage and routes:
• *Adult:* PO 100-200 mg/day in divided dose q12h; 50 mg q12h initially, then increase dose by 25 mg
increments q4d, max 400 mg/day
Available forms: Ext rel tabs 50,
75, 100 mg

Side effects/adverse reactions:
CV: **Dysrhythmias, CHF**
CNS: Headache, dizziness, light-
headedness
GI: Constipation, nausea
GU: Impotence
EENT: Blurred vision, diplopia

Contraindications: 2nd or 3rd degree AV block, right bundle branch
block, cardiogenic shock, hypersensitivity

Precautions: Severe CHF, hypokalemia, hyperkalemia, sick-sinus
syndrome, pregnancy (B), lactation, children, impaired hepatic or
renal disease

Pharmacokinetics:
Half-life 9-10 hr metabolized by
the liver; 63% of drug recovered in
urine

Interactions/incompatibilities:
• Increased effect of indecainide:
cimetidine
• Increased serum concentrations
of: digoxin

Lab test interferences:
Increase: CPK

NURSING CONSIDERATIONS
Assess:
• GI status: bowel pattern, number
of stools
• Cardiac rate: respiration, rate,
rhythm, character continuously
• Chest x-ray film, pulmonary
function test during treatment
• I&O ratio; check for decreasing
output
• B/P for fluctuations

• Lung fields; bilateral rales may
occur in CHF patient
• Increased respiration, increased
pulse; drug should be discontinued

Evaluate:
• Therapeutic response: absence of
dysrhythmias

Treatment of overdose: O_2, artificial ventilation, ECG, administer
dopamine for circulatory depression, diazepam or thiopental for
convulsions

**indomethacin/
indomethacin sodium
trihydrate**
(in-doe-meth'a-sin)
Indomethacin, Indocin, Indocin SR, Indocin IV
Func. class.: Nonsteroidal antiinflammatory (NSAID)
Chem. class.: Propionic acid
derivative

Action: Inhibits prostaglandin synthesis by decreasing enzyme
needed for biosynthesis; analgesic,
antiinflammatory, antipyretic

Uses: Rheumatoid arthritis, ankylosing rheumatoid spondylitis,
acute gouty arthritis, closure of patent ductus arteriosus in premature
infants

Dosage and routes:
Arthritis
• *Adult:* PO/REC 25 mg bid-tid;
may increase by 25 mg/day qwk,
not to exceed 200 mg/day; SUS
REL 75 mg qd, may increase to 75
mg bid
Acute arthritis
• *Adult:* PO/REC 50 mg tid; use
only for acute attack, then reduce
dose
Patent ductus arteriosus
• *Infant <2 days:* IV 0.2 mg/kg,
then 0.1 mg/kg q12-24h

italics = common side effects   ***bold italic*** = life threatening reactions

• *Infant 2-7 days:* IV 0.2 mg/kg, then 0.2 mg × 2 doses after 12, 24h
• *Infant >7 days:* IV 0.2 mg/kg, then 0.25 mg/kg × 2 doses after 12, 24 hr

Available forms: Caps 25, 50 mg; caps ext rel 75 mg; susp 25 mg/5 ml; rec supp 50 mg

Side effects/adverse reactions:

GI: Nausea, anorexia, vomiting, diarrhea, jaundice, ***cholestatic hepatitis,*** constipation, flatulence, cramps, dry mouth, peptic ulcer
CNS: Dizziness, drowsiness, fatigue, tremors, confusion, insomnia, anxiety, depression
CV: Tachycardia, peripheral edema, palpitations, dysrhythmias, hypertension
INTEG: Purpura, rash, pruritus, sweating
GU: ***Nephrotoxicity: dysuria, hematuria, oliguria, azotemia***
HEMA: ***Blood dyscrasias***
EENT: Tinnitus, hearing loss, blurred vision

Contraindications: Hypersensitivity, asthma, severe renal disease, severe hepatic disease, ulcer disease

Precautions: Pregnancy, lactation, children, bleeding disorders, GI disorders, cardiac disorders, hypersensitivity to other antiinflammatory agents, pregnancy (B) 1st and 2nd trimesters, depression

Pharmacokinetics:

PO: Onset 1-2 hr, peak 3 hr, duration 4-6 hr; metabolized in liver, kidneys; excreted in urine, bile, feces; crosses placenta; excreted in breast milk; 99% plasma protein binding

Interactions/incompatibilities:

• Increased action of: coumarin, phenytoin, sulfonamides
• Toxicity: lithium, methotrexate
• Decreased action of: triamterene
• Do not give with antacids

NURSING CONSIDERATIONS
Assess:

• Renal, liver, blood studies: BUN, creatinine, AST, ALT, Hgb, before treatment, periodically thereafter
• Audiometric, ophthalmic exam before, during, after treatment
• For eye, ear problems: blurred vision, tinnitus; may indicate toxicity
• For confusion, mood changes, hallucinations

Administer:

• IV after diluting 1 mg/ml or more normal saline or sterile H$_2$O for inj without preservative; give over 5-10 sec
• With food to decrease GI symptoms; however, best to take on empty stomach to facilitate absorption

Perform/provide:

• Storage at room temperature

Evaluate:

• Therapeutic response: decreased pain, stiffness in joints, decreased swelling in joints, ability to move more easily

Teach patient/family:

• To report blurred vision, ringing, roaring in ears; may indicate toxicity
• To avoid driving, other hazardous activities if dizziness, drowsiness occurs
• To report change in urine pattern, increased weight, edema, increased pain in joints, fever, blood in urine; indicate nephrotoxicity; to report mood changes: anxiety, depression
• That therapeutic antiinflammatory effects may take up to 1 mo
• To avoid alcohol, salicylates; bleeding may occur

---

* Available in Canada only

Influenza virus vaccine, trivalent A & B (whole virus/split virus)

Fluzone, Fluogen, Fluviral,* Influenza Virus vaccine, Trivalent

Func. class.: Vaccine

Action: Produces antibodies to influenza virus; split virus vaccine causes less adverse reactions

Uses: Prevention of Russian, Chile, Philippine influenza

Dosage and routes:
• *Adult and child >12 yr:* IM 0.5 ml in 1 dose
• *Child 3-12 yr:* IM 0.5 ml, repeat in 1 mo (split) unless 1978-1985 vaccine was given
• *Child 6 mo to 3 yr:* IM 0.25 ml, repeat in 1 mo (split) unless 1978-1985 vaccine was given

Available forms: Inj IM 100 μg/ml

Side effects/adverse reactions:
CNS: Fever, Guillain-Barré syndrome
INTEG: Urticaria, induration, erythema
SYST: Anaphylaxis, malaise
MS: Myalgia

Contraindications: Hypersensitivity, active infection, chicken, egg allergy, Guillain-Barré syndrome

Precautions: Elderly, immunosuppression, pregnancy

NURSING CONSIDERATIONS
Assess:
• For skin reactions: rash, induration, erythema
• For anaphylaxis: inability to breathe, bronchospasm

Administer:
• Only with epinephrine 1:1000 on unit to treat laryngospasm
• Only IM

Perform/provide:
• Written record of immunization

• At least 2 mo after measles virus vaccine; do not administer at same time as DPT

Evaluate:
• For history of allergies, skin conditions (eczema, psoriasis, dermatitis), reactions to vaccinations

Insulin, isophane suspension (NPH)

Beef NPH Iletin II, Humulin N, Iletin NPH,* Insulatard NPH, NPH Iletin I, Pork NPH Iletin II, Novolin N,* NPH Insulin, NPH Purified Pork

Func. class.: Antidiabetic
Chem. class.: Exogenous unmodified insulin

Action: Decreases blood sugar; indirectly increases blood pyruvate, lactate; decreases phosphate, potassium

Uses: Ketoacidosis, type I (IDDM), type II (NIDDM) diabetes mellitus, hyperkalemia

Dosage and routes:
• *Adult:* SC dosage individualized by blood, urine glucose, usual dose 7-26 U; may increase by 2-10 U/day if needed

Available forms: SC 100 U/ml

Side effects/adverse reactions:
CNS: Headache, lethargy, tremors, weakness, fatigue, delirium, sweating
CV: Tachycardia, palpitations
EENT: Blurred vision, dry mouth
GI: Hunger, nausea
META: Hypoglycemia
INTEG: Flushing, rash, urticaria, warmth, lipodystrophy, lipohypertrophy
SYST: Anaphylaxis

Contraindications: Hypersensitivity to protamine

Precautions: Pregnancy (B)

italics = common side effects   ***bold italic*** = life threatening reactions

Interactions/incompatibilities:

• Increased hypoglycemia: salicylate, alcohol, β-blockers, anabolic steroids, fenfluramine, phenylbutazone, sulfinpyrazone, guanethidine, oral hypoglycemics, MAOIs, tetracycline

• Decreased hypoglycemia: thiazides, thyroid hormones, oral contraceptives, corticosteroids, estrogens, dobutamine, epinephrine

Pharmacokinetics:

SC: Onset 1-2 hr, peak 4-12 hr, duration 18-24 hr

Metabolized by liver, muscle, kidneys; excreted in urine

Lab test interferences:

Increase: VMA

Decrease: K, Ca

Interference: Liver function studies, thyroid function studies

NURSING CONSIDERATIONS

Assess:

• Fasting blood glucose, 2 hr PP (80-150 mg/dl normal fasting level) (70-130 mg/dl-normal 2 hr level)

• Urine ketones during illness; insulin requirements may increase during stress, illness

• Hypoglycemic reaction that can occur during peak time

Administer:

• After warming to room temperature by rotating in palms to prevent injecting cold insulin

• Increased doses if tolerance occurs

• Human insulin to those allergic to beef or pork

Perform/provide:

• Storage at room temperature for <1 mo, keep away from heat and sunlight, refrigerate all other supply, do not use if discolored; do not freeze

• Rotation of injection sites within one area: abdomen, upper back, thighs, upper arm, buttocks; keep record of sites

Evaluate:

• Therapeutic response: decrease in polyuria, polydipsia, polyphagia, clear sensorium, absence of dizziness, stable gait

Teach patient/family:

• That blurred vision occurs; not to change corrective lens until vision is stabilized 1-2 mo

• To keep insulin, equipment available at all times

• That drug does not cure diabetes but controls symptoms

• To carry Medic Alert ID as diabetic

• Hypoglycemia reaction: headache, tremors, fatigue, weakness

• Dosage, route, mixing instructions, if any diet restrictions, disease process

• To carry candy or lump sugar to treat hypoglycemia; have glucagon emergency kit available

• Symptoms of ketoacidosis: nausea, thirst, polyuria, dry mouth, decreased B/P, dry, flushed skin, acetone breath, drowsiness, Kussmaul respirations

• That a plan is necessary for diet, exercise; all food on diet should be eaten; exercise routine should not vary

• To avoid OTC drugs unless directed by physician

Treatment of overdose: Glucose 25g IV, via dextrose 50% solution, 50 ml or 1 mg glucagon

Insulin, isophane suspension and regular insulin
Humulin 70/30, Mixtard, Novolin 70/30

Func. class.: Antidiabetic
Chem. class.: Exogenous unmodified insulin

Action: Decreases blood sugar, indirectly increases blood pyruvate, lactate, decreases phosphate, potassium
Uses: Ketoacidosis, type I (IDDM), type II (NIDDM) diabetes mellitus, hyperkalemia
Dosage and routes:
• *Adult:* SC individualized dose
Available forms: 70 U/ml isophane insulin with 30 U/ml regular insulin = 100 U/ml
Side effects/adverse reactions:
CNS: Headache, lethargy, tremors, weakness, fatigue, delirium, sweating
CV: Tachycardia, palpitations
EENT: Blurred vision, dry mouth
GI: Hunger, nausea
META: Hypoglycemia
INTEG: Flushing, rash, urticaria, warmth, lipodystrophy, lipohypertrophy
*SYST: **Anaphylaxis***
Contraindications: Hypersensitivity to protamine
Precautions: Pregnancy (B)
Interactions/incompatibilities:
• Increased hypoglycemia: salicylate, alcohol, β-blockers, anabolic steroids, fenfluramine, guanethidine, sulfinpyrazone, oral hypoglycemics, MAOIs, tetracycline
• Decreased hypoglycemia: thiazides, thyroid hormones, oral contraceptives, corticosteroids, estrogens, dobutamine, epinephrine, smoking, levothyroxine

Pharmacokinetics:
SC: Onset 30 min, peak 4-8 hr, duration 12-24 hr
Metabolized by liver, muscle, kidneys; excreted in urine
Lab test interferences:
Increase: VMA
Decrease: K, Ca
Interference: Liver function studies, thyroid function studies

NURSING CONSIDERATIONS
Assess:
• Fasting blood glucose, 2 hr PP (80-150 mg/dl normal fasting level) (70-130 mg/dl-normal 2 hr level)
• Urine ketones during illness; insulin requirement increases during stress, illness
• Hypoglycemic reaction that can occur during peak time
Administer:
• After warming to room temperature by rotating in palms to prevent injecting cold insulin
• Increased doses if tolerance occurs
• Human insulin to those allergic to beef or pork
Perform/provide:
• Storage at room temperature for <1 mo, keep cool and away from heat, refrigerate all other supply, do not use if discolored
• Rotation of injection sites within one area: abdomen, upper back, thighs, upper arm, buttocks; keep record of sites
Evaluate:
• Therapeutic response: decrease in polyuria, polydipsia, polyphagia, clear sensorium, absence of dizziness, stable gait
Teach patient/family:
• That blurred vision occurs; not to change corrective lens until vision is stabilized 1-2 mo

---

italics = common side effects   **bold italic** = life threatening reactions

• To keep insulin, equipment available at all times
• That drug does not cure diabetes but controls symptoms
• To carry Medic Alert ID as diabetic
• Hypoglycemia reaction: headache, tremors, fatigue, weakness
• Dosage, route, mixing instructions, if any diet restrictions, disease process
• To carry candy or lump sugar to treat hypoglycemia
• Symptoms of ketoacidosis: nausea, thirst, polyuria, dry mouth, decreased B/P, dry, flushed skin, acetone breath, drowsiness, Kussmaul respirations
• That a plan is necessary for diet, exercise; all food on diet should be eaten; exercise routine should not vary
• About urine glucose testing; make sure patient is able to determine glucose, acetone levels
• To avoid OTC drugs unless directed by physician

Treatment of overdose: Glucose 25 g IV, via dextrose 50% solution, 50cc or glucagon 1 mg

---

Insulin, regular

Beef Regular Iletin II, Humulin BR, Humulin R, Novolin R, Pork Regular Iletin II, Regular purified Pork, Novolin R PenFill, Velosulin

Func. class.: Antidiabetic
Chem. class.: Exogenous unmodified insulin

Action: Decreases blood sugar, indirectly increases blood pyruvate, lactate, decreases phosphate, potassium
Uses: Adult-onset diabetes, juvenile diabetes, ketoacidosis type I, II, NIDDM, IDDM, hyperkalemia

Dosage and routes:
Ketoacidosis
• *Adult:* IV/IM 5-10 U, then 5-10 U/hr until desired response, then switch to SC dose; IV/INF 2-12 U (50 U/500 ml of normal saline)
• *Child:* IV/IM 0.1 U/kg
Replacement
• *Adult:* SC dosage individualized by blood, urine glucose levels, up to qid given ½ hr before meals
Available forms: IV/IM/SC inj U 40, U 100/ml

Side effects/adverse reactions:
CNS: Headache, lethargy, tremors, weakness, fatigue, *delirium,* sweating
CV: Tachycardia, palpitations
EENT: Blurred vision, dry mouth
GI: Hunger, nausea
INTEG: Flushing, rash, urticaria, warmth, lipodystrophy, lipohypertrophy
META: Hypoglycemia
SYST: **Anaphylaxis**

Contraindications: Hypersensitivity
Precautions: Pregnancy (B)
Interactions/incompatibilities:
• Increased hypoglycemia: salicylate, alcohol, β-blockers, anabolic steroids, fenfluramine, guanethidine, oral hypoglycemics, MAOIs, tetracycline, sulfinpyrazone
• Decreased hypoglycemia: thiazides, thyroid hormones, oral contraceptives, corticosteroids, estrogens, dobutamine, epinephrine, dextrothyroxine, smoking
• Mask signs/symptoms of hypoglycemia: β-blocker
• Incompatible with aminophylline, amobarbital, chlorothiazide, dobutamine, heparin, penicillin G potassium, pentobarbital, phenobarbital, phenytoin, secobarbital,

---

*Available in Canada only

NaCO$_3$, thiopental, in sol or syringe

Pharmacokinetics:

SC: Onset 30-60 min, peak 2-3 hr, duration 5-7 hr .

IV: Onset 10-30 min, peak 30-60 min, duration 1-2 hr, half-life 3-5 min; metabolized by liver, muscle, kidneys, excreted in urine

Lab test interferences:

Increase: VMA

Decrease: K, Ca

Interference: Liver function studies, thyroid function studies

NURSING CONSIDERATIONS

Assess:

• Hypoglycemic/hyperglycemic reaction that can occur soon after meals

• Fasting blood glucose, 2 hr PP (60-100 mg/dl normal fasting level) (70-130 mg/dl-normal 2 hr level)

• Urine ketones during illness; insulin requirements increase during times of stress, illness

Administer:

• After warming to room temperature by rotating in palms to prevent lipodystrophy from injecting cold insulin

• SC at 90-degree angle (½″ needle), 45-degree angle (⅝″ needle); apply pressure; do not massage

• ½ hr ac, so peak action coincides with peak sugar level

• Increased doses if tolerance occurs

• Human insulin to those allergic to beef or pork

• IV undiluted through Y-tube or 3-way stopcock; give 50 U or less/min; may be diluted in 0.9% NS or 0.45% saline for INF; run at rate ordered; use infusion pump; drug rate should be decreased if serum glucose level is 250 mg/100 ml;

large single IV doses should not be given

Perform/provide:

• Storage at room temperature for 1 mo; keep in cool area; refrigerate all other supply; do not freeze; do not use discolored or cloudy sol; discard open vials not used for 1 mo

• Rotation of injection sites: abdomen, upper back, thighs, upper arm, buttocks; keep record of sites

Evaluate:

• Therapeutic response: decrease in polyuria, polydipsia, polyphagia; clear sensorium, absence of dizziness, stable gait

Teach patient/family:

• That blurred vision occurs; not to change corrective lenses until vision is stabilized 1-2 mo

• To keep insulin, equipment available at all times; provide instructions for using automatic injector if needed

• That drug does not cure diabetes, but controls symptoms

• To carry Medic Alert ID as diabetic

• Hypoglycemia reaction: headache, tremors, fatigue, weakness, sweating

• Dosage, route; mixing instructions if any diet restrictions; disease process

• To carry candy or lump sugar to treat hypoglycemia

• Symptoms of ketoacidosis: nausea, thirst, polyuria, dry mouth, decrease in B/P, dry flushed skin, acetone breath, drowsiness, Kussmaul respirations

• That a plan is necessary for diet, exercise; all food on diet should be eaten; exercise routine should not vary

• About urine glucose testing; make sure patient is able to deter-

mine glucose, acetone levels, also home blood glucose monitoring
• That pregnant patients should use glucose oxidase reagents
• To avoid OTC drugs unless directed by physician
• To identify lipotrophy; make chart of rotation sites
Treatment of overdose: Glucose 25 g IV, via dextrose 50% solution, 50 ml or 1 mg glucagon

---

Insulin, regular concentrated
Regular (concentrated) Iletin II U-500

Func. class.: Antidiabetic
Chem. class.: Exogenous unmodified insulin

Action: Decreases blood sugar, indirectly increases blood pyruvate, lactate, decreases phosphate, potassium

Uses: Treatment of diabetic patients with marked insulin resistance (>200 U/day)

Dosage and routes:
• *Adult:* SC/IM dosage individualized by blood, urine glucose qd-tid
Available forms: Inj SC, IM 500 U/ml

Side effects/adverse reactions:
CNS: Headache, lethargy, tremors, weakness, fatigue, delirium, sweating
CV: Tachycardia, palpitations
EENT: Blurred vision
GI: Hunger, nausea, dry mouth
META: Hypoglycemia
INTEG: Flushing, rash, urticaria, warmth, lipodystrophy, lipohypertrophy
SYST: Anaphylaxis
MISC: Thirst, leg pain, increased urination

Contraindications: Hypersensitivity
Precautions: Pregnancy (B)
Pharmacokinetics:
SC: Onset 30-60 min, peak 2-5 hr, duration 5-7 hr
Metabolized by liver, muscle, kidneys; excreted in urine
Interactions/incompatibilities:
• Increased hypoglycemia: salicylate, alcohol, β-blockers, anabolic steroids, fenfluramine, guanethidine, oral hypoglycemics, MAOIs, tetracycline, sulfinpyrazone
• Decreased hypoglycemia: thiazides, thyroid hormones, oral contraceptives, corticosteroids, estrogens, smoking, dextrothyroxine, dobutamine, epinephrine
Lab test interferences:
Increase: VMA
Decrease: K, Ca
Interference: Liver function studies, thyroid function studies
NURSING CONSIDERATIONS
Assess:
• Fasting blood glucose, 2 hr PP (60-100 mg/dl normal fasting level); (70-130 mg/dl-normal 2 hr level)
• Urine ketones during times of illness; insulin requirements increase during stress, illness
• Hypoglycemic/hyperglycemic reaction that can occur soon after meals or suddenly while on therapy
Administer:
• After warming to room temperature by rotating in palms, to prevent lipodystrophy from injecting cold insulin
• ½ hr ac, so peak action coincides with peak sugar level
• Increased doses if tolerance occurs
Perform/provide:
• Storage in refrigerator; do not

freeze; do not use discolored or cloudy solution
• Rotation of injection sites: abdomen, upper back, thighs, upper arms, buttocks; keep record of sites
Evaluate:
• Therapeutic response: decrease in polyuria, polydipsia, polyphagia; clear sensorium; absence of dizziness; stable gait
Teach patient/family:
• That blurred vision occurs; not to change corrective lenses until vision is stabilized 1-2 mo
• To keep insulin, equipment available at all times
• That drug does not cure diabetes but controls symptoms
• To carry Medic Alert ID as diabetic
• Hypoglycemia reaction: headache, tremors, fatigue, weakness
• Dosage, route, mixing instructions if any diet restrictions, disease process
• To carry candy or lump sugar to treat hypoglycemia
• Symptoms of ketoacidosis: nausea, thirst, polyuria, dry mouth, decrease B/P, dry, flushed skin, acetone breath, drowsiness, Kussmaul respirations
• That a plan is necessary for diet, exercise; all food on diet should be eaten; exercise routine should not vary
• About urine glucose testing; make sure patient is able to determine glucose, acetone levels
• To avoid OTC drugs unless directed by physician
Treatment of overdose: Glucose 25 g IV, via dextrose 50% solution, 50 ml or 1 mg glucagon

insulin, zinc suspension (Lente)

Humulin L, Lentard Monotard,* Lente Iletin II, Lente Insulin, Lente Iletin I, Lente Purified Pork Insulin, Novolin L
Func. class.: Antidiabetic
Chem. class.: Exogenous unmodified insulin

Action: Decreases blood sugar, indirectly increases blood pyruvate, lactate, decreases phosphate, potassium
Uses: Ketoacidosis, type I (IDDM), type II (NIDDM) diabetes mellitus, hyperkalemia
Dosage and routes:
• *Adult:* SC individualized
Available forms: SC 40 00 U/ml
Side effects/adverse reactions:
CNS: Headache, lethargy, tremors, weakness, fatigue, delirium, sweating
CV: Tachycardia, palpitations
EENT: Blurred vision, dry mouth
GI: Hunger, nausea
META: Hypoglycemia
INTEG: Flushing, rash, urticaria, warmth, lipodystrophy, lipohypertrophy
*SYST: **Anaphylaxis***
Contraindications: Hypersensitivity to protamine
Precautions: Pregnancy (B)
Pharmacokinetics:
SC: Onset 1-2½ hr, peak 7-15 hr, duration 12-24 hr
Metabolized by liver, muscle, kidneys; excreted in urine
Interactions/incompatibilities:
• Increased hypoglycemia: salicylate, alcohol, β-blockers, anabolic steroids, fenfluramine, guanethidine, oral hypoglycemics, MAOIs, tetracycline, sulfinpyrazone

---

italics = common side effects   ***bold italic*** = life threatening reactions

• Hyperglycemia: thiazides, thyroid hormones, oral contraceptives, corticosteroids, estrogens, dobutamine, epinephrine, smoking, levothyroxine

Lab test interferences:

Increase: VMA

Decrease: K, Ca

Interference: Liver function studies, thyroid function studies

NURSING CONSIDERATIONS

Assess:

• Fasting blood glucose, 2 hr PP (80-150 mg/dl normal fasting level); (70-130 mg/dl-normal 2 hr level)

• Urine ketones during illness; insulin requirements increase during illness, stress

• Hypoglycemic reaction that can occur during peak time

Administer:

• After warming to room temperature by rotating in palms to prevent injecting cold insulin

• Increased doses if tolerance occurs

• Human insulin to those allergic to beef or pork

Perform/provide:

• Storage at room temperature for <1 mo; keep in cool area; refrigerate all other supply; do not use if discolored

• Rotation of injection sites within one area: abdomen, upper back, thighs, upper arm, buttocks; keep record of sites

Evaluate:

• Therapeutic response: decrease in polyuria, polydipsia, polyphagia; clear sensorium, absence of dizziness, stable gait

Teach patient/family:

• That blurred vision occurs; not to change corrective lenses until vision is stabilized 1-2 mo

• To keep insulin, equipment available at all times

• That drug does not cure diabetes but controls symptoms

• To carry Medic Alert ID as diabetic

• About hypoglycemia reaction: headache, tremors, fatigue, weakness

• Dosage, route, mixing instructions; if any diet restrictions; disease process

• To carry candy or lump sugar to treat hypoglycemia

• Symptoms of ketoacidosis: nausea, thirst, polyuria, dry mouth, decreased B/P, dry, flushed skin, acetone breath, drowsiness, Kussmaul respirations

• That a plan is necessary for diet, exercise; all food on diet should be eaten; exercise routine should not vary

• About urine glucose testing, make sure patient is able to determine glucose, acetone levels

• To avoid OTC drugs unless directed by physician

Treatment of overdose: Glucose 25 g IV, via dextrose 50% solution, 50 ml or 1 mg glucagon

---

insulin, zinc suspension extended (Ultralente)

Ultralente,* Untralente Iletin I, Ultralente Insulin

Func. class.: Antidiabetic

Chem. class.: Exogenous unmodified insulin

Action: Decreases blood sugar, indirectly increases blood pyruvate, lactate, decreases phosphate, potassium

Uses: Ketoacidosis, type I

(IDDM), type II (NIDDM) diabetes mellitus, hyperkalemia

Dosage and routes:
• *Adult:* SC individualized
Available forms: SC 40, 100 U/ml

Side effects/adverse reactions:
CNS: Headache, lethargy, tremors, weakness, fatigue, delirium, sweating
CV: Tachycardia, palpitations
EENT: Blurred vision, dry mouth
GI: Hunger, nausea
META: Hypoglycemia
INTEG: Flushing, rash, urticaria, warmth, lipodystrophy, lipohypertrophy
*SYST: **Anaphylaxis***

Contraindications: Hypersensitivity to protamine

Precautions: Pregnancy (C)

Pharmacokinetics:
SC: Onset 4-8 hr, peak 10-30 hr, duration 7-36 hr
Metabolized by liver, muscle, kidneys, excreted in urine

Interactions/incompatibilities:
• Increased hypoglycemia: salicylate, alcohol, β-blockers, anabolic steroids, fenfluramine, guanethidine, oral hypoglycemics, MAOIs, tetracycline, sulfinpyrazone
• Decreased hypoglycemia: thiazides, thyroid hormones, oral contraceptives, corticosteroids, estrogens, dobutamine, epinephrine, smoking, levothyroxine

Lab test interferences:
Increase: VMA
Decrease: K, Ca
Interference: Liver function studies, thyroid function studies

NURSING CONSIDERATIONS
Assess:
• Fasting blood glucose, 2 hr PP (80-150 mg/dl normal fasting level); (70-130 mg/dl-normal 2 hr level)
• Urine ketones during illness; insulin requirements increase during stress, illness
• Hypoglycemic reaction that can occur during peak time

Administer:
• After warming to room temperature by rotating in palms to prevent injecting cold insulin
• Increased doses if tolerance occurs

Perform/provide:
• Storage at room temperature for <1 mo; refrigerate all other supply; do not use if discolored
• Rotation of injection sites within one area: abdomen, upper back, thighs, upper arm, buttocks; keep record of sites

Evaluate:
• Therapeutic response: decrease in polyuria, polydipsia, polyphagia; clear sensorium, absence of dizziness, stable gait

Teach patient/family:
• That blurred vision occurs; not to change corrective lenses until vision is stabilized 1-2 mo
• To keep insulin, equipment available at all times
• That drug does not cure diabetes but controls symptoms
• To carry Medic Alert ID as diabetic
• Hypoglycemia reaction: headache, tremors, fatigue, weakness
• Dosage, route, mixing instructions; if any diet restrictions; disease process
• To carry candy or lump sugar to treat hypoglycemia
• Symptoms of ketoacidosis: nausea, thirst, polyuria, dry mouth, decreased B/P, dry, flushed skin, acetone breath, drowsiness, Kussmaul respirations
• That a plan is necessary for diet, exercise; all food on diet should be

eaten; exercise routine should not vary
• About urine glucose testing; make sure patient is able to determine glucose, acetone levels
• That pregnant patients should use glucose oxidase reagents
• To avoid OTC drugs unless directed by physician
Treatment of overdose: Glucose 25 g IV, via dextrose 50% solution, 50 ml or 1 mg glucagon

---

insulin, zinc suspension, prompt (semilente)
Semilente Iletin I, Semilente Insulin
Func. class.: Antidiabetic
Chem. class.: Exogenous unmodified insulin

Action: Decreases blood sugar; indirectly increases blood pyruvate, lactate, decreases phosphate, potassium
Uses: Ketoacidosis, type I (IDDM), type II (NIDDM) diabetes mellitus, hyperkalemia
Dosage and routes:
• *Adult:* SC dosage individualized by blood, urine glucose qd-tid
Available forms: SC 40, 100 U/ml
Side effects/adverse reactions:
CNS: Headache, lethargy, tremors, weakness, fatigue, delirium, sweating
CV: Tachycardia, palpitations
EENT: Blurred vision, dry mouth
GI: Hunger, nausea
META: Hypoglycemia
INTEG: Flushing, rash, urticaria, warmth, lipodystrophy, lipohypertrophy
SYST: Anaphylaxis
Contraindications: Hypersensitivity to protamine
Precautions: Pregnancy (B)

Pharmacokinetics:
SC: Onset 1-1½ hr, peak 5-10 hr, duration 12-16 hr
Metabolized by liver, muscle, kidneys; excreted in urine
Interactions/incompatibilities:
• Increased hypoglycemia: salicylate, alcohol, β-blockers, anabolic steroids, fenfluramine, guanethidine, oral hypoglycemics, MAOIs, tetracycline, sulfinpyrazone
• Hyperglycemia: thiazides, thyroid hormones, oral contraceptives, corticosteroids, estrogens, dobutamine, epinephrine, smoking, levothyroxine
Lab test interferences:
Increase: VMA
Decrease: K, Ca
Interference: Liver function studies, thyroid function studies

NURSING CONSIDERATIONS
Assess:
• Fasting blood glucose, 2 hr PP (80-150 mg/dl normal fasting level); (70-130 mg/dl-normal 2 hr level)
• Urine ketones during illness; insulin requirements increase during stress, illness
• Hypoglycemic reaction that can occur during peak time
Administer:
• After warming to room temperature by rotating in palms, to prevent injecting cold insulin
• Increased doses if tolerance occurs
Perform/provide:
• Storage at room temperature for <1 mo in cool area; refrigerate all other supply; do not use if discolored
• Rotation of injection sites within one area: abdomen, upper back, thighs, upper arm, buttocks; keep record of sites

---

*Available in Canada only

Evaluate:
• Therapeutic response: decrease in polyuria, polydipsia, polyphagia; clear sensorium, absence of dizziness, stable gait

Teach patient/family:
• That blurred vision occurs; not to change corrective lenses until vision is stabilized 1-2 mo
• To keep insulin, equipment available at all times
• That drug does not cure diabetes but controls symptoms
• To carry Medic Alert ID as diabetic
• Hypoglycemia reaction: headache, tremors, fatigue, weakness
• Dosage, route, mixing instructions; if any diet restrictions; disease process
• To carry candy or lump sugar to treat hypoglycemia
• Symptoms of ketoacidosis: nausea, thirst, polyuria, dry mouth, decreased B/P, dry, flushed skin, acetone breath, drowsiness, Kussmaul respirations
• That a plan is necessary for diet, exercise; all food on diet should be eaten; exercise routine should not vary
• Urine glucose testing; make sure patient is able to determine glucose, acetone levels
• That pregnant patients should use glucose oxidase reagents
• To avoid OTC drugs unless directed by physician

Treatment of overdose: Glucose 25 g IV, via dextrose 50% solution, 50 ml or 1 mg glucagon

Interferon alfa-2a/interferon alfa-2b

(in-ter-ferón)
Roferon-a/Intron-a
Func. class.: Miscellaneous antineoplastic
Chem. class.: Protein product

Action: Antiviral action inhibits viral replication by reprogramming virus; antitumor action suppresses cell proliferation; immunomodulating action phagocytizes target cells

Uses: Hairy cell leukemia in persons >18 yr, condylomata acuminata, metastatic melanoma, AIDS

Dosage and routes:
• *Adult:* SC/IM (interferon alfa-2a) 3 million IU × 16-24 wk, then 3 million IU 3 × wk maintenance; hairy cell leukemia 2 million IU/m² 3 × wk; if severe adverse reactions occur, dose should be skipped or reduced by ½; condylomata acuminata 2b 1 million IU/lesion 3 × /wk × 3 wk; Kaposi's sarcoma 30 million IU/m² 3 × /wk

Available forms: alfa-2a inj 3, 18 million IU/vial; alfa-2b inj 3, 5, 10, 25 million IU/vial

Side effects/adverse reactions:
CNS: Dizziness, confusion, numbness, paresthesias, hallucinations, **convulsions, coma,** amnesia, anxiety, mood changes
CV: Edema, hypotension, hypertension, chest pain, palpitations, dysrhythmias, **CHF, MI, CVA**
INTEG: Rash, dry skin, itching, alopecia, flushing
GI: Weight loss, taste changes
GU: Impotence
MISC: Flulike syndrome; fever, fatigue, myalgias, headache, chills
Contraindications: Hypersensitivity

Precautions: Severe hypotension, dysrhythmia, tachycardia, pregnancy (C), lactation, children, severe renal or hepatic disease, convulsion disorder

Pharmacokinetics:
Half-life (interferon alfa-2a) 3.7-8.5 hr, peak 3-4 hr; half-life (interferon alfa-2b) 2-7 hr, peak 6-8 hr

Lab test interferences:
Interference: AST, ALT, LDH, alk phosphatase, WBC, platelets, granulocytes, creatinine

NURSING CONSIDERATIONS
Assess:
• For symptoms of infection; may be masked by drug fever
• CNS reaction: LOC, mental status, dizziness, confusion

Administer:
• IM/SC after reconstituting 3-5 million IU/1 ml, 10 million IU/2 ml, 25 million IU/5 ml, of diluent provided, mix gently
• Intralesional after reconstituting 10 million IU/1 ml bacteriostatic water for inj. No more than 5 lesions can safely be treated at a time
• At hs to minimize side effects
• Acetaminophen as ordered to alleviate fever and headache

Perform/provide:
• Storage of reconstituted solution for 1 mo in refrigerator
• Increased fluid intake to 2-3 L/day

Evaluate:
• Therapeutic response: decrease in tumor size, increase in ease of breathing

Teach patient/family:
• To avoid hazardous tasks, since confusion, dizziness may occur
• That brands of this drug should not be changed; each form is different, with different doses

• That fatigue is common; activity may have to be altered
• Not to become pregnant while taking drug; possible mutagenic effects
• To report signs of infection: sore throat, fever, diarrhea, vomiting
• That impotence may occur during treatment but is temporary
• Emotional lability is common; notify physician if severe or incapacitating

---

Interferon alfa-n 3
(in-ter-feer'on)
Alferon N
Func. class.: Antineoplastic
Chem. class.: Human interferon α-protein

Action: Binds interferon to membrane receptors on cell surface with high specificity; this produces protein synthesis, inhibition of virus replication, suppression of cell proliferide, and increased phagocytosis

Uses: Condylomata acuminata (veneral/genital warts)

Dosages and routes:
• *Adult:* 0.05 ml (250,000 IU) per wart, given 2 ×/wk × 8 wk; not to exceed 0.5 ml (2.5 million IU); inject into base of wart

Available forms: Inj 5 m IU/1 ml vial with 3.3 mg/ml phenol and 1 mg/ml human albumin

Side effects/adverse reactions:
CNS: Fever, headache, sweating, vasovagal reaction, chills, fatigue, dizziness, insomnia, sleepiness, depression
GI: Nausea, vomiting, heartburn, diarrhea, constipation, anorexia, stomatitis, dry mouth
MS: Myalgias, arthralgia, back pain

INTEG: Pain at injection site, pruritis

CV: Chest pain, hypotension

Contraindications: Hypersensitivity to this product, egg protein, IgG, neomycin

Precautions: Pregnancy (C), lactation, children, CHF, angina (unstable), COPD, diabetes mellitus with ketoacidosis, hemophilia, pulmonary embolism, thrombophlebitis, bone marrow depression, convulsive disorder

Pharmacokinetics: Unable to detect

Lab test interferences:

Interferences: AST, ALT, LDH, alk phosphatase, WBC, platelets, granulocytes, creatinine

NURSING CONSIDERATIONS

Assess:

• For symptoms of infection; may be masked by drug fever

• CNS reaction: LOC, mental status, dizziness, confusion

• For body image disturbance

Administer:

• Acetaminophen to alleviate fever and headache

Perform/provide:

• Storage of reconstituted solution for 1 mo in refrigerator

• Increased fluid intake to 2-3 L/day

Evaluate:

• Therapeutic response: decrease in wart size

Teach patient/family:

• To avoid hazardous tasks, since confusion, dizziness may occur

• That brands of this drug should not be changed; each form is different, with different doses

• That fatigue is common; activity may have to be altered

• Not to become pregnant while taking drug; possible mutagenic effects

• To report signs of infection: sore throat, fever, diarrhea, vomiting

• Signs of hypersensitivity: liver, urticaria, wheezing, dyspnea; notify physician immediately

interferon β-16
(in-ter-feer'on)
Betaseron
Func. class.: Multiple sclerosis agent
Chem. class.: E. coli derivative

Action: Antiviral, immunoregulatory; action not clearly understood; biologic response modifying properties mediated through specific receptors on cells, inducing expression of interferon-induced gene products

Uses: Ambulatory patients with relapsing or remitting multiple sclerosis; may be useful in treatment of AIDS, AIDS-related Kaposi's sarcoma, malignant melanoma, metastatic renal cell carcinoma, cutaneous T-cell lymphoma, acute non-A, non-B hepatitis

Dosage and routes:

Relapsing/remitting multiple sclerosis

Adult: SC 0.25 mg (8 IU) qod

Available forms: Powder for inj lyophilized 0.3 mg (9.6 mIU)

Side effects/adverse reactions:

CNS: Headache, fever, pain, chills, mental changes, hypertonia, **suicide attempts**

CV: Migraine, palpitations, hypertension, tachycardia, peripheral vascular disorders

EENT: Conjunctivitis, blurred vision

GI: Diarrhea, constipation, vomiting, abdominal pain

GU: Dysmenorrhea, irregular men-

ses, metrorrhagia, cystitis, breast pain
*HEMA: **Decreased lymphocytes, ANC, WBC;** lymphadenopathy*
INTEG: Sweating, inj site reaction
*MS: Myalgia, **myasthenia***
RESP: Sinusitis, dyspnea
Contraindications: Hypersensitivity to natural or recombinant interferon-β or human albumin
Precautions: Pregnancy (C), lactation, child <18 yr, chronic progressive MS, depression, mental disorders
NURSING CONSIDERATIONS
Assess:
• Blood, renal, hepatic studies: CBC, differential, platelet counts, BUN, creatinine ALT, urinalysis
• CNS symptoms: headache, fatigue, depression
• GI status: diarrhea or constipation, vomiting, abdominal pain
• Cardiac status: Increased B/P, tachycardia
Administer:
• Acetaminophen for fever, headache
• SC only; do not give IM or IV
Perform/provide:
• Storage in refrigerator; do not freeze
Evaluate:
• Therapeutic response: decreased symptoms of multiple sclerosis
Teach patient/family:
• To provide patient or family member with written, detailed information about the drug
• That blurred vision, sweating may occur
• Women patients that irregular menses, dysmenorrhea, or metrorrhagia as well as breast pain may occur

Interferon gamma-1b
(in-ter-fer'on)
Actimmune
Func. class.: Biologic response modifier
Chem. class.: Lymphokine, interleukin type

Action: Species-specific protein synthesized in response to viruses, potent phagocyte-activating effects; capable of mediating the killing of *S. aureus, T. gondii, L. donovani, L. monocytogenes, M. avium-intracellulare;* enhances oxidative metabolism of macrophages, enhances antibody-dependent cellular cytotoxicity
Uses: Serious infections associated with chronic granulomatous disease
Dosage and routes:
• *Adult:* SC 50 μg/m² (1.5 million U/m²) for patients with a surface area of >0.5 m²; 1.5 μg/kg/dose for patient with a surface area of <0.5/m²; give on Monday, Wednesday, Friday for 3×/wk dosing
Available forms: Inj 100 μg (3 million U) single-dose vial
Side effects/adverse reactions:
GI: Nausea, anorexia, abdominal pain, weight loss, diarrhea, vomiting
CNS: Headache, fatigue, depression, fever, chills
INTEG: Rash, pain at injection site
MS: Myalgia, arthralgia
Contraindications: Hypersensitivity to interferon gamma, *E. coli*–derived products
Precautions: Pregnancy (C), cardiac disease, seizure disorders, CNS disorders, myelosuppression, lactation, children

Pharmacokinetics:

SC: Dose absorbed 89%, elimination half-life 5.9 hr, peak 7 hr

Interactions/incompatibilities:

• Increased myelosuppression: other myelosuppressive agents

NURSING CONSIDERATIONS

Assess:

• Blood, renal, hepatic studies: CBC, differential, platelet counts, BUN, creatinine ALT, urinalysis

• CNS symptoms: headache, fatigue, depression

Administer:

• At HS to minimize adverse reactions; administer acetaminophen for fever, headache

• 50% of the dose if severe reactions occur or discontinue treatment until reactions subside

• Using sterilized glass or plastic disposable syringes

• In right and left deltoid and anterior thigh

• Warm to room temperature before use; do not leave at room temperature over 12 hr (unopened vial)

Perform/provide:

• Storage in refrigerator upon receipt; do not freeze; do not shake

Evaluate:

• Therapeutic response: decreased serious infections, improvement in existing infections and inflammatory conditions

Teach patient/family:

• Method of administration if family members will be giving medication

• To provide patient or family member with written, detailed information about the drug

---

iodinated glycerol

Iophen, Organidin, Par Glycerol, R-Gen

Func. class.: Expectorant
Chem. class.: Iodopropylidene glycerol isom

Action: Increases respiratory tract fluid by decreasing surface tension, adhesiveness, which increases removal of mucus

Uses: Bronchial asthma, emphysema, bronchitis

Dosage and routes:

• *Adult:* PO 60 mg qid; SOL 20 gtts qid; ELIX 5 ml qid

• *Child:* PO up to half adult dose, depending on weight

Available forms: Tabs 30 mg; sol 50 mg/ml, 60 mg/5 ml

Side effects/adverse reactions:

EENT: Burning mouth, throat, eye irritation, swelling of eyelids

GI: Gastric irritation

ENDO: Iodism, goiter, myxedema

RESP: Pulmonary edema

*INTEG: **Angioedema**,* rash

CNS: Frontal headache, ***CNS depression**,* fever, parkinsonism

Contraindications: Hypersensitivity to iodides, pulmonary TB, pregnancy (X), hyperthyroidism, hyperkalemia, newborns, lactation, acute bronchitis

Precautions: Hypothyroidism, cystic fibrosis, lactation

Pharmacokinetics: Excreted in urine

Interactions/incompatibilities:

• Increased hypothyroid effects: lithium, antithyroid drugs

• Dysrhythmias, hyperkalemia: K-sparing diuretics, K-containing medication

---

NURSING CONSIDERATIONS
Assess:
• Cough: type, frequency, character including sputum
Administer:
• Orally in solution or tablet form
Perform/provide:
• Increased fluids to liquefy secretions
Evaluate:
• Therapeutic response: absence of cough
Teach patient/family:
• Not to use if pregnant or if any potential for pregnancy
• Symptoms of iodism: eruptions, burning of oral cavity, eye irritation
• Symptoms of hyperthyroidism: CNS depression, fever, glomerulonephritis

---

Iodoquinol
(eye-oh-do-kwin'ole)
Diodoquin,* Yodoxin
Func. class.: Amebicide
Chem. class.: Dihalogenated derivative of 8-hydroxyquinoline

Action: Direct-acting amebicide; action occurs in intestinal lumen
Uses: Intestinal amebiasis
Dosage and routes:
• *Adult:* PO 630-650 mg tid × 20 days, not to exceed 2 g/day
• *Child:* PO 30-40 mg/kg/day in 2-3 divided doses × 20 days, not to exceed 1.95 g/24 hrs for 20 days; do not repeat treatment before 2-3 wk
Available forms: Tabs 210, 650 mg; powder
Side effects/adverse reactions:
*HEMA: **Agranulocytosis*** (rare)
INTEG: Rash; pruritus; discolored skin, hair, nails; alopecia

CNS: Malaise, headache, agitation, peripheral neuropathy
MISC: Fever, chills, vertigo, thyroid enlargement
EENT: Blurred vision, sore throat, retinal edema, subacute myelooptic neuropathy
GI: Anorexia, nausea, vomiting, diarrhea, epigastric distress, gastritis, constipation, abdominal cramps, rectal irritation, anal itching
Contraindications: Hypersensitivity to this drug or iodine, renal disease, hepatic disease, severe thyroid disease, preexisting optic neuropathy
Precautions: Pregnancy (C), lactation
Lab test interferences:
Interfere: Thyroid function test
False positive: PKU
Increase: PBI
Decrease: ^{131}I uptake test
NURSING CONSIDERATIONS
Assess:
• Stools during entire treatment; should be clear at end of therapy; stools should be free of parasites for 1 yr before patient is considered cured
• I&O, stools for number, frequency, character
• Iodism: skin eruption, urticaria, discoloring of hair, nails
• Allergic reaction: fever, rash, itching, chills; drug should be discontinued if these occur
• Blurred vision; patient should have periodic eye exams during treatment
• Superimposed infection, fever, monilial growth, fatigue, malaise
• Diarrhea for 2-3 days
Administer:
• PO after meals to avoid GI symptoms

---

* Available in Canada only

Perform/provide:
• Storage in tight container
Evaluate:
• Therapeutic response: decreased diarrhea, symptoms in amebiasis
Teach patient/family:
• Proper hygiene after BM: hand-washing technique
• To avoid contact of drug with eyes, mouth, nose, other mucous membranes
• About need for compliance with dosage schedule, duration of treatment

---

ipecac syrup
(ip′e-kak)

Func. class.: Emetic
Chem. class.: Cephaelis ipecacuanha derivative

Action: Acts on chemoreceptor trigger zone to induce vomiting; irritates gastric mucosa
Uses: In poisoning to induce vomiting
Dosage and routes:
• *Adult:* PO 15 ml, then 200-300 ml water
• *Child >1 yr:* PO 15 ml, then 200-300 ml water
• *Child <1 yr:* PO 5-10 ml, then 100-200 ml water; may repeat dose if needed
Available forms: Liq
Side effects/adverse reactions:
CNS: Depression, convulsions, coma
GI: Nausea, vomiting, bloody diarrhea
CV: Circulatory failure, atrial fibrillation, fatal myocarditis, dysrhythmias
Contraindications: Hypersensitivity, unconscious/semiconscious, depressed gag reflex, poisoning

with petroleum products or caustic substances, convulsions
Precautions: Lactation, pregnancy (C)
Pharmacokinetics:
PO: Onset 15-30 min
Interactions/incompatibilities:
• Do not administer with activated charcoal; effect will be decreased
NURSING CONSIDERATIONS
Assess:
• VS, B/P; check patients with cardiac disease more often
• Type of poisoning; do not administer if petroleum products or caustic substances have been ingested: kerosene, gasoline, lye, Drano
• Respiratory status before, during, after administration of emetic; check rate, rhythm, character; respiratory depression can occur rapidly with elderly or debilitated patients
Administer:
• **Ipecac *syrup*, not ipecac,** which is 14 times stronger; death may occur
• Then bounce child to increase emetic effect
• Activated charcoal if this drug doesn't work; may begin lavage after 10-15 min
Evaluate:
• Therapeutic response: vomiting

---

ipratropium bromide
(eye-pra-troep′ee-um)
Atrovent

Func. class.: Anticholinergic
Chem. class.: Synthetic quaternary ammonium compound

Action: Inhibits interaction of acetylcholine at receptor sites on the bronchial smooth muscle, resulting in bronchodilation

---

italics = common side effects   ***bold italic*** = life threatening reactions

Uses: Bronchodilation during bronchospasm in those with COPD

Dosage and routes:
• *Adult:* 2 INH 4 × day, not to exceed 12 INH/24 hr

Available forms: Aerosol 18 μg/actuation

Side effects/adverse reactions:
GI: Nausea, vomiting, cramps
EENT: Dry mouth, blurred vision
CNS: Anxiety, dizziness, headache, nervousness
RESP: Cough, worsening of symptoms, **bronchospasms**
INTEG: Rash
CV: Palpitation

Contraindications: Hypersensitivity to this drug, atropine, soya lecithin

Precautions: Pregnancy (B), lactation, children <12 yr, narrowangle glaucoma, prostatic hypertrophy, bladder neck obstruction

Pharmacokinetics:
Half-life 2 hr; does not cross bloodbrain barrier

NURSING CONSIDERATIONS
Assess:
• For palpitations; if severe, drug may have to be changed
• For tolerance over long-term therapy; dose may have to be increased or changed

Perform/provide:
• Storage at room temperature
• Hard candy, frequent drinks, sugarless gum to relieve dry mouth

Evaluate:
• Therapeutic response: ability to breathe adequately

Teach patient/family:
• That compliance is necessary with number of inhalations/24 hr, or overdose may occur
• To shake before using
• Correct method of inhalation and cleaning of equipment daily

---

iron dextran
Hydextran, Imferon, K-Feron
Func. class.: Hematinic
Chem. class.: Ferric hydroxide complex with dextran

Action: Iron is carried by transferrin to the bone marrow, where it is incorporated into hemoglobin

Uses: Iron deficiency anemia

Dosage and routes:
• *Adult and child:* IM 0.5 ml as a test dose by Z-track, then no more than the following per day
• *Adult <50 kg:* IM 100 mg
• *Adult >50 kg:* IM 250 mg
• *Infant <5 kg:* IM 25 mg
• *Child <9 kg:* IM 50 mg
• *Adult:* IV 0.5 ml test dose, then 100 mg qd after 2-3 days; IV 250/1000 ml of NaCl; give 25 mg test dose, wait 5 min, then infuse over 6-12 hr or follow equation

$$\frac{0.3 \times \text{wt (lb)} \times \frac{100\text{-Hgb (g/dl)} \times 100}{14.8}} = \text{mg iron}$$

<30 lb (66 kg) should be given 80% of above formula dose

Available forms: Inj IM/IV 50 mg/ml, inj IM only 50 mg/ml

Side effects/adverse reactions:
CNS: Headache, paresthesia, dizziness, shivering, weakness, *seizures*
GI: Nausea, vomiting, metallic taste, abdominal pain
INTEG: Rash, pruritus, urticaria, fever, sweating, chills, brown skin discoloration, pain at injection site, necrosis, sterile abscesses, phlebitis
CV: Chest pain, *shock,* hypotension, tachycardia
RESP: Dyspnea
HEMA: Leukocytosis
Other: Anaphylaxis

Contraindications: Hypersensitivity, all anemias excluding iron deficiency anemia, hepatic disease

Precautions: Acute renal disease, children, asthma, lactation, rheumatoid arthritis (IV), infants <4 mo, pregnancy (C)

Pharmacokinetics:

IM: Excreted in feces, urine, bile, breast milk; crosses placenta; most absorbed through lymphatics; can be gradually absorbed over weeks/months from fixed locations

Interactions/incompatibilities:

• Not to mix with other drugs in syringe or sol

• Decreased reticulocyte response: chloramphenicol

• Increased toxicity: oral iron—do not use

Lab test interferences:

False increase: Serum bilirubin

False decrease: Serum Ca

False positive: ^{99m}Tc diphosphate bone scan, iron test (large doses >2 ml)

NURSING CONSIDERATIONS

Assess:

• Blood studies: Hct, Hgb, reticulocytes, bilirubin before treatment, at least monthly

• Allergy: *anaphylaxis*, rash, pruritus, fever, chills

• Cardiac status: anginal pain, hypotension, tachycardia

• Nutrition: amount of iron in diet (meat, dark green leafy vegetables, dried beans, dried fruits, eggs)

• Cause of iron loss or anemia, including salicylates, sulfonamides

Administer:

• D/C oral iron before parenteral; only after test dose of 25 mg by preferred route; wait at least 1 hr before giving remaining portion

• IM deeply in large muscle mass; use Z-track method and a 19-20 G 2-3 inch needle; ensure needle is long enough to place drug deep in muscle

• IV after flushing with 10 ml of NS; give undiluted; may be diluted in 50-250 normal saline for infusion; give 1 ml (50 mg) or less over 1 min or more; flush line after use with 10 ml of 0.9% NaCl

• IV injection requires single-dose vial without preservative; verify on label IV use is approved

• Only with epinephrine available in case of anaphylactic reaction during dose

Perform/provide:

• Storage at room temperature in cool environment

• Recumbent position 30 min after IV injection to prevent orthostatic hypotension

Evaluate:

• Therapeutic response: increased serum iron levels

Teach patient/family:

• That iron poisoning may occur if increased beyond recommended level

• That delayed reaction may occur 1-2 days after administration and last 3-4 days (IV) 3-7 days (IM); report fever, chills, malaise, muscle, joint aches, nausea, vomiting, backache

Treatment of overdose:

Discontinue drug, treat allergic reaction, give diphenhydramine or epinephrine as needed, give iron-chelating drug in acute poisoning

---

isocarboxazid

(eye-soe-kar-box′a-zid)

Marplan

Func. class.: Antidepressant—MAOI

Chem. class.: Hydrazine

Action: Increases concentrations of

endogenous epinephrine, norepinephrine, serotonin, dopamine in storage sites in CNS by inhibition of MAO; increased concentration reduces depression

Uses: Depression when uncontrolled by other means

Dosage and routes:
• *Adult:* PO 30 mg/day in divided doses; reduce dose to lowest effective dose when condition improves

Available forms: Tabs 10 mg

Side effects/adverse reactions:
HEMA: Anemia
CNS: Dizziness, drowsiness, confusion, headache, anxiety, tremors, stimulation, weakness, hyperreflexia, mania, insomnia, fatigue, weight gain
GI: Constipation, dry mouth, nausea, vomiting, *anorexia,* diarrhea, weight gain
GU: Change in libido, frequency
INTEG: Rash, flushing, increased perspiration, jaundice
CV: Orthostatic hypotension, hypertension, dysrhythmias, hypertensive crisis
EENT: Blurred vision
*ENDO: **SIADH-like syndrome***

Contraindications: Hypersensitivity to MAOIs, elderly, hypertension, CHF, severe hepatic disease, pheochromocytoma, severe renal disease, severe cardiac disease

Precautions: Suicidal patients, convulsive disorders, severe depression, schizophrenia, hyperactivity, diabetes mellitus, pregnancy (C)

Pharmacokinetics:
PO: Duration up to 2 wk; metabolized by liver; excreted by kidneys

Interactions/incompatibilities:
• Increased pressor effects: guanethidine, clonidine, indirect-acting sympathomimetics (ephedrine)
• Increased effects of: direct-acting sympathomimetics (epinephrine), alcohol, barbiturates, benzodiazepines, CNS depressants, levodopa
• Hyperpyretic crisis, convulsions, hypertensive episode: tricyclic antidepressants, meperidine
• Hypoglycemic effect: increased insulin

NURSING CONSIDERATIONS
Assess:
• B/P (lying, standing), pulse; if systolic B/P drops 20 mm Hg, hold drug, notify physician
• Blood studies: CBC, leukocytes, cardiac enzymes if patient is receiving long-term therapy
• Hepatic studies: ALT, AST, bilirubin, creatinine; hepatotoxicity may occur
• Toxicity: increased headache, palpitation; discontinue drug immediately; prodromal signs of hypertensive crisis
• Mental status: mood, sensorium, affect, memory (long, short), increase in psychiatric symptoms
• Urinary retention, constipation, edema; take weight weekly
• Withdrawal symptoms: headache, nausea, vomiting, muscle pain, weakness

Administer:
• Increased fluids, bulk in diet if constipation, urinary retention occur
• With food or milk for GI symptoms
• Crushed if patient is unable to swallow medication whole
• Dosage hs if oversedation occurs during day
• Gum, hard candy, or frequent sips of water for dry mouth
• Phentolamine for severe hypertension

Perform/provide:
• Storage in tight container in cool environment, away from children

• Assistance with ambulation during beginning therapy, since drowsiness/dizziness occurs
• Safety measures, including side rails
• Checking to see PO medication swallowed

Evaluate:
• Therapeutic response: decreased depression

Teach patient/family:
• That therapeutic effects may take 1-4 wk
• To avoid driving or other activities requiring alertness; hypotension may be increased in the elderly
• To avoid alcohol ingestion, CNS depressants or OTC medications (cold, weight-control, hay fever, cough syrup)
• Not to discontinue medication quickly after long-term use
• To avoid high-tyramine foods: cheese (aged), sour cream, beer, wine, pickled products, liver, raisins, bananas, figs, avocados, meat tenderizers, chocolate, yogurt; increase caffeine
• Report headache, palpitation, neck stiffness

Treatment of overdose: Lavage, activated charcoal; monitor electrolytes, vital signs; diazepam IV, NaHCO$_3$

Isoetharine HCl/ isoetharine mesylate
(eye-soe-eth'a-reen)
Arm-a-Med Isoetharine HCl, Beta-2, Bronkometer, Bronkosol, Isoetharine HCl
Func. class.: Adrenergic β$_2$-agonist

Action: Causes bronchodilation by β$_2$ stimulation, resulting in increased levels of cAMP, causing relaxation of bronchial smooth muscle with very little effect on heart rate

Uses: Bronchospasm, asthma

Dosage and routes:
• *Adult:* INH 3-7 puffs undiluted, IPPB 0.5 ml diluted 1:3 with NS
Available forms: Sol for nebulization 0.06%, 0.08%, 0.1%, 0.125%, 0.17%, 0.2%, 0.25%, 0.5%, 10%

Side effects/adverse reactions:
CNS: Tremors, anxiety, insomnia, headache, dizziness, stimulation
CV: Palpitations, tachycardia, hypertension, ***cardiac arrest,*** dysrhythmias
GI: Nausea
• *META:* Hyperglycemia

Contraindications: Hypersensitivity to sympathomimetics, narrow-angle glaucoma

Precautions: Pregnancy (C), cardiac disorders, hyperthyroidism, diabetes mellitus, prostatic hypertrophy

Pharmacokinetics:
INH: Onset immediate, peak 5-15 min, duration 1-4 hr, metabolized in liver, GI tract, lungs, excreted in urine

Interactions/incompatibilities:
• Increased effects of both drugs: other sympathomimetics
• Decreased action when used with other β-blockers
• Hypertensive crisis: MAOIs

NURSING CONSIDERATIONS
Assess:
• Respiratory function: vital capacity, forced expiratory volume, ABGs, pulse, B/P
• Paresthesias and coldness of extremities; peripheral blood flow may decrease

Administer:
• 2 hr before hs to avoid sleeplessness

---

italics = common side effects   ***bold italic*** = life threatening reactions

Perform/provide:
• Storage at room temperature; do not use solution if brown or contains a precipitate

Evaluate:
• Therapeutic response: ease of breathing

Teach patient/family:
• Not to use OTC medications; extra stimulation may occur
• Use of inhaler; review package insert with patient
• To avoid getting aerosol in eyes
• To wash inhaler in warm water and dry qd
• About all aspects of drug; avoid smoking, smoke-filled rooms, persons with respiratory infections

Isoflurophate
(eye-soe-flure'oh-fate)
Floropryl
Func. class.: Miotic
Chem. class.: Cholinesterase inhibitor, irreversible

Action: Prevents breakdown of neurotransmitter acetylcholine, which then accumulates, causing enhancement, prolongation of its physiologic effects

Uses: Open-angle glaucoma, accommodative esotropia, conditions obstructing aqueous outflow

Dosage and routes:
• *Adult and child:* INSTILL ¼ in strip of 0.025% oint in conjunctival sac q8-72 hr for glaucoma or qhs × 2 wk for esotropia
Available forms: Only as ophthalmic ointment 0.025%

Side effects/adverse reactions:
CNS: Headache
CV: Hypotension, bradycardia, paradoxic tachycardia
*RESP: **Bronchospasm,** dyspnea, bronchoconstriction, wheezing

EENT: Blurred vision, lacrimation, conjunctival congestion, lid muscle twitching, stinging, burning
GU: Urinary incontinence
GI: Abdominal cramps, diarrhea, increased salivation, nausea, vomiting

Contraindications: Hypersensitivity, uveal inflammation

Precautions: History of retinal detachment, asthma, bradycardia, parkinsonism, peptic ulcer, recent MI, epilepsy, myasthenia gravis

Pharmacokinetics:
Miosis: Onset 5-10 min, duration 1-4 wk
Intraocular pressure: Peak 24 hr, duration 1 wk

Interactions/incompatibilities:
• Increased effects of both drugs: succinylcholine, systemic anticholinesterase

NURSING CONSIDERATIONS
Administer:
• Ointment to conjunctival sac with patient supine

Evaluate:
• Therapeutic response: decreased aqueous outflow

Teach patient/family:
• That top of tube must not come in contact with moisture; keep tube closed, dry, away from tears or cornea; to wash hands after application of ointment
• To report change in vision, blurring or loss of sight, trouble breathing, sweating, flushing
• That long-term therapy may be required
• That blurred vision will decrease with repeated use of drug
• To minimize effects of blurred vision, application should take place at bedtime
• To observe for signs/symptoms of systemic absorption (i.e., diarrhea, weakness)

- To observe eyes for irritation
- To monitor for cardiac, respiratory, or GI problems

Isoniazid (INH)
(eye-soe-nye'a-zid)
Isoniazid, Isotamine,* Laniazid, Laniazid C.T., Nydrazid, PMS-Isoniazid*

Func. class.: Antitubercular
Chem. class.: Isonicotinic acid hydrazide

Action: Bactericidal interference with lipid, nucleic acid biosynthesis

Uses: Treatment, prevention of tuberculosis

Dosage and routes:
Treatment
- *Adult:* PO/IM 5 mg/kg qd as single dose for 9 mo to 2 yr, not to exceed 300 mg/day
- *Child and infants:* PO/IM 10-20 mg/kg qd as single dose for 18-24 mo, not to exceed 300 mg/day

Prevention
- *Adult:* PO 300 mg qd as single dose $\times$ 12 mo
- *Child and infants:* PO/IM 10 mg/kg qd as single dose for 12 mo, not to exceed 300 mg/day

Available forms: Tabs 50, 100, 300 mg; inj 100 mg/ml; powder, syrup 50 mg/5 ml

Side effects/adverse reactions:
Hypersensitivity: fever, skin eruptions, lymphadenopathy, vasculitis
CNS: Peripheral neuropathy, memory impairment, ***toxic encephalopathy, convulsions,*** psychosis
EENT: Blurred vision, optic neuritis
HEMA: ***Agranulocytosis, hemolytic, aplastic anemia, thrombocytopenia,*** eosinophilia, methemoglobinemia
MISC: Dyspnea, B_6-deficiency, pellegra, hyperglycemia, metabolic acidosis, gynecomastia, rheumatic syndrome, SLE-like syndrome
GI: Nausea, vomiting, epigastric distress, ***jaundice, fatal hepatitis***

Contraindications: Hypersensitivity, optic neuritis

Precautions: Pregnancy (C), renal disease, diabetic retinopathy, cataracts, ocular defects, hepatic disease, child <13 yr

Pharmacokinetics:
PO: Peak 1-2 hr, duration 6-8 hr
IM: Peak 45-60 min
Metabolized in liver; excreted in urine (metabolites); crosses placenta; excreted in breast milk

Interactions/incompatibilities:
- Increased toxicity: alcohol, cycloserine, ethionamide, rifampin, carbamazepine
- Decreased absorption: aluminum antacids

NURSING CONSIDERATIONS
Assess:
- Liver studies qwk: ALT, AST, bilirubin
- Renal status: before, qmo: BUN, creatinine, output, sp gr, urinalysis
- Mental status often: affect, mood, behavioral changes; psychosis may occur
- Hepatic status: decreased appetite, jaundice, dark urine, fatigue

Administer:
- With meals to decrease GI symptoms; better to take on empty stomach 1 hr ac or 2 hr pc
- Antiemetic if vomiting occurs
- After C&S is completed; qmo to detect resistance

Evaluate:
- Therapeutic response: decreased symptoms of TB

Teach patient/family:
- That compliance with dosage schedule, duration is necessary
- That scheduled appointments

italics = common side effects   ***bold italic*** = life threatening reactions

must be kept or relapse may occur
• To avoid alcohol while taking drug
• That, if diabetic, use blood glucose monitor to obtain correct result
• To report weakness, fatigue, loss of appetite, nausea, vomiting, yellowing of skin or eyes, tingling/numbness of hands/feet

---

Isoproterenol HCl/isoproterenol sulfate

(eye-soe-proe-ter′e-nole)
Dispos-a-Med Isoproterenol HCl, Isuprel, Isoproterenol HCl, Isuprel Glossets, Isuprel Mistometer, Medihaler-Iso, Norisoprine Aerotrol

Func. class.: Adrenergic
Chem. class.: Catecholamine

Action: Has β_1 and β_2 action; relaxes bronchial smooth muscle and dilates the trachea and main bronchi by increasing levels of cAMP, which relaxes smooth muscles; causes increased contractility and heart rate by acting on β-receptors in heart

Uses: Bronchospasm, asthma, heart block, ventricular dysrhythmias, shock

Dosage and routes:
Asthma, bronchospasm
• *Adult:* SL 10-20 mg q6-8h; INH 1 puff, may repeat in 2-5 min, maintenance 1-2 puffs 4-6 × /day
• *Child:* SL 5-10 mg q6-8h; INH 1 puff, may repeat in 2-5 min, maintenance 1-2 puffs 4-6×/d
Heart block/ventricular dysrhythmias
• *Adult:* IV 0.02-0.06, then 0.01-0.2 mg or 5 µg/min HCl; IM 0.2 mg, then 0.02-1 mg as needed HCl

• *Child:* IV/IM ½ of beginning adult dose
Shock
• *Adult and child:* IV INF 0.5-5 µg/min 1 mg/500 ml D₅W, titrate to B/P, CVP, hourly urine output
Available forms: Sol for nebulization 1:400 (0.25%), 1:200 (0.5%), 1:100 (1%); aerosol 0.25%, 0.2%; powd for INH 0.1 mg/cart; inj 1:5000 (0.2 mg/ml) IV, IM; glossets (SL) 10 mg
Side effects/adverse reactions:
CNS: Tremors, anxiety, insomnia, headache, dizziness, stimulation
CV: Palpitations, tachycardia, hypertension, *cardiac arrest*
GI: Nausea, vomiting
RESP: Bronchial irritation, edema, dryness of oropharynx, **bronchospasms** (overuse)
META: Hyperglycemia
Contraindications: Hypersensitivity to sympathomimetics, narrow-angle glaucoma
Precautions: Pregnancy (C), cardiac disorders, hyperthyroidism, diabetes mellitus, prostatic hypertrophy
Pharmacokinetics:
IV: Onset rapid, duration 10 min
INH/SL: Onset 1-2 hr
REC: Onset 2-4 hr
Metabolized in liver, lungs, GI tract
Interactions/incompatibilities:
• Increased effects of both drugs: other sympathomimetics
• Decreased action when used with β-blockers
• Incompatible with aminophylline, barbiturates, carbenicillin, diazepam, epinephrine, lidocaine, NaCO₃ in sol or syringe
NURSING CONSIDERATIONS
Assess:
• Resp. function: B/P, pulse, lung sounds

---

*Available in Canada only

• Blood studies (CBC, WBC, differential), since blood dyscrasias may occur (rare)
• I&O ratio; check for urinary retention, frequency, hesitancy
• For paresthesias and coldness of extremities; peripheral blood flow may decrease
• Injection site: tissue sloughing; if this occurs, administer phentolamine mixed with NS

Administer:
• IV Direct dilute 0.2 mg/10 ml NS (1:50,000 sol); give over 1 min; IV INF 2 mg(1:5000 sol)/500 ml of D₅W; run each 1 ml (1:250,000) sol/min; may be increased; use infusion pump, intracardiac, 1:5000 sol undiluted
• With meals for GI symptoms

Perform/provide:
• Storage at room temperature; do not use discolored sol

Evaluate:
• Therapeutic response: increased B/P with stabilization, ease of breathing

Teach patient/family:
• To rinse mouth after use
• Use of inhaler; review package insert with patient
• To avoid getting aerosol in eyes
• To wash inhaler in warm water and dry qd
• About all aspects of drug; avoid smoking, smoke-filled rooms, persons with respiratory infections

Treatment of overdose: Administer a β-blocker

---

isosorbide
(eye-soe-sor′bide)
Ismotic
Func. class.: Miscellaneous ophthalmic agent

Action: Increases osmotic gradient between plasma and ocular fluids, which decreases intraocular pressure

Uses: Reduces intraocular pressure from glaucoma and cataract surgery

Dosage and routes:
• *Adult:* PO 1.5 g/kg, then increase to 1-3 g/kg bid-qid
Available forms: Sol 45%

Side effects/adverse reactions:
CNS: Headache, light-headedness, irritability, lethargy, syncope, confusion, dizziness, vertigo, disorientation
GI: Nausea, vomiting, anorexia, diarrhea, cramps, thirst
INTEG: Rash
META: Hypernatremia, hyperosmolarity

Contraindications: Hypersensitivity, anuria, severe renal disease, pulmonary edema, hemorrhagic glaucoma, dehydration

Precautions: Pregnancy (C), patients on Na-restricted diet

NURSING CONSIDERATIONS
Assess:
• I&O; report decrease in urinary output
• Electrolytes during treatment

Administer:
• After pouring over ice (oral)

Evaluate:
• Therapeutic response: decreased intraocular pressure

---

isosorbide dinitrate
(eye-soe-sor′bide)
Coronex,* Dilatrate-SR, Iso-Bid, Isordil Tembids, Isordil Titradose, Isosorbide Dinitrate, Isotrate Timecelles, Sorbitrate, Sorbitrate SA, Isordil, Isosorbide Dinitrate, Sorbitrate
Func. class.: Antianginal
Chem. class.: Nitrate

Action: Decreases preload, after-

---

italics = common side effects   ***bold italic*** = life threatening reactions

load, which is responsible for decreasing left ventricular end-diastolic pressure, systemic vascular resistance and reducing cardiac O_2 demand

Uses: Chronic stable angina pectoris, prophylaxis of angina pain

Dosage and routes:
• *Adult:* PO 5-40 mg qid; SL 2.5-10 mg, may repeat q2-3h; CHEW TAB 5-10 mg prn or q2-3h as prophylaxis, sus rel 40-80 mg q8-12h

Available forms: Caps ext rel 40 mg; caps 40; tabs 5, 10, 20, 30, 40; chew tabs 5, 10 mg; tabs ext rel 40 mg; SL tabs 2.5, 5, 10 mg

Side effects/adverse reactions:
MISC: Twitching, hemolytic anemia, *methemoglobinemia*
CV: Postural hypotension, tachycardia, *collapse,* syncope
GI: Nausea, vomiting
INTEG: Pallor, sweating, rash
CNS: Vascular headache, flushing, dizziness, weakness, faintness

Contraindications: Hypersensitivity to this drug or nitrates, severe anemia, increased intracranial pressure, cerebral hemorrhage, acute MI

Precautions: Postural hypotension, pregnancy (C), lactation, children

Pharmacokinetics:
SUS ACTION: Duration 6-8 hr
PO: Onset 15-30 min, duration 4-6 hr
SL: Onset 2-5 min, duration 1-4 hr
CHEW TAB: Onset 3 min, duration ½-3 hr; metabolized by liver, excreted in urine as metabolites (80%-100%)

Interactions/incompatibilities:
• Increased effects: β-blockers, diuretics, antihypertensives, alcohol products

NURSING CONSIDERATIONS
Assess:
• B/P, pulse, respirations during beginning therapy
• Pain: duration, time started, activity being performed, character
• Tolerance if taken over long period
• Headache, light-headedness, decreased B/P; may indicate a need for decreased dosage

Administer:
• After checking expiration date
• With 8 oz H_2O on empty stomach (oral tablet); do not crush SR or SL drug

Evaluate:
• Therapeutic response: decrease or prevention of anginal pain

Teach patient/family:
• To leave tabs in original container
• If 3 SL tabs in 15 min does not relieve pain, activate EMS
• To avoid alcohol products
• That drug may cause headache, but tolerance usually develops; taking with meals may reduce or eliminate headache
• That drug may be taken before stressful activity (exercise, sexual activity)
• That SL may sting when drug comes in contact with mucous membranes
• To avoid hazardous activities if dizziness occurs
• Importance of complying with complete medical regimen
• To make position changes slowly to prevent fainting
• Not to crush, chew SL or sus rel tabs

---

*Available in Canada only

isosorbide mononitrate

(eye-soe-sor′bide)
ISMO
Func. class.: Antianginal
Chem. class.: Nitrate

Action: Decreases preload, afterload, resulting in decreased left ventricular end-diastolic pressure, systemic vascular resistance

Uses: Prevention of angina pectoris due to coronary artery disease

Dosage and routes:
• *Adult:* PO 20 mg bid, 7 hr apart
Available forms: Tabs 20 mg

Side effects/adverse reactions:
MISC: Twitching, hemolytic anemia, methemoglobinemia
CV: Postural hypotension, tachycardia, *collapse,* syncope
GI: Nausea, vomiting
INTEG: Pallor, sweating, rash
CNS: Vascular headache, flushing, dizziness, weakness, faintness

Contraindications: Hypersensitivity to nitrates, severe anemia, increased intracranial pressure, cerebral hemorrhage, acute MI, closed-angle glaucoma

Precautions: Postural hypotension, pregnancy (C), lactation, children, glaucoma

Pharmacokinetics: Metabolized by the liver; excreted in urine as metabolites (80%-100%); half-life 4 hrs

Interactions/incompatibilities:
• Increased effects: β-blockers, diuretics, antihypertensives, alcohol, calcium channel blockers

NURSING CONSIDERATIONS
Assess:
• B/P, pulse, respirations during beginning therapy
• Headache, light-headedness, decreased B/P; may indicate a need for decreased dosage

Administer:
• With 8 oz H$_2$O on empty stomach (oral tablet)

Evaluate:
• Therapeutic response: absence of anginal pain

Teach patient/family:
• That drug may cause headache, but tolerance usually develops; taking with meals may reduce or eliminate headache
• To avoid hazardous activities if dizziness occurs
• To make position changes slowly to prevent fainting
• Not to use alcohol products

isotretinoin

(eye-soe-tret′i-noyn)
Accutane
Func. class.: Dermatologic
Chem. class.: Retinoic acid isomer, vitamin A derivative

Action: Decreases sebum secretion; improves cystic acne

Uses: Severe recalcitrant cystic acne

Dosage and routes:
• *Adult:* PO 0.5-2 mg/kg/day in 2 divided doses × 15-20 wk
Available forms: Caps 10, 20, 40 mg

Side effects/adverse reactions:
INTEG: Dry skin, pruritus, cheilosis, joint pain, hair loss, photosensitivity, urticaria, bruising, hirsutism, petechiae, hypo/hyperpigmentation, nail brittleness
MS: Hyperostosis, arthralgia, bone, joint, muscle pain
CV: Chest pain, palpitation, tachycardia
GI: Nausea, vomiting, anorexia, increased liver enzymes, regional

ileus, abdominal pain, weight loss
EENT: Eye irritation, conjunctivitis, epistaxis, dry nose, mouth, contact lens intolerance, optic neuritis, photophobia
GU: Hematuria, proteinuria, hypouricemia, white cells in urine
HEMA: Thrombocytopenia, decreased H&H, WBC, reticulocyte count
CNS: Lethargy, fatigue, headache, depression, *pseudotumor cerebri*
Contraindications: Hypersensitivity, inflamed skin, pregnancy (X)
Precautions: Lactation, diabetes, photosensitivity, hepatic disease, inflammatory bowel disease, obesity
Pharmacokinetics:
PO: Peak 2.9-3.2 hr, half-life 10-20 hr; metabolized in liver, excreted in urine, feces
Interactions/incompatibilities:
• Additive toxic effects: Vit A; do not use together
• Pseudotumor cerebri: minocycline or tetracycline
• Increased triglyceride levels: alcohol
Lab test interferences:
Increase: Sedimentation rate, triglyceride, liver function studies
Decrease: RBC/WBC count
NURSING CONSIDERATIONS
Assess:
• Triglyceride levels, AST, ALT, alk phosphatase before, during treatment
• Urinalysis qwk for protein, blood
• Blood glucose in diabetics periodically
• Area of body involved, including time involved, what helps or aggravates condition
• Pseudotumor cerebri: headache, vomiting, nausea, visual disturbance; discontinue drug

Administer:
• Whole; do not crush; give with meals
• Second course of treatment if needed after waiting 2 mo
Perform/provide:
• Storage in tight, light-resistant container
Evaluate:
• Therapeutic response: decrease in size and number of lesions
Teach patient/family:
• To avoid sunlight or wear sunscreen, since photosensitivity may occur
• That an increase in acne may occur during initial treatment, decrease in 4-6 wk
• Not to become pregnant while taking drug
• Not to take Vit A supplements; to take drug with meals
• Not to crush
• To minimize or eliminate alcohol consumption

Isoxsuprine HCl
(eye-sox'syoo-preen)
Isoxsuprine HCl, Vasodilan, Voxsuprine
Func. class.: Peripheral vasodilator
Chem. class.: Nylidrin-related agent

Action: α-Adrenoreceptor antagonist with β-adrenoreceptor stimulate properties; may also act directly on vascular smooth muscle; causes cardiac stimulation, uterine relaxation
Uses: Symptoms of cerebrovascular insufficiency, peripheral vascular disease including arteriosclerosis obliterans, thromboangiitis obliterans, Raynaud's disease

Dosage and routes:
• *Adult:* PO 10-20 mg tid or qid
Available forms: Tabs 10, 20 mg
Side effects/adverse reactions:
*CV: Hypotension, **tachycardia,*** palpitations, chest pain
CNS: Dizziness, weakness, tremors, anxiety
GI: Nausea, vomiting, abdominal pain, distention
INTEG: Severe rash, flushing
Contraindications: Hypersensitivity, postpartum, arterial bleeding
Precautions: Pregnancy (C), tachycardia
Pharmacokinetics:
PO: Peak 1 hr, duration 3 hr, half-life 1¼ hr; excreted in urine; crosses placenta

NURSING CONSIDERATIONS
Assess:
• B/P, pulse during treatment until stable; take B/P lying, standing; orthostatic hypotension is common
Administer:
• With meals to reduce GI upset
Perform/provide:
• Storage at room temperature
Evaluate:
• Therapeutic response: ability to walk without pain, increased pulse volume, increased temperature in extremities, improved orientation, long- and short-term memory
Teach patient/family:
• That medication is not cure; may have to be taken continuously depending on condition; therapeutic response may not be evident for 2-3 mo
• That it is necessary to quit smoking to prevent excessive vasoconstriction
• To avoid hazardous activities until stabilized on medication; dizziness may occur
• To make position changes slowly, or fainting will occur

• To discontinue drug, notify physician if rash develops
• To report palpitations, flushing if severe
• To avoid changes in temperature; extremities should be kept warm to promote better circulation

---

isradipine
(is-rad′-i-peen)
DynaCirc
Func. class.: Calcium channel blocker
Chem. class.: Dihydropyridine

Action: Inhibits calcium ion influx across cell membrane during cardiac depolarization; produces relaxation of coronary vascular smooth muscle, peripheral vascular smooth muscle; dilates coronary vascular arteries; increases myocardial oxygen delivery in patients with vasospastic angina

Uses: Essential hypertension, angina

Dosage and routes:
Hypertension:
Adult: PO 1.25 mg bid; increase at 3-4 wk intervals up to 10 mg bid
Angina
Adult: PO 2.5-7.5 mg tid
Available forms: Tabs 1.25 mg
Side effects/adverse reactions:
*HEMA: **Thrombocytopenia, leukopenia, anemia***
CV: Peripheral edema, tachycardia, hypotension, chest pain
GI: Nausea, vomiting, diarrhea, gastric upset, constipation, hepatitis
GU: Nocturia, polyuria, ***acute renal failure***
INTEG: Rash, pruritus, urticaria, photosensitivity, hair loss
CNS: Headache, fatigue, dizziness, fainting, sleep disturbances

---

italics = common side effects   ***bold italic*** = life threatening reactions

MISC: Flushing

Contraindications: Sick sinus syndrome, 2nd or 3rd degree heart block, hypotension less than 90 mm Hg systolic, hypersensitivity

Precautions: CHF, hypotension, hepatic disease, pregnancy (C), lactation, children, renal disease, elderly

Pharmacokinetics: Metabolized in liver; metabolites are excreted in urine and feces; secreted in breast milk, peak plasma levels at 2-3 hr

Interactions/incompatibilities:
• Increased effects of: digitalis, neuromuscular blocking agents, cyclosporine
• Increased effects of isradipine: cimetidine, carbamazepine

NURSING CONSIDERATIONS

Assess:
• B/P, pulse rate, chest pain; monitor ECG periodically during therapy
• Cardiac status: B/P, pulse, respiration, ECG

Evaluate:
• Therapeutic response: decreased anginal pain, decreased B/P

Teach patient/family:
• To avoid hazardous activities until stabilized on drug, dizziness is no longer a problem
• To limit caffeine consumption
• To avoid OTC drugs unless directed by physician
• Importance of compliance in all areas of medical regimen: diet, exercise, stress reduction, drug therapy
• To notify physician of irregular heartbeat, shortness of breath, swelling of feet and hands, pronounced dizziness, constipation, nausea, hypotension

Treatment of overdose: Defibrillation, β-agonists, IV Ca inotropic agents, diuretics, atropine for AV block, vasopressor for hypotension

itraconazole

(it-ra-con′-a-zol)
Sporanox

Func. class.: Antifungal
Chem. class.: Triazole derivative

Action: Alters cell membranes and inhibits several fungal enzymes

Uses: Systemic candidiasis, chronic mucocandidiasis, oral thrush, candiduria, coccidioidomycosis, histoplasmosis, chromomycosis, paracoccidioidomycosis, blastomycosis (pulmonary and extrapulmonary)

Dosage and routes:
• *Adult:* PO 200 mg qd with food; may increase to 400 mg qd if needed; divide doses over 200 mg in two doses

Available forms: Caps 100 mg

Side effects/adverse reactions:
GU: Gynecomastia, impotence, decreased libido
INTEG: Pruritus, fever, rash,
CNS: Headache, dizziness, insomnia, somnolence, depression
GI: Nausea, vomiting, anorexia, diarrhea, cramps, abdominal pain, flatulence, *GI bleeding, hepatotoxicity*
MISC: Edema, fatigue, malaise, hypertension, hypokalemia, tinnitus

Contraindications: Hypersensitivity, lactation, fungal meningitis, coadministration with terfenadine

Precautions: Hepatic disease, achlorhydria or hypochlorhydine (drug-induced), children, pregnancy (C)

Pharmacokinetics:
PO: Peak 3-5 hr, half-life 60 hr; metabolized in liver; excreted in

bile, feces; requires acid pH for absorption; distributed poorly to CSF; highly protein bound

Interactions/incompatibilities:

• Do not use with terfenadine: may result in rare instance of life-threatening dysrhythmias and death

• Hepatotoxicity: other hepatotoxic drugs

• Itraconazole increases levels of cyclosporine

• Decreased action of itraconazole: antacids, H₂-receptor antagonists, isoniazid, rifampin

• Increased anticoagulant effect: coumarin anticoagulants

• Severe hypoglycemia: oral hypoglycemics

• Concomitant administration with phenytoin may result in decreased levels of itraconazole; effects of phenytoin may be increased

NURSING CONSIDERATIONS

Assess:

• I&O ratio

• Liver studies (ALT, AST, bilirubin) if on long-term therapy

• For allergic reaction: rash, photosensitivity, urticaria, dermatitis

• For hepatotoxicity: nausea, vomiting, jaundice, clay-colored stools, fatigue

Administer:

• In the presence of acid products only; do not use alkaline products or antacids within 2 hr of drug; may give coffee, tea, acidic fruit juices

• With food to decrease GI symptoms

• With hydrochloric acid if achlorhydria is present

Perform/provide:

• Storage in tight container at room temperature

Evaluate:

• Therapeutic response: decreased fever, malaise, rash, negative C&S for infecting organism

Teach patient/family:

• That long-term therapy may be needed to clear infection (1 wk-6 mo depending on infection)

• To avoid hazardous activities if dizziness occurs

• To take 2 hr ac administration of other drugs that increase gastric pH (antacids, H₂-blockers, anticholinergics)

• Importance of compliance with drug regimen

• To notify physician if GI symptoms, signs of liver dysfunction (fatigue, nausea, anorexia, vomiting, dark urine, pale stools)

K

---

kanamycin sulfate
(kan-a-mye'sin)
Anamid,* Kanamycin Sulfate, Kantrex

Func. class.: Antibiotic
Chem. class.: Aminoglycoside

Action: Interferes with protein synthesis in bacterial cell by binding to ribosomal subunit, causing inaccurate peptide sequence to form in protein chain, causing bacterial death

Uses: Severe systemic infections of CNS, respiratory, GI, urinary tract, bone, skin, soft tissues caused by *E. coli, Enterobacter, Acinetobacter, Proteus, N. gonorrhoeae, H. influenzae, Shigella, K. pneumoniae, S. marcescens, Staphylococcus;* also used as adjunct in hepatic coma, peritonitis, preoperatively to sterilize bowel; decreases ammonia-producing bacteria in bowel and intraperitoneally after fecal spill during surgery

Dosage and routes:

Severe systemic infections

• *Adult and child:* IV INF 15 mg/kg/d in divided doses q8-12h; di-

---

luted 500 mg/200 ml of NS or D₅W given over 30-60 min, not to exceed 1.5 g/d; IM 15 mg/kg/d in divided doses q8-12h, not to exceed 1.5 g/d, irrigation not to exceed 1.5 g/d

Hepatic coma
• *Adult:* PO 8-12 g/d in divided doses

Preoperative bowel sterilization
• *Adult:* PO 1 g qh × 4 doses, then q6h × 36-72 hr

Available forms: Inj IM, IV 75, 500 mg/2ml, 1 g/3 ml; cap 500 mg

Side effects/adverse reactions:
GU: Oliguria, hematuria, renal damage, azotemia, renal failure, nephrotoxicity

CNS: Confusion, depression, numbness, tremors, *convulsions,* muscle twitching, *neurotoxicity*

RESP: Respiratory depression

EENT: Ototoxicity, deafness, visual disturbances, dizziness, vertigo, tinnitus

HEMA: Agranulocytosis, thrombocytopenia, leukopenia, eosinophilia, anemia

GI: Nausea, vomiting, anorexia, increased ALT, AST, bilirubin, hepatomegaly, *hepatic necrosis,* splenomegaly

CV: Hypotension

INTEG: Rash, burning, urticaria, dermatitis, alopecia

Contraindications: Bowel obstruction, severe renal disease, hypersensitivity

Precautions: Neonates, myasthenia gravis, hearing deficits, mild renal disease, pregnancy (D), lactation, Parkinson's disease

Pharmacokinetics:
IM: Onset rapid, peak 1-2 hr
IV: Onset immediate, peak 1-2 hr
Plasma half-life 2-3 hr; not metab-

olized; excreted unchanged in urine; crosses placenta

Interactions/incompatibilities:
• Increased ototoxicity, neurotoxicity, nephrotoxicity: other aminoglycosides, amphotericin B, polymyxin, vancomycin, ethacrynic acid, furosemide, mannitol, methoxyflurane, cisplatin, cephalosporins, bacitracin
• Do not mix in sol or syringe: carbenicillin, ticarcillin, amphotericin B, cephalothin, erythromycin, heparin
• Increased effects: nondepolarizing muscle relaxants, succinylcholine
• Decreased effects of: oral anticoagulants
• Incompatible with amphotericin B, ampicillin, carbenicillin, cefoxitin, cephalothin cephapirin, chlorpheniramine, colistimethate, heparin, hydrocortisone, methohexital, lincomycin, penicillins

NURSING CONSIDERATIONS
Assess:
• Weight before treatment; calculation of dosage is usually based on ideal body weight, but may be calculated on actual body weight
• I&O ratio, urinalysis daily for proteinuria, cells, casts; report sudden change in urine output
• VS during infusion, watch for hypotension, change in pulse
• IV site for thrombophlebitis, including pain, redness, swelling q30min; change site if needed; apply warm compresses to discontinued site
• Serum peak, drawn at 30-60 min after IV infusion or 60 min after IM injection; trough level drawn just before next dose; blood level should be 2-4 times bacteriostatic level; trough = 5-10 mEq/ml peak = <30 mEq/ml

• Urine pH if drug is used for UTI; urine should be kept alkaline

• Renal impairment by securing urine for CrCl testing, BUN, serum creatinine; lower dosage should be given in renal impairment (CrCl <80 ml/min)

• Deafness by audiometric testing, ringing, roaring in ears, vertigo; assess hearing before, during, after treatment

• Dehydration: high sp gr, decrease in skin turgor, dry mucous membranes, dark urine

• Overgrowth of infection: elevated temperature, malaise, redness, pain, swelling, perineal itching, diarrhea, stomatitis, change in cough, sputum

• C&S before starting treatment to identify infecting organism

• Vestibular dysfunction: nausea, vomiting, dizziness, headache; drug should be discontinued if severe

• Injection sites for redness, swelling, abscesses; use warm compresses at site

Administer:

• IV after diluting 500 mg or less/100 ml of D_5W, D_5/NaCl, NS or more; give 3-4 ml/min or less; flush line after use

• IM injection in large muscle mass; rotate injection sites

• Penicillins at least 1 hr before or after this drug

• Drug in evenly spaced doses to maintain blood level

• Bicarbonate to alkalinize urine if ordered in treating UTI, as drug is most active in alkaline environment

Perform/provide:

• Adequate fluids of 2-3 L/day unless contraindicated to prevent irritation of tubules

• Flush of IV line with NS or D_5W after infusion

• Supervised ambulation, other safety measures with vestibular dysfunction

Evaluate:

• Therapeutic effect: absence of fever, draining wounds, negative C&S after treatment

Teach patient/family:

• To report headache, dizziness, symptoms of overgrowth of infection, renal impairment

• To report loss of hearing, ringing, roaring in ears or feeling of fullness in head

Treatment of overdose: Hemodialysis; monitor serum levels of drug

K

kaolin, pectin
(kay'o-lynn)
Baropectin, Kaoparin, Kaopectate, Kapectin, Keotin, Pectokay
Func. class.: Antidiarrheal
Chem. class.: Hydrous magnesium aluminum silicate

Action: Decreases gastric motility, H_2O content of stool; adsorbent, demulcent

Uses: Diarrhea (cause undetermined)

Dosage and routes:

• *Adult:* PO 60-120 ml (45-90 ml conc) after each loose bowel movement

• *Child >12 yr:* PO 60 ml after each loose bowel movement

• *Child 6-12 yr:* PO 30-60 ml 30 ml conc after each loose bowel movement

• *Child 3-6 yr:* PO 15-30 ml 15 ml conc after each loose bowel movement

Available forms: Susp Kaolin 0.87 g/5ml, pectin 43 mg/5 ml; Kaolin 0.98 g/5 ml, pectin 21.7 mg/5 ml

---

italics = common side effects   **bold italic** = life threatening reactions

Side effects/adverse reactions:
GI: Constipation (chronic use)
Precautions: Pregnancy (C)
Interactions/incompatibilities:
• Decreased action of: all other drugs
NURSING CONSIDERATIONS
Assess:
• Bowel pattern before; for rebound constipation
• Dehydration in children
Administer:
• For 48 hr only
Evaluate:
• Therapeutic response: decreased diarrhea
Teach patient/family:
• Not to exceed recommended dose
• To shake well before administration

---

ketamine HCl
(keet'a-meen)
Ketalar

Func. class.: General anesthetic
Chem. class.: Phencyclidine derivative

Action: Acts on limbic system, cortex to provide anesthesia
Uses: Short anesthesia for diagnostic/surgical procedures
Dosage and routes:
• *Adult and child:* IV 1-4.5 mg/kg over 1 min
• *Adult and child:* IM 6.5-13 mg/kg
Available forms: Inj IM, IV 10, 50, 100 mg/ml vial
Side effects/adverse reactions:
CNS: Hallucinations, confusion, delirium, tremors, polyneuropathy, fasciculations, pseudoconvulsions
CV: Increased BP, hypotension, bradycardia
EENT: Diplopia, salivation, small increase in intraocular pressure

INTEG: Rash, pain at injection site
Contraindications: Hypersensitivity, CVA, increased intracranial pressure, severe hypertension, cardiac decompensation, child <2 yr
Precautions: Pregnancy (C), seizure disorders, elderly, psychiatric disorders
Pharmacokinetics:
IV: Peak 40 sec, duration 10 min
IM: Peak 3-8 min, duration 25 min
Interactions/incompatibilities:
• Increased action of ketamine: narcotics or atropine
• Respiratory depression: antihypertensives with CNS depressant effects
• Hypertension, tachycardia: thyroid hormones
• Increased action of: tubocurarine
• Incompatible with barbiturates, diazepam in sol or syringe
NURSING CONSIDERATIONS
Assess:
• VS q10min during IV administration, q30min after IM dose
• Hallucinations, delusions, separation from environment
• Extrapyramidal reactions: dystonia, akathisia
• Increasing heart rate or decreasing B/P; notify physician at once
Administer:
• IV after diluting 100 mg/ml with equal parts of D$_5$W, 0.9% NaCl, sterile H$_2$O for inj. give over 1 min; may be diluted 10 ml (50 mg/ml)/500 ml of normal saline or D$_5$W = 1 mg/ml; run at 1-2 mg/min titrate to patient response
• Anticholinergic preoperatively to decrease secretions
• Only with crash cart, resuscitative equipment nearby
• Narcotic or diazepam to control recovery symptoms
Perform/provide:
• Quiet environment for recovery to decrease psychotic symptoms

---

Evaluate:
• Therapeutic response: maintenance of anesthesia

---

ketoconazole
Nizoral
Func. class.: Antifungal
Chem. class.: Imidazole derivative

Action: Alters cell membranes and inhibits several fungal enzymes

Uses: Systemic candidiasis, chronic mucocandidiasis, oral thrush, candiduria, coccidioidomycosis, histoplasmosis, chromomycosis, paracoccidioidomycosis, blastomycosis

Dosage and routes:
• *Adult:* PO 200-400 mg once daily
• *Children:* >2 years: 3.3-6.6 mg/kg/day as single daily dose; <2 years, daily dose not established
Available forms: Caps 200 mg

Side effects/adverse reactions:
GU: Gynecomastia, impotence
INTEG: Pruritus, fever, chills, photophobia, rash, dermatitis, purpura, urticaria
CNS: Headache, dizziness, somnolence
SYST: Anaphylaxis
GI: Nausea, vomiting, anorexia, diarrhea, abdominal pain, hepatotoxicity
HEMA: Thrombocytopenia, leukopenia, hemolytic anemia

Contraindications: Hypersensitivity, lactation, fungal meningitis; coadministration with terfenadine

Precautions: Renal disease, hepatic disease, achlorhydria (drug-induced), pregnancy, children <2 years, other hepatotoxic agents including terfenadine

Pharmacokinetics:
PO: Peak 1-2 hr, half-life 2 hr, terminal 8 hr; metabolized in liver; excreted in bile, feces; requires acid pH for absorption; distributed poorly to CSF; highly protein bound

Interactions/incompatibilities:
• Do not use with terfenadine; may result in rare instances of life-threatening dysrhythmias and death
• Hepatotoxicity: other hepatotoxic drugs (including terfenadine)
• Ketoconazole increases concentration of cyclosporine and corticosteroids
• Decreased action of ketoconazole: antacids, H_2-receptor antagonists, isoniazid, rifampin
• Increased anticoagulant effect, coumarin anticoagulants
• Ketoconazole may decrease theophylline effect

NURSING CONSIDERATIONS
Assess:
• I&O ratio
• Liver studies (ALT, AST, bilirubin) if on long-term therapy
• For allergic reaction: rash, photosensitivity, urticaria, dermatitis
• For hepatotoxicity: nausea, vomiting, jaundice, clay-colored stools, fatigue

Administer:
• In the presence of acid products only; do not use alkaline products or antacids within 2 hr of drug; may give coffee, tea, acidic fruit juices
• With food to decrease GI symptoms
• With hydrochloric acid if achlorhydria is present

Perform/provide:
• Storage in tight containers at room temperature

Evaluate:
• Therapeutic response: decreased fever, malaise, rash, negative C&S for infecting organism

---

italics = common side effects   ***bold italic*** = life threatening reactions

Teach patient/family:
• That long-term therapy may be needed to clear infection (1 wk–6 mo depending on infection)
• To avoid hazardous activities if dizziness occurs
• To take 2 hr ac administration of other drugs that increase gastric pH (antacids, H₂-blockers, anticholinergics)
• Importance of compliance with drug regimen
• To notify physician of GI symptoms, signs of liver dysfunction (fatigue, nausea, anorexia, vomiting, dark urine, pale stools)

---

ketoprofen
(ke-to-proe′fen)
Ketoprofen, Orudis
Func. class.: Nonsteroidal antiinflammatory (NSAID)
Chem. class.: Propionic acid derivative

Action: Inhibits prostaglandin synthesis by decreasing enzyme needed for biosynthesis; analgesic, antiinflammatory, antipyretic
Uses: Mild to moderate pain, osteoarthritis, rheumatoid arthritis, dysmenorrhea
Dosage and routes:
• *Adult:* PO 150-300 mg in divided doses tid-qid, not to exceed 300 mg/day
Available forms: Caps 25, 50, 75 mg
Side effects/adverse reactions:
GI: Nausea, anorexia, vomiting, diarrhea, jaundice, *cholestatic hepatitis,* constipation, flatulence, cramps, dry mouth, peptic ulcer
CNS: Dizziness, drowsiness, fatigue, tremors, confusion, insomnia, anxiety, depression
CV: Tachycardia, peripheral

edema, palpitations, dysrhythmias, hypertension
INTEG: Purpura, rash, pruritus, sweating
GU: Nephrotoxicity: dysuria, hematuria, oliguria, azotemia
HEMA: Blood dyscrasias
EENT: Tinnitus, hearing loss, blurred vision
Contraindications: Hypersensitivity, asthma, severe renal disease, severe hepatic disease, ulcer disease
Precautions: Pregnancy (B), lactation, children, bleeding disorders, GI disorders, cardiac disorders, hypersensitivity to other antiinflammatory agents, elderly
Pharmacokinetics:
PO: Peak 2 hr, half-life 3-3½ hr; metabolized in liver; excreted in urine (metabolites); excreted in breast milk; 99% plasma protein binding
Interactions/incompatibilities:
• Increased action of: coumarin, streptokinase, probenecid
NURSING CONSIDERATIONS
Assess:
• Renal, liver, blood studies: BUN, creatinine, AST, ALT, Hgb, before treatment, periodically thereafter
• Audiometric, ophthalmic examination before, during, after treatment
• For eye, ear problems: blurred vision, tinnitus; may indicate toxicity
Administer:
• With food to decrease GI symptoms; however, best to take on empty stomach to facilitate absorption
Perform/provide:
• Storage at room temperature
Evaluate:
• Therapeutic response: decreased pain, stiffness in joints, decreased

---

swelling in joints, ability to move more easily

Teach patient/family:

• To report blurred vision, ringing, roaring in ears; may indicate toxicity

• To avoid driving, other hazardous activities if dizziness/drowsiness occurs, especially elderly

• To report change in urine pattern, increased weight, edema, increased pain in joints, fever, blood in urine; indicate nephrotoxicity

• That therapeutic effects may take up to 1 mo

• To avoid aspirin, alcohol, steroids

---

ketorolac
(kec'toe-role-ak)
Toradol
Func. class.: Nonsteroidal antiinflammatory
Chem. class.: Pyrrolo-pyrrole

Action: Inhibits prostaglandin synthesis by decreasing an enzyme needed for biosynthesis; analgesic, antiinflammatory, antipyretic

Uses: Mild to moderate pain

Dosage and routes:

• *Adult:* IM 30-60 mg loading dose, then 15-30 mg q6h ophth: 1 gtt (0.25 mg) QID

• *Adult:* PO prn; max 40 mg/day

Available forms: Inj 15, 30, 60 mg (prefilled syringes), ophth 0.5% sol, Tab 10 mg

Side effects/adverse reactions:

CV: Hypertension, flushing, syncope, pallor

CNS: Dizziness, drowsiness, tremors

EENT: Tinnitus, hearing loss, blurred vision

GI: Nausea, anorexia, vomiting, diarrhea, constipation, flatulence, cramps, dry mouth, peptic ulcer

*GU: **Nephrotoxicity: dysuria, hematuria, oliguria, azotemia***

*HEMA: **Blood dyscrasias***

INTEG: Purpura, rash, pruritus, sweating

Contraindications: Hypersensitivity, asthma, severe renal disease, severe hepatic disease, peptic ulcer disease

Precautions: Pregnancy (C), lactation, children, bleeding disorders, GI disorders, cardiac disorders, hypersensitivity to other antiinflammatory agents

Pharmacokinetics:

IM: Peak 50 min, half-life 6 hr

Interactions/incompatibilities:

• Increased action of ketorolac: phenytoin, sulfonamides

NURSING CONSIDERATIONS

Assess:

• Renal, liver, blood studies: BUN, creatinine, AST, ALT, Hgb before treatment, periodically thereafter

• Bleeding times; check for bruising, bleeding; test for occult blood in urine

• For eye, ear problems: blurred vision, tinnitus (may indicate toxicity)

• Hepatic dysfunction: jaundice, yellow sclera and skin, clay-colored stools

• Audiometric, ophthalmic exam before, during, after treatment

• GI condition, hypertension, cardiac conditions

Perform/provide:

• Storage at room temperature

Evaluate:

• Therapeutic response: decreased pain, stiffness, swelling in joints, ability to move more easily; decreased menstrual pain and cramping

Teach patient/family:

• To report blurred vision or ring-

---

italics = common side effects   ***bold italic*** = life threatening reactions

ing, roaring in ears (may indicate toxicity)
• To avoid driving, other hazardous activities if dizziness or drowsiness occurs
• To report change in urine pattern, weight increase, edema, pain increase in joints, fever, blood in urine (indicates nephrotoxicity)
• To avoid alcohol, ASA

labetalol
(la-bet′a-lole)
Normodyne, Trandate
Func. class.: Antihypertensive
Chem. class.: Nonselective β-blocker

Action: Produces falls in B/P without reflex tachycardia or significant reduction in heart rate through mixture of α-blocking, β-blocking effects; elevated plasma renins are reduced

Uses: Mild to moderate hypertension

Dosage and routes:
Hypertension
• *Adult:* PO 100 mg bid; may be given with a diuretic; may increase to 200 mg bid after 2 days; may continue to increase q1-3 days; max 400 mg bid
Hypertensive crisis
• *Adult:* IV INF 200 mg/160 ml D₅W, run at 2 ml/min; stop infusion after desired response obtained, repeat q6-8h as needed; IV BOL 20 mg over 2 min, may repeat 40-80 mg q10min, not to exceed 300 mg
Available forms: Tabs 100, 200, 300 mg, inj 5 mg/ml in 20 ml amps
Side effects/adverse reactions:
*CV: Orthostatic hypotension, bradycardia, **CHF,** chest pain,*

ventricular dysrhythmias, AV block
CNS: Dizziness, mental changes, drowsiness, fatigue, headache, catatonia, depression, anxiety, nightmares, paresthesias, lethargy
GI: Nausea, vomiting, diarrhea
INTEG: Rash, alopecia, urticaria, pruritus, fever
*HEMA: **Agranulocytosis, thrombocytopenia, purpura** (rare)*
EENT: Tinnitus, visual changes, sore throat, double vision, dry burning eyes
GU: Impotence, dysuria, ejaculatory failure
*RESP: **Bronchospasm,** dyspnea, wheezing*
Contraindications: Hypersensitivity to β-blockers, cardiogenic shock, heart block (2nd or 3rd degree), sinus bradycardia, CHF, bronchial asthma
Precautions: Major surgery, pregnancy (C), lactation, diabetes mellitus, renal disease, thyroid disease, COPD, well-compensated heart failure, CAD, nonallergic bronchospasm
Pharmacokinetics:
PO: Onset 1-2 hr, peak 2-4 hr, duration 8-12 hr
IV: Peak 5 min
Half-life 6-8 hr; metabolized by liver (metabolites inactive); excreted in urine, bile; crosses placenta; excreted in breast milk
Interactions/incompatibilities:
• Increased bronchodilation: β-adrenergic agonists
• Increased hypotension: diuretics, other antihypertensives, halothane, cimetidine, nitroglycerin
• Decreased effects: sympathomimetics, lidocaine, indomethacin, theophylline, cimetidine
• Increased hypoglycemia: insulin
• Incompatible with cefoperazone,

---

*Available in Canada only

nafcillin, $NaCO_3$ in sol or syringe; mixing with other drugs is not recommended

Lab test interferences:
False increase: Urinary catecholamines

NURSING CONSIDERATIONS
Assess:
• I&O, weight daily
• B/P during beginning treatment, periodically thereafter, pulse q4h; note rate, rhythm, quality
• Apical/radial pulse before administration; notify physician of any significant changes
• Baselines in renal, liver function tests before therapy begins
• Edema in feet, legs daily
• Skin turgor, dryness of mucous membranes for hydration status

Administer:
• IV undiluted or diluted in LR, D_5W, D_5 in 0.2%, 0.9%, 0.33% NaCl or Ringer's inj; give undiluted 20 mg or less/2 min; infusion is titrated to patient response; 200 mg of drug/160 ml sol = 1 mg/ml; 300 mg of drug/240 ml sol = 1 mg/ml; 200 mg of drug/250 ml sol = 2 mg/3 ml; use infusion pump
• PO ac, hs; tablet may be crushed or swallowed whole
• Reduced dosage in renal dysfunction
• IV, keep patient recumbent for 3 hr

Perform/provide:
• Storage in dry area at room temperature; do not freeze

Evaluate:
• Therapeutic response: decreased B/P after 1-2 wk

Teach patient/family:
• Not to discontinue drug abruptly; taper over 2 wk; may cause precipitate angina
• Not to use OTC products containing α-adrenergic stimulants (nasal decongestants, OTC cold preparations) unless directed by physician
• To report bradycardia, dizziness, confusion, depression, fever
• To take pulse at home, advise when to notify physician
• To avoid alcohol, smoking, Na intake
• To comply with weight control, dietary adjustments, modified exercise program
• To carry Medic Alert ID to identify drug you are taking, allergies
• To avoid hazardous activities if dizziness is present
• To report symptoms of CHF: difficult breathing, especially on exertion or when lying down, night cough, swelling of extremities
• To take medication at bedtime to prevent effect of orthostatic hypotension
• To wear support hose to minimize effects of orthostatic hypotension

Treatment of overdose: Lavage, IV atropine for bradycardia, IV theophylline for bronchospasm, digitalis, O_2, diuretic for cardiac failure; hemodialysis is useful for removal, hypotension; administer vasopressor (norepinephrine)

lactulose
(lak'tyoo-lose)
Cephulac, Cholac, Chronulac, Constilac, Constulose, Duphalac, Enulose
Func. class.: Ammonia detoxicant
Chem. class.: Lactose synthetic derivative

Action: Prevents absorption of ammonia in colon
Uses: Constipation, portal-sys-

temic encephalopathy in patients with hepatic disease

Dosage and routes:

Constipation

• *Adult:* PO 15-60 ml qd

Encephalopathy

• *Adult:* PO 20-30 g tid or qid until stools are soft; RET ENEMA 30-45 ml in 100 ml of fluid

Available forms: Oral sol, rec sol 3.33 g/5 ml

Side effects/adverse reactions:

GI: Nausea, vomiting, anorexia, cramps, diarrhea, flatulence

Contraindications: Hypersensitivity, low-galactose diet

Precautions: Pregnancy (C), lactation, diabetes mellitus

Pharmacokinetics: Metabolized in intestine, excreted by kidneys

Interactions/incompatibilities:

• Decreased effects of lactulose: neomycin, other oral antiinfectives

NURSING CONSIDERATIONS

Assess:

• Blood ammonia level (30-70 mg/ 100 ml)

• Blood, urine electrolytes if drug is used often by patient

• I&O ratio to identify fluid loss

• Cause of constipation; determine whether fluids, bulk, or exercise is missing from life-style

• Cramping, rectal bleeding, nausea, vomiting; if these symptoms occur, drug should be discontinued

• Clearing of confusion, lethargy, restlessness, irritability

Administer:

• With fruit juice, water, milk to increase palatability of oral form

• Retention enema by diluting 300 ml lactose/700 ml of water; administer by rectal balloon catheter

• Increase fluids to 2 L/day; do not give with other laxatives; if diarrhea occurs, reduce dosage

Evaluate:

• Therapeutic response: decreased constipation, decreased blood ammonia level

Teach patient/family:

• Not to use laxatives for long-term therapy; bowel tone will be lost

• To dilute with water or fruit juice to counteract sweet taste

• To store in cool environment; do not freeze

• Not to take other laxatives with this drug

• To take on an empty stomach for rapid action

---

leucovorin calcium (citrovorum factor/folinic acid)

(loo-koe-vor'in)

Leucovorin Calcium, Wellcovorin

Func. class.: Vitamin/folic acid antagonist antidote

Chem. class.: Tetrahydrofolic acid derivative

Action: Needed for normal growth patterns; prevents toxicity during antineoplastic therapy by protecting normal cells

Uses: Megaloblastic or macrocytic anemia caused by folic acid deficiency, overdose of folic acid antagonist, methotrexate toxicity, toxicity caused by pyrimethamine or trimethoprim, pneumocystosis, toxoplasmosis

Dosage and routes:

Megaloblastic anemia caused by enzyme deficiency

• *Adult and child:* IM 3-6 mg qd, then 1 mg PO for life

Megaloblastic anemia caused by deficiency of folate

• *Adult and child:* IM 1 mg or less qd until adequate response

---

* Available in Canada only

Methotrexate toxicity
• *Adult and child:* Given 6-36 hr after dose of methotrexate
Pyrimethamine toxicity
• *Adult and child:* PO/IM 5 mg qd
Trimethoprim toxicity
• *Adult and child:* PO IM 400 µg qd
Available forms: Tabs 5, 25 mg; inj IM 3, 5 mg/ml; powder for inj 10 mg/ml

Side effects/adverse reactions:
RESP: Wheezing
INTEG: Rash, pruritus, erythema, thrombocytosis, urticaria

Contraindications: Hypersensitivity, anemias other than megaloblastic not associated with B$_{12}$-deficiency

Precautions: Pregnancy (C)

Interactions/incompatibilities:
• Decreased folate levels: chloramphenicol
• Increased metabolism of: phenobarbitol, hydantoins

NURSING CONSIDERATIONS
Assess:
• CrCl before leucovorin rescue and qd to detect nephrotoxicity
• I&O; watch for nausea and vomiting
• Nutritional status: bran, yeast, dried beans, nuts, fruits, fresh vegetables, asparagus
• Drugs currently taken: alcohol, hydantoins, trimethoprim may cause increased folic acid use by body

Administer:
• Within 1 hr of folic acid antagonist
• After reconstituting with bacteriostatic H$_2$O for inj

Perform/provide:
• Increase fluid intake if used to treat folic acid inhibitor overdose
• Protection from light and heat

Evaluate:
• Therapeutic response: increased weight; improved orientation, well-being; absence of fatigue

Teach patient/family:
• To take drug exactly as prescribed
• To notify physician of side effects
• To report signs of hyposensitivity reaction immediately

---

leuprolide acetate
(loo-proe'-lide)
Lupron
Func. class.: Antineoplastic hormone
Chem. class.: Gonadotropin-releasing hormone

Action: Causes initial increase in circulating levels of LH, FSH; continuous administration results in decreased LH, FSH; in men, testosterone is reduced to castrate levels; in premenopausal women, estrogen is reduced to menopausal levels

Uses: Metastatic prostate cancer, management of endometriosis

Dosage and routes:
• *Adult:* SC 1 mg/day
Available forms: Inj IM 3.75 mg, 7.5 mg single dose, multiple dose vials

Side effects/adverse reactions:
GU: Edema, hot flashes, impotence, decreased libido, amenorrhea, vaginal dryness, gynecomastia

Contraindications: Hypersensitivity to GnRH or analogs, thromboembolic disorders, pregnancy (X), lactation, undiagnosed vaginal bleeding

Precautions: Edema, hepatic disease, CVA, MI, seizures, hypertension, diabetes mellitus

---

italics = common side effects   ***bold italic*** = life threatening reactions

NURSING CONSIDERATIONS
Assess:

• Liver function tests before, during therapy (bilirubin, AST, ALT, LDH) as needed or monthly

• Pituitary gonadotropic and gonadal function during therapy and 4-8 wk after therapy is decreased

• Worsening of signs and symptoms is normal during beginning therapy

• Fatigue, increased pulse, pallor, lethargy

• Food preferences; list likes, dislikes

• Edema in feet, joints; stomach pain; shaking

• Symptoms indicating severe allergic reaction: rash, pruritus, urticaria, purpuric skin lesions, itching, flushing

Perform/provide:

• Nutritious diet with iron, vitamin supplements as ordered

• Storage in tight container at room temperature

Evaluate:

• Therapeutic response: decreased tumor size. spread of malignancy

Teach patient/family:

• To notify physician if menstruation continues; menstruation should stop

• To use a nonhormonal method of contraception during therapy

• That bone pain will disappear after 1 wk

• To report any complaints, side effects to nurse or physician

• How to prepare, give; to rotate sites for SC injections

• To keep accurate records of dose

• That tumor flare may occur: increase in size of tumor, increased bone pain; will subside rapidly; may take analgesics for pain; premenopausal women must use mechanical birth control; ovulation may be induced

levamisole HCl
(lee-vam'i-sol)
Ergamisol
Func. class.: Immunomodulator

Action: May increase the action of macrophages, monocytes, and T cells, which will restore immune function; complete action is unknown

Uses: Treatment of Dukes' stage C colon cancer given with fluorouracil after surgical resection

Dosage and routes:

• *Adult:* PO 50 mg q8h × 3d; begin treatment at least 1 wk but no more than 4 wk after resection; given with fluorouracil 450 mg/m²/d; IV given daily × 5d beginning 21-34d after resection; maintenance is 50 mg q8h × 3d q2wk × 1 yr; given with fluorouracil 45 mg/m²/d by IV push qwk starting 28d after the initial 5-d course × 1 yr

Available forms: Tab 50 mg (base), IV

Side effects/adverse reactions:

CNS: Dizziness, headache, paresthesia, somnolence, depression, anxiety, fatigue, fever, mental changes, ataxia, insomnia

GI: Nausea, vomiting, anorexia, diarrhea, stomatitis, constipation, flatulence, dyspepsia, abdominal pain

INTEG: Rash, pruritus, alopecia, dermatitis, urticaria

*HEMA: **Granulocytopenia, leukopenia, thrombocytopenia***

CV: Chest pain, edema

META: Hyperbilirubinemia

EENT: Blurred vision, conjunctivitis

OTHER: Rigors, infection, altered sense of smell, arthralgia, myalgia

Contraindications: Hypersensitivity

Precautions: Pregnancy (C), lactation, children, blood dyscrasias

Pharmacokinetics: Peak 1.5-2 hr, elimination half-life 3-4 hr; metabolized by the liver

Interactions/incompatibilities:

• Increased plasma levels: phenytoin

• Disulfiram-like reaction: alcohol

NURSING CONSIDERATIONS
Assess:

• Kidney, liver function studies: BUN, creatinine, AST, ALT, alk phosphatase, bilirubin

• Baseline blood counts with differential, platelets, electrolyte, repeat q3mo for 1 yr; if platelets are <100,000/mm³ therapy, should be discontinued and restarted after recovery; fluorouracil should not be given if WBC is 2500-3500/mm³; after WBC is >3500/mm³, dose should be reduced by 20%; if WBC <2500/mm³ for 10 days, discontinue levamisole

• Stomatitis or GI symptoms: drug may have to be discontinued; then start fluorouracil 28 days after the start of 1st course

• Blood dyscrasias (anemia, granulocytopenia); bruising, fatigue, bleeding, poor healing

• Allergic reactions: dermatitis, exfoliative dermatitis, pruritus, urticaria

Administer:

• 7-20 days after surgery; start fluorouracil with 2nd course of levamisole; begin no sooner than 21d and no later than 35d after surgery; if levamisole therapy begins 21-30d after resection, fluorouracil should be given with 1st course; apply pressure to venipuncture sites for 10 min, especially if platelets are low

Evaluate:

• Therapeutic response: decrease in size and spread of tumor

Teach patient/family:

• To call physician if sore throat, swollen lymph nodes, malaise, fever occur, since other infections may occur

---

levodopa

(lee-voe-doe′pa)

Dopar, Larodopa

Func. class.: Antiparkinson agent

Chem. class.: Catecholamine

Action: Decarboxylation to dopamine, which increases dopamine levels in brain

Uses: Parkinsonism, carbon monoxide poisoning, chronic manganese intoxication, cerebral arteriosclerosis

Dosage and routes:

• *Adult:* PO 0.5-1 g qd divided bid-qid with meals; may increase by up to 0.75 g q3-7d to not exceed 8 g/d unless closely supervised

Available forms: Caps 100, 250, 500 mg; tabs 100, 250, 500 mg

Side effects/adverse reactions:

*HEMA: **Hemolytic anemia, leukopenia, agranulocytosis***

CNS: Involuntary choreiform movements, hand tremors, fatigue, headache, anxiety, twitching, numbness, weakness, confusion, agitation, insomnia, nightmares, psychosis, hallucination, hypomania, severe depression, dizziness

GI: Nausea, vomiting, anorexia, abdominal distress, dry mouth, flatulence, dysphagia, bitter taste, diarrhea, constipation

INTEG: Rash, sweating, alopecia

---

italics = common side effects   ***bold italic*** = life threatening reactions

CV: Orthostatic hypotension, tachycardia, hypertension, palpitation

EENT: Blurred vision, diplopia, dilated pupils

MISC: Urinary retention, incontinence, weight change, dark urine

Contraindications: Hypersensitivity, narrow-angle glaucoma, undiagnosed skin lesions

Precautions: Renal disease, cardiac disease, hepatic disease, respiratory disease, MI with dysrhythmias, convulsions, peptic ulcer, pregnancy (C), asthma, endocrine disease, affective disorders, psychosis, lactation, children <12 yr peptic ulcer

Pharmacokinetics:

PO: Peak 1-3 hr, excreted in urine (metabolites)

Interactions/incompatibilities:
- Hypertensive crisis: MAOIs, furazolidone
- Decreased effects of levodopa: anticholinergics, hydantoins, methionine, papaverine, pyridoxine, tricyclics, benzodiazepines
- Increased effects of levodopa: antacids, metoclopramide

Lab test interferences:

False positive: Urine ketones, urine glucose, Coombs' test

False negative: Urine glucose (glucose oxidase)

False increase: Uric acid, urine protein

Decrease: VMA

NURSING CONSIDERATIONS

Assess:
- B/P, respiration
- Mental status: affect, mood, behavioral changes, depression; complete suicide assessment

Administer:
- Drug until NPO before surgery
- Adjust dosage to patient response
- With meals; limit protein taken with drug
- Only after MAOIs have been discontinued for 2 wk

Perform/provide:
- Assistance with ambulation during beginning therapy
- Testing for diabetes mellitus, acromegaly if on long-term therapy

Evaluate:
- Therapeutic response: decrease in akathisia, increased mood

Teach patient/family:
- That therapeutic effects may take several weeks to a few months
- To change positions slowly to prevent orthostatic hypotension
- To report side effects: twitching, eye spasms; indicate overdose
- To use drug exactly as prescribed; if drug is discontinued abruptly, parkinsonian crisis may occur
- That urine, sweat may darken
- To avoid Vit B_6-preparations, vitamin-fortified foods containing B_6; these foods can reverse effects of levodopa

---

levomethydyle acetate HCl

(le'vo-meth'y-dyle)

ORLAMM

Func. class.: Narcotic agonist analgesics

Action: Depresses pain impulse transmission at the spinal cord level by interacting with opioid receptors

Uses: Management of opiate dependency

Dosage and routes:

Opiate withdrawal

Usually given 3×/wk (Monday, Wednesday, Friday or Tuesday, Thursday, Saturday)
- *Initial dose:* 20-40 mg each dose at 48 or 72 hr; may be adjusted in

---

increments of 5-10 mg until steady state occurs (1-2 wk)

Patients dependent on methadone may require larger doses

• *Maintenance:* 60-90 mg 3×/wk

• *Transfer to methadone:* Initial treatment given after 48 hr; may give increased or decreased (5-10 mg) in the daily methadone dose (symptoms of withdrawal)

Available forms: Oral sol 10 mg/ml

Side effects/adverse reactions:

CNS: Drowsiness, dizziness, confusion, headache, sedation, euphoria

CV: Palpitations, bradycardia, change in B/P

EENT: Tinnitus, blurred vision, miosis, diplopia

GI: Nausea, vomiting, anorexia, constipation, cramps, biliary tract spasm

GU: Increased urinary output, dysuria, urinary retention

INTEG: Rash, urticaria, bruising, flushing, diaphoresis, pruritus

*RESP: **Respiratory depression***

Contraindications: Hypersensitivity

Precautions: Addictive personality, pregnancy (B), lactation, increased intracranial pressure, MI (acute), severe heart disease, respiratory depression, hepatic disease, renal disease, child <18 yr

Pharmacokinetics:

PO: Onset 30-60 min, duration 6-8 hr, cumulative 22-48 hr

Metabolized by liver, excreted by kidneys, crosses placenta, excreted in breast milk

Interactions/incompatibilities:

• Increased effects with other CNS depressants: alcohol, narcotics, sedative/hypnotics, antipsychotics, skeletal muscle relaxants, rifampin, phenytoin

NURSING CONSIDERATIONS

Assess:

• I&O ratio; check for decreasing output; may indicate urinary retention

Administer:

• With antiemetic for nausea, vomiting

Perform/provide:

• Storage in light-resistant container at room temperature

Evaluate:

• Therapeutic response: decreased dependence on opiate

• CNS changes: dizziness, drowsiness, hallucinations, euphoria, LOC, pupil reaction

• Allergic reactions: rash, urticaria

• Respiratory dysfunction: depression, character, rate, rhythm

Teach patient/family:

• To report any symptoms of CNS changes, allergic reactions

• That physical dependency may result when used for extended periods

• That withdrawal symptoms may occur: nausea, vomiting, cramps, fever, faintness, anorexia

levonorgestrel implant

(lee-voe-nor-jess'trel)
Norplant System
Func. class.: Contraceptive system
Chem. class.: Synthetic progestin

Action: As a progestin, transforms proliferative endometrium into secretory endometrium; inhibits secretion of pituitary gonadotropins, which prevents follicular maturation and ovulation

Uses: Prevention of pregnancy for 5 yr

italics = common side effects   ***bold italic*** = life threatening reactions

Dosage and routes:
• *Adult:* 6 caps subdermally implanted in the upper arm during 1st 7 days after onset of menses
Available forms: Kit of 6 cap, 36 mg/cap
Side effects/adverse reactions:
CNS: Dizziness, headache, nervousness
GU: Amenorrhea, cervical erosion, breakthrough bleeding, dysmenorrhea, vaginal candidiasis, breast changes, vaginitis
GI: Nausea, abdominal discomfort
INTEG: Alopecia, dermatitis, hirsutism, acne, hypertrichosis, infection at site, pain/itching at site
OTHER: Change in appetite, weight gain
Contraindications: Hypersensitivity, pregnancy (X), thrombophlebitis, undiagnosed genital bleeding, liver tumors, breast carcinoma, liver disease
Precautions: Depression, psychosis, lactation, fluid retention, contact lens wearers
Pharmacokinetics: Max concentration at 24 hr
Interactions/incompatibilities:
• Decreased contraception: phenytoin, carbamazepine
NURSING CONSIDERATIONS
Assess:
• Blood studies: cholesterol, triglycerides; may be increased or decreased; sex hormone–binding globulin, thyroxine, T_3 uptake
• Menstrual irregularities: spotting, prolonged bleeding, amenorrhea; usually diminish
• For jaundice, thrombophlebitis, implants should be removed
• For acne, dermatitis, hirsutism, alopecia
Administer:
• 8 cm (3 in) above the crease of the elbow; implantation should be

during first 7 days after onset of menses; implantation should be fanlike, 15 degrees apart
Evaluate:
• Therapeutic response: absence of pregnancy
Teach patient/family:
• That if vision problems occur, an ophthalmologist should be seen
• That physical examinations are necessary

---

levorphanol tartrate
(lee-vor'fa-nole)
Levo-Dromoran
Func. class.: Narcotic analgesics
Chem. class.: Opiate, synthetic morphine derivative

Controlled Substance Schedule II
Action: Depresses pain impulse transmission at the spinal cord level by interacting with opioid receptors
Uses: Moderate to severe pain
Dosage and routes:
• *Adult:* PO/SC/IV 2-3 mg q6-8h prn
Available forms: Inj SC/IV 2 mg/ml; tabs 2 mg
Side effects/adverse reactions:
CNS: Drowsiness, dizziness, confusion, headache, sedation, euphoria
GI: Nausea, vomiting, anorexia, constipation, cramps
GU: Urinary retention, dysuria
INTEG: Rash, urticaria, diaphoresis, pruritus
EENT: Tinnitus, blurred vision, miosis, diplopia
CV: Palpitations, bradycardia, change in B/P
RESP: Respiratory depression
Contraindications: Hypersensitivity, addiction (narcotic)
Precautions: Addictive personality, pregnancy (B), lactation, in-

creased intracranial pressure, MI (acute), severe heart disease, respiratory depression, hepatic disease, renal disease, child <18 yr

Pharmacokinetics:

SC: Peak 1-½ hr, duration 6-8 hr
IV: Peak 20 min, duration 6-8 hr; metabolized by liver; excreted by kidneys; crosses placenta; excreted in breast milk; half-life 11 hr

Interactions/incompatibilities:

• Effects may be increased with other CNS depressants: alcohol, narcotics, sedative/hypnotics, antipsychotics, skeletal muscle relaxants

• Incompatible with aminophylline, ammonium chloride, amobarbital, chlorothiazide, heparin, methicillin, pentobarbital, phenobarbital, phenytoin, secobarbital, $NaCO_3$, sodium iodide, thiopental in sol or syringe

Lab test interferences:

Increase: Amylase

NURSING CONSIDERATIONS

Assess:

• I&O ratio; check for decreasing output; may indicate urinary retention

• CNS changes: dizziness, drowsiness, hallucinations, euphoria, LOC, pupil reaction

• Allergic reactions: rash, urticaria

• Respiratory dysfunction: respiratory depression, character, rate, rhythm; notify physician if respirations are <10/min

• Need for pain medication, physical dependence

Administer:

• With antiemetic if nausea, vomiting occur

• When pain is beginning to return; determine dosage interval by patient response

• IV directly after diluting each dose with 5 ml of sterile H_2O or

NaCl for inj, give through Y-tube or 3-way stopcock over 5 min

Perform/provide:

• Storage in light-resistant area at room temperature

• Assistance with ambulation

• Safety measures: side rails, nightlight, call bell within easy reach

Evaluate:

• Therapeutic response: decrease in pain

Teach patient/family:

• To report any symptoms of CNS changes, allergic reactions

• That physical dependency may result when used for extended periods

• Withdrawal symptoms may occur: nausea, vomiting, cramps, fever, faintness, anorexia

Treatment of overdose: Naloxone (Narcan) 0.2-0.8 IV, O_2, IV fluids, vasopressors

---

levothyroxine sodium (T_4, L-thyroxine sodium)

(lee-voe-thye-rox′een)

Levothroid, Levothyroxine Sodium, Levoxine, Synthroid

Func. class.: Thyroid hormone
Chem. class.: Levoisomer of thyroxine

Action: Increases metabolic rates, increases cardiac output, O_2 consumption, body temperature, blood volume, growth, development at cellular level

Uses: Hypothyroidism, myxedema coma, thyroid hormone replacement, cretinism, thyrotoxicosis

Dosage and routes:

Severe hypothyroidism

• *Adult:* PO 0.025-0.1 mg qd, increased by 0.05-0.1 mg q1-4 wk

---

italics = common side effects   ***bold italic*** = life threatening reactions

until desired response, maintenance dose 0.1-0.4 mg qd
• *Child:* PO 0.01-0.05 qd, may increase 0.025-0.05 mg q1-4 wk until desired response

Mild hypothyroidism
• Initial 50 μg qd; increase by 25-50 μg at interval of 2-4 wk

Cretinism
• *Child:* IV 0.025-0.05 mg qd, may increase by 0.05-0.1 mg PO q2-3wk

Myxedema coma
• *Adult:* IV 0.2-0.5 mg, may increase by 0.1-0.3 mg after 24 hr; place on oral medication as soon as possible

Available forms: Inj IV 200, 500 μg/vial; tabs 0.025, 0.05, 0.075, 0.088 mg, 0.1, 0.112 mg, 0.125, 0.15, 0.175, 0.2, 0.3 mg

Side effects/adverse reactions:
CNS: Anxiety, insomnia, tremors, headache, ***thyroid storm***
CV: Tachycardia, palpitations, angina, dysrhythmias, hypertension, ***cardiac arrest***
GI: Nausea, diarrhea, increased or decreased appetite, cramps
MISC: Menstrual irregularities, weight loss, sweating, heat intolerance, fever

Contraindications: Adrenal insufficiency, myocardial infarction, thyrotoxicosis

Precautions: Elderly, angina pectoris, hypertension, ischemia, cardiac disease, pregnancy (A), lactation

Pharmacokinetics:
IV/PO: Peak 12-48 hr, half-life 6-7 days; distributed throughout body tissues

Interactions/incompatibilities:
• Decreased absorption of levothyroxine: cholestyramine
• Increased effects of: anticoagulants, sympathomimetics, tricyclic antidepressants
• Decreased effects of: digitalis drugs, insulin, hypoglycemics
• Decreased effects of levothyroxine: estrogens
• Considered to be incompatible in syringe with all other drugs

Lab test interferences:
Increase: CPK, LDH, AST, PBI, blood glucose
Decrease: TSH, ^{131}I uptake test, uric acid, triglycerides

NURSING CONSIDERATIONS
Assess:
• B/P, pulse before each dose
• I&O ratio
• Weight qd in same clothing, using same scale, at same time of day
• Height, growth rate if given to a child
• T_3, T_4, FTIs, which are decreased; radioimmunoassay of TSH, which is increased; radio uptake, which is increased if patient is on too low a dose of medication
• Pro-time may require decreased anticoagulant, check for bleeding, bruising
• Increased nervousness, excitability, irritability, which may indicate too high dose of medication, usually after 1-3 wk of treatment
• Cardiac status: angina, palpitation, chest pain, change in VS

Administer:
• IV after diluting with provided diluent 0.5 mg/5 ml; shake; give through Y-tube or 3-way stopcock; give 0.1 mg or less over 1 min; do not add to IV inf; 0.1 mg = 1 ml
• In AM if possible as a single dose to decrease sleeplessness
• At same time each day to maintain drug level
• Only for hormone imbalances; not to be used for obesity, male in-

fertility, menstrual conditions, lethargy
• Lowest dose that relieves symptoms; lower dose to the elderly and in cardiac diseases

Perform/provide:
• Storage in tight, light-resistant container; sol should be discarded if not used immediately
• Removal of medication 4 wk before RAIU test

Evaluate:
• Therapeutic response: absence of depression; increased weight loss, diuresis, pulse, appetite; absence of constipation, peripheral edema, cold intolerance, pale, cool dry skin, brittle nails, alopecia, coarse hair, menorrhagia, night blindness, paresthesias, syncope, stupor, coma, rosy cheeks

Teach patient/family:
• That hair loss will occur in child, is temporary
• To report excitability, irritability, anxiety, which indicate overdose
• Not to switch brands unless approved by physician
• That drug may be discontinued after birth, thyroid panel evaluated after 1-2 mo
• That hypothyroid child will show almost immediate behavior/personality change
• That drug is not to be taken to reduce weight
• To avoid OTC preparations with iodine; read labels
• To avoid iodine food, iodized salt, soybeans, tofu, turnips, some seafood, some bread

lidocaine/lidocaine HCl (topical)

(lye'-doe-kane)
Anestacon, Lidocaine HCl, topical, Lidocaine Viscous, Xylocaine, Xylocaine Viscous

Func. class.: Topical anesthetic
Chem. class.: Aminoacylamide

Action: Inhibits nerve impulses from sensory nerves, which produces anesthesia

Uses: Pruritus, sunburn, toothache, sore throat, cold sores, oral pain

Dosage and routes:
• *Adult and child:* TOP apply q3-4h to affected area; INSTILL 15 ml (male) or 5 ml (female) into urethra

Available forms: Top sol

Side effects/adverse reactions:
INTEG: Rash, irritation, sensitization

Contraindications: Hypersensitivity, application to large areas

Precautions: Sepsis, pregnancy (B), denuded skin

NURSING CONSIDERATIONS

Assess:
• Allergy: rash, irritation, reddening, swelling
• Infection: if affected area is infected, do not apply

Administer:
• After cleansing and drying of affected area

Evaluate:
• Therapeutic response: absence of pain, itching of affected area

Teach patient/family:
• To report rash, irritation, redness, swelling
• How to apply ointment

---

italics = common side effects   ***bold italic*** = life threatening reactions

lidocaine HCl

(lye-doe-kane)
Lidopen Auto-Injector, Xylocaine HCl IM for Cardiac Arrythmias, Lidocaine HCl IV for Cardiac Arrhythmias, Xylocaine HCl IV for Cardiac Arrhythmias
Func. class.: Antidysrhythmic (Class IB)
Chem. class.: Aminoacyl amide

Action: Increases electrical stimulation threshold of ventricle, His-Purkinje system, which stabilizes cardiac membrane, decreases automaticity

Uses: Ventricular tachycardia, ventricular dysrhythmias during cardiac surgery, myocardial infarction, digitalis toxicity, cardiac catheterization

Dosage and routes:
• *Adult:* IV BOL 50-100 mg over 2-3 min, repeat q3-5min, not to exceed 300 mg in 1 hr; begin IV INF; IV INF 20-50 μg/kg/min; IM 200-300 mg in deltoid muscle
• *Elderly, CHF reduced liver function:* IV BOL give ½ adult dose
• *Child:* IV BOL 1 mg/kg, then IV INF 30 μg/kg/min
Available forms: IV INF 0.2%, 0.4%, 0.8%; IV Ad 4%, 10%, 20%; IV Dir 1%, 2%; IM 300 mg/ml, 10%

Side effects/adverse reactions:
CNS: Headache, dizziness, involuntary movement, confusion, tremor, drowsiness, euphoria, *convulsions*
EENT: Tinnitus, blurred vision
GI: Nausea, vomiting, anorexia
CV: Hypotension, bradycardia, heart block, cardiovascular collapse, arrest

RESP: Dyspnea, *respiratory depression*
INTEG: Rash, urticaria, edema, swelling
MISC: Febrile response, phlebitis at injection site

Contraindications: Hypersensitivity to amides, severe heart block, supraventricular dysrhythmias, Adams-Stokes syndrome, Wolff-Parkinson-White syndrome

Precautions: Pregnancy (B), lactation, children, renal disease, liver disease, CHF, respiratory depression, malignant hyperthermia

Pharmacokinetics:
IV: Onset 2 min, duration 20 min
IM: Onset 5-15 min, duration 1½ hr; half-life 8 min, 1-2 hr (terminal); metabolized in liver; excreted in urine; crosses placenta

Interactions/incompatibilities:
• Increased neuromuscular blockade of neuromuscular blockers, tubocurarine
• Increased effects of lidocaine: cimetidine, phenytoin, propranolol, metoprolol
• Decreased effects of lidocaine: barbiturates
• Incompatible with ampicillin, cefazolin, methohexital, phenytoin in syringe or sol; also incompatible with blood

Lab test interferences:
Increase: CPK

NURSING CONSIDERATIONS
Assess:
• ECG continuously to determine increased PR or QRS segments; if these develop, discontinue or reduce rate; watch for increased ventricular ectopic beats; may have to rebolus
• IV infusion rate using infusion pump; run at less than 4 mg/min
• Blood levels (therapeutic level: 1.5-6 μg/ml)

- B/P continuously for fluctuations
- I&O ratio, electrolytes (K, Na, Cl)
- Malignant hyperthermia: tachypnea, tachycardia, changes in B/P, increased temperature
- Cardiac rate, respiration: rate, rhythm, character, continuously
- Respiratory status: rate, rhythm, lung fields for rales, watch for respiratory depression
- CNS effects: dizziness, confusion, psychosis, paresthesias, convulsions; drug should be discontinued
- Lung fields, bilateral rales may occur in CHF patient
- Increased respiration, increased pulse; drug should be discontinued

Administer:
- IV bolus undiluted; give 50 mg or less over 1 min or dilute 1 g/250-500 ml of D₅W; titrate to patient response; use infusion pump; pediatric inf is 120 mg of lidocaine/100 ml D₅W; 1-2.5 ml/kg/hr = 20-50 µg/kg/min; use only 1%, 2% sol for IV bol
- IM injection in deltoid; aspirate to avoid intravascular administration; check site daily for infiltration or extravasation

Evaluate:
- Therapeutic response: decreased dysrhythmias

Teach patient/family:
- Use of automatic lidocaine injection device if ordered

Treatment of overdose: O₂, artificial ventilation, ECG; administer dopamine for circulatory depression, diazepam or thiopental for convulsions; decrease drug if needed

lidocaine HCl (local)

(lye'doe-kane)

Dalcaine, Dilocaine, Duo-Trach Kit, L-Caine, Lidocaine HCl, Lidoject-1, Lidoject-2, Nervocaine 1%, Nervocaine 2%, Octocaine HCl, Xylocaine HCl

Func. class.: Local anesthetic
Chem. class.: Amide

Action: Competes with calcium for sites in nerve membrane that control sodium transport across cell membrane; decreases rise of depolarization phase of action potential

Uses: Peripheral nerve block; caudal anesthesia; epidural, spinal, surgical anesthesia

Dosage and routes:
Varies by route of anesthesia
Available forms: Inj 0.5%, 1%, 1.5%, 2%, 4%, 5%; inj with epinephrine 0.5%, 1%, 1.5%, 2%

Side effects/adverse reactions:
CNS: Anxiety, restlessness, ***convulsions, loss of consciousness,*** drowsiness, disorientation, tremors, shivering

*CV: **Myocardial depression, cardiac arrest, dysrhythmias,*** bradycardia, hypotension, hypertension, fetal bradycardia

GI: Nausea, vomiting

EENT: Blurred vision, tinnitus, pupil constriction

INTEG: Rash, urticaria, allergic reactions, edema, burning, skin discoloration at injection site, tissue necrosis

*RESP: **Status asthmaticus, respiratory arrest, anaphylaxis***

Contraindications: Hypersensitivity, child <12 yr, elderly, severe liver disease

---

italics = common side effects   ***bold italic*** = life threatening reactions

Precautions: Elderly, severe drug allergies, pregnancy (C)
Pharmacokinetics:
Onset 4-17 min, duration 3-6 hr; metabolized by liver, excreted in urine (metabolites)
Interactions/incompatibilities:
• Dysrhythmias: epinephrine, halothane, enflurane
• Hypertension: MAOIs, tricyclic antidepressants, phenothiazines
• Decreased action of lidocaine: chloroprocaine
NURSING CONSIDERATIONS
Assess:
• B/P, pulse, respiration during treatment
• Fetal heart tones if drug is used during labor
• For allergic reactions: rash, urticaria, itching
• Cardiac status: ECG for dysrhythmias, pulse, B/P during anesthesia
Administer:
• Only with crash cart, resuscitative equipment nearby
• Only drugs without preservatives for epidural or caudal anesthesia
Perform/provide:
• Use of new solution; discard unused portions
Evaluate:
• Therapeutic response: anesthesia necessary for procedure
Treatment of overdose: Airway, O₂, vasopressor, IV fluids, anticonvulsants for seizures

---

lincomycin HCl
(lin-koe-mye´sin)
Lincocin, Lincorex
Func. class.: Antibacterial
Chem. class.: Lincomycin derivative

Action: Binds to 50S subunit of bacterial ribsomes, suppresses protein synthesis
Uses: Infections caused by group A β-hemolytic streptococci, pneumococci, staphylococci (respiratory tract, skin, soft tissue, urinary tract infections, osteomyelitis, septicemia)
Dosage and routes:
• *Adult:* PO 500 mg q6-8h, not to exceed 8 g/d; IM 600 mg/d or q12h; IV 600 mg-1 g q8-12h; dilute in 100 ml IV sol; infuse over 1 hr, not to exceed 8 g/day
• *Child >1 mo:* PO 30-60 mg/kg/d in divided doses q6-8h; IM 10 mg/kg/d q12h; IV 10-20 mg/kg/d in divided doses q8-12h; dilute to 100 ml IV sol; infuse over 1 hr
Available forms: Caps 500 mg; caps pediatric 250 mg; inj IM, IV 300 mg/ml
Side effects/adverse reactions:
HEMA: Leukopenia, eosinophilia, agranulocytosis, thrombocytopenia
GI: Nausea, vomiting, abdominal pain, tenesmus, diarrhea, pseudomembranous colitis
GU: Increased AST, ALT, bilirubin, alk phosphatase, jaundice, *vaginitis,* urinary frequency
EENT: Rash, urticaria, pruritus, erythema, pain, abscess at injection site
Contraindications: Hypersensitivity, ulcerative colitis/enteritis, infants <1 mo
Precautions: Renal disease, liver disease, GI disease, elderly, pregnancy (C), lactation
Pharmacokinetics:
PO: Peak 2-4 hr, duration 6 hr
IM: Peak 30 min, duration 8-12 hr
Half-life 4-6 hr; metabolized in liver; excreted in urine, bile, feces as active, inactive metabolites;

crosses placenta; excreted in breast milk

Interactions/incompatibilities:
• Increased neuromuscular blockage: nondepolarizing muscle relaxants
• Decreased absorption of lincomycin: kaolin
• Decreased action of: chloramphenicol, erythromycin
• Incompatible with ampicillin, carbenicillin, kanamycin, novobiocin, phenytoin, in sol or syringe; incompatible after 4 hr with penicillin

Lab test interferences:
Increase: Alk phosphatase, bilirubin, CPK, AST/ALT

NURSING CONSIDERATIONS
Assess:
• Signs of infection
• Any patient with compromised renal system; drug is excreted slowly in poor renal system function; toxicity may occur rapidly
• Liver studies: AST, ALT
• Blood studies: WBC, RBC, Hct, Hgb, platelets, serum iron, reticulocytes; drug should be discontinued if bone marrow depression occurs
• Renal studies: urinalysis, protein, blood, BUN, creatinine
• C&S before drug therapy; drug may be taken as soon as culture is taken
• Drug level in impaired hepatic, renal systems
• B/P, pulse in patient receiving drug parenterally
• Bowel pattern before, during treatment
• Skin eruptions, itching, dermatitis
• Respiratory status: rate, character, wheezing, tightness in chest
• Allergies before treatment, reaction of each medication; place allergies on chart, Kardex in bright red letters; notify all people giving drugs

Administer:
• IV by infusion only; do not administer bolus dose; dilute 1g or less/100 ml or more D₅W, D₁₀W, 0.9% NaCl, RL, not to exceed 100 ml/hr; if more than 4 g of drug is to be given, add to 500 ml of sol
• IM deep injection; rotate sites
• Orally with at least 8 oz H₂O on empty stomach

Perform/provide:
• Storage at room temperature (capsules) and up to 2 wk (reconstituted solution)
• Adrenalin, suction, tracheostomy set, endotracheal intubation equipment on unit
• Adequate intake of fluids (2 L) during diarrhea episodes

Evaluate:
• Therapeutic response: decreased temperature, negative C&S

Teach patient/family:
• To take oral drug with full glass of water; may give with food if GI symptoms occur
• Aspects of drug therapy: complete entire course of medication to ensure organism death (10-14 days); culture may be taken after completed course of medication
• To report sore throat, fever, fatigue; may indicate superimposed infection
• That drug must be taken in equal intervals around clock to maintain blood levels
• To notify nurse of diarrhea

Treatment of hypersensitivity: Withdraw drug; maintain airway; administer epinephrine, aminophylline, O₂, IV corticosteroids

---

italics = common side effects   ***bold italic*** = life threatening reactions

lindane (gamma benzene hexachloride)

(lin-dane)

gBh,* G-Well, Kwell, Kwellada,* Lindane, Scabene

Func. class.: Scabicide/Pediculicide

Chem. class.: Chlorinated hydrocarbon (synthetic)

Action: Stimulates nervous system of arthropods, resulting in seizures, death of organism

Uses: Scabies, lice (head/pubic), nits

Dosage and routes:

• *Adult and child:* CREAM/LOTION wash area with soap, water; remove visible crusts; apply to skin surfaces; remove with soap, water in 8-12 hr; may reapply in 1 wk if needed; shampoo using 30 ml: work into lather, rub for 5 min, rinse, dry with towel; comb with fine-toothed comb to remove nits

Available forms: Lotion, shampoo, cream (1%)

Side effects/adverse reactions:

INTEG: Pruritus, rash, irritation, contact dermatitis

GI: Nausea, vomiting, diarrhea, liver damage (inhalation of vapors)

*HEMA: **Aplastic anemia*** (chronic inhalation of vapors)

*CV: **Ventricular fibrillation*** (chronic inhalation of vapors)

*GU: **Kidney damage*** (chronic inhalation of vapors)

CNS: Tremors, ***convulsions,*** stimulation, dizziness (chronic inhalation of vapors)

Contraindications: Hypersensitivity; premature neonate; patients with known seizure disorders, inflammation of skin, abrasions, or breaks in skin

Precautions: Pregnancy (B), avoid contact with eyes, children <10 yr, infants, lactation

Interactions/incompatibilities:

• Oils may enhance absorption; if an oil-based hair dressing is used, shampoo, rinse, dry hair before applying lindane shampoo

NURSING CONSIDERATIONS

Administer:

• To body areas, scalp only; do not apply to face, lips, mouth, eyes, any mucous membrane, anus, or meatus

• Topical corticosteroids as ordered to decrease contact dermatitis

• Antihistamines

• Lotions of menthol or phenol to control itching

• Topical antibiotics for infection

Perform/provide:

• Isolation until areas on skin, scalp have cleared and treatment is completed

• Removal of nits by using a fine-toothed comb rinsed in vinegar after treatment; use gloves

Evaluate:

• Therapeutic response: decreased crusts, nits, brownish trails on skin, itching papules in skin folds, decreased itching after several weeks

Teach patient/family:

• To wash all inhabitants' clothing, using insecticide; preventive treatment may be required of all persons living in same house, using lotion or shampoo to decrease spread of infection; use rubber gloves when applying drug

• That itching may continue for 4-6 wk

• That drug must be reapplied if accidently washed off, or treatment will be ineffective

• Not to apply to face; if accidental contact with eyes occurs, flush with water

---

* Available in Canada only

• To treat sexual contacts simultaneously

Treatment of ingestion: Gastric lavage, saline laxatives, IV diazepam (Valium) for convulsions

---

liothyronine sodium (T₃)

(lye-oh-thye'roe-neen)

Cytomel, Liothyronine Sodium, Triostat

Func. class.: Thyroid hormone
Chem. class.: Synthetic T₃

Action: Increases metabolic rates, cardiac output, O_2 consumption, body temperature, blood volume, growth, development at cellular level

Uses: Hypothyroidism, myxedema coma, thyroid hormone replacement, cretinism, nontoxic goiter, T₃ suppression test

Dosage and routes:
• *Adult:* PO 25 µg qd, increased by 12.5-25 µg q1-2wk until desired response, maintenance dose 25-75 µg qd

Cretinism
• *Child >3 yr:* PO 50-100 µg qd
• *Child <3 yr:* PO 5 µg qd, increased by 5 µg q3-4d titrated to response

Myxedema
• *Adult:* PO 5 µg qd; may increase by 5-10 µg q1-2 wk; maintenance dose 50-100 µg qd

Nontoxic goiter
• *Adult:* PO 5 µg qd, increased by 12.5-25 µg q1-2 wk; maintenance dose 75 µg qd

Suppression test
• *Adult:* PO 75-100 µg qd × 1 wk
Available forms: Tabs 5, 25, 50 µg

Side effects/adverse reactions:
CNS: Insomnia, tremors, headache, ***thyroid storm***

CV: Tachycardia, palpitations, angina, dysrhythmias, hypertension, cardiac arrest

GI: Nausea, diarrhea, increased or decreased appetite, cramps

MISC: Menstrual irregularities, weight loss, sweating, heat intolerance, fever

Contraindications: Adrenal insufficiency, myocardial infarction, thyrotoxicosis

Precautions: Elderly, angina pectoris, hypertension, ischemia, cardiac disease, pregnancy (A), lactation

Pharmacokinetics:
PO: Peak 12-48 hr, half-life 6-7 days

Interactions/incompatibilities:
• Decreased absorption of liothyronine: cholestyramine
• Increased effects of: anticoagulants, sympathomimetics, tricyclic antidepressants
• Decreased effects of: digitalis drugs, insulin, hypoglycemics
• Decreased effects of liothyronine: estrogens

Lab test interferences:
Increase: CPK, LDH, AST, PBI, blood glucose
Decrease: TSH, ¹³¹I uptake test, uric acid, triglycerides

NURSING CONSIDERATIONS
Assess:
• B/P, pulse before each dose
• I&O ratio
• Weight qd in same clothing, using same scale, at same time of day
• Height, growth rate if given to a child
• T₃, T₄, which are decreased; radioimmunoassay of TSH, which is increased; radio uptake, which is increased if patient is on too low a dose of medication
• Pro-time may require decreased

---

anticoagulant; check for bleeding, bruising

• Increased nervousness, excitability, irritability, which may indicate too high dose of medication, usually after 1-3 wk of treatment

• Cardiac status: angina, palpitation, chest pain, change in VS

Administer:

• In AM if possible as a single dose to decrease sleeplessness

• At same time each day to maintain drug level

• Only for hormone imbalances; not to be used for obesity, male infertility, menstrual conditions, lethargy

• Lowest dose that relieves symptoms

• Liothyronine after discontinuing other thyroid preparation

Perform/provide:

• Removal of medication 4 wk before RAIU test

Evaluate:

• Therapeutic response: absence of depression; increased weight loss, diuresis, pulse, appetite; absence of constipation, peripheral edema, cold intolerance, pale, cool dry skin, brittle nails, alopecia, coarse hair, menorrhagia, night blindness, paresthesia, snycope, stupor, coma, rosy cheeks

Teach patient/family:

• That hair loss will occur in child but is temporary

• To report excitability, irritability, anxiety, which indicates overdose

• Not to switch brands unless approved by physician

• That hypothyroid child will show almost immediate behavior/personality change

• That drug is not to be taken to reduce weight

• To avoid OTC preparations with iodine; read labels

• To avoid iodine food, iodized salt, soybeans, tofu, turnips, some seafood, some bread

---

liotrix

(lye'oh-trix)
Euthroid, Thyrolar
Func. class.: Thyroid hormone
Chem. class.: Levothyroxine/liothyronine (synthetic T₄, T₃)

Action: Increases metabolic rates, cardiac output, O_2 consumption, body temperature, blood volume, growth, development at cellular level

Uses: Hypothyroidism, thyroid hormone replacement

Dosage and routes:

• *Adult and child:* PO 15-30 mg qd, increased by 15-30 mg q1-2wk until desired response; may increase by 15-30 mg q2wk in child

• *Geriatric:* PO 15-30 mg, double dose q6-8wk until desired response

Available forms: Tabs 15, 30, 60, 120, 180 mg as thyroid equivalent

Side effects/adverse reactions:

CNS: Insomnia, tremors, headache, thyroid storm

CV: Tachycardia, palpitations, angina, dysrhythmias, hypertension, cardiac arrest

GI: Nausea, diarrhea, increased or decreased appetite, cramps

MISC: Menstrual irregularities, weight loss, sweating, heat intolerance, fever

Contraindications: Adrenal insufficiency, myocardial infarction, thyrotoxicosis

Precautions: Elderly, angina pectoris, hypertension, ischemia, cardiac disease, pregnancy (A), lactation

Pharmacokinetics:

PO: Peak 12-48 hr, half-life 6-7 days

---

*Available in Canada only

Interactions/incompatibilities:
• Decreased absorption of liotrix: cholestyramine
• Increased effects of: anticoagulants, sympathomimetics, tricyclic antidepressants, catecholamines
• Decreased effects of: digitalis drugs, insulin, hypoglycemics
• Decreased effects of liotrix: estrogens

Lab test interferences:
Increase: CPK, LDH, AST, PBI, blood glucose
Decrease: TSH, ^{131}I uptake test, uric acid, triglycerides

NURSING CONSIDERATIONS
Assess:
• B/P, pulse before each dose
• I&O ratio
• Weight qd in same clothing, using same scale, at same time of day
• Height, growth rate if given to a child
• T_3, T_4 FTIs, which are decreased; radioimmunoassay of TSH, which is increased; radio uptake, which is increased if patient is on too low a dose of medication
• Pro-time may require decreased anticoagulant; check for bleeding, bruising
• Increased nervousness, excitability, irritability, which may indicate too high dose of medication, usually after 1-3 wk of treatment
• Cardiac status: angina, palpitation, chest pain, change in VS

Administer:
• In AM if possible as a single dose to decrease sleeplessness
• At same time each day to maintain drug level
• Only for hormone imbalances; not to be used for obesity, male infertility, menstrual conditions, lethargy
• Lowest dose that relieves symptoms

Perform/provide:
• Removal of medication 4 wk before RAIU test

Evaluate:
• Therapeutic response: absence of depression; increased weight loss, diuresis, pulse, appetite; absence of constipation, peripheral edema, cold intolerance, pale, cool dry skin, brittle nails, coarse hair, menorrhagia, night blindness, paresthesias, syncope, stupor, coma, rosy cheeks

Teach patient/family:
• That hair loss will occur in child, is temporary
• To report excitability, irritability, anxiety, which indicate overdose
• Not to switch brands unless approved by physician
• That hypothyroid child will show almost immediate behavior/personality change
• That drug is not to be taken to reduce weight
• To avoid OTC preparations with iodine; read labels
• To avoid iodine food, iodized salt, soybeans, tofu, turnips, some seafood, some bread

---

lisinopril
(lyse-in'oh-pril)
Prinivil, Zestril

Func. class.: Angiotensin converting enzyme (ACE) inhibitor
Chem. class.: Enalaprilat lysine analog

Action: Selectively suppresses renin-angiotensin-aldosterone system; inhibits ACE, preventing conversion of angiotensin I to angiotensin II
Uses: Mild to moderate hypertension, adjunctive therapy of CHF

---

italics = common side effects   ***bold italic*** = life threatening reactions

Dosage and routes:
• *Adult:* PO 10-40 mg qd; may increase to 80 mg qd if required
CHF
• Adult PO 5 mg initially with diuretics/digitalis
Available forms: Tabs 5, 10, 20 mg
Side effects/adverse reactions:
GI: Nausea, vomiting, anorexia, constipation, flatulence, GI irritation
GU: Proteinuria, renal insufficiency, sexual dysfunction, impotence
INTEG: Rash, pruritus
CNS: Vertigo, depression, stroke, insomnia, paresthesias, headache, fatigue, asthenia
EENT: Blurred vision, nasal congestion
RESP: Cough, dyspnea
Contraindications: Hypersensitivity
Precautions: Pregnancy (C), lactation, renal disease, hyperkalemia
Pharmacokinetics:
Peak 6-8 hr, excreted unchanged in urine
Interactions/incompatibilities:
• Increased hypotensive effect: diuretics, other hypertensives, probenecid
• Decreased effects of lisinopril: aspirin, indomethacin
• Increased K levels: K salt substitutes, K-sparing diuretics, K supplements
• Increased effects of: antihypertensives, reserpine, diuretics
• Increased hypersensitivity reactions: allopurinol
Lab test interferences:
Interfere: Glucose/insulin tolerance tests
NURSING CONSIDERATIONS
Assess:
• B/P, pulse q4h; note rates rhythm, quality

• Electrolytes: K, Na, Cl
• Apical/pedal pulse before administration; notify physician of any significant changes
• Baselines in renal, liver function tests before therapy begins
• Edema in feet, legs daily
• Skin turgor, dryness of mucous membranes for hydration status
• Symptoms of CHF: edema, dyspnea, wet rales
Evaluate:
• Therapeutic response: decreased B/P
Teach patient/family:
• Not to discontinue drug abruptly
• To rise slowly to sitting or standing position to minimize orthostatic hypotension
Treatment of overdose: Lavage, IV atropine for bradycardia, IV theophylline for bronchospasm, digitalis, O_2, diuretic for cardiac failure, hemodialysis

---

lithium carbonate

(li'thee-um)
Carbolith,* Duralith, Eskalith, Eskalith CR, Lithane, Lithium Carbonate, Lithobid, Lithonate, Lithotabs
Func. class.: Antimanic
Chem. class.: Alkali metal ion salt

Action: May alter sodium, potassium ion transport across cell membrane in nerve, muscle cells; may balance biogenic amines of norepinephrine, serotonin in CNS areas involved in emotional responses
Uses: Manic-depressive illness (manic phase), prevention of bipolar manic-depressive psychosis
Dosage and routes:
• *Adult:* PO 300-600 mg tid, maintenance 300 mg tid or qid; slow rel

tabs 300 mg bid; dose should be individualized to maintain blood levels at 0.5-1.5 mEq/L

Available forms: Caps 150, 300 mg; tabs 300 mg; tabs ext rel 300, 450 mg; syrup 300 mg/5ml

Side effects/adverse reactions:

CNS: Headache, drowsiness, dizziness, tremors, twitching, ataxia, *seizure,* slurred speech, restlessness, confusion, stupor, memory loss, clonic movements

GI: Dry mouth, anorexia, nausea, vomiting, diarrhea, incontinence, abdominal pain, metallic taste

*GU: **Polyuria, glycosuria, proteinuria, albuminuria,*** urinary incontinence, polydipsia, edema

CV: Hypotension, ECG changes, dysrhythmias, *circulatory collapse, edema*

INTEG: Drying of hair, alopecia, rash, pruritus, hyperkeratosis

*HEMA: **Leukocytosis***

EENT: Tinnitus, blurred vision

ENDO: Hyponatremia

MS: Muscle weakness

Contraindications: Hepatic disease, renal disease, brain trauma, OBS, pregnancy (D), lactation, children <12 yr, schizophrenia, severe cardiac disease, severe renal disease, severe dehydration

Precautions: Elderly, thyroid disease, seizure disorders, diabetes mellitus, systemic infection, urinary retention

Pharmacokinetics:

PO: Onset rapid, peak ½-4 hr, half-life 18-36 hr depending on age; crosses blood-brain barrier; 80% of filtered lithium is reabsorbed by the renal tubules, excreted in urine; crosses placenta; enters breast milk; well absorbed by oral method

Interactions/incompatibilities:

• Increased hypothyroid effects: antithyroid effects, calcium iodide,

potassium iodide, iodinated glycerol

• Brain damage: haloperidol, thioridazine

• Increased effects of: neuromuscular blocking agents, phenothiazines

• Increased renal clearance: sodium bicarbonate, acetazolamide, mannitol, aminophylline

• Increased toxicity: indomethacin, diuretics, nonsteroidal antiinflammatories

• Decreased effects of lithium: theophyllines, urea, urinary alkalinizers

Lab test interferences:

Increase: K excretion, urine glucose, blood glucose, protein, BUN

Decrease: VMA, T_3, T_4, PBI, ^{131}I

NURSING CONSIDERATIONS

Assess:

• Weight daily; check for edema in legs, ankles, wrists; report if present

• Na intake; decreased Na intake with decreased fluid intake may lead to lithium retention; increased Na and fluids may decrease lithium retention

• Skin turgor at least daily

• Urine for albuminuria, glycosuria, uric acid during beginning treatment, q2mo thereafter

• Neuro status: LOC, gait, motor reflexes, hand tremors

• Serum lithium levels weekly initially, then q2mo (therapeutic level: 0.5-1.5 mEq/L)

Administer:

• Reduced dose to elderly

• With meals to avoid GI upset

• Adequate fluids (2-3 L/day) to prevent dehydration during initial treatment, 1-2 L/day during maintenance

Evaluate:

• Therapeutic response: decrease in excitement, manic phase

---

italics = common side effects   ***bold italic*** = life threatening reactions

Teach patient/family:
• Symptoms of minor toxicity: vomiting, diarrhea, poor coordination, fine motor tremors, weakness, lassitude; major toxicity: coarse tremors, severe thirst, tinnitus, dilute urine
• To monitor urine specific gravity, emphasize need for follow-up care to determine lithium levels
• That contraception is necessary, since lithium may harm fetus
• Not to operate machinery until lithium levels are stable
• That beneficial effects may take 1-3 wks
• Provide a list of drugs that interact with lithium and discuss need for adequate salt and fluid intake
Treatment of overdose: Induce emesis or lavage, maintain airway, respiratory function; dialysis for severe intoxication

---

Iodoxamide tromethamine
(Io-dox'-a-mide)
Alomide
Func. class.: Antiallergic, ophthalmic
Chem. class.: Mast-cell stabilizer

Action: Inhibits increase in cutaneous vascular permeability (IgE, antigen-mediated reactions), prevents release of mast-cell inflamatory mediators, inhibits eosinophil chemotaxis
Uses: Vernal keratoconjunctivitis, conjunctivitis, keratitis
Dosage and routes:
• *Adult and Child >2 yrs:* 1-2 gtts in affected eye qid × 3 mo
Available forms: Sol 0.1%
Side effects/adverse reactions:
EENT: Burning, stinging, itching, pruritus, blurred vision, dry eye, tearing, corneal ulcers, scales on the eyelid, ocular fatigue, corneal abrasion
SYST: Headache, dizziness, nausea, sneezing, dry nose, rash, heat sensation
Contraindications: Hypersensitivity
Precautions: Soft contact lens wearers, pregnancy (B), lactation, children <2 yr
Pharmacokinetics: Elimination half-life 8½ hr, excreted in urine
NURSING CONSIDERATIONS
Evaluate:
• Eye pain; notify physician
Teach patient/family:
• To report change in vision, with blurring or loss of sight, burning, stinging, itching, swelling, ulcers, scales
• Method of instillation, including pressure on lacrimal sac for 1 min, and not to touch dropper to eye
• That soft contact lenses should not be worn during treatment
• Not to use by any other route than ophthalmic

---

lomefloxacin HCl
(lome-flock'a-sin)
Maxaquin
Func. class.: Antiinfective
Chem. class.: Fluoroquinolone

Action: Interferes with conversion of intermediate DNA fragments into high-molecular-weight DNA in bacteria; DNA gyrase inhibitor
Uses: Treatment of lower respiratory tract infections (pneumonia, bronchitis), genitourinary infections (prostatitis, UTIs), preoperatively to reduce urinary tract infec-

tions in transurethral surgical procedures

Dosage and routes:
• *Adult:* PO 400 mg/d 7-14d depending on type of infection
In renal impairment
• *Adult:* PO 200 mg/dose
Prophylaxis of UTI
• *Adult:* PO 400 mg 2-6 hr before surgery
Available forms: Tabs 400

Side effects/adverse reactions:
CNS: Dizziness, headache, somnolence, depression, insomnia, nervousness, confusion, agitation
GI: Diarrhea, nausea, vomiting, anorexia, flatulence, heartburn, dry mouth, increased AST, ALT, constipation, abdominal pain, oral thrush, glossitis, stomatitis
INTEG: Rash, pruritus, urticaria, photosensitivity
EENT: Visual disturbances

Contraindications: Hypersensitivity to quinolones

Precautions: Pregnancy (C), lactation, children, elderly, renal disease, seizure disorders, excessive exposure to sunlight

Pharmacokinetics:
PO: Peak 1-2 hr, half-life 6-8 hr; excreted in urine as active drug, metabolites

Interactions/incompatibilities:
• Decreased effects of lomefloxacin: antacids, nitrofurantoin, sucralfate, iron salts, zinc salts
• Increased lomefloxacin levels: probenecid, cimetidine
• Increased levels of: cyclosporine, warfarin

NURSING CONSIDERATIONS
Assess:
• Kidney, liver function studies: BUN, creatinine, AST, ALT
• I&O ratio, urine pH; <5.5 is ideal
• CNS symptoms: insomnia, vertigo, headache, agitation, confusion
• Allergic reactions: rash, flushing, urticaria, pruritus

Administer:
• After clean-catch urine is obtained for C&S

Perform/provide:
• Limited intake of alkaline foods, drugs; milk, dairy products, peanuts, vegetables, alkaline actacids, sodium bicarbonate

Evaluate:
• Therapeutic response: negative C&S

Teach patient/family:
• That fluids must be increased to 3L/day to avoid crystallization in kidneys
• That if dizziness or light-headedness occurs, to ambulate, perform activities with assistance
• To complete full course of drug therapy
• To contact physician if adverse reactions occur
• To avoid iron- or mineral-containing supplements within 2 hr before and after dosing
• That photosensitivity may occur and sunscreen should be used

---

lomustine (CCNU)
(loe-mus'teen)
CeeNU
Func. class.: Antineoplastic alkylating agent
Chem. class.: Nitrosourea

Action: Responsible for cross-linking DNA strands, which leads to cell death; activity is not cell cycle phase specific
Uses: Hodgkin's disease, lymphomas, melanomas, multiple myeloma; brain, lung, bladder, kidney, colon cancer

---

Dosage and routes:
• *Adult:* PO 130 mg/m² as a single dose q6wk; titrate dose to WBC level; do not give repeat dose unless WBCs are >4000/mm³, platelet count >100,000/mm³

Available forms: Cap 10, 40, 100 mg

Side effects/adverse reactions:
*HEMA: **Thrombocytopenia, leukopenia, myelosuppression, anemia***
*GI: Nausea, vomiting, anorexia, stomatitis, **hepatotoxicity***
*GU: **Azotemia, renal failure***
INTEG: Burning at injection site
*RESP: **Fibrosis, pulmonary infiltrate***

Contraindications: Hypersensitivity, leukopenia, thrombocytopenia, pregnancy (D)

Precautions: Radiation therapy

Pharmacokinetics:
Metabolized in liver, excreted in urine; half-life 16-48 hr; 50% protein bound; crosses blood-brain barrier; appears in breast milk

Interactions/incompatibilities:
• Increased toxicity: barbiturates, phenytoin, chloral hydrate
• Increased metabolism of lomustine: phenobarbital
• Potentiation of lomustine: succinylcholine
• Increased bone marrow depression: allopurinol

NURSING CONSIDERATIONS
Assess:
• CBC, differential, platelet count weekly; withhold drug if WBC is <4000 or platelet count is <75,000; notify physician of results
• Pulmonary function tests, chest x-ray films before, during therapy; chest film should be obtained q2wk during treatment
• Renal function studies: BUN, serum uric acid, urine CrCl before, during therapy
• I&O ratio; report fall in urine output of 30 ml/hr
• Monitor temperature q4h (may indicate beginning infection); no rectal temperatures
• Liver function tests before, during therapy (bilirubin, AST, ALT, LDH) as needed or monthly
• Bleeding: hematuria, guaiac, bruising or petechiae, mucosa or orifices q8h
• Dyspnea, rales, unproductive cough, chest pain, tachypnea
• Food preferences; list likes, dislikes
• Yellowing of skin and sclera, dark urine, clay-colored stools, itchy skin, abdominal pain, fever, diarrhea
• Inflammation of mucosa, breaks in skin
• Buccal cavity q8h for dryness, sores or ulceration, white patches, oral pain, bleeding, dysphagia
• Local irritation, pain, burning, discoloration at injection site
• Symptoms indicating severe allergic reaction: rash, pruritus, urticaria, purpuric skin lesions, itching, flushing

Administer:
• Antiemetic 30-60 min before giving drug to prevent vomiting
• Antibiotics for prophylaxis of infection
• Topical or systemic analgesics for pain
• Local or systemic drugs for infection

Perform/provide:
• Storage in tight container at room temperature
• Strict medical asepsis, protective isolation if WBC levels are low
• Special skin care
• Deep-breathing exercises with

patient tid-qid; place in semi-Fowler's position

• Increase fluid intake to 2-3 L/day to prevent urate deposits, calculi formation

• Rinsing of mouth tid-qid with water, club soda; brushing of teeth bid-tid with soft brush or cotton-tipped applicators for stomatitis; use unwaxed dental floss

Evaluate:

• Therapeutic response: decreased tumor size, spread of malignancy

Teach patient/family:

• Of protective isolation precautions

• To report any changes in breathing or coughing

• To avoid foods with citric acid, hot or rough texture if buccal inflammation is present

• To report any bleeding, white spots or ulcerations in mouth to physician; tell patient to examine mouth qd

• To report signs of infection: fever, sore throat, flu symptoms

• To report signs of anemia: fatigue, headache, faintness, shortness of breath, irritability

• To avoid use of razors, commercial mouthwash

• To avoid use of aspirin products or ibuprofen

---

loperamide HCl

(loe-per'a-mide)

Loperamide solution, Imodium, Imodium A-D, Imodium A-D Caplet, Loperamide

Func. class.: Antidiarrheal
Chem. class.: Piperidine derivative

Action: Direct action on intestinal muscles to decrease GI peristalsis

Uses: Diarrhea (cause undetermined), chronic diarrhea, ileostomy discharge

Dosage and routes:

• *Adult:* PO 4 mg, then 2 mg after each loose stool, not to exceed 16 mg/d

• *Child 2-5 yr:* PO 1 mg then 1, 0.1 mg/kg after each loose stool

• *Child 5-8 yr:* PO 2 mg bid on day 1, then 0.1 mg/kg after each loose stool

• *Child 8-12 yr:* PO 2 mg tid on day 1, then 0.1 mg/kg after each loose stool

Available forms: Caps 2 mg; liq 1 mg/5 ml

Side effects/adverse reactions:

CNS: Dizziness, drowsiness, fatigue, fever

GI: Nausea, dry mouth, vomiting, constipation, abdominal pain, anorexia, ***toxic megacolon***

INTEG: Rash

*RESP: **Respiratory depression***

Contraindications: Hypersensitivity, severe ulcerative colitis, pseudomembranous colitis, acute diarrhea associated with *E. coli*

Precautions: Pregnancy (B), lactation, children <2 yr, liver disease, dehydration, bacterial disease

Pharmacokinetics:

PO: Onset ½-1 hr, duration 4-5 hr, half-life 7-14 hr; metabolized in liver; excreted in feces as unchanged drug; small amount in urine

Interactions/incompatibilities:

• Do not mix oral solution with other solutions

NURSING CONSIDERATIONS
Assess:

• Electrolytes (K, Na, Cl) if on long-term therapy

• Skin turgor q8h if dehydration is suspected

• Bowel pattern before; for rebound constipation

L

• Response after 48 hr; if no response, drug should be discontinued
• Dehydration in children
• Abdominal distention, toxic megacolon; may occur in ulcerative colitis

Administer:
• For 48 hr only, cont INF

Perform/provide:
• Storage in tight containers

Evaluate:
• Therapeutic response: decreased diarrhea

Teach patient/family:
• To avoid OTC products unless directed by physician
• That ostomy patient may take this drug for extended time
• That if drowsiness occurs, not to operate machinery
• To use hard candy, sips of water for dry mouth

---

loracarbef
(lor-a-kar'bef)
Lorabid
Func. class.: Antibiotic
Chem. class.: Carbacephem

Action: Inhibits bacterial cell wall synthesis, which renders cell wall osmotically unstable

Uses: Gram-negative: *H. influenzae, E. coli, P. mirabilis, Klebsiella;* gram-positive: *S. pneumoniae, S. pyogenes, S. aureus;* upper and lower respiratory tract, urinary tract, skin infections; otitis media

Dosage and routes:
• *Adult:* PO UTI 200 mg qd × 7d
• *Child:* PO Acute otitis media 15 mg/kg bid × 10d

Available forms: Caps 200 mg; 100, 200 mg/5 ml suspension

Side effects/adverse reactions:
CNS: Dizziness, headache, fatigue, paresthesia, fever, chills, confusion
GI: Diarrhea, nausea, vomiting, anorexia, dysgeusia, glossitis, bleeding, increased AST, ALT, bilirubin, LDH, alk phosphatase, abdominal pain, loose stools, flatulence, heartburn, stomach cramps, colitis, jaundice
INTEG: Rash, urticaria, dermatitis, *anaphylaxis*
GU: Vaginitis, pruritus, candidiasis, increased BUN, *nephrotoxicity, renal failure,* pyuria, dysuria, reversible interstitial nephritis
HEMA: **Leukopenia, thrombocytopenia, agranulocytosis,** anemia, **neutropenia, lymphocytosis, eosinophilia, pancytopenia, hemolytic anemia, leukocytosis, granulocytopenia**
RESP: Dyspnea

Contraindications: Hypersensitivity to cephalosporins or related antibiotics, seizures

Precautions: Pregnancy (B), lactation, children, renal disease

Pharmacokinetics:
PO: Peak 1 hr, half-life 1 hr; excreted in urine as unchanged drug

Interactions/incompatibilities:
• Decreased effects: tetracyclines, erythromycins
• Increased effect/toxicity: aminoglycosides, furosemide, probenecid, ethacrynic acid, vancomycin

Lab test interferences:
Increase (false): Creatinine (serum urine), urinary 17-KS
False positive: Urinary protein, direct Coombs' test, urine glucose
Interference: Cross-matching

NURSING CONSIDERATIONS
Assess:
• Nephrotoxicity: increased BUN, creatinine
• I&O ratio
• Blood studies: AST, ALT, CBC, Hct, bilirubin, LDH, alk phospha-

tase, Coombs' test monthly if patient is on long-term therapy
• Electrolytes: K, Na, Cl monthly if patient is on long-term therapy
• Bowel pattern qd; if severe diarrhea occurs, drug should be discontinued; may indicate pseudomembranous colitis
• Urine output; if decreasing, notify physician (may indicate nephrotoxicity)
• Allergic reactions: rash, flushing, urticaria, pruritus
• Bleeding: ecchymosis, bleeding gums, hematuria, stool guaiac daily
• Overgrowth of infection: perineal itching, fever, malaise, redness, pain, swelling, drainage, rash, diarrhea, change in cough sputum

Administer:
• 1 hr before or 2 hr after a meal
• After C&S is completed
• For 7 days to ensure organism death, prevent superimposed infection

Evaluate:
• Therapeutic response: negative C&S

Teach patient/family:
• If diabetic, to use Clinistix or Keto-Diastix
• Not to drink alcohol or take meds with alcohol or reaction may occur
• Complete full course of drug therapy
• Take on an empty stomach 1 hr before or 2 hr after a meal
• Notify physician if breastfeeding or of any side effects

Treatment of overdose: Epinephrine, antihistamines; resuscitate if needed (anaphylaxis)

loratidine
(loer-at-i-deen)
Claritin
Func. class.: Antihistamine
Chem. class.: Selective histamine$_1$ (H$_1$) receptor antagonist

Action: Binds to peripheral histamine receptors, which provides antihistamine action without sedation
Uses: Seasonal rhinitis
Dosage and routes:
• *Adult:* PO 10 mg qd
Available forms: Tabs 10 mg
Side effects/adverse reactions:
CNS: Sedation (more common with increased doses) Blurred vision
Contraindications: Hypersensitivity, acute asthma attacks, lower respiratory tract disease
Precautions: Pregnancy (B), increased intraocular pressure, bronchial asthma
Pharmacokinetics:
Peak 1½ hr, elimination half-life 14½ hr; metabolized in liver to active metabolites, excreted in urine
Interactions/incompatibilities:
• Additive CNS depressant effects: alcohol, other CNS depressants
NURSING CONSIDERATIONS
Perform/provide:
• Storage in tight container at room temperature
Evaluate:
• Therapeutic response: absence of running or congested nose
Teach patient/family:
• To avoid driving or other hazardous activities if drowsiness occurs

L

---

lorazepam

(lor-a'ze-pam)

Ativan, Alzapam, Loraz, Lorazepam, Lorazepam Intensol, Novolorazem,*

Func. class.: Antianxiety
Chem. class.: Benzodiazepine

Controlled Substance Schedule IV

Action: Potentiates the actions of GABA, especially in system and reticular formation

Uses: Anxiety, irritability in psychiatric or organic disorders, preoperatively, insomnia, acute alcohol withdrawal symptoms, anticonvulsant, adjunct in endoscopic procedures

Dosage and routes:

Anxiety

• Adult: PO 2-6 mg/day in divided doses, not to exceed 10 mg/day

Insomnia

• Adult: PO 2-4 mg hs; only minimally effective after 2 wk continuous therapy

Preoperatively

• Adult: IM/IV 2-4 mg

Available forms: Tabs 0.5, 1, 2 mg; IM/IV inj 2, 4 mg/ml

Side effects/adverse reactions:

CNS: Dizziness, drowsiness, confusion, headache, anxiety, tremors, stimulation, fatigue, depression, insomnia, hallucinations, weakness, unsteadiness

GI: Constipation, dry mouth, nausea, vomiting, anorexia, diarrhea

INTEG: Rash, dermatitis, itching

*CV: Orthostatic hypotension, **ECG changes, tachycardia,*** hypotension

EENT: Blurred vision, tinnitus, mydriasis

Contraindications: Hypersensitivity to benzodiazepines, narrow-angle glaucoma, psychosis, pregnancy (D), child <12 yr, history of drug abuse, COPD

Precautions: Elderly, debilitated, hepatic disease, renal disease

Pharmacokinetics:

PO: Peak 1-3 hr, duration 3-6 hr; metabolized by liver; excreted by kidneys; crosses placenta, breast milk; half-life 14 hr

Interactions/incompatibilities:

• Decreased effects of lorazepam: oral contraceptives, valproic acid

• Increased effects of lorazepam: CNS depressants, alcohol, disulfiram, oral contraceptives

• Incompatible with all drugs except cimetidine, ranitidine in sol or syringe

Lab test interferences:

Increase: AST/ALT, serum bilirubin

Decrease: RAIU

False increase: 17-OHCS

NURSING CONSIDERATIONS

Assess:

• B/P (lying, standing), pulse; if systolic B/P drops 20 mm Hg, hold drug, notify physician; respirations q5-15 min if given IV

• Blood studies: CBC during long-term therapy; blood dyscrasias have occurred rarely

• Hepatic studies: AST, ALT, bilirubin, creatinine, LDH, alk phosphatase

• Mental status: mood, sensorium, affect, sleeping pattern, drowsiness, dizziness

• Physical dependency, withdrawal symptoms: headache, nausea, vomiting, muscle pain, weakness, tremors, convulsions, after long-term, excessive use

• Suicidal tendencies

Administer:

• With food or milk for GI symptoms

---

*Available in Canada only

• Crushed if patient is unable to swallow medication whole
• Sugarless gum, hard candy, frequent sips of water for dry mouth
• IV after diluting in an equal volume of sterile water, 5% dextrose or 0.9% NaCl for inj; give through Y-tube or 3-way stopcock; give at 2 mg or less over 1 min
• Deep into large muscle mass (IM inj)

Perform/provide:
• Assistance with ambulation during beginning therapy, since drowsiness/dizziness occurs
• Safety measures, including side rails
• Check to see whether PO medication has been swallowed
• Store parenteral form in refrigerator

Evaluate:
• Therapeutic response: decreased anxiety, restlessness, insomnia

Teach patient/family:
• That drug may be taken with food
• Not to be used for everyday stress or used longer than 4 mo unless directed by physician
• Not to take more than prescribed amount; may be habit forming
• To avoid OTC preparations (cough, cold, hay fever) unless approved by physician
• To avoid driving, activities that require alertness, since drowsiness may occur
• To avoid alcohol ingestion, other psychotropic medications, unless prescribed by physician
• Not to discontinue medication abruptly after long-term use
• To rise slowly or fainting may occur, especially elderly
• That drowsiness may worsen at beginning of treatment
• To use birth control if child-bearing age

Treatment of overdose: Lavage, VS, supportive care, flumazenil

---

lovastatin
(lo'va-sta-tin)
Mevacor
Func. class.: Cholesterol-lowering agent
Chem. class.: Aspergillus terreus strain derivative

Action: Inhibits HMG-COA reductase enzyme, which reduces cholesterol synthesis
Uses: As an adjunct in primary hypercholesterolemia (types IIa, IIb), mixed hyperlipidemia
Dosage and routes:
(Patient should first be placed on a cholesterol-lowering diet)
• *Adult:* PO 20 mg qd with evening meal; may increase to 20-80 mg/d in single or divided doses, not to exceed 80 mg/d; dosage adjustments should be made qmo
Available forms: Tabs 20 mg
Side effects/adverse reactions:
GI: Nausea, constipation, diarrhea, dyspepsia, flatus, abdominal pain, heartburn, liver dysfunction
MS: Muscle cramps, myalgia, myositis, rhabdomyolysis
CNS: Dizziness, headache
INTEG: Rash, pruritus
EENT: Blurred vision, dysgeusia, lens opacities
Contraindications: Pregnancy (X), lactation, active liver disease
Precautions: Past liver disease, alcoholics, severe acute infections, trauma, hypotension, uncontrolled seizure disorders, severe metabolic disorders, electrolyte imbalances
Pharmacokinetics:
PO: Peak 2-4 hr, metabolized in liver (metabolites), highly protein bound, excreted in urine, feces,

crosses placenta, excreted in breast milk

Interactions/incompatibilities:

• Increased effects: bile acid sequestrants, coumadin

• Increased myalgia, myositis: cyclosporine, gemfibrozil, niacin

Lab test interferences:

Increase: CPK, liver function tests

NURSING CONSIDERATIONS

Assess:

• Cholesterol levels periodically during treatment

• Liver function studies q1-2mo during the first 1½ yr of treatment; AST, ALT, liver function tests may increase

• Renal function in patients with compromised renal system: BUN, creatinine, I&O ratio

• Eyes with slit lamp before, 1 mo after treatment begins, annually, lens opacities may occur

Administer:

• In evening with meal; if dose is increased, take with breakfast and evening meal

Perform/provide:

• Storage in cool environment in tight light-resistant container

Evaluate:

• Therapeutic response: decrease in cholesterol to desired level after 8 wk

Teach patient/family:

• That treatment will take several years

• That blood work and eye exam will be necessary during treatment

• To report blurred vision, severe GI symptoms, dizziness, headache

• That previously prescribed regimen will continue: low-cholesterol diet, exercise program

---

loxapine succinate/ loxapine HCl

(lox'a'peen)

Loxapax,* Loxapine Succinate, Loxitane IM, Loxitane/Loxitane-C

Func. class.: Antipsychotic/ neuroleptic

Chem. class.: Dibenzoxazepine

Action: Depresses cerebral cortex, hypothalamus, limbic system, which control activity and aggression; blocks neurotransmission produced by dopamine at synapse; exhibits strong α-adrenergic, anticholinergic blocking action; mechanism for antipsychotic effects is unclear

Uses: Psychotic disorders

Dosage and routes:

• *Adult:* PO 10 mg bid-qid initially, may be rapidly increased depending on severity of condition, maintenance 60-100 mg/day; IM 12.5-50 mg q4-6hr or more until desired response, then start PO form

Available forms: Caps 5, 10, 25, 50 mg; conc 25 mg/ml; inj IM 50 mg/ml

Side effects/adverse reactions:

*RESP: **Laryngospasm,** dyspnea, **respiratory depression***

*CNS: Extrapyramidal symptoms: pseudoparkinsonism, akathisia, dystonia, tardive dyskinesia, drowsiness, headache, **seizures,** confusion*

*HEMA: **Anemia, leukopenia, leukocytosis, agranulocytosis***

INTEG: Rash, photosensitivity, dermatitis

EENT: Blurred vision, glaucoma

GI: Dry mouth, nausea, vomiting, anorexia, constipation, diarrhea, jaundice, weight gain

---

GU: Urinary retention, urinary frequency, enuresis, impotence, amenorrhea, gynecomastia

*CV: Orthostatic hypotension, **cardiac arrest,** ECG changes, tachycardia*

Contraindications: Hypersensitivity, blood dyscrasias, coma, child, brain damage, bone marrow depression, alcohol and barbiturate withdrawal states

Precautions: Pregnancy (C), lactation, seizure disorders, hepatic disease, cardiac disease, prostatic hypertrophy, cardiac conditions child <16 yr

Pharmacokinetics:

PO: Onset 20-30 min, peak 2-4 hr, duration 12 hr

IM: Onset 15-30 min, peak 15-20 min, duration 12 hr

Metabolized by liver; excreted in urine; crosses placenta; enters breast milk; initial half-life 5 hr; terminal half-life 19 hr

Interactions/incompatibilities:

• Toxicity: epinephrine
• Increased extrapyramidal effect: other antipsychotics
• Decreased effects: guanadrel, guanethidine
• Increased CNS depression: MAOIs, antidepressants

NURSING CONSIDERATIONS
Assess:

• Mental status before initial administration
• Swallowing of PO medication; check for hoarding or giving of medication to other patients
• I&O ratio; palpate bladder if low urinary output occurs
• Bilirubin, CBC, liver function studies monthly
• Urinalysis is recommended before and during prolonged therapy
• Affect, orientation, LOC, reflexes, gait, coordination, sleep pattern disturbances
• B/P standing and lying; take pulse and respirations q4h during initial treatment; establish baseline before starting treatment; report drops of 30 mm Hg
• Dizziness, faintness, palpitations, tachycardia on rising
• Extrapyramidal symptoms including akathisia (inability to sit still, no pattern to movements), tardive dyskinesia (bizarre movements of the jaw, mouth, tongue, extremities), pseudoparkinsonism (rigidity, tremors, pill rolling, shuffling gait)
• Skin turgor daily
• For neuroleptic malignant syndrome: muscle rigidity, increased CPK, altered mental status, hyperthermia
• Constipation, urinary retention daily; if these occur, increase bulk, water in diet

Administer:

• Reduced dose to elderly
• Antiparkinsonian agent if extrapyramidal symptoms occur
• IM injection into large muscle mass
• Concentrate mixed in orange or grapefruit juice

Perform/provide:

• Decreased noise input by dimming lights, avoiding loud noises
• Supervised ambulation until stabilized on medication; do not involve in strenuous exercise program because fainting is possible; patient should not stand still for long periods
• Increased fluids to prevent constipation
• Sips of water, candy, gum for dry mouth
• Storage in tight, light-resistant container

italics = common side effects   ***bold italic*** = life threatening reactions

Evaluate:

• Therapeutic response: decrease in emotional excitement, hallucinations, delusions, paranoia; reorganization of patterns of thought, speech

Teach patient/family:

• That orthostatic hypotension may occur and to rise from sitting or lying position gradually

• To remain lying down after IM injection for at least 30 min

• To avoid hot tubs, hot showers, tub baths, since hypotension may occur

• To avoid abrupt withdrawal of this drug, or EPS may result; drug should be withdrawn slowly

• To avoid OTC preparations (cough, hay fever, cold) unless approved by physician, since serious drug interactions may occur; avoid use with alcohol or CNS depressants; increased drowsiness may occur

• To avoid hazardous activities until stabilized on medication

• To use a sunscreen during sun exposure to prevent burns

• Regarding compliance with drug regimen; warn patient about avoiding OTC preparations

• About necessity for meticulous oral hygiene, since oral candidiasis may occur

• To report impaired vision, jaundice, tremors, muscle twitching

• That in hot weather heat stroke may occur; take extra precautions to stay cool

Treatment of overdose: Lavage if orally ingested; provide an airway

lypressin
(lye-press'in)
Diapid
Func. class.: Pituitary hormone
Chem. class.: Lysine vasopressin

Action: Promotes reabsorption of water by action on renal tubular epithelium

Uses: Nonnephrogenic diabetes insipidus

Dosage and routes:

• *Adult:* INTRANASAL 1-2 sprays in one or both nostrils qid, an extra dose hs if needed

Available forms: Intranasal 0.185 mg/ml

Side effects/adverse reactions:

EENT: Nasal irritation, congestion, rhinitis, conjunctivitis, rhinorrhea

CNS: Headache

GI: Nausea, heartburn, cramps

MISC: Chest tightness, cough, dyspnea

Precautions: CAD, pregnancy (B)

Pharmacokinetics:

NASAL: Onset 1 hr, duration 3-8 hr, half-life 15 min; metabolized in liver, kidneys, excreted in urine

NURSING CONSIDERATIONS

Assess:

• Nares for irritation

• I&O ratio; weight daily; check for edema in extremities; if water retention is severe, diuretic may be prescribed

• Water intoxication: lethargy, behavioral changes, disorientation, neuromuscular excitability

Perform/provide:

• Storage at room temperature

Evaluate:

• Therapeutic response: absence of severe thirst, decreased urine output, osmolality

Teach patient/family:
• To clear nasal passages before using drug, not to inhale spray
• To carry drug at all times

---

mafenide acetate (topical)
(ma'fe-nide)
Sulfamylon
Func. class.: Local antiinfective
Chem. class.: Sulfonamide

Action: Interferes with bacterial cell wall synthesis
Uses: Adjunctive treatment in burns (2nd, 3rd degree)
Dosage and routes:
• *Adult and child:* TOP apply 1/16 in to affected area qd-bid, reapply as needed
Available forms: Cream 85 mg/g as acetate
Side effects/adverse reactions:
INTEG: Rash, urticaria, stinging, burning, bleeding, excoriation of new skin, superinfections, pruritus, blisters, facial edema, hives, erythema
OTHER: Metabolic acidosis, tachypnea, ***bone marrow suppression, fatal hemolytic anemia, eosinophilia***
Contraindications: Hypersensitivity, inhalation injury
Precautions: Pregnancy (C), impaired pulmonary function, lactation, impaired renal function
• Allergic reaction: burning, stinging, swelling, redness
• Fluid loss: decreased urinary output
NURSING CONSIDERATIONS
Administer:
• Analgesic before application if needed
• Enough medication to cover burns completely; the [...] covered at all times
• After cleansing debris from bu[...] before each application
• Using aseptic technique to debrided areas
Perform/provide:
• Storage at room temperature in dry place
Evaluate:
• Therapeutic response: appearance of granulation tissue
Teach patient/family:
• That therapy will continue until area is ready for grafting
• About signs of superimposed infection
• About changes in respiratory activity

---

magaldrate (hydroxy-magnesium aluminate)
(mag' al-drate)
Lowsium, Riopan, Riopan Extra Strength
Func. class.: Antacid
Chem. class.: Aluminum/magnesium hydroxide

Action: Neutralizes gastric acidity
Uses: Antacid
Dosage and routes:
• *Adult:* PO 1-2 (480-1080 mg) between meals, hs, not to exceed 20 tabs/d; chew tab 1-2 (480-960 mg) between meals, hs, not to exceed 20 tabs/d; susp 5-10 ml (400-800 mg) with H_2O between meals, hs, not to exceed 100 ml/d
Available forms: Tabs 480 mg; chew tabs 480 mg; susp 540 mg/5 ml, 480 mg/5 ml, 1080 mg/5 ml
Side effects/adverse reactions:
GI: Constipation, diarrhea
META: Hypermagnesium

---

italics = common side effects   ***bold italic*** = life threatening reactions

...sitiv-
...n prod-

...uid restric-
...tility, GI ob-
...on, renal dis-
ea...   ...ed diets, pregnancy

Pharmacokinetics:
PO: Duration 60 min
Interactions/incompatibilities:
• Decreased effectiveness of: tetracyclines, ketoconazole
• Decreased absorption of: anticholinergics, chlordiazepoxide, cimetidine, corticosteroids, iron salts, phenothiazines, phenytoin, salicylates

NURSING CONSIDERATIONS
Assess:
• Serum Mg^{++} levels with impaired renal function
• Constipation: increase bulk in diet if needed
Administer:
• Laxatives or stool softeners if constipation occurs
• After shaking; give between meals and hs
Evaluate:
• Therapeutic response: absence of pain, decreased acidity
Teach patient/family:
• To separate enteric-coated drugs and antacid by 1 hr

---

magnesium carbonate

Func. class.: Antacid
Chem. class.: Magnesium product

Action: Neutralizes gastric acidity
Uses: Antacid, constipation
Dosage and routes:
• *Adult:* PO 0.5-2 g between meals with water

Laxative
• *Adult:* PO 8 g with water hs
Available forms: Powder
Side effects/adverse reactions:
GI: Diarrhea, flatulence, cramps, belching, nausea, vomiting, impaction, *obstruction,* pain
META: Hypermagnesia: *weakness, lethargy, depression, decreased B/P, increased pulse, respiratory depression, coma*
Contraindications: Hypersensitivity
Precautions: Severe renal disease, GI bleeding, diarrhea, intestinal obstruction, pregnancy (C)
Pharmacokinetics:
PO: Excreted in urine
Interactions/incompatibilities:
• Decreased effectiveness of: tetracyclines
• Decreased absorption of: anticholinergics, chlordiazepoxide, cimetidine, corticosteroids, iron salts

NURSING CONSIDERATIONS
Assess:
Lab test interferences:
Increase: Urinary pH, gastrin
Decrease: K^+
Administer:
• After mixing with water
Evaluate:
• Therapeutic response: absence of pain, decreased acidity
Teach patient/family:
• Not to change antacids unless directed by physician
• To store in tightly covered container

---

magnesium oxide
Mag-Ox, Maox, Uro-Mag
Func. class.: Antacid
Chem. class.: Magnesium product

Action: Neutralizes gastric acidity

Uses: Constipation, hypomagnesemia, antacid
Dosage and routes:
• *Adult:* PO 250 mg-1 g pc, hs with 4-8 oz water
Laxative
• *Adult:* PO 2-4 g with water hs
Hypomagnesemia
• *Adult:* PO 650-1.3 g qd
Available forms: Caps 140; tabs 400, 420 mg
Side effects/adverse reactions:
GU: Renal stones
GI: Diarrhea, flatulence, cramps, belching, nausea, vomiting
META: Hypermagnesemia: *weakness, lethargy, depression, decreased B/P, increased pulse, respiratory depression, coma*
Contraindications: Hypersensitivity
Precautions: Severe renal disease, GI bleeding, diarrhea, intestinal obstruction, pregnancy (C)
Pharmacokinetics:
PO: Excreted in urine
Interactions/incompatibilities:
• Decreased effectiveness of: tetracyclines, ketoconazole
• Decreased absorption of: anticholinergics, chlordiazepoxide, cimetidine, corticosteroids, iron salts, phenothiazines, phenytoin
Lab test interferences:
Increase: Urinary pH, gastrin
Decrease: K+

NURSING CONSIDERATIONS
Assess:
• Decreased constipation, characteristics of stools
Perform/provide:
• Storage in airtight container
Evaluate:
• Therapeutic response: absence of pain, decreased acidity
Teach patient/family:
• Not to change antacids unless directed by physician

| **magnesium salicylate** |
| Doan's pills, Magan, Mobidin |
| *Func. class.:* Nonnarcotic analgesic |
| *Chem. class.:* Salicylate |

Action: Blocks pain impulses in CNS that occur in response to inhibition of prostaglandin synthesis; antipyretic action results from inhibition of hypothalamic heat-regulating center to produce vasodilation to allow heat dissipation
Uses: Mild to moderate pain or fever including arthritis, juvenile rheumatoid arthritis
Dosage and routes:
Arthritis
• *Adult:* PO not to exceed 4.8 g/d in divided doses
Pain/fever
• *Adult:* PO 600 mg tid or qid
Available forms: Tabs 325, 545, 600 mg
Side effects/adverse reactions:
HEMA: **Thrombocytopenia, agranulocytosis, leukopenia, neutropenia, hemolytic anemia,** increased pro-time
CNS: Stimulation, drowsiness, dizziness, confusion, **convulsion,** headache, flushing, hallucinations, coma
GI: Nausea, vomiting, GI bleeding, diarrhea, heartburn, anorexia, **hepatitis**
INTEG: Rash, urticaria, bruising
EENT: Tinnitus, hearing loss
CV: Rapid pulse, **pulmonary edema**
RESP: Wheezing, hyperpnea
ENDO: Hypoglycemia, hyponatremia, hypokalemia
Contraindications: Hypersensitivity to salicylates, GI bleeding, bleeding disorders, children <12 yr, Vit K deficiency

M

---

italics = common side effects   **bold italic** = life threatening reactions

Precautions: Anemia, hepatic disease, renal disease, Hodgkin's disease, pregnancy (C), lactation

Pharmacokinetics:

PO: Onset 15-30 min, peak 1-2 hr, duration 4-6 hr; metabolized by liver; excreted by kidneys; crosses placenta; excreted in breast milk; half-life 1-3½ hr

Interactions/incompatibilities:

• Decreased effects of magnesium salicylate: antacids, steroids, urinary alkalizers

• Increased blood loss: alcohol, heparin

• Increased effects of: anticoagulants, insulin, methotrexate

• Decreased effects of: probenecid, spironolactone, sulfinpyrazone, sulfonylmides

• Toxic effects: PABA

• Decreased blood sugar levels: salicylates

Lab test interferences:

Increase: Coagulation studies, liver function studies, serum uric acid, amylase, CO_2, urinary protein

Decrease: Serum K, PBI, cholesterol, blood glucose

Interfere: Urine catecholamines, pregnancy test

NURSING CONSIDERATIONS

Assess:

• Liver function studies: AST, ALT, bilirubin, creatinine if patient is on long-term therapy

• Renal function studies: BUN, urine creatinine if patient is on long-term therapy

• Blood studies: CBC, Hct, Hgb, pro-time if patient is on long-term therapy

• I&O ratio; decreasing output may indicate renal failure (long-term therapy)

• Hepatotoxicity: dark urine, clay-colored stools, yellowing of skin and sclera, itching, abdominal pain, fever, diarrhea if patient is on long-term therapy

• Allergic reactions: rash, urticaria; if these occur, drug may have to be discontinued

• Renal dysfunction: decreased urine output

• Ototoxicity: tinnitus, ringing, roaring in ears; audiometric testing is needed before, after long-term therapy

• Visual changes: blurring, halos, corneal and retinal damage

• Edema in feet, ankles, legs

• Prior drug history; there are many drug interactions

Administer:

• To patient crushed or whole; chewable tablets may be chewed

• With food or milk to decrease gastric symptoms; give 30 min before or 2 hr after antacids

• With full glass of water

Evaluate:

• Therapeutic response: decreased pain, fever

Teach patient/family:

• To report any symptoms of hepatotoxicity, renal toxicity, visual changes, ototoxicity, allergic reactions, bleeding (long-term therapy)

• Not to exceed recommended dosage; acute poisoning may result

• To read label on other OTC drugs; many contain aspirin

• That therapeutic response takes 2 wk (arthritis)

• To avoid alcohol ingestion; GI bleeding may occur

• That if anticoagulants are given with this drug, both should be discontinued 2 wk before surgery

Treatment of overdose: Lavage, activated charcoal, monitor electrolytes, VS

---

magnesium salts

Concentrated Phillip's Milk of Magnesia, Milk of Magnesia, Phillip's Milk of Magnesia

Func. class.: Laxative, saline

Action: Increases osmotic pressure, draws fluid into colon neutralizes HCl

Uses: Constipation, bowel preparation before surgery or examination

Dosage and routes:
• *Adult:* PO 30-60 ml hs (Milk of Magnesia), 300 mg
• *Adult and child >6 yr:* PO 15 g in 8 oz H_2O (magnesium sulfate); PO 10-20 ml (concentrated Milk of Magnesia); PO 5-10 oz hs (magnesium citrate)
• *Child 2-6 yr:* 5-15 ml (Milk of Magnesia)

Available forms: Oral sol, susp 77.5 mg/g; tabs 300, 600 mg

Side effects/adverse reactions:
CNS: Muscle weakness, flushing, sweating, confusion, sedation, depressed reflexes, ***flaccid, paralysis,*** hypothermia
GI: Nausea, vomiting, anorexia, cramps
CV: Hypotension, heart block, ***circulatory collapse***
META: Electrolyte, fluid imbalances

Contraindications: Hypersensitivity, renal diseases, abdominal pain, nausea/vomiting, obstruction, acute surgical abdomen, rectal bleeding

Precautions: Pregnancy (B)

Pharmacokinetics:
PO: Peak 1-2 hr; excreted in feces

Interactions/incompatibilities:
• Increased CNS depression: CNS depressants, barbiturates, narcotics, anesthetics

NURSING CONSIDERATIONS

Assess:
• I&O ratio; check for decrease in urinary output
• Cause of constipation; identify whether fluids, bulk, or exercise is missing from life-style
• Cramping, rectal bleeding, nausea, vomiting; if these symptoms occur, drug should be discontinued
• Mg toxicity: thirst, confusion, decrease in reflexes

Administer:
• With 8 oz H_2O

Evaluate:
• Therapeutic response: decreased constipation

Teach patient/family:
• Not to use laxatives for long-term therapy; bowel tone will be lost
• Chilling helps the taste of magnesium citrate
• Shake suspension well
• Do not give at hs as a laxative; may interfere with sleep
• Give citrus fruit after administering to counteract unpleasant taste

M

magnesium sulfate

Func. class.: Anticonvulsant
Chem. class.: Magnesium product

Action: Decreases acetylcholine in motor nerve terminals, which is responsible for anticonvulsant properties; osmotically retains fluid, which increases amount of water in feces when used as laxative; reduces SA node impulse formation, prolongs conduction time in myocardium

Uses: Hypomagnesemic seizures, control of seizures in pregnancy-induced hypertension, seizures in acute nephritis

italics = common side effects   ***bold italic*** = life threatening reactions

Dosage and routes:

Hypomagnesemic seizures
• *Adult:* IV 1-2 g over 15 min, then 1 g IM q4-6h, depending on response

Nephritis
• *Child:* IM 20-40 mg/kg in 20% sol, repeat as needed

Preeclampsia/eclampsia
• *Adult:* IV 4 g/250 ml D₅W and 4 g IM, then 4 g IM q4h prn; or 4 g IV loading dose, then 1-4 g IV inf hourly, not to exceed 3 ml/min

Available forms: Inj IV, IM 10%, 50%, 12.5%, 25%; granules

Side effects/adverse reactions:
CNS: *Sweating, depressed deep tendon reflexes, flushing,* drowsiness, flaccid paralysis, hypothermia, weakness, sedation
RESP: ***Paralysis***
CV: *Hypotension,* **circulatory collapse, heart block,** decreased cardiac function

Contraindications: Hypersensitivity, myocardial infarction, renal disease

Precaution: Pregnancy (C)

Pharmacokinetics:
IV: Onset 1-5 min, duration 30 min
IM: Onset 1 hr, duration 3-4 hr
Excreted by kidneys

Interactions/incompatibilities:
• Increased CNS depression: barbiturates, general anesthetics, narcotics, antipsychotics
• Increased effects of: neuromuscular blockers
• Incompatible with alkalies, alcohol, calcium gluconate, chlorpromazine, clindamycin, dobutamine, hydrocortisone, phosphates, polymyxin B, phytonadione, procaine, salicylates, NaCO₃, tobramycin, Vit B complex, IV fat emulsion 10%

NURSING CONSIDERATIONS
Assess:
• VS q15min after IV dose; do not exceed 150 mg/min
• Cardiac function: monitoring, Mg levels
• Timing of contractions; determine intensity; monitor fetal heart rate, reactivity; may decrease with this drug if using during labor
• I&O: should remain at 30 ml/hr or more; if less than this, notify physician
• Urine output before each dose; output should be 100 ml/4 hr or more
• Mental status: mood, sensorium, affect, memory (long, short)
• Respiratory dysfunction: respiratory depression, character, rate, rhythm; hold drug if respirations are <16/min
• Hypermagnesemia: depressed patellar reflex, flushing, polydipsia, confusion, weakness, flaccid paralysis, hypothermia, dyspnea begin to appear at blood levels of 4 mEq/L
• Respiratory rate, rhythm of newborn if drug was given 24 hr before delivery or less; check reflexes of newborn whose mother received this drug before delivery
• Reflexes: knee jerk, patellar; decrease signals Mg⁺⁺ toxicity; mild depression will occur in therapeutic range

Administer:
• Only when calcium gluconate available for magnesium toxicity
• IV undiluted 1.5 ml of 10% sol over 1 min; may dilute to 20% sol, infuse over 3 hr
• IV at less than 150 mg/min; circulatory collapse may occur
• IV as a single dose infused/3 hr in hypomagnesemia

*Available in Canada only

Perform/provide:

• Seizure precautions: placing in dark room with decreased stimuli, padded side rails

Evaluate:

• Therapeutic response; absence of seizures

Teach patient/family:

• Symptoms of hypermagnesemia

Treatment of overdose: Stop drug; administer calcium gluconate; monitor reflexes, magnesium levels; ECG monitoring if Ca is administered

---

magnesium trisilicate
Trisomin

Func. class.: Antacid

Chem. class.: Magnesium product

Action: Neutralizes gastric acidity

Uses: Constipation, hypomagnesemia

Dosage and routes:

• *Adult:* PO 1-4 g qid with 4 oz of water

Available forms: Powder, tabs 488 mg

Side effects/adverse reactions:

GI: Diarrhea, flatulence, cramps, belching, nausea, vomiting

META: Hypermagnesemia: *weakness, lethargy, depression, decreased B/P, increased pulse, **respiratory depression, coma***

Contraindications: Hypersensitivity to this drug

Precautions: Severe renal disease, pregnancy (C)

Pharmacokinetics:

PO: Excreted in urine

Interactions/incompatibilities:

• Decreased effectiveness of: tetracyclines, ketoconazole

• Decreased absorption of: anticholinergics, chlordiazepoxide, cimet-

---

idine
phen
Lab t
Increa
Decre

NURS

Assess:

• Decrea
teristics of s......

Administer:

• After mixing with H_2O

Evaluate:

• Therapeutic response; absence of pain, decreased acidity

Teach patient/family:

• Not to change antacids unless directed by physician

• That tabs must be chewed before swallowing

• That drug has a delayed reaction

• To separate doses of other drugs by 1 hr

---

mannitol
(man'i-tole)

Mannitol, Osmitrol, Resectial

Func. class.: Osmotic diuretic

Chem. class.: Hexahydric alcohol

Action: Acts by increasing osmolarity of glomerular filtrate, which raises osmotic pressure of fluid in renal tubules; there is a decrease in reabsorption of water electrolytes, increase in urinary output, sodium, chloride excretion

Uses: Edema, promote systemic diuresis, decrease in cerebral edema, decrease intraocular pressure, improve renal function in acute renal failure, chemical poisoning

Dosage and routes:

Oliguria, prevention

• *Adult:* IV 50-100 g of a 5%-25% sol

mannitol

Oliguria, treat

• *Adult:* IV

20%-25%

20%

In

654

M

300-400 mg/kg of a
sol up to 100 g of a 15%-
sol

*raocular pressure/intracranial
pressure*
• *Adult:* IV 1.5-2 g/kg of a 15%-
25% sol over ½-1 hr
Renal failure
• *Adult:* IV 50-200 g/24 hr, adjusted to maintain output of 30-50 mg/hr
Diuresis in drug intoxication
• *Adult and child >12 yr:* 5%-10% sol continuously up to 200 g IV, while maintaining 100-500 ml output/hr
Available forms: Inj IV 5%, 10%, 15%, 20%, 25%

Side effects/adverse reactions:
GU: Marked diuresis, urinary retention, thirst
CNS: Dizziness, headache, **convulsions,** rebound increased ICP, confusion
GI: Nausea, vomiting, dry mouth, diarrhea
CV: Edema, thrombophlebitis, hypotension, hypertension, tachycardia, angina-like chest pains, fever, chills
RESP: Pulmonary congestion
ELECT: Fluid, electrolyte imbalances, acidosis, electrolyte loss, dehydration
EENT: Loss of hearing, blurred vision, nasal congestion, decreased intraocular pressure
Contraindications: Active intracranial bleeding, hypersensitivity, anuria, severe pulmonary congestion, edema, severe dehydration
Precautions: Dehydration, pregnancy (C), severe renal disease, CHF, lactation
Pharmacokinetics:
IV: Onset 30-60 min for diuresis, ½-1 hr for intraocular pressure, 25 min for cerebrospinal fluid; duration 4-6 hr for intraocular pressure, 3-8 hr for cerebrospinal fluid; excreted in urine

Interactions/incompatibilities:
• Decreased effect: lithium
• Increased effects of: EDTA
• Incompatible with whole blood, KCl, NaCl

Lab test interferences:
Interference: Inorganic phosphorus, ethylene glycol

NURSING CONSIDERATIONS
Assess:
• Weight, I&O daily to determine fluid loss; effect of drug may be decreased if used qd; output hourly if needed
• Rate, depth, rhythm of respiration, effect of exertion
• B/P lying, standing; postural hypotension may occur
• Electrolytes: K, Na, Cl; include BUN, CBC, serum creatinine, blood pH, ABGs
• Signs of metabolic acidosis: drowsiness, restlessness
• Signs of hypokalemia: postural hypotension, malaise, fatigue, tachycardia, leg cramps, weakness
• Rashes, temperature elevation qd
• Confusion, especially in elderly; take safety precautions if needed
• Hydration including skin turgor, thirst, dry mucous membranes
Administer:
• IV in 15%-25% solutions with filter; give over ½-1½ hr; rapid infusion may worsen CHF; warm in hot water and shake to dissolve crystals before giving
• Test dose in severe oliguria, 0.2 g/kg over 3-5 min; if no urine increase, give 2nd test dose; if no response, reassess patient
Evaluate:
• Therapeutic response: improvement in edema of feet, legs, sacral

area daily if medication is being used in CHF

Teach patient/family:
• To increase fluid intake to 2-3 L/day unless contraindicated; to rise slowly from lying or sitting position

Treatment of overdose: Discontinue infusion; correct fluid, electrolyte imbalances; hemodialysis; monitor hydration, CV, renal function

---

maprotiline HCl
(ma-proe′ti-leen)
Ludiomil, Maprotiline HCl
Func. class.: Antidepressant
Chem. class.: Tetracyclic

Action: Blocks reuptake of norepinephrine, serotonin into nerve endings, increasing action of norepinephrine, serotonin in nerve cells

Uses: Depression, dysthymic disorder, bipolar disorder—depressed, agitated depression

Dosage and routes:
• *Adult:* PO 75 mg/day in moderate depression, may increase to 150 mg/day; not to exceed 225 mg in hospitalized patients; severely depressed patients who are hospitalized may be given 300 mg/day
• *Elderly:* 50-75 mg/day

Available forms: Tabs 25, 50, 75 mg

Side effects/adverse reactions:
*HEMA: **Agranulocytosis, thrombocytopenia, eosinophilia, leukopenia***
CNS: Dizziness, drowsiness, confusion, headache, anxiety, tremors, stimulation, weakness, insomnia, nightmares, EPS (elderly), increased psychiatric symptoms, *seizures*
GI: Diarrhea, dry mouth, nausea, vomiting, ***paralytic ileus,*** increased appetite, cramps, epigastric distress, jaundice, ***hepatitis,*** stomatitis
*GU: Retention, **acute renal failure***
INTEG: Rash, urticaria, sweating, pruritus, photosensitivity
*CV: Orthostatic hypotension, ECG changes, tachycardia, **hypertension,*** palpitations
EENT: Blurred vision, tinnitus, mydriasis

Contraindications: Hypersensitivity to tricyclic antidepressants, recovery phase of myocardial infarction, convulsive disorders, prostatic hypertrophy

Precautions: Suicidal patients, severe depression, increased intraocular pressure, narrow-angle glaucoma, urinary retention, cardiac disease, hepatic disease, hypothyroidism, hyperthyroidism, electroshock therapy, elective surgery, elderly, pregnancy (B)

Pharmacokinetics:
PO: Onset 15-30 min, peak 12 hr, duration up to 3 wk, steady state 6-10 days; metabolized by liver; excreted by kidneys, feces; crosses placenta; half-life 21-25 hr

Interactions/incompatibilities:
• Decreased effects of: guanethidine, clonidine, indirect-acting sympathomimetics (ephedrine)
• Increased effects of: direct-acting sympathomimetics (epinephrine), alcohol, barbiturates, benzodiazepines, CNS depressants
• Hyperpyretic crisis, convulsions, hypertensive episode: MAOI (pargyline [Eutonyl])

Lab test interferences:
Increase: Serum bilirubin, blood glucose, alk phosphatase
False increase: Urinary catecholamines
Decrease: VMA, 5-HIAA

---

italics = common side effects   ***bold italic*** = life threatening reactions

NURSING CONSIDERATIONS
Assess:

• B/P (lying, standing), pulse q4h; if systolic B/P drops 20 mm Hg, hold drug, notify physician; take vital signs q4h in patients with cardiovascular disease

• Blood studies: CBC, leukocytes, differential, cardiac enzymes if patient is receiving long-term therapy

• Hepatic studies: AST, ALT, bilirubin, creatinine

• Weight qwk; appetite may increase with drug

• ECG for flattening of T wave, bundle branch block, AV block, dysrhythmias in cardiac patients

• EPS primarily in elderly: rigidity, dystonia, akathisia

• Mental status: mood, sensorium, affect, suicidal tendencies, increase in psychiatric symptoms: depression, panic

• Urinary retention, constipation; constipation is more likely to occur in children

• Withdrawal symptoms: headache, nausea, vomiting, muscle pain, weakness; do not usually occur unless drug was discontinued abruptly

• Alcohol consumption; if alcohol is consumed, hold dose until morning

Administer:

• Increased fluids, bulk in diet if constipation occurs, especially elderly

• With food or milk for GI symptoms

• Dosage hs if oversedation occurs during day; may take entire dose hs; elderly may not tolerate once/day dosing

• Gum, hard candy, or frequent sips of water for dry mouth

• Concentrate with fruit juice, water, or milk to disguise taste

Perform/provide:

• Storage in tight container at room temperature; do not freeze

• Assistance with ambulation during beginning therapy, since drowsiness/dizziness occurs

• Safety measures, including side rails, primarily in elderly

• Checking to see PO medication swallowed

Evaluate:

• Therapeutic response: decreased depression

Teach patient/family:

• That therapeutic effects may take 2-3 wk

• Use of caution in driving, other activities requiring alertness, because of drowsiness, dizziness, blurred vision

• To avoid alcohol ingestion, other CNS depressants

• Not to discontinue medication quickly after long-term use; may cause nausea, headache, malaise

• To wear sunscreen or large hat, since photosensitivity occurs

Treatment of overdose: ECG monitoring, induce emesis; lavage, activated charcoal; administer anticonvulsant

---

masoprocol
(mas-o-proe'-cole)
Actinex
Func. class.: Miscellaneous topical product

Action: Unknown
Uses: Actinic keratoses
Dosage and routes:
• *Adult:* Top apply to lesion bid × 2-4 wk
Available forms: Cream 10%
Side effects/adverse reactions:
INTEG: Irritation, redness, flaking,

itching, burning, tightness of the skin, edema, dryness, soreness
Contraindications: Hypersensitivity, children
Precautions: Avoid occlusive dressings, pregnancy (B), lactation
Pharmacokinetics: <2% absorption over 96-hr period
NURSING CONSIDERATIONS
Assess:
• Number and severity of lesions; inflammation, erythema, flaking, itching, burning, tightness, bleeding, edema
Administer:
• By covering lesion with cream; do not cover
Perform/provide:
• Storage out of reach of children
Evaluate:
• Therapeutic response: decrease in size and number of lesions
Teach patient/family:
• To avoid all other medications unless prescribed by physician

---

mazindol
(may'zin-dole)
Mazanor, Sanorex
Func. class.: Anorexiant
Chem. class.: Imidazoisoindole derivative

Controlled Substance Schedule IV
Action: Acts on central adrenergic and dopaminergic pathways to stimulate satiety center in hypothalamic, limbic regions
Uses: Exogenous obesity
Dosage and routes:
• *Adult:* PO 1 mg ac, or 2 mg 1 hr ac lunch
Available forms: Tabs 1, 2 mg
Side effects/adverse reactions:
*HEMA: **Bone marrow depression, leukopenia, agranulocytosis***

EENT: Mydriasis, blurred vision, eye irritation
MISC: Hair loss, muscle pain, flushing, fever
CNS: Hyperactivity, insomnia, restlessness, dizziness, headache, stimulation, irritability, drowsiness, weakness, tremor, fatigue, malaise, euphoria, depression, confusion
GI: Nausea, anorexia, dry mouth, diarrhea, constipation, vomiting
GU: Impotence, change in libido, dysuria, menstrual irregularities, testicular pain, urinary frequency
CV: Palpitations, tachycardia, hypertension, dysrhythmias, pulmonary hypertension
INTEG: Urticaria, rash, pallor, shivering, sweating
Contraindications: Hypersensitivity to sympathomimetic amine, glaucoma, drug abuse, cardiovascular disease, children <12 yr, hypertension, severe arteriosclerosis, agitated states, hyperthyroidism
Precautions: Diabetes mellitus, convulsive disorders, pregnancy (C), lactation
Pharmacokinetics:
PO: Onset ½-1 hr, duration 8-15 hr; metabolized by liver, excreted by kidneys
Interactions/incompatibilities:
• Hypertensive crisis: MAOIs or within 14 days of MAOIs, furazolidone
• Decreased effects of mazindol: tricyclics
• Decreased effects of: guanethidine
• Increased effects of: insulin
NURSING CONSIDERATIONS
Assess:
• VS, B/P, since this drug may reverse antihypertensives; check patients with cardiac disease more often

---

italics = common side effects   ***bold italic*** = life threatening reactions

• CBC, urinalysis, in diabetes: blood sugar, urine sugar; insulin changes may have to be made, since eating will decrease

• Height, growth rate in children; growth rate may be decreased

• Mental status: mood, sensorium, affect, stimulation, insomnia, aggressiveness

• Physical dependency: should not be used for extended time; dose should be discontinued gradually; tolerance will occur after long-term use

• Withdrawal symptoms: headache, nausea, vomiting, muscle pain, weakness

Administer:

• At least 6 hr before hs to avoid sleeplessness, 1 hr ac meals

• For obesity only if patient is on weight reduction program including dietary changes, exercise; patient will develop tolerance, and weight loss won't occur without additional methods

• Gum, hard candy, frequent sips of water for dry mouth

Evaluate:

• Therapeutic response: decreased weight

Teach patient/family:

• To take with meals to avoid GI symptoms

• To decrease caffeine consumption (coffee, tea, cola, chocolate), which may increase irritability, stimulation

• Not to take more frequently than prescribed

• To avoid OTC preparations unless approved by physician

• To taper off drug over several weeks, or depression, increased sleeping, lethargy may ensue

• To avoid alcohol ingestion

• To avoid hazardous activities until patient is stabilized on medication

• To get needed rest; patient will feel more tired at end of day

Treatment of overdose: Administer fluids, chlorpromazine 1 mg/kg; antihypertensive for increased B/P; ammonium Cl for increased excretion

---

measles, mumps, and rubella virus vaccine, live

M-M-R-II

Func. class.: Vaccine

Action: Produces antibodies to measles, mumps, rubella

Uses: Prevention of measles, mumps, rubella

Dosage and routes:

• *Children >15 mos and adults:* SC 0.5 ml

Available forms: Inj SC measles 1000 $TCID_{50}$, mumps 20,000 $TCID_{50}$, rubella 1000 $TCID_{50}$ (0.5 ml)

Side effects/adverse reactions:

CNS: Fever, *subacute sclerosing panencephalitis and blindness associated with optic neuritis,* paresthesias

INTEG: Urticaria, erythema, burning, stinging at injection site

SYST: Lymphadenitis, *anaphylaxis,* malaise, sore throat, headache

MS: Osteomyelitis, arthralgia, arthritis

Contraindications: Hypersensitivity, blood dyscrasias, anemia, active infection, immunosuppression, egg, chicken allergy, pregnancy, febrile illness, neomycin allergy, neoplasms

Precautions: Elderly, lactation, children with TB

Interactions/incompatibilities:
• Decreased response to: TB skin test
• Other live virus vaccines
NURSING CONSIDERATIONS
Assess:
• For skin reactions: rash, induration, erythema
• For anaphylaxis: inability to breathe, bronchospasm
Administer:
• Only with epinephrine 1:1000 on unit to treat laryngospasm
• Only SC
Perform/provide:
• Storage at 39° F (4° C); protect from heat and light; do not give within 1 month of other live virus vaccines
• Written record of immunization
Evaluate:
• For history of allergies, skin disorders (eczema, psoriasis, dermatitis), reactions to vaccinations
Teach patient/family:
• That fever may occur 5-12 days after vaccine given
• That joint pains, tingling in extremities may occur 5-12 days after vaccine given
• That pain and inflammation may occur
• To take acetaminophen for fever

mebendazole
(me-ben'da-zole)
Vermox
Func. class.: Anthelmintic
Chem. class.: Carbamate

Action: Inhibits glucose uptake, degeneration of cytoplasmic microtubules in the cell; interferes with absorption, secretory function
Uses: Pinworms, roundworms, hookworms, whipworms, threadworms, pork tapeworms, dwarf tapeworms, beef tapeworms, hydatid cyst
Dosage and routes:
• *Adult and child >2 yr:* PO 100 mg as a single dose or bid × 3 days, depending on type of infection; course may be repeated in 3 wk if needed
Available forms: Tabs, chewable 100 mg
Side effects/adverse reactions:
CNS: Dizziness, fever
GI: Transient diarrhea, abdominal pain
Contraindications: Hypersensitivity
Precautions: Child <2 yr, lactation, pregnancy (1st trimester) (C)
Pharmacokinetics:
PO: Peak ½-7 hr; excreted in feces primarily (metabolites), small amount in urine (unchanged); highly bound to plasma proteins
Interactions/incompatibilities:
• Decreased effect of mebendazole: carbamazine, hydantoins
NURSING CONSIDERATIONS
Assess:
• Stools during entire treatment; specimens must be sent to lab while still warm
• For allergic reaction: rash (rare)
• For diarrhea during expulsion of worms; avoid self-contamination with patient's feces
• For infection in other family members, since infection from person to person is common
Administer:
• May be crushed, chewed if unable to swallow whole
• PO after meals to avoid GI symptoms, since absorption is not altered by food
• Second course after 3 wk if needed; usually recommended
Perform/provide:
• Storage in tight container

italics = common side effects   ***bold italic*** = life threatening reactions

Evaluate:
• Therapeutic response: expulsion of worms and 3 negative stool cultures after completion of treatment
Teach patient/family:
• Proper hygiene after BM, including hand-washing technique; tell patient to avoid putting fingers in mouth; clean fingernails
• That infected person should sleep alone; do not shake bed linen, change bed linen qd, wash in hot water, change and wash undergarments daily
• To clean toilet qd with disinfectant (green soap solution)
• Need for compliance with dosage schedule, duration of treatment
• To wear shoes, wash all fruits and vegetables well before eating

---

mecamylamine HCl
(mek-a-mill′a-meen)
Inversine
Func. class.: Antihypertensive
Chem. class.: Ganglionic blocker

Action: Occupies receptor site, prevents acetylcholine from attaching to postsynaptic nerve ending in sympathetic and parasympathetic ganglia
Uses: Moderate to severe hypertension, malignant hypertension
Dosage and routes:
• *Adult:* PO 2.5 mg bid, may increase in increments of 2.5 mg × 2 days until desired response; maintenance 25 mg/day in 3 divided doses
Available forms: Tabs 2.5 mg
Side effects/adverse reactions:
CV: Postural hypotension, irregular heart rate, *CHF*
CNS: Drowsiness, *sedation*, headache, tremors, weakness, syncope,

paresthesia, dizziness, *convulsions*
EENT: Blurred vision, nasal congestion, dry mouth, dilated pupils
GU: Impotence, urinary retention, decreased libido
GI: Anorexia, glossitis, nausea, vomiting, constipation, *paralytic ileus*
Contraindications: Hypersensitivity, myocardial infarction, coronary insufficiency, renal disease, glaucoma, organic pyloric stenosis, uremia, uncooperative patients, mild/labile hypertension
Precautions: CVA, prostatic hypertrophy, bladder neck obstruction, urethral stricture, renal dysfunction (elevated BUN), cerebral dysfunction, pregnancy (C)
Pharmacokinetics:
PO: Onset ½-2 hr, duration 6-12 hr; excreted in urine, feces, breast milk; crosses placenta
Interactions/incompatibilities:
• Increased effects: thiazide diuretics, antihypertensives, CNS depressants (alcohol, anesthetics, MAOIs), bethanechol
NURSING CONSIDERATIONS
Assess:
• B/P lying and standing, other VS throughout treatment
• Weight daily, I&O
• Edema in feet, legs daily
• Skin turgor, dryness of mucous membranes for hydration status
• Tolerance to drug that occurs with prolonged use
• Constipation: number of stools, consistency; give stool softener as ordered or increase bulk in diet
Administer:
• Whole; do not chew or crush tablets
• After meals for better absorption; give larger dose at noon and evening, smaller dose in AM

• Gum, frequent rinsing of mouth, hard candy for dry mouth
Evaluate:
• Therapeutic response: decreased B/P
Teach patient/family:
• To notify physician if tremor, seizure, or signs of paralytic ileus occur
• To avoid OTC preparations unless directed by physician
• To rise slowly from sitting or lying position; orthostatic hypotension may occur
• That impotence may occur but is reversible after discontinuing drug
Treatment of overdose: Administer gastric lavage, discontinue drug, administer small doses of pressor amines for hypotension

---

mechlorethamine HCl (nitrogen mustard)
(me-klor-eth'a-meen)
Mustargen
Func. class.: Antineoplastic alkylating agent
Chem. class.: Nitrogen mustard

Action: Responsible for cross-linking DNA strands leading to cell death; rapidly degraded, a vesicant; activity is not cell cycle specific
Uses: Hodgkin's disease, lymphomas, lymphosarcoma; ovarian, breast, lung cancer; neoplastic effusions
Dosage and routes:
• *Adult:* IV 0.4 mg/kg or 10 mg/m² as 1 dose or 2-4 divided doses over 2-4 days; second course after 3 wk depending on blood cell count
Neoplastic effusions
• *Adult:* Intracavity 10-20 mg
Available forms: Inj IV, intracavity 10 mg; powder for inj

Side effects/adverse reactions:
EENT: Tinnitus, hearing loss
HEMA: **Thrombocytopenia, leukopenia, agranulocytosis,** anemia
GI: Nausea, vomiting, diarrhea, stomatitis, weight loss, colitis, **hepatotoxicity**
CNS: Headache, dizziness, drowsiness, paresthesia, peripheral neuropathy, **coma**
INTEG: Alopecia, pruritus, herpes zoster
Contraindications: Lactation, pregnancy (1st trimester) (D), myelosuppression, acute herpes zoster
Precautions: Radiation therapy, chronic lymphocytic leukopenia
Pharmacokinetics:
Metabolized in liver, excreted in urine
Interactions/incompatibilities:
• Increased toxicity: antineoplastics, radiation
• Blood dyscrasias: amphotericin B
• Incompatible with any drug in syringe or sol

M

NURSING CONSIDERATIONS
Assess:
• CBC, differential, platelet count weekly; withhold drug if WBC is <4000 or platelet count is <75,000; notify physician of results
• Renal function studies: BUN, serum uric acid, urine CrCl before, during therapy
• I&O ratio; report fall in urine output of 30 ml/hr
• Monitor temperature q4h (may indicate beginning infection); no rectal temperatures
• Liver function tests before, during therapy (bilirubin, AST, ALT, LDH) as needed or monthly
• Bleeding: hematuria, guaiac, bruising or petechiae, mucosa or orifices q8h

---

italics = common side effects **bold italic** = life threatening reactions

• Food preferences; list likes, dislikes
• Yellowing of skin and sclera, dark urine, clay-colored stools, itchy skin, abdominal pain, fever, diarrhea
• Effects of alopecia on body image; discuss feelings about body changes
• Inflammation of mucosa, breaks in skin
• Buccal cavity q8h for dryness, sores, ulceration, white patches, oral pain, bleeding, dysphagia
• Local irritation, pain, burning, discoloration at injection site
• Symptoms indicating severe allergic reaction: rash, pruritus, urticaria, purpuric skin lesions, itching, flushing

Administer:
• After using guidelines for preparation of cytotoxic drugs
• Antiemetic 30-60 min before giving drug to prevent vomiting and prn
• Antibiotics for prophylaxis of infection
• IV after diluting 10 mg/10 ml sterile H_2O or NaCl; leave needle in vial, shake, withdraw dose, give through Y-tube or 3-way stopcock or directly
• Slow IV infusion using 21-, 23-, 25-gauge needle, watch for infiltration. If infiltration occurs, infiltrate area with isotonic sodium thiosulfate or 1% lidocaine. Apply ice for 6-12 hr
• Topical or systemic analgesics for pain
• Local or systemic drugs for infection

Perform/provide:
• Storage at room temperature in dry form
• Strict medical asepsis, protective isolation if WBC levels are low
• Special skin care
• Increase fluid intake to 2-3 L/day to prevent urate deposits, calculi formation
• Diet low in purines: organ meats (kidney, liver), dried beans, peas to maintain alkaline urine
• Preparation under hood using gloves and mask
• Rinsing of mouth tid-qid with water, club soda; brushing of teeth bid-tid with soft brush or cotton-tipped applicators for stomatitis; use unwaxed dental floss
• Warm compresses at injection site for inflammation

Evaluate:
• Therapeutic response: decreased tumor size, spread of malignancy

Teach patient/family:
• About protective isolation precautions
• That sterility, amenorrhea can occur; reversible after discontinuing treatment
• That hair may be lost during treatment; a wig or hairpiece may make patient feel better; new hair may be different in color, texture
• To avoid foods with citric acid, hot or rough texture
• To report any bleeding, white spots, or ulcerations in mouth to physician; tell patient to examine mouth qd
• To report signs of infection: increased temperature, sore throat, flu symptoms
• To report signs of anemia: fatigue, headache, faintness, shortness of breath, irritability
• To avoid use of razors or commercial mouthwash
• To avoid use of aspirin products or ibuprofen

meclizine HCl

(mek'li-zeen)
Antivert, Antivert/25, Antivert/
25 Chewable, Antivert-50, An-
trizine, Bonamine,* Bonine,
Dizmiss, Meclizine HCl, Meni-
D, Ru-Vert-M
Func. class.: Antiemetic, anti-
histamine, anticholinergic
Chem. class.: H₁-receptor an-
tagonist, piperazine derivative

Action: Acts centrally by blocking
chemoreceptor trigger zone, which
in turn acts on vomiting center
Uses: Dizziness, motion sickness
Dosage and routes:
• *Adult:* PO 25-100 mg qd in di-
vided doses or 1 hr before traveling
Available forms: Tabs 12.5, 25, 50
mg; chew tabs 25 mg; tabs film
coated 25 mg
Side effects/adverse reactions:
CNS: Drowsiness, fatigue, restless-
ness, headache, insomnia
GI: Nausea, anorexia
EENT: Dry mouth, blurred vision
Contraindications: Hypersensitiv-
ity to cyclizines, shock, lactation
Precautions: Children, narrow-an-
gle glaucoma, glaucoma, urinary
retention, lactation, prostatic hy-
pertrophy, elderly, pregnancy (B)
Pharmacokinetics:
PO: Duration 8-24 hr, half-life 6 hr
Interactions/incompatibilities:
• Increased effect of: alcohol, tran-
quilizers, narcotics
Lab test interferences:
False negative: Allergy skin testing
NURSING CONSIDERATIONS
Assess:
• VS, B/P
• Signs of toxicity of other drugs
or masking of symptoms of disease:
brain tumor, intestinal obstruction

• Observe for drowsiness, dizziness, LOC
Administer:
• Tablets may be swallowed whole,
chewed, or allowed to dissolve
Evaluate:
• Therapeutic response: absence of
dizziness, vomiting
Teach patient/family:
• That a false-negative result may
occur with skin testing; these procedures should not be scheduled for
4 days after discontinuing use
• To avoid hazardous activities, activities requiring alertness; dizziness may occur; instruct patient to
request assistance with ambulation
• To avoid alcohol, other depressants

meclofenamate

(me-kloe-fen-am'ate)
Meclofenamate, Meclomen
Func. class.: Nonsteroidal an-
tiinflammatory
Chem. class.: Anthranilic acid
derivative

Action: Inhibits prostaglandin synthesis by decreasing an enzyme
needed for biosynthesis; analgesic,
antiinflammatory, antipyretic
Uses: Mild to moderate pain, osteoarthritis, rheumatoid arthritis
Dosage and routes:
• *Adult:* PO 200-400 mg/day in divided doses tid-qid
Available forms: Caps 50, 100 mg
Side effects/adverse reactions:
GI: Nausea, anorexia, vomiting,
diarrhea, jaundice, ***cholestatic hepatitis,*** constipation, flatulence,
cramps, dry mouth, peptic ulcer,
ulceration, perforation
CNS: Dizziness, drowsiness, fatigue, tremors, confusion, insomnia, anxiety, depression

italics = common side effects   ***bold italic*** = life threatening reactions

CV: Tachycardia, hypertension, peripheral edema, palpitations, dysrhythmias

INTEG: Purpura, rash, pruritus, sweating

*GU: **Nephrotoxicity: dysuria, hematuria, oliguria, azotemia***

*HEMA: **Blood dyscrasias***

EENT: Tinnitus, hearing loss, blurred vision

Contraindications: Hypersensitivity, asthma, severe renal disease, severe hepatic disease, ulcer disease

Precautions: Pregnancy (B), lactation, children, bleeding disorders, GI disorders, cardiac disorders, hypersensitivity to other antiinflammatory agents

Pharmacokinetics:

PO: Peak 2 hr, half-life 3-3½ hr; metabolized in liver, excreted in urine (metabolites), excreted in breast milk

Interactions/incompatibilities:

• Increased action of: coumarin, phenytoin, sulfonamides

NURSING CONSIDERATIONS
Assess:

• Renal, liver, blood studies: BUN, creatinine, AST, ALT, Hgb, Hct before treatment, periodically thereafter

• Audiometric and ophthalmic exam before, during, after treatment

• For history of peptic ulcer disease

• For eye, ear problems: blurred vision, tinnitus (may indicate toxicity)

Administer:

• With food to decrease GI symptoms; best to take on empty stomach to facilitate absorption

Perform/provide:

• Storage at room temperature

Evaluate:

• Therapeutic response: decreased pain, stiffness, swelling in joints, ability to move more easily

Teach patient/family:

• To report increased GI symptoms; dose may have to be reduced

• To report blurred vision, ringing, roaring in ears (may indicate toxicity)

• To avoid driving, other hazardous activities if dizziness or drowsiness occurs

• To report change in urine pattern, weight increase, edema, pain increase in joints, fever, blood in urine (indicates nephrotoxicity)

• That therapeutic effects may take up to 1 mo

• To take with full glass water

• To avoid other NSAIDs, alcohol, steroids

---

medium-chain triglycerides
MCT Oil
Func. class.: Caloric

Action: Needed for energy in body; more rapidly hydrolyzed than fat

Uses: Inadequate dietary fat intake or absorption

Dosage and routes:

• *Adult:* PO 15 ml tid-qid, not to exceed 100 ml/day

Available forms: Oil (115 calories/15 ml)

Side effects/adverse reactions:

CNS: Loss of consciousness (reversible)

GI: Nausea, vomiting, anorexia, cramps, diarrhea, distention

Contraindications: Hypersensitivity, severe hepatic disease, lipoproteinemia

Precautions: Portacaval shunts, pregnancy (C), pancreatitis, hyperlipemia

---

*Available in Canada only

NURSING CONSIDERATIONS
Assess:
• Triglycerides, free-fatty-acid levels, platelet counts daily to prevent fat overload, thrombocytopenia
• Liver function: AST, ALT
• Nutritional status: calorie count by dietitian
Evaluate:
• Therapeutic response: increased weight
Teach patient/family:
• Reason for use of lipids
• Methods of incorporating drug in food or beverages (salad dressings, chilled fruit juices)

---

medroxyprogesterone acetate

(me-drox′ee-proe-jess′te-rone)
Amen, Curretab, Cycrin, Depo-Provera, Medroxyprogesterone Acetate, Provera

Func. class.: Progestogen
Chem. class.: Progesterone derivative

Action: Inhibits secretion of pituitary gonadotropins, which prevents follicular maturation and ovulation; stimulates growth of mammary tissue; antineoplastic action against endometrial cancer

Uses: Uterine bleeding (abnormal), secondary amenorrhea, endometrial cancer, renal cancer, contraceptive

Dosage and routes:
Secondary amenorrhea
• *Adult:* PO 5-10 mg qd × 5-10 days
Endometrial/renal cancer
• *Adult:* 1M 400-1000 mg/wk
Uterine bleeding
• *Adult:* PO 5-10 mg qd × 5-10 days starting on 16th day of menstrual cycle
Contraceptive
• *Adult:* injected q3mo
Available forms: Tabs 2.5, 10 mg; inj susp 100, 400 mg/ml, contraceptive injectable

Side effects/adverse reactions:
CNS: Dizziness, headache, migraines, depression, fatigue
CV: Hypotension, thrombophlebitis, edema, *thromboembolism, stroke, pulmonary embolism, myocardial infarction*
GI: Nausea, vomiting, anorexia, cramps, increased weight, *cholestatic jaundice*
EENT: Diplopia
GU: Amenorrhea, cervical erosion, breakthrough bleeding, dysmenorrhea, vaginal candidiasis, breast changes, *gynecomastia, testicular atrophy, impotence,* endometriosis, *spontaneous abortion*
INTEG: Rash, urticaria, acne, hirsutism, alopecia, oily skin, seborrhea, purpura, melasma, photosensitivity
META: Hyperglycemia

Contraindications: Breast cancer, hypersensitivity, thromboembolic disorders, reproductive cancer, genital bleeding (abnormal, undiagnosed), pregnancy (X)

Precautions: Lactation, hypertension, asthma, blood dyscrasias, gallbladder disease, CHF, diabetes mellitus, bone disease, depression, migraine headache, convulsive disorders, hepatic disease, renal disease, family history of cancer of breast or reproductive tract

Pharmacokinetics:
PO: Duration 24 hr, excreted in urine and feces, metabolized in liver

Lab test interferences:
Increase: Alk phosphatase, N

M

italics = common side effects   **bold italic** = life threatening reactions

(urine), pregnanediol, amino acids
Decrease: GTT, HDL

NURSING CONSIDERATIONS
Assess:
• Weight daily; notify physician of weekly weight gain >5 lb
• B/P at beginning of treatment and periodically
• I&O ratio; be alert for decreasing urinary output, increasing edema
• Liver function studies: ALT, AST, bilirubin, periodically during long-term therapy
• Edema, hypertension, cardiac symptoms, jaundice
• Mental status: affect, mood, behavioral changes, depression
• Hypercalcemia

Administer:
• Titrated dose; use lowest effective dose
• Oil solution deeply in large muscle mass (IM), rotate sites
• In one dose in AM
• With food or milk to decrease GI symptoms
• After warming to dissolve crystals

Perform/provide:
• Storage in dark area

Evaluate:
• Therapeutic response: decreased abnormal uterine bleeding, absence of amenorrhea

Teach patient/family:
• To avoid sunlight or use sunscreen; photosensitivity can occur
• About cushingoid symptoms
• To report breast lumps, vaginal bleeding, edema, jaundice, dark urine, clay-colored stools, dyspnea, headache, blurred vision, abdominal pain, numbness or stiffness in legs, chest pain; male to report impotence or gynecomastia
• To report suspected pregnancy

---

mefenamic acid
(me-fe-nam'-ik)
Ponstel
Func. class.: Nonsteroidal antiinflammatory
Chem. class.: Anthranilic acid derivative

Action: Inhibits prostaglandin synthesis by decreasing an enzyme needed for biosynthesis and interferes with prostaglandins at receptor sites; analgesic, antiinflammatory, antipyretic
Uses: Mild to moderate pain, dysmenorrhea, inflammatory disease
Dosage and routes:
• *Adult and child >14 yr:* PO 500 mg, then 250 mg q6h, use not to exceed 1 wk
Available forms: Caps 250 mg
Side effects/adverse reactions:
GI: Nausea, anorexia, vomiting, diarrhea, jaundice, ***cholestatic hepatitis,*** constipation, flatulence, cramps, dry mouth, peptic ulcer, ***ulceration, perforation***
CNS: Dizziness, drowsiness, fatigue, tremors, confusion, insomnia, anxiety, depression
CV: Tachycardia, peripheral edema, palpitations, dysrhythmias
INTEG: Purpura, rash, pruritus, sweating
*GU: **Nephrotoxicity: dysuria, hematuria, oliguria, azotemia***
*HEMA: **Blood dyscrasias***
EENT: Tinnitus, hearing loss, blurred vision
Contraindications: Hypersensitivity, asthma, severe renal disease, severe hepatic disease, ulcer disease
Precautions: Pregnancy (C), lactation, children, bleeding disorders, GI disorders, cardiac disor-

ders, hypersensitivity to other antiinflammatory agents

Pharmacokinetics:

PO: Peak 2 hr, half-life 3-3½ hr; metabolized in liver, excreted in urine (metabolites), excreted in breast milk, extensive protein binding

Interactions/incompatibilities:

• Increased action of: coumarin, phenytoin, sulfonamides

NURSING CONSIDERATIONS

Assess:

• Renal, liver, blood studies: BUN, creatinine, AST, ALT, Hgb before treatment, periodically thereafter

• Audiometric, ophthalmic exam before, during, after treatment

• For eye, ear problems: blurred vision, tinnitus (may indicate toxicity)

Administer:

• With food to decrease GI symptoms; take on empty stomach to facilitate absorption

Perform/provide:

• Storage at room temperature

Evaluate:

• Therapeutic response: decreased pain, stiffness, swelling in joints, ability to move more easily

Teach patient/family:

• To report blurred vision or ringing, roaring in ears (may indicate toxicity)

• To avoid driving, other hazardous activities if dizziness or drowsiness occurs

• To report change in urine pattern, weight increase, edema, pain increase in joints, fever, blood in urine (indicates nephrotoxicity)

• That therapeutic effects may take up to 1 mo

• To report diarrhea or skin rash: drug may be discontinued

• To take with full glass of water

• To avoid ASA, alcohol, steroids

---

mefloquine HCl

(me-flow′quine)

Lariam

Func. class.: Antimalarial

Chem. class.: Analog of quinine

Action: Exact mechanism not known; blood schizonticide

Uses: Treatment and prevention of *P. falciparum* malaria, *P. vivax*

Dosage and routes:

• *Adult:* PO 1250 mg as a single dose (treatment); 250 mg qwk × 4 wk, then 250 mg q2wk (prevention)

Available forms: Tabs 250 mg

Side effects/adverse reactions:

CV: Bradycardia, extrasystole

CNS: Dizziness, headache, syncope, *neuropsychiatric disturbances: disorientation, hallucinations,* **coma, convulsions**

GI: Nausea, vomiting, loss of appetite, diarrhea, abdominal pain

INTEG: Itching, rash

MISC: Myalgia

Contraindications: Hypersensitivity, pregnancy (C)

Precautions: Cardiac dysrhythmias, neurologic disease, lactation, children

Pharmacokinetics:

Protein binding 98%, excreted in breast milk and urine, half-life 21 days (adults)

Interactions/incompatibilities:

• Increased ECG abnormalities, possible cardiac arrest: β-blockers, quinine, quinidine

• Increased potential for convulsions: chloroquine, valproic acids

NURSING CONSIDERATIONS

Assess:

• B/P, pulse; watch for bradycardia

• Neuropsychiatric symptoms: disorientation, hallucinations; drug should be discontinued

M

---

italics = common side effects   ***bold italic*** = life threatening reactions

• Liver studies weekly: ALT, AST, bilirubin

Administer:

• Do not take on an empty stomach; take medication with at least 8 oz water

Perform/provide:

• Storage in tight, light-resistant container

Evaluate:

• Therapeutic response: decreased symptoms of malaria

Teach patient/family:

• Do not take on empty stomach

---

megestrol acetate

(me-jess'trole)
Megace, Megestrol Acetate
Func. class.: Antineoplastic
Chem. class.: Hormone, progestin

Action: Affects endometrium by antiluteinizing effect; this is thought to bring about cell death

Uses: Breast, endometrial cancer, renal cell cancer

Dosage and routes:

• *Adult:* PO 40-320 mg/day in divided doses

Available forms: Tabs 20, 40 mg

Side effects/adverse reactions:

GI: Nausea, vomiting, anorexia, diarrhea, abdominal cramps

GU: Gynecomastia, fluid retention, **hypercalcemia**

CV: **Thrombophlebitis**

INTEG: Alopecia, rash, pruritus, purpura, itching

CNS: Mood swings

Contraindications: Hypersensitivity, pregnancy (X)

Pharmacokinetics:

PO: Duration 1-3 days, half-life 60 min; metabolized in liver; excreted in feces, breast milk

Lab test interferences:

Increase: Alk phosphatase, urinary N, urinary pregnanediol, plasma amino acids

False positive: Urine glucose

Decrease: HDL, glucose tolerance test

NURSING CONSIDERATIONS

Assess:

• I&O ratio; weights
• Serum Ca levels
• Homan's sign
• Food preferences; list likes, dislikes
• Effects of alopecia on body image; discuss feelings about body changes
• Symptoms indicating severe allergic reaction: rash, pruritus, urticaria, purpuric skin lesions, itching, flushing
• Frequency of stools, characteristics: cramping, acidosis, signs of dehydration (rapid respirations, poor skin turgor, decreased urine output, dry skin, restlessness, weakness)
• Mood swings
• Anorexia, nausea, vomiting, constipation, weakness, loss of muscle tone

Administer:

• Antispasmodic
• Diuretics for increased fluids

Perform/provide:

• Increase fluid intake to 2-3 L/day to prevent dehydration and maintain normal Ca
• Nutritious diet with iron, vitamin supplements as ordered
• Limitation of Ca (dairy products)
• Storage in tight container at room temperature

Evaluate:

• Therapeutic response: decreased tumor size, spread of malignancy

Teach patient/family:

• To report any complaints or side effects to nurse or physician

---

*Available in Canada only

• That gynecomastia can occur; reversible after discontinuing treatment
• To recognize and report signs of fluid retention, thromboemboli, hepatotoxicity

---

melphalan
(mel'fa-lan)
Alkeran, Alkeran IV
Func. class.: Antineoplastic alkylating agent
Chem. class.: Nitrogen mustard

Action: Responsible for cross-linking DNA strands leading to cell death; activity is not cell cycle specific
Uses: Multiple myeloma, breast cancer, reticulum cell sarcoma, testicular seminoma, malignant melanoma, advanced ovarian cancer
Dosage and routes:
• *Adult:* PO 6 mg qd × 2-3 wk; stop drug for 4 wk or until WBC level begins to rise; do not administer if WBC <3000/mm³ or platelets <100,000/mm³; may be given 0.15 mg/kg/day × 7 days; wait until platelets and WBCs rise, then 0.05 mg/kg/day
• *Adult:* IV Inf 16 mg/m², reduce in renal insufficiency, give over 15-20 mins, give at 2 wk intervals × 4 doses, then at 4 wk intervals
Available forms: Tabs 2 mg, powder for Inj (IV)
Side effects/adverse reactions:
*HEMA: **Thrombocytopenia, neutropenia, myelosuppression,** anemia*
GI: Nausea, vomiting, stomatitis
GU: Amenorrhea, hyperuricemia
INTEG: Rash, urticaria
*RESP: **Fibrosis, dysplasia***

Contraindications: Lactation, pregnancy (D)
Precautions: Radiation therapy, bone marrow depression
Pharmacokinetics:
Metabolized in liver, excreted in urine, half-life 1½ hr
Interactions/incompatibilities:
• Increased toxicity: antineoplastics, radiation
NURSING CONSIDERATIONS
Assess:
• CBC, differential, platelet count weekly; withhold drug if WBC is <4000 or platelet count is <75,000; notify physician of results
• Renal function studies: BUN, serum uric acid, urine CrCl before, during therapy
• I&O ratio; report fall in urine output of 30 ml/hr
• Monitor temperature q4h (may indicate beginning infection); no rectal temperatures
• Liver function tests before, during therapy (bilirubin, AST, ALT, LDH) as needed or monthly
• Bleeding: hematuria, guaiac, bruising or petechiae, mucosa or orifices q8h
• Food preferences; list likes, dislikes
• Yellowing of skin and sclera, dark urine, clay-colored stools, itchy skin, abdominal pain, fever, diarrhea
• Inflammation of mucosa, breaks in skin
• Buccal cavity q8h for dryness, sores, ulceration, white patches, oral pain, bleeding, dysphagia
• Local irritation, pain, burning, discoloration at injection site
• Symptoms indicating severe allergic reaction: rash, pruritus, urticaria, purpuric skin lesions, itching, flushing

M

---

italics = common side effects   ***bold italic*** = life threatening reactions

Administer:
• Antiemetic 30-60 min before giving drug to prevent vomiting
• Antibiotics for prophylaxis of infection
• Topical or systemic analgesics for pain
• Local or systemic drugs for infection

Perform/provide:
• Storage in tight, light-resistant container
• Strict medical asepsis, protective isolation if WBC levels are low
• Special skin care
• Increase fluid intake to 2-3 L/day to prevent urate deposits, calculi formation
• Diet low in purines: organ meats (kidney, liver), dried beans, peas to maintain alkaline urine
• Rinsing of mouth tid-qid with water, club soda; brushing of teeth bid-tid with soft brush or cotton-tipped applicators for stomatitis; use unwaxed dental floss
• Warm compresses at injection site for inflammation

Evaluate:
• Therapeutic response: decreased tumor size, spread of malignancy

Teach patient/family:
• Of protective isolation precautions
• That sterility, amenorrhea can occur; reversible after discontinuing treatment
• To avoid foods with citric acid, hot or rough texture
• To report any bleeding, white spots, or ulcerations in mouth to physician; tell patient to examine mouth qd
• To report signs of infection: increased temperature, sore throat, flu symptoms
• To report signs of anemia: fatigue, headache, faintness, shortness of breath, irritability
• To avoid use of razors, commercial mouthwash
• To avoid use of aspirin products, ibuprofen

---

menadione/menadiol sodium diphosphate (vitamin K₃)
(men-a-dye'one)
Synkavite,* Synkayvite
Func. class.: Vitamin, fat soluble

Action: Needed for adequate blood clotting (factors II, VII, IX, X)

Uses: Vit K malabsorption, hypoprothrombinemia

Dosage and routes:
• *Adult:* PO 2-10 mg (menadione)
• *Adult:* PO/IM/IV 5-15 mg (menadiol sodium diphosphate)

Available forms: Tabs 5 mg; inj 5, 10, 37.5 mg/ml

Side effects/adverse reactions:
CNS: Headache, *brain damage* (large doses)
GI: Nausea, decreased liver function tests
HEMA: Hemolytic anemia, hemoglobinuria, hyperbilirubinemia
INTEG: Rash, urticaria

Contraindications: Hypersensitivity, severe hepatic disease, last few weeks of pregnancy (X)

Precautions: Neonates

Pharmacokinetics: Metabolized, crosses placenta

Interactions/incompatibilities:
• Decreased action of menadione: oral antibiotics, cholestyramine, mineral oil
• Decreased action of: oral anticoagulants
• Incompatible with alkaloids, co-

deine, levarterenol, levorphanol, meperidine, methadone, procaine

NURSING CONSIDERATIONS
Assess:

• Pro-time during treatment (2 sec deviation from control time, bleeding time, and clotting time), monitor for bleeding, pulse, and BP

• Nutritional status: liver (beef), spinach, tomatoes, coffee, asparagus, broccoli, cabbage, lettuce, greens

Administer:

• Deep IM, IV slowly over 7 min; may be given IV undiluted or added to infusions

Evaluate:

• Therapeutic response: decreased bleeding tendencies, decreased pro-time, decreased clotting time

Teach patient/family:

• Not to take other supplements unless directed by physician

• Necessary foods to be included in diet

• To avoid use of mineral oil

• To avoid IM injections and activities leading to injury. Use soft tooth brush, don't floss, and use electric razor until coagulation defect corrected

• Not to take OTC drugs, especially those containing aspirin or alcohol

• Importance of frequent lab tests to monitor coagulation factors

---

menotropins

(men-oh-troe′pin)

Pergonal

Func. class.: Gonadotropin
Chem. class.: Exogenous gonadotropin

Action: In women, increases follicular growth, maturation; in men, when given with HCG, stimulates spermatogenesis

Uses: Infertility, anovulation in women, stimulates spermatogenesis in men

Dosage and routes:
Infertility

• *Adult (men):* IM 1 amp 3 × wk with HCG 2000 U 2 × wk × 4 mo

• *Adult (women):* IM 75 IU of FSH, LH qd × 9-12 days, then 10,000 U HCG 1 day after these drugs; repeat × 2 menstrual cycles, then increase to 150 IU of FSH, LH qd × 9-12 days, then 10,000 U HCG 1 day after these drugs × 2 menstrual cycles

Anovulation

• *Adult (women):* IM 75 IU FSH, LH qd × 9-12d, then 10,000 U HCG 1d after last dose of these drugs; repeat × 1-3 menstrual cycles

Available forms: Powder for inj 17 IU/amp

Side effects/adverse reactions:

CNS: Fever

CV: Hypovolemia

GI: *Nausea,* vomiting, diarrhea, anorexia

GU: Ovarian enlargement, abdominal distention/pain, multiple births, ovarian hyperstimulation: sudden ovarian enlargement, ascites with or without pain, pleural effusion, gynecomastia in men

*HEMA: **Hemoperitoneum, arterial thromboembolism***

Contraindications: Primary ovarian failure, abnormal bleeding, thyroid/adrenal dysfunction, organic intracranial lesion, ovarian cysts, primary testicular failure

Precautions: Pregnancy (C)

NURSING CONSIDERATIONS
Assess:

• Weight qd; notify physician if weight gain increases rapidly

---

italics = common side effects   ***bold italic*** = life threatening reactions

- Estrogen excretion level; if >100 µg/24 hr, drug is withheld; hyperstimulation syndrome may occur
- I&O ratio; be alert for decreasing urinary output
- Ovarian enlargement, abdominal distention/pain; report symptoms immediately

Administer:
- After reconstituting with 1-2 ml sterile saline injection; use immediately

Evaluate:
- Therapeutic response: ovulation, pregnancy

Teach patient/family:
- That multiple births are possible; if pregnancy occurs, usually 4-6 wk after start of treatment
- To keep appointment during treatment qd × 2 wk
- That daily intercourse is necessary from day preceding administration of gonadotropin until ovulation occurs

---

mepenzolate bromide
(me-pen'zoe'late)
Cantil
Func. class.: GI anticholinergic
Chem. class.: Synthetic quaternary ammonium antimuscarinic

Action: Inhibits muscarinic actions of acetylcholine at postganglionic parasympathetic neuroeffector sites
Uses: Treatment of peptic ulcer disease, irritable bowel syndrome in combination with other drugs; for other GI disorders
Dosage and routes:
- *Adult:* PO 25-50 mg qid with meals, hs; titrate to patient response
Available forms: Tabs 25 mg
Side effects/adverse reactions:
CNS: Confusion, stimulation in elderly, headache, insomnia, dizziness, drowsiness, anxiety, weakness, hallucination
*GI: Dry mouth, constipation, **paralytic ileus,** heartburn, nausea, vomiting, dysphagia, absence of taste
GU: Hesitancy, retention, impotence
CV: Palpitations, tachycardia
EENT: Blurred vision, photophobia, mydriasis, cycloplegia, increased ocular tension
INTEG: Urticaria, rash, pruritus, anhidrosis, fever, allergic reactions
Contraindications: Hypersensitivity to anticholinergics, narrow-angle glaucoma, GI obstruction, myasthenia gravis, paralytic ileus, GI atony, toxic megacolon
Precautions: Hyperthyroidism, coronary artery disease, dysrhythmias, CHF, ulcerative colitis, hypertension, hiatal hernia, hepatic disease, renal disease, pregnancy (C), elderly, urinary retention, prostatic hypertrophy
Pharmacokinetics:
PO: Onset 1 hr, duration 3-4 hr; metabolized by liver, excreted in urine
Interactions/incompatibilities:
- Increased anticholinergic effect: amantadine, tricyclic antidepressants, MAOIs
- Decreased effect of: phenothiazines, levodopa, ketoconazole
NURSING CONSIDERATIONS
Assess:
- VS, cardiac status: checking for dysrhythmias, increased rate, palpitations
- I&O ratio; check for urinary retention or hesitancy
- GI complaints: pain, bleeding (frank or occult), nausea, vomiting, anorexia
Administer:
- ½-1 hr ac for better absorption
- Decreased dose to elderly pa-

tients; their metabolism may be slowed

• Gum, hard candy, frequent rinsing of mouth for dryness of oral cavity

Perform/provide:

• Storage in tight container protected from light

• Increased fluids, bulk, exercise to patient's life-style to decrease constipation

Evaluate:

• Therapeutic response: absence of epigastric pain, bleeding, nausea, vomiting

Teach patient/family:

• Avoid driving, other hazardous activities until stabilized on medication

• Avoid alcohol, other CNS depressants; will enhance sedating properties of this drug

• To avoid hot environments; stroke may occur; drug suppresses perspiration

• Use sunglasses when outside to prevent photophobia; may cause blurred vision

• To drink plenty of fluids

• To report dysphagia

---

meperidine HCl
(me-per′i-deen)
Demerol, Meperidine HCl, Pethidine
Func. class.: Narcotic analgesic
Chem. class.: Opiate, phenyl-piperidine derivative

Controlled Substance Schedule II
Action: Depresses pain impulse transmission at the spinal cord level by interacting with opioid receptors
Uses: Moderate to severe pain, preoperatively
Dosage and routes:
Pain
• *Adult:* PO/SC/IM 50-150 mg q3-4h prn; dose should be decreased if given IV

• *Child:* PO/SC/IM 1 mg/kg q4-6h prn, not to exceed 100 mg q4hr
Preoperatively
• *Adult:* IM/SC 50-100 mg q30-90 min before surgery; dose should be reduced if given IV

• *Child:* IM/SC 1-2.2 mg/kg 30-90 min before surgery
Available forms include: Inj SC, IM, IV 25, 50, 75, 100 mg/ml; tabs 50, 100 mg; syr 50 mg/5 ml
Side effects/adverse reactions:
CNS: Drowsiness, dizziness, confusion, headache, sedation, euphoria, **increased intracranial pressure**
CV: Palpitations, bradycardia, change in B/P, tachycardia (IV)
EENT: Tinnitus, blurred vision, miosis, diplopia, depressed corneal reflex
GI: Nausea, vomiting, anorexia, constipation, cramps
GU: Urinary retention, dysuria
INTEG: Rash, urticaria, bruising, flushing, diaphoresis, pruritus
RESP: **Respiratory depression**
Contraindications: Hypersensitivity, addiction (narcotic)
Precautions: Addictive personality, pregnancy (B), lactation, increased intracranial pressure, MI (acute), severe heart disease, respiratory depression, hepatic disease, renal disease, child <18 yr
Pharmacokinetics:
Absorption 50% (PO), well absorbed IM, SC
PO: Onset 15 min, peak 1 hr, duration 4-5 hr
SC/IM: Onset 10 min, peak 1 hr, duration 4-5 hr
IV: Onset 5 min, duration 2 hr
Metabolized by liver (to active/inactive metabolites), excreted by kidneys; crosses placenta, excreted

---

italics = common side effects   ***bold italic*** = life threatening reactions

in breast milk; half-life 3-6 hr; toxic by-product can result from regular use

Interactions/incompatibilities:
• Increased effects with other CNS depressants: alcohol, narcotics, sedative/hypnotics, antipsychotics, skeletal muscle relaxants, MAOIs, chlorpromazine
• Incompatible with aminophylline, amobarbital, furosemide, heparin, hydrocortisone, methicillin, methylprednisolone, morphine, pentobarbital, phenobarbital, secobarbital, phenytoin, $NaCO_3$, thiopental

Lab test interferences:
Increase: Amylase, lipase

NURSING CONSIDERATIONS
Assess:
• Pain: location, type, character; give dose before pain becomes extreme
• I&O ratio; check for decreasing output; may indicate urinary retention
• Need for drug
• For constipation; increase fluids, bulk in diet
• CNS changes: dizziness, drowsiness, hallucinations, euphoria, LOC, pupil reactions
• Allergic reactions: rash, urticaria
• Respiratory dysfunction: depression, character, rate, rhythm; notify physician if respirations are <12/min

Administer:
• IV after diluting with 5 ml or more sterile H_2O or NS; give directly over 4-5 min; may be further diluted in sol to 1 mg/ml during anesthesia in D_5W or NS; if diluted in NS, may be given through patient-controlled inf device
• With antiemetic for nausea, vomiting
• When pain is beginning to return;

determine dosage interval by patient response
• In gradually decreasing dose after long-term use; withdrawal symptoms may occur

Perform/provide:
• Storage in light-resistant container at room temperature
• Assistance with ambulation
• Safety measures: side rails, nightlight, call bell within easy reach

Evaluate:
• Therapeutic response: decrease in pain

Teach patient/family:
• To report any symptoms of CNS changes, allergic reactions
• That physical dependency may result when used for extended periods
• That drowsiness, dizziness may occur; to call for assistance
• Withdrawal symptoms may occur: nausea, vomiting, cramps, fever, faintness, anorexia
• To make position changes slowly; orthostatic hypotension can occur
• To avoid OTC medications, alcohol unless directed by physician

Treatment of overdose: Naloxone (Narcan) 0.2-0.8 IV, O_2, IV fluids, vasopressors

---

mephentermine sulfate
(me-fen'ter-meen)
Wyamine
Func. class.: Adrenergic, direct and indirect acting
Chem. class.: Substituted phenylethylamine

Action: Causes increased contractility and heart rate by acting on β-receptors in heart; also, acts on α-receptors, causing vasoconstriction in blood vessels; cardiac output is in blood vessels; cardiac output is elevated and systolic and diastolic pressures are increased

Uses: Shock and hypotension following variety of procedures

Dosage and routes:

Hypotension

• *Adult:* IV 15-45 mg depending on procedure

Hypotension/shock

• *Adult:* IV 0.5 mg/kg

• *Child:* IV 0.4 mg/kg

Available forms: Inj IV 15, 30 mg/ml

Side effects/adverse reactions:

CV: Palpitations, tachycardia, hypertension

CNS: Tremors, drowsiness, confusion, incoherence

Contraindications: Hypersensitivity to sympathomimetics

Precautions: Pregnancy (B), cardiac disorders, hyperthyroidism, diabetes mellitus, prostatic hypertrophy

Pharmacokinetics:

IV: Onset immediate, duration ½-1 hr; metabolized in liver, excreted in urine

Interactions/incompatibilities:

• Do not use with MAOIs or tricyclic antidepressants; hypertensive crisis may occur

• Decreased effect of mephentermine: methyldopa, urinary acidifiers, rauwolfia alkaloids

• Increased effect of mephentermine: urinary alkalizers

• Dysrhythmias: halothane, cyclopropane, digitalis

• Incompatible with epinephrine, hydralazine

NURSING CONSIDERATIONS

Assess:

• I&O ratio; notify physician if output is <30 ml/hr

• ECG during administration con-

tinuo[us] ... decre[ase]

• B/[P] ... route ...

• CV[P] ... possib[le]

Admi[n]

• Plasm[a] ... mia

• IV undiluted 30 mg or less/1 min, or diluted 600 mg/500 ml D_5W, titrate to patient response, check site for extravasation; use an infusion pump

Perform/provide:

• Storage of reconstituted solution if refrigerated for no longer than 24 hr

• Do not use discolored solutions

Evaluate:

• Therapeutic response: increased B/P with stabilization

Teach patient/family:

• Reason for drug administration

mephenytoin

(me-fen'i-toyn)

Mesantoin

Func. class.: Anticonvulsant

Chem. class.: Hydantoin derivative

Action: Reduces electrical discharges in motor cortex, reducing seizures; increases AV conduction velocity, prolongs refractory period

Uses: Generalized tonic-clonic, complex-partial seizures

Dosage and routes:

• *Adult:* PO 50-100 mg/day, may increase by 50-100 mg q7d, up to 200 mg tid

• *Child:* PO 50-100 mg/day or 100-450 mg/m²/day in 3 divided doses, initially; then increase 50-100 mg q7d, up to 200 mg tid in divided doses q8h

Available forms: Tabs 100 mg

italics = common side effects   ***bold italic*** = life threatening reactions

...oin

...verse reactions:
...nulocytosis, leuko-
...utropenia, pancytope-
...sinophilia, lymphadenop-

...WS: Drowsiness, dizziness, fatigue, irritability, tremors, insomnia, depression
GI: Nausea, vomiting
INTEG: Rash, exfoliative dermatitis
EENT: Photophobia, conjunctivitis, nystagmus, diplopia
RESP: Pulmonary fibrosis

Contraindications: Hypersensitivity to hydantoins, sinus bradycardia, heart block, Adams-Stokes syndrome

Precautions: Alcoholism, hepatic disease, renal disease, blood dyscrasias, CHF, elderly, pregnancy (C), respiratory depression, diabetes mellitus

Pharmacokinetics:
PO: Onset 30 min, duration 24-48 hr, metabolized by liver, excreted by kidneys, half-life 144 hr

Interactions/incompatibilities:
• Decreased effects: rifampin, chronic alcohol use, barbiturates, antihistamines, antacids, other anticonvulsants antineoplastics, Ca products, folic acid, oxacillin
• Increased effects: benzodiazepines, cimetidine, salicylates, sulfonamide, pyrazolones, phenothiazines, estrogens, disulfiram, chloramphenicol, anticoagulants
• Seizures: valproic acid
• Myocardial depression: lidocaine, propanolol, sympathomimetics

NURSING CONSIDERATIONS
Assess:
• Blood studies: CBC, platelets q2 wk until stabilized, then qmo × 12, then q3mo; discontinue drug if neutrophils are <1600/mm³, liver function tests with long-term use

• Drug level: therapeutic level 25-40 μg/ml
• Blood glucose may be increased
• Mental status: mood, sensorium, affect, behavioral changes; if mental status changes, notify physician
• Eye problems: need for ophthalmic examinations before, during, after treatment (slit lamp, fundoscopy, tonometry)
• Allergic reaction: red raised rash; if this occurs, drug should be discontinued
• Blood dyscrasias: fever, sore throat, bruising, rash, jaundice
• Toxicity: bone marrow depression, nausea, vomiting, ataxia, diplopia, cardiovascular collapse, Stevens-Johnson syndrome

Evaluate:
• Therapeutic response: decreased seizure activity

Teach patient/family:
• Not to discontinue drug quickly; should be tapered
• To avoid activities that require alertness if drowsiness, dizziness occurs
• That use of alcohol may decrease effects of drug
• To inform dentist; use good oral hygiene

mephobarbital
(me-foe-bar'bi-tal)
Mebaral
Func. class.: Anticonvulsant
Chem. class.: Barbiturate

Controlled Substance Schedule IV

Action: Depresses sensory cortex, motor activity; inhibits ascending conduction in reticular formation of thalamus

Uses: Generalized tonic-clonic

(grand mal), absence (petit mal) seizures

Dosage and routes:

• *Adult:* PO 400-600 mg/day or in divided doses

• *Child:* PO 6-12 mg/kg/day in divided doses q6-8h

Available forms: Tabs 32, 50, 100, 200 mg

Side effects/adverse reactions:

HEMA: ***Thrombocytopenia, agranulocytosis, megaloblastic anemia***

CNS: Dizziness, headache, hangover, paradoxic stimulation, drowsiness, increased pain

GI: Nausea, vomiting, epigastric pain

INTEG: Rash, urticaria, purpura, erythema multiforme, facial edema

EENT: Tinnitus, hearing loss

CV: Hypotension, bradycardia

RESP: Wheezing, hyperpnea

ENDO: Hypoglycemia, hyponatremia, hypokalemia

Contraindications: Hypersensitivity to barbiturates, pregnancy (D)

Precautions: Hepatic disease, renal disease, lactation, alcoholism, drug abuse, hyperthyroidism

Pharmacokinetics:

PO: Onset 20-60 min, duration 6-8 hr

Interactions/incompatibilities:

• Increased effects: CNS depressants, chloramphenicol, valproic acid, disulfiram, nondepolarizing skeletal muscle relaxants, sulfonamides

• Increased orthostatic hypotension: furosemide

NURSING CONSIDERATIONS

Assess:

• Drug level, CBC, BUN, creatinine

• Mental status: mood, sensorium, affect, memory (long, short)

• Respiratory depression: respiration <10/min, shallow

• Blood dyscrasias: fever, sore throat, bruising, rash, jaundice

Perform/provide:

• Storage in light-resistant container

Evaluate:

• Therapeutic response: decreased seizure activity

Teach patient/family:

• Never to withdraw drug abruptly; notify physician if side effects occur

• To avoid hazardous activities until stabilized on drug

• That dreaming may increase when drug is discontinued

Treatment of overdose: Administer calcium gluconate IV

---

mepivacaine HCl

(meep-ee-va-kane)

Carbocaine, Carbocaine with Neo-Cobefrin, Isocaine HCl, Mepivicane HCl, Polocaine

Func. class.: Local anesthetic

Chem. class.: Amide

M

Action: Competes with calcium for sites in nerve membrane that control sodium transport across cell membrane; decreases rise of depolarization phase of action potential

Uses: Nerve block, caudal anesthesia, epidural, pain relief, paracervical block, transvaginal block or infiltration

Dosage and routes:

Varies with route of anesthesia

Available forms: Inj 1%, 1.5%, 2%, 3%

Side effects/adverse reactions:

CNS: Anxiety, restlessness, ***convulsions, loss of consciousness,*** drowsiness, disorientation, tremors, shivering

CV: ***Myocardial depression, car-***

---

diac arrest, dysrhythmias, bradycardia, hypotension, hypertension,
fetal bradycardia
GI: Nausea, vomiting
EENT: Blurred vision, tinnitus, pupil constriction
INTEG: Rash, urticaria, allergic reactions, edema, burning, skin discoloration at injection site, tissue
necrosis
*RESP: Status asthmaticus, respi-
ratory arrest, anaphylaxis*
Contraindications: Hypersensitivity, child <12 yr, elderly, severe
liver disease
Precautions: Elderly, severe drug
allergies, pregnancy (C)
Pharmacokinetics:
Onset 15 min, duration 3 hr; metabolized by liver, excreted in urine
(metabolites)
Interactions/incompatibilities:
• Dysrhythmias: epinephrine,
halothane, enflurane
• Hypertension: MAOIs, tricyclic
antidepressants, phenothiazines
• Decreased action of mepivacaine:
chloroprocaine
NURSING CONSIDERATIONS
Assess:
• B/P, pulse, respiration during
treatment
• Fetal heart tones if drug is used
during labor
• Allergic reactions: rash, urti-
caria, itching
• Cardiac status: ECG for dys-
rhythmias, pulse, B/P during an-
esthesia
Administer:
• Only with crash cart, resuscita-
tive equipment nearby
• Only drugs without preservatives
for epidural or caudal anesthesia
Perform/provide:
• Use of new solution; discard un-
used portions

Evaluate:
• Therapeutic response: anesthesia
necessary for procedure
Treatment of overdose: Airway,
O_2, vasopressor, IV fluids, anticonvulsants for seizures

---

meprobamate
(me-proe-ba′mate)
Equanil, Meditran,* Meprobamate, Meprospan, Miltown,
Miltown 600, Neo-Tran,* No-
vomepro,* Saronil, Sedaba-
mate, Tranhep
Func. class.: Sedative/hyp-
notic
Chem. class.: Propanediol carbamate derivative

**Controlled Substance Schedule
IV**
Action: Widespread depression of
the CNS
Uses: Anxiety
Dosage and routes:
• *Adult:* PO 1.2-1.6 g in 2-3 di-
vided doses, not to exceed 2.4
g/day
• *Child 6-12 yr:* PO 100-200 mg
bid-tid
Available forms: Tabs 200, 400,
600 mg; caps 400 mg sust rel caps
200, 400 mg
Side effects/adverse reactions:
*HEMA: Thrombocytopenia, leuko-
penia, eosinophilia*
CNS: Dizziness, drowsiness, head-
ache, *convulsions,* ataxia
GI: Nausea, vomiting, anorexia,
diarrhea, stomatitis
INTEG: Urticaria, pruritus, macu-
lopapular rash
CV: Hypotension, tachycardia, palpitations, *hyperthermia*
EENT: Blurred vision, tinnitus, mydriasis, slurred speech
Contraindications: Hypersensitiv-

ity, renal failure, porphyria, pregnancy (D), history of drug abuse or dependence

Precautions: Suicidal patients, severe depression, renal disease, hepatic disease, elderly

Pharmacokinetics:

PO: Onset 1 hr; metabolized by liver; excreted by kidneys, in feces; crosses placenta, breast milk; half-life 6-16 hr

Interactions/incompatibilities:
• Increased effects of meprobamate: CNS depressants, alcohol, tricyclic antidepressants

Lab test interferences:
False increase: 17-OHCS
False positive: Phentolamine test

NURSING CONSIDERATIONS
Assess:
• B/P (lying, standing), pulse; if systolic B/P drops 20 mm Hg, hold drug, notify physician
• Blood studies: CBC during long-term therapy; blood dyscrasias have occurred rarely
• Therapeutic blood levels 0.5-2 mg/100 ml
• Hepatic studies: AST, ALT, bilirubin, creatinine, LDH, alk phosphatase
• Mental status: mood, sensorium, affect, sleeping pattern, drowsiness, dizziness
• Physical dependency, withdrawal symptoms: headache, nausea, vomiting, muscle pain, weakness, hyperthermia, death, convulsions after long-term use
• Suicidal tendencies

Administer:
• With food or milk for GI symptoms
• Crushed tabs if patient is unable to swallow medication whole
• Sugarless gum, hard candy, frequent sips of water for dry mouth

Perform/provide
• Assistance with ambulation during beginning therapy, since drowsiness/dizziness occurs
• Safety measures, including side rails
• Check to see PO medication has been swallowed

Evaluate:
• Therapeutic response: decreased anxiety, restlessness, insomnia

Teach patient/family:
• That drug may be taken with food
• Not to be used for everyday stress or used longer than 4 months unless directed by physician; not to take more than prescribed amount; may be habit forming
• To avoid OTC preparations (alcohol, cold, hay fever) unless approved by physician
• To avoid driving, activities that require alertness, since drowsiness may occur
• To avoid alcohol ingestion, other psychotropic medications unless prescribed by physician
• Not to discontinue medication abruptly after long-term use
• To rise slowly or fainting may occur, especially elderly
• That drowsiness may worsen at beginning of treatment

Treatment of overdose: Lavage, VS, supportive care

---

mercaptopurine (6-MP)
(mer-kap-toe-pyoor'een)
Purinethol
Func. class.: Antineoplastic-antimetabolite
Chem. class.: Purine analog

Action: Inhibits purine metabolism at multiple sites, which inhibits

DNA and RNA synthesis S phase of cell cycle specific

Uses: Chronic myelocytic leukemia, acute lymphoblastic leukemia in children, acute myelogenous leukemia

Dosage and routes:
• *Adult and child:* PO 2.5 mg/kg/day, not to exceed 5 mg/kg/day; maintenance 1.5-2.5 mg/kg/day
• *Child:* 70 mg/m^2/day

Available forms: Tabs 50 mg

Side effects/adverse reactions:
CNS: Fever, headache, weakness
HEMA: **Thrombocytopenia, leukopenia, myelosuppression, anemia**
GI: Nausea, vomiting, anorexia, diarrhea, stomatitis, **hepatotoxicity** (with high doses), jaundice, gastritis
GU: **Renal failure,** hyperuricemia, **oliguria,** crystalluria, **hematuria**
INTEG: Rash, dry skin, urticaria

Contraindications: Patients with prior drug resistance, leukopenia (<2500/mm^3), thrombocytopenia (<100,000/mm^3), anemia, pregnancy (D)

Precautions: Renal disease

Pharmacokinetics: Incompletely absorbed when taken orally; metabolized in liver, excreted in urine

Interactions/incompatibilities:
• Increased toxicity: radiation or other antineoplastics
• Increased bone marrow depression: allopurinol
• Reversal of neuromuscular blockade: nondepolarizing muscle relaxants

NURSING CONSIDERATIONS
Assess:
• CBC, differential, platelet count weekly; withhold drug if WBC is <3500 or platelet count is <100,000; notify physician of these results; drug should be discontinued

• Renal function studies: BUN, serum uric acid, urine CrCl, electrolytes before, during therapy
• I&O ratio; report fall in urine output to <30 ml/hr
• Monitor temperature q4h; fever may indicate beginning infection; no rectal temperatures
• Liver function tests before, during therapy: bilirubin, alk phosphatase, AST, ALT, qwk during beginning therapy
• Bleeding: hematuria, guaiac, bruising, petechiae, mucosa or orifices q8h
• Food preferences; list likes, dislikes
• Inflammation of mucosa, breaks in skin
• Buccal cavity q8h for dryness, sores, ulceration, white patches, oral pain, bleeding, dysphagia
• Symptoms indicating severe allergic reaction: rash, urticaria, itching, flushing

Administer:
• Antacid before oral agent; give drug after evening meal before bedtime
• Allopurinol or sodium bicarbonate to maintain uric acid levels, alkalinization of urine
• Antibiotics for prophylaxis of infection
• Topical or systemic analgesics for pain
• Transfusion for anemia

Perform/provide:
• Strict medical asepsis, protective isolation if WBC levels are low
• Increase fluid intake to 2-3 L/day to prevent urate deposits, calculi formation, unless contraindicated
• Diet low in purines: absence of organ meats (kidney, liver), dried beans, peas to maintain alkaline urine
• Rinsing of mouth tid-qid with

water, club soda; brushing of teeth bid-tid with soft brush or cotton-tipped applicators for stomatitis; use unwaxed dental floss
• Nutritious diet with iron, vitamin supplements as ordered
• Storage in tightly closed container in cool environment

Evaluate:
• Therapeutic response: decreased size of tumor, spread of malignancy

Teach patient/family:
• To avoid foods with citric acid, hot or rough texture if stomatitis is present
• To report stomatitis: any bleeding, white spots, ulcerations in mouth; tell patient to examine mouth qd, report symptoms
• Contraceptive measures are recommended during therapy
• To drink 10-12 (8 oz) glasses of fluid/day
• Notify physician of fever, chills, sore throat, nausea, vomiting, anorexia, diarrhea, bleeding, bruising, which may indicate blood dyscrasias
• To report signs of infection: increased temperature, sore throat, flu symptoms
• To report signs of anemia: fatigue, headache, faintness, shortness of breath, irritability
• To report bleeding: avoid use of razors, commercial mouthwash
• To avoid use of aspirin products, ibuprofen

---

mesalamine
(mez-al'a-meen)
Asacol, Rowasa
Func. class.: GI antiinflammatory
Chem. class.: 5-aminosalicylic acid

Action: May diminish inflammation by blocking cyclooxygenase, inhibiting prostaglandin production in colon

Uses: Mild to moderate active distal ulcerative colitis, proctosigmoiditis, proctitis

Dosage and routes:
• *Adult:* REC 60 ml (4 g) hs, retained for 8 hr × 3-6 wk PO 800 mg tid for 6 wk SUPP: 500 mg bid for 3-6 wk

Available forms: Rec susp 4 g/60 ml supp 500 mg, tab del rel 400 mg

Side effects/adverse reactions:
CV: Pericarditis, myocarditis
GI: Cramps, gas, nausea, diarrhea, rectal pain, constipation
CNS: Headache, fever, dizziness, insomnia, asthenia, weakness, fatigue
INTEG: Rash, itching, acne
SYST: Flu, malaise, back pain, peripheral edema, leg and joint pain, arthralgia, dysmenorrhea
EENT: Sore throat, cough, pharyngitis, rhinitis

Contraindications: Hypersensitivity to this drug or salicylates

Precautions: Renal disease, pregnancy (B), lactation, children, sulfite sensitivity

Pharmacokinetics:
REC: Primarily excreted in feces but some in urine as metabolite; half-life 1 hr, metabolite half-life 5-10 hr

NURSING CONSIDERATIONS
Assess:
• GI symptoms: cramps, gas, nausea, diarrhea, rectal pain; if severe, the drug should be discontinued

Administer:
• May give orally; tablets should be swallowed whole
• Rectally; drug should be given hs, retained until morning

M

---

italics = common side effects   **bold italic** = life threatening reactions

Perform/provide:
• Storage at room temperature
Evaluate:
• Therapeutic response: absence of pain, bleeding from GI tract, decrease in number of diarrhea stools
Teach patient/family:
• That usual course of therapy is 3-6 wk
• To shake bottle well
• Method of rectal administration
• To inform physician of GI symptoms
• Do not crush tabs

---

mesoridazine besylate
(mez-oh-rid'a-zeen)
Serentil
Func. class.: Antipsychotic/neuroleptic
Chem. class.: Phenothiazine, piperidine

Action: Depresses cerebral cortex, hypothalamus, limbic system, which control activity, aggression; blocks neurotransmission produced by dopamine at synapse; exhibits strong α-adrenergic, anticholinergic blocking action; mechanism for antipsychotic effects is unclear
Uses: Psychotic disorders, schizophrenia, anxiety, alcoholism, behavioral problems in mental deficiency, chronic brain syndrome
Dosage and routes:
Schizophrenia
• *Adult:* PO 50 mg tid, optimum dose 100-400 mg/day; IM 25 mg may repeat ½-1 hr; dosage range 25-200 mg/day
Behavior problems
• *Adult:* PO 25 mg tid; optimum dose 75-300 mg/day;
Alcoholism
• *Adult:* PO 25 mg bid; optimum dose 50-200 mg/day

Schizoaffective disorders
• *Adult:* PO 10 mg tid; optimum dose 30-150 mg/day
Available forms: Tabs 10, 25, 50, 100 mg; conc 25 mg/ml; inj IM 25 mg/ml
Side effects/adverse reactions:
RESP: **Laryngospasm,** dyspnea, *respiratory depression*
CNS: Extrapyramidal symptoms: pseudoparkinsonism, akathisia, dystonia, tardive dyskinesia, drowsiness, headache,
HEMA: **Anemia, leukopenia, leukocytosis, agranulocytosis**
INTEG: Rash, photosensitivity, dermatitis
EENT: Blurred vision, glaucoma
GI: Dry mouth, nausea, vomiting, anorexia, constipation, diarrhea, jaundice, weight gain
GU: Urinary retention, urinary frequency, enuresis, impotence, amenorrhea, gynecomastia
CV: Orthostatic hypotension, hypertension, **cardiac arrest,** ECG changes, tachycardia
Contraindications: Hypersensitivity, circulatory collapse, liver damage, cerebral arteriosclerosis, coronary disease, severe hypertension/hypotension, blood dyscrasias, coma, brain damage, bone marrow depression, narrow-angle glaucoma
Precautions: Pregnancy (C), lactation, seizure disorders, hypertension, hepatic disease, cardiac disease, prostatic hypertrophy, intestinal obstruction, respiratory conditions
Pharmacokinetics:
PO: Onset erratic, peak 2 hr, duration 4-6 hr
IM: Onset 15-30 min, peak 30 min, duration 6-8 hr; metabolized by liver, excreted in urine, crosses placenta, enters breast milk

---

* Available in Canada only

Interactions/incompatibilities:
• Oversedation: other CNS depressants, alcohol, barbiturate anesthetics
• Toxicity: epinephrine
• Decreased absorption: aluminum hydroxide, magnesium hydroxide antacids
• Decreased effects of: lithium, levodopa
• Increased effects of both drugs: β-adrenergic blockers, alcohol
• Increased anticholinergic effects: anticholinergics

Lab test interferences:
Increase: Liver function tests, cardiac enzymes, cholesterol, blood glucose, prolactin, bilirubin, PBI, cholinesterase, ^{131}I
Decrease: Hormones (blood, urine)
False positive: Pregnancy tests, PKU
False negative: Urinary steroids, 17-OHCS

NURSING CONSIDERATIONS
Assess:
• Mental status before initial administration
• Swallowing of PO medication; check for hoarding or giving of medication to other patients
• I&O ratio; palpate bladder if low urinary output occurs
• Bilirubin, CBC, liver function studies monthly
• Urinalysis is recommended before, during prolonged therapy
• Affect, orientation, LOC, reflexes, gait, coordination, sleep pattern disturbances
• B/P standing and lying; also include pulse and respirations; take these q4h during initial treatment; establish baseline before starting treatment; report drops of 30 mm Hg

• Dizziness, faintness, palpitations, tachycardia on rising
• Extrapyramidal symptoms including akathisia (inability to sit still, no pattern to movements), tardive dyskinesia (bizarre movements of jaw, mouth, tongue, extremities), pseudoparkinsonism (rigidity, tremors, pill rolling, shuffling gait)
• For neuroleptic malignant syndrome: hyperthermia, altered mental status, muscle rigidity, increased CPK
• Skin turgor daily
• Constipation, urinary retention daily; if these occur increase bulk, water in diet

Administer:
• Antiparkinsonian agent after securing order from physician, to be used if extrapyramidal symptoms occur
• Concentrate mixed in distilled water, orange, grape juice; do not prepare, store bulk dilutions
• IM injection into large muscle mass; do not use if precipitate present

Perform/provide:
• Decreased noise input by dimming lights, avoiding loud noises
• Supervised ambulation until stabilized on medication; do not involve in strenuous exercise program because fainting is possible; patient should not stand still for long periods
• Increased fluids to prevent constipation
• Sips of water, candy, gum for dry mouth
• Storage in tight, light-resistant container

Evaluate:
• Therapeutic response: decrease in emotional excitement, hallucinations, delusions, paranoia, and re-

organization of patterns of thought, speech

Teach patient/family:

• That orthostatic hypotension occurs commonly, and to rise from sitting or lying position gradually; to avoid hazardous activities until stabilized on medication

• To remain lying down for at least 30 min after IM injection

• To avoid hot tubs, hot showers, tub baths, since hypotension may occur

• To avoid abrupt withdrawal of mesoridazine, or extrapyramidal symptoms may result; drugs should be withdrawn slowly

• To avoid OTC preparations (cough, hay fever, cold) unless approved by physician, since serious drug interactions may occur; to avoid use with alcohol, CNS depressants increased drowsiness may occur

• To use sunscreen during sun exposure to prevent burns

• Regarding compliance with drug regimen

• About necessity for meticulous oral hygiene, since oral candidiasis may occur

• To report sore throat, malaise, fever, bleeding, mouth sores; if these occur, a CBC should be drawn and drug discontinued

• That in hot weather heat stroke may occur; take extra precautions to stay cool

Treatment of overdose: Lavage if orally ingested; provide an airway; *do not induce vomiting*

metaproterenol sulfate

(met-a-proe-ter′e-nole)
Alupent, Arm-A-Med Metaproterenol Sulfate, Dey-Dose Metaproterenol Sulfate, Dey-Lute Metaproterenol Sulfate, Metaprel, Prometa

Func. class.: Selective β_2-agonist

Action: Relaxes bronchial smooth muscle by direct action on β_2-adrenergic receptors

Uses: Bronchial asthma, bronchospasm

Dosage and routes:

• *Adult and child>12 yr:* INH 2-3 puffs; may repeat q3-4h, not to exceed 12 puffs/day

Asthma/bronchospasm

• *Adult:* PO 20 mg q6-8h

• *Child >9 yr or >27 kg:* PO 20 mg q6-8h or 0.4-0.9 mg/kg tid

• *Child 6-9 yr or <27 kg:* PO 10 mg q6-8h or 0.4-0.9 mg/kg tid

Available forms include: Tabs 10, 20 mg; aerosol 0.65 mg/dose; syrup 10 mg/5 ml; sol nebulizer 0.6%, 5%

Side effects/adverse reactions:

CNS: Tremors, anxiety, insomnia, headache, dizziness, stimulation

CV: Palpitations, tachycardia, hypertension, dysrhythmias, *cardiac arrest*

GI: Nausea

RESP: Dyspnea

Contraindications: Hypersensitivity to sympathomimetics, narrowangle glaucoma

Precautions: Pregnancy (C), cardiac disorders, hyperthyroidism, diabetes mellitus, prostatic hypertrophy

Pharmacokinetics:

Well absorbed (PO)

PO: Onset 15-30 min, peak 1 hr, duration 4 hr, excreted in urine as metabolites

Inh: Onset 5 min, peak 1 hr, duration 4 hr

Interactions/incompatibilities:

• Increased effects of both drugs: other sympathomimetics

• Decreased action of β-blockers, oral hypoglycemics

Lab Test Interferences:

Decrease: K

NURSING CONSIDERATIONS

Assess:

• Respiratory function: vital capacity, forced expiratory volume, ABGs; also B/P; lung sounds, secretion before and after treatment

• Tolerance over long-term therapy; dose may have to be changed; check for rebound bronchospasm

Administer:

• 2 hr before hs to avoid sleeplessness

• PO with food for GI upset

Perform/provide:

• Storage at room temperature; do not use discolored solutions

Evaluate:

• Therapeutic response: absence of dyspnea, wheezing

Teach patient/family:

• To increase fluid intake to liquefy secretions

• Not to use OTC medications; extra stimulation may occur

• To notify physician of headaches, chest pain, weakness, dizziness, anxiety

• Use of inhaler; review package insert with patient

• To avoid getting aerosol in eyes

• To wash inhaler in warm water and dry qd

• On all aspects of drug; avoid smoking, smoke-filled rooms, persons with respiratory infections

---

methadone HCl

(meth'a-done)

Dolophine HCl, Methadone HCl, Methadone HCl Diskets, Methadone HCl Intensol

Func. class.: Narcotic analgesics

Chem. class.: Opiate, synthetic diphenylheptane derivative

Controlled Substance Schedule II

Action: Depresses pain impulse transmission at the spinal cord level by interacting with opioid receptors

Uses: Severe pain, narcotic withdrawal

Dosage and routes:

Pain

• *Adult:* PO/SC/IM 2.5-10 mg q4-12h prn

Narcotic withdrawal

• *Adult:* PO 15-40 mg/day individualized initially, then 20-120 mg/day titrated to patient response

Available forms: Inj SC, IM 10 mg/ml; tabs 5, 10 mg; oral sol 5, 10 mg/5 ml; dispersible tabs 40 mg

Side effects/adverse reactions:

CNS: Drowsiness, dizziness, confusion, headache, sedation, euphoria

GI: Nausea, vomiting, anorexia, constipation, cramps, biliary tract spasm

GU: Increased urinary output, dysuria, urinary retention

INTEG: Rash, urticaria, bruising, flushing, diaphoresis, pruritus

EENT: Tinnitus, blurred vision, miosis, diplopia

CV: Palpitations, bradycardia, change in B/P

*RESP: **Respiratory depression***

Contraindications: Hypersensitivity, addiction (narcotic)

Precautions: Addictive personality, pregnancy (B), lactation, in-

---

creased intracranial pressure, MI (acute), severe heart disease, respiratory depression, hepatic disease, renal disease, child <18 yr

Pharmacokinetics:

PO: Onset 30-60 min, duration 6-8 hr, cumulative 22-48 hr

SC/IM: Onset 10-20 min, peak 1 hr, duration 6-8 hr, cumulative 22-48 hr

Metabolized by liver; excreted by kidneys; crosses placenta; excreted in breast milk; half-life 1-1½ days; 90% bound to plasma proteins

Interactions/incompatibilities:

• Increased effects with other CNS depressants: alcohol, narcotics, sedative/hypnotics, antipsychotics, skeletal muscle relaxants, rifampin, phenytoin

Lab test interferences:

Increase: Amylase

NURSING CONSIDERATIONS

Assess:

• I&O ratio; check for decreasing output; may indicate urinary retention

• CNS changes: dizziness, drowsiness, hallucinations, euphoria, LOC, pupil reaction

• Allergic reactions: rash, urticaria

• Respiratory dysfunction: respiratory depression, character, rate, rhythm; notify physician if respirations are <10/min

• Need for pain medication, physical dependence

Administer:

• With antiemetic if nausea/vomiting occurs

• When pain is beginning to return; determine dosage interval by patient response

• Rotating injection sites

Perform/provide:

• Storage in light-resistant area at room temperature

• Assistance with ambulation

• Safety measures: side rails, nightlight, call bell within easy reach

Evaluate:

• Therapeutic response: decrease in pain

Teach patient/family:

• To report any symptoms of CNS changes, allergic reactions

• That physical dependency may result when used for extended periods

• Withdrawal symptoms may occur: nausea, vomiting, cramps, fever, faintness, anorexia

Treatment of overdose: Narcan 0.2-0.8 IV, O_2, IV fluids, vasopressors

---

methamphetamine HCl

(meth-am-fet′a-meen)

Desoxyn, Desoxyn Gradumet

Func. class.: Cerebral stimulants

Chem. class.: Amphetamine

Controlled Substance Schedule II

Action: Increases release of norepinephrine and dopamine in cerebral cortex to reticular activating system

Uses: Exogenous obesity, minimal brain dysfunction, attention deficit disorder with hyperactivity

Dosage and routes:

Attention deficit disorder

• *Child >6 yr:* 2.5-5 mg qd or bid increasing by 5 mg/wk

Obesity

• *Adult:* PO 2.5-5 mg, 30 min ac or 10-15 mg long-acting tab qd in AM

Available forms: Tabs 5; tabs long-acting 5, 10, 15 mg

Side effects/adverse reactions:

CNS: Hyperactivity, insomnia, restlessness, talkativeness, dizziness,

---

headache, chills, stimulation, dysphoria, irritability, aggressiveness, tremor

GI: Anorexia, dry mouth, diarrhea, constipation, weight loss, metallic taste, cramps

GU: Impotence, change in libido

CV: Palpitations, tachycardia, hypertension, decreased heart rate, dysrhythmia

INTEG: Urticaria

Contraindications: Hypersensitivity to sympathomimetic amines, hyperthyroidism, hypertension, glaucoma hypertrophy, severe arteriosclerosis, drug abuse, cardiovascular disease, anxiety

Precautions: Gilles de la Tourette's disorder, pregnancy (C), lactation, child <3 years

Pharmacokinetics:

PO: Duration 3-6 hr, metabolized by liver, excreted by kidneys, crosses blood-brain barrier

Interactions/incompatibilities:

• Hypertensive crisis: MAOIs or within 14 days of MAOIs

• Increased effect of methamphetamine: acetazolamide, antacids, sodium bicarbonate

• Decreased effects of methamphetamine: barbiturates, tricyclics, ascorbic acid, ammonium chloride

• Decreased effects of: guanethidine

NURSING CONSIDERATIONS
Assess:

• VS, B/P, since this drug may reverse antihypertensives; check patients with cardiac disease more often

• CBC, urinalysis, in diabetes: blood sugar, urine sugar; insulin changes may have to be made, since eating will decrease

• Height, growth rate in children; growth rate may be decreased

• Mental status: mood, sensorium,

affect, stimulation, insomnia, aggressiveness

• Physical dependency: should not be used for extended time; dose should be discontinued gradually; tolerance will occur after long-term use

• Withdrawal symptoms: headache, nausea, vomiting, muscle pain, weakness

Administer:

• At least 6 hr before hs to avoid sleeplessness

• For obesity only if patient is on weight reduction program including dietary changes, exercise; patient will develop tolerance; loss of weight won't occur without additional methods; give 2 hr before meals

• Gum, hard candy or frequent sips of water for dry mouth

Evaluate:

• Therapeutic response: decreased weight, decreased hyperactivity

Teach patient/family:

• To decrease caffeine consumption (coffee, tea, cola, chocolate), which may increase irritability, stimulation

• To avoid OTC preparations unless approved by physician

• To taper off drug over several weeks, or depression, increased sleeping, lethargy may ensue

• To avoid alcohol ingestion

• To avoid hazardous activities until patient is stabilized on medication

• To get needed rest; patients will feel more tired at end of day

• Not to chew or crush sus rel forms

Treatment of overdose: Administer fluids, hemodialysis or peritoneal dialysis; antihypertensive for increased B/P; ammonium Cl for increased excretion.

M

---

italics = common side effects   ***bold italic*** = life threatening reactions

methantheline bromide

(meth-an'tha-leen)
Banthine
Func. class.: GI anticholinergic
Chem. class.: Synthetic quaternary ammonium antimuscarinic

Action: Inhibits muscarinic actions of acetylcholine at postganglionic parasympathetic neuroeffector sites

Uses: Treatment of peptic ulcer disease, irritable bowel syndrome, pancreatitis, gastritis, biliary dyskinesia, pylorospasm, reflex neurogenic bladder in children

Dosage and routes:
• *Adult:* PO 50-100 mg q6h
• *Child >1 yr:* PO 12.5-50 mg qid
• *Child <1 yr:* PO 12.5-25 mg qid
• *Neonate:* PO 12.5 mg bid-tid
Available forms: Tabs 50 mg

Side effects/adverse reactions:
CNS: Confusion, stimulation in elderly, headache, insomnia, dizziness, drowsiness, anxiety, weakness, hallucination
GI: Dry mouth, constipation, paralytic ileus, heartburn, nausea, vomiting, dysphagia, absence of taste
GU: Hesitancy, retention, impotence
CV: Palpitations, tachycardia
EENT: Blurred vision, photophobia, mydriasis, cycloplegia, increased ocular tension
INTEG: Urticaria, rash, pruritus, anhidrosis, fever, allergic reactions

Contraindications: Hypersensitivity to anticholinergics, narrow-angle glaucoma, GI obstruction, myasthenia gravis, paralytic ileus, GI atony, toxic megacolon

Precautions: Hyperthyroidism, coronary artery disease, dysrhythmias, CHF, ulcerative colitis, hypertension, hiatal hernia, hepatic disease, renal disease, pregnancy (C), urinary retention, prostatic hypertrophy

Pharmacokinetics:
PO: Onset 30-45 min, duration 4-6 hr; metabolized by liver, excreted in urine, bile

Interactions/incompatibilities:
• Increased anticholinergic effect: amantadine, tricyclic antidepressants, MAOIs, H_1 antihistamines
• Increased effect of: nitrofurantoin
• Decreased effect of: phenothiazines, levodopa

NURSING CONSIDERATIONS

Assess:
• VS, cardiac status: checking for dysrhythmias, increased rate, palpitations
• I&O ratio; check for urinary retention, hesitancy
• GI complaints: pain, bleeding (frank or occult), nausea, vomiting, anorexia

Administer:
• ½-1 hr ac for better absorption
• Decreased dose to elderly patients; their metabolism may be slowed
• Gum, hard candy, frequent rinsing of mouth for dryness of oral cavity

Perform/provide:
• Storage in tight container protected from light
• Increased fluids, bulk, exercise to patient's life-style to decrease constipation

Evaluate:
• Therapeutic response: absence of epigastric pain, bleeding, nausea, vomiting

Teach patient/family:
• To avoid driving or other hazardous activities until stabilized on medication

---

*Available in Canada only

• To avoid alcohol or other CNS depressants; will enhance sedating properties of this drug
• That drug may cause blurred vision

---

methazolamide
(meth-a-zoe′la-mide)
Neptazane
Func. class.: Carbonic anhydrase inhibitor diuretic
Chem. class.: Sulfonamide derivative

Action: Decreases production of aqueous humor in eye, which lowers intraocular pressure
Uses: Open-angle glaucoma or preoperatively in narrow-angle glaucoma; can be used with miotic, osmotic agents
Dosage and routes:
• *Adult:* PO 50-100 mg bid or tid
Available forms: Tabs 25, 50 mg
Side effects/adverse reactions:
GU: Frequency, hypokalemia, polyuria, uremia, **glucosuria, hematuria,** dysuria, renal calculi
CNS: Drowsiness, paresthesia, anxiety, depression, headache, dizziness, confusion, stimulation, fatigue, **convulsions,** sedation, nervousness
GI: Nausea, vomiting, anorexia, constipation, diarrhea, melena, weight loss, hepatic insufficiency, metallic taste in mouth
EENT: Myopia, tinnitus
INTEG: Rash, pruritus, urticaria, fever, photosensitivity, Stevens-Johnson syndrome
ENDO: Hyperglycemia
*HEMA: **Aplastic anemia, hemolytic anemia, leukopenia, agranulocytosis, thrombocytopenia, purpura, pancytopenia***
Contraindications: Hypersensitivity to sulfonamides, severe renal disease, severe hepatic disease, electrolyte imbalances (hyponatremia, hypokalemia), hyperchloremic acidosis, Addison's disease, COPD
Precautions: Hypercalciuria, pregnancy (C), diabetes mellitus
Pharmacokinetics:
PO: Onset 2-4 hr, peak 6-8 hr, duration 10-18 hr; excreted in urine, crosses placenta
Interactions/incompatibilities:
• Decreased effectiveness of: lithium, barbiturates
• Increased action of: amphetamines, procainamide, quinidine, flecainide, ephedrine, pseudoephedrine
• Hypokalemia: with other diuretics, corticosteroids, amphotericin B
• Toxicity: salicylates
Lab test interferences:
False positive: Urinary protein
NURSING CONSIDERATIONS
Assess:
• Weight, I&O daily to determine fluid loss; effect of drug may be decreased if used qd
• Rate, depth, rhythm of respiration, effect of exertion
• B/P lying, standing; postural hypotension may occur
• Electrolytes: K, Na, Cl; include BUN, blood sugar, CBC, serum creatinine, blood pH, ABGs, liver function tests
• Signs of metabolic acidosis: drowsiness, restlessness
• Signs of hypokalemia: postural hypotension, malaise, fatigue, tachycardia, leg cramps, weakness
• Rashes, temperature elevation qd
• Confusion, especially in elderly; take safety precautions if needed
Administer:
• In AM to avoid interference with sleep

---

italics = common side effects   ***bold italic*** = life threatening reactions

• K replacement if K is less than 3.0
• With food if nausea occurs; absorption may be decreased slightly

Evaluate:
• Therapeutic response: decrease in aqueous humor

Teach patient/family:
• To increase fluid intake to 2-3 L/day unless contraindicated; to rise slowly from lying or sitting position
• To use sunscreen for photosensitivity
• To notify physician if sore throat, unusual bleeding, bruising, paresthesias, tremors, flank pain, or skin rash occurs
• To avoid hazardous activities if drowsiness occurs

Treatment of overdose: Lavage if taken orally; monitor electrolytes; administer dextrose in saline; monitor hydration, CV, renal status

---

methenamine hippurate/methenamine mandelate

(meth-en'a-meen hip'yoo-rate)
Hiprex, Hip-Rex,* Urex, Mandameth, Mandelamine, Methenamine Mandelate
Func. class.: Urinary antiinfective
Chem. class.: Methenamine, mandelic acid

Action: In acid urine, hydrolyzed to ammonia, formaldehyde, which are bactericidal

Uses: UTIs caused by *E. coli, Klebsiella, Enterobacter, P. mirabilis, P. morganii, Serratia, Citrobacter*

Dosage and routes:
• *Adult and child >12 yr:* PO 1 g q12h, maximum: 4 g/24 hr

• *Child 6-12 yr:* PO 500 mg-1g q12h

Neurogenic bladder
• *Adult:* PO 1 g qid pc
• *Child 6-12 yr:* PO 500 mg qid pc
• *Child <6 yr:* PO 50 mg/kg in 4 divided doses pc

Available forms: Tabs 500 mg, 1 g; oral sol 500 mg, 1 g; susp 250, 500 mg/5 ml; tabs, enteric-coated 250, 500 mg, 1g; tabs, film-coated 500 mg, 1g

Side effects/adverse reactions:
CNS: Headache
INTEG: Pruritus, rash, urticaria
GI: Nausea, vomiting, anorexia, abdominal pain, increase AST, ALT
GU: Dysuria, bladder irritation, *albuminuria, hematuria,* crystalluria
EENT: Tinnitus, stomatitis

Contraindications: Hypersensitivity, severe dehydration, renal insufficiency

Precautions: Renal disease, pregnancy (C), lactation

Pharmacokinetics:
PO: Excreted in urine, half-life 4 hr

Interactions/incompatibilities:
• Insoluble precipitate in urine: sulfonamides
• Do not use with silver, iron, mercury salts

Lab test interferences:
Interfere: VMA, urinary catecholamines
False decrease: Urine estriol, 5HIAA
False increase: 17-OHCS

NURSING CONSIDERATIONS
Assess:
• I&O ratio; urine pH <5.5 is ideal; monitor for hematuria indicating crystalluria
• Periodic liver function test: AST, ALT, alk phosphatase

---

* Available in Canada only

• C&S before treatment, after completion
• Allergy: fever, flushing, rash, urticaria, pruritus

Administer:
• After clean-catch urine is obtained for C&S
• Two daily doses if urine output is high or if patient has diabetes
• Up to 12 g of Vit C if needed to acidify urine; cranberry, prune juice may be used

Perform/provide:
• Storage protected from high temperature
• Limited intake of alkaline foods or drugs: milk, dairy products, peanuts, vegetables, alkaline antacids, sodium bicarbonate

Evaluate:
• Therapeutic response: decreased pain, frequency, urgency, negative C&S, absence of infection

Teach patient/family:
• To keep urine acidic by eating food that acidifies urine (meats, eggs, fish, gelatin products, prunes, plums, cranberries)
• That fluids must be increased to 3 L/day to avoid crystallization in kidneys
• To complete full course of drug therapy; to take drug at evenly spaced intervals around clock for best results

---

methicillin sodium

(meth-i-sill'in)
Staphcillin
Func. class.: Broad-spectrum antibiotic
Chem. class.: Penicillinase-resistant penicillin

Action: Interferes with cell wall replication of susceptible organisms; osmotically unstable cell wall swells, bursts from osmotic pressure

Uses: Effective for gram-positive cocci *(S. aureus, S. pyogenes, S. viridans, S. faecalis, S. bovis, S. pneumoniae)*, infections caused by penicillinase-producing *Staphylococcus*

Dosage and routes:
• *Adult:* IM/IV 4-12 g/day in divided doses q4-6h
• *Child:* IM/IV 50-300 mg/kg/day in divided doses q4-12h
Available forms: Powder for inj IM, IV 1, 4, 6, 10 g; IV INF only 1 g

Side effects/adverse reactions:
HEMA: Anemia, increased bleeding time, *bone marrow depression, granulocytopenia*
GI: Nausea, vomiting, diarrhea, increased AST, ALT, abdominal pain, glossitis, colitis, interstitial nephritis
GU: Oliguria, *proteinuria, hematuria, vaginitis, moniliasis, glomerulonephritis*
CNS: Lethargy, hallucinations, anxiety, depression, twitching, *coma, convulsions*

Contraindications: Hypersensitivity to penicillins

Precautions: Pregnancy (B), hypersensitivity to cephalosporins, neonates

Pharmacokinetics:
IM: Peak ½-1 hr, duration 4 hr
IV: Peak 15 min, duration 2 hr; metabolized in liver; excreted in urine, bile, breast milk; crosses placenta

Interactions/incompatibilities:
• Decreased antimicrobial effectiveness of methicillin: tetracyclines, erythromycins
• Increased methicillin concentrations: aspirin, probenecid
• Incompatible in solution with

M

---

italics = common side effects   ***bold italic*** = life threatening reactions

amikacin, hydrocortisone, tetracyclines, vancomycin, heparin, lincomycin, chloramphenicol, codeine, levorphanol, methadone, methohexital, morphine, promethazine, NaCO$_3$, vancomycin

Lab test interferences:

False positive: Urine glucose, urine protein

NURSING CONSIDERATIONS
Assess:
• I&O ratio; report hematuria, oliguria, since penicillin in high doses is nephrotoxic
• Any patient with compromised renal system, since drug is excreted slowly in poor renal system function; toxicity may occur rapidly
• Liver studies: AST, ALT
• Blood studies: WBC, RBC, H&H, bleeding time
• Renal studies: urinalysis, protein, blood
• C&S before drug therapy; drug may be given as soon as culture is taken
• Bowel pattern before, during treatment
• Skin eruptions after administration of penicillin to 1 wk after discontinuing drug
• For thrombophlebitis at IV site, change IV site q48hr
• Respiratory status: rate, character, wheezing, tightness in chest
• Allergies before initiation of treatment, reaction of each medication; highlight allergies on chart, Kardex

Administer:
• IV after diluting 1 g/1.8 ml sterile H$_2$O; further dilute each 500 mg/25 ml or more NaCl; give directly at rate of 10 ml/min, added to D$_5$W, NS, LR, or by inf over ½-8 hr
• Drug after C&S has been completed

Perform/provide:
• Adrenalin, suction, tracheostomy set, endotracheal intubation equipment
• Adequate fluid intake (2 L) during diarrhea episodes
• Scratch test to assess allergy after securing order from physician; usually done when penicillin is only drug of choice
• Storage at room temperature; reconstituted solution is stable for 8 hr

Evaluate:
• Therapeutic response: absence of fever, draining wounds

Teach patient/family:
• That culture may be taken after completed course of medication
• To report sore throat, fever, fatigue (may indicate superimposed infection)
• To wear or carry Medic Alert ID if allergic to penicillins
• To notify nurse of diarrhea

Treatment of overdose: Withdraw drug; maintain airway; administer epinephrine, aminophylline, O$_2$, IV corticosteroids for anaphylaxis

---

methimazole

(meth-im'a-zole)

Tapazole

Func. class.: Antithyroid hormone

Chem. class.: Thioamide

Action: Inhibits synthesis of thyroid hormones by decreasing iodine use in manufacture of thyroglobin and iodothyronine; does not affect already formed hormones

Uses: Hyperthyroidism, preparation for thyroidectomy, thyrotoxic crisis, thyroid storm

Dosage and routes:

Hyperthyroidism
• *Adult:* PO 5-20 mg tid depending

on severity of condition; continue until euthyroid; maintenance dose 5-10 mg qd-tid, maximal dose 150 mg qd

• *Child:* PO 0.4 mg/kg/day in divided doses q8h; continue until euthyroid maintenance dose 0.2 mg/kg/day in divided doses q8h

Preparation for thyroidectomy
• *Adult and child:* PO same as above; iodine may be added × 10 days before surgery

Thyrotoxic crisis
• *Adult and child:* PO same as hyperthyroidism with iodine and propranolol

Available forms: Tabs 5, 10 mg

Side effects/adverse reactions:
ENDO: Enlarged thyroid
INTEG: Rash, urticaria, pruritus, alopecia, hyperpigmentation, lupuslike syndrome
GU: Nephritis
CNS: Drowsiness, headache, vertigo, fever, paresthesias, neuritis
*HEMA: **Agranulocytosis, leukopenia, thrombocytopenia, hypothrombinemia, lymphadenopathy,*** bleeding, vasculitis
*GI: Nausea, diarrhea, vomiting, **jaundice, hepatitis,*** loss of taste
MS: Myalgia, arthralgia, nocturnal muscle cramps

Contraindications: Hypersensitivity, pregnancy (3rd trimester) (D), lactation

Precautions: Infection, bone marrow depression, hepatic disease, pregnancy (1st, 2nd trimester), >40 yr

Pharmacokinetics:
PO: Onset 30-40 min, duration 2-4 hr, half-life 1-2 hr, excreted in urine, bile, breast milk, crosses placenta

Lab test interferences:
Increase: Pro-time, AST/ALT, alk phosphatase

NURSING CONSIDERATIONS
Assess:
• Pulse, B/P, temperature
• I&O ratio; check for edema: puffy hands, feet, periorbits; indicate hypothyroidism
• Weight qd; same clothing, scale, time of day
• T_3, T_4, which are increased; serum TSH, which is decreased; free thyroxine index, which is increased if dosage is too low; discontinue drug 3-4 wk before RAIU
• Blood work: CBC for blood dyscrasias: leukopenia, thrombocytopenia, agranulocytosis; LFTs
• Overdose: peripheral edema, heat intolerance, diaphoresis, palpitations, dysrhythmias, severe tachycardia, increased temperature, delirium, CNS irritability
• Hypersensitivity: rash, enlarged cervical lymph nodes; drug may have to be discontinued
• Hypoprothrombinemia: bleeding, petechiae, ecchymosis
• Clinical response: after 3 wk should include increased weight, pulse; decreased T_4
• Bone marrow depression: sore throat, fever, fatigue
Administer:
• With meals to decrease GI upset
• At same time each day to maintain drug level
• Lowest dose that relieves symptoms; discontinue before RAI
Perform/provide:
• Storage in light-resistant container
• Fluids to 3-4 L/day, unless contraindicated
Evaluate:
• Therapeutic response: weight gain, decreased pulse, decreased T_4, B/P
Teach patient/family:
• To abstain from breastfeeding after delivery

italics = common side effects   ***bold italic*** = life threatening reactions

- To take pulse daily
- To report redness, swelling, sore throat, mouth lesions, which indicate blood dyscrasias
- To keep graph of weight, pulse, mood
- To avoid OTC products that contain iodine
- That seafood, other iodine products may be restricted
- Not to discontinue this medication abruptly; thyroid crisis may occur; stress patient response
- That response may take several months if thyroid is large
- Symptoms/signs of overdose: periorbital edema, cold intolerance, mental depression
- Symptoms of inadequate dose: tachycardia, diarrhea, fever, irritability

---

methocarbamol

(meth-oh-kar'ba-mole)
Marbaxin 750, Methocarbamol, Robaxin, Robaxin-750, Robomol-500, Robomol-750, Tresortil*

Func. class.: Skeletal muscle relaxant
Chem. class.: Carbamate derivative

Action: Depresses multisynaptic pathways in the spinal cord
Uses: Adjunct for relief of spasm and pain in musculoskeletal conditions, tetanus management
Dosage and routes:
Pain
- *Adult:* PO 1.5 g × 2-3 days, then 1 g qid; IM 500 mg in each gluteal region, may repeat q8h; IV BOL 1-3 g/day at 3 ml/min; IV INF 1 gm/250 ml D₅W or NS, not to exceed 3 g/day

Tetanus
- *Adult:* IV INF 1-3 g/L of solution q6h; IV BOL 1-2 g injected into running IV
- *Child:* IV 15 mg/kg q6h
Available forms: Tabs 500, 750 mg; inj IM, IV 100 mg/ml
Side effects/adverse reactions:
CNS: Dizziness, weakness, drowsiness, headache, tremor, depression, insomnia, *seizures*
HEMA: Hemolysis, increased hemoglobin (IV only)
EENT: Diplopia, temporary loss of vision, blurred vision, nystagmus
CV: Postural hypotension, bradycardia
GI: Nausea, vomiting, hiccups, anorexia, metallic taste
GU: Brown, black, green urine
INTEG: Rash, pruritus, fever, facial flushing, urticaria
Contraindications: Hypersensitivity, child <12 yr, intermittent porphyria
Precautions: Renal disease, hepatic disease, addictive personalities, pregnancy (C), myasthenia gravis, epilepsy
Pharmacokinetics:
PO: Onset ½ hr, peak 1-2 hr, half-life 1-2 hr, metabolized in liver, excreted in urine (unchanged), crosses placenta
Interactions/incompatibilities:
- Increased CNS depression: alcohol, tricyclic antidepressants, narcotics, barbiturates, sedatives, hypnotics
- Considered incompatible with any drug in sol or syringe
Lab test interferences:
False increase: VMA, urinary 5-HIAA
NURSING CONSIDERATIONS
Assess:
- Blood studies: CBC, WBC, dif-

---

ferential; blood dyscrasias may occur
• During and after injection: CNS effects, rash, conjunctivitis, and nasal congestion may occur
• Liver function studies: AST, ALT, alk phosphatase; hepatitis may occur
• ECG in epileptic patients; poor seizure control has occurred with patients taking this drug
• Allergic reactions: rash, fever, respiratory distress
• Severe weakness, numbness in extremities
• Psychologic dependency: increased need for medication, more frequent requests for medication, increased pain
• CNS depression: dizziness, drowsiness, psychiatric symptoms
Administer:
• With meals for GI symptoms
• IV undiluted over 1 min or more, give 300 mg or less/1 min or longer; may be diluted in 250 ml or less D₅ or isotonic NaCl sol
• By slow IV to prevent phlebitis; keep recumbent for 15 min to prevent orthostatic hypotension; check for extravasation
• IM deeply in large muscle mass; rotate sites
Perform/provide:
• Storage in tight container at room temperature
• Assistance with ambulation if dizziness/drowsiness occurs
Evaluate:
• Therapeutic response: decreased pain, spasticity
Teach patient/family:
• Not to discontinue medication quickly; insomnia, nausea, headache, spasticity, tachycardia will occur; drug should be tapered off over 1-2 wk

• That urine may turn green, black or brown
• Not to take with alcohol, other CNS depressants
• To avoid altering activities while taking this drug
• To avoid hazardous activities if drowsiness, dizziness occurs
• To avoid using OTC medication: cough preparations, antihistamines, unless directed by physician
Treatment of overdose: Induce emesis of conscious patient, lavage, dialysis; have epinephrine, antihistamines, and corticosteroids available

---

methohexital sodium
(meth-oh-hex′i-tal)
Brevital Sodium, Brietal Sodium*
Func. class.: General anesthetic
Chem. class.: Barbiturate

Controlled Substance Schedule IV

Action: Acts in reticular-activating system to produce anesthesia
Uses: General anesthesia for electroshock therapy, reduction of fractures
Dosage and routes:
• *Adult and child:* IV 50-100 mg given 1 ml/5 sec
Maintenance
• *Adult and child:* IV 20-40 mg q4-7 min of a 0.1% sol; cont IV 1 gtt/sec of a 0.2% solution
Available forms: Inj IV 500 mg, 2.5, 5g
Side effects/adverse reactions:
*RESP: **Respiratory depression, bronchospasm***
CNS: Retrograde amnesia, prolonged somnolence
CV: Tachycardia, hypotension,

myocardial depression, dysrhythmias
EENT: Sneezing, coughing
INTEG: Chills, *shivering,* necrosis, pain at injection site
MS: Muscle irritability
Contraindications: Hypersensitivity, status asthmaticus, hepatic/intermittent porphyrias, pregnancy (D)
Precautions: Severe cardiovascular disease, renal disease, hypotension, liver disease, myxedema, myasthenia gravis, asthma, increased intracranial pressure
Pharmacokinetics:
IV: Onset 30-40 sec; half-life 11.5 hr; crosses placenta
Interactions/incompatibilities:
• Increased action: CNS depressants
• Do not mix with atropine or silicone in solution or syringe
NURSING CONSIDERATIONS
Assess:
• VS q3-5min during IV administration, after dose, q4hr postoperatively
• Extravasation; if it occurs, use chloroprocaine to decrease pain, increase circulation
• Dysrhythmias or myocardial depression
Administer:
• After preparation with sterile water 0.9%, NaCl or 5% dextrose
• Only with crash cart, resuscitative equipment nearby
• IV slowly only by qualified persons
Evaluate:
• Therapeutic response: induction of anesthesia

methotrexate/methotrexate sodium (amethopterin, MTX)

(meth-oh-trex′ate)
Folex PFS, Methotrexate, Methotrexate LPF, Rheumatrex Dose Pack
Func. class.: Antineoplastic-antimetabolite
Chem. class.: Folic acid antagonist

Action: Inhibits an enzyme that reduces folic acid, which is needed for nucleic acid synthesis in all cells; S phase of cell cycle specific
Uses: Acute lymphocytic leukemia, in combination for breast, lung, head, neck cancer, lymphosarcoma, psoriasis, gestational choriocarcinoma, hydatidiform mole
Dosage and routes:
Leukemia
• *Adult and child:* PO 3.3 mg/m²/day, maintenance 30 mg/m²/day 2×/wk; IV 2.5 mg/kg q2wk
Choriocarcinoma
• *Adult and child:* PO 15-30 mg/m² qd × 5 days, then off 1 wk; may repeat
Available forms: Tabs, 2.5 mg; inj IV 25 mg/ml; powder for inj IV 20, 25, 50, 100, 250 mg; sodium inj IV 2.5, 25 mg/ml
Side effects/adverse reactions:
HEMA: Leukopenia, thrombocytopenia, myelosuppression, anemia
GI: Nausea, vomiting, anorexia, diarrhea, stomatitis, hepatotoxicity, cramps, ulcer, gastritis, *GI hemorrhage,* abdominal pain, hematemesis
GU: Urinary retention, *renal failure,* menstrual irregularities, defective spermatogenesis, *hematuria, azotemia, uric acid nephropathy*

INTEG: Rash, alopecia, dry skin, urticaria, photosensitivity, folliculitis, vasculitis, petechiae, ecchymosis, acne, alopecia

CNS: Dizziness, **convulsions,** headache, confusion, hemiparesis, malaise, fatigue, chills, fever

Contraindications: Hypersensitivity, leukopenia ($<2500/mm^3$), thrombocytopenia ($<100,000/mm^3$), anemia, psoriatic patients with severe renal/hepatic disease, pregnancy (D)

Precautions: Renal disease, lactation

Pharmacokinetics:

PO: Readily absorbed when taken orally, peak 1-4 hr

IV/IM: Peak ½-2 hr

Not metabolized; excreted in urine (unchanged); crosses placenta, blood-brain barrier; 50% plasma protein bound

Interactions/incompatibilities:

• Increased toxicity: aspirin, sulfa drugs, other antineoplastics, radiation, alcohol, probenecid, phenytoin, phenylbutazone, pyrimethamine

• Decreased effect of: oral digoxin

• Increased hypoprothrombinemia: oral anticoagulants

• Decreased effect of methotrexate: folic acid supplements

• Possible fatal interactions: nonsteroidal antiinflammatory drugs

• Incompatible with bleomycin, fluorouracil, metoclopramide, prednisolone

NURSING CONSIDERATIONS

Assess:

• CBC, differential, platelet count weekly; withhold drug if WBC is $<3500/mm^3$ or platelet count is $<100,000/mm^3$; notify physician of these results; drug should be discontinued

• Renal function studies: BUN, serum uric acid, urine CrCl, electrolytes before, during therapy

• I&O ratio; report fall in urine output to <30 ml/hr

• Monitor temperature q4h; fever may indicate beginning infection; no rectal temperatures

• Liver function tests before and during therapy: bilirubin, alk phosphatase, AST, ALT; liver biopsy should be done before start of therapy (psoriasis patients)

• Bleeding time, coagulation time during treatment

• Bleeding: hematuria, guaiac, bruising or petechiae, mucosa or orifices q8h

• Food preferences; list likes, dislikes

• Effects of alopecia on body image; discuss feelings about body changes

• Hepatotoxicity: yellowing of skin and sclera, dark urine, clay-colored stools, pruritus, abdominal pain, fever, diarrhea

• Buccal cavity q8h for dryness, sores, ulceration, white patches, oral pain, bleeding, dysphagia

• Symptoms indicating severe allergic reaction: rash, urticaria, itching, flushing

Administer:

• IV after diluting 5 mg/2 ml of sterile H_2O for inj; give through Y-tube or 3-way stopcock at 10 mg or less/min

• Antacid before oral agent; give drug after evening meal before bedtime

• Antiemetic 30-60 min before giving drug to prevent vomiting

• Allopurinol or sodium bicarbonate to maintain uric acid levels, alkalinization of urine, adequate fluids

• Leucovorin Ca within 12 hr of

M

---

italics = common side effects   ***bold italic*** = life threatening reactions

this drug to prevent tissue damage; check agency policy
• Antibiotics for prophylaxis of infection
• Topical or systemic analgesics for pain
• Transfusion for anemia

Perform/provide:
• Strict medical asepsis and protective isolation if WBC levels are low
• Liquid diet: carbonated beverage, Jell-O; dry toast, crackers may be added when patient is not nauseated or vomiting
• Increased fluid intake to 2-3 L/day to prevent urate deposits, calculi formation, unless contraindicated
• Diet low in purines: absence of organ meats (kidney, liver), dried beans, peas to maintain alkaline urine
• Rinsing of mouth tid-qid with water, club soda; brushing of teeth bid-tid with soft brush or cotton-tipped applicators for stomatitis; use unwaxed dental floss
• Nutritious diet with iron, vitamin supplements
• Storage in tightly closed container in cool environment; store injection, powder for injection in dark, dry area

Evaluate:
• Therapeutic response: decreased tumor size, spread of malignancy

Teach patient/family:
• Why protective isolation precautions are needed
• To report any complaints, side effects to nurse or physician: black tarry stools, chills, fever, sore throat, bleeding, bruising, cough, shortness of breath, dark or bloody urine
• That hair may be lost during treatment; wig or hairpiece may make patient feel better; tell patient that new hair may be different in color, texture (alopecia is rare)
• To avoid foods with citric acid, hot or rough texture if stomatitis is present
• To report stomatitis: any bleeding, white spots, ulcerations in mouth to physician; tell patient to examine mouth qd, report symptoms to nurse
• That contraceptive measures are recommended during therapy for at least 8 wk following cessation of therapy
• To drink 10-12 glasses of fluid/day
• To avoid alcohol, salicylates
• To avoid use of razors, commercial mouthwash

---

methotrimeprazine HCl
(meth-oh-trye-mep'ra-zeen)
Levoprome, Nozinan*
Func. class.: Nonnarcotic analgesic
Chem. class.: Aliphatic (propylamine-phenothiazine derivative)

Action: Depresses cerebral cortex, hypothalamus, limbic system; blocks neurotransmission produced by dopamine at synapse; exhibits strong α-adrenergic, anticholinergic blocking action, antihistamine

Uses: Sedation, analgesia, preoperative and postoperative analgesia, obstetric analgesia in nonambulatory patients

Dosage and routes:
Analgesia/sedation
• *Adult and child >12 yr:* IM 10-20 mg q4-6h prn
• *Elderly:* IM 5-10 mg q4-6h
Preoperative medication
• *Adult and child >12 yr:* IM 2-20

mg 45 min to 3 hr before surgery
Postoperative medication
• *Adult and child >12 yr:* IM 2.5-7.5 mg q4-6h titrated to patient's needs
Obstetric analgesia
• *Adult:* 15-20 mg, may be repeated
Available forms: Inj IM 20 mg/ml
Side effects/adverse reactions:
HEMA: ***Thrombocytopenia, agranulocytosis, leukopenia, neutropenia, hemolytic anemia*** (long-term, high dose)
CNS: Weakness, dizziness, drowsiness, confusion, delirium, euphoria, headache, sedation, EPS
GI: Nausea, vomiting, abdominal pain, dry mouth, jaundice (long-term use)
GU: ***Hematuria,*** dysuria, hesitancy, retention, uterine inertia (rare)
INTEG: Pain, edema at injection site, fever, chills
EENT: Nasal congestion, blurred vision, slurred speech
CV: Orthostatic hypotension, palpitations, tachycardia, bradycardia
Contraindications: Hypersensitivity to this drug, phenothiazines, bisulfite; seizures; severe hepatic disease; severe renal disease; severe cardiac disease; coma
Precautions: Elderly, pregnancy (C)
Pharmacokinetics:
IM: Onset 20-30 min, peak 1-2 hr, duration 4 hr; metabolized by liver, excreted by kidneys and in feces, crosses placenta, excreted in breast milk
Interactions/incompatibilities:
• Mix only with scopolamine or atropine; not to be mixed in syringe or sol with any other drugs
• Increased sedation: CNS depressants, alcohol, barbiturates, reser-

pine, narcotics, general anesthetics, meprobamate
NURSING CONSIDERATIONS
Assess:
• Blood studies: CBC, ALT, AST, bilirubin
• VS q10min for 30 min; watch for decreasing B/P with increased pulse that may occur 10-30 min after injection; continue to monitor closely for 6-12 hr after several injections
• Effect on uterine contractions, fetal heart tones if using for labor
Administer:
• After removal of cigarettes to prevent fires
• IM injection in deep large muscle mass to prevent tissue sloughing; rotate sites
• Lowest dose, then gradually increase; lower doses are required after general anesthesia
Perform/provide:
• Bed rest for several hours after injection if orthostatic hypotension occurs
• Safety measure: side rails, nightlight, call bell within easy reach
• Storage in darkness; expires after 5 yr
• Assistance with ambulation for 6 hr after injection
Evaluate:
• Therapeutic response: decrease in pain, grimacing, absence of change in VS, ability to cough and breathe deep after surgery
Teach patient/family:
• To avoid ambulation without assistance for 6 hr after drug is given
Treatment of overdose: Monitor electrolytes, vital signs

M

---

italics = common side effects   ***bold italic*** = life threatening reactions

methoxsalen

(meth-ox′a-len)
8-Mop, Oxsoralen, Oxsoralen Ultra

Func. class.: Pigmenting agent
Chem. class.: Psoralen derivative

Action: Decreases cell turnover by combining with epidermal cell DNA, causing photo damage when used with ultraviolet rays

Uses: Vitiligo, psoriasis

Dosage and routes:

Vitiligo

• *Adult and child >12 yr:* PO 20 mg qd 2-4 hr before exposure to therapeutic ultraviolet rays; administer on alternate days; TOP apply 1-2 hr before exposure to UVA light; treatment intervals regulated by erythema response

Psoriasis

Adult PO: Dosage individualized according to weight; taken 2 hr before exposure to therapeutic ultraviolet rays

Available forms: Lotion 1%; hard caps 10 mg; soft caps 10 mg; contains tartrazine

Side effects/adverse reactions:

CNS: Headache, depression, restlessness, anxiety, nervousness, vertigo, insomnia, malaise

GI: Nausea

INTEG: Rash, pruritus, burning, peeling, erythema, edema, urticaria, hypopigmentation

MISC: Leg cramps, hypotension, herpes simplex

Contraindications: Hypersensitivity, melanoma, LE, albinism, sunburn, cataracts, squamous cell cancer, child ≤12 yr, diseases associated with photosensitivity

Precautions: Hepatic disease, cardiac disease, children, lactation, pregnancy (C); contains tartrazine (FD&C #5), photosensitizing agents

Pharmacokinetics:

PO: Duration 8 hr, half-life 2 hr, metabolized in liver, excreted in urine

Interactions/incompatibilities:

• Increased effects of methoxsalen: other photosensitizing agents, phenothiazines, thiazides, tetracyclines, griseofulvin, halogenated salicylanides, sulfonamides, coal tar derivatives, nalidixic acid

NURSING CONSIDERATIONS

Assess:

• Hepatic test (AST, ALT, bilirubin), renal test (BUN, protein), antinuclear antibodies during treatment

Administer:

• With food or milk to prevent GI upset

• To prevent extensive phototoxicity, qod

• Lotion to small areas; use systemic treatment for large areas

Perform/provide:

• Protection to eyes, lips during treatment

• Use of finger cot or gloves to apply lotion

Evaluate:

• Therapeutic response: increased pigmentation in vitiligo, decreased psoriatic areas

Teach patient/family:

• To avoid UVA exposure for at least 24 hr after topical application and 8 hr after PO dose

• That sunscreen may be used if exposure to sunlight occurs after treatment

• That repigmentation may require 6-9 mo

• Avoid furocoumarin-containing

foods: limes, figs, parsley, parsnips, mustard, carrots, celery

---

methscopolamine bromide

(meth-skoe-pol′a-meen)
Pamine
Func. class.: GI anticholinergic
Chem. class.: Synthetic quaternary ammonium antimuscarinic

Action: Inhibits muscarinic actions of acetylcholine at postganglionic parasympathetic neuroeffector sites
Uses: Treatment of peptic ulcer disease
Dosage and routes:
• *Adult:* PO 2.5-5 mg ½ hr ac, hs
Available forms: Tabs 2.5 mg
Side effects/adverse reactions:
CNS: Confusion, stimulation in elderly, headache, insomnia, dizziness, drowsiness, anxiety, weakness, hallucination
*GI: Dry mouth, constipation, **paralytic ileus,*** heartburn, nausea, vomiting, dysphagia, absence of taste
GU: Hesitancy, retention, impotence
CV: Palpitations, tachycardia
EENT: Blurred vision, photophobia, mydriasis, cycloplegia, increased ocular tension
INTEG: Urticaria, rash, pruritus, anhidrosis, fever, allergic reactions
Contraindications: Hypersensitivity to anticholinergics, narrow-angle glaucoma, GI obstruction, myasthenia gravis, paralytic ileus, GI atony, toxic megacolon
Precautions: Hyperthyroidism, coronary artery disease, dysrhythmias, CHF, ulcerative colitis, hypertension, hiatal hernia, hepatic disease, renal disease, pregnancy (C), urinary retention, pros pertrophy
Pharmacokinetics:
PO: Onset 1 hr, duration 6-8 hr; metabolized by liver, excreted in urine
Interactions/incompatibilities:
• Increased anticholinergic effect: amantadine, tricyclic antidepressants, MAOIs, H₁ antihistamines
• Decreased effect of: phenothiazines, levodopa, ketoconazole
NURSING CONSIDERATIONS
Assess:
• VS, cardiac status: checking for dysrhythmias, increased rate, palpitations
• I&O ratio; check for urinary retention or hesitancy
• GI complaints: pain, bleeding (frank or occult), nausea, vomiting, anorexia
Administer:
• ½-1 hr ac for better absorption
• Decreased dose to elderly patients; their metabolism may be slowed
• Gum, hard candy, frequent rinsing of mouth for dryness of oral cavity
Perform/provide:
• Storage in tight container protected from light
• Increased fluids, bulk, exercise to patient's life-style to decrease constipation
Evaluate:
• Therapeutic response: absence of epigastric pain, bleeding, nausea, vomiting
Teach patient/family:
• To avoid driving or other hazardous activities until stabilized on medication
• To avoid alcohol or other CNS depressants; will enhance sedating properties of this drug
• To drink plenty of fluids
• To report dysphagia

---

italics = common side effects   ***bold italic*** = life threatening reactions

...se blurred vi-

Celontin, Kapseals

Func. class.: Anticonvulsant
Chem. class.: Succinimide

Action: Inhibits spike, wave formation in absence seizures (petit mal), decreases amplitude, frequency, duration, spread of discharge in minor motor seizures

Uses: Refractory absence seizures (petit mal)

Dosage and routes:
• *Adult and child:* PO 300 mg/day; may increase by 300 mg/wk, not to exceed 1.2 g/day in divided doses

Available forms: Caps, half-strength 150 mg; caps 300 mg

Side effects/adverse reactions:
*HEMA: **Agranulocytosis, aplastic anemia, thrombocytopenia, leukocytosis, eosinophilia, pancytopenia***
CNS: Drowsiness, dizziness, fatigue, euphoria, lethargy, irritability, depression, insomnia, anxiety, aggressiveness, ataxia, headache, confusion
GI: Nausea, vomiting, heartburn, anorexia, diarrhea, abdominal pain, cramps, constipation, gum hypertrophy, tongue swelling
GU: Vaginal bleeding, ***hematuria, renal damage***
INTEG: Urticaria, pruritic erythema, hirsutism, ***Stevens-Johnson syndrome***, systemic lupus erythematosus
EENT: Myopia, blurred vision

Contraindications: Hypersensitivity to succinimide derivatives

Precautions: Hepatic disease, re-nal disease, pregnancy (C), lactation

Pharmacokinetics:
PO: Onset 15-30 min, peak 1-2 hr, duration 4-6 hr
REC: Onset slow, duration 4-6 hr; metabolized by liver, excreted by kidneys, half-life 2⅗-4 hr

Interactions/incompatibilities:
• Antagonist effect: tricyclic antidepressants
• Decreased effects of: estrogens, oral contraceptives

Lab test interferences:
Increase: Coombs' test

NURSING CONSIDERATIONS
Assess:
• Renal studies: urinalysis, BUN, urine creatinine
• Blood studies: CBC, Hct, Hgb, reticulocyte counts qwk for 4 wk then qmo
• Hepatic studies: ALT, AST, bilirubin, creatinine
• Drug levels during initial treatment, therapeutic range (10-40 μg/ml)
• Mental status: mood, sensorium, affect, behavioral changes; if mental status changes notify physician
• Eye problems; need for ophthalmic exams before, during, after treatment (slit lamp, fundoscopy, tonometry)
• Allergic reaction: red raised rash; if this occurs, drug should be discontinued
• Blood dyscrasias: fever, sore throat, bruising, rash, jaundice
• Toxicity: bone marrow depression, nausea, vomiting, ataxia, diplopia

Administer:
• With food, milk to decrease GI symptoms

Perform/provide:
• Hard candy, frequent rinsing of mouth, gum for dry mouth

• Assistance with ambulation during early part of treatment; dizziness occurs

Evaluate:
• Therapeutic response: decreased seizure activity, document on patient's chart

Teach patient/family:
• To avoid driving, other activities that require alertness
• To avoid alcohol ingestion, CNS depressants; increased sedation may occur
• Not to discontinue medication quickly after long-term use
• To call physician promptly if lupuslike syndrome occurs (enlarged lymph nodes, fever, bruising, sore throat)
• That drug may change urine to pink or brown

Treatment of overdose: Lavage, activated charcoal; monitor electrolytes, VS

---

methylcellulose
(meth-ill-sell'yoo-lose)
Citrucel
Func. class.: Laxative, bulk
Chem. class.: Hydrophilic semisynthetic cellulose derivative

Action: Attracts water, expands in intestine to increase peristalsis; also absorbs excess water in stool; decreases diarrhea
Uses: Constipation
Dosage and routes:
• *Adult:* PO 5-20 ml tid with 8 oz H_2O
• *Child:* PO 5-10 ml qd or bid with H_2Oor 500 mg tid with 8 oz H_2O
Available forms: Powder 105 mg/g; sol 450 mg/5 ml; tab 500 mg
Side effects/adverse reactions:
*GI: **Obstruction,*** abdominal distention

Contraindications: Hypersensitivity, GI obstruction, hepatitis
Pharmacokinetics:
PO: Onset 12-24 hr, peak 1-3 days
Interactions/incompatibilities:
• Decreased absorption: antibiotics, digitalis, nitrofurantoin, salicylates, tetracyclines, oral anticoagulants
NURSING CONSIDERATIONS
Assess:
• Blood, urine electrolytes if drug is used often by patient
• I&O ratio to identify fluid loss
• Cause of constipation; identify whether fluids, bulk, or exercise is missing from life-style
• Cramping, rectal bleeding, nausea, vomiting; if these symptoms occur, drug should be discontinued
Administer:
• Alone for better absorption; do not take within 1 hr of other drugs
• In morning or evening (oral dose)
Evaluate:
• Therapeutic response: decrease in constipation
Teach patient/family:
• To swallow tabs whole; do not chew, increase fluid intake
• That normal bowel movements do not always occur daily
• Not to use in presence of abdominal pain, nausea, vomiting
• To notify physician if constipation unrelieved or if symptoms of electrolyte imbalance occur: muscle cramps, pain, weakness, dizziness, excessive thirst

M

---

italics = common side effects **bold italic** = life threatening reactions

methyldopa/methyl-dopate

(meth-ill-doe'pa)

Aldomet, Amodopa, Dopa-met,* Medimet,* Methyldopa/Methyldopate HCl, Novomedopa*

Func. class.: Antihypertensive
Chem. class.: Centrally acting adrenergic inhibitor

Action: Stimulates central inhibitory α-adrenergic receptors or acts as false transmitter, resulting in reduction of arterial pressure

Uses: Hypertension

Dosage and routes:

• *Adult:* PO 250 mg bid or tid, then adjusted q2d as needed, 0.5-3 g qd in 2-4 divided doses (maintenance), not to exceed 3 g/day; IV 250 mg-500 mg in 100 ml D_5W q6h, run over 30-60 min, not to exceed 1 g q6h

• *Child:* PO 10 mg/kg/day in 2-4 divided doses, not to exceed 65 mg/kg or 3 g/day, whichever is less; IV 20-40 mg/kg/day in 4 divided doses, not to exceed 65 mg/kg

Available forms: Tabs 125, 250, 500 mg; oral susp 250 mg/5ml; inj IV 50 mg/ml

Side effects/adverse reactions:

GI: Nausea, vomiting, diarrhea, constipation, hepatic dysfunction

CV: Bradycardia, myocarditis, orthostatic hypotension, angina, edema, weight gain

CNS: Drowsiness, weakness, dizziness, sedation, headache, depression, psychosis

EENT: Nasal congestion, eczema

HEMA: Leukopenia, thrombocytopenia, hemolytic anemia, positive Coombs' test

INTEG: Lupuslike syndrome

GU: Impotence, failure to ejaculate

Contraindications: Active hepatic disease, hypersensitivity, blood dyscrasias

Precautions: Pregnancy (C), liver disease, eclampsia, severe cardiac disease

Pharmacokinetics:

PO: Peak 2-4 hr, duration 12-24 hr

IV: Peak 2 hr, duration 10-16 hr; metabolized by liver, excreted in urine

Interactions/incompatibilities:

• Increased pressor effect: sympathomimetic amines (norepinephrine, phenylpropanolamine)

• Increased hypotension: levodopa

• Increased sedation: haloperidol

• Increased action of: anesthetics

NURSING CONSIDERATIONS

Assess:

• Blood studies: neutrophils, decreased platelets

• Baselines in renal, liver function tests before therapy begins

• B/P during beginning treatment, periodically thereafter

• Allergic reaction: rash, fever, pruritus, urticaria; drug should be discontinued if antihistamines fail to help

• Symptoms of CHF: edema, dyspnea, wet rales, B/P

• Renal symptoms: polyuria, oliguria, frequency

Administer:

• IV after diluting with 100-200 ml of D_5W run over ½-1 hr

Perform/provide:

• Storage of tablets in tight containers

Evaluate:

• Therapeutic response: decrease in B/P in hypertension

Teach patient/family:

• To avoid hazardous activities

• To administer 1 hr before meals

---

* Available in Canada only

• Not to discontinue drug abruptly, or withdrawal symptoms may occur: anxiety, increased B/P, headache, insomnia, increased pulse, tremors, nausea, sweating
• Not to use OTC (cough, cold, allergy) products unless directed by physician
• To avoid sunlight or wear sunscreen if in sunlight; photosensitivity may occur
• To comply with dosage schedule even if feeling better
• To rise slowly to sitting or standing position to minimize orthostatic hypotension
• To notify physician of mouth sores, sore throat, fever, swelling of hands or feet, irregular heartbeat, chest pain, signs of angioedema
• That excessive perspiration, dehydration, vomiting, diarrhea may lead to fall in blood pressure; consult physician if these occur
• That dizziness, fainting, lightheadedness may occur during 1st few days of therapy
• That compliance is necessary; not to skip or stop drug unless directed by physician
• That drug may cause skin rash or impaired perspiration

---

methylene blue
(meth'i-leen)
Methylene Blue, Urolene Blue
Func. class.: Urinary tract antiseptic
Chem. class.: Antiseptic dye

Action: Oxidation-reduction; has opposite action on hemoglobin depending on concentration; with increased concentration, converts ferrous ion of reduced hemoglobin to ferric form methemoglobin is thus produced; prolonged administration accelerates destruction of erythrocytes

Uses: Oxalate urinary tract calculi; urinary tract infections caused by *E. coli, Klebsiella, Enterobacter, P. mirabilis, P. vulgaris, P. morganii, Serratia, Citrobacter,* cyanide poisoning, methemoglobinemia

Dosage and routes:
• *Adult:* PO 65-130 mg pc with full glass of water
Cyanide poisoning/methemoglobinemia
• *Adult and child:* IV 1-2 mg/kg of 1% sol; inject slowly over 5 min or more
Available forms: Tabs 65 mg, inj 10 mg/ml

Side effects/adverse reactions:
CV: Cyanosis, CV abnormalities
INTEG: Pruritus, rash, urticaria, photosensitivity, profuse sweating
CNS: Dizziness, headache, drowsiness, mental confusion, fever with large doses
GI: Nausea, vomiting, abdominal pain, diarrhea
GU: Bladder irritation

Contraindications: Hypersensitivity to this drug, renal insufficiency

Precautions: Anemia, renal disease, hepatic disease, G-6-PD deficiency, pregnancy (C)

Pharmacokinetics:
PO/IV: Excreted in urine, bile, feces

NURSING CONSIDERATIONS
Assess:
• For cyanosis
• I&O ratio; urine pH <5.5 is ideal
• Hct, Hgb
• CNS symptoms: insomnia, headache, drowsiness, confusion
• Allergic reactions: fever, flushing, rash, urticaria, pruritus

M

---

italics = common side effects   **bold italic** = life threatening reactions

Administer:

• After clean-catch urine is obtained for C&S

• Two daily doses if urine output is high or if patient has diabetes

Perform/provide:

• Limited intake of alkaline foods, drugs: milk, dairy products, peanuts, vegetables, alkaline antacids, sodium bicarbonate

Evaluate:

• Therapeutic response: decreased pain, frequency, urgency, C&S absence of infection

Teach patient/family:

• That anemia may result with continued administration

• That drug turns urine, sometimes stool, blue-green

• To notify physician if symptoms do not improve

• To notify physician of any sign/symptoms of side effects or adverse reactions

---

methylergonovine maleate

(meth-ill-er-goe-noe′veen)
Methergine, Methylergobasine*

Func. class.: Oxytocic
Chem. class.: Ergot alkaloid

Action: Stimulates uterine contractions, decreases bleeding

Uses: Treatment of hemorrhage associated with postpartum or postabortion

Dosage and routes:

• *Adult:* IM 0.2 mg q2-5h, not to exceed 5 doses; IV 0.2 mg given over 1 min; PO 0.2-0.4 mg q6-12h × 2-7 days after initial IM or IV dose

Available forms Inj IM, IV 0.2 mg/ml; tabs 0.2 mg

Side effects/adverse reactions:

CNS: Headache, dizziness
GI: Nausea, vomiting
CV: Chest pain, palpitation, hypertension
EENT: Tinnitus
INTEG: Sweating, rash

Contraindications: Hypersensitivity to ergot preparations, indication of labor, before delivery of placenta, hypertension, pelvic inflammatory disease (PID), respiratory disease, cardiac disease, peripheral vascular disease

Precautions: Pregnancy (C), severe hepatic disease, severe renal disease, jaundice, diabetes mellitus, convulsive disorders

Pharmacokinetics:

PO: Onset 5-25 min, duration 3 hr
IM: Onset 2-5 min, duration 3 hr
IV: Onset immediate, duration 45 min

Metabolized in liver, excreted in urine

Interactions/incompatibilities:

• Incompatible in sol or syringe with any other drug

NURSING CONSIDERATIONS
Assess:

• B/P, pulse, character and amount of vaginal bleeding; watch for changes that may indicate hemorrhage

• Respiratory rate, rhythm, depth; notify physician of abnormalities

• For uterine relaxation; observe for severe cramping

• Ergot toxicity: tinnitus, hypertension, palpitations, chest pain

Administer:

• IV undiluted through Y-tube or 3-way stopcock; give 0.2 mg or less/min

• Only during fourth stage of labor; not to be used to augment labor

• IM in deep muscle mass; rotate

injection sites if additional doses are given

• With crash cart available on unit; IV route used only in emergencies

Evaluate:

• Therapeutic response: absence of postpartum, postabortion hemorrhage

Teach patient/family:

• To report increased blood loss, severe abdominal cramps, increased temperature or foul-smelling lochia

---

methylphenidate HCl

(meth-ill-fen'i-date)

Methidate, Ritalin, Ritalin SR

Func. class.: Cerebral stimulant

Chem. class.: Piperidine derivative

Controlled Substance Schedule II

Action: Increases release of norepinephrine, dopamine in cerebral cortex to reticular activating system; exact action not known

Uses: Attention deficit disorder with hyperactivity, narcolepsy

Dosage and routes:

Attention deficit disorder

• *Child >6 yr:* 5 mg before breakfast and lunch, increasing by 5-10 mg/wk, not to exceed 60 mg/day

Narcolepsy

• *Adult:* PO 10 mg bid-tid, 30-45 min before meals, may increase up to 40-60 mg/day

Available forms: Tabs 5, 10, 20 mg; tabs sus rel 20 mg

Side effects/adverse reactions:

MISC: fever, arthralgia, scalp hair loss

CNS: Hyperactivity, insomnia, restlessness, talkativeness, dizziness, headache, akathisia, dyskinesia, Gilles de la Tourette's syndrome

GI: Nausea, anorexia, dry mouth, weight loss, abdominal pain

CV: Palpitations, tachycardia, B/P changes, angina, dysrhythmias, ***thrombocytopenic purpura***

*INTEG: **Exfoliative dermatitis,*** urticaria, rash, erythema-multiforme

ENDO: Growth retardation

*GU: **Uremia***

HEMA: Leukopenia, anemia

Contraindications: Hypersensitivity, anxiety, history of Gilles de la Tourette's syndrome; children <6 yrs., glaucoma

Precautions: Hypertension, depression, pregnancy (C), seizures, lactation, drug abuse

Pharmacokinetics:

PO: Onset ½-1 hr, duration 4-6 hr, metabolized by liver, excreted by kidneys

Interactions/incompatibilities:

• Hypertensive crisis: MAOIs or within 14 days of MAOIs, vasopressors

• Decreased effects of: guanethidine

NURSING CONSIDERATIONS

Assess:

• VS, B/P, since this drug may reverse antihypertensives; check patients with cardiac disease more often

• CBC, urinalysis, in diabetes: blood sugar, urine sugar; insulin changes may have to be made, since eating will decrease

• Height, growth rate in children; growth rate may be decreased

• Mental status: mood, sensorium, affect, stimulation, insomnia, aggressiveness

• Withdrawal symptoms: headache, nausea, vomiting, muscle pain, weakness

---

italics = common side effects   ***bold italic*** = life threatening reactions

Administer:
• At least 6 hr before hs to avoid sleeplessness
• Gum, hard candy, frequent sips of water for dry mouth

Evaluate:
• Therapeutic response: decreased hyperactivity or ability to stay awake

Teach patient/family:
• To decrease caffeine consumption (coffee, tea, cola, chocolate); may increase irritability, stimulation
• Not to chew or crush timed-released medication
• To avoid OTC preparations unless approved by physician
• To taper off drug over several weeks, or depression, increased sleeping, lethargy will ensue
• To avoid alcohol ingestion
• To avoid hazardous activities until patient is stabilized on medication
• To get needed rest; patients will feel more tired at end of day

Treatment of overdose: Administer fluids; hemodialysis or peritoneal dialysis; antihypertensive for increased B/P; administer short-acting barbiturate before lavage

---

methylprednisolone/ methylprednisolone acetate/methylprednisolone sodium succinate
(meth-il-pred-niss'-oh-lone)
Medrol/Depo-Medrol, Duralone, Medralone, Rep-Pred/A-Methapred, Solu-Medrol
Func. class.: Corticosteroid
Chem. class.: Glucocorticoid, immediate acting

Action: Decreases inflammation by suppression of migration of polymorphonuclear leukocytes, fibroblasts, reversal of increased capillary permeability and lysosomal stabilization

Uses: Severe inflammation, shock, adrenal insufficiency, collagen disorders

Dosage and routes:
Adrenal insufficiency/inflammation
• *Adult:* PO 2-60 mg in 4 divided doses; IM 40-80 mg (acetate); IM/IV 10-250 mg (succinate); intra-articular: 4-30 mg (acetate)
• *Child:* IV 117 μg-1.66 mg/kg in 3-4 divided doses (succinate)
Shock
• *Adult:* IV 100-250 mg q2-6h (succinate)

Available forms: Tabs 2, 4, 6, 8, 16, 24, 32 mg; inj 20, 40, 80 mg/ml acetate; inj 40, 125, 500, 1000 mg/vial succinate

Side effects/adverse reactions:
CNS: Depression, flushing, sweating, headache, mood changes
CV: Hypertension, *circulatory collapse, thrombophlebitis, embolism,* tachycardia
EENT: Fungal infections, increased intraocular pressure, blurred vision
GI: Diarrhea, nausea, abdominal distention, GI hemorrhage, increased appetite, pancreatitis
HEMA: Thrombocytopenia
INTEG: Acne, poor wound healing, ecchymosis, petechiae
MS: Fractures, osteoporosis, weakness

Contraindications: Psychosis, hypersensitivity, idiopathic thrombocytopenia, acute glomerulonephritis, amebiasis, fungal infections, nonasthmatic bronchial disease, child <2 yr, AIDS, TB

Precautions: Pregnancy (C), diabetes mellitus, glaucoma, osteo-

porosis, seizure disorders, ulcerative colitis, CHF, myasthenia
gravis, renal disease, esophagitis,
peptic ulcer
Pharmacokinetics: Well absorbed
PO, IM
PO: Peak 1-2 hr, duration 1½ day
IM: Peak 4-8 days, duration 1-4 wk
INTRAARTICULAR: Peak 1 wk
Half-life >3½ hr; crosses placenta,
enters breast milk in small
amounts; metabolized in liver, excreted by the kidneys (unchanged)
Interactions/incompatibilities:
• Decreased action of methylprednisolone: cholestyramine, colestipol, barbiturates, rifampin, ephedrine, phenytoin, theophylline
• Decreased effects of: anticoagulants, anticonvulsants, antidiabetics, ambenonium, neostigmine,
isoniazid, toxoid, vaccines, anticholinesterases, salicylates, somatrem
• Increased side effects: alcohol,
salicylates, indomethacin, amphotericin B, digitalis, cyclosporine,
diuretics
• Increased action of methylprednisolone: salicylates, estrogens, indomethacin, oral contraceptives,
ketoconazole, macrolide antibiotics
• Incompatible with aminophylline, calcium gluconate, cephalothin, chlorpromazine, cytarabine,
digitoxin, diphenhydramine, glycopyrrolate, insulin, meperidine,
metaraminol, nafcillin, penicillin
G, promethazine, tetracycline,
thiopental, tolazine
Lab test interferences:
Increase: Cholesterol, Na, blood
glucose, uric acid, Ca, urine glucose
Decrease: Ca, K, T₄, T₃, thyroid
¹³¹I uptake test, urine 17-OHCS,
17-KS, PBI
False negative: Skin allergy tests

NURSING CONSIDERATIONS
Assess:
• K depletion: parethesias, fatigue,
nausea, vomiting, depression,
polyuria, dysrhythmias, weakness
• Edema, hypertension, cardiac
symptoms
• Mental status: affect, mood, behavioral changes, aggression
• K, blood sugar, urine glucose
while on long-term therapy; hypokalemia and hyperglycemia
• Joint mobility, pain, edema if
given intraarticularly
• Weight daily; notify physician of
weekly gain >5 lb
• B/P q4hr, pulse; notify physician
of chest pain, rales
• I&O ratio; be alert for decreasing
urinary output and increasing
edema
• Adrenal insufficiency: weight
loss, nausea, vomiting, confusion,
anxiety, hypotension, weakness
• Plasma cortisol levels during
long-term therapy (normal level:
138-635 nmol/L SI units when
drawn at 8 AM)
• Growth in children on long-term
treatment
Administer:
• IV after diluting with diluent provided; agitate slowly; give 500 mg
or less/1 min or longer; may be
given as IV infusion in its own diluent over 10-20 min
• Titrated dose; use lowest effective dose
• IM inj deeply in large mass; rotate sites; avoid deltoid; use 21G
needle; after shaking suspension
(parenteral)
• In one dose in AM to prevent adrenal suppression; avoid SC administration; may damage tissue
• With food or milk to decrease GI
symptoms (PO)

M

---

italics = common side effects   ***bold italic*** = life threatening reactions

Perform/provide:
• Assistance with ambulation in patient with bone tissue disease to prevent fractures

Evaluate:
• Therapeutic response: ease of respirations, decreased inflammation; decreased symptoms of adrenal insufficiency
• Infection: increased temperature, WBC, even after withdrawal of medication; drug masks symptoms of infection

Teach patient/family:
• To increase intake of K, Ca, protein
• That ID as steroid user should be carried
• To notify physician if therapeutic response decreases; dosage adjustment may be needed
• Not to discontinue this medication abruptly, or adrenal crisis can result
• To avoid OTC products: salicylates, alcohol in cough products, cold preparations unless directed by physician; to avoid vaccinations, since immunosuppression occurs
• About cushingoid symptoms
• Symptoms of adrenal insufficiency: nausea, anorexia, fatigue, dizziness, dyspnea, weakness, joint pain

---

methylprednisolone acetate

(meth-ill-pred-niss'oh-lone)
Depo-Medrol

Func. class.: Topical corticosteroid
Chem. class.: Synthetic non-fluorinated agent, group VI potency

Action: Antipruritic, antiinflammatory

Uses: Psoriasis, eczema, contact dermatitis, pruritus

Dosage and routes:
• *Adult and child:* Apply to affected area qd-qid
Available forms: Oint 0.25%, 1%

Side effects/adverse reactions:
INTEG: Burning, dryness, itching, irritation, acne, folliculitis, hypertrichosis, perioral dermatitis, hypopigmentation, atrophy, striae, miliaria, allergic contact dermatitis, secondary infection

Contraindications: Hypersensitivity to corticosteroids, fungal infections

Precautions: Pregnancy (C), lactation, viral or bacterial infections

NURSING CONSIDERATIONS

Assess:
• Temperature: if fever develops, drug should be discontinued
• For systemic absorption: increased temperature, inflammation, irritation

Administer:
• Only to affected areas; do not get in eyes
• Medication, then cover with occlusive dressing (only if prescribed), seal to normal skin, change q12h; systemic absorption may occur; use gloves for application
• Only to dermatoses; do not use on weeping, denuded, or infected area

Perform/provide:
• Cleansing before application of drug
• Treatment for a few days after area has cleared
• Storage at room temperature

Evaluate:
• Therapeutic response: absence of severe itching, patches on skin, flaking

Teach patient/family:
• To avoid sunlight on affected area; burns may occur

---

*Available in Canada only

methyprylon
(meth-i-prye'lon)
Noludar
Func. class.: Sedative-hypnotic
Chem. class.: Piperidine derivative

Controlled Substance Schedule III (USA), Schedule F (Canada)
Action: Acts at level of thalamus to produce CNS mood alterations by interfering with nerve impulse transmission in sensory cortex by increasing threshold of arousal centers; suppresses REM sleep
Uses: Insomnia
Dosage and routes:
• *Adult:* PO 200-400 mg 15-30 min before hs
• *Child >12 yrs:* PO 50 mg hs; may increase to 200 mg
Available forms: Caps 300 mg, tabs 50, 200 mg
Side effects/adverse reactions:
CNS: Residual sedation, dizziness, ataxia, stimulation, headache, pyrexia, nightmares, depression; REM rebound after discharge
GI: Nausea, vomiting, diarrhea, esophagitis, constipation
INTEG: Rash, pruritus
Contraindications: Hypersensitivity to piperidine derivatives, severe pain, severe renal or hepatic disease, porphyria
Precautions: Depression, suicidal individuals, drug abuse, cardiac dysrhythmias, narrow-angle glaucoma, prostatic hypertrophy, stenosed peptic ulcer, pyloroduodenal/bladder neck obstruction, pregnancy (B)
Pharmacokinetics:
PO: Onset 45 min, peak 1-2 hr, duration 5-8 hr; metabolized by the liver, excreted by the kidneys, crosses placenta, excreted in breast milk; half-life 3-6 hr
Interactions/incompatibilities:
• Increased CNS depression: alcohol, barbiturates, narcotics and other CNS depressants

NURSING CONSIDERATIONS
Assess:
• Blood studies: Hct, Hgb, RBCs (long-term therapy)
• Hepatic studies: AST, ALT, bilirubin (long-term therapy)
• Mental status: mood, sensorium, affect, memory (long, short)
• Type of sleep problem: falling asleep, staying asleep
• Physical dependency, including more frequent requests for medication, shakes, anxiety
• Withdrawal: nausea, vomiting, anxiety, hallucinations, insomnia, tachycardia, fever, cramps, tremors, seizures
• Allergic reaction: rash; discontinue drug if rash occurs
Administer:
• After removal of cigarettes to prevent fires
• After trying conservative measures for insomnia
• ½-1 hr before hs for sleeplessness
• On empty stomach for fast onset, but may be taken with food if GI symptoms occur
• Overdosing symptoms: respiratory depression, hypotension, confusion, coma, constricted pupils
Perform/provide:
• Assistance with ambulation after receiving dose
• Safety measures: side rails, nightlight, call bell within easy reach
• Checking to see PO medication has been swallowed; watch depressed, drug-dependent patients for hoarding, self-overdosing
• Storage in tight, light-resistant container in cool environment

italics = common side effects   ***bold italic*** = life threatening reactions

Evaluate:
• Therapeutic response: ability to sleep at night, decreased amount of early morning awakening if taking drug for insomnia

Teach patient/family:
• To avoid driving or other activities requiring alertness until drug stabilizes
• To avoid alcohol ingestion or CNS depressants; serious CNS depression may result
• Not to discontinue medication quickly after long-term use; drug should be tapered over 1-2 wk
• That effects may take 2 nights for benefits to be noticed
• Alternate measures to improve sleep: reading, exercise several hours before hs, warm bath, warm milk, TV, self-hypnosis, deep breathing
• That hangover is common in elderly, but less common than with barbiturates

Treatment of overdose: Lavage, activated charcoal; monitor electrolytes, vital signs

---

methysergide maleate
(meth-i-ser'jide)
Sansert
Func. class.: Serotonin antagonist
Chem. class.: Ergot derivative

Action: Competitively blocks serotonin HT receptors in CNS and periphery; potent vasoconstrictor
Uses: Prophylaxsis for migraine and other vascular headaches

Dosage and routes:
• *Adult:* PO 2 mg bid with meals
Available forms: Tabs 2 mg

Side effects/adverse reactions:
CNS: Tremors, anxiety, insomnia, headache, dizziness, euphoria, confusion, depersonalization, hallucination, paresthesias, drowsiness
CV: Retroperitoneal fibrosis, valvular thickening, palpitations, tachycardia, postural hypertension, angina, thrombophlebitis, ECG changes, *cardiac fibrosis*
GI: Nausea, vomiting, weight gain
MS: Arthralgia, myalgia
INTEG: Flushing, rash, alopecia
HEMA: Blood dyscrasias

Contraindications: Hypersensitivity to ergot, tartrazine, occlusion (peripheral, vascular), CAD, hepatic disease, renal disease, peptic ulcer, hypertension, connective tissue disease, fibrotic pulmonary disease

Precautions: Pregnancy (C), lactation, children

Pharmacokinetics:
PO: Half-life 10 hr, metabolized by liver, excreted in urine (metabolites/unchanged drug)

Interactions/incompatibilities:
• Increased vasoconstriction: β-blockers
• Decreased effect of: narcotic analgesics

NURSING CONSIDERATIONS
Assess:
• Weight daily, check for peripheral edema in feet, legs, B/P
• For stress level, activity, recreation, coping mechanisms of patient
• Neurologic status: LOC, blurring vision, nausea, vomiting, tingling in extremities that occur preceding headache
• Ingestion of tyramine foods (pickled products, beer, wine, aged cheese), food additives, preservatives, colorings, artificial sweeteners, chocolate, caffeine may precipitate these types of headaches

Administer:

• At beginning of headache; dose must be titrated to patient response

• Give with or after meals to avoid GI symptoms

• Only to women who are not pregnant; harm to fetus may occur

Perform/provide:

• Storage in dark area

• Quiet, calm environment with decreased stimulation for noise, bright light, or excessive talking

Evaluate:

• Therapeutic response: decrease in frequency, severity of headache

Teach patient/family:

• Not to use OTC medications; serious drug interactions may occur

• To maintain dose at approved level, not to increase even if drug does not relieve headache

• To report side effects: increased vasoconstriction starting with cold extremities, then paresthesia, weakness

• That an increase in headaches may occur when this drug is discontinued after long-term use

• To keep drug out of reach of children; death may occur

• To report at once: dyspnea, paresthesias, urinary problems, pain in abdomen, chest, back, legs

• To use drug for less than 6 months

• That drug may cause drowsiness

---

metipranolol HCl

(met-ee-pran'oh-lole)

Optipranolol

Func. class.: β-Adrenergic blocker

Chem. class.: I-isomer

Action: Reduces production of aqueous humor by unknown mechanism

Uses: Ocular hypertension, chronic open-angle glaucoma

Dosage and routes:

• *Adult:* Instill 1 gtt bid

Available forms: Sol 0.3%

Side effects/adverse reactions:

CNS: Weakness, fatigue, depression, anxiety, headache, confusion

GI: Nausea, anorexia, dyspepsia

EENT: Eye irritation, conjunctivitis, keratitis

INTEG: Rash, urticaria

*CV: **Bradycardia,** hypertension, **MI, atrial fibrillation, angina, palpitations***

RESP: Bronchospasm, dyspnea, bronchitis, coughing, rhinitis

Contraindications: Hypersensitivity, asthma, 2nd or 3rd degree heart block, right ventricular failure, congenital glaucoma (infants)

Pharmacokinetics:

INSTILL: Onset 15-30 min, peak 1-2 hr, duration 24 hr

Interactions/incompatibilities:

• Increased effect: propranolol, metoprolol

NURSING CONSIDERATIONS

Evaluate:

• Therapeutic response: decreased intraocular pressure

Teach patient/family:

• To report change in vision (blurring or loss of sight), trouble breathing, sweating, flushing

• Method of instillation, including pressure on lacrimal sac for 1 min, and not to touch dropper to eye

• That long-term therapy may be required

• That blurred vision will decrease with continued use of drug

M

---

italics = common side effects   ***bold italic*** = life threatening reactions

metoclopramide HCl

(met-oh-kloe-pra' mide)
Clopra, Maxeran,* Maxolon,
Metoclopramide, Metoclorpramide HCl, Octamide PFS,
Reclomide, Reglan

Func. class.: Cholinergic
Chem. class.: Central dopamine receptor antagonist

Action: Enhances response to acetylcholine of tissue in upper GI tract, which causes contraction of gastric muscle, relaxes pyloric, duodenal segments, increases peristalsis without stimulating secretions

Uses: Prevention of nausea, vomiting induced by chemotherapy, radiation, delayed gastric emptying, gastroesophageal reflux

Dosage and routes:
Nausea/vomiting
• *Adult:* IV 2 mg/kg q2h × 5 doses 30 min before administration of chemotherapy

Delayed gastric emptying
• *Adult:* PO 10 mg 30 min ac, hs × 2-8 wk

Gastroesophageal reflux
• *Adult:* PO 10-15 mg qid 30 min ac

Available forms: Tabs 5, 10 mg; syr 5 mg/5 ml; inj IV 5 mg/ml

Side effects/adverse reactions:
CNS: Sedation, fatigue, restlessness, headache, sleeplessness, dystonia, dizziness, drowsiness

GI: Dry mouth, constipation, nausea, anorexia, vomiting

GU: Decreased libido, prolactin secretion, amenorrhea, galactorrhea

CV: Hypotension, supraventricular tachycardia

INTEG: Urticaria, rash

Contraindications: Hypersensitivity to this drug or procaine or procainamide, seizure disorder, pheochromocytoma, breast cancer (prolactin-dependent), GI obstruction

Precautions: Pregnancy (B), lactation, GI hemorrhage, CHF

Pharmacokinetics:
IV: Onset 1-3 min, duration 1-2 hr
PO: Onset ½-1 hr, duration 1-2 hr
IM: Onset 10-15 min, duration 1-2 hr

Metabolized by liver, excreted in urine, half-life 4 hr

Interactions/incompatibilities:
• Decreased action of metoclopramide: anticholinergics, opiates
• Increased sedation: alcohol, other CNS depressants
• Incompatible with ampicillin, calcium gluconate, cephalothin, chloramphenicol, cisplatin, erythromycin, methotrexate, penicillin G, $NaCO_3$, tetracycline

Lab test interferences:
Increase: Prolactin, aldosterone, thyrotropin

NURSING CONSIDERATIONS
Assess:
• GI complaints: nausea, vomiting, anorexia, constipation

Administer:
• IV undiluted if dose is <10 mg; give over 2 min; 10 mg or more may be diluted in 50 ml or more D_5W, NaCl, Ringer's, LR and given over 15 min or more
• ½-1 hr before meals for better absorption
• Gum, hard candy, frequent rinsing of mouth for dryness of oral cavity

Perform/provide:
• Protect from light with aluminum foil during infusion
• Discard open ampules

Evaluate:
• Therapeutic response: absence of

nausea, vomiting, anorexia, fullness

Teach patient/family:
• To avoid driving, other hazardous activities until patient is stabilized on this medication
• To avoid alcohol, other CNS depressants that will enhance sedating properties of this drug

---

metocurine iodide
(met-oh-kyoo′reen)
Metubine Iodide
Func. class.: Neuromuscular blocker (nondepolarizing)
Chem. class.: Methyl analog of tubocurarine

Action: Inhibits transmission of nerve impulses by binding with cholinergic receptor sites, antagonizing action of acetylcholine

Uses: Facilitation of endotracheal intubation, skeletal muscle relaxation during mechanical ventilation, surgery, or general anesthesia, reduction of fractures/dislocations

Dosage and routes:
• *Adult:* IV 2-4 mg if given cyclopropane as an anesthetic; 1.5-3 mg if given ether as an anesthetic; 4-7 mg if given nitrous oxide
Available forms: Inj IV 2 mg/ml

Side effects/adverse reactions:
CV: Bradycardia, tachycardia, increased, decreased B/P
*RESP: **Prolonged apnea, bronchospasm, cyanosis, respiratory depression***
EENT: Increased secretions
INTEG: Rash, flushing, pruritus, urticaria

Contraindications: Hypersensitivity to iodides

Precautions: Pregnancy (C), cardiac disease, hepatic disease, renal disease, lactation, children <2 yr, electrolyte imbalances, dehydration, neuromuscular disease (myasthenia gravis), respiratory disease, or when histamine release is a definite hazard (e.g., asthma)

Pharmacokinetics:
IV: Peak 3-5 min, duration 35-90 min, half-life 3½ hr; excreted in urine, bile (½ unchanged); crosses placenta

Interactions/incompatibilities:
• Increased neuromuscular blockade: aminoglycosides, clindamycin, lincomycin, quinidine, local anesthetics, polymyxin antibiotics, lithium, narcotic analgesics, thiazides, enflurane, isoflurane, magnesium sulfate
• Dysrhythmias: theophylline
• Do not mix with barbiturates in sol or syringe; unstable in alkaline sol

NURSING CONSIDERATIONS
Assess:
• For electrolyte imbalances (K, Mg); may lead to increased action of this drug
• Vital signs (B/P, pulse, respirations, airway) until fully recovered; rate, depth, pattern of respirations (keep airway clear), strength of hand grip
• I&O ratio; check for urinary retention, frequency, hesitancy
• Recovery: decreased paralysis of face, diaphragm, leg, arm, rest of body
• Allergic reactions: rash, fever, respiratory distress, pruritus; drug should be discontinued

Administer:
• Using nerve stimulator by anesthesiologist to determine neuromuscular blockade
• Anticholinesterase to reverse neuromuscular blockade
• By slow IV over 1-2 min (only

M

by qualified person, usually an anesthesiologist)
• Only slightly discolored solution
Perform/provide:
• Storage in light-resistant, cool area
• Reassurance if communication is difficult during recovery from neuromuscular blockade
Evaluate:
• Therapeutic response: paralysis of jaw, eyelid, head, neck, rest of body
Treatment of overdose: Edrophonium or neostigmine, atropine; monitor VS; may require mechanical ventilation
Teach patient/family: That postoperative stiffness is normal and will subside

---

metolazone
(me-tole'a-zone)
Diulo, Mykrox, Zaroxolyn
Func. class.: Diuretic
Chem. class.: Thiazide-like quinazoline derivative

Action: Acts on distal tubule by increasing excretion of water, sodium, chloride, potassium, magnesium
Uses: Edema, hypertension, CHF
Dosage and routes:
Edema
• *Adult:* PO 5-20 mg/day
Hypertension
• *Adult:* PO 2.5-5 mg/day
Available forms: Tabs 0.5, 2.5, 5, 10 mg
Side effects/adverse reactions:
GU: Frequency, polyuria, ***uremia, glucosuria***
CNS: Drowsiness, paresthesia, anxiety, depression, headache, *dizziness, fatigue, weakness*
GI: Nausea, vomiting, anorexia,

constipation, diarrhea, cramps, pancreatitis, GI irritation, ***hepatitis***
EENT: Blurred vision
INTEG: Rash, urticaria, purpura, photosensitivity, fever
META: Hyperglycemia, hyperuricemia, increased creatinine, BUN
*HEMA: **Aplastic anemia, hemolytic anemia, leukopenia, agranulocytosis, thrombocytopenia,*** neutropenia
CV: Irregular pulse, orthostatic hypotension, palpitations, volume depletion
ELECT: Hypokalemia, hypomagnesemia, hypercalcemia, hyponatremia, hypochloremia
Contraindications: Hypersensitivity to thiazides or sulfonamides, anuria, pregnancy (D), lactation
Precautions: Hypokalemia, renal disease, hepatic disease, gout, COPD, lupus erythematosus, diabetes mellitus
Pharmacokinetics:
PO: Onset 1 hr, peak 2 hr, duration 12-24 hr; excreted unchanged by kidneys; crosses placenta; enters breast milk; half-life 8 hr
Interactions/incompatibilities:
• Synergism: furosemide
• Increased toxicity of: lithium, nondepolarizing skeletal muscle relaxants
• Decreased effects of: antidiabetics, methenamine
• Decreased absorption of: thiazides, cholestyramine, colestipol
• Decreased hypotensive response: indomethacin
• Hyperglycemia, hyperuricemia, hypotension: diazoxide
Lab test interferences:
Increase: BSP retention, Ca, amylase, parathyroid test
Decrease: PBI, PSP
NURSING CONSIDERATIONS
Assess:
• Weight, I&O daily to determine

---

* Available in Canada only

fluid loss; effect of drug may be decreased if used qd

• Rate, depth, rhythm of respiration, effect of exertion

• B/P lying, standing; postural hypotension may occur

• Electrolytes: K, Mg, Na, Cl; include BUN, blood sugar, CBC, serum creatinine, blood pH, ABGs, uric acid, Ca

• Glucose in urine if patient is diabetic

• Improvement in edema of feet, legs, sacral area daily if medication is being used in CHF

• Improvement in CVP q8h

• Signs of metabolic alkalosis: drowsiness, restlessness

• Signs of hypokalemia: postural hypotension, malaise, fatigue, tachycardia, leg cramps, weakness

• Rashes, temperature elevation qd

• Confusion, especially in elderly; take safety precautions if needed

Administer:

• In AM to avoid interference with sleep if using drug as a diuretic

• K replacement if K is less than 3.0

• With food; if nausea occurs, absorption may be decreased slightly

Evaluate:

• Therapeutic response: decreased edema, B/P

Teach patient/family:

• To increase fluid intake to 2-3 L/ day unless contraindicated, to rise slowly from lying or sitting position

• To notify physician of muscle weakness, cramps, nausea, dizziness

• That drug may be taken with food or milk

• To use sunscreen for photosensitivity

• That blood sugar may be increased in diabetics

• To take ea
turia
Treatment of
taken orally; m
administer dextro.
itor hydration, CV,

---

metoprolol tartrate

(met-oh′proe-lole)
Betaloc,* Lopresor,* Lopressor
Func. class.: Antihypertensive
Chem. class.: β₁-blocker

Action: Lowers B/P by β-blocking effects; elevated plasma renins are reduced; blocks β₂-adrenergic receptors in bronchial, vascular smooth muscle only at high doses

Uses: Mild to moderate hypertension, acute myocardial infarction to reduce cardiovascular mortality, angina pectoris

Dosage and routes:

Hypertension

• *Adult:* PO 50 mg bid, or 100 mg qd; may give up to 200-450 mg in divided doses

Myocardial infarction

• *Adult:* (early treatment) IV bol 5 mg q2min × 3, then 50 mg PO 15 min after last dose and q6h × 48 hr; (late treatment) PO maintenance 100 mg bid for 3 mo

Available forms: Tabs 50, 100 mg; inj IV 1 mg/ml

Side effects/adverse reactions:

CV: Hypotension, *bradycardia, CHF: Palpitations,* dysrhythmias, ***cardiac arrest, AV block***

CNS: Insomnia, dizziness, mental changes, hallucinations, ***depression,*** anxiety, headaches, nightmares, confusion, fatigue

GI: Nausea, vomiting, colitis, cramps, ***diarrhea,*** constipation, flatulence, dry mouth, ***hiccups***

---

italics = common side effects   ***bold italic*** = life threatening reactions

Rash, purpura, alopecia, skin, urticaria, pruritus

*HEMA: **Agranulocytosis, eosinophilia, thrombocytopenia, purpura***

EENT: Sore throat, dry burning eyes

GU: Impotence

*RESP: **Bronchospasm,** dyspnea, wheezing*

Contraindications: Hypersensitivity to β-blockers, cardiogenic shock, heart block (2nd, 3rd degree), sinus bradycardia, CHF, bronchial asthma

Precautions: Major surgery, pregnancy (C), lactation, diabetes mellitus, renal disease, thyroid disease, COPD, heart failure, CAD, nonallergic bronchospasm, hepatic disease

Pharmacokinetics:

PO: Peak 2-4 hr, duration 13-19 hr; half-life 3-4 hr; metabolized in liver (metabolites); excreted in urine; crosses placenta; enters breast milk

Interactions/incompatibilities:

• Increased hypotension, bradycardia: reserpine, hydralazine, methyldopa, prazosin

• Decreased antihypertensive effects: indomethacin, sympathomimetics

• Increased hypoglycemic effects: insulin

• Decreased bronchodilation: theophyllines β-agonists

• Incompatible with any drug in syringe or sol

Lab test interferences:

Increase: Liver function tests, renal function tests

NURSING CONSIDERATIONS

Assess:

• ECG directly when giving IV during initial treatment

• I&O, weight daily

• B/P during initial treatment, periodically thereafter; pulse q4h; note rate, rhythm, quality

• Apical/radial pulse before administration; notify physician of any significant changes

• Baselines in renal, liver function tests before therapy begins

• Edema in feet, legs daily

• Skin turgor, dryness of mucous membranes for hydration status

Administer:

• PO ac, hs, tablet may be crushed or swallowed whole

• IV, undiluted, give over 1 min, keep patient recumbent for 3 hr

Perform/provide:

• Storage in dry area at room temperature, do not freeze

Evaluate:

• Therapeutic response: decreased B/P after 1-2 wk

Teach patient/family:

• To take with or immediately after meals

• Not to discontinue drug abruptly; taper over 2 wk; may cause precipitate angina

• Not to use OTC products containing α-adrenergic stimulants (nasal decongestants, OTC cold preparations) unless directed by physician

• To report bradycardia, dizziness, confusion, depression, fever, sore throat, shortness of breath to physician

• To take pulse at home; advise when to notify physician

• To avoid alcohol, smoking, Na intake

• To comply with weight control, dietary adjustments, modified exercise program

• To carry Medic Alert ID to identify drug you are taking, allergies

• To avoid hazardous activities if dizziness is present

• To report symptoms of CHF: difficult breathing, especially on exertion or when lying down, night cough, swelling of extremities

• To take medication hs to prevent effect of orthostatic hypotension

• To wear support hose to minimize effects of orthostatic hypotension

Treatment of overdose: Lavage, IV atropine for bradycardia, IV theophylline for bronchospasm, digitalis, O₂, diuretic for cardiac failure, hemodialysis, hypotension administer vasopressor (norepinephrine)

---

metronidazole/metronidazole HCl

(me-troe-ni′da-zole)

Apo-Metronidazole,* Femazole, Flagyl, Flagyl IV, Flagyl IV RTU, Metro IV, Metronidazole, Metronidazole Redi-Infusion, Metryl, Neo-Tric,* Novonidazole,* PMS-Metronidazole,* Protostat, Trikacide*

Func. class.: Trichomonacide, amebicide

Chem. class.: Nitroimidazole derivative

Action: Direct-acting amebicide/trichomonacide binds, degrades DNA in organism

Uses: Intestinal amebiasis, amebic abscess, trichomoniasis, refractory trichomoniasis, bacterial anaerobic infections, giardiasis

Dosage and routes:

Trichomoniasis

• *Adult:* PO 250 mg tid × 7 days or 2 g in single dose; do not repeat treatment for 4-6 wk

Refractory trichomoniasis

• *Adult:* PO 250 mg bid × 10 days

Amebic abscess

• *Adult:* PO 500-750 mg tid × 5-10 days

• *Child:* PO 35-50 mg/kg/day in 3 divided doses × 10 days

Intestinal amebiasis

• *Adult:* PO 750 mg tid × 5-10 days

• *Child:* PO 35-50 mg/kg/day in 3 divided doses × 10 days; then oral iodoquinol

Anaerobic bacterial infections

• *Adult:* IV INF 15 mg/kg over 1 hr, then 7.5 mg/kg IV or PO q6h, not to exceed 4 g/day; first maintenance dose should be administered 6 hr following loading dose

Giardiasis

• *Adult:* PO 250 mg tid × 5 days

• *Child:* PO 5 mg/kg tid × 5 days

Available forms: Tabs 250, 500 mg; film-coated tabs 250, 1500 mg; inj IV 5 mg/vial; HCl inj IV 500 mg

Side effects/adverse reactions:

CV: Flat T waves

CNS: Headache, dizziness, confusion, irritability, restlessness, ataxia, depression, fatigue, drowsiness, insomnia, paresthesia, peripheral neuropathy, *convulsions,* incoordination, depression

EENT: Blurred vision, sore throat, retinal edema, dry mouth, metallic taste, furry tongue, glossitis, stomatitis

GI: Nausea, vomiting, diarrhea, epigastric distress, anorexia, constipation, abdominal cramps, metallic taste, *pseudomembranous colitis*

GU: Darkened urine, vaginal dryness, polyuria, *albuminuria,* dysuria, cystitis, decreased libido, *neurotoxicity,* incontinence, dyspareunia

HEMA: Leukopenia, bone marrow, depression, aplasia

INTEG: Rash, pruritus, urticaria, flushing

Contraindications: Hypersensitiv-

M

---

italics = common side effects   ***bold italic*** = life threatening reactions

ity to this drug, renal disease, hepatic disease, contracted visual or color fields, blood dyscrasias, pregnancy (1st trimester), lactation, CNS disorders

Precautions: Candida infections, pregnancy (2nd, 3rd trimesters) (B)

Pharmacokinetics:

IV: Onset immediate, peak end of inf

PO: Peak 1-2 hr, half-life 6-11 hr, crosses placenta, enters breast milk, excreted in feces; absorbed PO (80%-85%)

Interactions/incompatibilities:

• Disulfiram reaction: alcohol
• May increase action of: warfarin
• Decreased action of metronidazole: phenobarbital
• Incompatible with any drug in syringe or sol

Lab test interferences:

Decrease: AST, ALT

NURSING CONSIDERATIONS
Assess:

• For infection: WBC, wound symptoms, fever, skin or vaginal secretions; start treatment after C&S
• Stools during entire treatment; should be clear at end of therapy; stools should be free of parasites for 1 yr before patient is considered cured (amebiasis)
• Vision by ophthalmic exam during, after therapy; vision problems frequent
• I&O; weight daily; stools for number, frequency, character
• Neurotoxicity: peripheral neuropathy, seizures, dizziness, incoordination, pruritus, joint pains; may be discontinued
• Allergic reaction: fever, rash, itching, chills; drug should be discontinued if these symptoms occur
• Superimposed infection: fever, monilial growth, fatigue, malaise

• Renal and reproductive dysfunction: dysuria, polyuria, impotence, dyspareunia, decreased libido

Administer:

• IV prediluted; Flagyl IV, dilute with 4.4 ml sterile H_2O or 0.9% NaCl; must be diluted further with 8 mg/ml or more 0.9% NaCl, D_5W, or Lactated Ringer's sol; must neutralize with 5 mEq Na_2CO_3/500 mg; CO_2 gas will be generated and may require venting; run over 1 hr; primary IV must be discontinued; may be given as continuous infusion; do not use aluminum products; IV may require venting
• PO with or after meals to avoid GI symptoms, metallic taste; crush tabs if needed

Perform/provide:

• Storage in light-resistant container; do not refrigerate

Evaluate:

• Therapeutic response: decreased symptoms of infection

Teach patient family:

• That urine may turn dark-reddish brown
• Proper hygiene after BM; handwashing technique
• To avoid hazardous activities, since dizziness can occur
• Need for compliance with dosage schedule, duration of treatment
• To use condoms if treatment for trichomoniasis, or cross-contamination may occur
• To use frequent sips of water, sugarless gum for dry mouth
• That treatment of both partners is necessary in trichomoniasis
• Not to drink alcohol or use preparations containing alcohol; disulfiram reaction can occur

metyrosine

(me-tye'roe-seen)

Demser

Func. class.: Antihypertensive

Chem. class.: Adrenergic blocker

Action: Inhibits enzyme tyrosine hydroxylase, resulting in decreased levels of catecholamines

Uses: Pheochromocytoma

Dosage and routes:

• *Adult and child >12 yr:* PO 250 mg qid, may increase by 250-500 mg qd to a max of 4 g/day in divided doses

Available forms: Caps 250 mg

Side effects/adverse reactions:

CNS: Sedation, drowsiness, dizziness, headache, depression, EPS, hallucinations, psychosis, agitation

INTEG: Rash, urticaria

EENT: Dry mouth, nasal stuffiness

GU: Dysuria, **oliguria, hematuria,** enuresis, impotence

GI: Nausea, vomiting, anorexia, diarrhea, abdominal pain

MISC: Breast swelling

Contraindications: Hypersensitivity, essential hypertension, children <12 yr

Precautions: Pregnancy (C), lactation, hepatic disease, renal disease

Pharmacokinetics:

PO: Onset 2 days, duration 3-4 days; half-life 3.4-3.7 hr, excreted in urine

Interactions/incompatibilities:

• Increased sedation: CNS depressants: alcohol, barbiturates, antipsychotics

• Decreased effects of: levodopa

• Extrapyramidal effects: phenothiazines, haloperidol

Lab test interferences:

False increase: Urinary catecholamines

NURSING CONSIDERATIONS

Assess:

• Electrolytes: K, Na, Cl, CO_2

• Renal function studies: catecholamines, BUN, creatinine

• Hepatic function studies: AST, ALT, alk phosphatase

• B/P, ECG other VS throughout treatment

• Weight daily, I&O

• Change in behavior or personality: psychosis, anxiety, hallucinations, EPS

• Nausea, vomiting, diarrhea

• Edema in feet, legs daily

• Skin turgor, dryness of mucous membranes for hydration status

Administer:

• Antiemetic or antidiarrheals for vomiting, diarrhea

Perform/provide:

• Fluids to 2 L/day to prevent crystallization by kidneys

Evaluate:

• Therapeutic response: decreased B/P, decreased levels of catecholamines

Teach patient/family:

• To take each dose with a full glass of water; maintain sufficient daily intake

• Not to drive or perform hazardous tasks if behavioral changes, dizziness, or drowsiness occurs

• To avoid alcohol or other CNS depressants

• To notify physician if any of following occur: jaw stiffness, drooling, speech difficulty, tremors, disorientation, diarrhea, painful urination

Treatment of overdose: Administer vasopressors, discontinue drug

mexiletine HCl
(mex-il'e-teen)
Mexitil
Func. class.: Antidysrhythmic
(Class IB)
Chem. class.: Lidocaine analog

Action: Increases electrical stimulation threshold of ventricle, His-Purkinje system, which stabilizes cardiac membrane

Uses: Ventricular tachycardia, ventricular dysrhythmias during cardiac surgery, myocardial infarction

Dosage and routes:
• *Adult:* PO 200-400 mg q8h
Available forms: Caps 150, 200, 250 mg

Side effects/adverse reactions:
CNS: Headache, dizziness, confusion, *convulsions,* tremors, psychosis, nervousness, paresthesias, weakness, fatigue, coordination difficulties, change in sleep habits
EENT: Blurred vision, hearing loss, tinnitus
GI: Nausea, vomiting, anorexia, diarrhea, abdominal pain, *hepatitis,* dry mouth, peptic ulcer, altered taste, GI bleeding
CV: Hypotension, bradycardia, angina, PVCs, *heart block, cardiovascular collapse, arrest,* sinus node slowing, *left ventricular failure,* syncope, *cardiogenic shock*
RESP: Dyspnea, *fibrosis, embolism,* pneumonia
INTEG: Rash, alopecia, dry skin
HEMA: Thrombocytopenia, leukopenia, agranulocytosis, hypoplastic anemia, systemic lupus erythematosus syndrome
GU: Urinary hesitancy, decreased libido
MISC: Edema, arthralgia, fever

Contraindications: Hypersensitivity to amides, cardiogenic shock, blood dyscrasias, severe heart block

Precautions: Pregnancy (C), lactation, children, renal disease, liver disease, CHF, respiratory depression, myasthenia gravis

Pharmacokinetics:
PO: Peak 2-3 hr; half-life 12 hr, metabolized by liver, excreted unchanged by kidneys (10%), excreted in breast milk

Interactions/incompatibilities:
• Decreased effects: cimetidine
• Decreased levels of mexiletine: phenytoin, phenobarbital, rifampin

Lab test interferences:
Increase: CPK

NURSING CONSIDERATIONS
Assess:
• ECG continuously to determine increased PR or QRS segments; if these develop, discontinue or reduce rate; watch for increased ventricular ectopic beats; may have to rebolus
• Blood levels (therapeutic level 0.5-2 μg/ml)
• B/P continuously for fluctuations
• I&O ratio, electrolytes (K, Na, Cl), liver enzymes
• Malignant hyperthermia: tachypnea, tachycardia, changes in B/P, increased temperature
• Cardiac rate, respiration: rate, rhythm, character
• Respiratory status: rate, rhythm, lung fields for rales, watch for respiratory depression
• CNS effects: dizziness, confusion, psychosis, paresthesias, convulsions; drug should be discontinued
• Lung fields, bilateral rales may occur in CHF patient
• Increased respiration, increased pulse; drug should be discontinued

Evaluate:
• Therapeutic response: decreased dysrhythmias

Treatment of overdose: O₂, artificial ventilation, ECG; administer dopamine for circulatory depression; administer diazepam or thiopental for convulsions, to acidify urine

---

mezlocillin sodium
(mez-loe-sill'in)
Mezlin
Func. class.: Broad-spectrum antibiotic
Chem. class.: Extended-spectrum penicillin

Action: Interferes with cell wall replication of susceptible organisms; osmotically unstable cell wall swells, bursts from osmotic pressure

Uses: Effective for gram-positive cocci (*S. aureus, S. viridans, S. faecalis, S. pneumoniae*), gram-negative cocci *(N. gonorrhoeae)*, gram-positive bacilli, *C. perfringens, C. tetani*, gram-negative bacilli (*Bacteroides, E. coli, H. influenzae, Klebsiella, P. mirabilis, Peptococcus, Peptostreptococcus, M. morganii, Enterobacter, Serratia, Pseudomonas, P. vulgaris, P. rettgeri, Shigella, Citrobacter, Veillonella*)

Dosage and routes:
• *Adult:* IM/IV 200-300 mg/kg/day in divided doses q4-6h; may give up to 24 g/day for severe infections
• *Child:* IM/IV 50 mg/kg q4-6h
• *Infants >8 days;* >2000 g: 75 mg/kg q6h; <2000 g: 75 mg/kg q8h
• *Infants <8 days:* 75 mg/kg q12h
Available forms: Powder for inj

IM, IV 1, 2, 3, 4 g; IV INF 2, 3, 4 g

Side effects/adverse reactions:
HEMA: Anemia, increased bleeding time, **bone marrow depression, granulocytopenia**
GI: Nausea, vomiting, diarrhea, increased AST, ALT, abdominal pain, glossitis, colitis, abnormal taste
GU: Oliguria, proteinuria, hematuria, (vaginitis, moniliasis), **glomerulonephritis,** increased BUN, creatinine
CNS: Lethargy, hallucinations, anxiety, depression, twitching, **coma, convulsions**
META: Hyperkalemia, hypokalemia, alkalosis, hypernatremia

Contraindications: Hypersensitivity to penicillins

Precautions: Pregnancy (B), hypersensitivity to cephalosporins, neonates

Pharmacokinetics:
IM: Peak 45 min
IV: Peak 5 min
Half-life 50-55 min; partially metabolized in liver; excreted in urine, bile, breast milk (small amount); crosses placenta

Interactions/incompatibilities:
• Decreased effectiveness of: aminoglycosides
• Decreased antimicrobial effectiveness of mezlocillin: tetracyclines, erythromycins
• Increased mezlocillin concentrations: aspirin, probenecid
• Incompatible in sol with aminoglycosides, ciprofloxacin, meperidine, verapamil

Lab test interferences:
False positive: Urine glucose, urine protein

NURSING CONSIDERATIONS
Assess:
• I&O ratio; report hematuria, oli-

M

---

guria, since penicillin in high doses is nephrotoxic
• Any patient with compromised renal system, since drug is excreted slowly in poor renal system function; toxicity may occur rapidly
• Liver studies: AST, ALT
• Blood studies: WBC, RBC, H&H, bleeding time
• Renal studies: urinalysis, protein, blood
• C&S before drug therapy; drug may be given as soon as culture is taken
• Bowel pattern before and during treatment
• Skin eruptions after administration of penicillin to 1 wk after discontinuing drug
• Respiratory status: rate, character, wheezing, and tightness in chest
• Check IV site for thrombophlebitis
• WBC, differential, liver, renal studies periodically for patients on long-term therapy
• Allergies before initiation of treatment, and reaction of each medication; highlight allergies on chart, Kardex

Administer:
• IV after diluting 1g or less/10 ml of sterile H_2O, D_5, or 0.9% NaCl for inj; shake, dilute further with D_5W or 0.45 NaCl, and give over 3-5 min; may be given by intermittent INF over ½ hr
• Drug after C&S has been completed

Perform/provide:
• Adrenalin, suction, tracheostomy set, endotracheal intubation equipment
• Adequate fluid intake (2 L) during diarrhea episodes
• Scratch test to assess allergy after securing order from physician; usu-

ally done when penicillin is only drug of choice
• Storage at room temperature; reconstituted solution is stable for 24 hr refrigerated

Evaluate:
• Therapeutic response: absence of fever, draining wounds

Teach patient/family:
• That culture may be taken after completed course of medication
• To report sore throat, fever, fatigue (may indicate superimposed infection)
• To wear or carry Medic Alert ID if allergic to penicillins
• To notify nurse of diarrhea, symptoms of *Candida* vaginitis

Treatment of overdose: Withdraw drug, maintain airway, administer epinephrine, aminophylline, O_2, IV corticosteroids for anaphylaxis

---

miconazole

(mi-kon′a-zole)
Monistat, Monistat IV
Func. class.: Antifungal
Chem. class.: Imidazole

Action: Alters cell membranes, inhibits fungal enzymes
Uses: Coccidioidomycosis, candidiasis, cryptococcoses, paracoccidioidomycosis, chronic mucocutaneous candidiasis, fungal meningitis; IV used for severe infections only

Dosage and routes:
• *Adult:* IV INF 200-3600 mg/day; may be divided in 3 infusions 200-1200 mg/infusion; may have to repeat course; intrathecal 20 mg given simultaneously with IV for fungal meningitis q3-7d
• *Child:* IV 20-40 mg/kg/day, not to exceed 15 mg/kg/day

Available forms: Inj IV 10 mg/ml; aerosol 2%

Side effects/adverse reactions:

CV: Tachycardia, dysrhythmias (rapid IV)

CNS: Drowsiness, headache, laziness

GI: Nausea, vomiting, anorexia, diarrhea, cramps

GU: Vulvovaginal burning, itching, hyponatremia, pelvic cramps (topical forms)

HEMA: Decreased Hct, thrombocytopenia, hyperlipidemia

INTEG: Pruritus, rash, fever, flushing, *anaphylaxis,* hives

Contraindications: Hypersensitivity

Precautions: Renal disease, hepatic disease, pregnancy (B)

Pharmacokinetics:

IV: Onset immediate; peak end of inf; half-life triphasic 0.4, 2.1, 24.1 hr; metabolized in liver; excreted in feces, urine (inactive metabolites); >90% protein binding

Interactions/incompatibilities:

• Increased action of: anticoagulants

• Decreased action of both drugs: amphotericin

• Considered incompatible in syringe or sol

Lab test interferences:

False positive: Urine glucose, urine protein

NURSING CONSIDERATIONS

Assess:

• Cardiac system: B/P, pulse, ECG; watch for increasing pulse, cardiac dysrhythmias; drug should be discontinued

• Blood studies: WBC, RBC, H & H bleeding time

• Renal studies: urinalysis, protein, blood

• C&S before drug therapy; drug may be given as soon as culture is taken; monitor signs of infection prior to and throughout treatment

• Bowel pattern before and during treatment; diarrhea is common

• Skin eruptions after administration of drug to 1 wk after discontinuing drug

• Respiratory status: rate, character, wheezing, tightness in chest

• IV site for thrombophlebitis

• WBC and differential liver and renal studies periodically for patients on long-term therapy

• Allergies before initiation of treatment, and reaction of each medication; highlight allergies on chart, Kardex

Administer:

• 200 mg initially to prevent severe hypersensitive reaction

• IV after diluting 1 g or less/10 ml of sterile H_2O, D_5W or 0.45% NaCl; give over 3-5 min; may be given by intermittent INF over ½ hr

• Drug after C&S has been completed

Perform/provide:

• Adrenalin, suction, tracheostomy set, endotracheal intubation equipment

• Adequate fluid intake (2 L) during diarrhea episodes

• Scratch test to assess allergy after securing order from physician; usually done when penicillin is only drug of choice

• Storage at room temperature; reconstituted solution is stable for 24 hr refrigerated

Evaluate:

• Therapeutic response: absence of fever, draining wounds

Teach patient/family:

• That culture may be taken after completed course of medication

• To report sore throat, fever, fa-

tigue (may indicate superimposed infection)
• To wear or carry Medic Alert ID if allergic to drug
• To notify nurse of diarrhea, symptoms of *Candida* vaginitis
Treatment of overdose:
Withdraw drug; maintain airway; administer epinephrine, aminophylline, O₂, IV corticosteroids for anaphylaxis

---

miconazole nitrate (topical)

(mi-kon'a-zole)
Micatin, Miconazole Nitrate, Micatin Liquid, Monistat-Derm, Monistat 3, Monistat 7, Monistat Dual-Pak
Func. class.: Local antiinfective
Chem. class.: Antifungal

Action: Interferes with fungal cell membrane, which increases permeability, leaking of nutrients
Uses: Tinea pedis, tinea cruris, tinea corporis, tinea versicolor, vaginal or vulvae *Candida albicans*
Dosage and routes:
• *Adult and child:* TOP apply to affected area bid × 2-4 wk
• *Adult:* Intra vag give 1 applicator or suppository ×7 days hs
Available forms: Cream, lotion, powder, spray 2%; vag cream 2%; vag supp 100, 200 mg
Side effects/adverse reactions:
GU: Vulvovaginal burning, itching, pelvic cramps
INTEG: Rash, urticaria, stinging, burning, contact dermatitis
Contraindications: Hypersensitivity
Precautions: Child <2 yr, pregnancy (B), lactation

NURSING CONSIDERATIONS
Assess:
• Allergic reaction: burning, stinging, swelling, redness
Administer:
• Enough medication to cover lesions completely
• After cleansing with soap, water before each application; dry well
Perform/provide:
• Storage at room temperature in dry place
Evaluate:
• Therapeutic response: decrease in size, number of lesions
Teach patient/family:
• To use medical asepsis (hand washing) before, after each application
• To apply with glove to prevent further infection
• To avoid use of OTC creams, ointments, lotions unless directed by physician
• To avoid contact with eyes
• To avoid use of occlusive dressings
• To notify physician if no improvement in condition in 4 wk or if symptoms return in 2 months; pregnancy or a serious medical condition may be the cause
• To use for full prescribed treatment time

---

microfibrillar collagen hemostat

Avitene
Func. class.: Hemostatic
Chem. class.: Purified cattle collagen

Action: Platelets adhere to hemostat, cause aggregation to and formation of thrombi
Uses: For hemostasis in surgery

when ligature is ineffective/impractical

Dosage and routes:
• *Adult and child:* TOP apply to bleeding area after drying with sponge; compress for 1-5 min; may reapply if needed
• *Available forms:* Fibrous form, nonwoven web form

Side effects/adverse reactions:
INTEG: Rash, abscess, allergic reactions, infection, wound dehiscence
HEMA: Hematoma

Contraindications: Hypersensitivity, closure of skin incision

Precautions: Pregnancy (C)

NURSING CONSIDERATIONS
Assess:
• Possible infection: hematoma, abscess
• Allergy: rash, itching

Administer:
• Dry, do not moisten
• Using gloves with forceps; area must be dry for drug to work
• Only new product; do not resterilize

Evaluate:
• Therapeutic response: decreased bleeding in surgery

---

midazolam HCl
(mid′-az-zoe-lam)
Versed
Func. class.: General anesthetic
Chem. class.: Benzodiazepine, short-acting

Controlled Substance Schedule IV

Action: Depresses subcortical levels in CNS; may act on limbic system, reticular formation; may potentiate γ-aminobenzoic acid (GABA) by binding to specific benzodiazepine receptors

Uses: Preoperative sedation, general anesthesia induction, sedation for diagnostic endoscopic procedures, intubation

Dosage and routes:
Preoperative sedation
Adult: IM 0.07-0.08 mg/kg ½-1 hr before general anesthesia
Induction of general anesthesia
Adult: IV (unpremedicated patients) 0.3-0.35 mg/kg over 30 sec, wait 2 min, follow with 25% of initial dose if needed; (premedicated patients) 0.15-0.35 mg/kg over 20-30 sec, allow 2 min for effect

Available forms: Inj 1, 5 mg/ml

Side effects/adverse reactions:
CNS: Retrograde amnesia, euphoria, confusion, headache, anxiety, insomnia, slurred speech, paresthesia, tremors, weakness, chills
RESP: Coughing, **apnea, bronchospasm, laryngospasm,** dyspnea
CV: Hypotension, PVCs, tachycardia, bigeminy, nodal rhythm
EENT: Blurred vision, nystagmus, diplopia, blocked ears, loss of balance
GI: Nausea, vomiting, increased salivation, hiccups
INTEG: Urticaria, pain, swelling at injection site, rash, pruritus

Contraindications: Pregnancy (D), hypersensitivity to benzodiazepines, shock, coma, alcohol intoxication, acute narrow-angle glaucoma

Precautions: COPD, CHF, chronic renal failure, chills, elderly, debilitated

Pharmacokinetics:
IM: Onset: 15 min, peak ½-1 hr
IV: Onset: 3-5 min, onset of anesthesia 1½-2½ min; protein binding 97%; half-life 1.2-12.3 hr; metab-

---

italics = common side effects   ***bold italic*** = life threatening reactions

olized in liver; metabolites excreted in urine; crosses placenta, blood-brain barrier

Interactions/incompatibilities:

• Prolonged respiratory depression: other CNS depressants, alcohol, barbiturates

• Increased hypnotic effect: fentanyl, narcotic agonists, analgesics, droperidol

• Incompatible with dimenhydrinate, pentobarbital, perphenazine, prochlorperazine, rantidine

NURSING CONSIDERATIONS
Assess:

• Injection site for redness, pain, swelling

• Degree of amnesia in elderly; may be increased

• Anterograde amnesia

• Vital signs for recovery period in obese patient, since half-life may be extended

Administer:

• IV after diluting with D$_5$W or 0.9% NaCl to a concentration of 0.25 mg/ml; give over 2 min (conscious sedation) or over 30 sec (anesthesia induction)

• IM deep into large muscle mass

Perform/provide:

• Assistance with ambulation until drowsy period relieved

• Storage at room temperature

• Immediate availability of resuscitation equipment, O$_2$ to support airway; do not give by rapid bolus

Evaluate:

• Therapeutic response: induction of sedation, general anesthesia

Teach patient/family:

• To avoid hazardous activities until drowsiness, weakness subside

• That amnesia occurs; events may not be remembered

Treatment of overdose: O$_2$, vasopressors, physostigmine, resuscitation

---

milrinone lactate
(mill-re'-none)
Primacor
Func. class.: Inotropic/vasodilator agent with phosphodiesterase activity
Chem. class.: Bipyridine derivative

Action: Positive inotropic agent with vasodilator properties; reduces preload and afterload by direct relaxation on vascular smooth muscle

Uses: Short-term management of CHF that has not responded to other medication; can be used with digitalis

Dosage and routes:

• *Adult:* IV BOL 50 μg/kg given over 10 min; start infusion of 0.375-0.75 μg/kg/min; reduce dose in renal impairment

Available forms: Inj 1 mg/ml

Side effects/adverse reactions:

HEMA: **Thrombocytopenia**

MISC: Headache, hypokalemia, tremor

CV: Dysrhythmias, hypotension, chest pain

GI: Nausea, vomiting, anorexia, abdominal pain, *hepatotoxicity*, jaundice

Contraindications: Hypersensitivity to this drug, severe aortic disease, severe pulmonic valvular disease, acute myocardial infarction

Precautions: Lactation, pregnancy (C), children, renal disease, hepatic disease, atrial flutter/fibrillation, elderly

Pharmacokinetics:

IV: Onset 2-5 min, peak 10 min, duration variable; half-life 4-6 hr; metabolized in liver; excreted in urine as drug and metabolites 60%-90%

---

*Available in Canada only

Interactions/incompatibilities:
• Excessive hypotension: antihypertensives

NURSING CONSIDERATIONS
Assess:
• B/P and pulse q5min during infusion; if B/P drops 30 mm Hg, stop infusion and call physician
• Electrolytes: K, Na, Cl, Ca; renal function studies: BUN, creatinine; blood studies: platelet count
• ALT, AST, bilirubin daily
• I&O ratio and weight qd; diuresis should increase with continuing therapy
• If platelets are <150,000/mm³ drug is usually discontinued and another drug started
• Extravasation, change site q48h

Administer:
• Into running dextrose infusion through Y-connector or directly into tubing; dilute with NS to concentration of 1-3 mg/ml; do not mix with glucose for long-term infusion
• By infusion pump for doses other than bolus
• K supplements if ordered for K levels <3.0

Evaluate:
• Therapeutic response: increased cardiac output, decreased PCWP, adequate CVP, decreased dyspnea, fatigue, edema, ECG

Treatment of overdose: Discontinue drug, support circulation

---

mineral oil

Agoral Plain, Fleet Mineral Oil
Enema, Kondremul, Milkinol,
Neo-Cultol, Petrogalar Plain,
Zymenol

Func. class.: Laxative
Chem. class.: Petroleum hydrocarbon

Action: Eases passage of stool by decreasing water absorption from feces; acts as lubricant

Uses: Constipation, preparation for bowel surgery or examination

Dosage and routes:
• *Adult:* PO 15-30 ml hs; enema 4 oz
• *Child:* PO 5-15 ml hs; enema 1-2 oz

Available forms: Oil, enema; jelly 55%; susp 1.4, 2.5, 2.75 mg/5 ml

Side effects/adverse reactions:
CNS: Muscle weakness
GI: Nausea, vomiting, anorexia, diarrhea, pruritus ani, hepatic infiltration
META: **Hypoprothrombinemia**
RESP: Lipoid pneumonia

Contraindications: Hypersensitivity, intestinal obstruction, abdominal pain, nausea/vomiting

Precautions: Pregnancy (C)

Pharmacokinetics: Excreted in feces

Interactions/incompatibilities:
• Increased effect of: oral anticoagulants
• Decreased absorption: fat-soluble vitamins (A, D, E, K) if used for prolonged time

NURSING CONSIDERATIONS
Assess:
• Blood, urine electrolytes if drug is used often by patient
• I&O ratio to identify fluid loss
• Cause of constipation; identify whether fluids, bulk, or exercise is missing from life-style
• Cramping, rectal bleeding, nausea, vomiting; if these symptoms occur, drug should be discontinued

Administer:
• Alone for better absorption
• In morning or evening (oral dose)
• Cautiously in elderly to prevent aspiration

Evaluate:
• Therapeutic response: decrease in constipation

---

italics = common side effects   ***bold italic*** = life threatening reactions

Teach patient/family:
• Not to use laxatives for long-term therapy; bowel tone will be lost
• That normal bowel movements do not always occur daily
• Not to use in presence of abdominal pain, nausea, vomiting
• To notify physician if constipation unrelieved or if symptoms of electrolyte imbalance occur: muscle cramps, pain, weakness, dizziness, excessive thirst
• Not to use with food or vitamin preparations; delays digestion and absorption of fat-soluble vitamins

---

minocycline HCl
(mi-noe-sye′kleen)
Dynacin, Minocin, Minocin IV
Func. class.: Broad-spectrum antibiotic
Chem. class.: Tetracycline

Action: Inhibits protein synthesis, phosphorylation in microorganisms by binding to 30S ribosomal subunits, reversibly binding to 50S ribosomal subunits; bacteriostatic
Uses: Syphilis, chlamydia trachomatis, gonorrhea, lymphogranuloma venereum, rickettsial infections, inflammatory acne, *Mycobacterium marinum, Neisseria* meningitis carriers
Dosage and routes:
• *Adult:* PO/IV 200 mg, then 100 mg q12h or 50 mg q6h, not to exceed 400 mg/24h IV
• *Child >8 yr:* PO/IV 4 mg/kg then 4 mg/kg/day PO in divided doses q12h
Gonorrhea
• *Adult:* PO 200 mg, then 100 mg q12h × 4 days
Chlamydia trachomatis
• *Adult:* PO 100 mg bid × 7 days

Syphilis
• *Adult:* PO 200 mg, then 100 mg q12h × 10-15 days
Available forms: Tabs 50, 100 mg; caps 50, 100 mg oral susp 50 mg/5 ml; powder for inj IV 100 mg/vial
Side effects/adverse reactions:
CNS: Dizziness, fever, light-headedness, vertigo
*HEMA: **Eosinophilia, neutropenia, thrombocytopenia, hemolytic anemia***
EENT: Dysphagia, glossitis, decreased calcification of deciduous teeth, oral candidiasis
GI: Nausea, abdominal pain, *vomiting, diarrhea,* anorexia, enterocolitis, **hepatotoxicity,** flatulence, abdominal cramps, epigastric burning, stomatitis
CV: Pericarditis
GU: Increased BUN, polyuria, polydipsia, *renal failure, nephrotoxicity*
INTEG: Rash, urticaria, *photosensitivity, increased pigmentation,* **exfoliative dermatitis,** pruritus, angioedema, blue-gray color of skin, mucous membranes
Contraindications: Hypersensitivity to tetracyclines, children <8 yr, pregnancy (D)
Precautions: Hepatic disease, lactation
Pharmacokinetics:
PO: Peak 2-3 hr half-life 11-17 hr; excreted in urine, feces; crosses placenta; excreted in breast milk, 55%-88% protein bound
Interactions/incompatibilities:
• Decreased effect of minocycline: antacids, NaHCO₃, alkali products, iron, kaolin/pectin, cimetidine
• Increased effect of: anticoagulants
• Decreased effect of: penicillins, oral contraceptives

• Nephrotoxicity: methoxyflurane
• Do not mix with other drugs

Lab test interferences:
False negative: Urine glucose with Clinistix or Tes-Tape

NURSING CONSIDERATIONS
Assess:
• I&O ratio
• Blood studies: PT, CBC, AST, ALT, BUN, creatinine
• Signs of anemia: Hct, Hgb, fatigue
• Allergic reactions: rash, itching, pruritus, angioedema
• Nausea, vomiting, diarrhea; administer antiemetic, antacids as ordered
• Overgrowth of infection: increased temperature, malaise, redness, pain, swelling, drainage, perineal itching, diarrhea, changes in cough or sputum

Administer:
• IV after diluting 100 mg/5 ml sterile H_2O for inj; further dilute in 500-1000 ml of NaCl, dextrose sol, LR; Ringer's sol; run 100 mg/6 hr
• After C&S obtained
• 2 hr before or after laxative or ferrous products; 3 hr after antacid or kaolin-pectin product

Perform/provide:
• Storage in tight, light-resistant container at room temperature

Evaluate:
• Therapeutic response: decreased temperature, absence of lesions, negative C&S

Teach patient/family:
• To avoid sun exposure, since burns may occur; sunscreen does not seem to decrease photosensitivity
• That diabetics should avoid use of Clinistix, Diastix, or Tes-Tape for urine glucose testing
• That all prescribed medication

must be taken to prevent superimposed infection
• To take with a full glass of water; may take with food or milk if GI symptoms occur

---

minoxidil
(mi-nox-i-dill)
Loniten, Minodyl, Minoxidil, Rogaine
Func. class.: Antihypertensive
Chem. class.: Vasodilator—peripheral

Action: Directly relaxes arteriolar smooth muscle, causing vasodilation
Uses: Severe hypertension not responsive to other therapy (use with diuretic); topically to treat alopecia
Dosage and routes:
• *Adult:* PO 5 mg/day not to exceed 100 mg daily, usual range 10-40 mg/day in single doses
• *Child <12 yr:* (initial) 0.2 mg/kg/day; (effective range) 0.25-1 mg/kg/day; (max) 50 mg/day
Alopecia
• *Adult:* Apply topically, rub into scalp daily
Available forms: Tabs 2.5, 10 mg, top 20 mg/ml
Side effects/adverse reactions:
CV: Severe rebound hypertension, tachycardia, angina, increased T wave, ***CHF, pulmonary edema, pericardial effusion,*** edema, sodium, water retention
CNS: Drowsiness, dizziness, sedation, headache, depression, fatigue
GI: Nausea, vomiting
GU: Gynecomastia, breast tenderness
INTEG: Pruritus, ***Stevens-Johnson syndrome,*** rash, hirsutism
HEMA: Hct, Hgb, erythrocyte count may decrease initially

M

Contraindications: Acute MI, dissecting aortic aneurysm, hypersensitivity, pheochromocytoma

Precautions: Pregnancy (C), lactation, children, renal disease, CAD, CHF

Pharmacokinetics:

PO: Onset 30 min, peak 2-3 hr, duration 75 hr; half-life 4.2 hr; metabolized in liver; metabolites excreted in urine, feces

Interactions/incompatibilities:

• Orthostatic hypotension: guanethidine

Lab test interferences:

Increase: Renal function studies

Decrease: Hgb/Hct/RBC

NURSING CONSIDERATIONS

Assess:

• Nausea, edema in feet, legs daily
• Skin turgor, dryness of mucous membranes for hydration status
• Rales, dyspnea, orthopnea

Monitor:

• Electrolytes: K, Na, Cl, CO_2
• Renal function studies: catecholamines, BUN, creatinine
• Hepatic function studies: AST, ALT, alk phosphatase
• B/P, pulse
• Weight daily, I&O

Administer:

• With meals for better absorption, to decrease GI symptoms
• With β-blocker and/or diuretic

Evaluate:

• Therapeutic response: decreased B/P or increased hair growth

Teach patient/family:

• That body hair will increase but is reversible after discontinuing treatment
• Not to discontinue drug abruptly
• To report pitting edema, dizziness, weight gain >5 lb, shortness of breath, bruising or bleeding, heart rate >20 beats/min over normal, severe indigestion, dizziness,

light-headedness, panting, new or aggravated symptoms of angina
• To take drug exactly as prescribed, or serious side effects may occur

Treatment of overdose: Administer normal saline IV, vasopressors

---

misoprostol

(mye-soe-prost′ ole)

Cytotec

Func. class.: Gastric mucosa protectant

Chem. class.: Prostaglandin E_1 analog

Action: Inhibits gastric acid secretion; may protect gastric mucosa; can increase bicarbonate, mucus production

Uses: Prevention of nonsteroidal antiinflammatory drug–induced gastric ulcers

Dosage and routes:

• *Adult:* PO 200 μg qid with food for duration of nonsteroidal antiinflammatory therapy; if 200 μg is not tolerated, 100 μg may be given

Available forms: Tabs 200 μg

Side effects/adverse reactions:

GI: Diarrhea, nausea, vomiting, flatulence, constipation, dyspepsia, abdominal pain

GU: Spotting, cramps, hypermenorrhea, menstrual disorders

Contraindications: Hypersensitivity, pregnancy (X)

Precautions: Lactation, children, elderly, renal disease

Pharmacokinetics:

PO: Peak 12 min, plasma steady state achieved within 2 days, excreted in urine

NURSING CONSIDERATIONS

Assess:

• Gastric pH (>5 should be maintained)
• I&O ratio, BUN, creatinine

Perform/provide:
• Storage at room temperature
Evaluate:
• Therapeutic response: absence of pain or GI complaints
Teach patient/family:
• To take only as directed
• Not to take if pregnant (can cause miscarriage) and do not become pregnant while taking this medication; if pregnancy occurs during therapy, discontinue drug, notify physician; not to administer to nursing mothers
• Not to give drug to anyone else or take for more than 4 wk unless directed by physician

---

mitomycin
(mye-toe-mye'sin)
Mutamycin
Func. class.: Antineoplastic, antibiotic

Action: Inhibits DNA synthesis, primarily; derived from *Streptomyces caespitosus;* appears to cause cross-linking of DNA, a vesicant

Uses: Pancreas, stomach cancer, head and neck or breast cancer

Dosage and routes:
• *Adult:* IV 2 mg/m²/day × 5 days, stop drug for 2 days, then repeat cycle; or 10-20 mg/m² as a single dose, repeat cycle in 6-8 wk; stop drug if platelets are <75,000/mm³ or WBC is <3000/mm³

Available forms: Inj IV 5, 20, 40 mg/vial

Side effects/adverse reactions:
HEMA: Thrombocytopenia, leukopenia, anemia
GI: Nausea, vomiting, anorexia, stomatitis, *hepatotoxicity,* diarrhea
GU: Urinary retention, *renal failure,* edema

INTEG: Rash, alopecia, *extravasation*
RESP: Fibrosis, pulmonary infiltrate, dyspnea
CNS: Fever, headache, confusion, drowsiness, syncope, fatigue
EENT: Blurred vision, drowsiness, syncope

Contraindications: Hypersensitivity, pregnancy (1st trimester) (D), as a single agent, thrombocytopenia, coagulation disorders

Precautions: Renal disease, bone marrow depression

Pharmacokinetics: Half-life 17 min, metabolized in liver, 10% excreted in urine (unchanged)

Interactions/incompatibilities:
• Increased toxicity: other antineoplastics (vinca alkaloids) or radiation
• Incompatible with bleomycin

NURSING CONSIDERATIONS
Assess:
• CBC, differential, platelet count weekly; withhold drug if WBC is <4000/mm³ or platelet count is <75,000/mm³; notify physician of these results
• Pulmonary function tests, chest x-ray before, during therapy; chest x-ray should be obtained q2wk during treatment
• Renal function studies: BUN, serum uric acid, urine CrCl, electrolytes before, during therapy
• I&O ratio; report fall in urine output to <30 ml/hr
• Monitor temperature q4h; fever may indicate beginning infection
• Liver function tests before, during therapy: bilirubin, AST, ALT, alk phosphatase as needed or monthly
• Alkalosis if severe vomiting is present
• Bleeding: hematuria, guaiac,

M

---

italics = common side effects   ***bold italic*** = life threatening reactions

bruising, petechiae, mucosa or orifices q8h
• Dyspnea, rales, unproductive cough, chest pain, tachypnea, fatigue, increased pulse, pallor, lethargy
• Food preferences; list likes, dislikes
• Effects of alopecia on body image; discuss feelings about body changes
• Inflammation of mucosa, breaks in skin
• Yellowing of skin and sclera, dark urine, clay-colored stools, itchy skin, abdominal pain, fever, diarrhea
• Buccal cavity q8h for dryness, sores, ulceration, white patches, oral pain, bleeding, dysphagia
• Local irritation, pain, burning at injection site
• GI symptoms: frequency of stools, cramping
• Acidosis, signs of dehydration: rapid respirations, poor skin turgor, decreased urine output, dry skin, restlessness, weakness

Administer:
• Sodium thiosulfate for extravasation, apply ice compress
• Antiemetic 30-60 min before giving drug to prevent vomiting
• IV after diluting 5 mg/10 ml sterile H$_2$O for inj; allow to stand, give through Y-tube or 3-way stopcock; give over 5-10 min
• Transfusion for anemia
• Antispasmodic for GI symptoms

Perform/provide:
• Liquid diet: carbonated beverages, gelatin may be added if patient is not nauseated or vomiting
• Rinsing of mouth tid-qid with water; brushing of teeth with baking soda bid-tid with soft brush or cotton-tipped applicators for stomatitis; use unwaxed dental floss

• Storage at room temperature for 1 wk after reconstituting or 2 wk refrigerated

Evaluate:
• Therapeutic response: decreased tumor size, spread of malignancy

Teach patient/family:
• To report any complaints, side effects to nurse or physician
• That hair may be lost during treatment and wig or hairpiece may make the patient feel better; tell patient that new hair may be different in color, texture
• To avoid foods with citric acid, hot or rough texture
• To report any bleeding, white spots, ulcerations in mouth; tell patient to examine mouth qd
• To avoid crowds, people with infections if granulocyte count is low

---

mitotane
(mye'toe-tane)
Lysodren
Func. class.: Antineoplastic
Chem. class.: Hormone, adrenal cytotoxic agent

Action: Cytotoxic and suppressive activity without cellular destruction in the adrenal cortex
Uses: Adrenocortical carcinoma
Dosage and routes:
• *Adult:* PO 9-10 g/day in divided doses tid or qid; may have to decrease dose if severe reactions occur
Available forms: Tabs 500 mg
Side effects/adverse reactions:
GI: Nausea, vomiting, anorexia, diarrhea
*GU: **Proteinuria, hematuria***
INTEG: Rash
*RESP: **Fibrosis, pulmonary infiltrate***

CV: Hypertension, orthostatic hypotension

CNS: Light-headedness, flushing, sedation, vertigo

EENT: Lethargy, blurring, retinopathy

Contraindications: Hypersensitivity

Precautions: Lactation, hepatic disease, pregnancy (C)

Pharmacokinetics: Adequately absorbed orally (40%), excreted in urine, bile

Interactions/incompatibilities:
• Decreased effects of: corticosteroids

Lab test interferences:
Decrease: PBI, urinary 17-OHCS

NURSING CONSIDERATIONS
Assess:
• Adrenal insufficiency: fatigue, orthostatic hypotension, weight loss, weakness, nausea, vomiting, diarrhea
• Pulmonary function tests, chest x-ray films before, during therapy; chest film should be obtained q2wk during treatment
• Renal function studies: BUN, serum uric acid, urine CrCl electrolytes before, during therapy
• I&O ratio
• Urinary 17-OHCS before, during treatment
• Dyspnea, chest pain, tachypnea, fatigue, increased pulse, pallor, lethargy
• Food preferences; list likes, dislikes
• Muscular weakness, fatigue, oliguria, hypoglycemia
• Frequency of stools, characteristics: cramping, acidosis, signs of dehydration (rapid respirations, poor skin turgor, decreased urine output, dry skin, restlessness, weakness)
• Symptoms indicating severe allergic reactions: rash, pruritus, itching, flushing
• Signs of infection: increased temperature, cough, fatigue, malaise

Administer:
• Antacid before oral agent, give drug after evening meal, before bedtime
• Antiemetic 30-60 min before giving drug to prevent vomiting
• Antispasmodic

Perform/provide:
• Increase fluid intake to 2-3 L/day to prevent dehydration if not contraindicated
• HOB raised to facilitate breathing
• Nutritious diet with iron, vitamin supplements as ordered
• Storage in tight, light-resistant container

Evaluate:
• Therapeutic response: decreased tumor size, spread of malignancy

Teach patient/family:
• To report any complaints, side effects to nurse or physician
• To report any changes in breathing, coughing
• To avoid driving, other activities requiring alertness

---

mitoxantrone HCl
(mye-toe-zan´trone)
Novantrone
Func. class.: Antineoplastic
Chem. class.: Synthetic anthraquinone

Action: DNA reactive agent, cytocidal effect on both proliferating and nonproliferating cells, suggesting lack of cell cycle phase specificity (vesicant)

Uses: Acute nonlymphocytic leukemia (adult), relapsed leukemia, breast cancer

---

italics = common side effects   ***bold italic*** = life threatening reactions

Dosage and routes:
• *Adult:* IV inf 12 mg/m^2/day on days 1-3, and 100 mg/m^2 cytosine arabinoside × 7 days as a continuous 24hr infusion

Available forms: Inj 2 mg/ml

Side effects/adverse reactions:
GI: Nausea, vomiting, diarrhea, anorexia, mucositis, hepato-toxicity

HEMA: Thrombocytopenia, leukopenia, myelosuppression, anemia

INTEG: Rash, necrosis at injection site, dermatitis, thrombophlebitis at injection site, alopecia

CV: CHF, cardiopathy, dysrhythmias

MISC: Fever

RESP: Cough, dyspnea

Contraindications: Hypersensitivity

Precautions: Myelosuppression, lactation, cardiac disease, children, pregnancy (D), renal, hepatic disease, gout

Pharmacokinetics:
Highly bound to plasma proteins, metabolized in liver, excreted via renal, hepatobiliary systems; half-life 24-72 hr

Interactions/incompatibilities:
• Do not mix with heparin; precipitate will form; considered incompatible in syringe or sol

NURSING CONSIDERATIONS
Assess:
• CBC, differential, platelet count weekly; withhold drug if WBC is <4000/mm^3 or platelet count is <75,000/mm^3; notify physician of these results
• Liver function test before, during therapy: bilirubin, AST, ALT, alk phosphatase prn or monthly
• Renal function studies: BUN, serum uric acid, urine CrCl, electrolytes before, during therapy
• Bleeding, hematuria, guaiac,

bruising or petechiae, mucosa or orifices q8h
• Food preferences; list likes, dislikes
• Yellowing of skin and sclera, dark urine, clay-colored stools, itchy skin, abdominal pain, fever, diarrhea
• Acidosis, signs of dehydration: rapid respirations, poor skin turgor, decreased urine output, dry skin, restlessness, weakness

Administer:
• Medications by oral route if possible; avoid IM, SC, IV routes to prevent infections
• Antiemetic 30-60 min before giving drug to prevent vomiting
• IV after diluting with 50 ml or more normal saline or D$_5$W; give over 3-5 min, running IV of D$_5$W or NS; may be diluted further in D$_5$W, NS and run over 15-30 min; check for extravasation

Perform/provide:
• Liquid diet: carbonated beverages, Jell-O; dry toast, crackers may be added if patient is not nauseated or vomiting
• Rinsing of mouth tid-qid with water, club soda, brushing of teeth bid-qid with soft brush or cotton-tipped applicators for stomatitis; use unwaxed dental floss

Evaluate:
• Therapeutic response: decreased tumor size, spread of malignancy

Teach patient/family:
• To report side effects to nurse or physician
• To avoid foods with citric acid, rough texture, or hot
• To report any bleeding, white spots, ulcerations in mouth; tell patient to examine mouth daily

*Available in Canada only

mivacurium chloride
(miv-a-kure'ee-um)
Mivacron
Func. class.: Nondepolarizing neuromuscular blocker

Action: Inhibits transmission of nerve impulses by binding competitively with cholinergic receptor sites, antagonizing the action of acetylcholine

Uses: Facilitation of endotracheal intubation, skeletal muscle relaxation during mechanical ventilation, surgery, or general anesthesia

Dosage and routes:
• *Adult:* IV 0.15 mg/kg; maintenance q15min
• *Child:* 2-12 IV 0.2 mg/kg for a 10 min block

Available forms: 5, 10 ml single-use vial (2 mg/ml); premixed infusion in D_5W 50 ml flex container

Side effects/adverse reactions:
CV: Decreased B/P, bradycardia, tachycardia
*RESP: **Prolonged apnea, bronchospasm, wheezing, respiratory depression***
EENT: Diplopia
MS: Weakness, prolonged skeletal muscle relaxation, *paralysis*
INTEG: Rash, urticaria

Contraindications: Hypersensitivity

Precautions: Pregnancy (C), renal or hepatic disease, lactation, children <3 mo, fluid and electrolyte imbalances, neuromuscular disease, respiratory disease, obesity, elderly

Pharmacokinetics: Rapidly hydrolyzed by plasma cholinesterases, peak 2-3 min, reversal within 15-30 min

Interactions/incompatibilities:
• Increased neuromuscular block-ade: aminoglycosides, quinidine, local anesthetics, polymyxin antibiotics, enflurane, isoflurane, tetracyclines, halothane, Mg, colistin, procainamide, bacitracin, lincomycin, clindamycin, lithium

NURSING CONSIDERATIONS
Assess
• For electrolyte imbalances (K, Mg); may lead to increased action of this drug
• Vital signs (B/P, pulse, respirations, airway) until fully recovered; rate, depth, pattern of respirations, strength of hand grip
• I&O ratio; check for urinary retention, frequency, hesitancy
• Recovery: decreased paralysis of face, diaphragm, leg, arm, rest of body
• Allergic reactions: rash, fever, respiratory distress, pruritus; drug should be discontinued

Administer:
• Using nerve stimulator by anesthesiologist to determine neuromuscular blockade
• Anticholinesterase to reverse neuromuscular blockade
• By slow IV over 1-2 min (only by qualified persons, usually an anesthesiologist)
• Only fresh solution

Perform/provide:
• Storage at room temperature; do not freeze
• Reassurance if communication is difficult during recovery from neuromuscular blockade
• Frequent (q2h) instillation of artificial tears and covering eyes to prevent drying of cornea

Evaluate:
• Therapeutic response: paralysis of jaw, eyelid, head, neck, rest of body

Treatment of overdose: Neostig-

M

mine, monitor VS; may require mechanical ventilation

---

molindone HCl
(moe-lin'done)
Moban
Func. class.: Antipsychotic/neuroleptic
Chem. class.: Dihydroindolone

Action: Depresses cerebral cortex, hypothalamus, limbic system, which control activity, aggression; blocks neurotransmission produced by dopamine at synapse; exhibits strong α-adrenergic, anticholinergic blocking action; mechanism for antipsychotic effects is unclear
Uses: Psychotic disorders
Dosage and routes:
• *Adult:* PO 50-75 mg/day increasing to 225 mg/day if needed
Available forms: Tabs 5, 10, 25, 50, 100 mg; conc 20 mg/ml
Side effects/adverse reactions:
*RESP: **Laryngospasm,** dyspnea, **respiratory depression***
CNS: Extrapyramidal symptoms: pseudoparkinsonism, akathisia, dystonia, tardive dyskinesia, drowsiness, headache, seizures
*HEMA: **Anemia, leukopenia, leukocytosis, agranulocytosis***
INTEG: Rash, photosensitivity, dermatitis
EENT: Blurred vision, glaucoma
GI: Dry mouth, nausea, vomiting, anorexia, constipation, diarrhea, jaundice, weight gain
GU: Urinary retention, urinary frequency, enuresis, impotence, amenorrhea, gynecomastia
CV: Orthostatic hypotension, hypertension, **cardiac arrest,** ECG changes, **tachycardia**
Contraindications: Hypersensitivity, coma, child

Precautions: Pregnancy (C), lactation, hypertension, hepatic disease, cardiac disease, Parkinson's disease, brain tumor, glaucoma, urinary retention, diabetes mellitus, respiratory disease, prostatic hypertrophy
Pharmacokinetics:
PO: Onset erratic, peak 1½ hr, duration 24-36 hr; metabolized by liver, excreted in urine and feces, may cross placenta, enters breast milk, half-life 1½ hr
Interactions/incompatibilities:
• Increased sedation: other CNS depressants
• Increased EPS: other antipsychotics, lithium
Lab test interferences:
Alterations in: BUN, RBC, serum glucose, WBC
Increase: Serum prolactin levels
NURSING CONSIDERATIONS
Assess:
• Mental status before initial administration
• Swallowing of PO medication; check for hoarding or giving of medication to other patients
• I&O ratio; palpate bladder if low urinary output occurs
• Bilirubin, CBC, liver function studies monthly
• Urinalysis is recommended before, during prolonged therapy
• Affect, orientation, LOC, reflexes, gait, coordination, sleep pattern disturbances
• B/P standing and lying; also include pulse, respirations; take these q4h during initial treatment; establish baseline before starting treatment; report drops of 30 mm Hg, watch for ECG changes
• Dizziness, faintness, palpitations, tachycardia on rising
• Extrapyramidal symptoms including akathisia (inability to sit

---

*Available in Canada only

still, no pattern to movements), tardive dyskinesia (bizarre movements of the jaw, mouth, tongue, extremities), pseudoparkinsonism (rigidity, tremors, pill rolling, shuffling gait)
• For neuroleptic malignant syndrome: hyperthermia, increased CPK, altered mental status, muscle rigidity
• Skin turgor daily
• Constipation, urinary retention daily; if these occur, increase bulk and water in diet

Administer:
• Reduced dose in elderly
• Antiparkinsonian agent, after securing order from physician, to be used if extrapyramidal symptoms occur
• Concentrate mixed in orange or grapefruit juice

Perform/provide:
• Decreased noise input by dimming lights, avoiding loud noises
• Supervised ambulation until stabilized on medication; do not involve in strenuous exercise program because fainting is possible; patient should not stand still for a long time
• Increased fluids to prevent constipation
• Sips of water, candy, gum for dry mouth
• Storage in tight, light-resistant container

Evaluate:
• Therapeutic response: decrease in emotional excitement, hallucinations, delusions, paranoia, reorganization of patterns of thought, speech

Teach patient/family:
• That orthostatic hypotension may occur and to rise from sitting or lying position gradually
• To avoid hot tubs, hot showers,

tub baths, since hypotension may occur
• To avoid abrupt withdrawal of this drug, or EPS may result; drug should be withdrawn slowly
• To avoid OTC preparations (cough, hay fever, cold) unless approved by physician, since serious drug interactions may occur; avoid use with alcohol, CNS depressants; increased drowsiness may occur
• To avoid hazardous activities if drowsiness or dizziness occurs
• To use sunscreen during sun exposure to prevent burns
• Regarding compliance with drug regimen
• About necessity for meticulous oral hygiene, since oral candidiasis may occur
• To report impaired vision, jaundice, tremors, muscle twitching
• In hot weather, that heat stroke may occur; take extra precautions to stay cool

Treatment of overdose: Lavage if orally ingested; provide an airway; *do not induce vomiting*

moricizine
(mor iss' i-zeen)
Ethmozine
Func. class.: Antidysrhythmic, type I
Chem. class.: Phenothiazine

Action: Decreased rate of rise of action potential, prolonging refractory period and shortening the action potential duration; depression of inward influx if sodium mediates the effects; drug may slow atrial and AV nodal conduction
Uses: Symptomatic ventricular and life-threatening dysrhythmias
Dosage and routes:
Adult: PO 10-15 mg/kg/day in 2-3 divided doses

Available forms: Film-coated tabs 200, 250, 300 mg

Side effects/adverse reactions:

GI: Nausea, abdominal pain, vomiting, diarrhea

CNS: Dizziness, headache, fatigue, perioral numbness, euphoria, nervousness, sleep disorders, depression, tinnitus, fatigue

RESP: Dyspnea, hyperventilation, *apnea,* asthma, pharyngitis, cough

GU: Sexual dysfunction, difficult urination, dysuria, incontinence

CV: Palpitations, chest pain, *CHF,* hypertension, syncope, dysrythmias, bradycardia, *MI,* thrombophlebitis

MISC: Sweating, musculoskeletal pain

Contraindications: 2-3 degree AV block, right bundle branch block, cardiogenic shock, hypersensitivity

Precautions: CHF, hypokalemia, hyperkalemia, sick sinus syndrome, pregnancy (B), lactation, children, impaired hepatic and renal function, cardiac dysfunction

Pharmacokinetics: Half-life 1.5-3.5 hr; peak 0.5-2.2 hr; metabolized by the liver; metabolites are excreted in feces and urine, protein binding >90%

Interactions/incompatibilities:

• Increased plasma levels of moricizine: amantadine

• Digoxin or propranolol may enhance some of cardiac effects of moricizine; moricizine may decrease effects of theophylline

Lab test interferences:

Increase: CPK

NURSING CONSIDERATIONS

Assess:

• GI status: bowel pattern, number of stools

• Cardiac status: rate, rhythm, quality

• Chest x-ray, pulmonary function test during treatment

• I&O ratio; check for decreasing output

• B/P for fluctuations

• Lung fields: bilateral rales may occur in CHF patient

• Increased respiration, increased pulse; drug should be discontinued

• Toxicity: fine tremors, dizziness

• Cardiac rate: respiration, rate, rhythm, character continuously

Evaluate:

• Therapeutic response: absence of dysrhythmias

Treatment of overdose: O_2 artificial ventilation, ECG; administer dopamine for circulatory depression; administer diazepam or thiopental for convulsions

---

morphine sulfate

(mor'feen)

Astramorph PF, Duramorph, Infumorph 200, Infumorph 500, Morphine Sulfate, MS Contin, MSIR, OMS Concentrate, Oramorph SR, RMS, Roxanol, Roxanol 100, Roxanol Rescudose, Roxanol SR

Func. class.: Narcotic analgesic

Chem. class.: Opiate

Controlled Substance Schedule II

Action: Depresses pain impulse transmission at the spinal cord level by interacting with opioid receptors

Uses: Severe pain

Dosage and routes:

• *Adult:* SC/IM 4-15 mg q4h prn; PO 10-30 mg q4h prn; EXT REL q8-12h; REC 10-20 mg q4h prn; IV 4-10 mg diluted in 4-5 ml H_2O for injection, over 5 min

• *Child:* SC 0.1-0.2 mg/kg, not to exceed 15 mg

Available forms: Inj SC, IM, IV 2, 4, 5, 8, 10, 15 mg/ml; sol tabs 10, 15, 30 mg; oral sol 10, 20 mg/5 ml, 20 mg/10 ml, 20 mg/ml; oral tabs 15, 30 mg; rec supp 5, 10, 20 mg; ext rel tabs 300 mg

Side effects/adverse reactions:
CNS: Drowsiness, dizziness, confusion, headache, sedation, euphoria
CV: Palpitations, bradycardia, change in B/P
EENT: Tinnitus, blurred vision, miosis, diplopia
GI: Nausea, vomiting, anorexia, constipation, cramps, biliary tract pressure
GU: Urinary retention
INTEG: Rash, urticaria, bruising, flushing, diaphoresis, pruritus
*RESP: **Respiratory depression***

Contraindications: Hypersensitivity, addiction (narcotic), hemorrhage, bronchial asthma, increased intracranial pressure

Precautions: Addictive personality, pregnancy (B), lactation, acute MI, severe heart disease, elderly, respiratory depression, hepatic disease, renal disease, child <18 yr

Pharmacokinetics:
PO: Onset variable, peak variable, duration variable
SC: Onset 15-20 min, peak 50-90 min, duration 3-5 hr
IV: Peak 20 min; metabolized by liver, excreted by kidneys, crosses placenta, excreted in breast milk, half-life 2½-3 hr

Interactions/incompatibilities:
• Increased effects with other CNS depressants: alcohol, narcotics, sedative/hypnotics, antipsychotics, skeletal muscle relaxants
• Incompatible with aminophylline, amobarbital, chlorothiazide, heparin, meperidine, methicillin, pentobarbital, phenobarbital, phenytoin, NaCO₃, thiopental

Lab test interferences:
Increase: Amylase

NURSING CONSIDERATIONS
Assess:
• Bowel status; constipation frequent
• Pain: type, location, intensity, characteristics
• I&O ratio; check for decreasing output; may indicate urinary retention
• B/P, pulse, respirations (character, depth, rate)
• CNS changes: dizziness, drowsiness, hallucinations, euphoria, LOC, pupil reaction
• Allergic reactions: rash, urticaria
• Respiratory dysfunction: depression, character, rate, rhythm; notify physician if respirations are <10/min
• Need for pain medication, physical dependence

Administer:
• IV after diluting with 5 ml sterile H₂O or NS; give 15 mg or less over 4-5 min; give through Y-tube or 3-way stopcock; may be added to IV sol, each 0.1-1 mg diluted in 1 ml D₅W, given with inf pump titrated to patient response
• With antiemetic for nausea, vomiting
• When pain is beginning to return; determine dosage interval by patient response

Perform/provide:
• Storage in light-resistant container at room temperature
• Assistance with ambulation
• Safety measures: side rails, nightlight, call bell within easy reach
• Gradual withdrawal after long-term use

Evaluate:
• Therapeutic response; decrease in pain intensity

M

---

italics = common side effects   ***bold italic*** = life threatening reactions

Teach patient/family:
• To change position slowly; orthostatic hypotension may occur
• To report any symptoms of CNS changes, allergic reactions
• That physical dependency may result when used for extended periods
• To avoid use of alcohol, CNS depressants
• That withdrawal symptoms may occur: nausea, vomiting, cramps, fever, faintness, anorexia

Treatment of overdose: Naloxone (Narcan) 0.2-0.8 IV, O₂, IV fluids, vasopressors

---

moxalactam disodium
(mox′a-lak-tam)
Moxam
Func. class.: Antibiotic, broad-spectrum
Chem. class.: Cephalosporin (3rd generation)

Action: Inhibits bacterial cell wall synthesis, rendering cell wall osmotically unstable and leading to cell death
Uses: Gram-negative organisms: *H. influenzae, E. coli, P. mirabilis, Klebsiella, Citrobacter, Salmonella, Shigella, Serratia;* gram-positive organisms: *S. pneumoniae, S. pyogenes, S. aureus;* serious lower respiratory tract, urinary tract, skin, bone infections, septicemia, meningitis, intraabdominal infections
Dosage and routes:
• *Adult:* IM/IV 2-4 g q8-12h
Mild infections
• *Adult:* IM/IV 250-500 mg q8-12h
Severe infections
• *Adult:* IM/IV 2-6 g q8h
• *Child:* IM/IV 50 mg/kg q6-8h

• Dosage reduction indicated even for mild renal impairment (CrCl < 80 ml/min)
Available forms: Powder for inj IM, IV 1, 2, 10 g
Side effects/adverse reactions:
CNS: Headache, dizziness, weakness, paresthesia, fever, chills
GI: Nausea, vomiting, diarrhea, anorexia, pain, glossitis, bleeding, increased AST, ALT, bilirubin, LDH, alk phosphatase, abdominal pain
GU: Proteinuria, vaginitis, pruritus, candidiasis, increased BUN, *nephrotoxicity, renal failure*
HEMA: Leukopenia, thrombocytopenia, agranulocytosis, anemia, neutropenia, lymphocytosis, eosinophilia, pancytopenia, hemolytic anemia, bleeding, hypoprothrombinemia
INTEG: Rash, urticaria, dermatitis, *anaphylaxis*
RESP: Dyspnea
Contraindications: Hypersensitivity to cephalosporins
Precautions: Hypersensitivity to penicillins, pregnancy (C), lactation, renal disease
Pharmacokinetics:
IV: Peak 5 min
IM: Peak ½-2 hr
Half-life 1½-2½ hr, 25% bound by plasma proteins; 60%-97% eliminated unchanged in urine in 24 hr; crosses placenta, blood-brain barrier; excreted in breast milk; not metabolized
Interactions/incompatibilities:
• Incompatible with tetracyclines, erythromycins, aminoglycosides in same parenteral fluid
• Decreased effects of: tetracyclines, erythromycins
• Increased toxicity: aminoglycosides, furosemide, probenecid, sulfinpyrazone, colistin, etha-

crynic acid, vancomycin, agents affecting platelet function
• Disulfiram reaction: ethanol

Lab test interferences:
Increase (false): Urinary 17-KS
False positive: Urinary protein, direct Coombs' test, urine glucose
Interference: Cross-matching

NURSING CONSIDERATIONS
Assess:
• Nephrotoxicity: increased BUN, creatinine
• I&O daily
• Blood studies: AST, ALT, CBC, Hct, bilirubin, LDH, alk phosphatase, Coombs' test pro-time monthly if patient is on long-term therapy
• Electrolytes: potassium, sodium, chloride monthly if patient is on long-term therapy
• Bowel pattern qd; if severe diarrhea occurs, drug should be discontinued; may indicate pseudomembranous colitis
• IV site for extravasation, phlebitis; change site q72h
• Urine output: if decreasing, notify physician; may indicate nephrotoxicity
• Allergic reactions: rash, urticaria, pruritus, chills, fever, joint pain, angioedema; may occur few days after therapy begins
• Bleeding: ecchymosis, bleeding gums, hematuria, stool guaiac daily
• Overgrowth of infection: perineal itching, fever, malaise, redness, pain, swelling, drainage, rash, diarrhea, change in cough, sputum

Administer:
• For 10-14 days to ensure organism death, prevent superimposed infection
• IV after diluting 1 g/10 ml sterile H$_2$O, D$_5$, 0.9% NaCl; give through Y-tube over 3-5 min; may be further diluted 1 g/20 ml in D$_5$, 0.9%

NaCl, give over ½ hr; may be added 500-1000, give over 6-24 hr
• Vit K for bleeding (10 mg/wk)
• After C&S

Evaluate:
• Therapeutic response: decreased fever, malaise, chills

Teach patient/family:
• To report sore throat, bruising, bleeding, joint pain; may indicate blood dyscrasias (rare)
• Not to drink alcohol while taking this drug

Treatment of overdose: Epinephrine, antihistamines; resuscitate if needed (anaphylaxis)

---

multivitamins
Many brands
Func. class.: Vitamin

M

Action: Needed for adequate metabolism
Uses: Prevention and treatment of vitamin deficiencies

Dosage and routes:
• *Adult and child:* PO depends on brand
Available forms: Many forms available

Side effects/adverse reactions:
None known

Precautions: Pregnancy (A)

Interactions/incompatibilities:
• Check each vitamin for specific interactions

NURSING CONSIDERATIONS
Assess:
• Vitamin deficiency: usually more than one vitamin is deficient

Evaluate:
• Therapeutic response: check each individual vitamin for guidelines

Teach patient/family:
• That adequate nutrition must be maintained to prevent further deficiencies

---

italics = common side effects   ***bold italic*** = life threatening reactions

• Drug interaction that should be avoided
• To comply with regimen
• To avoid using flavored multivitamins as candy; child may overdose
• To store out of children's reach

---

mupirocin

(mew-per'-o-sen)
Bactroban
Func. class.: Topical antiinfective
Chem. class.: Pseudomonic acid A

Action: Inhibits bacterial protein synthesis, shows no cross-resistance to most antibiotics
Uses: Impetigo caused by *S. aureus,* β-hemolytic *Streptococcus, S. pyogenes*
Dosage and routes:
Apply small amount to affected area tid
Available forms: Oint 2% (20 mg/g)
Side effects/adverse reactions:
INTEG: Burning, stinging, itching, rash, dry skin, swelling, contact dermatitis, erythema, tenderness, increased exudate
Contraindications: Hypersensitivity
Precautions: Pregnancy (B), lactation
NURSING CONSIDERATIONS
Assess:
• Affected area for continuing infection: increased size, number of lesions
Administer:
• Then cover with 2 × 2 in gauze if needed
Perform/provide:
• Storage at room temperature

• Isolation (wound) for hospitalized child (2-5 days)
• Washing of hands after applying ointment
Evaluate:
• Therapeutic response: reduction in size, number of lesions
Teach patient/family:
• To wash hands after applying ointment
• To trim fingernails to prevent scratching
• To report irritation, worsening of rash, itching, pain at site; if no improvement within 3-5 days, report to physician

---

muromonab-CD3

(mur-oo-mone'ab)
Orthoclone OKT3
Func. class.: Immunosuppressive
Chem. class.: Murine monoclonal antibody

Action: Reverses graft rejection by blocking T-cell function
Uses: Acute allograft rejection in renal, cardiac/hepatic transplant patients
Dosage and routes:
• *Adult:* IV BOL 5 mg/day × 10-14 days; usually methylprednisolone Na succinate, 1 mg/kg IV is given before muromonab-CD3, 100 mg IV hydrocortisone Na succinate is given ½ hr after muromonab-CD3
Cardiac/hepatic allograft rejection, steroid resistant
• *Adult:* IV BOL 5 mg/day × 10-14 days; begin when it is known that rejection has not been reversed by steroids
Available forms: Inj 5 mg/5 ml
Side effects/adverse reactions:
CNS: Pyrexia, chills, tremors

---

*RESP: Dyspnea, wheezing, **pulmonary edema***
CV: Chest pain
GI: Vomiting, nausea, diarrhea
MISC: Infection
Contraindications: Hypersensitivity to murine origin, fluid overload
Precautions: Pregnancy (C), child <2 yr, fever
Pharmacokinetics:
Trough level steady state 3-14 days
Interactions/incompatibilities:
• Incompatible with any drug in syringe or sol
NURSING CONSIDERATIONS
Assess:
• Blood studies: Hgb, WBC, platelets during treatment monthly; if leukocytes are <3000/mm³, drug should be discontinued
• Liver function studies: alk phosphatase, AST, ALT, bilirubin
• Hepatotoxicity: dark urine, jaundice, itching, light-colored stools; drug should be discontinued
Administer:
• IV undiluted; withdraw with a 0.2-0.22 low protein-binding μm filter, discard and use new needle for administration; give over 1 min
• For several days before transplant surgery
• All medications PO if possible; avoid IM injection, since infection may occur
Evaluate:
• Therapeutic response: decreased tumor size, spread of malignancy
Teach patient/family:
• To report fever, chills, sore throat, fatigue, since serious infection may occur
• To use contraceptive measures during treatment, for 12 wk after ending therapy; possible mutagenic effects

nabumetone
(nay-bume'tone)
Relafen
Func. class.: Nonsteroidal antiinflammatory
Chem. class.: Acetic acid derivative

Action: May inhibit prostaglandin synthesis by decreasing enzyme needed for biosynthesis; analgesic, antiinflammatory, antipyretic
Uses: Osteoarthritis, rheumatoid arthritis, acute or chronic treatment
Dosage and routes:
• *Adult:* PO 1 g as a single dose; may increase to 1.5-2 g/day if needed; may give qd or bid
Available forms: Tabs 500, 750 mg
Side effects/adverse reactions:
CNS: Dizziness, headache, drowsiness, fatigue, tremors, confusion, insomnia, anxiety, depression, nervousness
*GU: **Nephrotoxicity, dysuria, hematuria, oliguria, azotemia,** cystitis*
GI: Nausea, anorexia, vomiting, diarrhea, jaundice, ***cholestatic hepatitis,*** constipation, flatulence, cramps, dry mouth, peptic ulcer, gastritis, ***ulceration, perforation***
CV: Tachycardia, peripheral edema, palpitations, dysrhythmias, CHF
INTEG: Purpura, rash, pruritus, sweating, photosensitivity
*HEMA: **Blood dyscrasias***
EENT: Tinnitus, hearing loss, blurred vision
RESP: Dyspnea, pharyngitis, ***bronchospasm***
Contraindications: Hypersensitivity to this drug or aspirin, iodides, NSAIDs, asthma, severe renal disease, severe

---

italics = common side effects   ***bold italic*** = life threatening reactions

Precautions: Pregnancy (B) 1st and 2nd trimester, lactation, children, bleeding disorders, GI disorders, cardiac disorders, renal disorders, hepatic dysfunction, elderly

Pharmacokinetics:

PO: Peak 2½-4 hr, plasma protein binding >90%, half-life 22-30 hr; metabolized in liver to active metabolite; excreted in urine (metabolites), breast milk

Interactions/incompatibilities:

• May increase the action or increased toxicity of: coumarin, cyclosporine, phenytoin, methotrexate, probenecid

• May decrease effects of nabumetone: salicylates

NURSING CONSIDERATIONS

Assess:

• Renal, liver, blood studies: BUN, creatinine, AST, ALT, Hgb, before treatment, periodically thereafter

• Audiometric, ophthalmic exam before, during, after treatment

• For eye, ear problems: blurred vision, tinnitus; may indicate toxicity

Administer:

• With food to decrease GI symptoms

• Avoid alcoholic beverages and aspirin

Perform/provide:

• Storage at room temperature

Evaluate:

• Therapeutic response: decreased pain and stiffness in joints

Teach patient/family:

• To report blurred vision, ringing, roaring in ears; may indicate toxicity

• To avoid driving, other hazardous activities if dizziness, drowsiness occur

• To report change in urine pattern, increased weight, edema, increased pains in joints, fever, blood in urine; indicates nephrotoxicity

• That therapeutic effects may take up to 1 mo

• To take with a full glass of water to enhance absorption

• To report dark stools; may indicate GI bleeding

---

nadolol

(nay-doe'-lole)

Corgard

Func. class.: Antihypertensive, antianginal

Chem. class.: β-adrenergic receptor blocker

Action: Long-acting, nonselective β-adrenergic receptor blocking agent; mechanism is similar to that of propranolol

Uses: Chronic stable angina pectoris, mild to moderate hypertension, prophylaxis of migraine headaches

Dosage and routes:

• *Adult:* PO 40 mg qd, increase by 40-80 mg q3-7d; maintenance 40-240 mg/day for angina, 40-320 mg/day for hypertension

Available forms: Oral tabs 20, 40, 80, 120, 160 mg

Side effects/adverse reactions:

RESP: Dyspnea, respiratory dysfunction, ***bronchospasm,*** cough, wheezing, nasal stuffiness, pharyngitis, ***laryngospasm***

*CV: Bradycardia, hypotension, **CHF,*** palpitations, AV block, chest pain, peripheral ischemia, flushing, edema, vasodilation, conduction disturbances

*HEMA: **Agranulocytosis, thrombocytopenia***

GI: Nausea, vomiting, diarrhea, colitis, constipation, cramps, dry mouth, flatulence, hepatomegaly, pancreatitis, taste distortion

INTEG: Rash, pruritus, fever

CNS: Depression, hallucinations, dizziness, fatigue, lethargy, paresthesias, headache
EENT: Sore throat

Contraindications: Hypersensitivity to this drug, cardiac failure, cardiogenic shock, 2nd or 3rd degree heart block, bronchospastic disease, sinus bradycardia, CHF, COPD

Precautions: Diabetes mellitus, pregnancy (C), renal disease, lactation, hyperthyroidism, peripheral vascular disease, myasthenia gravis

Pharmacokinetics:
PO: Onset variable, peak 3-4 hr, duration 17-24 hr; half-life 16-20 hr; not metabolized; excreted in urine (unchanged), bile, breast milk

Interactions/incompatibilities:
• Increased effects of: reserpine, digitalis, ergots, neuromuscular blocking agents, calcium channel blockers
• Increased hypotensive effects: other hypotensive agents, diuretics, phenothiazines
• Decreased effects of: norepinephrine, xanthines, isoproterenol, thyroid

Lab test interferences:
Increase: Serum K, serum uric acid, ALT/AST, alk phosphatase, LDH blood glucose, cholesterol

NURSING CONSIDERATIONS
Assess:
• B/P, pulse, respirations during beginning therapy
• Weight qd; report gain of 5 lb
• I&O ratio, CrCl if kidney damage is diagnosed
• Qd, note need to be administered more often
• Pain: duration, time started, activity being performed, character
• Tolerance if taken over long time
• Headache, light-headedness, de-

creased B/P; may indicate a need for decreased dosage
Administer:
• With 8 oz water
Evaluate:
• Therapeutic response: decreased B/P, symptoms of angina
Teach patient/family:
• That drug may mask signs of hypoglycemia or alter blood glucose in diabetics
• Not to discontinue abruptly
• To avoid OTC drugs unless physician approves
• To avoid hazardous activities if dizziness occurs
• To comply with complete medical regimen

---

nafarelin acetate
Synarel
Func. class.: Gonadotropin
Chem. class.: Analog of gonadotropin-releasing hormone

Action: Stimulates the release of LH and FSH, which increases ovarian steroid production; repeated dosing prevents stimulation of the pituitary gland

Uses: Endometriosis gonadotropin-dependent precocious puberty

Doses and routes: 400 µg/day as one spray (200 µg) into one nostril in morning and one spray into other nostril in evening; start treatment between days 2 and 4 of menstrual cycle; may increase to 800 µg/day (one spray into each nostril twice a day); recommended duration of treatment is 6 months

Available forms: Nasal sol 2 mg/ml

Side effects/adverse reactions:
GU: Decreased libido, vaginal dryness, breast tenderness, increased pubic hair

---

italics = common side effects   ***bold italic*** = life threatening reactions

CNS: Headache, flushing, depression, insomnia, emotional lability, hot flashes
INTEG: Nasal irritation, acne
MISC: Body odor, seborrhea, rhinitis
SENSITIVITY: Shortness of breath, chest pain, urticaria pruritis
Contraindications: Hypersensitivity, pregnancy (X), lactation, undiagnosed abnormal vaginal bleeding
Precautions: Children
Pharmacokinetics: Rapidly absorbed, peak 10-40 min, half-life 3 hr; 80% bound to plasma proteins
NURSING CONSIDERATIONS
Assess:
• Test results: pituitary/hypothalamus dysfunction (decreased LH); postmenopausal (increased LH)
Administer:
• Repeated doses may be necessary to elevate pituitary gonadotropin reserve
Perform/provide:
• Storage at room temperature; protect from light
Evaluate:
• Therapeutic response: decreased symptoms of endometriosis

---

nafcillin sodium

(naf-sill'-in)
Nafcil, Nafcillin Sodium, Nallpen, Unipen
Func. class.: Broad-spectrum antibiotic
Chem. class.: Penicillinase-resistant penicillin

Action: Interferes with cell wall replication of susceptible organisms; osmotically unstable cell wall swells, bursts from osmotic pressure
Uses: Effective for gram-positive cocci *(S. aureus, S. viridans, S. pneumoniae)*, infections caused by penicillinase-producing *Staphylococcus*

Dosage and routes:
• *Adult:* IM/IV 2-6 g/day in divided doses q4-6h; PO 2-6 g/day in divided doses q4-6h
• *Child:* IM 25 mg/kg q12h; PO 25-50 mg/kg/day in divided doses q6h
• *Neonates* IM 10 mg/kg bid
Available forms: Caps 250 mg; tabs 500 mg; powder for oral susp 250 mg/5 ml; powder for inj IM, IV 500 mg, 1, 2, 10 g; IV 1, 1.5, 2, 4 g

Side effects/adverse reactions:
HEMA: Anemia, increased bleeding time, *bone marrow depression, granulocytopenia*
GI: Nausea, vomiting, diarrhea, increased AST, ALT, abdominal pain, glossitis, colitis
GU: Oliguria, *proteinuria, hematuria, vaginitis, moniliasis, glomerulonephritis,* interstitial nephritis
CNS: Lethargy, hallucinations, anxiety, depression, twitching, *coma, convulsions*
Contraindications: Hypersensitivity to penicillins
Precautions: Pregnancy (B), hypersensitivity to cephalosporins, neonates
Pharmacokinetics:
IM/PO: Peak 30-60 min, duration 4-6 hr, half-life 1 hr, metabolized by the liver, excreted in bile, urine
Interactions/incompatibilities:
• Decreased antimicrobial effectiveness of nafcillin: tetracyclines, erythromycins
• Increased nafcillin concentrations: aspirin, probenecid
• Incompatible in sol with ami-

---

*Available in Canada only

nophylline, aztreonam, methylprednisolone, droperidol, innovar

Lab test interferences:

False positive: Urine glucose, urine
protein

NURSING CONSIDERATIONS

Assess:

• I&O ratio; report hematuria, oliguria, since penicillin in high doses
is nephrotoxic

• Any patient with compromised
renal system, since drug is excreted
slowly in poor renal system function; toxicity may occur rapidly

• Liver studies: AST, ALT

• Blood studies: WBC, RBC,
H&H, bleeding time

• Renal studies: urinalysis, protein,
blood

• C&S before drug therapy; drug
may be given as soon as culture is
taken

• Bowel pattern before and during
treatment

• Skin eruptions after administration of penicillin to 1 wk after discontinuing drug

• Respiratory status: rate, character, wheezing, and tightness in
chest

• Allergies before initiation of
treatment and reaction of each medication; highlight allergies on chart,
Kardex

• Differential WBC in patients on
long-term therapy

Administer:

• IV after diluting 500 mg/1.7 ml
of sterile H$_2$O for inj; further dilute
each 500 mg/15-30 ml sterile water
or NS sol; give through Y-tube or
stopcock 500 mg or less/5-10 min;
may be further diluted and run over
24 hr

• IM give deep IM in gluteal muscle

• Drug after C&S has been completed

• Divided oral doses on empty
stomach before meals; oral absorption is erratic

Perform/provide:

• Adrenalin, suction, tracheostomy
set, endotracheal intubation equipment

• Adequate fluid intake (2 L) during diarrhea episodes

• Scratch test to assess allergy after
securing order from physician; usually done when penicillin is only
drug of choice

• Storage in tight container; refrigerate reconstituted solution

Evaluate:

• Therapeutic response: absence
of fever, draining wounds

Teach patient/family:

• Aspects of drug therapy, including need to complete course of
medication to ensure organism
death (10-14 days); culture may be
taken after completed course

• To report sore throat, fever, fatigue (may indicate superimposed
infection)

• To wear or carry Medic Alert ID
if allergic to penicillins

• To notify nurse of diarrhea

Treatment of overdose: Withdraw
drug; maintain airway; administer
epinephrine, aminophylline, O$_2$, IV
corticosteroids for anaphylaxis

---

naftifine HCl

(naf-tee-fin)

Naftin

Func. class.: Topical antifungal

Chem. class.: Synthetic allylamine derivative

Action: Interferes with cell membrane permeability in fungi such as
*T. rubrum, T. mentagrophytes, T.
tonsurans, E. floccosum, M. canis,
M. audouinii, M. gypseum, Can-*

---

italics = common side effects   ***bold italic*** = life threatening reactions

dida; broad-spectrum antifungal

Uses: Tinea cruris, tinea corporis

Dosage and routes:

Massage into affected area, surrounding area bid, continue for 7-14 days

Available forms: Cream 1%

Side effects/adverse reactions:

INTEG: Burning, stinging, dryness, itching, local irritation

Contraindications: Hypersensitivity

Precautions: Pregnancy (B), lactation, children

NURSING CONSIDERATIONS

Assess:

• For continuing infection: increased size, number of lesions

Administer:

• To affected area, surrounding area; do not cover with occlusive dressings

Perform/provide:

• Storage below 30° C (86° F)

Evaluate:

• Therapeutic response: decrease in size, number of lesions

Teach patient/family:

• To wear cotton clothing

• To use clean towel, dry well

• To avoid contact with mucous membranes

• Not to cover areas unless directed to by physician

• To report excessive itching, burning

• How to apply; massage cream into affected area and surrounding skin in AM, PM; effects observed within 1 wk, continue 1-2 wk after symptoms decrease; wash hands after application

---

nalbuphine HCl

(nal'byoo-feen)

Nubain, Nalbuphine HCl

Func. class.: Narcotic agonist

Chem. class.: Synthetic narcotic agonist

Controlled Substance Schedule II

Action: Depresses pain impulse transmission at the spinal cord level by interacting with opioid receptors

Uses: Moderate to severe pain

Dosage and routes:

• *Adult:* SC/IM/IV 10-20 mg q3-6h prn, not to exceed 160 mg/day

Available forms: Inj SC, IM, IV 10, 20 mg/ml

Side effects/adverse reactions:

CNS: Drowsiness, dizziness, confusion, headache, sedation, euphoria, dysphoria (high doses)

GI: Nausea, vomiting, anorexia, constipation, cramps

GU: Increased urinary output, dysuria, urinary retention

INTEG: Rash, urticaria, bruising, flushing, diaphoresis, pruritus

EENT: Tinnitus, blurred vision, miosis, diplopia

CV: Palpitations, bradycardia, change in B/P

RESP: Respiratory depression

Contraindications: Hypersensitivity, addiction (narcotic)

Precautions: Addictive personality, pregnancy (B), lactation, increased intracranial pressure, MI (acute), severe heart disease, respiratory depression, hepatic disease, renal disease

Pharmacokinetics:

SC/IM/IV: Duration 3-6 hr; metabolized by liver, excreted by kidneys, half-life 5 hr

Interactions/incompatibilities:

• Increased effects with other CNS

---

depressants: alcohol, narcotics, sedative/hypnotics, antipsychotics, skeletal muscle relaxants
• Incompatible with diazepam, pentobarbital

Lab test interferences:
Increase: Amylase

NURSING CONSIDERATIONS
Assess:
• I&O ratio; check for decreasing output; may indicate urinary retention
• For withdrawal reactions in narcotic-dependent individuals: pulmonary embolus, vascular occlusion; abscesses, ulcerations, nausea, vomiting, convulsions
• CNS changes: dizziness, drowsiness, hallucinations, euphoria, LOC, pupil reaction
• Allergic reactions: rash, urticaria
• Respiratory dysfunction: respiratory depression, character, rate, rhythm; notify physician if respirations are <10/min
• Need for pain medication by pain sedation scoring, physical dependence

Administer:
• IV undiluted 10 mg or less over 3-5 min
• With antiemetic if nausea, vomiting occur
• When pain is beginning to return; determine dosage interval by patient response

Perform/provide:
• Storage in light-resistant area at room temperature
• Assistance with ambulation
• Safety measures: side rails, nightlight, call bell within easy reach

Evaluate:
• Therapeutic response: decrease in pain

Teach patient/family:
• To report any symptoms of CNS changes, allergic reactions

• That physical dependency may result when used for extended periods
• Withdrawal symptoms may occur: nausea, vomiting, cramps, fever, faintness, anorexia

Treatment of overdose: (Narcan) 0.2-0.8 IV, O_2, IV fluids, vasopressors

---

nalidixic acid
(nal-i-dix'ik)
NegGram, NegGram Caplets
Func. class.: Urinary tract anti-infective
Chem. class.: Synthetic naphthyridine derivative

N

Action: Appears to inhibit DNA polymerization, primary target being single-stranded DNA precursors in late stages of chromosomal replication

Uses: Urinary tract infections (acute/chronic) caused by *E. coli, Klebsiella, Enterobacter, P. mirabilis, P. vulgaris, P. morganii*

Dosage and routes:
• *Adult:* PO 1 g qid × 1-2 wk, 2 g/day for long-term treatment
• *Child >3 mo:* PO 55 mg/kg/day in 4 divided doses for 1-2 wk; 33 mg/kg/day in 4 divided doses for long-term treatment

Available forms: Tabs 100, 250, 500 mg, 1 g susp 250 mg/5 ml

Side effects/adverse reactions:
INTEG: Pruritus, rash, urticaria, photosensitivity
CNS: Dizziness, headache, drowsiness, insomnia, ***convulsions***
GI: Nausea, vomiting, abdominal pain, diarrhea
EENT: Sensitivity to light, blurred vision, change in color perception

Contraindications: Hypersensitivity, CNS damage, liver disease,

---

italics = common side effects   ***bold italic*** = life threatening reactions

liver failure, infants <3 months
Precautions: Elderly, renal disease, hepatic disease, pregnancy (B)
Pharmacokinetics:
PO: Peak 1-2 hr, metabolized in liver, excreted in urine (unchanged/conjugates), crosses placenta, enters breast milk
Interactions/incompatibilities:
• Increased effects of: oral coagulants
• Decreased effects of: antacids
Lab test interferences:
False positive: Urinary glucose
False increase: 17-OHCS, VMA

NURSING CONSIDERATIONS
Assess:
• Blood count for patients on chronic therapy
• I&O ratio; urine pH <5.5 is ideal
• Renal, hepatic function
• Photosensitivity: if present, drug should be discontinued
• CNS symptoms: insomnia, vertigo, headache, drowsiness, convulsions
• Allergy: fever, flushing, rash, urticaria, pruritus
Administer:
• After clean-catch urine is obtained for C&S
• Two daily doses if urine output is high or if patient has diabetes
Perform/provide:
• Limited intake of alkaline foods, drugs: milk, dairy products, peanuts, vegetables, alkaline antacids, sodium bicarbonate
• Protection from freezing
Evaluate:
• Therapeutic response: decreased dysuria, negative culture
Teach patient/family:
• That photosensitivity occurs; that patient should avoid sunlight or use sunscreen to prevent burns

• To take medication with food or milk to decrease GI irritation
• To protect suspension from freezing, shake well before taking
• That drug may cause drowsiness; instruct client to seek aid in walking, other activities; advise client not to drive or operate machinery while on medication
• That diabetics should use Keto-Diastix to measure blood glucose level

naloxone HCl
(nal-oks'one)
Naloxone HCl, Narcan
Func. class.: Narcotic antagonist
Chem. class.: Thebaine derivative

Action: Competes with narcotics at narcotic receptor sites
Uses: Respiratory depression induced by narcotics, pentazocine, propoxyphene
Dosage and routes:
Narcotic-induced respiratory depression
• *Adult:* IV/SC/IM 0.4-2 mg; repeat q2-3 min if needed
Postoperative respiratory depression
• *Adult:* IV 0.1-0.2 mg q2-3 min prn
• *Child:* IV/IM/SC 0.01 mg/kg q2-3 min prn
Asphyxia neonatorum
• *Neonates:* IV 0.01 mg/kg given into umbilical vein after delivery; may repeat in q2-3 min × 3 doses
Available forms: Inj IV, IM, SC 0.02, 0.4, 1 mg/ml
Side effects/adverse reactions:
CNS: Drowsiness, nervousness
CV: Rapid pulse, increased systolic B/P (high doses)

GI: Nausea, vomiting
RESP: Hyperpnea
Contraindications: Hypersensitivity, respiratory depression
Precautions: Pregnancy (B), children
Pharmacokinetics:
Well absorbed IM, SC
Metabolized by liver, excreted by kidneys, crosses placenta, excreted in breast milk, half-life 1 hr
IV: Onset 1 min, duration 45 min
IM/SC: Onset 2-5 min, duration 45-60 min
Interactions/incompatibilities:
• Incompatible with alkaline drugs, bisulfites, sulfites
Lab test interferences:
Interferences: Urine VMA, 5-HIAA, urine glucose

NURSING CONSIDERATIONS
Assess:
• Withdrawal: cramping, hypertension, anxiety, vomiting
• VS q3-5 min
• ABGs including Po_2, Pco_2
• Signs of withdrawal in drug-dependent individuals
• Cardiac status: tachycardia, hypertension; monitor ECG
• Respiratory dysfunction: respiratory depression, character, rate, rhythm; if respirations are <10/min, administer naloxone; probably due to narcotic overdose, not naloxone; monitor LOC
Administer:
• IV undiluted with sterile H_2O for inj; may be further diluted with NS or D_5 and given as an inf; give 0.4 mg or less over 15 sec or titrate inf to response
• Only with resuscitative equipment, O_2 nearby
• Only sol prepared within 24 hr
Perform/provide:
• Storage at room temperature in darkness

Evaluate:
• Therapeutic response: reversal of respiratory depression; LOC-alert

---

naltrexone HCl
(nal-trex'one)
Trexan
Func. class.: Narcotic antagonist
Chem. class.: Thebaine derivative

Action: Competes with narcotics at narcotic receptor sites
Uses: Blockage of opioid analgesics, used in treatment of opiate addiction
Dosage and routes:
• *Adult:* PO 25 mg, may give 25 mg after 1 hr if there are no withdrawal symptoms; 50-150 mg may be given qd depending on patient need, maintenance 50 mg q24h; 100-150 mg may be given on alternate days or 3 days 1 wk
Available forms: Tabs 50 mg
Side effects/adverse reactions:
MISC: Increased thirst, chills, fever
MS: Joint and muscle pain
GU: Delayed ejaculation, decreased potency
CNS: Stimulation, drowsiness, dizziness, confusion, convulsion, headache, flushing, hallucinations, nervousness, irritability
GI: Nausea, vomiting, diarrhea, heartburn, anorexia, **hepatitis,** constipation
INTEG: Rash, urticaria, bruising, oily skin, acne, pruritis
EENT: Tinnitus, hearing loss, blurred vision
CV: Rapid pulse, pulmonary edema, hypertension
RESP: Wheezing, hyperpnea, nasal congestion, rhinorrhea, sneezing, sore throat

N

---

italics = common side effects   ***bold italic*** = life threatening reactions

Contraindications: Hypersensitivity, opioid dependence, hepatic failure, hepatitis

Precautions: Pregnancy (C), hepatic disease, lacation, children

Pharmacokinetics:
PO: Onset 15-30 min, peak 1-2 hr, duration is dose dependent
Metabolized by liver, excreted by kidneys; crosses placenta, excreted in breast milk; half-life 4 hr; extensive first-pass metabolism

NURSING CONSIDERATIONS
Assess:
• VS q3-5min
• ABGs including PO_2, PCO_2
• Signs of withdrawal in drug-dependent individuals
• Cardiac status: tachycardia, hypertension
• Respiratory dysfunction: respiratory depression, character, rate, rhythm; if respirations are <10/min, respiratory stimulant should be administered

Administer:
• Only if resuscitative equipment is nearby

Perform/provide:
• Storage in tight container

Evaluate:
• Therapeutic response: blocking narcotic ingestion

nandrolone decanoate/nandrolone phenpropionate
(nan'droe-lone)
Androlone-D 200, Deca-Durabolin, Hybolin Decanoate-50, Hybolin Decanoate-100, Nandrolone Decanoate, Neo-Durabolic, Durabolin, Hybolin Improved, Nandrobolic, Nandrolone Phenpropionate

Func. class.: Androgenic anabolic steroid
Chem. class.: Halogenated testosterone derivative

Action: Increases weight by building body tissue, increases potassium, phosphorus, chloride, nitrogen levels, increases bone development

Uses: Tissue building, severe disease, refractory anemias, metastatic breast cancer

Dosage and routes:
Tissue building (possibly effective)
• *Adult:* IM 50-100 mg q3-4wk (decanoate)
• *Child 2-13 yr:* IM 25-50 mg q3-4wk (decanoate)
Severe disease/refractory anemias
• *Adult:* IM 100-200 mg qwk (decanoate)
Breast cancer
• *Adult:* IM 50-100 mg qwk (phenpropionate)
Available forms: Phenpropionate inj IM 25, 50 mg/ml; decanoate inj IM 50, 100, 200 mg/ml

Side effects/adverse reactions:
INTEG: Rash, acneiform lesions, oily hair, skin, flushing, sweating, acne vulgaris, alopecia, hirsutism
CNS: Dizziness, headache, fatigue, tremors, paresthesias, flushing,

sweating, anxiety, lability, insomnia, carpal tunnel syndrome
MS: Cramps, spasms
CV: Increased B/P
GU: **Hematuria,** amenorrhea, vaginitis, decreased libido, decreased breast size, clitoral hypertrophy, testicular atrophy
GI: Nausea, vomiting, constipation, weight gain, ***cholestatic jaundice***
EENT: Conjunctival edema, nasal congestion
ENDO: Abnormal GTT
Contraindications: Severe renal disease, severe cardiac disease, severe hepatic disease, hypersensitivity, pregnancy (X), lactation, abnormal genital bleeding, males with Cancer of breast, prostate
Precautions: Diabetes mellitus, CV disease, MI
Pharmacokinetics:
IM: Metabolized in liver, excreted in urine, crosses placenta, excreted in the breast milk
Interactions/incompatibilities:
• Increased effects of: oral antidiabetics, oxyphenbutazone
• Increased PT: anticoagulants
• Edema: ACTH, adrenal steroids
• Decreased effects of: insulin
Lab test interferences:
Increase: Serum cholesterol, blood glucose, urine glucose
Decrease: Serum Ca, serum K, T_4, T_3, thyroid ^{131}I uptake test, urine 17-OHCS, 17-KS, PBI, BSP
NURSING CONSIDERATIONS
Assess:
• Weight daily; notify physician if weekly weight gain is >5 lb
• B/P q4h
• I&O ratio; be alert for decreasing urinary output, increasing edema
• Growth rate in children, since growth rate may be uneven (linear/

bone growth) when used for extended periods
• Electrolytes: K, Na, Cl, Ca; cholesterol
• Liver function studies: ALT, AST, bilirubin
• Edema, hypertension, cardiac symptoms, jaundice
• Mental status: affect, mood, behavioral changes, aggression
• Signs of masculinization in female: increased libido, deepening of voice, breast tissue, enlarged clitoris, menstrual irregularities; male: gynecomastia, impotence, testicular atrophy
• Hypercalcemia: lethargy, polyuria, polydipsia, nausea, vomiting, constipation, drug may need to be decreased
• Hypoglycemia in diabetics, since oral antidiabetic action is increased
Administer:
• Titrated dose; use lowest effective dose
Perform/provide:
• Diet with increased calories, protein; decrease Na if edema occurs
Evaluate:
• Therapeutic response: increased appetite, increased stamina
Teach patient/family:
• That drug must to be combined with complete health plan: diet, rest, exercise
• To notify physician if therapeutic response decreases
• Not to discontinue medication abruptly
• About changes in sex characteristics
• That females should report menstrual irregularities
• That 1-3 mo course is necessary for response in breast cancer
• Procedure for use of buccal tablets: requires 30-60 min to dissolve, change absorption site with each

N

---

italics = common side effects   ***bold italic*** = life threatening reactions

dose; do not eat, drink, chew, or smoke while tablet is in place

---

naphazoline HCl
(naf-az′oh-leen)
Privine
Func. class.: Nasal decongestant
Chem. class.: Sympathomimetic amine

Action: Produces vasoconstriction (rapid, long-acting) of arterioles, thereby decreasing fluid exudation, mucosal engorgement
Uses: Nasal congestion
Dosage and routes:
• *Adult:* Instill 2 gtts or sprays to nasal mucosa q3-4h
• *Child 6-12 yr:* Instill 1-2 gtts or sprays, repeat q3-4h prn, not to exceed 5 days
Available forms: Sol 0.025, 0.05%
Side effects/adverse reactions:
GI: Nausea, vomiting, anorexia
EENT: Irritation, burning, sneezing, stinging, dryness, rebound congestion
INTEG: Contact dermatitis
CNS: Anxiety, restlessness, tremors, weakness, insomnia, dizziness, fever, headache
Contraindications: Hypersensitivity to sympathomimetic amines
Precautions: Child <6 yr, elderly, diabetes, cardiovascular disease, hypertension, hyperthyroidism, increased ICP, prostatic hypertrophy, pregnancy (C), glaucoma
Interactions/incompatibilities:
• Hypertension: MAOIs, β-adrenergic blockers
• Hypotension: methyldopa, mecamylamine, reserpine
NURSING CONSIDERATIONS
Assess:
• Redness, swelling, pain in nasal passages

Administer:
• No more than q4h
• For <4 consecutive days
Perform/provide:
• Environmental humidification to decrease nasal congestion, dryness
• Storage in light-resistant containers; do not expose to high temperatures or let sol come into contact with aluminum
Evaluate:
• Therapeutic response: decreased nasal congestion
Teach patient/family:
• That stinging may occur for several applications; drying of mucosa may be decreased by environmental humidification
• To notify physician if irregular pulse, insomnia, dizziness, or tremors occur
• Proper administration to avoid systemic absorption
• To rinse dropper with very hot water to prevent contamination

---

naphazoline HCl
(naf-az′oh-leen)
AK-Con Ophthalmic, Allerest Eye Drops, Albalon Liquifilm Ophthalmic, Clear Eyes, Comfort Eye Drops, Degest 2, Nafazair, Naphazoline HCl, Naphcon, Naphcon Forte, Opcon, Vasoclear, Vasocon Regular, Estivin II
Func. class.: Ophthalmic vasoconstrictor
Chem. class.: Direct imidazoline derivative

Action: Vasoconstriction of eye arterioles; decreases eye engorgement by stimulation of α-adrenergic receptors
Uses: Relieves hyperemia, irrita-

---

tion in superficial corneal vascularity

Dosage and routes:
• *Adult:* Instill 1-2 gtts q3-4h
Available forms: Sol 0.1%, 0.02%, 0.025%, 0.05%, 0.03%, 0.012%

Side effects/adverse reactions:
CNS: Headache, dizziness, sedation, anxiety, weakness, sweating (systemic absorption)
CV: Hypertension, dysrhythmias, tachycardia, *CV collapse* (systemic absorption)
EENT: Pupil dilation, increased intraocular pressure, photophobia

Contraindications: Hypersensitivity, glaucoma (narrow-angle)

Precautions: Hypertension, hyperthyroidism, elderly, severe arteriosclerosis, cardiac disease, pregnancy (C)

Pharmacokinetics:
Instill: Duration 2-3 hr

Interactions/incompatibilities:
• Increased pressor effects: MAOIs, tricyclic antidepressants

NURSING CONSIDERATIONS
Perform/provide:
• Storage in tight, light-resistant container

Evaluate:
• Therapeutic response: vasoconstriction of the eye

Teach patient/family:
• To report change in vision, blurring, or loss of sight; breathing trouble, sweating, flushing, anxiety, weakness
• Method of instillation; tilt head backward, hold dropper over eye, drop medication inside lower lid, using pressure on inside corner of eye hold 1 min, do not touch dropper to eye
• That blurred vision will decrease with repeated use of drug
• To notify physician if headache,

spots, redness, pain occur; discontinue use

naproxen/naproxen sodium

(na-prox'en)
Naprosyn/Anaprox, Anaprox DS

Func. class.: Nonsteroidal antiinflammatory
Chem. class.: Propionic acid derivative

Action: Inhibits prostaglandin synthesis by decreasing an enzyme needed for biosynthesis; analgesic, antiinflammatory, antipyretic

Uses: Mild to moderate pain, osteoarthritis, rheumatoid, gouty arthritis, juvenile arthritis primary dysmenorrhea

Dosage and routes:
• *Adult:* PO 250-500 mg bid, not to exceed 1 g/day (base); 525 mg, then 275 mg q6-8h prn, not to exceed 1475 mg (sodium)
• *Children:* PO 10 mg/kg in 2 divided doses
Available forms: Tabs 250, 275, 375, 500 mg; susp 125 mg/5 ml

Side effects/adverse reactions:
GI: Nausea, anorexia, vomiting, diarrhea, jaundice, *cholestatic hepatitis,* constipation, flatulence, cramps, dry mouth, peptic ulcer, *GI ulceration, bleeding, perforation*
CNS: Dizziness, drowsiness, fatigue, tremors, confusion, insomnia, anxiety, depression
CV: Tachycardia, peripheral edema, palpitations, dysrhythmias
INTEG: Purpura, rash, pruritus, sweating
GU: Nephrotoxicity: dysuria, hematuria, oliguria, azotemia
HEMA: Blood dyscrasias

N

---

italics = common side effects   **bold italic** = life threatening reactions

EENT: Tinnitus, hearing loss, blurred vision

Contraindications: Hypersensitivity, asthma, severe renal disease, severe hepatic disease, ulcer disease

Precautions: Pregnancy (B), lactation, children < 2 yrs, bleeding disorders, GI disorders, cardiac disorders, hypersensitivity to other antiinflammatory agents, elderly

Pharmacokinetics:
PO: Peak 2-4 hr, half-life 3-3½ hr; metabolized in liver, excreted in urine (metabolites), excreted in breast milk, 99% protein binding

Interactions/incompatibilities:
• May increase action of: heparin
• Increased lithium toxicity: lithium

Laboratory test interferences:
Increase: BUN, alk phosphatase
False increase: 5-HIAA, 17KGS

NURSING CONSIDERATIONS
Assess:
• Renal, liver, blood studies: BUN, creatinine, AST, ALT, Hgb before treatment, periodically thereafter
• Audiometric, ophthalmic exam before, during, after treatment
• For eye, ear problems: blurred vision, tinnitus (may indicate toxicity)

Administer:
• With food to decrease GI symptoms; best to take on empty stomach to facilitate absorption

Perform/provide:
• Storage at room temperature

Evaluate:
• Therapeutic response: decreased pain, stiffness, swelling in joints, ability to move more easily

Teach patient/family:
• To report blurred vision, ringing, roaring in ears (may indicate toxicity)
• To avoid driving, other hazardous

activities if dizziness or drowsiness occurs
• To report change in urine pattern, weight increase, edema (face, lower extremities), pain increase in joints, fever, blood in urine (indicates nephrotoxicity)
• That therapeutic effects may take up to 1 mo
• To avoid ASA, alcohol, steroids

natamycin (ophthalmic)

(na-ta-mye'sin)
Natacyn
Func. class.: Antiinfective/antifungal
Chem. class.: Tetraene polyene compound

Action: Inhibits transport functions and cell permeability in organism

Uses: Fungal blepharitis, conjunctivitis, keratitis

Dosage and routes:
• *Adult and child:* Instill 1 gtt q1-2h × 3-4 days, then decrease to 1 gtt 8 × /day, duration of therapy, 14-21 days

Available forms: Susp 5%

Side effects/adverse reactions:
EENT: Temporary visual haze, overgrowth of nonsusceptible organisms

Contraindications: Hypersensitivity

Precautions: Antibiotic hypersensitivity, pregnancy (C); failure of keratitis to improve after 7-10 days suggests infection not caused by susceptible organism
• Allergy: itching, lacrimation, redness, swelling, eye pain

NURSING CONSIDERATIONS
Administer:
• After washing hands; cleanse

crusts or discharge from eye before application
Perform/provide:
• Storage at room temperature or refrigerate
Evaluate:
• Therapeutic response: absence of redness, inflammation, tearing, photophobia
Teach patient/family:
• To use drug exactly as prescribed, to shake well before using
• Not to use eye makeup, towels, washcloths, eye medication of others; reinfection may occur
• That drug container tip should not be touched to eye
• To report itching, increased redness, burning, stinging, swelling; drug should be discontinued

nedocromil inhaler
(ned-o-kroe'-mill)
Tilade
Func. class.: Antiasthmatic
Chem. class.: Mast cell stabilizer

Action: Stabilizes the membrane of the sensitized mast cell, preventing release of chemical mediators after an antigen-IgE interaction
Uses: Severe perennial bronchial asthma, exercise-induced bronchospasm (prevention), prevention of acute bronchospasm induced by environmental pollutants; *not* for treatment of acute asthma attacks
Dosage and routes:
Bronchospasm
• *Adult and child >12 yr:* 2 inhalations 2-4× a day at regular intervals to provide 14 g/day
Bronchial asthma
• *Adult and child >12 yr:* same as above
Available forms: 1.75 mg nedo-

cromil Na per activation in 16.2 g canisters providing at least 112 metered inhalations
Side effects/adverse reactions:
EENT: Throat irritation, cough, nasal congestion, burning eyes, rhinitis
CNS: Headache, dizziness, neuritis, dysphonia
GI: Nausea, vomiting, anorexia, dry mouth, bitter taste
Contraindications: Hypersensitivity to this drug or lactose, status asthmaticus
Precautions: Pregnancy (B), lactation, children
Pharmacokinetics:
INH: Peak 15 min, duration 4-6 hr; excreted unchanged in urine; half-life 80 min

NURSING CONSIDERATIONS
Assess:
• Eosinophil count during treatment
• Respiratory status: respiratory rate, rhythm, characteristics, cough, wheezing, dyspnea
Administer:
• By inhalation only
• Gargle, sip of water to decrease irritation in throat
Evaluate:
• Therapeutic response: decrease in asthmatic symptoms, congested runny nose
Teach patient/family:
• To clear mucus before using
• Proper inhalation technique: exhale; using inhaler, inhale deeply with head tipped back to open airway; remove, hold breath, exhale, repeat until all of drug is inhaled
• That therapeutic effect may take up to 4 wk
• That drug is preventive only, not restorative

neomycin sulfate
(nee-oh-mye'sin)
Mycifradin Sulfate, Neobiotic
Func. class.: Antibiotic
Chem. class.: Aminoglycoside

Action: Inferferes with protein synthesis in bacterial cell by binding to ribosomal subunit, causing inaccurate peptide sequence to form in protein chain, causing bacterial death

Uses: Severe systemic infections of CNS, respiratory, GI, urinary tract, eye, bone, skin, soft tissues caused by *P. aeruginosa, E. coli, Enterobacter, K. pneumoniae, P. vulgaris;* also used for hepatic coma, preoperatively to sterilize bowel, infectious diarrhea caused by enteropathogenic *E. coli*

Dosage and routes:
Severe systemic infections
• *Adult:* IM 15 mg/kg/day in 4 divided doses, not to exceed 1 g/day
Hepatic coma
• *Adult:* PO 4-12 g/day in divided doses × 5-6 days
• *Child:* 50-100 mg/kg/day in divided doses
Preoperative bowel sterilization
• *Adult:* PO on 3rd day of a 3-day regimen, give 1 g early PM, repeat in 1 hr, repeat at hs (given with erythromycin); give saline cathartic before giving this drug
Available forms: Tabs 500 mg; top, inj IM 500 mg; ophthalmic oint, oral sol 125 mg/5 ml

Side effects/adverse reactions:
GU: Oliguria, hematuria, renal damage, azotemia, renal failure, nephrotoxicity
CNS: Confusion, depression, numbness, tremors, *convulsions,* muscle twitching, *neurotoxicity,* dizziness, vertigo

EENT: Ototoxicity, deafness, visual disturbances, tinnitus
HEMA: Agranulocytosis, thrombocytopenia, leukopenia, eosinophilia, anemia
GI:Nausea, vomiting, anorexia, increased ALT, AST, bilirubin, hepatomegaly, *hepatic necrosis,* splenomegaly
CV: Hypotension, hypertension, palpitation
INTEG: Rash, burning, urticaria, photosensitivity, dermatitis, alopecia

Contraindications: Bowel obstruction (oral use), severe renal disease, hypersensitivity, infants, children

Precautions: Mild renal disease, pregnancy (C), hearing deficits, lactation, myasthenia gravis, Parkinson's disease

Pharmacokinetics:
PO: Onset rapid, peak 1-2 hr
Plasma half-life 2-3 hr; not metabolized, excreted unchanged in urine, crosses placental barrier

Interactions/incompatibilities:
• Increased ototoxicity, neurotoxicity, nephrotoxicity: other aminoglycosides, amphotericin B, polymyxin, vancomycin, ethacrynic acid, furosemide, mannitol, methoxyflurane, cisplatin, cephalosporins, bacitracin
• Do not mix in sol or syringe: carbenicillin, ticarcillin, amphotericin B, cephalothin, erythromycin, heparin
• Increased effects: nondepolarizing muscle relaxants, succinylcholine, oral anticoagulants when given with oral neomycin
• Decreased effects of: digoxin, penicillin V when given with oral neomycin

NURSING CONSIDERATIONS
Assess:
• Weight before treatment; calcu-

lation of dosage is usually based on ideal body weight, but may be calculated on actual body weight
• I&O ratio, urinalysis daily for proteinuria, cells, casts; report sudden change in urine output
• Urine pH if drug is used for UTI; urine should be kept alkaline
• Renal impairment by securing urine for CrCl testing, BUN, serum creatinine; lower dosage should be given in renal impairment (CrCl <80 ml/min)
• Deafness by audiometric testing, ringing, roaring in ears, vertigo; assess hearing before, during, after treatment
• Dehydration: high sp gr, decrease in skin turgor, dry mucous membranes, dark urine
• Overgrowth of infection: increased temperature, malaise, redness, pain, swelling, perineal itching, diarrhea, stomatitis, change in cough, sputum
• C&S before starting treatment to identify infecting organism
• Vestibular dysfunction: nausea, vomiting, dizziness, headache; drug should be discontinued if severe
• Injection sites for redness, swelling, abscesses; use warm compresses at site

Administer:
• IM injection in large muscle mass; rotate injection sites
• Drug in evenly spaced doses to maintain blood level
• Bicarbonate to alkalinize urine if ordered in treating UTI, as drug is most active in alkaline environment

Perform/provide:
• Adequate fluids of 2-3 L/day unless contraindicated to prevent irritation of tubules
• Supervised ambulation, other

safety measures, with vestibular dysfunction

Evaluate:
• Therapeutic response: absence of fever, draining wounds, negative C&S after treatment

Teach patient/family:
• To report headache, dizziness, symptoms of overgrowth of infection, renal impairment
• To report loss of hearing, ringing, roaring in ears or a feeling of fullness in head

Treatment of overdose: Hemodialysis; monitor serum levels of drug

---

neomycin sulfate
(nee-oh-mye′sin)
Drotic, Otocort
Func. class.: Otic antibiotic
Chem. class.: Aminoglycoside

Action: Inhibits protein synthesis in susceptible microorganisms
Uses: Ear infection (external), short-term use

Dosage and routes:
• *Adult and child:* Instill 2-5 gtt tid-qid
Available forms: Otic sol in combination with neomycin, hydrocortisone 0.25%, 0.5%

Side effects/adverse reactions:
EENT: Itching, irritation in ear
INTEG: Rash, urticaria

Contraindications: Hypersensitivity, perforated eardrum
Precautions: Pregnancy (C)

NURSING CONSIDERATIONS
Assess:
• For redness, swelling, fever, pain in ear, which indicates superimposed infection

Administer:
• After removing impacted cerumen by irrigation

---

italics = common side effects   **bold italic** = life threatening reactions

• After cleaning stopper with alcohol
• After restraining child if necessary
• Warming solution

Evaluate:
• Therapeutic response: decreased ear pain

Teach patient/family:
• Method of instillation using aseptic technique, including not touching dropper to ear
• That dizziness may occur after instillation

---

neomycin sulfate (topical)

(nee-oh-mye'sin)
Myciguent, Neomycin Sulfate
Func. class.: Local antibacterial
Chem. class.: Aminoglycoside

Action: Interferes with bacterial protein synthesis
Uses: Skin infections, minor burns, wounds, skin grafts, primary pyodemas, otitis externa
Dosage and routes:
• *Adult and child:* TOP rub into affected area bid-tid
Available forms: Oint, cream 0.5%
Side effects/adverse reactions:
INTEG: Rash, urticaria, scaling, redness
OTHER: Possible nephrotoxicity, ototoxicity, neuromuscular blockade
Contraindications: Hypersensitivity, large areas, burns, ulcerations
Precautions: Pregnancy (C), lactation, impaired renal function, external ear of perforated eardrum
NURSING CONSIDERATIONS
Assess:
• Allergic reaction: burning, stinging, swelling, redness

• For signs of nephrotoxicity or ototoxicity
Administer:
• Enough medication to cover lesions completely
• After cleansing with soap, water before each application; dry well
• To less than 20% of body surface area when patient has impaired renal function
Perform/provide:
• Storage at room temperature in dry place
Evaluate:
• Therapeutic response: decrease in size, number of lesions
Teach patient/family:
• To use medical asepsis (hand washing) before, after each application
• To apply with glove to prevent further infection
• To avoid use of OTC creams, ointments, lotions unless directed by physician
• To notify physician if condition worsens
• That prolonged use may lead to overgrowth of susceptible organisms
• To avoid use of occlusive dressings

---

neostigmine bromide/ neostigmine methylsulfate

(nee-oh-stig'meen)
Neostigmine Bromide, Neostigmine Methylsulfate, Prostigmin
Func. class.: Cholinergic stimulant
Chem. class.: Quaternary compound

Action: Inhibits destruction of ace-

---

tylcholine, which increases concentration at sites where acetylcholine is released; this facilitates transmission of impulses across myoneural junction

Uses: Myasthenia gravis, nondepolarizing neuromuscular blocker, antagonist, bladder distention, postoperative ileus

Dosage and routes:

Myasthenia gravis

• *Adult:* PO 15-375 mg/day; IM/IV 0.5-2 mg q1-3h

• *Child:* PO 2 mg/kg/day q3-4h

Tubocurarine antagonist

• *Adult:* IV 0.5-2 mg slowly, may repeat if needed (give 0.6-1.2 mg atropine before this drug)

Abdominal distention/postoperative ileus

• *Adult:* IM/SC 0.25-1 mg q4-6h depending on condition

Available forms: Tabs 15 mg; inj IM, SC, IV 1:1000, 1:2000, 1:4000

Side effects/adverse reactions:

INTEG: Rash, urticaria, flushing

CNS: Dizziness, headache, sweating, weakness, *convulsions,* incoordination, *paralysis,* drowsiness, LOC

GI: Nausea, diarrhea, vomiting, cramps, increased peristalsis, salivary and gastric secretions

CV: Tachycardia, dysrhythmias, bradycardia, hypotension, AV block, ECG changes, *cardiac arrest,* syncope

GU: Frequency, incontinence, urgency

RESP: Respiratory depression, bronchospasm, constriction, laryngospasm, respiratory arrest, dyspnea

EENT: Miosis, blurred vision, lacrimation, visual changes

Contraindications: Obstruction of intestine, renal system, pregnancy (C), bromide sensitivity, peritonitis

Precautions: Bradycardia, hypotension, seizure disorders, bronchial asthma, coronary occlusion, hyperthyroidism, dysrhythmias, peptic ulcer, megacolon, poor GI motility, lactation, children

Pharmacokinetics:

PO: Onset 45-75 min, duration 2½-4 hr

IM/SC: Onset 10-30 min, duration 2½-4 hr

IV onset 4-8 min; duration 2-4 hr; metabolized in liver, excreted in urine

Interactions/incompatibilities:

• Decreased action of: gallamine, metocurine, pancuronium, tubocurarine, atropine

• Increased action of: decamethonium, succinylcholine

• Decreased action of neostigmine: aminoglycosides, anesthetics, procainamide, quinidine, mecamylamine, polymyxin, magnesium

• Considered incompatible with drugs in sol or syringe

NURSING CONSIDERATIONS

Assess:

• VS, respiration q8h

• I&O ratio; check for urinary retention or incontinence

• Bradycardia, hypotension, bronchospasm, headache, dizziness, convulsions, respiratory depression; drug should be discontinued if toxicity occurs

Administer:

• IV undiluted, give through Y-tube or 3-way stopcock; give 0.5 mg or less over 1 min

• Only with atropine sulfate available for cholinergic crisis

• Only after all other cholinergics have been discontinued

• Increased doses if tolerance occurs

• Larger doses after exercise or fatigue

• On empty stomach for better absorption
Perform/provide:
• Storage at room temperature
Evaluate:
• Therapeutic response: increased muscle strength, hand grasp, improved gait, absence of labored breathing (if severe)
Teach patient/family:
• That drug is not a cure; it only relieves symptoms
• To wear Medic Alert ID specifying myasthenia gravis, drugs taken
Treatment of overdose:
Respiratory support, atropine 1-4 mg (IV)

---

netilmicin sulfate
(ne-til-mye′sin)
Netromycin
Func. class.: Antibiotic
Chem. class.: Aminoglycoside

Action: Interferes with protein synthesis in bacterial cell by binding to ribosomal subunit, causing inaccurate peptide sequence to form in protein chain, causing bacterial death
Uses: Severe systemic infections of CNS, respiratory, GI, urinary tract, bone, skin, soft tissues caused by *P. aeruginosa, E. coli, Enterobacter, Citrobacter, Staphylococcus, K. pneumoniae, P. mirabilis, Serratia, Shigella, Salmonella, Acinetobacter, Neisseria*
Dosage and routes:
Normal renal function
• *Adult and child >12 yr:* IM/IV 3-6.5 mg/kg/day; may give q8-12h for severe infections
• *Child and infant 6 wk-12 yr:* IM/IV 5.5-8 mg/kg/day in divided doses q8-12h

• *Neonate <6 wk:* IM/IV 4-6.5 mg/kg/day in divided doses q12h
Available forms: Inj IM, IV 10, 25, 100 mg/ml
Side effects/adverse reactions:
GU: Oliguria, hematuria, renal damage, azotemia, renal failure, nephrotoxicity
CNS: Confusion, depression, numbness, tremors, *convulsions,* muscle twitching, *neurotoxicity,* dizziness, vertigo
EENT: Ototoxicity, deafness, visual disturbances, tinnitus
HEMA: Agranulocytosis, thrombocytopenia, leukopenia, eosinophilia, anemia
GI: Nausea, vomiting, anorexia, increased ALT, AST, bilirubin, hepatomegaly, *hepatic necrosis,* splenomegaly
CV: Hypotension, hypertension, palpitations
INTEG: Rash, burning, urticaria, dermatitis
Contraindications: Severe renal disease, hypersensitivity
Precautions: Neonates, mild renal disease, pregnancy (D), children <12 yr, lactation, myasthenia gravis, hearing deficit, Parkinson's disease, severe burns, cystic fibrosis
Pharmacokinetics:
IM: Onset rapid, peak 1-2 hr
IV: Onset immediate, peak 1-2 hr
Plasma half-life 2-3 hr, not metabolized, excreted unchanged in urine, crosses placental barrier
Interactions/incompatibilities:
• Increased ototoxicity, neurotoxicity, nephrotoxicity: other aminoglycosides, amphotericin B, polymyxin, vancomycin, ethacrynic acid, furosemide, mannitol, methoxyflurane, cisplatin, cephalosporins, bacitracin
• Incompatible with carbenicillin,

ticarcillin, amphotericin B, cephalothin, erythromycin, heparin, furosemide, dopamine, cefamandole
• Increased effects: nondepolarizing muscle relaxants, succinylcholine

NURSING CONSIDERATIONS
Assess:
• Weight before treatment; calculation of dosage is usually based on ideal body weight, but may be calculated on actual body weight
• Daily I&O ratio, urinalysis for proteinuria, cells, casts; report sudden change in urine output
• VS during infusion, watch for hypotension, change in pulse
• IV site for thrombophlebitis, including pain, redness, swelling q30 min; change site if needed; apply warm compresses to discontinued site
• Serum peak, drawn at 30-60 min after IV infusion or 60 min after IM injection; trough level drawn just before next dose; blood level should be 2-4 times bacteriostatic level; trough = 0.5-2mEq/ml, peak = 6-10mEq/ml
• Urine pH if drug is used for UTI; urine should be kept alkaline
• Renal impairment by securing urine for CrCl testing, BUN, serum creatinine; a lower dosage should be given in renal impairment (CrCl <80 ml/min)
• Deafness by audiometric testing, ringing, roaring in ears, vertigo; assess hearing before, during, after treatment
• Dehydration: high sp gr, decrease in skin turgor, dry mucous membranes, dark urine
• Overgrowth of infection: increased temperature, malaise, redness, pain, swelling, perineal itching, diarrhea, stomatitis, change in cough or sputum

• C&S before starting treatment to identify infecting organism
• Vestibular dysfunction: nausea, vomiting, dizziness, headache; drug should be discontinued if severe
• Injection sites for redness, swelling, abscesses; use warm compresses at site
Administer:
• IM injection in large muscle mass; rotate injection sites
• Drug in evenly spaced doses to maintain blood level
• Bicarbonate to alkalinize urine if ordered in treating UTI, as drug is most active in alkaline environment
• IV diluted in 50-200 ml D_5W, 0.9% NaCl; saline infuse over ½-2 hr
Perform/provide:
• Adequate fluids of 2-3 L/day unless contraindicated to prevent irritation of tubules
• Flush of IV line with NS or D_5W after infusion
• Supervised ambulation, other safety measures, with vestibular dysfunction
Evaluate:
• Therapeutic response: absence of fever, draining wounds, negative C&S after treatment
Teach patient/family:
• To report headache, dizziness, symptoms of overgrowth of infection, renal impairm ent
• To report loss o f hearing, ringing, roaring in ears or feeling of fullness in head
Treatment of overdose: Hemodialysis; monitor serum levels of drug

N

---

italics = common side effects   ***bold italic*** = life threatening reactions

niacin (vitamin B₃/ nicotinic acid)/niacinamide (nicotinamide)

(nye'a-sin) (nye-a-sin'a-mide)
Nia-Bid, Niac, Niacels, Niacin TD, SpaN Niacin, Niacin TR Niacor, Nico-400, Nicobid, Nicolar, Nicotinex, Nicotinic Acid, Novaniacin*, Slo-Niacin

Func. class.: Vitamin B₃
Chem. class.: Water-soluble vitamin

Action: Needed for conversion of fats, protein, carbohydrates, by oxidation reduction; acts directly on vascular smooth muscle, causing vasodilation; high doses decrease serum lipids

Uses: Pellagra, hyperlipidemias, peripheral vascular disease

Dosage and routes:
Adjunct in hyperlipidemia
• *Adult:* PO 1.5-3 g qd in 3 divided doses after meals, may be increased to 6 g/day
Pellagra
• *Adult:* PO 300-500mq, qd in divided doses
Child: Po 100-300 mg qd in divided doses
Peripheral vascular disease
• *Adult:* PO 250-800 mg qd in divided doses

Available forms: Nicotinic acid— tabs 20, 25, 50, 100, 500 mg; caps time release 125, 250, 300, 400, 500 mg; tabs time release 150 mg; elix 50 mg/5 ml; inj 100 mg/ml; nicotinamide—tabs 50, 100, 500 mg; tabs time release 1000 mg

Side effects/adverse reactions:
CNS: Paresthesias, headache, dizziness, anxiety
GI: Nausea, vomiting, anorexia, flatulence, xerostomia, *jaundice,* diarrhea, peptic ulcer

GU: Hyperuricemia, *glycosuria, hypoalbuminemia*
CV: Postural hypotension, vasovagal attacks, dysrhythmias, vasodilation
EENT: Blurred vision, ptosis
INTEG: Flushing, dry skin, rash, pruritus
RESP: Wheezing

Contraindications: Hypersensitivity, peptic ulcer, hepatic disease, lactation, hemorrhage, severe hypotension

Precautions: Glaucoma, cardiovascular disease, CAD, diabetes mellitus, gout, schizophrenia, pregnancy (A)

Pharmacokinetics:
PO: Peak 30-70 min, half-life 45 min; metabolized in liver; 30% excreted unchanged in urine

Interactions/incompatibilities:
• Increased action of: ganglionic blockers
• Incompatible with alkali, erythromycin, kanamycin

Lab test interferences:
Increase: Bilirubin, alk phosphatase, liver enzymes, LDH, uric acid
Decrease: Cholesterol
False increase: Urinary catecholamines
False positive: Urine glucose

NURSING CONSIDERATIONS

Assess:
• Liver function studies: AST, ALT, bilirubin, alk phosphatase; blood glucose before and during treatment
• Niacin levels while taking this drug
• Cardiac status: rate, rhythm, quality; postural hypotension, dysrhythmias
• Nutritional status: liver, yeast, legumes, organ meat, lean poultry
• Liver dysfunction: clay-colored stools, itching, dark urine, jaundice

• CNS symptoms: headache, paresthesias, blurred vision

Administer:

• With meals for GI symptoms

Evaluate:

• Therapeutic response: decreased lipids, warm extremities, absence of numbness in extremities

Teach patient/family:

• That flushing and increase in feelings of warmth will occur several hours after taking drug (PO); time-release product will minimize flushing

• To remain recumbent if postural hypotension occurs

• To abstain from alcohol if drug is prescribed for hyperlipidemia

• To avoid sunlight if skin lesions are present

---

nicardipine HCl
(nye-card'i-peen)
Cardene, Cardene IV, Cardene SR
Func. class.: Calcium channel blocker
Chem. class.: Dihydropyridine

Action: Inhibits calcium ion influx across cell membrane during cardiac depolarization; produces relaxation of coronary vascular smooth muscle, peripheral vascular smooth muscle; dilates coronary vascular arteries; increases myocardial oxygen delivery in patients with vasospastic angina

Uses: Chronic stable angina pectoris, hypertension

Dosage and routes:

Angina

Adult: PO 20 mg tid initially, may increase after 3 days (range 20-40 mg tid)

Hypertension

Adult: PO 20 mg tid initially, then increase after 3 days (range 20-40 mg tid); IV dilute to 0.1 mg/ml, give 5 mg/hr initially, then increase by 2.5 mg/hr q15 min to a maximum of 15 mg/hr

Available forms: Caps 20, 30 mg; caps SR 30, 45, 60 mg; inj 2.5 mg/ml (10 ml)

Side effects/adverse reactions:

CV: Dysrhythmia, edema, CHF, bradycardia, hypotension, palpitations, *MI, pulmonary edema*

GI: Nausea, vomiting, diarrhea, gastric upset, constipation, *hepatitis,* abdominal cramps

GU: Nocturia, polyuria, *acute renal failure*

INTEG: Rash, pruritus, urticaria, photosensitivity, hair loss

CNS: Headache, fatigue, drowsiness, dizziness, anxiety, depression, weakness, insomnia, confusion, paresthesia, somnolence

OTHER: Blurred vision, flushing, nasal congestion, sweating, shortness of breath, gynecomastia, hyperglycemia, sexual difficulties

Contraindications: Sick sinus syndrome, 2nd or 3rd degree heart block, hypotension less than 90 mm Hg systolic, hypersensitivity

Precautions: CHF, hypotension, hepatic injury, pregnancy (C), lactation, children, renal disease, elderly

Pharmacokinetics:

PO: Onset 10 min, peak 1-2 hr, half-life 2-5 hr; metabolized by liver, excreted in urine (98% as metabolites)

Interactions/incompatibilities:

• Increased effects of: digitalis, neuromuscular blocking agents, theophylline

• Increased effects of nicardipine: cimetidine

NURSING CONSIDERATIONS
Assess:
• Cardiac status: B/P, pulse, respiration, ECG
Administer:
• ac, hs
• IV after diluting ampule in NS or D₅W before use
Evaluate:
• Therapeutic response: decreased anginal pain, decreased B/P
Teach patient/family:
• To avoid hazardous activities until stabilized on drug, dizziness is no longer a problem
• To limit caffeine consumption, no alcohol products
• To avoid OTC drugs unless directed by physician
• To comply in all areas of medical regimen: diet, exercise, stress reduction, drug therapy
• To notify physician of irregular heart beat, shortness of breath, swelling of feet and hands, pronounced dizziness, constipation, nausea, hypotension
Treatment of overdose: Defibrillation, β-agonists, IV Ca, diuretics, atropine for AV block, vasopressor for hypotension

---

niclosamide
(ni-kloe'sa-mide)
Niclocide
Func. class.: Anthelmintic
Chem. class.: Salicylanilide derivative

Action: Inhibits synthesis of ATP in mitochondria; leads to destruction in intestine, where worm may be digested, removed in feces; not effective for ova or larval stage
Uses: Regular, dwarf tapeworms
Dosage and routes:
• *Adult:* PO 2 g chewed as a single dose for *T. saginata* and *D. latum*; 2g × 7 days for *Hymenolepis nana*
• *Child >34 kg:* PO 1.5 g chewed as a single dose for *T. saginata* and *D. latum*; 1.5 g as single dose on day 1 followed by 1 g × 6 days for *H. nana*
• *Child <34 kg:* PO 1 g chewed as a single dose for *T. saginata* and *D. latum*; 1 g on day 1, then 0.5 g × 6 days for *H. nana*
Available forms: Tabs, chewable 500 mg
Side effects/adverse reactions:
INTEG: Rash, pruritus, pruritus ani, alopecia
CNS: Dizziness, headache, drowsiness, restlessness, sweating, fever
EENT: Bad taste, oral irritation
GI: Nausea, vomiting, anorexia, diarrhea, constipation, rectal bleeding
Contraindications: Hypersensitivity
Precautions: Child <2 yr, pregnancy (B), lactation
NURSING CONSIDERATIONS
Assess:
• Stools during entire treatment, 1, 3 mo after treatment; specimens must be sent to lab while still warm
• For allergic reaction: rash, itching in anal area
• For diarrhea during expulsion of worms
• For infection in other family members; since infection from person to person is common
Administer:
• May be crushed, mixed with water if unable to swallow whole
• Laxatives if constipated; not needed for drug to work
• After breakfast; tab must be chewed, not swallowed whole
Perform/provide:
• Storage in tight, light-resistant

container in cool environment; do not freeze

Evaluate:

• Therapeutic response: expulsion of worms, 3 negative stool cultures after completion of treatment

Teach patient/family:

• Proper hygiene after BM, 5 including hand-washing technique; tell patient to avoid putting fingers in mouth

• That infected person should sleep alone; do not shake bed linen; change bed linen qd; wash in hot water

• To clean toilet qd; with disinfectant (green soap solution)

• Need for compliance with dosage schedule, duration of treatment

• To drink fruit juice to remove mucus that intestinal tapeworms burrow in; aids in expulsion of worms (dwarf tapeworms only)

Treatment of overdose: Enemas, laxatives; do not induce vomiting

---

nicotine resin complex

(nik'o-teen)
Nicorette, Nicorette DS
Func. class.: Smoking deterrent
Chem. class.: Ganglionic cholinergic agonist

Action: Agonist at nicotinic receptors in the peripheral and central nervous systems; acts at sympathetic ganglia; on chemoreceptors of the aorta and carotid bodies; also affects adrenalin-releasing catecholamines

Uses: Deter cigarette smoking

Dosage and routes:

• *Adult:* Gum 1 piece chewed × ½ hr as needed to abstain from smoking, not to exceed 30/day

Available forms: Gum 2 mg/piece of gum

Side effects/adverse reactions:

RESP: Breathing difficulty, cough, hoarseness, sneezing, wheezing

EENT: Jaw ache, irritation in buccal cavity

CNS: Dizziness, vertigo, insomnia, headache, confusion, convulsions, depression, euphoria, numbness, tinnitus

GI: Nausea, vomiting, anorexia, indigestion, diarrhea, abdominal pain, constipation, eructation

CV: Dysrhythmias, tachycardia, palpitations, edema, flushing, hypertension

Contraindications: Hypersensitivity, immediate post MI recovery period, severe angina pectoris, pregnancy (X)

Precautions: Vasospastic disease, dysrhythmias, diabetes mellitus, children, hyperthyroidism, pheochromocytoma, coronary disease, esophagitis, peptic ulcer, lactation, children, hepatic/renal disease

Pharmacokinetics:

Onset 15-30 min, metabolized in liver, excreted in urine, half-life 2-3 hr, 30-120 hr, (terminal)

Interactions/incompatibilities:

• Decreased absorption: glutethimide

• Increased absorption: SC insulin

• Decreased metabolism of: propoxyphene

• Smoking cessation increases diuretic effects of: furosemide

• Increased blood levels with cessation of smoking: caffeine, theophylline, petazocine, imipramine, oxazepam, propranolol, acetaminophen

NURSING CONSIDERATIONS

Assess:

• Adverse reaction: irritation of

N

buccal cavity, dislike of taste, jaw ache

Evaluate:
• Therapeutic response: decrease in urge to smoke, decreased need for gum after 3-6 mo

Teach patient/family:
• To chew gum slowly for 30 min to promote buccal absorption of the drug; do not chew over 45 min
• To begin drug withdrawal after 3 mo use; not to exceed 6 mo
• All aspects of drug; give package insert to patient and explain
• That gum will not stick to dentures, dental appliances
• That gum is as toxic as cigarette; it is to be used only to deter smoking
• Not to use during pregnancy; birth defects may occur

---

nicotine transdermal system
Habitrol, Nicoderm, Nicotrol, Prostep
Func. class.: Smoking deterrent
Chem. class.: Ganglionic cholinergic agonist

Action: Binds to acetylcholine receptors at autonomic ganglia in the adrenal medulla, at neuromuscular junctions, and in the brain
Uses: Deter cigarette smoking
Dosage and routes:
• *Nicotrol:* 15 mg/day × 12 wk; 10 mg/day × 2 wk; 5 mg/day × 2 wk
Prostep: 22 mg/day × 4-8 wk 11 mg/day × 2-4 wk
Available forms: Transdermal patch delivering 7, 14, 21 mg, 15 mg, 10 mg, 5 mg, 22 mg, & 11 mg/day patches depending on product

Side effects/adverse reactions:
RESP: Cough, pharyngitis, sinusitis
MISC: Back pain, pain, chest pain
INTEG: Erythema, pruritus, burning at application site, cutaneous hypersensitivity, sweating, rash
GI: Diarrhea, dyspepsia, constipation, nausea, abdominal pain, vomiting
MS: Arthralgia, myalgia
EENT: Dry mouth, abnormal taste
CNS: Abnormal dreams, insomnia, nervousness, headache, dizziness, paresthesia
Contraindications: Hypersensitivity, children, pregnancy (D), nonsmokers, during immediate post-myocardial infarction period, life-threatening dysrhythmias, severe or worsening angina pectoris
Precautions: Skin disease, angina pectoris, myocardial infarction, renal or hepatic insufficiency, peptic ulcer, accelerated hypertension, serious cardiac dysrhythmias, hyperthyroidism, pheochromocytoma, insulin-dependent diabetes, elderly
Pharmacokinetics: Half-life 3-4 hr, protein binding <5%, 30% is excreted unchanged in urine
Interactions/incompatibilities:
• Decreased absorption: glutethimide
• Decreased dose at cessation of smoking: acetaminophen, caffeine, imipramine, oxazepam, pentazocine, propranolol, theophylline, insulin, adrenergic antagonists
• Increased dose at cessation of smoking: adrenergic agonists
• Decreased metabolism of: propoxyphene
• Increased diuretic effects of: furosemide
• Increased absorption: SC insulin
NURSING CONSIDERATIONS
Assess:
• Adverse reactions: irritation, pruritus, burning at patch site

---

* Available in Canada only

Perform/provide:
• Storage below 86° F (30° C)
Evaluate:
• Therapeutic response: decrease in urge to smoke, absence of nicotine withdrawal symptoms
Teach patient/family:
• All aspects of drug; give package insert to patient and explain
• That patch is as toxic as cigarettes; it is to be used only to deter smoking
• Not to use during pregnancy; birth defects may occur
• To keep used and unused system out of reach of children and pets
• To apply once a day to a non-hairy, clean, dry area of skin on upper body or upper outer arm
• To stop smoking immediately when beginning treatment with patch
• To apply promptly after removing from protective patch; system may lose strength

---

nifedipine

(nye-fed'i-peen)
Adalat, Nifedipine, Procardia, Procardia XL
Func. class.: Calcium-channel blocker
Chem. class.: Dihydropyridine

Action: Inhibits calcium ion influx across cell membrane during cardiac depolarization; relaxes coronary vascular smooth muscle; dilates coronary arteries; increases myocardial oxygen delivery in patients with vasospastic angina; dilates peripheral arteries
Uses: Chronic stable angina pectoris, vasospastic angina, hypertension (sus rel only)
Dosage and routes:
• *Adult PO immediate release:* 10

mg tid, increase in 10 mg increments q4-6h, not to exceed 180 mg/24h or single dose of 30 mg
• *Adult PO sus rel:* 30-60 mg/qd, may increase q7-14d, doses >120 mg not recommended
Available forms: Caps 10, 20 mg, tabs sus rel 30, 60, 90 mg
Side effects/adverse reactions:
CNS: Headache, fatigue, drowsiness, dizziness, anxiety, depression, weakness, insomnia, lightheadedness, paresthesia, tinnitus, blurred vision, nervousness
CV: Dysrhythmias, *edema,* CHF, hypotension, palpitations, *MI, pulmonary edema,* tachycardia
GI: Nausea, vomiting, diarrhea, gastric upset, constipation, increased liver function studies, dry mouth
GU: Nocturia, polyuria
INTEG: Rash, pruritus, flushing, photosensitivity, hair loss
MISC: Flushing, sexual difficulties, cough, fever, chills
Contraindications: Hypersensitivity
Precautions: CHF, hypotension, sick sinus syndrome, 2nd or 3rd degree heart block, hypotension less than 90 mm Hg systolic, hepatic injury, pregnancy (C), lactation, children, renal disease
Pharmacokinetics:
Well absorbed PO
PO-SR: Duration 24 hrs
PO: Onset 20 min, peak 0.5-6 hr, duration 6-8 hrs, half-life 2-5 hr; metabolized by liver, excreted in urine (98% as metabolites)
Interactions/incompatibilities:
• Increased effects of: theophylline, β-blockers, antihypertensives, digitalis
• Increased nifedipine level: cimetidine
• Decreased effects: quinidine

---

italics = common side effects   ***bold italic*** = life threatening reactions

NURSING CONSIDERATIONS
Assess:
• Cardiac status: B/P, pulse, respiration, ECG
Administer:
• SL: Use sterile needle to puncture liquid capsules, squeeze into buccal area
• Before meals, hs
Evaluate:
• Therapeutic response: decreased anginal pain, B/P, activity tolerance
Teach patient/family:
• To avoid hazardous activities until stabilized on drug, dizziness is no longer a problem
• To limit caffeine consumption; no alcohol products
• To avoid OTC drugs unless directed by a physician
• To comply with all areas of medical regimen: diet, exercise, stress reduction, drug therapy
• To change position slowly; orthostatic hypotension is common
• Not to chew, divide, or crush sus rel tablets
• To notify physician of dyspnea, edema of extremities, nausea, vomiting, severe ataxia
Treatment of overdose: Defibrillation, atropine for AV block, vasopressor for hypotension

nitrofurantoin/nitrofurantoin macrocrystals
(nye-troe-fyoor'an-toyn)
Furadantin, Furalan, Furanite, Macrobid, Nephronex,* Nitrofan, Nitrofurantoin, Novofuran,* Macrodantin
Func. class.: Urinary tract antiinfective
Chem. class.: Synthetic nitrofuran derivative

Action: Appears to inhibit bacterial enzymes
Uses: Urinary tract infections caused by *E. coli, Klebsiella, Pseudomonas, P. vulgaris, P. morganii, Serratia, Citrobacter, S. aureus*
Dosage and routes:
• *Adult and child >12 yr:* PO 50-100 mg qid pc or 50-100 mg hs for long-term treatment
• *Child 1 mo-3 yr:* PO 5-7 mg/kg/day in 4 divided doses; 1-3 mg/kg/day for long-term treatment
Available forms include: Caps 25, 50, 100 mg; tabs 50, 100 mg; susp 25 mg/5 ml
Side effects/adverse reactions:
INTEG: Pruritus, rash, urticaria, angioedema, alopecia, tooth staining
CNS: Dizziness, headache, drowsiness, peripheral neuropathy
GI: Nausea, vomiting, abdominal pain, diarrhea, **cholestatic jaundice**
Contraindications: Hypersensitivity, anuria, severe renal disease
Precautions: Pregnancy (B), lactation
Pharmacokinetics:
PO: Half-life 20-60 min; crosses blood-brain barrier, placenta; enters breast milk; excreted as inactive metabolites in liver

Interactions/incompatibilities:
• Increased levels of nitrofurantoin: probenecid
• Antagonistic effect: nalidixic acid
• Decreased absorption of: Mg trisilicate antacid

NURSING CONSIDERATIONS
Assess:
• Blood count for patients on chronic therapy
• I&O ratio; urine pH <5.5 is ideal
• Renal and hepatic function
• CNS symptoms: insomnia, vertigo, headache, drowsiness, convulsions
• Allergy: fever, flushing, rash, urticaria, pruritus

Administer:
• After clean-catch urine is obtained for C&S
• Two daily doses if urine output is high or if patient has diabetes

Evaluate:
• Therapeutic response: decreased dysuria, fever

Teach patient/family:
• To take medication with food or milk
• To protect susp from freezing and shake well before taking
• That drug may cause drowsiness; instruct client to seek aid in walking and other activities; advise client not to drive or operate machinery while on medication
• That diabetics should use Keto-Diastix, blood glucose level
• That drug may turn urine rust-yellow to brown

---

nitrofurazone (topical)
(nye-troe-fyoor´a-zone)
Furacin, Nitrofurazone
Func. class.: Local antibacterial
Chem. class.: Synthetic nitrofuran

Action: A broad-spectrum, mostly bactericidal agent for aerobic, anaerobic gram-positive organisms; may interfere with enzyme systems needed for carbohydrate metabolism; antibacterial action

Uses: Adjunctive treatment in burns (2nd, 3rd degree), prevention of skin allograft rejection

Dosage and routes:
• *Adult and child:* TOP apply to affected area qd or qod
Available forms: Sol, oint (soluble dressing), cream 0.2%

Side effects/adverse reactions:
INTEG: Rash, urticaria, stinging, burning, superinfections, photosensitivity, local edema
GU: Renal toxicity

Contraindications: Hypersensitivity, G-6-PD deficiency

Precautions: Pregnancy (C), lactation; superinfection may result in bacterial or fungal overgrowth

NURSING CONSIDERATIONS
Assess:
• Allergic reaction: burning, stinging, swelling, redness

Administer:
• Analgesic before application if needed
• Enough medication to cover burns completely
• After cleansing debris from area before each application
• Using sterile technique

Perform/provide:
• Storage at room temperature in dry place

N

---

italics = common side effects   **bold italic** = life threatening reactions

Evaluate:

• Therapeutic response: development of granulation tissue

Teach patient/family:

• That drug may be used until grafting is possible

• To avoid sunlight or ultraviolet light

• To stop drug and notify physician if rash or irritation occurs

---

nitroglycerin

(nye-troe-gli'ser-in)

Nitro-Bid IV, Nitroglycerin, Tridil, Nitrostat, Nitro-Bid Plateau Caps, Nitrocine Timecaps, Nitroglyn, Nitrong, Nitro-Bid, Nitrol, Deponit, Minitran, Nitrodisc, Nitro-Dur, Nitroglycerin Transdermal, Nitrocine, Transderm-Nitro, Nitrolingual, Nitrogard

Func. class.: Coronary vasodilator

Chem. class.: Nitrate

Action: Decreases preload, afterload, which is responsible for decreasing left ventricular end-diastolic pressure, systemic vascular resistance

Uses: Chronic stable angina pectoris, prophylaxis of angina pain, CHF associated with acute MI, controlled hypotension in surgical procedures

Dosage and routes:

• *Adult:* SL dissolve tablet under tongue when pain begins; may repeat q5min until relief occurs; take no more than 3 tabs/15 min; use 1 tab prophylactically 5-10 min before activities; Sus cap q6-12h on empty stomach; TOP 1-2 in q8h, increase to 4 in q4h as needed; IV 5 μg/min, then increase by 5 μg/min q3-5min; if no response after 20 μg/min, increase by 10-20 μg/min until desired response; trans apply a pad qd to a site free of hair

Available forms: Buccal tabs 1, 2, 3 mg; aero 0.4 mg/meter spray; caps 2.5, 6.5, 9 mg; tabs ext rel 2.6, 6.5, 9 mg; inj 0.5, 0.8, 5, 10 mg/ml; SL tabs 0.15, 0.3, 0.4, 0.6 mg; top oint 2%; trans derm syst 2.5, 5, 7.5, 10, 15 mg/24 hr

Side effects/adverse reactions:

CV: Postural hypotension, tachycardia, *collapse,* syncope

GI: Nausea, vomiting

INTEG: Pallor, sweating, rash

CNS: Headache, flushing, dizziness

Contraindications: Hypersensitivity to this drug or nitrites, severe anemia, increased intracranial pressure, cerebral hemorrhage

Precautions: Postural hypotension, pregnancy (C), lactation

Pharmacokinetics:

SUS REL: Onset 20-45 min, duration 3-8 hr

SL: Onset 1-3 min, duration 30 min

TRANS DER: Onset ½-1 hr, duration 12-24 hr

IV: Onset immediately, duration variable

TRANSMUC: Onset 3 min, duration 10-30 min

AEROSOL: Onset 2 min, duration 30-60 min

TOP OINT: Onset 30-60 min, duration 2-12 hr

Metabolized by liver, excreted in urine

Interactions/incompatibilities:

• Increased effects: β-blockers, diuretics, antihypertensives, anticoagulants, alcohol

• Decreased heparin: IV nitroglycerin

• Incompatible with any drug in sol or syringe

NURSING CONSIDERATIONS
Assess:
• Orthostatic B/P, pulse
• Pain: duration, time started, activity being performed, character
• Tolerance if taken over long period of time
• Headache, light-headedness, decreased B/P; may indicate a need for decreased dosage
Administer:
• IV diluted in amount specified D$_5$ or NS for infusion; use glass infusion bottles, nonpolyvinyl chloride infusion tubing; titrate to patient response; do not use filters
• With 8 oz H$_2$O on empty stomach (oral tablet)
Evaluate:
• Therapeutic response: decrease, prevention of anginal pain
Teach patient/family:
• To place buccal tab between lip and gum above incisors or between cheek and gum; sus rel must be swallowed whole, do not chew; SL should be dissolved under tongue, do not swallow; aerosol should be sprayed under tongue, do not inhale
• To use inhaler only when lying down
• Not to inhale spray
• To keep tabs in original container
• If 3 SL tabs in 15 min do not relieve pain, activate EMS
• To avoid alcohol
• That drug may cause headache; tolerance usually develops; use nonnarcotic analgesic
• That drug may be taken before stressful activity: exercise, sexual activity
• That SL may sting when drug comes in contact with mucous membranes
• To avoid hazardous activities if dizziness occurs

• To comply with complete medical regimen
• To make position changes slowly to prevent fainting

---

nitroprusside sodium
(nye-troe-pruss'ide)
Nitropress, Sodium Nitroprusside
Func. class.: Antihypertensive
Chem. class.: Peripheral vasodilator

Action: Directly relaxes arteriolar, venous smooth muscle, resulting in reduction in cardiac preload, afterload

Uses: Hypertensive crisis, to decrease bleeding by creating hypotension during surgery, acute CHF

Dosage and routes:
• *Adult:* IV INF dissolve 50 mg in 2-3 ml of D$_5$W, then dilute in 250-1000 ml of D$_5$W; run at 0.5-8 µg/kg/min

Available forms: Inj IV 50 mg

Side effects/adverse reactions:
GI: Nausea, vomiting, abdominal pain
CNS: Dizziness, headache, agitation, twitching, decreased reflexes, **LOC,** restlessness
EENT: Tinnitus, blurred vision
GU: Impotence
INTEG: Pain, irritation at injection site, sweating
CV: Palpitation, severe hypotension, dyspnea
MISC: Cyanide, thiocyanate toxicity

Contraindications: Hypersensitivity, hypertension (compensatory)

Precautions: Pregnancy (C), lactation, children, fluid, electrolyte imbalances, hepatic disease, renal disease, hypothyroidism, elderly

N

Pharmacokinetics:
IV: Onset 1-2 min, duration 1-10 min half-life 4 days in patients with abnormal renal function; metabolized in liver, excreted in urine
Interactions/incompatibilities:
• Severe hypotension: ganglionic blockers, volatile liquid anesthetics, halothane, enflurane, circulatory depressants
• Incompatible with any drug in syringe or sol
NURSING CONSIDERATIONS
Assess:
• Electrolytes: K, Na, Cl, CO_2
• Renal function studies: catecholamines, BUN, creatinine
• Hepatic function studies: AST, ALT, alk phosphatase
• B/P by direct means if possible; check ECG continuously
• Weight daily, I&O
• Thiocyanate levels qd if on long-term treatment
• Nausea, vomiting, diarrhea
• Edema in feet, legs daily
• Skin turgor, dryness of mucous membranes for hydration status
• Rales, dyspnea, orthopnea q30 min
Administer:
• Depending on B/P reading q15 min
• IV after diluting 50 mg/2-3 ml of D_5W, further dilute in 250 ml of D_5W; use an infusion pump only; wrap bottle with aluminum foil to protect from light; observe for color change in the infusion; discard if highly discolored (blue, green, dark red); titrate to patient response
Evaluate:
• Therapeutic response: decreased B/P, absence of bleeding
Treatment of overdose: Administer amyl nitrite inhalation until 3% sodium nitrate solution can be prepared for IV administration, then inject sodium thiosulfate IV, correct drop in BP with vasopressor

norepinephrine injection
(nor-ep-i-nef′rin)
Levophed
Func. class.: Adrenergic
Chem. class.: Catecholamine

Action: Causes increased contractility and heart rate by acting on β-receptors in heart; also, acts on α-receptors, causing vasoconstriction in blood vessels; B/P is elevated, coronary blood flow improves, cardiac output increases, B/P elevates
Uses: Acute hypotension
Dosage and routes:
• *Adult:* IV INF 8-12 μg/min titrated to B/P
Available forms: Inj IV 1 mg/ml
Side effects/adverse reactions:
CNS: Headache, anxiety, dizziness, insomnia, restlessness, tremor
CV: Palpitations, tachycardia, hypertension, ectopic beats, angina
GI: Nausea, vomiting
INTEG: Necrosis, tissue sloughing with extravasation, *gangrene*
RESP: Dyspnea
GU: Decreased urine output
Contraindications: Hypersensitivity, ventricular fibrillation, tachydysrhythmias, pheochromocytoma, pregnancy (D)
Precautions: Lactation, arterial embolism, peripheral vascular disease, hypertension, hyperthyroidism, elderly, heart disease
Pharmacokinetics:
IV: Onset 1-2 min; metabolized in liver; excreted in urine (inactive metabolites); crosses placenta
Interactions/incompatibilities:
• Do not use within 2 wk of

MAOIs, or hypertensive crisis may result
• Dysrhythmias: general anesthetics
• Decreased action of norepinephrine: α-blockers
• Increased B/P: oxytocics
• Increased pressor effect: tricyclic antidepressant, MAOIs
• Incompatible with alkaline solutions: Na, HCO₃

NURSING CONSIDERATIONS
Assess:
• I&O ratio; notify physician if output <30 ml/hr
• ECG during administration continuously; if B/P increases, drug is decreased
• B/P and pulse q5min after parenteral route
• CVP or PWP during infusion if possible
• For paresthesias and coldness of extremities; peripheral blood flow may decrease
• Injection site: tissue sloughing; if this occurs, administer phentolamine mixed with NS
Administer:
• Plasma expanders for hypovolemia
• IV after diluting with 500-1000 ml D₅W or NS; average dilution is 4 ml/1000 ml diluent; give as infusion 2-3 ml/min; titrate to patient response
• Using 2-bottle setup so drug may be discontinued while IV is still running; use infusion pump
Perform/provide:
• Storage of reconstituted solution if refrigerated for no longer than 24 hr
• Do not use discolored sol
Evaluate:
• Therapeutic response: increased B/P with stabilization

Teach patient/family:
• Reason for drug administration
Treatment of overdose: Administer fluids, electrolyte replacement

---

norethindrone
(nor-eth-in'drone)
Micronor, Norlutin, Nor-QD
Func. class.: Progestogen
Chem. class.: Progesterone derivative

Action: Inhibits secretion of pituitary gonadotropins, which prevents follicular maturation, ovulation; stimulates growth of mammary tissue; antineoplastic action against endometrial cancer
Uses: Uterine bleeding (abnormal), amenorrhea, endometriosis
Dosage and routes:
• Adult: PO 5-20 mg qd days 5-25 of menstrual cycle
Endometriosis
• Adult: PO 10 mg qd × 2 wk, then increased by 5 mg qd × 2 wk, up to 30 mg qd
Available forms: Tabs 5 mg
Side effects/adverse reactions:
CNS: Dizziness, headache, migraines, depression, fatigue
CV: Hypotension, thrombophlebitis, edema, ***thromboembolism, stroke, pulmonary embolism, myocardial infarction***
GI: Nausea, vomiting, anorexia, cramps, increased weight, ***cholestatic jaundice***
EENT: Diplopia
GU: Amenorrhea, cervical erosion, breakthrough bleeding, dysmenorrhea, vaginal candidiasis, breast changes, (gynecomastia, testicular atrophy, impotence), endometriosis, ***spontaneous abortion***
INTEG: Rash, urticaria, acne, hir-

N

sutism, alopecia, oily skin, seborrhea, purpura, melasma

META: Hyperglycemia

Contraindications: Breast cancer, hypersensitivity, thromboembolic disorders, reproductive cancer, genital bleeding (abnormal, undiagnosed), pregnancy (X)

Precautions: Lactation, hypertension, asthma, blood dyscrasias, gallbladder disease, CHF, diabetes mellitus, bone disease, depression, migraine headache, convulsive disorders, hepatic disease, renal disease, family history of breast or reproductive tract cancer

Pharmacokinetics:

PO: Duration 24 hr, excreted in urine, feces, metabolized in liver

Lab test interferences:

Increase: Alk phosphatase, nitrogen (urine), pregnanediol, amino acids, factors VII, VIII, IX, X

Decrease: GTT, HDL

NURSING CONSIDERATIONS

Assess:

• Weight daily: notify physician of weekly weight gain >5 lb

• B/P at beginning of treatment and periodically

• I&O ratio; be alert for decreasing urinary output, increasing edema

• Liver function studies: ALT, AST, bilirubin, periodically during long-term therapy

• Edema, hypertension, cardiac symptoms, jaundice

• Mental status: affect, mood, behavioral changes, depression

• Hypercalcemia

Administer:

• Titrated dose; use lowest effective dose

• Oil solution deeply in large muscle mass (IM), rotate sites

• In one dose in AM

• With food or milk to decrease GI symptoms

• After warming to dissolve crystals

Perform/provide:

• Storage in dark area

Evaluate:

• Therapeutic response: decreased abnormal uterine bleeding, absence of amenorrhea

Teach patient/family:

• About cushingoid symptoms

• To report breast lumps, vaginal bleeding, edema, jaundice, dark urine, clay-colored stools, dyspnea, headache, blurred vision, abdominal pain, numbness or stiffness in legs, chest pain; male to report impotence or gynecomastia

• To report suspected pregnancy

---

norethindrone acetate

(nor-eth-in′drone)

Aygestin, Norlutate

Func. class.: Progestogen

Chem. class.: Progesterone derivative

Action: Inhibits secretion of pituitary gonadotropins, which prevents follicular maturation, ovulation; stimulates growth of mammary tissue; antineoplastic action against endometrial cancer

Uses: Uterine bleeding (abnormal), amenorrhea, endometriosis

Dosage and routes:

• *Adult:* PO 2.5-10 mg qd days 5-25 of menstrual cycle

Endometriosis

• *Adult:* PO 5 mg qd × 2 wk, then increased by 2.5 mg qd × 2 wk, up to 15 mg qd

Available forms: Tabs 5 mg

Side effects/adverse reactions:

CNS: Dizziness, headache, migraines, depression, fatigue

CV: Hypotension, thrombophlebitis, edema, **_thromboembolism, stroke, pulmonary embolism, myocardial infarction_**

GI: Nausea, vomiting, anorexia, cramps, increased weight, **_cholestatic jaundice_**

EENT: Diplopia

GU: Amenorrhea, cervical erosion, breakthrough bleeding, dysmenorrhea, vaginal candidiasis, breast changes, *gynecomastia, testicular atrophy, impotence,* endometriosis, **_spontaneous abortion_**

INTEG: Rash, urticaria, acne, hirsutism, alopecia, oily skin, seborrhea, purpura, melasma

META: Hyperglycemia

Contraindications: Breast cancer, hypersensitivity, thromboembolic disorders, reproductive cancer, genital bleeding (abnormal, undiagnosed), cerebral hemorrhage, pregnancy (X)

Precautions: Lactation, hypertension, asthma, blood dyscrasias, gallbladder disease, CHF, diabetes mellitus, bone disease, depression, migraine headache, convulsive disorders, hepatic disease, renal disease, family history of breast or reproductive tract cancer

Pharmacokinetics:

PO: Duration 24 hr, excreted in urine, feces, metabolized in liver

Lab test interferences:

Increase: Alk phosphatase, nitrogen (urine), pregnanediol, amino acids, factors VII, VIII, IX, X

Decrease: GTT, HDL

NURSING CONSIDERATIONS
Assess:

• Weight daily; notify physician of weekly weight gain >5 lb

• B/P at beginning of treatment and periodically

• I&O ratio; be alert for decreasing urinary output, increasing edema

• Liver function studies: ALT, AST, bilirubin, periodically during long-term therapy

Administer:

• Titrated dose; use lowest effective dose

• Oil solution deeply in large muscle mass (IM); rotate sites

• In one dose in AM

• With food or milk to decrease GI symptoms

• After warming to dissolve crystals

• Edema, hypertension, cardiac symptoms, jaundice

• Mental status: affect, mood, behavioral changes, depression

• Hypercalcemia

Perform/provide:

• Storage in dark area

Evaluate:

• Therapeutic response: decreased abnormal uterine bleeding, absence of amenorrhea

Teach patient/family:

• About cushingoid symptoms

• To report breast lumps, vaginal bleeding, edema, jaundice, dark urine, clay-colored stools, dyspnea, headache, blurred vision, abdominal pain, numbness or stiffness in legs, chest pain; male to report impotence or gynecomastia

• To monitor blood sugar if diabetic

• To report suspected pregnancy

---

norfloxacin
(nor-flox'-a-sin)
Noroxin
Func. class.: Urinary antiinfective
Chem. class.: Fluoroquinolone antibacterial

Action: Interferes with conversion of intermediate DNA fragments into high-molecular-weight DNA

---

in bacteria, inhibits DNA gyrase
Uses: Adult urinary tract infections (including complicated) caused by *E. coli, E. cloacae, P. mirabilis, K. pneumoniae,* group D strep, indole-positive *Proteus, C. freundii, S. aureus*
Dosage and routes:
Uncomplicated
• *Adult:* 400 mg bid × 7-10 days 1 hr before or 2 hr after meals
Complicated
• *Adult:* 400 mg bid × 10-21 days; 400 mg qd × 7-10 days in impaired renal function
Available forms: Tabs 400 mg
Side effects/adverse reactions:
CNS: Headache, dizziness, fatigue, somnolence, depression, insomnia
GI:Nausea, constipation, increased ALT, AST, flatulence, heartburn, vomiting, diarrhea, dry mouth
INTEG: Rash
EENT: Visual disturbances
Contraindications: Hypersensitivity to quinolones
Precautions: Pregnancy (C), lactation, children, renal disease, seizure disorders
Pharmacokinetics:
Peak 1 hr, half-life 3-4 hr; steady state 2 days; excreted in urine as active drug, metabolites
Lab test interferences:
Increase: AST, ALT, BUN, creatinine, alk phosphatase
NURSING CONSIDERATIONS
Assess:
• Kidney, liver function studies: BUN, creatinine, AST, ALT
• I&O ratio, urine pH; <5.5 is ideal
• CNS symptoms: insomnia, vertigo, headache, agitation, confusion
• Allergic reactions: fever, flushing, rash, urticaria, pruritus

Administer:
• After clean-catch urine is obtained for C&S
• Two daily doses if urine output is high or if patient has diabetes
Perform/provide:
• Limited intake of alkaline foods, drugs: milk, dairy products, peanuts, vegetables, alkaline antacids, sodium bicarbonate
Evaluate:
• Therapeutic response: decreased pain, frequency, urgency, C&S, absence of infection
Teach patient/family:
• Fluids must be increased to 3 L/day to avoid crystallization in kidneys
• If dizziness occurs, to ambulate, perform activities with assistance
• Complete full course of drug therapy
• To contact physician if adverse reaction occurs
• To take 1 hr before or 2 hr after meals; not to take antacids with or within 2 hr of this drug use sips of water or hard candy for dry mouth

---

norgestrel
(nor-jess'trel)
Ovrette, Ovral*
Func. class.: Progestogen
Chem. class.: Progesterone derivative

Action: Inhibits secretion of pituitary gonadotropins, which prevents follicular maturation, ovulation, stimulates growth of mammary tissue, antineoplastic action against endometrial cancer
Uses: Female contraception
Dosage and routes:
• *Adult:* PO 1 tablet qd
Available forms: Tabs 0.35, 0.075 mg

Side effects/adverse reactions:

CNS: Dizziness, headache, migraines, depression, fatigue

CV: Hypotension, thrombophlebitis, edema, ***thromboembolism, stroke, pulmonary embolism, myocardial infarction***

GI: Nausea, vomiting, anorexia, cramps, increased weight, ***cholestatic jaundice***

EENT: Diplopia

GU: Amenorrhea, cervical erosion, breakthrough bleeding, dysmenorrhea, vaginal candidiasis, breast changes, *gynecomastia, testicular atrophy, impotence,* endometriosis, ***spontaneous abortion***

INTEG: Rash, urticaria, acne, hirsutism, alopecia, oily skin, seborrhea, purpura, melasma

META: Hyperglycemia

Contraindications: Breast cancer, hypersensitivity, thromboembolic disorders, reproductive cancer, genital bleeding (abnormal, undiagnosed), cerebral hemorrhage, pregnancy (X)

Precautions: Lactation, hypertension, asthma, blood dyscrasias, gallbladder disease, CHF, diabetes mellitus, bone disease, depression, migraine headache, convulsive disorders, hepatic disease, renal disease, family history of breast or reproductive tract cancer

Pharmacokinetics:

PO: Duration 24 hr; excreted in urine and feces; metabolized in liver

Lab test interferences:

Increase: Alk phosphatase, nitrogen (urine), pregnanediol, amino acids, factors VII, VIII, IX, X

Decrease: GTT, HDL

NURSING CONSIDERATIONS

Assess:

• Weight daily; notify physician of weekly weight gain >5 lb

• B/P at beginning of treatment and periodically

• I&O ratio; be alert for decreasing urinary output, increasing edema

• Liver function studies: ALT, AST, bilirubin, periodically during long-term therapy

• Edema, hypertension, cardiac symptoms, jaundice

• Mental status: affect, mood, behavioral changes, depression

• Hypercalcemia

Administer:

• Titrated dose; use lowest effective dose

• Oil solution deeply in large muscle mass (IM); rotate sites

• In one dose in AM

• With food or milk to decrease GI symptoms

• After warming to dissolve crystals

Perform/provide:

• Storage in dark area

Evaluate:

• Therapeutic response: absence of pregnancy

Teach patient/family:

• About cushingoid symptoms

• To report breast lumps, vaginal bleeding, edema, jaundice, dark urine, clay-colored stools, dyspnea, headache, blurred vision, abdominal pain, numbness or stiffness in legs, chest pain

• To report suspected pregnancy

• To monitor blood sugar; if diabetic

---

nortriptyline HCl

(nor-trip′ti-leen)

Aventyl HCl, Pamelor

Func. class.: Antidepressant—tricyclic

Chem. class.: Dibenzocycloheptene—secondary amine

Action: Blocks reuptake of norepinephrine, serotonin into nerve endings, increasing action of norepinephrine, serotonin in nerve cells

Uses: Major depression

Dosage and routes:

• *Adult:* PO 25 mg tid or qid; may increase to 150 mg/day; may give daily dose hs

Available forms: Caps 10, 25, 50, 75 mg; sol 10 mg/5 ml

Side effects/adverse reactions:

*HEMA: **Agranulocytosis, thrombocytopenia, eosinophilia, leukopenia***

CNS: Dizziness, drowsiness, confusion, headache, anxiety, tremors, stimulation, weakness, insomnia, nightmares, EPS (elderly), increased psychiatric symptoms

GI: Constipation, dry mouth, nausea, vomiting, ***paralytic ileus,*** increased appetite, cramps, epigastric distress, jaundice, ***hepatitis,*** stomatitis

*GU: Retention, **acute renal failure***

INTEG: Rash, urticaria, sweating, pruritus, photosensitivity

*CV: Orthostatic hypotension, ECG changes, tachycardia, **hypertension,*** palpitations

EENT: Blurred vision, tinnitus, mydriasis

Contraindications: Hypersensitivity to tricyclic antidepressants, recovery phase of myocardial infarction, convulsive disorders, prostatic hypertrophy

Precautions: Suicidal patients, severe depression, increased intraocular pressure, narrow-angle glaucoma, urinary retention, cardiac disease, hepatic disease, hyperthyroidism, electroshock therapy, elective surgery, pregnancy (C)

Pharmacokinetics:

PO: Steady state 4-19 days; metabolized by liver; excreted by kidneys; crosses placenta; excreted in breast milk; half-life 18-28 hr

Interactions/incompatibilities:

• Decreased effects of: guanethidine, clonidine, indirect-acting sympathomimetics (ephedrine)

• Increased effects of: direct-acting sympathomimetics (epinephrine), alcohol, barbiturates, benzodiazepines, CNS depressants

• Hyperpyretic crisis, convulsions, hypertensive episode: MAOI

Lab test interferences:

Increase: Serum bilirubin, blood glucose, alk phosphatase

False increase: Urinary catecholamines

Decrease: VMA, 5-HIAA

NURSING CONSIDERATIONS

Assess:

• B/P (lying, standing), pulse q4h; if systolic B/P drops 20 mm Hg, hold drug, notify physician; take vital signs q4h in patients with cardiovascular disease

• Blood studies: CBC, leukocytes, differential, cardiac enzymes if patient is receiving long-term therapy

• Hepatic studies: AST, ALT, bilirubin

• Weight qwk; appetite may increase with drug

• ECG for flattening of T wave, bundle branch block, AV block, dysrhythmias in cardiac patients

• EPS primarily in elderly: rigidity, dystonia, akathisia

• Mental status changes: mood, sensorium, affect, suicidal tendencies, increase in psychiatric symptoms, depression, panic

• Urinary retention, constipation; constipation is more likely to occur in children

• Withdrawal symptoms: headache, nausea, vomiting, muscle pain, weakness; do not usually occur unless drug was discontinued abruptly

• Alcohol consumption; if alcohol is consumed, hold dose until morning

Administer:
• Increased fluids, bulk in diet if constipation occurs
• With food or milk for GI symptoms
• Dosage hs if oversedation occurs during day; may take entire dose hs; elderly may not tolerate once/day dosing
• Gum, hard candy, or frequent sips of water for dry mouth
• Concentrate with fruit juice, water, or milk to disguise taste

Perform/provide:
• Storage in tight, light-resistant container at room temperature
• Assistance with ambulation during beginning therapy, since drowsiness/dizziness occurs
• Safety measures including side rails, primarily for elderly
• Checking to see PO medication swallowed

Evaluate:
• Therapeutic response: decreased depression

Teach patient/family:
• That therapeutic effects may take 2-3 wk
• To use caution in driving or other activities requiring alertness because of drowsiness, dizziness, blurred vision
• To avoid alcohol ingestion, other CNS depressants
• Not to discontinue medication quickly after long-term use; may cause nausea, headache, malaise
• To wear sunscreen or large hat, since photosensitivity occurs

Treatment of overdose: ECG monitoring; induce emesis; lavage,

italics = common side effects

activated charcoal; administer anticonvulsant

nylidrin HCl
(nye'li-drin)
Arlidin, Rolidrin
Func. class.: Peripheral vasodilator, β-adrenergic agonist
Chem. class.: β-Adrenergic agonist—phenylisopropylamine

Action: Acts on β-adrenergic receptors to dilate arterioles in skeletal muscles; increases cardiac output; may have direct vasodilatory effect on vascular smooth muscle

Uses: Arteriosclerosis obliterans, thromboangiitis obliterans, diabetic vascular disease, night leg cramps, Raynaud's disease, ischemic ulcer, frostbite, acrocyanosis, acroparesthesia, thrombophlebitis, primary cochlear cell ischemia, cochlear stria ischemia, muscular or ampullar ischemia, other disturbances from labyrinth artery spasm or obstruction

Dosage and routes:
• *Adult:* PO 3-12 mg tid or qid
Available forms: Tabs 6, 12 mg

Side effects/adverse reactions:
CV: Postural hypotension, palpitations
CNS: Dizziness, anxiety, tremors, weakness, nervousness
GI: Nausea, vomiting
INTEG: Flushing

Contraindications: Hypersensitivity, paroxysmal tachycardia, progressive angina pectoris, thyrotoxicosis, MI

Precautions: CHF, pregnancy (C)

Pharmacokinetics:
PO: Onset 10 min, peak 30 min, duration 2 hr; slowly metabolized in liver; excreted in urine; thera-

bold italic = life threatening reactions

...ke several

...patibilities:
...nsion: phenothi-
a...   ...sodilators, antihy-
perten...

NURSING CONSIDERATIONS
Assess:
• B/P, pulse during treatment until stable; take B/P lying, standing; orthostatic hypotension is common
Administer:
• With meals to reduce GI upset
Perform/provide:
• Storage at room temperature
Evaluate:
• Therapeutic response: ability to walk without pain, increased pulse volume, increased temperature in extremities or orientation, long- and short-term memory
Teach patient/family:
• That medication is not cure, may have to be taken continuously depending on condition; therapeutic response may not be evident for 2-3 mo
• That it is necessary to quit smoking to prevent excessive vasoconstriction
• To avoid hazardous activities until stabilized on medication; dizziness may occur
• That palpitations should subside as therapy continues

---

nystatin
(nye-stat'in)
Mycostatin, Mycostatin Pastilles, Nadostine,* Nilstat Oral, Nystatin
Func. class.: Antifungal
Chem. class.: Amphoteric polyene

Action: Interferes with fungal DNA replication; binds sterols in fungal cell membrane, which increases permeability, leaking of cell nutrients

Uses: *Candida* species causing oral, vaginal, intestinal infections
Dosage and routes:
Oral infection
• *Adult:* SUSP 400,000-600,000 U qid
• *Child and infants >3 mo:* SUSP 250,000-500,000 U qid
• *Newborn and premature infants:* susp 100,000 U qid
GI infection
• *Adult:* PO 500,000-1,000,000 U tid
Available forms: Tabs 500,000 U; powder 50 mill, 150 mill, 500 mill, 1 bill, 2 bill, 5 bill U; susp 100,000 U
Side effects/adverse reactions:
INTEG: Rash, urticaria (rare)
GI: Nausea, vomiting, anorexia, diarrhea, cramps
Contraindications: Hypersensitivity
Precautions: Pregnancy (B)
Pharmacokinetics:
PO: Little absorption, excreted in feces

NURSING CONSIDERATIONS
Assess:
• For allergic reaction: rash, urticaria; drug may have to be discontinued
• For predisposing factors: antibiotic therapy, pregnancy, diabetes mellitus, sexual partner infection (vaginal infections)
Administer:
• Oral suspension dose by placing ½ in each cheek, then swallow
• Topical dose after cleansing area; mouth may be swabbed
Perform/provide:
• Storage in refrigerator, oral susp, tabs in tight, light-resistant containers at room temperature

---

*Available in Canada only

Evaluate:
• Therapeutic response: culture negative for *Candida*

Teach patient/family:
• That long-term therapy may be needed to clear infection; to complete entire course of medication
• Proper hygiene: changing socks if feet are infected; using no commercial mouthwashes for mouth infection
• To avoid getting preparation on hands
• To wear light-day pad for vaginal preparations
• To avoid tight shoes, bandages when using for feet infection
• To avoid sexual contact during treatment to minimize reinfection
• To notify physician if irritation occurs; drug may have to be discontinued
• That relief from itching may occur after 24-72 hr

---

nystatin (topical)
(nye-stat'in)
Mycostatin, Nilstat, Nystatin, Nystex, O-V Statin
Func. class.: Local antiinfective
Chem. class.: Antifungal

Action: Interferes with fungal DNA replication; binds sterols in fungal cell membrane, which increases permeability, leaking of cell nutrients

Uses: Cutaneous vulvovaginal candidiasis, mucocutaneous fungal infections, infant eczema, pruritis ani and vulvae

Dosage and routes:
• *Adult and child:* TOP apply to affected area bid-tid × 14 days; vag 1-2 tabs (100,000 U each) inserted into vagina

Available forms: Cream, oint, powder, spray, vag tabs 100,000 U

Side effects/adverse reactions:
INTEG: Rash, urticaria, stinging, burning

Contraindications: Hypersensitivity

Precautions: Pregnancy (B), lactation

NURSING CONSIDERATIONS
Assess:
• Allergic reaction: burning, stinging, swelling, redness

Administer:
• To moist lesions with a swab
• Vaginal tablets by inserting high into vagina with applicator provided
• Enough medication to cover lesions completely
• In gravid client 3-6 wk before term to decrease candidiasis in the newborn
• After cleansing with soap, water before each application; dry well

Perform/provide:
• Storage at room temperature in dry place; protect from light, air, heat

Evaluate:
• Therapeutic response: decrease in size, number of lesions, decreased itching, white patches on vulva

Teach patient/family:
• To discontinue use and notify physician if irritation occurs
• To apply with glove to prevent further infection; drug may stain, pads may protect clothing
• Not to use occlusive dressings
• To avoid use of OTC creams, ointments, lotions unless directed by physician
• To use medical asepsis (hand washing) before, after each application
• To complete treatment regimen

N

---

italics = common side effects   ***bold italic*** = life threatening reactions

ofloxacin
(o-flox′a-sin)
Floxin, Floxin IV
Func. class.: Antiinfective
Chem. class.: Fluoroquinolone

Action: Interferes with conversion of intermediate DNA fragments into high-molecular-weight DNA in bacteria, inhibits DNA gyrase

Uses: Treatment of lower respiratory tract infections (pneumonia, bronchitis), genitourinary infections (prostatitis, UTIs) caused by *E. coli, K. pneumoniae, C. trachomatis, N. gonorrhoeae;* skin and skin structure infections

Dosage and routes:
Lower respiratory tract infections/ skin and skin structure infections
• *Adult:* PO, IV 400 mg q12h × 10 days
Cervicitis, urethritis
• *Adult:* PO, IV 300 mg q12h × 7 days
Prostatitis
• *Adult:* PO, IV 300 mg q12h × 6 wk
Acute, uncomplicated gonorrhea
• *Adult:* PO, IV 400 mg as a single dose
Available forms: Tabs 200, 300, 400 mg; 4 mg/ml (IV)

Side effects/adverse reactions:
CNS: Dizziness; headache, fatigue, somnolence, depression, insomnia, lethargy, malaise
GI: Diarrhea, nausea, vomiting, anorexia, flatulence, heartburn, dry mouth, increased AST, ALT, abdominal pain, constipation
INTEG: Rash, pruritus
EENT: Visual disturbances

Contraindications: Hypersensitivity to quinolones

Precautions: Pregnancy (C), lactation, children, elderly, renal disease, seizure disorders, excessive sunlight

Pharmacokinetics:
PO: Peak 1-2 hr, half-life 9 hr, steady state 2 days; excreted in urine as active drug, metabolites; 90%-95%, bioavailability

Interactions/incompatibilities:
• Decreased effects of ofloxacin: antacids, nitrofurantoin, sucralfate, iron salts, zinc salts
• Increased ofloxacin levels: probenecid
• Increased effects of: warfarin, cyclosporine

NURSING CONSIDERATIONS
Assess:
• Kidney, liver function studies: BUN, creatinine, AST, ALT
• I&O ratio; urine pH <5.5 is ideal
• CNS symptoms: insomnia, vertigo, headache, agitation, confusion
• Allergic reactions: rash, flushing, urticaria, pruritus

Administer:
• After clean-catch urine is obtained for C&S

Perform/provide:
• Limited intake of alkaline foods, drugs; milk, dairy products, peanuts, vegetables, alkaline antacids, sodium bicarbonate

Evaluate:
• Therapeutic response: negative C&S

Teach patient/family:
• That fluids must be increased to 3L/day to avoid crystallization in kidneys
• That if dizziness or light-headedness occurs, ambulate, perform activities with assistance
• To complete full course of drug therapy
• To contact physician if adverse reactions occur

*Available in Canada only

• To avoid iron- or mineral-containing supplements within 2 hr before or after dose

---

olsalazine sodium

(ohl-sal'ah-zeen)

Dipentum

Func. class.: Antiinflammatory
Chem. class.: Salicylate derivative

Action: Bioconverted to 5-aminosalicylic acid, which decreases inflammation

Uses: Maintenance of remission of ulcerative colitis in patients intolerant to sulfasalazine

Dosage and routes:
Adult: PO 1 g/day in 2 divided doses

Available forms: Tabs 250 mg

Side effects/adverse reactions:
EENT: Dry mouth, dry eyes, watery eyes, blurred vision

SYST: **Anaphylaxis**

GI: Nausea, vomiting, abdominal pain, stomatitis, hepatitis, pancreatitis, diarrhea, bloating

CNS: Headache, insomnia, hallucinations, depression, vertigo, fatigue, drug fever, chills, dizziness, drowsiness, tremors

HEMA: **Leukopenia, neutropenia, thrombocytopenia, agranulocytosis, anemia**

INTEG: Rash, dermatitis, urticaria, **Stevens-Johnson syndrome,** erythema, photosensitivity, alopecia

GU: Frequency, dysuria, hematuria, impotence

CV: Allergic myocarditis, 2nd degree heart block, hypertension, peripheral edema, chest pain, palpitations

RESP: **Bronchospasm,** shortness of breath

Contraindications: Hypersensitivity to salicylates

Precautions: Pregnancy (C), child <14 yr, lactation, impaired hepatic renal function, severe allergy, bronchial asthma

Pharmacokinetics:
PO: Partially absorbed, peak 1½ hr, half-life 5-10 hr, excreted in urine as 5-aminosalicylic acid and metabolites, crosses placenta

Lab test interferences:
False positive: Urinary glucose test

NURSING CONSIDERATIONS
Assess:
• I&O ratio: note color, character, pH of urine if drug is administered for UTIs; output should be 800 ml less than intake; if urine is highly acidic, alkalization may be needed
• Kidney function studies: BUN, creatinine, urinalysis if on long-term therapy
• Blood dyscrasias: skin rash, fever, sore throat, bruising, bleeding, fatigue, joint pain
• Allergic reaction: rash, dermatitis, urticaria, pruritus, dyspnea, bronchospasm

Administer:
• With food in evenly divided doses
• Medication after C&S; repeat C&S after full course of medication completed
• With resuscitative equipment available; severe allergic reactions may occur
• Total daily dose in evenly spaced doses to help minimize GI intolerance

Perform/provide:
• Storage in tight, light-resistant containers at room temperature

Evaluate:
• Therapeutic response: absence of fever, mucus in stools

---

italics = common side effects   ***bold italic*** = life threatening reactions

omeprazole
(om-ee-pray-zole)
Prilosec
Func. class.: Antisecretory
compound
Chem. class.: Benzimidazole

Action: Suppresses gastric secretion by inhibiting hydrogen/potassium ATPase enzyme system in the gastric parietal cell; characterized as a gastric acid pump inhibitor, since it blocks the final step of acid production

Uses: Gastroesophageal reflux disease (GERD), severe erosive esophagitis, poorly responsive systemic GERD, pathologic hypersecretory conditions (Zollinger-Ellison syndrome, systemic mastocytosis, multiple endocrine adenomas); possibly effective for treatment of duodenal ulcers

Dosage and routes:
Severe erosine esophagitis/poorly responsive gastroesophageal reflux disease
• *Adult:* PO 20 mg gd × 4-8 wk
Pathologic hypersecretory conditions
• *Adult:* PO 60 mg/day; may increase to 120 mg tid; daily doses >80 mg should be divided
Available forms: Cap, sus rel 20 mg

Side effects/adverse reactions
CNS: Headache, dizziness, asthenia
GI: Diarrhea, abdominal pain, vomiting, nausea, constipation, flatulence, acid regurgitation, abdominal swelling, anorexia, irritable colon, esophageal candidiasis, dry mouth
RESP: Upper respiratory infections, cough, epistaxis
INTEG: Rash, dry skin, urticaria, pruritus, alopecia

META: Hypoglycemia, increased hepatic enzymes, weight gain
EENT: Tinnitus, taste perversion
CV: Chest pain, angina, tachycardia, bradycardia, palpitations, peripheral edema
GU: UTI, frequency, increased creatinine, *proteinuria, hematuria,* testicular pain, glycosuria
HEMA: Pancytopenia, thrombocytopenia, neutropenia, leukocytosis, anemia
MISC: Back pain, fever, fatigue, malaise

Contraindications: Hypersensitivity

Precautions: Pregnancy (C), lactation, children

Pharmacokinetics:
Peak ½-3½ hr, half-life ½-1 hr, protein binding 95%, eliminated in urine as metabolites and in feces; in the elderly the elimination rate is decreased, bioavailability is increased

Interactions/incompatibilities:
• Increased serum levels: diazepam, phenytoin
• Possible increased bleeding: warfarin

NURSING CONSIDERATIONS
Assess:
• GI system: bowel sounds q8h, abdomen for pain, swelling, anorexia
• Hepatic enzymes: AST, ALT during treatment
Administer:
• Before eating; swallow capsule whole; do not open, chew, or crush
Evaluate:
• Therapeutic response: absence of epigastric pain, swelling, fullness
Teach patient/family:
• To report severe diarrhea; drug may have to be discontinued
• That the diabetic patient should

be aware that hypoglycemia may occur

ondansetron HCl
(on-dan-see'tron)
Zofran
Func. class.: Antiemetic
Chem. class.: 5-HT3 receptor antagonist

Action: Prevents nausea, vomiting by blocking serotonin peripherally, centrally, and in the small intestine
Uses: Prevention of nausea, vomiting associated with cancer chemotherapy and prevention of postoperative nausea, vomiting
Dosage and routes:
• *Adult:* IV 0.15 mg/kg infused over 15 min, 30 min before the start of cancer chemotherapy; 0.15 mg/kg is given 4 hr and 8 hr after first dose; dilute 50 ml of D$_5$W or 0.9% NaCl before giving
Prevention of nausea/vomiting associated with cancer chemotherapy
Adult: PO 8 mg tid; give first dose ½ hr before chemotherapy, subsequent doses 4, 8 hrs after first dose; give 8 mg tid × 1-2 days after chemotherapy completion
Prevention of postoperative nausea/vomiting
Adult: IV 4 mg undiluted over >30 sec
Available forms: Inj 2 mg/ml, tabs 4, 8 mg
Side effects/adverse reactions:
GI: Diarrhea, constipation, increased AST, ALT
CNS: Headache
MISC: Rash, ***bronchospasm***
Contraindications: Hypersensitivity
Precautions: Pregnancy (B), lactation, children, elderly

Pharmacokinetics:
IV: Mean elimination half-life 3.5-4.7 hr, plasma protein binding 70%-76%; extensively metabolized in the liver
Interactions/incompatibilities:
• Incompatibility unknown
NURSING CONSIDERATIONS
Assess:
• For absence of nausea, vomiting during chemotherapy
• Hypersensitive reaction: rash, bronchospasm
Administer:
• IV after diluting a single dose in 50 ml NS or D$_5$W, 0.45% or NS and given over 15 min
Perform/provide:
• Storage at room temperature for 48 hr after dilution
Evaluate:
• Therapeutic response: absence of nausea, vomiting during cancer chemotherapy
Teach patient/family:
• To report diarrhea, constipation, rash, or changes in respirations

opium tincture/camphorated opium tincture
(oh'pee-um)
Opium Tincture Deodorized, Pantopan, Paregoric, Paregorique*
Func. class.: Antidiarrheal
Chem. class.: Opium/opium and morphine

Controlled Substance Schedule III/II (depending on amount of opium)
Action: Antiperistaltic activity
Uses: Diarrhea (cause undetermined); to treat withdrawal symptoms in infants born to addicted mothers

italics = common side effects   ***bold italic*** = life threatening reactions

Dosage and routes:
• *Adult:* PO 0.3-1 ml qid, not to exceed 6 ml/day (tincture) or 5-10 ml qd-qid (camphorated)
• *Child:* PO 0.25-0.5 ml/kg qd-qid (camphorated)
Withdrawal
• *Neonates:* PO 1:25 dilution, 3-6 gtt q3-6hr (tincture), dosage adjustment is made to control symptoms
Available forms: Liq 2 mg morphine equivalent per 5 ml
Side effects/adverse reactions:
CNS: Dizziness, drowsiness, fainting, flushing, physical dependency
CNS depression
GI: Nausea, vomiting, constipation, abdominal pain
Contraindications: Hypersensitivity, severe ulcerative colitis, pseudomembranous colitis
Precautions: Liver disease, addiction-prone individuals, prostatic hypertrophy (severe), pregnancy (B)
Pharmacokinetics:
PO: Duration 4 hr, half-life 2-3 hr; metabolized in liver; excreted in urine
Interactions/incompatibilities:
• Increased action of both drugs: other CNS depressants
• Increased CNS toxicity: cimetidine
NURSING CONSIDERATIONS
Assess:
• Electrolytes (K, Na, Cl) if on long-term therapy
• Skin turgor q8h if dehydration is suspected
• Bowel pattern before; for rebound constipation
• Response after 48 hr; if no response, drug should be discontinued
• Dehydration in children
• Abdominal distention; toxic megacolon may occur in ulcerative colitis
Administer:
• Undiluted with water
• For 48 hr only
Evaluate:
• Therapeutic response: decreased diarrhea
Teach patient/family:
• To avoid OTC products (cough, cold, hay fever preparations) unless directed by physician
• Not to exceed recommended dose
• That drug may be habit-forming
• To avoid hazardous activities, drowsiness may occur

---

oral contraceptives
Func. class.: Hormone
Chem. class.: Estrogen/progestin combinations

Action: Prevents ovulation by suppressing follicle stimulating, luteinizing hormone
Uses: To prevent pregnancy, endometriosis, hypermenorrhea
Dosage and routes:
• *Adult:* PO 1 qd starting on day 5 of menstrual cycle; day 1 is 1st day of period
20/21 tablet packs
• *Adult:* PO 1 qd starting on day 7 of menstrual cycle; day 1 is 1st day of period, then on 20 or 21 days, off 7 days
28 tablet packs
• *Adult:* PO 1 qd continuously
Biphasic
• *Adult:* 1 qd × 10 days, then next color 1 qd × 11 days
Triphasic
• *Adult:* 1 qd; check package insert for each new brand
Endometriosis
• *Adult:* PO 1 qd × 20 days from day 5 to 24 of cycle

• *Adult:* PO 1 qd; check package insert for specific instructions
Available forms: Check specific brand
Side effects/adverse reactions:
GI: Nausea, vomiting, cramps, diarrhea, bloating, constipation, change in appetite, ***cholestatic jaundice***
INTEG: Chloasma, melasma, acne, rash, urticaria, erythema, pruritus, hirsutism, alopecia, photosensitivity
CV: Increased B/P, thromboembolic conditions, fluid retention, edema
ENDO: Decreased glucose tolerance, increased TBG, PBI, T_4, T_3
GU: Breakthrough bleeding, amenorrhea, spotting, dysmenorrhea, galactorrhea, endocervical hyperplasia, vaginitis, cystitis-like syndrome, breast change
CNS: Depression, fatigue, dizziness, nervousness, anxiety, headache
EENT: Optic neuritis, retinal thrombosis, cataracts
HEMA: Increased fibrinogen, clotting factor
Contraindications: Pregnancy (X), lactation, reproductive cancer, thrombophlebitis, MI, hepatic tumors, hepatic disease, CAD, women 40 and over, CVA
Precautions: Depression, hypertension, renal disease, seizure disorders, lupus erythematosus, rheumatic disease, migraine headache, amenorrhea, irregular menses, breast cancer (fibrocystic), gallbladder disease, diabetes mellitus, heavy smoking, acute mononucleosis, sickle cell disease
Pharmacokinetics: Excreted in breast milk
Interactions/incompatibilities:
• Decreased effectiveness of oral contraceptives: anticonvulsants, rifampin, analgesics, antibiotics, antihistamines, chenodiol, griseofulvin
• Decreased action of: oral anticoagulants
• Increased clotting: aminocaproic acid
Lab test interferences:
Increase: Pro-time, clotting factors VII, VIII, IX, X, TBG, PBI, T_4, platelet aggregability, BSP, triglycerides, bilirubin, AST, ALT
Decrease: T_3, antithrombin III, folate, metyrapone test, GTT, 17-OHCS
NURSING CONSIDERATIONS
Assess:
• Glucose, thyroid function, liver function tests
• Reproductive changes: change in breasts, tumors, positive Pap smear; drug should be discontinued if changes occur
Evaluate:
• Therapeutic response: absence of pregnancy, endometriosis, hypermenorrhea
Teach patient/family:
• About detection of clots using Homan's sign
• To use sunscreen or avoid sunlight; photosensitivity can occur
• To take at same time each day to ensure equal drug level
• To report GI symptoms that occur after 4 mo
• To use another birth control method during 1st week of oral contraceptive use
• To take another tablet as soon as possible if one is missed
• That after drug is discontinued, pregnancy may not occur for several months
• To report abdominal pain, change in vision, shortness of breath, change in menstrual flow, spotting,

breakthrough bleeding, breast lumps, swelling, headache, severe leg pain
• That continuing medical care is needed: PAP smear and gynecologic examinations q6mo
• To notify physician and dentist of oral contraceptive use

---

orphenadrine citrate

(or-fen′a-dreen)

Banflex, Flexoject, Flexon, Marflex, Myolin, Neocyten, Norflex, O-Flex, Orphenadrine Citrate, Orphenate

Func. class.: Skeletal muscle relaxant, central acting; anticholinergic

Chem. class.: Tertiary amine

Action: Acts centrally on skeletal muscle to relax, inhibit muscle spasm

Uses: Pain in musculoskeletal conditions

Dosage and routes:
• *Adult:* PO 100 mg bid; IM/IV 60 mg q12h

Available forms: Tabs 100 mg; tabs sus rel 100 mg; inj IM, IV 30 mg/ml

Side effects/adverse reactions:

HEMA: Aplastic anemia

CNS: Dizziness, weakness, fatigue, drowsiness, headache, disorientation, insomnia, stimulation, hallucination, agitation

EENT: Nasal congestion, blurred vision, increased intraocular pressure, mydriasis

CV: Orthostatic hypotension, tachycardia

GI: Nausea, vomiting, constipation, dry mouth

GU: Urinary frequency, hesitancy, retention

INTEG: Rash, pruritus, urticaria

Contraindications: Hypersensitivity, narrow-angle glaucoma, GI obstruction, myasthenia gravis, stenosing peptic ulcer, bladder neck obstruction, cardiospasm

Precautions: Pregnancy (C), children, cardiac disease, tachycardia

Pharmacokinetics:

PO: Peak 2 hr, duration 4-6 hr, half-life 14 hr; metabolized in liver, excreted in urine (unchanged)

Interactions/incompatibilities:
• Increased CNS effects: propoxyphene, other anticholinergics, oral contraceptives
• Incompatibility unknown

NURSING CONSIDERATIONS

Assess:
• Monitor vital signs q10-15min during administration
• Blood studies: CBC, WBC, differential; blood dyscrasias may occur (rare)
• I&O ratio; check for urinary retention, frequency, hesitancy
• Dosage: even slight overdose can cause toxicity
• Allergic reactions: rash, fever, respiratory distress
• Blood dyscrasias: temperature, bleeding, fatigue (rare)
• CNS symptoms: dizziness, drowsiness, psychiatric symptoms

Administer:
• With meals for GI symptoms
• IV undiluted, or diluted in 5-10 ml sterile H_2O for inj; give 60 mg or less over 5 min
• When giving IV, may cause paradoxical initial bradycardia; usually disappears in 2 min

Perform/provide:
• Assistance with ambulation if dizziness/drowsiness occurs

Evaluate:
• Therapeutic response: decreased rigidity, spasms

Teach patient/family:
• Not to discontinue medication quickly; insomnia, nausea, headache will occur
• Not to take with alcohol, other CNS depressants
• To avoid altering activities while taking this drug
• To avoid hazardous activities if drowsiness/dizziness occurs
• To avoid using OTC medication: cough preparations, antihistamines, unless directed by physician
• To use gum, frequent sips of water for dry mouth

---

oxacillin sodium

(ox-a-sill'in)
Bactocill, Oxacillin Sodium, Prostaphilin
Func. class.: Broad-spectrum antibiotic
Chem. class.: Penicillinase-resistant penicillin

Action: Interferes with cell wall replication of susceptible organisms; osmotically unstable cell wall swells, bursts from osmotic pressure

Uses: Effective for gram-positive cocci *(S. aureus, S. pneumoniae)*, infections caused by penicillinase-producing *Staphylococcus*

Dosage and routes:
• *Adult:* PO 2-6 g/day in divided doses q4-6h; IM/IV 2-12 g/day in divided doses q4-6h
• *Child:* PO 50-100 mg/kg/day in divided doses q6h; IM/IV 50-100 mg/kg/day in divided doses q4-6h
Available forms include: Caps 250, 500 mg; powder for oral susp 250 mg/5 ml; powder for inj IM, IV 250, 500 mg, 1, 2, 4, 10 g; IV INF 1, 2 g

Side effects/adverse reactions:
HEMA: Anemia, increased bleeding time, **bone marrow depression, granulocytopenia**
GI:Nausea, vomiting, diarrhea, increased AST, ALT, abdominal pain, glossitis, colitis
GU: **Oliguria, proteinuria, hematuria,** *vaginitis, moniliasis,* **glomerulonephritis**
CNS: Lethargy, hallucinations, anxiety, depression, twitching, **coma, convulsions**

Contraindications: Hypersensitivity to penicillins

Precautions: Pregnancy (B), hypersensitivity to cephalosporins, neonates

Pharmacokinetics:
PO/IM: Peak 30-60 min, duration 4-6 hr
IV: Peak 5 min, duration 4-6 hr, half-life 30-60 min, metabolized in the liver, excreted in urine, bile, breast milk, crosses placenta

Interactions/incompatibilities:
• Decreased antimicrobial effectiveness of oxacillin: tetracyclines, erythromycins
• Increased oxacillin concentrations: aspirin, probenecid
• Incompatible in solution with amikacin, levarterenol, metaraminol, tetracycline, verapamil

Lab test interferences:
False positive: Urine glucose, urine protein

NURSING CONSIDERATIONS
Assess:
• I&O ratio; report hematuria, oliguria, since penicillin in high doses is nephrotoxic
• Any patient with compromised renal system, since drug is excreted slowly in poor renal system function; toxicity may occur rapidly
• Liver studies: AST, ALT

---

italics = common side effects   ***bold italic*** = life threatening reactions

---

794 **oxacillin sodium**

- Blood studies: WBC, RBC, Hct/Hgb, bleeding time
- Renal studies: urinalysis, protein, blood
- C&S before drug therapy; drug may be given as soon as culture is taken
- Bowel pattern before and during treatment
- Skin eruptions after administration of penicillin to 1 wk after discontinuing drug
- Respiratory status: rate, character, wheezing, tightness in chest
- Allergies before initiation of treatment, and reaction of each medication; highlight allergies on chart, Kardex

Administer:
- IV after diluting 500 mg or less/5 ml sterile H$_2$O or NaCl for inj; may dilute further in D$_5$W, or saline, NS, LR and give 1 g/10 min; may be given as infusion over 6 hr
- Drug after C&S has been completed
- PO with full glass of water 1 hr before or 2 hr after meals
- IM deep in gluteal muscle

Perform/provide:
- Adrenalin, suction, tracheostomy set, endotracheal intubation equipment
- Scratch test to assess allergy, after securing order from physician; usually done when penicillin is only drug of choice
- Storage in tight container; refrigerate reconstituted solution up to 2 wk

Evaluate:
- Therapeutic response: absence of fever, draining wounds

Teach patient/family:
- Aspects of drug therapy, including need to complete course of medication to ensure organism death (10-14 days); culture may be taken after completed course
- To report sore throat, fever, fatigue (may indicate superimposed infection)
- To wear or carry Medic Alert ID if allergic to penicillins
- To take on empty stomach with a full glass of water

Treatment of overdose: Withdraw drug, maintain airway, administer epinephrine, aminophylline, O$_2$, IV corticosteroids for anaphylaxis

---

oxamniquine
(ox-am′ni-kwin)
Vansil
Func. class.: Anthelmintic
Chem. class.: Tetrahydroquinone derivative

Action: Causes paralysis, contraction, leading to dislodgement of suckers; they are carried to liver, where phagocytosis takes place
Uses: Schistosomiasis
Dosage and routes:
- *Adult and child >30 kg:* PO 12-15 mg/kg as single dose
- *Child <30 kg:* PO 20 mg/kg in 2 divided doses q2-8h
Available forms: Caps 250 mg
Side effects/adverse reactions:
INTEG: Rash, pruritus, urticaria
CNS: Dizziness, headache, drowsiness, insomnia, *convulsions,* hallucination, personality changes, stimulation
EENT: Bad taste, oral irritation
GI: Nausea, vomiting, anorexia, abdominal pain
HEMA: Increased sed rate, reticulocyte count, increase or decrease in leukocytes
Contraindications: Hypersensitivity

Precautions: Pregnancy (C), lactation, seizure disorders

Pharmacokinetics:

PO: Peak 1-1½ hr, half-life 1-2½ hr; excreted in urine (unchanged/metabolites)

Lab test interferences:

Interferences: Urinalysis

NURSING CONSIDERATIONS

Assess:

• Stools during entire treatment, 1, 3 mo after treatment; specimens must be sent to lab while still warm

• For allergic reaction: rash, itching, urticaria

• For infection in other family members, since infection from person to person is common

Administer:

• PO after meals to avoid GI symptoms

Perform/provide:

• Storage in tight container, cool environment

Evaluate:

• Therapeutic response: expulsion of worms, 3 negative stool cultures after completion of treatment

Teach patient/family:

• Proper hygiene after BM, including hand-washing technique; tell patient to avoid putting fingers in mouth

• That infected person should sleep alone; do not shake bed linen; change bed linen daily; wash in hot water

• To clean toilet qd with disinfectant (green soap solution)

• Need for compliance with dosage schedule, duration of treatment

• That urine may turn orange or red

• To avoid hazardous activities since drowsiness occurs

• That seizures may recur in patient who is controlled on medication

---

oxandrolone

(ox-an′droe-lone)

Oxandrin, Oxandrolone

Func. class.: Androgenic anabolic steroid

Chem. class.: Halogenated testosterone derivative

Action: Increases weight by building body tissue, increases potassium, phosphorus, chloride, nitrogen levels, increases bone development

Uses: Tissue building after steroid therapy, osteoporosis, prolonged immobility

Dosage and routes:

• *Adult:* PO 2.5 mg bid-qid, not to exceed 20 mg qd × 2-3 wk

• *Child:* PO 0.25 mg/kg/day × 2-4 wk, not to exceed 3 mo

Available forms: Tabs 2.5 mg

Side effects/adverse reactions:

INTEG: Rash, acneiform lesions, oily hair, skin, flushing, sweating, acne vulgaris, alopecia, hirsutism

CNS: Dizziness, headache, fatigue, tremors, paresthesias, flushing, sweating, anxiety, lability, insomnia

MS: Cramps, spasms

CV: Increased B/P

GU: **Hematuria,** amenorrhea, vaginitis, decreased libido, decreased breast size, clitoral hypertrophy, testicular atrophy

GI: Nausea, vomiting, constipation, weight gain, ***cholestatic jaundice***

EENT: Carpal tunnel syndrome, conjunctival edema, nasal congestion

ENDO: Abnormal GTT

Contraindications: Severe renal disease, severe cardiac disease, severe hepatic disease, hypersensitiv-

---

italics = common side effects   ***bold italic*** = life threatening reactions

ity, pregnancy (X), lactation, genital bleeding (abnormal)

Precautions: Diabetes mellitus, CV disease, MI

Pharmacokinetics:
PO: Metabolized in liver, excreted in urine, crosses placenta, excreted in breast milk

Interactions/incompatibilities:
• Increased effects of: oral antidiabetics, oxyphenbutazone
• Increased PT: anticoagulants
• Edema: ACTH, adrenal steroids
• Decreased effects of: insulin

Lab test interferences:
Increase: Serum cholesterol, blood glucose, urine glucose
Decrease: Serum Ca, serum K, T_4, T_3, thyroid ^{131}I uptake test, urine 17-OHCS, 17-KS, PBI, BSP

NURSING CONSIDERATIONS
Assess:
• Weight daily; notify physician if weekly weight gain is >5 lb
• B/P q4h
• I&O ratio; be alert for decreasing urinary output, increasing edema
• Growth rate in children, since growth rate may be uneven (linear/bone growth) when used for extended time
• Electrolytes: K, Na, Cl, Ca; cholesterol
• Liver function studies: ALT, AST, bilirubin
• Edema, hypertension, cardiac symptoms, jaundice
• Mental status: affect, mood, behavioral changes, aggression
• Signs of masculinization in female: increased libido, deepening of voice, decreased breast tissue, enlarged clitoris, menstrual irregularities; male: gynecomastia, impotence, testicular atrophy
• Hypercalcemia: lethargy, polyuria, polydipsia, nausea, vomiting,

constipation; drug may have to be decreased
• Hypoglycemia in diabetics, since oral anticoagulant action is decreased

Administer:
• Titrated dose; use lowest effective dose

Perform/provide:
• Diet with increased calories and protein; decrease Na if edema occurs
• Supportive drug of anemia

Evaluate:
• Therapeutic response: occurs in 4-6 wk in osteoporosis

Teach patient/family:
• That drug must be combined with complete health plan: diet, rest, exercise
• To notify physician if therapeutic response decreases
• Not to discontinue this medication abruptly
• About change in sex characteristics
• Women to report menstrual irregularities
• That 1-3 mo course is necessary for response in breast cancer
• Procedure for use of buccal tablets (requires 30-60 min to dissolve, change absorption site with each dose; do not eat, drink, chew, or smoke while tablet is in place)

---

oxaprozin
(ox-a-pro-zin)
Daypro
Func. class.: Nonsteroidal antiinflammatory
Chem. class.: Propionic acid derivative

Action: May inhibit prostaglandin synthesis by decreasing enzyme needed for biosynthesis; analgesic, antiinflammatory, antipyretic

Uses: Acute and long-term management of osteoarthritis, rheumatoid arthritis

Dosage and routes:
• *Adult:* PO 600-1200 mg qd; maximum dose 1800 mg/day or 26 mg/kg, whichever is lower

Available forms: Tablets 600 mg

Side effects/adverse reactions:
GI: Nausea, anorexia, vomiting, diarrhea, jaundice, ***cholestatic hepatitis***, constipation, flatulence, cramps, dry mouth, peptic ulcer
CNS: Dizziness, headache, drowsiness, fatigue, tremors, confusion, insomnia, anxiety, depression
CV: Tachycardia, peripheral edema, palpitations, dysrhythmias
INTEG: Purpura, rash, pruritus, sweating
*GU: **Nephrotoxicity: dysuria, hematuria, oliguria, azotemia***
*HEMA: **Blood dyscrasias***
EENT: Tinnitus, hearing loss, blurred vision

Contraindications: Hypersensitivity, asthma, patients in whom aspirin and iodides have induced symptoms of allergic reactions or asthma

Precautions: Pregnancy (B) 1st and 2nd trimester, lactation, children, bleeding disorders, GI disorders, cardiac disorders, hypersensitivity to other antiinflammatory agents, severe renal and hepatic disease, elderly

Pharmacokinetics:
PO: Peak 2 hr, half-life 3-3½ hr; metabolized in liver; excreted in urine (metabolites), breast milk; 99% plasma protein binding

Interactions/incompatibilities:
• Oxaprozin may decrease effects of: loop diuretics and β-blockers
• May increase the action or tox-icity of: coumarin, phenytoin, lithium, methotrexate
• May increase effects of oxaprozin: phenobarbital, probenecid
• Salicylates may decrease plasma levels of oxaprozin

NURSING CONSIDERATIONS
Assess:
• Renal, liver, blood studies: BUN, creatinine, AST, ALT, Hgb, before treatment, periodically thereafter
• Audiometric: ophthalmic examination before, during, after treatment
• For eye, ear problems: blurred vision, tinnitus; may indicate toxicity

Administer:
• With food to decrease GI symptoms

Perform/provide:
• Storage at room temperature

Evaluate:
• Therapeutic response: decreased pain, stiffness in joints, decreased swelling in joints, ability to move more easily

Teach patient/family:
• To report blurred vision, ringing, roaring in ears; may indicate toxicity
• To avoid driving, other hazardous activities if dizziness/drowsiness occurs
• To report change in urine pattern, increased weight, edema, increased pain in joints, fever, blood in urine; indicates nephrotoxicity
• That therapeutic effects may take up to 1 mo
• To take with a full glass of water to enhance absorption

---

italics = common side effects   ***bold italic*** = life threatening reactions

oxazepam

(ox-a'ze-pam)
Apo-Oxazepam,* Novoxa-
pam,* Oxazepam, Ox-Pam,*
Serax, Zapex*
Func. class.: Antianxiety
Chem. class.: Benzodiazepine

Controlled Substance Schedule IV

Action: Potentiates the actions of GABA, especially in limbic system and reticular formation

Uses: Anxiety, alcohol withdrawal

Dosage and routes:

Anxiety
• *Adult:* PO 10-30 mg tid-qid
Alcohol withdrawal
• *Adult:* PO 15-30 mg tid-qid

Available forms: Caps 10, 15, 30 mg, tabs 10, 15, 30 mg

Side effects/adverse reactions:

CNS: Dizziness, drowsiness, confusion, headache, anxiety, tremors, fatigue, depression, insomnia, hallucinations, paradoxical excitement, transient amnesia

GI: Nausea, vomiting, anorexia

INTEG: Rash, dermatitis, itching

CV: Orthostatic hypotension, ECG changes, tachycardia, hypotension

EENT: Blurred vision, tinnitus, mydriasis

Contraindications: Hypersensitivity to benzodiazepines, narrow-angle glaucoma, psychosis, pregnancy (D), child <12 yr

Precautions: Elderly, debilitated, hepatic disease, renal disease

Pharmacokinetics:

PO: Peak 2-4 hr, metabolized by liver, excreted by kidneys, half-life 5-15 hr

Interactions/incompatibilities:

• Decreased effects of oxazepam:

oral contraceptives, valproic acid
• Increased effects of oxazepam: CNS depressants, alcohol, disulfiram, oral contraceptives

Lab test interferences:

Increase: AST/ALT, serum bilirubin
Decrease: RAIU
False increase: 17-OHCS

NURSING CONSIDERATIONS

Assess:

• B/P (lying, standing), pulse; if systolic B/P drops 20 mm Hg, hold drug, notify physician
• Blood studies: CBC during long-term therapy; blood dyscrasias have occurred rarely
• Hepatic studies: AST, ALT, bilirubin, creatinine, LDH, alk phosphatase
• Mental status: mood, sensorium, affect, sleeping pattern, drowsiness, dizziness
• Physical dependency, withdrawal symptoms: headache, nausea, vomiting, muscle pain, weakness, tremors, *convulsions* after long-term use
• Suicidal tendencies

Administer:

• With food or milk for GI symptoms
• Sugarless gum, hard candy, frequent sips of water for dry mouth

Perform/provide:

• Assistance with ambulation during beginning therapy; drowsiness/dizziness occurs
• Safety measures, including side rails
• Check to see PO medication has been swallowed

Evaluate:

• Therapeutic response: decreased anxiety, restlessness, insomnia

Teach patient/family:

• That drug may be taken with food
• Not to be used for everyday stress

or used longer than 4 mo unless directed by physician; not to take more than prescribed dose; may be habit forming
• To avoid OTC preparations (cough, cold, hay fever) unless approved by physician
• To avoid driving, activities that require alertness, since drowsiness may ocur
• To avoid alcohol ingestion, other psychotropic medications unless prescribed by physician
• Not to discontinue medication abruptly after long-term use
• To rise slowly, or fainting may occur, especially elderly
• That drowsiness may worsen at beginning of treatment
Treatment of overdose: Lavage, VS, supportive care, flumazenil

---

oxidized cellulose
Oxycel, Surgicel
Func. class.: Hemostatic
Chem. class.: Cellulose product

Action: Absorbs blood, acts as an artificial clot
Uses: Hemostasis in surgery, oral surgery, exodontia
Dosage and routes:
Adult and child: TOP apply using sterile technique as needed, remove after bleeding stops, if possible, or leave in place if needed
Available forms: TOP knitted fabric as strips, pads, pledgets
Side effects/adverse reactions:
EENT: Sneezing, burning in epistaxis
INTEG: Burning, stinging, encapsulation of fluid, foreign bodies
CNS: Headache in epistaxis
Contraindications: Hypersensitivity, large artery hemorrhage, ooz-

ing surfaces, implantation in bone deficit, placement around optic nerve, and chiasm
NURSING CONSIDERATIONS
Assess:
• Allergy: fever, rash, itching, burning, stinging
Administer:
• Dry; use only amount needed to control bleeding
• Loosely; remove excess before closure in surgery; irrigate first, then remove using sterile technique
• Using sterile technique; cannot be resterilized
Evaluate:
• Therapeutic response: decreased bleeding in surgery

---

oxtriphylline
(ox-trye'fi-lin)
Choledyl, Choledyl SA, Novo-triphyl,* Oxtriphylline
Func. class.: Bronchodilator, spasmolytic
Chem. class.: Choline salt of theophylline

Action: Relaxes smooth muscle of respiratory system by blocking phosphodiesterase, which increases cyclic AMP; 64% theophylline
Uses: Acute bronchial asthma, reversible bronchospasm in chronic bronchitis and COPD
Dosage and routes:
• *Adult and child >12 yr:* PO 200 mg qid
• *Child 2-12 yr:* PO 4 mg/kg q6h; may be increased to desired response, therapeutic level
Available forms: Elix 100 mg/5 ml; syr 50 mg/5 ml; tabs 100, 200, 400, 600 mg
Side effects/adverse reactions:
CNS: Anxiety, restlessness, insom-

---

*nia, dizziness, **convulsions,*** headache, light-headedness
CV: Palpitations, sinus tachycardia, hypotension
GI: Nausea, vomiting, anorexia, diarrhea, bitter taste, dyspepsia
RESP: Increased rate
INTEG: Flushing, urticaria, alopecia
Contraindications: Hypersensitivity to xanthines, tachydysrhythmias
Precautions: Elderly, CHF, cor pulmonale, hepatic disease, active peptic ulcer disease, diabetes mellitus, hyperthyroidism, hypertension, children, pregnancy (C), glaucoma, prostatic hypertrophy
Pharmacokinetics:
SOL: Peak 1 hr; metabolized in liver; excreted in urine, breast milk; crosses placenta
Interactions/incompatibilities:
• Increased action of oxtriphylline: cimetidine, erythromycin, troleandomycin, oral contraceptive, propranolol
• May increase effects of: anticoagulants, coffee (caffeine items)
• Cardiotoxicity: β-blockers
• Decreased effect of: lithium
• Decreased theophylline level: rifampin, phenytoin
NURSING CONSIDERATIONS
Assess:
• Therapeutic blood levels; toxicity may occur with small increase above therapeutic level
• Therapeutic theophylline levels: 11-20
• Smoking reduces effects of theophyllines, requiring larger doses
• Respiratory rate, rhythm, depth; auscultate lung fields bilaterally; notify physician of abnormalities
• Allergic reactions: rash, urticaria; if these occur, drug should be discontinued

Administer:
• PO after meals to decrease GI symptoms; absorption may be affected
• After meals, hs
Perform/provide:
• Storage in closed container away from heat; protect elixir from light
Evaluate:
• Therapeutic response: absence of dyspnea, wheezing
Teach patient/family:
• Tablets should not be chewed or crushed
• To check OTC medications, current prescription medications for ephedrine, which will increase stimulation
• To avoid hazardous activities; dizziness may occur
• If GI upset occurs, to take drug with 8 oz water; avoid food; absorption may be decreased
• To notify physician of toxicity: nausea, vomiting, anxiety, convulsions, insomnia, rapid pulse
• To notify physician of change in smoking habit; may need to change dose; encourage not to smoke

oxybutynin chloride

(ox-i-byoo'ti-nin)
Ditropan, Oxybutynin chloride
Func. class.: Spasmolytic
Chem. class.: Synthetic tertiary amine

Action: Relaxes smooth muscles in urinary tract
Uses: Antispasmodic for neurogenic bladder
Dosage and routes:
• *Adult:* PO 5 mg bid-tid, not to exceed 5 mg qid
• *Child >5 yr:* PO 5 mg bid, not to exceed 5 mg tid

Available forms: Sol 5 mg/5 ml;
tabs 5 mg

Side effects/adverse reactions:

*HEMA: **Leukopenia, eosinophilia***

CNS: Anxiety, restlessness, *dizziness, **convulsions,*** headache,
drowsiness, confusion

CV: Palpitations, sinus tachycardia, hypotension

GI: Nausea, vomiting, anorexia,
abdominal pain, constipation

GU: Dysuria, retention, hesitancy

INTEG: Urticaria, dermatitis

EENT: Blurred vision, increased intraocular tension, dry mouth, throat

Contraindications: Hypersensitivity, GI obstruction, GI hemorrhage,
GU obstruction, glaucoma, severe
colitis, myasthenia gravis, unstable
CV status in acute hemorrhage

Precautions: Pregnancy (C), lactation, suspected glaucoma, children <12 yr

Pharmacokinetics: Onset ½-1 hr,
peak 3-4 hr, duration 6-10 hr; metabolized by liver, excreted in urine

NURSING CONSIDERATIONS

Assess:

• Allergic reactions: rash, urticaria;
if these occur, drug should be discontinued

Evaluate:

• Urinary status: dysuria, frequency, nocturia, incontinence

Teach patient/family:

• To avoid hazardous activities;
dizziness may occur

---

oxycodone HCl

(ox-i-koe'done)

Supeudol,* Roxicodone, Roxicoden, Intensol; **Combinations**—Codoxy, Percocet,*
Percocet-Demi, Percodan, Tylox **(check each for specific ingredients)**

Func. class.: Narcotic analgesics

Chem. class.: Opiate, semisynthetic derivative

Controlled Substance Schedule II

Action: Inhibits ascending pain
pathways in CNS, increases pain
threshold, alters pain perception

Uses: Moderate to severe pain

Dosage and routes:

• *Adult:* REC 1-3 supp/day prn
(Supeubol)

• *Child:* PO ¼-½ tab q6h prn (Percodan-Demi)

• *Adult:* PO 1-2 tab q6h prn (Combinations)

Available forms: Tabs 5 mg; sol 5
mg/5ml

Side effects/adverse reactions:

CNS: Drowsiness, dizziness, confusion, headache, sedation, euphoria

*GI: Nausea, vomiting, anorexia,
constipation, cramps*

GU: Increased urinary output, dysuria, urinary retention

INTEG: Rash, urticaria, bruising,
flushing, diaphoresis, pruritus

EENT: Tinnitus, blurred vision,
miosis, diplopia

CV: Palpitations, bradycardia,
change in B/P

*RESP: **Respiratory depression***

Contraindications: Hypersensitivity, addiction (narcotic)

Precautions: Addictive personality, pregnancy (B), lactation, increased intracranial pressure, MI

---

italics = common side effects   ***bold italic*** = life threatening reactions

(acute), severe heart disease, respiratory depression, hepatic disease, renal disease, child <18 yr

Pharmacokinetics:
PO: Onset 10-15 min, peak ½-1 hr, duration 4-5 hr; detoxified by liver, excreted in urine, crosses placenta, excreted in breast milk

Interactions/incompatibilities:
• Increased effects with other CNS depressants: alcohol, narcotics, sedative/hypnotics, antipsychotics, skeletal muscle relaxants

Lab test interferences:
Increase: Amylase

NURSING CONSIDERATIONS
Assess:
• I&O ratio; check for decreasing output; may indicate urinary retention
• CNS changes: dizziness, drowsiness, hallucinations, euphoria, LOC, pupil reaction
• Allergic reactions: rash, urticaria
• Respiratory dysfunction: respiratory depression, character, rash, rhythm; notify physician if respirations are <10/min
• Need for pain medication by pain, sedation scoring; physical dependence

Administer:
• With antiemetic if nausea, vomiting occur
• When pain is beginning to return; determine dosage interval by patient response

Perform/provide:
• Storage in light-resistant area at room temperature
• Assistance with ambulation
• Safety measures: side rails, nightlight, call bell within easy reach

Evaluate:
• Therapeutic response: decrease in pain

Teach patient/family:
• To report any symptoms of CNS changes, allergic reactions

• That physical dependency may result when used for extended periods
• That withdrawal symptoms may occur: nausea, vomiting, cramps, fever, faintness, anorexia

Treatment of overdose: Naloxone (Narcan) 0.2-0.8 IV, O$_2$, IV fluids, vasopressors

---

oxymetazoline HCl (nasal)

(ox-i-met-az'oh-leen)
Afrin, Afrin Children's Nose Drops, Allerest 12-Hour Nasal, Chlorphed-LA, Coricidin Nasal Mist, Dristan Long Lasting, Duramist Plus, Duration, Genasal, NTZ Long-Acting Nasal, Nafrine,* Neo-Synephrine 12 Hour, Nōstrilla, Oxymetazoline HCl, Sinarest 12-Hour, Sinex Long-Acting, Twice-A-Day Nasal, 4-Way Long Acting Nasal
Func. class.: Nasal decongestant
Chem. class.: Sympathomimetic amine

Action: Produces vasoconstriction (rapid, long-acting) of arterioles, thereby decreasing fluid exudation, mucosal engorgement

Uses: Nasal congestion

Dosage and routes:
• *Adult and child >6 yr:* instill 2-3 gtts or sprays to each nostril bid
• *Child 2-6 yr:* instill 2-3 gtts or sprays 0.025% sol bid, not to exceed 3 days

Available forms: Sol 0.025%, 0.05%

Side effects/adverse reactions:
GI: Nausea, vomiting, anorexia
EENT: Irritation, burning, sneezing, stinging, dryness, rebound congestion

INTEG: Contact dermatitis

CNS: Anxiety, restlessness, tremors, weakness, insomnia, dizziness, fever, headache

Contraindications: Hypersensitivity to sympathomimetic amines

Precautions: Child <6 yr, elderly, diabetes, cardiovascular disease, hypertension, hyperthyroidism, increased ICP, prostatic hypertrophy, pregnancy (C), glaucoma

Interactions/incompatibilities:

• Hypertension: MAOIs, β-adrenergic blockers

• Hypotension: methyldopa, mecamylamine, reserpine

NURSING CONSIDERATIONS
Assess:

• For redness, swelling, pain in nasal passages

Administer:

• No more than q4h

• For <3 consecutive days

Perform/provide:

• Environmental humidification to decrease nasal congestion, dryness

• Storage in light-resistant container; do not expose to high temperatures

Evaluate:

• Therapeutic response: decreased nasal congestion

Teach patient/family:

• That stinging may occur for a few applications; drying of mucosa may be decreased by environmental humidification

• To notify physician if irregular pulse, insomnia, dizziness, or tremors occur

• Proper administration to avoid systemic absorption

---

oxymetholone
(ox-i-meth'oh-lone)
Anadrol-50, Anapolon 50*
Func. class.: Androgenic anabolic steroid
Chem. class.: Halogenated testosterone derivative

Action: Increases weight by building body tissue, increases potassium, phosphorus, chloride, and nitrogen levels, increases bone development

Uses: Tissue building after steroid therapy, osteoporosis, aplastic anemia, anemias caused by deficient RBC production

Dosage and routes:
Aplastic anemia

• *Adult and child:* PO 1-5 mg/kg/day, titrated to patient response, not to exceed 3 months

Osteoporosis/tissue building (possible indication)

• *Adult:* PO 5-15 mg/day, not to exceed 30 mg/day or 3 mo

• *Child >6 yr:* PO up to 10 mg/day, not to exceed 1 mo

• *Child <6 yr:* PO 1.25 mg qd-qid, not to exceed 1 mo

Available forms: Tabs 50 mg

Side effects/adverse reactions:

INTEG: Rash, acneiform lesions, oily hair, skin, flushing, sweating, acne vulgaris, alopecia, hirsutism

CNS: Dizziness, headache, fatigue, tremors, paresthesias, flushing, sweating, anxiety, lability, insomnia

MS: Cramps, spasms

CV: Increased B/P

GU: **Hematuria,** amenorrhea, vaginitis, decreased libido, decreased breast size, clitoral hypertrophy, testicular atrophy

GI: Nausea, vomiting, constipa-

---

italics = common side effects   **bold italic** = life threatening reactions

tion, weight gain, *cholestatic jaundice*

EENT: Carpal tunnel syndrome, conjunctional edema, nasal congestion

ENDO: Abnormal GTT

Contraindications: Severe renal disease, severe cardiac disease, severe hepatic disease, hypersensitivity, pregnancy (X), lactation, genital bleeding (abnormal)

Precautions: Diabetes mellitus, CV disease, MI

Pharmacokinetics:

PO: Metabolized in liver, excreted in urine, crosses placenta, excreted in breast milk

Interactions/incompatibilities:

• Increased effects of: oral antidiabetics, oxyphenbutazone
• Increased PT: anticoagulants
• Edema: ACTH, adrenal steroids
• Decreased effects of: Insulin

Lab test interferences:

Increase: Serum cholesterol, blood glucose, urine glucose

Decrease: Serum Ca, serum K, T_4, T_3, thyroid ^{131}I uptake test, urine 17-OHCS, 17-KS, PBI, BSP

NURSING CONSIDERATIONS
Assess:

• Weight daily, notify physician if weekly weight gain is >5 lb
• B/P q4h
• I&O ratio; be alert for decreasing urinary output, increasing edema
• Growth rate in children, since growth rate may be uneven (linear/bone growth) when used for extended period
• Electrolytes: K, Na, Cl, Ca; cholesterol
• Liver function studies: ALT, AST, bilirubin
• Edema, hypertension, cardiac symptoms, jaundice

• Mental status: affect, mood, behavioral changes, aggression
• Signs of masculinization in female: increased libido, deepening of voice, breast tissue, enlarged clitoris, menstrual irregularities; male: gynecomastia, impotence, testicular atrophy
• Hypercalcemia: lethargy, polyuria, polydipsia, nausea, vomiting, constipation; drug may have to be decreased
• Hypoglycemia in diabetics since oral antidiabetic action is increased

Administer:

• Titrated dose; use lowest effective dose

Perform/provide:

• Diet with increased calories and protein; decrease Na if edema occurs
• Supportive drug of anemia

Evaluate:

• Therapeutic response: occurs in 4-6 wk in osteoporosis

Teach patient/family:

• That drug needs to be combined with complete health plan: diet, rest, exercise
• To notify physician if therapeutic response decreases
• Not to discontinue this medication abruptly
• About changes in sex characteristics
• That women should report menstrual irregularities
• That 1-3 mo course is necessary for response in breast cancer
• Procedure for use of buccal tablets (requires 30-60 min to dissolve; change absorption site with each dose; do not eat, drink, chew, or smoke while tablet is in place)

oxymorphone HCl

(ox-i-mor-fone)
Numorphan, Numorphan H.P.
Func. class.: Narcotic analgesic
Chem. class.: Opiate, semisynthetic phenanthrene derivative

Controlled Substance Schedule II
Action: Inhibits ascending pain pathways in CNS, increases pain threshold, alters pain perception
Uses: Moderate to severe pain
Dosage and routes:
• *Adult:* IM/SC 1-1.5 mg q4-6h prn; IV 0.5 mg q4-6h prn; REC 2.5-5 mg q4-6h prn
Available forms: Inj SC, IM, IV 1, 1.5 mg/ml; supp 5 mg
Side effects/adverse reactions:
CNS: Drowsiness, dizziness, confusion, headache, sedation, euphoria
GI: Nausea, vomiting, anorexia, constipation, cramps
GU: Increased urinary output, dysuria, urinary retention
INTEG: Rash, urticaria, bruising, flushing, diaphoresis, pruritus
EENT: Tinnitus, blurred vision, miosis, diplopia
CV: Palpitations, bradycardia, change in B/P
*RESP: **Respiratory depression***
Contraindications: Hypersensitivity, addiction (narcotic)
Precautions: Addictive personality, pregnancy (B), lactation, increased intracranial pressure, MI (acute), severe heart disease, respiratory depression, hepatic disease, renal disease, child <18 yr
Pharmacokinetics:
SC/IM: Onset 10-15 min, peak 1-½ hr, duration 2-6 hr
IV: Onset 5-10 min, peak 1-½ hr, duration 3-6 hr

REC: Onset 15-30 min, duration 3-6 hr
Metabolized by liver, excreted in urine, crosses placenta
Interactions/incompatibilities:
• Increased effects with other CNS depressants: alcohol, narcotics, sedative/hypnotics, antipsychotics, skeletal muscle relaxants
• Incompatiblity not known
Lab test interferences:
Increase: Amylase
NURSING CONSIDERATIONS
Assess:
• I&O ratio; check for decreasing output; may indicate urinary retention
• CNS changes: dizziness, drowsiness, hallucinations, euphoria, LOC, pupil reaction
• Allergic reactions: rash, urticaria
• Respiratory dysfunction: respiratory depression, character, rate, rhythm; notify physician if respirations are <10/min
• Need for pain medication, physical dependence
Administer:
• IV after diluting with 5 ml sterile H₂O or NS for inj; give over 2-5 min through Y-tube or 3-way stopcock
• With antiemetic if nausea, vomiting occur
• When pain is beginning to return; determine dosage interval by patient response
Perform/provide:
• Storage in light-resistant area at room temperature
• Assistance with ambulation
• Safety measures: side rails, nightlight, call bell within easy reach
Evaluate:
• Therapeutic response: decrease in pain
Teach patient/family:
• To report any symptoms of CNS changes, allergic reactions

italics = common side effects   ***bold italic*** = life threatening reactions

• That physical dependency may result when used for extended periods
• That withdrawal symptoms may occur: nausea, vomiting, cramps, fever, faintness, anorexia
Treatment of overdose: Naloxone (Narcan) 0.2-0.8 IV, O$_2$, IV fluids, vasopressors

---

oxyphenbutazone
(ox-i-fen-byoo′ta-zone)
Oxybutazone,* Oxyphenbutazone
Func. class.: Nonsteroidal antiinflammatory
Chem. class.: Pyrazolone derivative

Action: Inhibits prostaglandin synthesis by decreasing an enzyme needed for biosynthesis; analgesic, antiinflammatory, antipyretic
Uses: Mild to moderate pain, osteoarthritis, rheumatoid arthritis
Dosage and routes:
Pain
• *Adult:* PO 100-200 mg tid-qid
Acute arthritis
• *Adult:* PO 400 mg, then 100 mg q4h × 4 days or until desired response
Available forms: Tabs 100 mg
Side effects/adverse reactions:
GI: Nausea, anorexia, vomiting, diarrhea, jaundice, *cholestatic hepatitis,* constipation, flatulence, cramps, dry mouth, peptic ulcer
CNS: Dizziness, drowsiness, fatigue, tremors, confusion, insomnia, anxiety, depression
CV: Tachycardia, peripheral edema, palpitations, dysrhythmias, hypertension, cardiac decompensation
INTEG: Purpura, rash, pruritus, sweating

GU: Nephrotoxicity: dysuria, hematuria, oliguria, azotemia
HEMA: Blood dyscrasias, bone marrow suppression
EENT: Tinnitus, hearing loss, blurred vision
Contraindications: Hypersensitivity, asthma, severe renal disease, severe hepatic disease, pregnancy (D), children <14 yr, ulcer disease
Precautions: Lactation, children, bleeding disorders, GI disorders, cardiac disorders, hypersensitivity to other antiinflammatory agents
Pharmacokinetics:
PO: Peak 2 hr, half-life 3-3½ hr; metabolized in liver, excreted in urine (metabolites), excreted in breast milk
Interactions/incompatibilities:
• Increased action of: coumarin, phenytoin, sulfonamides
NURSING CONSIDERATIONS
Assess:
• Renal, liver, blood studies: BUN, creatinine, AST, ALT, Hgb before treatment, periodically thereafter
• Audiometric, ophthalmic exam before, during, after treatment
• For eye, ear problems: blurred vision, tinnitus (may indicate toxicity)
Administer:
• With food to decrease GI symptoms; best to take on empty stomach to facilitate absorption
Perform/provide:
• Storage at room temperature
Evaluate:
• Therapeutic response: decreased pain, stiffness, swelling in joints, ability to move more easily
Teach patient/family:
• To report blurred vision, or ringing, roaring in ears (may indicate toxicity)
• To avoid driving, other hazardous

---

activities if dizziness or drowsiness occurs
• To report change in urine pattern, weight increase, edema, pain increase in joints, fever, blood in urine (indicates nephrotoxicity)
• That therapeutic effects may take up to 1 mo

---

oxytetracycline HCl
(ox-i-tet-ra-sye′kleen)
Oxytetracycline HCl, Terramycin, Terramycin IM, Uri-Tet
Func. class.: Broad-spectrum antibiotic/antiinfective
Chem. class.: Tetracycline

Action: Inhibits protein synthesis, phosphorylation in microorganisms by binding to 30S ribosomal subunits, reversibly binding to 50S ribosomal subunits; bacteriostatic
Uses: Syphilis, chlamydia trachomatis, gonorrhea, lymphogranuloma venereum, uncommon gram-positive/negative organisms, rickettsial infections
Dosage and routes:
• *Adult:* PO 250-500 mg q6h; IM 100 mg q8h or 150 mg q12h IV 250-500 mg q12h, 250 mg q24h
• *Child >8 yr:* PO 25-50 mg/kg/day in divided doses q6h; IM 15-25 mg/kg/day in divided doses q8-12h; IV 10-20 mg/kg/day in divided doses q12h
Gonorrhea
• *Adult:* PO 1.5 g, then 500 mg qid for a total of 9 g
Chlamydia trachomatis
• *Adult:* PO 500 mg qid × 7 days
Syphilis
• *Adult:* PO 2-3 g in divided doses × 10-15 days up to 30-40 g total
• Dosage adjustment necessary in renal impairment
Available forms: Tabs 250 mg;

caps 125, 250 mg; powder for inj IV 250, 500 mg; inj IM 50, 125 mg/ml
Side effects/adverse reactions:
CNS: Fever
HEMA: **Eosinophilia, neutropenia, thrombocytopenia, leukocytosis, hemolytic anemia**
EENT: Dysphagia, glossitis, decreased calcification of deciduous teeth, oral candidiasis
GI: Nausea, abdominal pain, *vomiting, diarrhea,* anorexia, enterocolitis, *hepatotoxicity,* flatulence, abdominal cramps, epigastric burning, stomatitis
CV: Pericarditis
GU: Increased BUN
INTEG: Rash, urticaria, photosensitivity, increased pigmentation, **exfoliative dermatitis,** pruritus, angioedema, pain at injection site
Contraindications: Hypersensitivity to tetracyclines, children <8 yr, pregnancy (D)
Precautions: Renal disease, hepatic disease, lactation
Pharmacokinetics:
PO: Peak 2-4 hr, half-life 6-12 hr; excreted in urine, bile, feces in active form; crosses placenta; 20%-40% protein bound
Interactions/incompatibilities:
• Decreased effect of oxytetracycline: antacids, $NaHCO_3$, dairy products, alkali products, iron, kaolin/pectin, cimetidine
• Increased effect: anticoagulants
• Decreased effect: penicillins, oral contraceptives
• Nephrotoxicity: methoxyflurane
• Do not mix with other drugs
Lab test interferences:
False negative: Urine glucose with Clinistix or Tes-Tape
False increase; Urinary catecholamines

---

italics = common side effects   **bold italic** = life threatening reactions

NURSING CONSIDERATIONS
Assess:
• I&O ratio
• Blood studies: PT, CBC, AST, ALT, BUN, creatinine
• Signs of anemia: Hct, Hgb, fatigue
• Allergic reactions: rash, itching, pruritus, angioedema
• Nausea, vomiting, diarrhea; administer antiemetic, antacids as ordered
• Overgrowth of infection: increased temperature, malaise, redness, pain, swelling, drainage, perineal itching, diarrhea, changes in cough or sputum
Administer:
• PO with a full glass of water
• IM, deep only
• IV after diluting 250 mg or less/10 ml of sterile H₂O for inj; further dilute with at least 100 ml of D₅W or NS for inj; give 100 mg or less/5 min or more; use within 12 hr, decrease rate or increase volume of diluent if vein irritation occurs; do not give SC
• After C&S obtained
• 2 hr before or after laxative or ferrous products, 3 hr after antacid
Perform/provide:
• Storage in tight, light-resistant container at room temperature
Evaluate:
• Therapeutic response: decreased temperature, absence of lesions, negative C&S
Teach patient/family:
• To avoid sun exposure, since burns may occur; sunscreen does not seem to decrease photosensitivity
• If diabetic to avoid use of Clinistix, Diastix, Tes-Tape for urine glucose testing
• That all prescribed medication must be taken to prevent superimposed infection
• To avoid milk products, to take with a full glass of water

oxytocin, synthetic injection
(ox-i-toe'sin)
Pitocin, Syntocinon
Func. class.: Oxytocic
Chem. class.: Hormone

Action: Acts directly on myofibrils, producing uterine contraction; stimulates milk ejection by the breast
Uses: Stimulation, induction of labor; missed or incomplete abortion; postpartum bleeding
Dosage and routes:
Stimulation of labor
• *Adult:* IV INF 1 ml/1 L D₅W or 0.9% NaCl over 1-2 mU/min; may increase q15-30 min, not to exceed 20 mU/min
Incomplete abortion
• *Adult:* IV INF 10 U/500 ml D₅W or 0.9% NaCl given at 20-40 mU/min
Available forms: Inj IV 10 U/ml
Side effects/adverse reactions:
CNS: Hypertension, *convulsions, tetanic contractions*
CV: Hypotension, dysrhythmias, increased pulse, bradycardia, tachycardia, PVC
FETUS: Dysrhythmias, jaundice, hypoxia, *intracranial hemorrhage*
GI: Anorexia, nausea, vomiting, constipation
GU: **Abruptio placentae, decreased uterine blood flow**
HEMA: Increased hyperbilirubinemia
INTEG: Rash
RESP: Asphyxia
Contraindications: Hypersensitiv-

ity, serum toxemia, cephalopelvic disproportion, fetal distress, hypertonic uterus

Precautions: Cervical/uterine surgery, uterine sepsis, primipara >35 yr, 1st, 2nd stage of labor

Pharmacokinetics:

IM: Onset 3-7 min, duration 1 hr, half-life 12-17 min

IV: Onset 1 min, duration 30 min, half-life 12-17 min

Interactions/incompatibilities:

• Hypertension: vasopressors

• Incompatible with levarterenol, prochlorperazine, warfarin

NURSING CONSIDERATIONS

Assess:

• I&O ratio

• Respiration

• B/P, pulse; watch for changes that may indicate hemorrhage

• Respiratory rate, rhythm, depth; notify physician of abnormalities

• Length, intensity, duration of contraction; notify physician of contractions lasting over 1 min or absence of contractions; turn patient on her side

• FHTs, fetal distress; watch for acceleration, deceleration; notify physician if problems occur; fetal presentation, pelvic dimensions; turn patient on left side if FHT change in rate

• For signs and symptoms of water intoxication; confusion, anuria, drowsiness, headache

Administer:

Labor induction

• IV after diluting 10 U/L of 0.9% NS or D₅ NS run at 1-2 mU/min at 15-30 min intervals to begin normal labor; dilute 10-40 mU/min, titrate to control postpartum bleeding; dilute 10 U/500 ml of solution; run 10 U-20 mU/ml; administer by only 1 route at a time; use inf pump;

rotate inf to provide mixing; do not shake

Control of postpartum bleeding

• IV: Dilute 10-40 U/1 L of sol, run at 10-20 mU 1 min; adjust rate as needed

• With crash cart available on unit (Mg⁺, SO₄ at bedside)

Evaluate:

• Therapeutic response: stimulation of labor, control of postpartum bleeding

Teach patient/family:

• To report increased blood loss, abdominal cramps, increased temperature or foul-smelling lochia

• That contractions will be similar to menstrual cramps, gradually increasing in intensity

---

oxytocin, synthetic nasal

(ox-i-toe'sin)

Func. class.: Oxytocic hormone

Action: Acts directly on myofibrils, producing uterine contraction; stimulates milk ejection by the breast

Uses: Postpartum breast engorgement, initial milk letdown

Dosage and routes:

• *Adult:* Nas spray 1 spray into one or both nostrils q2-3min before breast-feeding; nas drops 3 gtts into one or both nostrils q2-3min before breast-feeding

Available forms: Nas spray 40 U/ml; nas drops

Side effects/adverse reactions: None

Pharmacokinetics:

Onset 5-10 min, half-life 1 min

Interactions/incompatibilities:

• Hypertension: vasopressors

italics = common side effects   ***bold italic*** = life threatening reactions

NURSING CONSIDERATIONS
Assess:
• I&O ratio
• Environment conducive to let-down reflex
Evaluate
• Therapeutic response: stimulation of milk ejection
Teach patient/family:
• To blow nose before administering; not to touch dropper to inside of nares
• To rinse dropper with warm water after each use
• Not to overuse

---

paclitaxel
(pack-lye′-tax-el)
Taxol
Func. class.: Misc. antineoplastic
Chem. class.: Natural diterpene

Action: Inhibits the reorganization of the microtubule network needed for interphase and mitotic cellular functions; also causes abnormal bundles of microtubules during cell cycle and multiple esters of microtubules during mitosis
Uses: Metastatic carcinoma of the ovary
Dosage and routes:
• *Adult:* IV INF 135/m² given over 24 hrs q 3 wks
Available forms: 30 mg (5 ml) vial (IV)
Side effects/adverse reactions:
*HEMA: **Neutropenia, leutropenia, thrombocytopenia, anemia,** bleeding, infections*
SYST: Hypersensitivity reactions
CV: Bradycardia, hypotension, abnormal ECG
NEURO: Peripheral neuropathy
MS: Arthralgia, myalgia
GI: Nausea, vomiting, diarrhea,
mucositis, increased bilirubin, alk phosphatase, AST
INTEG: Alopecia
Contraindications: Hypersensitivity to paclitaxel or other drugs with polyoxyethylated castor oil, neutropenia of <1500/mm³, pregnancy (D)
Precautions: Children, lactation, hepatic, cardiovascular disease, CNS disorder
Pharmacokinetics: 89%-98% of drug is serum protein bound, metabolized in liver, excreted in bile and urine; terminal half-life 5.3–17.4 hr
Interactions/incompatibilities:
• Increased myelosuppression: cisplatin
• Decreased metabolism of paclitaxel: ketoconazole
NURSING CONSIDERATIONS
Assess:
• CBC, differential, platelet count weekly; withhold drug if WBC is <4000 or platelet count is 100,000, neutrophil is <1500/mm³; notify physician of results
• Monitor temperature q4h (may indicate beginning infection)
• Liver function tests before, during therapy (bilirubin, AST, alk phosphatase) as needed or monthly
• Vital signs during first hour of infusion
• Hypersensitive reactions including hypotension, dyspnea, angioedema, generalized urticaria; discontinued infusion immediately if these occur
• Bleeding: hematuria, guaiac, bruising or petechiae, mucosa or orifices q8h; obtain prescription for viscous lidocaine (Xylocaine)
• Food preferences; list likes, dislikes
• Effects of alopecia on body im-

age; discuss feelings about body changes

Administer:

• IV after diluting in 0.9% NaCl, D₅, D₅ and 0.9% NaCl, D₅LR to a concentration of 0.3-1.2 mg/ml
• Using an in-line filter <0.22 μm
• After premedicating with dexamethasone 20 mg PO 12 hr and 6 hr before paclitaxel or diphenhydramine 50 mg IV ½-1 hr before paclitaxel and cimetidine 300 mg or ranitidine 50 mg IV ½-1 hr before paclitaxel
• Using only glass bottles, polypropylene, polyolefin bags and administration sets; do not use PVC infusion bags or sets
• Using gloves and cytotoxic handling precautions
• Antiemetic 30-60 min before giving drug to prevent vomiting, and prn
• Antibiotics for prophylaxis of infection

Perform/provide:

• Storage of prepared sol up to 27 hr in refrigeration

Evaluate:

• Therapeutic response: decreased tumor size, spread of malignancy

Teach patient/family:

• To report signs of infection: increased temperature, sore throat, flu symptoms
• To report signs of anemia: fatigue, headache, faintness, shortness of breath, irritability
• To report bleeding; avoid use of razors, commercial mouthwash
• To avoid use of aspirin, ibuprofen
• To report any complaints or side effects to nurse or physician
• That hair may be lost during treatment; a wig or hairpiece may make patient feel better; new hair may be different in color, texture

---

pamidronate
(pam-i-drone'ate)
Aredia
Func. class.: Bone-resorption inhibitor
Chem. class.: Bisphosphonate

Action: Absorbs calcium phosphate crystals in bone and may directly block dissolution of hydroxyappetite crystals of bone; inhibits bone resorption, apparently without inhibiting bone formation and mineralization

Uses: Moderate to severe hypercalcemia associated with malignancy with or without bone metastases

Dosage and routes:

• *Adult:* IV INF 60-90 mg in moderate hypercalcemia, 90 mg in severe hypercalcemia given over 24 hr

Available forms: Inj 30 mg pamidronate disodium and 470 mg of mannitol

Side effects/adverse reactions:

INTEG: Redness, swelling, induration, pain on palpitation at site of catheter insertion
META: Anemia, hypokalemia, hypomagnesemia, hypophosphatemia
GI: Abdominal pain, anorexia, constipation, nausea, vomiting
MS: Bone pain
CV: Hypertension
GU: UTI, fluid overload

Contraindications: Hypersensitivity to biphosphonates

Precautions: Children, nursing mothers, pregnancy (C), renal dysfunction

Pharmacokinetics: Rapidly cleared from circulation and taken up mainly by bones, eliminated primarily by kidneys

P

---

italics = common side effects   ***bold italic*** = life threatening reactions

Interactions/incompatibilities:
• Do not mix with Ca-containing infusion solutions such as Ringer's solutions

NURSING CONSIDERATIONS
Assess:
• Renal studies and Ca, P, Mg, K
Administer:
• After reconstituting by adding 10 ml of sterile water for inj to each vial, then adding to 1000 ml of sterile 0.45%, 0.9% NaCl, D₅W, run over 24 hr
Perform/provide:
• Storage of infusion solution for up to 24 hr at room temperature
• Reconstituted solution with sterile water may be stored under refrigeration for up to 24 hr
Evaluate:
• Therapeutic response: decreased Ca levels

---

pancreatin
(pan'kree-a-tin)
Elzyme 303 Enseals
Func. class.: Digestant
Chem. class.: Pancreatic enzyme concentrate—bovine/porcine

Action: Pancreatic enzyme needed for proper pancreatic functioning
Uses: Exocrine pancreatic secretion insufficiency, cystic fibrosis (digestive aid)
Dosage and routes:
• *Adult:* PO 8000-24,000 USP U with meals
Available forms: Tab 650, 2000, 12,000 U
Side effects/adverse reactions:
GI: Anorexia, nausea, vomiting, diarrhea, glossitis, anal soreness
GU: Hyperuricuria, hyperuricemia
INTEG: Rash, hypersensitivity
EENT: Buccal soreness

Contraindications: Hypersensitivity to pork, chronic pancreatic disease
Precautions: Pregnancy (C), lactation
Interactions/incompatibilities:
• Decreased absorption: cimetidine, antacids, oral iron
NURSING CONSIDERATIONS
Assess:
• I&O ratio; watch for increasing urinary output
• Fecal fat, N, pro-time, Ca during treatment
• For polyuria, polydipsia, polyphagia (may indicate diabetes mellitus)
Administer:
• After antacid or H₂ blockers; decreased pH inactivates drug
• Whole; not to be crushed, chewed (enteric coated)
• Low-fat diet to decrease GI symptoms
Perform/provide:
• Storage in tight container at room temperature
Evaluate:
• For allergy to pork

---

pancrelipase
(pan-kre-li'pase)
Cotazym Capsules, Cotazym-S Capsules, Creon Capsules, Entolase-HP, Festal II Tablets, Ilozyme Tables, Ku-Zyme HP Capsules, Pancrease Capsules, Pancrease MT 4, Pancrease MT 10, Pancrease MT 16, Pancrease MT 25, Ultrase MT 12, Ultrase MT 20, Ultrase MT 24, Viokase Powder, Viokase Tablets, Zymase
Func. class.: Digestant
Chem. class.: Pancreatic enzyme—bovine/porcine

Action: Pancreatic enzyme needed

for proper pancreatic functioning
Uses: Exocrine pancreatic secretion insufficiency, cystic fibrosis (digestive aid), steatorrhea, pancreatic enzyme deficiency
Dosage and routes:
• *Adult and child:* PO 1-3 caps/tabs ac or with meals, or 1 caps/tab with snack or 1-2 pdr pkt ac
Available forms: Tab 8000, 11,000, 30,000 U; caps 8000, 30,000 U; enteric coated caps 4000, 5000, 20,000, 25,000 U; powd 16,800 U
Side effects/adverse reactions:
GI: Anorexia, nausea, vomiting, diarrhea
GU: Hyperuricuria, hyperuricemia
Contraindications: Allergy to pork, chronic pancreatic disease
Precautions: Pregnancy (C)
Interactions/incompatibilities:
• Decreased absorption: cimetidine, antacids, oral iron
NURSING CONSIDERATIONS
Assess:
• I&O ratio; watch for increasing urinary output
• Fecal fat, nitrogen, pro-time during treatment
• For polyuria, polydipsia, polyphagia (may indicate diabetes mellitus)
Administer:
• After antacid or cimetidine; decreased pH inactivates drug
• Powder mixed in prepared fruit for infants, children
• Whole, not crushed or chewed (enteric coated)
• Low-fat diet to decrease GI symptoms
• Powder mixed with pureed fruit; take tabs with or before food
Perform/provide:
• Storage in tight container at room temperature

italics = common side effects

Evaluate:
• For allergy to pork

pancuronium bromide
(pan-kyoo-roe'nee-um)
Pancuronium Bromide, Pavulon
Func. class.: Neuromuscular blocker (nondepolarizing)
Chem. class.: Synthetic curariform

Action: Inhibits transmission of nerve impulses by binding with cholinergic receptor sites, antagonizing action of acetylcholine
Uses: Facilitation of endotracheal intubation, skeletal muscle relaxation during mechanical ventilation, surgery, or general anesthesia
Dosage and routes:
• *Adult:* IV 0.04-0.1 mg/kg, then 0.01 mg/kg q½-1hr
• *Child >10 yr:* IV 0.04-0.1 mg/kg, then ⅕ initial dose q½-1hr
Available forms: Inj IV, IM, 1, 2 mg/ml
Side effects/adverse reactions:
CV: Bradycardia; tachycardia; increased, decreased B/P; ventricular extra systoles
*RESP: **Prolonged apnea, bronchospasm, cyanosis, respiratory depression***
EENT: Increased secretions
MS: Weakness to prolonged skeletal muscle relaxation
INTEG: Rash, flushing, pruritus, urticaria, sweating, salivation
Contraindications: Hypersensitivity to bromide ion
Precautions: Pregnancy (C), renal disease, cardiac disease, lactation, children <2 yr, electrolyte imbalances, dehydration, neuromuscular disease, respiratory disease

bold italic = life threatening reactions

Pharmacokinetics:
IV: Onset 30-45 sec, peak 3-5 min; metabolized (small amounts), excreted in urine (unchanged), crosses placenta

Interactions/incompatibilities:
• Increased neuromuscular blockade: aminoglycosides, clindamycin, lincomycin, quinidine, local anesthetics, polymyxin antibiotics, lithium, narcotic analgesics, thiazides, enflurane, isoflurane
• Dysrhythmias: theophylline
• Incompatible with barbiturates in solution or syringe

Lab test interferences:
Decrease: Cholinesterase

NURSING CONSIDERATIONS
Assess:
• For electrolyte imbalances (K, Mg); may lead to increased action of this drug
• Vital signs (B/P, pulse, respirations, airway) until fully recovered; rate, depth, pattern of respirations, strength of hand grip
• I&O ratio; check for urinary retention, frequency, hesitancy
• Recovery: decreased paralysis of face, diaphragm, leg, arm, rest of body; allow to recover fully before completing a neuro assessment
• Allergic reactions: rash, fever, respiratory distress, pruritus; drug should be discontinued

Administer:
• With diazepam or morphine when used for therapeutic paralysis; this drug provides no sedation alone
• Using nerve stimulator by anesthesiologist to determine neuromuscular blockade
• Atropine to counteract muscarinic effects
• After succinylcholine effects subside

• Anticholinesterase to reverse neuromuscular blockade
• IV undiluted, give over 1-2 min (only by qualified persons)

Perform/provide:
• Storage in refrigerator; do not store in plastic container or syringe; use only fresh solution
• Reassurance if communication is difficult during recovery from neuromuscular blockade
• Frequent (q2h) instillation of artificial tears and covering eyes to prevent drying of cornea

Evaluate:
• Therapeutic response: paralysis of jaw, eyelid, head, neck, rest of body

Treatment of overdose: Edrophonium or neostigmine, atropine, monitor VS; may require mechanical ventilation

---

papaverine HCl
(pa-pav'er-een)
Cerespan, Genabid, Papaverine HCl, Pavabid HP Capsulets, Pavabid Plateau Caps, Pavarine Spancaps, Pavased, Pavatine, Pavatym, Paverolan Lanacaps
Func. class.: Peripheral vasodilator
Chem. class.: Opium alkaloid (no narcotic activity)

Action: Relaxes all smooth muscle; inhibits cyclic nucleotide phosphodiesterase, which increases intracellular cAMP, causing vasodilation

Uses: Arterial spasm resulting in cerebral and peripheral ischemia; myocardial ischemia associated with vascular spasm or dysrhythmias; angina pectoris; peripheral pulmonary embolism; visceral spasm as in ureteral, biliary, GI colic PVD

Dosage and routes:

• *Adult:* PO 100-300 mg 3-5 times day; sus rel 150-300 mg q8-12h; IM/IV 30-120 mg q3h prn

Available forms: Cap time-release 150, 200, 300 mg; tabs 30, 60, 100, 150, 200, 300 mg; inj IM/IV 30 mg/ml

Side effects/adverse reactions:

CV: Tachycardia, increased B/P

RESP: Increased depth of respirations

CNS: Headache, dizziness, drowsiness, sedation, vertigo, malaise

GI: Nausea, anorexia, abdominal pain, constipation, diarrhea, jaundice, altered liver enzymes, *hepatotoxicity*

INTEG: Flushing, sweating, rash

Contraindications: Hypersensitivity, complete AV heart block

Precautions: Cardiac dysrhythmias, glaucoma, pregnancy (C), lactation, drug dependency, children

Pharmacokinetics:

PO: Onset 30 sec, peak 1-2 hr, duration 3-4 hr

SUS REL: Onset erratic

90% bound to plasma proteins, metabolized in liver, excreted in urine (inactive metabolites)

Interactions/incompatibilities:

• Decreased effect of: levodopa

• Increased hypotension: antihypertensives, vasodilators, diazoxide, alcohol

• Incompatible with alkaline sol, aminophylline, iodides, bromides

NURSING CONSIDERATIONS

Assess:

• B/P, pulse, respiratory rate, rhythm, character during treatment until stable; take B/P lying, standing; orthostatic hypotension is common

• Hepatic tests: AST, ALT, bilirubin; liver enzymes may increase

• Hepatic hypersensitivity reaction: nausea, vomiting, jaundice; drug should be discontinued if this occurs

Administer:

• With meals to reduce GI upset

• An ordered analgesic if headache develops

• IV undiluted or diluted in equal amount of sterile H_2O; give 30 mg or less/2 min through Y-tube or 3-way stopcock

Perform/provide:

• Storage at room temperature

Evaluate:

• Therapeutic response: ability to walk without pain, increased pulse volume, increased temperature in extremities or orientation, long- and short-term memory

Teach patient/family:

• That medication is not cure, may have to be taken continuously depending on condition; therapeutic response may not be evident for 2-3 mo

• That it is necessary to quit smoking to prevent excessive vasoconstriction

• To avoid hazardous activities until stabilized on medication; dizziness may occurs

• To notify physician if nausea, flushing, sweating, headache, or jaundice occurs

Treatment of overdose: Discontinue medication

---

paraldehyde

(par-al′de-hyde)

Paral, Paraldehyde

Func. class.: Anticonvulsant

Chem. class.: Cyclic ether

Controlled Substance Schedule IV

Action: CNS depressant; exact

P

---

italics = common side effects

bold italic = life threatening reactions

mechanism of action is unknown

Uses: Refractory seizures, status epilepticus, sedation, insomnia, alcohol withdrawal, tetanus, eclampsia

Dosage and routes:

Seizures

• *Adult:* IM 5-10 ml; divide 10 ml into 2 inj; IV 0.2-0.4 ml/kg in NS inj

• *Child:* IM 0.15 ml/kg; REC 0.3 ml/kg q4-6h or 1 ml/yr of age, not to exceed 5 ml; may repeat in 1 hr prn; IV 5 ml/90 ml NS inj; begin infusion at 5 ml/hr; titrate to patient response

Alcohol withdrawal

• *Adult:* PO/REC 5-10 ml, not to exceed 60 ml; IM 5 ml q4-6h × 24 hr, then q6h on following days, not to exceed 30 ml

Sedation

• *Adult:* PO/REC 4-10 ml; IM 5 ml; IV 3-5 ml to be used in emergency only

• *Child:* PO/REC/IM 0.15 ml/kg

Tetanus

• *Adult:* IV 4-5 ml or 12 ml by gastric tube q4h diluted with water; IM 5-10 ml prn

Available forms: Inj IM, IV; oral and rectal liquid

Side effects/adverse reactions:

*HEMA: **Thrombocytopenia, agranulocytosis, leukopenia, neutropenia, hemolytic anemia,*** increased pro-time

CNS: Stimulation, drowsiness, dizziness, confusion, ***convulsion,*** headache, flushing, hallucinations, coma

*GI: **Foul breath,*** irritation

GU: Nephrosis

*INTEG: **Rash, erythema,*** local pain, sloughing fat necrosis

CV: Pulmonary edema, ***pulmonary hemorrhage, circulatory collapse, respiratory depression***

Contraindications: Hypersensitivity, gastroenteritis with ulceration

Precautions: Asthma, hepatic disease, pulmonary disease, pregnancy (C)

Pharmacokinetics:

PO: Onset 10-15 min, peak 1-2 hr, duration 6-8 hr

REC: Onset slow, duration 4-6 hr; metabolized by liver; excreted by kidneys, lungs; crosses placenta; half-life 7.5 hr

Interactions/incompatibilities:

• Increased blood levels of paraldehyde: alcohol, CNS depressants, general anesthetics, disulfiram

• Increase crystallization in kidneys: sulfonamides

• Incompatible with chlorpromazine, prochlorperazine, plastics; do not mix in syringe or sol with any drug

Lab test interferences:

False positive: Ketones (serum)(urine), interference, 17-OHCS

NURSING CONSIDERATIONS

Assess:

• VS q30min after parenteral route

• Blood studies: Hct, Hgb, RBCs, serum folate, Vit D if on long-term therapy

• Hepatic studies: AST, ALT, bilirubin, creatinine, failure

• For signs of jaundice, hepatitis

• Mental status: mood, sensorium, affect, memory (long, short)

• Respiratory dysfunction; respiratory depression, character, rate, rhythm; hold drug if respirations are >10/min or if pupils are dilated

Administer:

• IV after diluting 1 ml/20 ml of NaCl for inj; give 21 ml or less over 3-5 min

• IM injection in deep large muscle

mass; use Z-track method to prevent tissue sloughing; maximum of 5 ml at any one site
• After conservative measures have been tried for insomnia
• Rectal after diluting in cottonseed or olive oil as retention enema or 200 ml NS for enema
• Keep patient's room well ventilated to remove exhaled drug
• Orally with juice or milk to cover taste/smell, decrease GI symptoms
• Using fresh supply; don't expose to air, don't use if brown or if odor is vinegary or if container opened >24 hr
• Using glass container only; reacts with plastic

Perform/provide:
• Ventilation of room

Evaluate:
• Therapeutic response: increased sedation, decreased seizures

Teach patient/family:
• That physical dependency may result when used for extended periods
• To avoid driving, other activities that require alertness
• Not to discontinue medication quickly after long-term use; taper over several weeks

---

paramethadione
(par-a-meth-a-dye′one)
Paradione
Func. class.: Anticonvulsant
Chem. class.: Oxazolidinedione

Action: Increases seizure threshold in cortex and basal ganglia; decreases synaptic stimulation to low-frequency impulses

Uses: Refractory absence (petit mal) seizures

Dosage and routes:
• *Adult:* PO 300 mg tid; may increase by 300 mg/wk, not to exceed 600 mg qid
• *Child >6 yr:* PO 0.9 g/day in divided doses tid or qid
• *Child 2-6 yr:* PO 0.6 g/day in divided doses tid or qid
• *Child <2 yr:* PO 0.3 g/day in divided doses tid or qid
Available forms: Caps 150, 300 mg; sol 300 mg/ml

Side effects/adverse reactions:
HEMA: **Thrombocytopenia, agranulocytosis, leukopenia, neutropenia, hemolytic anemia,** increased pro-time
CNS: Drowsiness, dizziness, fatigue, paresthesia, irritability, headache
GU/GYN: Vaginal bleeding, albuminuria, nephrosis
GI: Nausea, vomiting, abdominal pain, weight loss, bleeding gums, abnormal liver function tests
INTEG: **Exfoliative dermatitis,** rash, alopecia, petechiae, erythema
EENT: Photophobia, diplopia, epistaxis, retinal hemorrhage
CV: Hypertension, hypotension

Contraindications: Hypersensitivity, blood dyscrasias, pregnancy (D)

Precautions: Hepatic disease, renal disease, retinal or optic nerve damage

Pharmacokinetics:
PO: Onset 15-30 min, peak 1-2 hr, duration 4-6 hr
REC: Onset slow, duration 4-6 hr, metabolized by the liver, excreted by the kidneys, crosses placenta, excreted in breast milk, half-life 1-3½ hr

NURSING CONSIDERATIONS
Assess:
• Blood studies: Hct, Hgb, RBCs, serum folate, Vit D if on long-term

P

---

italics = common side effects   ***bold italic*** = life threatening reactions

therapy; discontinue drug if neutrophil count falls below 2500/mm³
- Hepatic studies: ALT, AST, bilirubin
- Skin: If rash occurs, withhold drug
- Mental status: mood, sensorium, affect, memory (long, short)

Administer:
- After diluting oral solution with water
- Oral with juice or milk to cover taste/smell, to decrease GI symptoms

Perform/provide:
- Ventilation of room

Evaluate:
- Therapeutic response: decreased seizures

Teach patient/family:
- To avoid driving, other activities that require alertness
- Not to discontinue medication quickly after long-term use; convulsions may result
- To obtain liver function tests and urinalysis monthly
- To notify physician if sore throat, fever, malaise, bruises, petechiae, or epistaxis occurs
- To wear dark glasses if photosensitivity occurs
- To take drug with food, milk to decrease GI symptoms

---

paramethasone acetate
(par-a-meth'a-sone)
Haldrone
Func. class.: Corticosteroid
Chem. class.: Glucocorticoid, long acting

Action: Decreases inflammation by suppression of migration of polymorphonuclear leukocytes, fibroblasts, reversal to increase capillary permeability and lysosomal stabilization

Uses: Severe inflammation, collagen disorders, respiratory, dermatologic disorders, adrenal insufficiency

Dosage and routes:
- *Adult:* PO 0.5-6 mg tid-qid
- *Child:* PO 58-800 μg/kg/day in divided doses tid-qid

Available forms: Tabs 2 mg

Side effects/adverse reactions:
INTEG: Acne, poor wound healing, ecchymosis, petechiae
CNS: Depression, flushing, sweating, headache, mood changes
*CV: Hypertension, **circulatory collapse, thrombophlebitis, embolism,** tachycardia, edema
*HEMA: **Thrombocytopenia***
MS: Fractures, osteoporosis, weakness
GI: Diarrhea, nausea, abdominal distention, ***GI hemorrhage,*** increased appetite, ***pancreatitis***
EENT: Fungal infections, increased intraocular pressure, blurred vision

Contraindications: Psychosis, hypersensitivity, idiopathic thrombocytopenia, acute glomerulonephritis, amebiasis, fungal infections, nonasthmatic bronchial disease, child <2 yr, AIDS, TB

Precautions: Pregnancy (C), diabetes mellitus, glaucoma, osteoporosis, seizure disorders, ulcerative colitis, CHF, myasthenia gravis, renal disease, esophagitis, peptic ulcer

Pharmacokinetics:
PO: Peak 1-2 hr, duration 2 days
IM: Peak 3-45 hr

Interactions/incompatibilities:
- Decreased action of paramethasone: cholestyramine, colestipol, barbiturates, rifampin, ephedrine, phenytoin, theophylline

---

*Available in Canada only

• Decreased effects of: anticoagulants, anticonvulsants, antidiabetics, ambenonium, neostigmine, isoniazid, toxoids, vaccines
• Increased side effects: alcohol, salicylates, indomethacin, amphotericin B, digitalis preparations
• Increased action of paramethasone: salicylates, estrogens, indomethacin

Lab test interferences:
Increase: Cholesterol, Na, blood glucose, uric acid, Ca, urine glucose
Decrease: Ca, K, T_4, T_3, thyroid ^{131}I uptake test, urine 17-OHCS, 17-KS, PBI
False negative: Skin allergy tests

NURSING CONSIDERATIONS
Assess:
• K, blood sugar, urine glucose while on long-term therapy; hypokalemia and hyperglycemia
• Weight daily; notify physician of weekly gain >5 lb
• B/P q4h, pulse; notify physician if chest pain occurs
• I&O ratio; be alert for decreasing urinary output and increasing edema
• Plasma cortisol levels during long-term therapy (normal level: 138-635 nmol/L SI units when drawn at 8 AM)
• Infection: increased temperature, WBC, even after withdrawal of medication; drug masks symptoms of infection
• K, depletion: paresthesias, fatigue, nausea, vomiting, depression, polyuria, dysrhythmias, weakness
• Edema, hypertension, cardiac symptoms
• Mental status: affect, mood, behavioral changes, aggression

Administer:
• Titrated dose; use lowest effective dose

• In one dose in AM to prevent adrenal suppression; avoid SC administration may damage tissue
• With food or milk to decrease GI symptoms

Perform/provide:
• Assistance with ambulation in patient with bone tissue disease to prevent fractures

Evaluate:
• Therapeutic response: ease of respirations, decreased inflammation

Teach patient/family:
• That ID as steroid user should be carried
• To notify physician if therapeutic response decreases; dosage adjustment may be needed
• Not to discontinue this medication abruptly or adrenal crisis can result
• To avoid OTC products: salicylates, alcohol in cough products, cold preparations unless directed by physician
• About cushingoid symptoms
• Symptoms of adrenal insufficiency: nausea, anorexia, fatigue, dizziness, dyspnea, weakness, joint pain

P

---

pargyline HCl
(par'gi-leen)
Eutonyl
Func. class.: Antihypertensive
Chem. class.: MAOI

Action: Inhibits monoamine oxidase, decreasing B/P
Uses: Moderate to severe hypertension

Dosage and routes:
• *Adult:* PO 25 mg daily; increase by 10 mg q7d, not to exceed 200 mg; maintenance dosage: 25-50 mg daily

---

italics = common side effects   ***bold italic*** = life threatening reactions

Available forms: Tabs 10, 25, 50 mg

Side effects/adverse reactions:

CV: Orthostatic hypotension, tachycardia, chest pain, bradycardia, fluid retention, ***CHF***

CNS: Drowsiness, dizziness, sedation, headache, depression, insomnia, weakness, fatigue, confusion, blurred vision, EPS

GI: Nausea, vomiting, anorexia, constipation, weight gain

EENT: Dry mouth

GU: Impotence

MS: Arthralgia

MISC: Sweating, increased appetite, hypoglycemia

Contraindications: Hypersensitivity, malignant hypertension, paranoid schizophrenia, severe pulmonary failure, pheochromocytoma, hyperthyroidism, advanced renal failure, children <12 yr

Precautions: Pregnancy (C), lactation, impaired renal function, liver disease, CAD, parkinsonism, diabetes mellitus

Pharmacokinetics:

Excreted in urine, therapeutic response may take 4 days–3 weeks

Interactions/incompatibilities:

• Hypertensive crisis: amphetamine, cyclopentamide, ephedrine, pseudoephedrine, metaraminol, methylphenidate, phenylpropanolamine, levodopa, methyldopa, reserpine, tryptamine, tyramine foods

• Hypotension and increased sedation: barbiturates, alcohol, narcotics, CNS depressants, antihypertensive agents

• May potentiate effects: doxapram, narcotics, phenothiazines, other psychotropic agents, tricyclic antidepressants

NURSING CONSIDERATIONS

Assess:

• Electrolytes: K, Na, Cl, CO_2

• Renal function studies: catecholamines, BUN, creatinine

• Hepatic function studies: AST, ALT, alk phosphatase

• Weight daily, I&O

• B/P lying, standing before starting treatment

• Nausea, vomiting, diarrhea

• Edema in feet, legs daily

• Skin turgor, dryness of mucous membranes for hydration status

Administer:

• Gum, frequent rinsing of mouth or hard candy for dry mouth

Evaluate:

• Therapeutic response: lower B/P

Teach patient/family:

• To report dizziness, palpitations, fainting

• To change position slowly, or fainting may occur

• To take drug exactly as prescribed

• Not to eat tyramine-rich foods: beer, wine, pickled products, yeast products, aged cheeses, avocados, chocolate

• That drug may cause drowsiness

• To avoid all OTC products unless directed by physician

Treatment of overdose: Induce emesis or gastric lavage, support respiration; severe hypertension—administer α-blocker, treat CNS stimulation with IV diazepam, maintain fluid, electrolyte balance

paromomycin sulfate

(par-oh-moe-mye'sin)

Humatin

Func. class.: Amebicide

Chem. class.: Aminoglycoside antibiotic

Action: Direct action in intestinal lumen

Uses: Intestinal amebiasis, adjunct in hepatic coma

Dosage and routes:

Intestinal amebiasis

• *Adult and child:* PO 25-35 mg/kg/day in 3 divided doses × 5-10 days pc

Hepatic coma

• *Adult:* 4 g qd in divided doses × 5-6 days

Available forms: Caps 250 mg

Side effects/adverse reactions:

EENT: Ototoxicity

GI: Nausea, vomiting, diarrhea, epigastric distress, anorexia, steatorrhea, pruritus ani, hypocholesterolemia

GU: Nephrotoxicity, hematuria

Contraindications: Hypersensitivity, renal disease, GI obstruction

Precautions: GI ulcerations, pregnancy (C), children, lactation

Pharmacokinetics:

PO: Excreted in feces, urine, slowly

Lab test interferences:

Decrease: Serum cholesterol

NURSING CONSIDERATIONS

Assess:

• Stools during entire treatment; should be clear at end of therapy; stools should be free of parasite for 1 yr before patient is considered cured

• I&O, stools for number, frequency, character

• Allergic reaction: rash, itching; drug should be discontinued if these occur

• Diarrhea for 2-3 days

Administer:

• Cleansing enema if ordered before beginning treatment

• PO after meals to avoid GI symptoms

Perform/provide:

• Storage in tight container

Evaluate:

• Therapeutic response: decreased diarrhea, stools clear on culture

Teach patient/family:

• Proper hygiene after BM: handwashing technique

• Avoid contact of drug with eyes, mouth, nose, other mucous membranes

• Need for compliance with dosage schedule, duration of treatment

paroxetine

(par-oh'xe-teen)

Paxil

Func. class.: Antidepressant, serotonin re-uptake inhibitor

Chem. class.: Phenylpiperidine derivative

Action: Inhibits CNS neuron uptake of serotonin but not of norepinephrine

Uses: Major depressive disorder

Dosage and routes:

• *Adult:* PO 20 mg qd in AM; after 4 wk if no clinical improvement is noted, dose may be increased by 10 mg/day qwk to desired response, not to exceed 50 mg/day

Available forms: Tabs 20, 30 mg

Side effects/adverse reactions:

CNS: Headache, nervousness, insomnia, drowsiness, anxiety, tremor, dizziness, fatigue, sedation, abnormal dreams, agitation,

P

apathy, euphoria, hallucinations, delusions, psychosis
GI: Nausea, diarrhea, dry mouth, anorexia, dyspepsia, constipation, cramps, vomiting, taste changes, flatulence, decreased appetite
INTEG: Sweating, rash
RESP: Infection, pharyngitis, nasal congestion, sinus headache, sinusitis, cough, dyspnea
CV: Vasodilation, postural hypotension, palpitations
MS: Pain, arthritis, myalgia, myopathy, myosthenia
GU: Dysmenorrhea, decreased libido, urinary frequency, urinary tract infection, amenorrhea, cystitis, impotence, abnormal ejaculation
EENT: Visual changes
SYST: Asthenia, fever
Contraindications: Hypersensitivity, patients taking MAO inhibitors
Precautions: Pregnancy (B), lactation, children, elderly, seizure history, patients with history of mania, renal and hepatic disease
Pharmacokinetics:
PO: Peak 6-8 hr; metabolized in liver, unchanged drugs and metabolites excreted in feces and urine; half-life 2-7 days
Interactions/incompatibilities:
• When used with warfarin: increased bleeding
• Do not use with MAOIs
• Cimetidine increases paroxetine plasma levels
• Increased agitation: L-tryptophan
• Phenobarbital and phenytoin decrease paroxetine levels
• Increased side effects: highly protein-bound drugs
• Paroxetine may increase digoxin levels
Lab test interferences:
• *Increase:* Serum bilirubin, blood glucose, alk phosphatase
• *Decrease:* VMA, 5-HIAA
• *False increase:* Urinary catecholamines

NURSING CONSIDERATIONS
Assess:
• Mental status: mood, sensorium, affect, suicidal tendencies, increase in psychiatric symptoms, depression, panic
• B/P (lying/standing), pulse q4h; if systolic B/P drops 20 mm Hg, hold drug, notify physician; take vital signs q4h in patients with cardiovascular disease
• Blood studies: CBC, leukocytes, differential, cardiac enzymes if patient is receiving long-term therapy
• Hepatic studies: AST, ALT, bilirubin, creatinine
• Weight qwk; appetite may decrease with drug
• ECG for flattening of T wave, bundle branch, AV block, dysrhythmias in cardiac patients
• EPS primarily in elderly, rigidity, dystonia, akathisia
• Urinary retention, constipation
• Withdrawal symptoms: headache, nausea, vomiting, muscle pain, weakness; do not usually occur unless drug was discontinued abruptly
• Alcohol consumption; if alcohol is consumed, hold dose until morning
Administer:
• Increased fluids, bulk in diet if constipation, urinary retention occur
• With food or milk for GI symptoms
• Crushed if patient is unable to swallow medication whole
• Dosage hs if oversedation occurs during the day; may take entire dose hs; elderly may not tolerate once/day dosing

• Gum, hard candy, frequent sips of water for dry mouth

Perform/provide:

• Storage at room temperature; do not freeze

• Assistance with ambulation during therapy, since drowsiness, dizziness occur

• Safety measures including side rails, primarily in elderly

• Checking to see PO medication swallowed

Evaluate:

• Therapeutic response: decreased depression

Teach patient/family:

• That therapeutic effect may take 2-3 wk

• To use caution in driving, other activities requiring alertness because of drowsiness, dizziness, or blurred vision

• Not to discontinue medication quickly after long-term use, may cause nausea, headache, malaise

• To avoid alcohol ingestion, other CNS depressants

---

pemoline
(pem'oh-leen)
Cylert, Cylert Chewable
Func. class.: Cerebral stimulant
Chem. class.: Oxazolidinone derivative

Controlled Substance Schedule IV

Action: Exact mechanism unknown; may act through dopaminergic mechanisms

Uses: Attention deficit disorder with hyperactivity

Dosage and routes:

• *Child >6 yr:* 37.5 mg in AM, increasing by 18.75 mg/wk, not to exceed 112.5 mg/day

Available forms: Tabs 18.75, 37.5, 75 mg; chewable tabs 37.5 mg

Side effects/adverse reactions:

MISC: Rashes, growth suppression in children

CNS: Hyperactivity, insomnia, restlessness, dizziness, depression, headache, stimulation, irritability, aggressiveness, hallucinations, *seizures, Gilles de la Tourette's disorder,* drowsiness, dyskinetic movements

GI: Nausea, anorexia, diarrhea, abdominal pain, increased liver enzymes, hepatitis, jaundice

Contraindications: Hypersensitivity, hepatic insufficiency

Precautions: Renal disease, pregnancy (B), lactation, drug abuse, child <6

Pharmacokinetics:

PO: Peak 2-4 hr, duration 8 hr, metabolized (50%) by liver, excreted (40%) by kidneys, half-life 12 hr

NURSING CONSIDERATIONS

Assess:

• Hepatic function studies: ALT, AST, bilirubin, creatinine

• Child for height, growth rate, since growth retardation occurs

• Mental status: mood, sensorium, affect, stimulation, insomnia, aggressiveness

Administer:

• At least 6 hr before hs

Evaluate:

• Therapeutic response: decreased hyperactivity

Teach patient/family:

• To decrease caffeine consumption (coffee, tea, cola, chocolate), which may increase irritability, stimulation

• To avoid OTC preparations unless approved by physician

• To taper off drug over several weeks

• To avoid alcohol ingestion

---

italics = common side effects   **bold italic** = life threatening reactions

- To avoid hazardous activities until patient is stabilized on medication
- That therapeutic effect may take 2-4 wk

---

penicillin G benzathine
(pen-i-sill'in)
Bicillin L-A, Megacillin,* Permapen, Bicillin C-R, Bicillin C-R 900/300
Func. class.: Broad-spectrum antibiotic
Chem. class.: Natural penicillin

Action: Interferes with cell wall replication of susceptible organisms; osmotically unstable cell wall swells, bursts from osmotic pressure

Uses: Respiratory infections, scarlet fever, erysipelas, otitis media, pneumonia, skin and soft tissue infections, gonorrhea; effective for gram-positive cocci *(Staphylococcus, S. pyogenes, S. viridans, S. faecalis, S. bovis, S. pneumoniae)*, gram-negative cocci *(N. gonorrhoeae)*, gram-positive bacilli *(B. anthracis, C. perfringens, C. tetani, C. diphtheriae, L. monocytogenes)*, gram-negative bacilli *(E. coli, P. mirabilis, Salmonella, Shigella, Enterobacter, S. moniliformis)*, spirochetes *(T. pallidum)*, Actinomyces

Dosage and routes:
Early syphilis
- *Adult:* IM 2.4 million U in single dose
Congenital syphilis
- *Child <2 yr:* IM 50,000 U/kg in single dose
Prophylaxis of rheumatic fever, glomerulonephritis
- *Adult and child >60 lb:* IM 1.2

million U in single dose qmo or 600,000 U q2wk
- *Child <60 lb:* IM 600,000 U in single dose
Upper respiratory infections (group A streptococcal)
- *Adult:* IM 1.2 million U in single dose, PO 400,000-600,000 U q4-6h
- *Child >27 kg:* IM 900,000 U in single dose
- *Child <27 kg:* IM 50,000 U/kg in single dose
Available forms: Inj IM 300,000, 600,000 U/ml; tabs 200,000 U
Side effects/adverse reactions:
HEMA: Anemia, increased bleeding time, *bone marrow depression, granulocytopenia*
GI: Nausea, *vomiting, diarrhea,* increased AST, ALT, abdominal pain, glossitis, colitis
GU: Oliguria, proteinuria, hematuria, vaginitis, moniliasis, glomerulonephritis
CNS: Lethargy, hallucinations, anxiety, depression, twitching, *coma, convulsions*
META: Hyperkalemia, hypokalemia, alkalosis, hypernatremia
MISC: Local pain, tenderness and fever with IM injection
Contraindications: Hypersensitivity to penicillins; neonates
Precautions: Hypersensitivity to cephalosporins, pregnancy (B)
Pharmacokinetics:
IM: Very slow absorption, duration 21-28 days, half-life 30-60 min; excreted in urine, feces, breast milk; crosses placenta
Interactions/incompatibilities:
- Decreased antimicrobial effect of penicillin: tetracyclines, erythromycins
- Increased penicillin concentrations: aspirin, probenecid

---

* Available in Canada only

Lab test interferences:

False positive: Urine glucose, urine protein

NURSING CONSIDERATIONS
Assess:

• I&O ratio; report hematuria, oliguria, since penicillin in high doses is nephrotoxic

• Any patient with compromised renal system, since drug is excreted slowly in poor renal system function; toxicity may occur rapidly

• Liver studies: AST, ALT

• Blood studies: WBC, RBC, H&H, bleeding time

• Renal studies: urinalysis, protein, blood

• C&S before drug therapy; drug may be given as soon as culture is taken

• Bowel pattern before and during treatment

• Skin eruptions after administration of penicillin to 1 wk after discontinuing drug

• Respiratory status: rate, character, wheezing, tightness in chest

• Allergies before initiation of treatment, reaction of each medication; highlight allergies on chart, Kardex; because of prolonged duration of action, allergic reaction may be prolonged and severe

Administer:

• Orally on an empty stomach for best absorption

• Drug after C&S has been completed

• After shaking well, deep IM inj in large muscle masses; avoid intravascular inj, aspirate

Perform/provide:

• Adrenalin, suction, tracheostomy set, endotracheal intubation equipment

• Adequate fluid intake (2 L) during diarrhea episodes

• Scratch test to assess allergy after securing order from physician; usually done when penicillin is only drug of choice

• Storage in tight container; refrigerate injection

Evaluate:

• Therapeutic response: absence of fever, purulent drainage, redness, inflammation

Teach patient/family:

• To take oral penicillin on empty stomach with full glass of water

• That culture may be taken after completed course of medication

• To report sore throat, fever, fatigue; (may indicate superimposed infection)

• To wear or carry Medic Alert ID if allergic to penicillins

• To notify nurse of diarrhea

Treatment of hypersensitivity: Withdraw drug; maintain airway; administer epinephrine, aminophylline, O_2, IV corticosteroids for anaphylaxis

---

penicillin G potassium
Acrocillin, Burcillin-G, Deltapen, Megacillin,* Novopen G,* Pentids, Pfizerpen

Func. class.: Broad-spectrum antibiotic—penicillin
Chem. class.: Natural penicillin

Action: Interferes with cell wall replication of susceptible organisms; osmotically unstable cell wall swells, bursts from osmotic pressure

Uses: Emphysema, gangrene, anthrax, gonorrhea, mastoiditis, meningitis, osteomyelitis, pneumonia, tetanus, urinary tract infections, prophylactically in rheumatic fever; effective for non–penicillinase-producing gram-positive cocci *(S.*

---

aureus, S. pyogenes, S. viridans, S. faecalis, S. bovis, S. pneumoniae), gram-negative cocci *(N. gonorrhoeae, N. meningitidis),* gram-positive bacilli *(B. anthracis, C. perfringens, C. tetani, C. diphtheriae, L. monocytogenes),* gram-negative bacilli *(Bacteroides, F. nucleatum, P. multiocida, S. minor, S. moniliformis),* spirochetes *(T. pallidum, T. pertenue, B. recurrentis, L. icterohaemorrhagiae), Actinomyces*

Dosage and routes:

Pneumococcal/streptococcal infections (mild to moderate)

• *Adult:* PO 400,000-500,000 U q6-8h × 10 days (streptococcal infections) or afebrile × 2 days (pneumococcal infections)

• *Child <12 yr:* PO 25,000-90,000 U/kg/day in 3-6 divided doses

Prevention of recurrence of rheumatic fever

• *Adult:* PO 200,000-250,000 U bid continuously

• *Child <12 yr:* PO 25,000-90,000 U/kg/day in 3-6 divided doses

Vincent's gingivitis/pharyngitis

• *Adult:* PO 400,000-500,000 U q6-8h

Available forms: Tabs 200,000, 250,000, 400,000, 500,000, 800,000 U; powder for oral sol 200,000, 400,000 U/5 ml

Side effects/adverse reactions:

CNS: Lethargy, hallucinations, anxiety, depression, twitching, *coma, convulsions*

GI: Nausea, vomiting, diarrhea, increased AST and ALT, abdominal pain, glossitis, colitis

HEMA: Anemia, *increased bleeding time, bone marrow depression, granulocytopenia*

META: Hyperkalemia, hypokalemia, alkalosis, hypernatremia

Contraindications: Hypersensitivity to penicillins; neonates

Precautions: Hypersensitivity to cephalosporins, pregnancy (B)

Pharmacokinetics:

IV: Peak immediate

IM: Peak ¼-½ hr

PO: Duration 6 hr, peak 1 hr, excreted in urine unchanged, excreted in breast milk, crosses placenta

Interactions/incompatibilities:

• Decreased antimicrobial effectiveness of penicillin: tetracyclines, erythromycins

• Decreased absorption: cholestyramine, colestipol

• Increased penicillin concentrations: aspirin, probenecid

• Incompatible in sol with dextran 40, fat emulsion, aminophylline, cephalothin, tetracyclines, metoclopramide

Lab test interferences:

Decrease: Uric acid

False positive: Urine glucose, urine protein

NURSING CONSIDERATIONS

Assess:

• I&O ratio; report hematuria, oliguria, since penicillin in high doses is nephrotoxic

• For infection: draining wounds, color of sputum, condition of urine, VS, cough

• Any patient with compromised renal system, since drug is excreted slowly in poor renal system function; toxicity may occur rapidly

• Liver studies: AST, ALT; liver enzyme may increase

• Blood studies: WBC, RBC, H & H, bleeding time

• Renal studies: urinalysis, protein, blood

• C&S before drug therapy; drug may be given as soon as culture is taken

---

*Available in Canada only

• Bowel pattern before and during treatment
• Skin eruptions after administration of penicillin to 1 wk after discontinuing drug; rash, pruritus, wheezing, laryngeal spasm
• Respiratory status: rate, character, wheezing, tightness in chest

Administer:
• Orally on an empty stomach for best absorption; avoid acidic or carbonate beverages for 1 hr before and after taking PO form
• Drug after C&S

Perform/provide:
• Adrenalin, suction, tracheostomy set, endotracheal intubation equipment
• Adequate fluid intake (2 L) during diarrhea episodes
• Scratch test to assess allergy after securing order from physician; usually done when penicillin is only drug of choice
• Storage in dry, tight container; oral susp refrigerated 2 wk, 1 wk at room temperature

Evaluate:
• Therapeutic response: absence of fever, draining wounds
• Allergies before initiation of treatment, reaction of each medication; highlight allergies on chart; hypersensitivity reaction may be delayed

Teach patient/family:
• Aspects of drug therapy, including need to complete course of medication to ensure organism death (10-14 days); culture may be taken after completed course
• To report sore throat, fever, fatigue (may indicate superimposed infection)
• To wear or carry Medic Alert ID if allergic to penicillins

• To report diarrhea, prevent dehydration

Treatment of overdose: Withdraw drug, maintain airway, administer epinephrine, aminophylline, O_2, IV corticosteroids for anaphylaxis

penicillin G procaine
Crysticillin A.S., Duracillin A.S., Wycillin, Pfizerpen-AS

Func. class.: Broad-spectrum long-acting antibiotic
Chem. class.: Natural penicillin

Action: Interferes with cell wall replication of susceptible organisms; osmotically unstable cell wall swells, bursts from osmotic pressure

Uses: Empyema, gangrene, anthrax, gonorrhea, mastoiditis, meningitis, osteomyelitis, pneumonia, tetanus, UTIs, prophylactically in rheumatic fever; effective for gram-positive cocci *(S. aureus, S. pyogenes, S. viridans, S. faecalis, S. bovis, S. pneumoniae)*, gram-negative cocci *(N. gonorrhoeae, N. meningitidis)*, gram-positive bacilli *(B. anthracis, C. perfringens, C. tetani, C. diphtheriae, L. monocytogenes)*, gram-negative bacilli *(Bacteroides, F. nucleatum, P. multocida, S. minor, S. moniliformis)*, spirochetes *(T. pallidum, T. pertenue, B. recurrentis, L. icterohaemorrhagiae)*, Actinomyces

Dosage and routes:
Moderate to severe infections
• *Adult and child:* IM 600,000-1.2 million U in one or two doses/day for 10 days to 2 wk
• *Newborn:* 50,000 U/kg IM once daily
Gonorrhea
• *Adult and child >12 yr:* IM 4.8

million units in two injections given 30 min after probenecid 1 g

Pneumonia (pneumococcal)
• *Adult and child >12 yr:* IM 300,000-600,000 U q6-12h

Available forms: Inj IM 300,000, 500,000, 600,000 U/ml, 600,000 U/1.2 ml, 1,200,000 U/dose, 2,400,000 U/dose

Side effects/adverse reactions:
HEMA: Anemia, increased bleeding time, *bone marrow depression, granulocytopenia*
GI: Nausea, vomiting, diarrhea, increased AST, ALT, abdominal pain, glossitis, colitis
GU: Oliguria, proteinuria, hematuria, vaginitis, moniliasis, glomerulonephritis
CNS: Lethargy, hallucinations, anxiety, depression, twitching, *coma, convulsions*
META: Hyperkalemia, hypokalemia, alkalosis, hypernatremia

Contraindications: Hypersensitivity to penicillins, procaine nates

Precautions: Hypersensitivity to cephalosporins, pregnancy (B)

Pharmacokinetics:
IM: Peak 1-4 hr, duration 15 hr, excreted in urine

Interactions/incompatibilities:
• Decreased antimicrobial effect of penicillin: tetracyclines, erythromycins
• Increased penicillin concentrations: aspirin, probenecid

Lab test interferences:
False positive: Urine glucose, urine protein

NURSING CONSIDERATIONS
Assess:
• I&O ratio; report hematuria, oliguria, since penicillin in high doses is nephrotoxic
• Any patient with compromised renal system, since drug is excreted

slowly in poor renal system function; toxicity may occur rapidly
• Liver studies: AST, ALT
• Blood studies: WBC, RBC, H&H, bleeding time
• Renal studies: urinalysis, protein, blood
• C&S before drug therapy; drug may be given as soon as culture is taken
• Bowel pattern before and during treatment
• Skin eruptions after administration of penicillin to 1 wk after discontinuing drug
• Respiratory status: rate, character, wheezing, tightness in chest
• Allergies before initiation of treatment, reaction of each medication; highlight allergies on chart, Kardex
• For transient toxic reaction to procaine, which may occur immediately and subside after 15-30 min

Administer:
• Drug after C&S has been completed
• Deep IM, avoid intravascular inj, aspirate

Perform/provide:
• Adrenalin, suction, tracheostomy set, endotracheal intubation equipment
• Adequate fluid intake (2 L) during diarrhea episodes
• Scratch test to assess allergy after securing order from physician; usually done when penicillin is only drug of choice
• Storage in refrigerator

Evaluate:
• Therapeutic response: absence of fever, purulent drainage, redness, inflammation

Teach patient/family:
• That culture may be taken after completed course of medication

---

*Available in Canada only

• To report sore throat, fever, fatigue (may indicate superimposed infection)

• To wear or carry Medic Alert ID if allergic to penicillins; be aware that allergic reaction may be prolonged because of drug's long duration

• To notify nurse of diarrhea

Treatment of hypersensitivity: Withdraw drug; maintain airway; administer epinephrine, aminophylline, O_2, IV corticosteroids for anaphylaxis

---

penicillin G sodium

Crystapen,* Pfizerpen

Func. class.: Broad-spectrum antibiotic

Chem. class.: Natural penicillin

Action: Acts by interfering with cell wall replication of susceptible organisms; osmotically unstable cell wall swells and bursts from osmotic pressure

Uses: Empyema, gangrene, anthrax, gonorrhea, mastoiditis, meningitis, osteomyelitis, pneumonia, tetanus, urinary tract infections, prophylactically in rheumatic fever; effective for non–penicillinase-producing gram-positive cocci *(S. aureus, S. pyogenes, S. viridans, S. faecalis, S. bovis, S. pneumoniae)*, gram-negative cocci *(N. gonorrhoeae, N. meningitidis)*, gram-positive bacilli *(B. anthracis, C. perfringens, C. tetani, C. diphtheriae, L. monocytogenes)*, gram-negative bacilli *(Bacteroides, E. nucleatum, P. multocida, S. minor, S. moniliformis)*, spirochetes *(T. pallidum, T. pertenue, B. recurrentis, L. icterohaemorrhagiae)*, *Actinomyces*

Dosage an
Moderate to
• *Adult:* IM/\
lion U/day in\
• *Child:* IM/I\
U/day in divided\

Dental surgery prop\ ...s for endocarditis

• *Adult:* IM/IV 2 million U ½-1 hr before procedure, then 1 million U 6 hr after procedure

Available forms: Inj IM, IV 1 million, 5 million, 20 million U

Side effects/adverse reactions:

HEMA: Anemia, increased bleeding time, *bone marrow depression, granulocytopenia*

GI: Nausea, vomiting, diarrhea, increased AST, ALT, abdominal pain, glossitis, colitis

GU: Oliguria, proteinuria, hematuria, vaginitis, moniliasis, *glomerulonephritis*

CNS: Lethargy, hallucinations, anxiety, depression, twitching, *convulsions*

META: Hyperkalemia, hypokalemia, alkalosis, hypernatremia

Contraindications: Hypersensitivity to penicillins; neonates

Precautions: CHF caused by Na retention, pregnancy (B)

Pharmacokinetics:

IM: Peak 1-3 hr, duration 6 hr; excreted in urine

Interactions/incompatibilities:

• Decreased antimicrobial effect of penicillin: tetracyclines, erythromycins

• Increased penicillin concentrations: aspirin, probenecid

• Decreases bacterial action when mixed with acids, alkalines, aminophylline, amphotericin B, cephalothin, chlorpromazine, dopamine, heparin, lincomycin, pentobarbital, phenytoin, prochlorperazine, promazine, promethazine,

P

italics = common side effects   ***bold italic*** = life threatening reactions

..., thiopental, trifluoper-
..., vancomycin, Vit C, Vit B
...n C

Lab test interferences:
False positive: Urine glucose, urine protein

NURSING CONSIDERATIONS
Assess:
• I&O ratio; report hematuria, oliguria, since penicillin in high doses is nephrotoxic
• Any patient with a compromised renal system, since drug is excreted slowly in poor renal system function; toxicity may occur rapidly
• Liver studies: AST, ALT
• Blood studies: WBC, RBC, H&H, bleeding time
• Renal studies: urinalysis, protein, blood
• C&S before drug therapy; drug may be given as soon as culture is taken
• Bowel pattern before, during treatment
• Skin eruptions after administration of penicillin to 1 wk after discontinuing drug
• Respiratory status: rate, character, wheezing, tightness in chest
• Allergies before initiation of treatment, reaction of each medication; highlight allergies on chart, Kardex; hypersensitivity reaction may be delayed

Administer:
• IV after diluting with sterile H_2O; shake; follow manufacturers' instructions for dilution; may be added to 0.9% NaCl; give by continuous inf, usually over 12 hr
• Drug after C&S has been completed

Perform/provide:
• Adrenalin, suction, tracheostomy set, endotracheal intubation equipment
• Adequate fluid intake (2 L) during diarrhea episodes
• Scratch test to assess allergy after securing order from physician; usually done when penicillin is only drug of choice
• Storage of sterile sol in refrigerator for 1 wk, IV sol at room temperature for 24 hr

Evaluate:
• Therapeutic response: absence of fever, purulent drainage, redness, inflammation

Teach patient family:
• That culture may be taken after completed course of medication
• To report sore throat, fever, fatigue (may indicate superimposed infection)
• To wear or carry Medic Alert ID if allergic to penicillins
• To notify nurse of diarrhea

Treatment of overdose: Withdraw drug, maintain airway, administer epinephrine, aminophylline, O_2, IV corticosteroids for anaphylaxis

---

penicillin V potassium
Pen-Vee K*, Deltapen-VK, V-Cillin K, Veetids, PVFK,* Apo-Pen-VK,* Novopen-VK,* Ledercillin-VK, Uticillin-VK, Betapen-VK, Penapar-VK, Robicillin-VK

Func. class.: Broad-spectrum antibiotic
Chem. class.: Natural penicillin

Action: Interferes with cell wall replication of susceptible organisms; osmotically unstable cell wall swells, bursts from osmotic pressure.

Uses: Effective for gram-positive cocci (*S. aureus, S. pyogenes, S. viridans, S. faecalis, S. bovis, S. pneumoniae*), gram-negative cocci

(N. gonorrhoeae, N. meningitidis),
gram-positive bacilli *(B. anthracis,*
C. perfringens, C. tetani, C. diph-
theriae, L. monocytogenes), gram-
negative bacilli *(S. moniliformis),*
spirochetes *(T. pallidum),* Actinomyces

Dosage and routes:
Pneumococcal/staphylococcal in-
fections
• *Adult:* PO 250-500 mg q6h
• *Child <12 yr:* PO 15-50 mg/kg/
day in divided doses q6-8hr
Streptococcal infections
• *Adult:* PO 125-250 mg q6-8h ×
10 days
Prevention of recurrence of rheu-
matic fever/chorea
• *Adult:* PO 125-250 mg bid con-
tinuously
Vincent's infection of oropharynx
• *Adult:* PO 500 mg q6h
Available forms: Tabs 125, 250,
500 mg; film-coated tabs 250, 500
mg; powder for oral susp 125, 250
mg/5 ml

Side effects/adverse reactions:
HEMA: Anemia, increased bleeding
time, *bone marrow depression,*
granulocytopenia
GI:Nausea, vomiting, diarrhea, increased AST, ALT, abdominal
pain, glossitis, colitis
GU: Oliguria, proteinuria, hema-
turia, vaginitis, moniliasis, *glo-*
merulonephritis
CNS: Lethargy, hallucinations, anxiety, *depression,* twitching, *coma,*
convulsions
META: Hyperkalemia, hypokalemia, alkalosis
Contraindications: Hypersensitivity to penicillins; neonates
Precautions: Hypersensitivity to
cephalosporins, pregnancy (B)
Pharmacokinetics:
PO: Peak 30-60 min, duration 6-8

hr, half-life 30 min, excreted in
urine, breast milk
Interactions/incompatibilities:
• Decreased antimicrobial effec-
tiveness of penicillin: tetracyclines,
erythromycins
• Increased penicillin concentra-
tions: aspirin, probenecid
Lab test interferences:
False positive: Urine glucose, urine
protein
NURSING CONSIDERATIONS
Assess:
• I&O ratio; report hematuria, oliguria, since penicillin in high doses
is nephrotoxic
• Any patient with compromised
renal system, since drug is excreted
slowly in poor renal system function; toxicity may occur rapidly
• Liver studies: AST, ALT
• Blood studies: WBC, RBC,
H&H, bleeding time
• Renal studies: urinalysis, protein,
blood
• C&S before drug therapy; drug
may be given as soon as culture is
taken
• Bowel pattern before and during
treatment
• Skin eruptions after administration of penicillin to 1 wk after discontinuing drug
• Respiratory status: rate, character, wheezing, tightness in chest
• Allergies before initiation of
treatment, reaction of each medi-
cation; highlight allergies on chart,
Kardex
Administer:
• Orally with food for best absorption
• Drug after C&S has been completed
Perform/provide:
• Adrenalin, suction, tracheostomy
set, endotracheal intubation equipment

P

---

italics = common side effects   ***bold italic*** = life threatening reactions

• Adequate fluid intake (2 L) during diarrhea episodes
• Scratch test to assess allergy after securing order from physician; usually done when penicillin is only drug of choice
• Storage in tight container; after reconstituting, refrigerate for up to 2 wk

Evaluate:
• Therapeutic response: absence of fever, draining wounds

Teach patient/family:
• Aspects of drug therapy, including need to complete entire course of medication to ensure organism death (10-14 days); culture may be taken after completed course
• To report sore throat, fever, fatigue; (may indicate superimposed infection)
• To wear or carry Medic Alert ID if allergic to penicillins
• To notify nurse of diarrhea

Treatment of overdose: Withdraw drug, maintain airway, administer epinephrine, aminophylline, O_2, IV corticosteroids for anaphylaxis

---

pentaerythritol tetranitrate
(pen-ta-er-ith'ri-tole)
Duotrate, Duotrate 45, P.E.T.N., Pentylan, Peritrate, Peritrate SA
Func. class.: Vasodilatory, coronary
Chem. class.: Nitrate

Action: Decreases preload, afterload, which is responsible for decreasing left ventricular end-diastolic pressure, systemic vascular resistance

Uses: Chronic stable angina pectoris, prophylaxis of angina pain

Dosage and routes:
• *Adult:* PO 10-20 mg tid or qid,

max 40 mg qid; sus rel 30-80 mg q12h

Available forms: Caps ext rel 30, 45, 80 mg; tabs 10, 20, 40, 80 mg; tabs ext rel 80 mg

Side effects/adverse reactions:
CV: Postural hypotension, palpitations, tachycardia, *collapse,* syncope
GI: Nausea, vomiting, abdominal pain
INTEG: Pallor, sweating, rash
CNS: Headache, flushing, dizziness, restlessness, weakness, faintness
MISC: Muscle twitching, *hemolytic anemia, methemoglobinemia*

Contraindications: Hypersensitivity to this drug or nitrates, severe anemia, increased intracranial pressure, cerebral hemorrhage, acute MI

Precautions: Postural hypotension, pregnancy (C), lactation, children

Pharmacokinetics:
PO: Onset 30 min, duration 4-5 hr
SUS REL: Onset 30 min, duration 12 hr
Metabolized by liver, excreted in urine, half-life 10 min

Interactions/incompatibilities:
• Increased effects: β-blockers, diuretics, antihypertensives, alcohol

NURSING CONSIDERATIONS
Assess:
• B/P, pulse, respirations during beginning therapy
• Pain: duration, time started, activity being performed, character
• Tolerance if taken over long period of time
• Headache, light-headedness, decreased B/P; may indicate a need for decreased dosage

Administer:
• With 8 oz of water on empty stomach

Evaluate:
• Therapeutic response: decrease, prevention of anginal pain

Teach patient/family:
• To keep tabs in original container; do not crush or chew sus rel preparations
• To avoid alcohol products
• That drug may cause headache; tolerance usually develops
• That drug may be taken before stressful activity: exercise, sexual activity
• To avoid hazardous activities if dizziness occurs
• To comply with complete medical regimen
• To make position changes slowly to prevent fainting

---

pentamidine isethionate
(pen-tam′i-deen)
Pentam 300, Pentacarinat,* Nebu Pent
Func. class.: Antiprotozoal
Chem. class.: Aromatic diamide derivative

Action: Interferes with DNA/RNA synthesis in protozoa

Uses: *P. carinii* infections

Dosage and routes:
• *Adult and child:* IV/IM 4 mg/kg/day × 2 wk: Neb 600 mg/6ml NS via specific nebulizer given q4wk for prevention

Available forms: Inj IV, IM, aerosol 300 mg/vial

Side effects/adverse reactions:
CV: Hypotension, ventricular tachycardia, ECG abnormalities
HEMA: Anemia, *leukopenia, thrombocytopenia*
INTEG: Sterile abscess, pain at injection site, pruritus, urticaria, rash
GU: Acute renal failure, increased serum creatinine, renal toxicity
GI: Nausea, vomiting, anorexia, increased AST, ALT, *acute pancreatitis,* metallic taste
CNS: Disorientation, hallucinations, dizziness, confusion
RESP: Cough, shortness of breath, *bronchospasm* (with aerosol)
MISC: Fatigue, chills, night sweats
META: Hyperkalemia, hypocalcemia, hypoglycemia

Precautions: Blood dyscrasias, hepatic disease, renal disease, diabetes mellitus, cardiac disease, hypocalcemia, pregnancy (C), hypertension, hypotension, lactation, children

Pharmacokinetics: Excreted unchanged in urine (66%)

Interactions/incompatibilities
• Nephrotoxicity: aminoglycosides, amphotericin B, colistin, cisplatin, methoxyflurane, polymyxin B, vancomycin
• Considered incompatible with any drug in sol or syringe

NURSING CONSIDERATIONS
Assess:
• Blood studies, blood glucose, CBC, platelets
• I&O ratio; report hematuria, oliguria
• ECG for cardiac dysrhythmias
• Patient should be lying down when receiving drug; severe hypotension may develop; monitor BP during administration and several times after until BP stable
• Any patient with compromised renal system; drug is excreted slowly in poor renal system function; toxicity may occur rapidly
• Liver studies: AST, ALT
• Renal studies: urinalysis, BUN, creatinine; nephrotoxicity may occur
• Signs of infection, anemia

P

italics = common side effects   ***bold italic*** = life threatening reactions

• Bowel pattern before, during treatment
• Sterile abscess, pain at injection site
• Respiratory status: rate, character, wheezing, dyspnea
• Dizziness, confusion, hallucination
• Allergies before treatment, reaction of each medication; place allergies on chart, Kardex in bright red letters; notify all people giving drugs

Administer:
• IV by intermittent inf over 60 min
• Inhalation through nebulizer; mix contents in 6 ml of sterile H_2O; do not use low pressure (<20 psi); flow rate should be 5-7 L/min (40-50 psi) air or O_2 source over 30-45 min until chamber is empty
• IM diluted in 3 ml sterile H_2O; give deep IM; painful by this route

Perform/provide:
• Storage in refrigerator protected from light

Evaluate:
• Therapeutic response: decreased temperature, ability to breathe

Teach patient/family:
• To report sore throat, fever, fatigue; may indicate superimposed infection

---

pentazocine HCl/ pentazocine lactate
(pen-taz'oh-seen)
Talwin
Func. class.: Narcotic analgesic, antagonist
Chem. class.: Synthetic benzomorphan

Controlled Substance Schedule IV
Action: Inhibits ascending pain pathways in CNS, increases pain threshold, alters pain perception
Uses: Moderate to severe pain

Dosage and routes:
• *Adult:* PO 50-100 mg q3-4h prn, not to exceed 600 mg/day; IV/IM/SC 30 mg q3-4h prn, not to exceed 360 mg/day
Available forms: SC, IM, IV 30 mg/ml; tabs 50 mg

Side effects/adverse reactions:
CNS: Drowsiness, dizziness, confusion, headache, sedation, euphoria, hallucinations
GI: Nausea, vomiting, anorexia, constipation, cramps
GU: Increased urinary output, dysuria
INTEG: Rash, urticaria, bruising, flushing, diaphoresis, pruritus, severe irritation at injection sites
EENT: Tinnitus, blurred vision, miosis, diplopia
CV: Palpitations, bradycardia, change in B/P, tachycardia, increased B/P (high doses)
RESP: Respiratory depression
Contraindications: Hypersensitivity, addiction (narcotic)
Precautions: Addictive personality, pregnancy (B), lactation, increased intracranial pressure, MI (acute), severe heart disease, respiratory depression, hepatic disease, renal disease, seizure disorder, child <18 yr

Pharmacokinetics:
SC/IM: Onset 15-30 min, peak 1-2 hr, duration 2-4 hr
IV: Onset 2-3 min, duration 4-6 hr; metabolized by liver, excreted by kidneys, crosses placenta, half-life 2-3 hr, extensive first-pass metabolism with less than 20% entering circulation

Interactions/incompatibilities:
• Increased effects: CNS depressants; alcohol, sedative/hypnotics,

antipsychotics, skeletal muscle relaxants
• Decreased effects: narcotics
• Incompatible with barbiturates, aminophylline, glycopyrrolate, $NaCO_3$

Lab test interferences:
Increase: Amylase

NURSING CONSIDERATIONS
Assess:
• I&O ratio; check for decreasing output; may indicate urinary retention
• For withdrawal symptoms in narcotic-dependent patients
• Pulmonary embolism, abscesses, ulcerations, vascular occlusion, WBC
• CNS changes: dizziness, drowsiness, hallucinations, euphoria, LOC, pupil reaction
• Allergic reactions: rash, urticaria
• Respiratory dysfunction: respiratory depression, character, rate, rhythm; notify physician if respirations are <10/min
• Need for pain medication, physical dependence

Administer:
• IV undiluted or diluted 5 mg/ml of sterile H_2O for inj; give 5 mg or less over 1 min
• With antiemetic if nausea, vomiting occur
• When pain is beginning to return; determine dosage interval by patient response

Perform/provide:
• Storage in light-resistant area at room temperature
• Assistance with ambulation
• Safety measures: side rails, nightlight, call bell within easy reach

Evaluate:
• Therapeutic response: decrease in pain

Teach patient/family:
• To report any symptoms of CNS changes, allergic reactions

• That physical dependency may result when used for extended periods
• That withdrawal symptoms may occur: nausea, vomiting, cramps, fever, faintness, anorexia

Treatment of overdose: Naloxone (Narcan) 0.2-0.8 IV, O_2, IV fluids, vasopressors

---

pentobarbital/pentobarbital sodium

(pen-toe-bar'bi-tal)
Nembutal, Nembutal Sodium, Nembutal Sodium Solution, Nova-Rectal,* Pentobarbital Sodium, Pentogen*

Func. class.: Sedative/hypnotic barbiturate
Chem. class.: Barbitone, short acting

P

Controlled Substance Schedule II (USA), Schedule G (Canada)
Action: Depresses activity in brain cells, primarily in reticular activating system in brain stem; selectively depresses neurons in posterior hypothalamus, limbic structures
Uses: Insomnia, sedation, preoperative medication, increased intracranial pressure, dental anesthetic

Dosage and routes:
• *Adult:* PO 100-200 mg hs; IM 150-200 mg hs; IV 100 mg initially, then up to 500 mg; REC 120-200 mg hs
• *Child:* IM 3-5 mg, not to exceed 100 mg
• *Child 2 mo-1 yr:* REC 30 mg
• *Child 1-4 yr:* REC 30-60 mg
• *Child 5-12 yr:* REC 60 mg
• *Child 12-14 yr:* REC 60-120 mg
Available forms: Caps 50, 100 mg; elix 18.2 mg/5 ml; powder, rec

---

italics = common side effects   **bold italic** = life threatening reactions

supp 30, 60, 120, 200 mg; inj IM, IV 50 mg/ml

Side effects/adverse reactions:

CNS: Lethargy, drowsiness, hangover, dizziness, paradoxical stimulation in elderly and children, light-headedness, dependence, *CNS depression,* mental depression, slurred speech

GI: Nausea, vomiting, diarrhea, constipation

INTEG: Rash, urticaria, pain, abscesses at injection site, angioedema, thrombophlebitis, *Stevens-Johnson syndrome*

CV: Hypotension, bradycardia

RESP: Depression, apnea, laryngospasm, bronchospasm

HEMA: Agranulocytosis, thrombocytopenia, megaloblastic anemia (long-term treatment)

Contraindications: Hypersensitivity to barbiturates, respiratory depression, addiction to barbiturates, severe liver, renal impairment, porphyria, uncontrolled pain

Precautions: Anemia, pregnancy (D), lactation, hepatic disease, renal disease, hypertension, elderly, acute/chronic pain

Pharmacokinetics:

PO: Onset 15-30 min, duration 4-6 hr

REC: Onset slow, duration 4-6 hr

Metabolized by liver, excreted by kidneys (metabolites); half-life 15-48 hr

Interactions/incompatibilities:

• Incompatible with atropine, benzquinamide, brompheniramine, butorphanol, cefazolin, cephalothin, chlordiazepoxide chlorpheniramine, chlorpromazine, cimetidine, clindamycin, codeine, dimenhydrate, droperidol, erythromycin, glycopyrrolate, hydrocortisone, insulin, kanamycin, levarterenol, levorphanol, meperidine, methadone, midazolam, morphine, nalbuphine, opium, penicillins, pentazocine, phenytoin, prochlorperazine, promazine, promethazine, ranitidine, streptomycin, succinylcholine, tetracycline, triflupromazine, vancomycin, NaCO₃, fructose sol

• Increased CNS depression: alcohol, MAOIs, sedatives, narcotics

• Decreased effect of: oral anticoagulants, corticosteroids, griseofulvin, quinidine

• Increased half-life of: doxycycline

Lab test interferences:

False increase: Sulfobromophthalein

NURSING CONSIDERATIONS

Assess:

• VS q30min after parenteral route for 2 hr

• Blood studies: Hct, Hgb, RBCs, serum folate, Vit D (if on long-term therapy); pro-time in patients receiving anticoagulants

• Hepatic studies: AST, ALT, bilirubin; if increased, drug is usually discontinued

• Mental status: mood, sensorium, affect, memory (long, short)

• Physical dependency: more frequent requests for medication, shakes, anxiety

• Barbiturate toxicity: hypotension; pupillary constriction; cold, clammy skin; cyanosis of lips; insomnia; nausea; vomiting; hallucinations; delirium; weakness; coma; mild symptoms may occur in 8-12 hr without drug

• Respiratory dysfunction: respiratory depression, character, rate, rhythm; hold drug if respirations are <10/min or if pupils are dilated

• Blood dyscrasias: fever, sore throat, bruising, rash, jaundice, epistaxis

---

* Available in Canada only

Administer:
• After removal of cigarettes to prevent fires
• IM injection in deep large muscle mass to prevent tissue sloughing and abscesses; do not inject more than 5 ml in one site
• After trying conservative measures for insomnia
• After mixing with sterile water for injection, inject within 30 min of preparation
• IV undiluted or dilute in sterile H_2O, LR, NaCl, give 50 mg or less/min; titrate to patient response; use only clear sol; avoid extravasation
• IV only with resuscitative equipment available; administer at <100 mg/min (only by qualified personnel)
• ½-1 hr before hs for sleeplessness
• On empty stomach for best absorption
• For <14 days, since not effective after that; tolerance develops
• Crushed or whole
• Alone; do not mix with other drugs or inject if there is precipitate
Perform/provide:
• Assistance with ambulation after receiving dose
• Safety measure: side rails, nightlight, call bell within easy reach
• Checking to see PO medication has been swallowed
• Storage of suppositories in refrigerator; do not use aqueous solutions that contain precipitate
Evaluate:
• Therapeutic response: ability to sleep at night, decreased amount of early morning awakening if taking drug for insomnia, or decrease in number, severity of seizures if taking drug for seizure disorder
Teach patient/family:
• That morning hangover is common

• That drug is indicated only for short-term treatment of insomnia and is probably ineffective after 2 wk
• That physical dependency may result when used for extended periods (45-90 days depending on dose)
• To avoid driving, other activities requiring alertness
• To avoid alcohol ingestion, CNS depressants; serious CNS depression may result
• Not to discontinue medication quickly after long-term use; drug should be tapered over 1-2 wk
• To tell all prescribers that a barbiturate is being taken
• That withdrawal insomnia may occur after short-term use; do not start using drug again; insomnia will improve in 1-3 nights
• That effects may take 2 nights for benefits to be noticed
• Alternate measures to improve sleep (reading, exercise several hours before hs, warm bath, warm milk, TV, self-hypnosis, deep breathing)
Treatment of overdose: Lavage, activated charcoal, warming blanket, vital signs, hemodialysis, I&O ratio

pentostatin
(pen-toe-sta'-tin)
Nipent
Func. class.: Antineoplastic antibiotic
Chem. class.: Streptomyces antibioticus derivative

Action: Inhibits the enzyme adenosine deaminase (ADA), which is able to block DNA synthesis and some RNA synthesis

italics = common side effects   ***bold italic*** = life threatening reactions

Uses: Alpha-interferon-refractory hairy cell leukemia

Dosage and routes:
• *Adult:* IV 4 mg/m² every other week; may be given IV BOL, or diluted in a larger volume and given over 20-30 min

Available forms: Powder for inj 10 mg/vial

Side effects/adverse reactions:
CNS: Headache, anxiety, confusion, depression, dizziness, insomnia, nervousness, paresthesia

RESP: Cough, upper respiratory infection, bronchitis, dyspnea, epistaxis, pneumonia, pharyngitis, rhinitis, sinusitis

SYST: Fever, infection, fatigue, pain, allergic reaction, chills, *death, sepsis,* chest pain, flu syndrome

HEMA: **Leukopenia, anemia, thrombocytopenia, ecchymosis, lymphadenopathy,** petechia

GI: Nausea, vomiting, anorexia, diarrhea, constipation, flatulence, stomatitis, elevated liver function tests

INTEG: Rash, eczema, dry skin, pruritus, sweating, herpes simplex/zoster

GU: **Hematuria,** dysuria, increased BUN/creatinine

Contraindications: Hypersensitivity

Precautions: Renal disease, pregnancy (C), lactation, children, bone marrow depression

Pharmacokinetics:
IV: Elimination half-life 5.7 hr, low protein binding, 90% excreted in urine as unchanged drug or metabolites

Interactions/incompatibilities:
• Fatal pulmonary toxicity: fludarabine
• Increased adverse reactions: vidarabine

Lab test interferences:
Increase: Uric acid

NURSING CONSIDERATIONS
Assess:
• CBC, differential, platelet count weekly; withhold drug if WBC is 4000/mm³ or platelet count is <75,000/mm³; notify physician of these results
• Renal function studies; BUN, serum uric acid, urine CrCl, electrolytes before, during therapy
• I&O ratio; report fall in urine output to <30 ml/hr
• Monitor temperature q4h; fever may indicate beginning infection
• Liver function tests before, during therapy: bilirubin, AST, ALT, alk phosphatase, as needed or monthly
• Bleeding: hematuria, guaiac stools, bruising, petechiae, mucosa or orifices q8h
• Effects of alopecia on body image; discuss feelings about body changes
• Inflammation of mucosa, breaks in skin
• Yellowing of skin and sclera, dark urine, clay-colored stools, itchy skin, abdominal pain, fever, diarrhea
• Buccal cavity q8h for dryness, sores, ulceration, white patches, oral pain, bleeding, dysphagia
• Local irritation, pain, burning at injection site
• Symptoms indicating severe allergic reaction: rash, pruritus, urticaria, purpuric skin lesions, itching, flushing
• GI symptoms: frequency of stools, cramping
• Acidosis, signs of dehydration; rapid respiration, poor skin turgor, decreased urine output, dry skin, restlessness, weakness

*Available in Canada only

Administer:

• Antiemetic 30-60 min before giving drug to prevent vomiting

• Antibiotics as ordered for prophylaxis of infection

• After diluting, use with 5 ml sterile water for injection and mix thoroughly (2 mg/ml); may be given by bolus or diluted in 25-50 ml of 5% dextrose, or 0.9% NaCl (0.33 or 0.18 mg/ml)

Perform/provide:

• Hydrocortisone, sodium thiosulfate to infiltration area, and ice compress after stopping infusion

• Strict hand-washing technique, gloves, protective covering

• Liquid diet: carbonated beverages; gelatin may be added if patient is not nauseated or vomiting

• Rinsing of mouth tid-qid with water, club soda; brushing of teeth bid-qid with soft brush or cotton-tipped applicators for stomatitis; use unwaxed dental floss

• Storage in refrigerator; reconstituted or diluted solution may be stored at room temperature for no longer than 8 hr

Evaluate:

• Therapeutic response: decrease in tumor size and spread of malignancy

Teach patient/family:

• To report any complaints, side effects to nurse or physician

• That hair may be lost during treatment and wig or hairpiece may make patient feel better; tell patient that new hair may be different in color, texture

• To avoid foods with citric acid, hot or rough texture

• To report any bleeding, white spots, ulcerations in mouth to physician; tell patient to examine mouth qd

• To avoid crowds and sources of infection when granulocyte count is low

---

pentoxifylline
(pen-tox-i'-leen)
Trental
Func. class.: Hemorrheologic agent
Chem. class.: Dimethylxanthine derivative

Action: Decreases blood viscosity, stimulates prostacyclin formation, increases blood flow by increasing flexibility of RBCs; decreases RBC hyperaggregation; reduces platelet aggregation, decreases fibrinogin concentration

Uses: Intermittent claudication related to chronic occlusive vascular disease

Dosage and routes:

• *Adult:* PO 400 mg tid with meals

Available forms: Tabs, controlled-release 400 mg

Side effects/adverse reactions:

MISC: Epistaxis, flulike symptoms, laryngitis, nasal congestion, leukopenia, malaise, weight changes

EENT: Blurred vision, earache, increased salivation, sore throat, conjunctivitis

CNS: Headache, anxiety, tremors, confusion, dizziness

GI: Dyspepsia, nausea, vomiting, anorexia, bloating, belching, constipation, cholecystitis, dry mouth, thirst, bad taste

INTEG: Rash, pruritus, urticaria, brittle fingernails

CV: Angina, dysrhythmias, palpitation, hypotension, chest pain, dyspnea, edema

Contraindications: Hypersensitivity to this drug or xanthines

Precautions: Pregnancy (C), angina pectoris, cardiac disease, lac-

P

---

tation, children, impaired renal function

Pharmacokinetics:

PO: Peak 1 hr, half-life ½-1 hr, degradation in liver, excreted in urine

Interactions/incompatibilities:

Increased PT: warfarin

NURSING CONSIDERATIONS

Assess:

• B/P, respirations of patient taking antihypertensives also

Administer:

• With meals

Evaluate:

• Therapeutic response: decreased pain, cramping, increased ambulation

Teach patient/family:

• That therapeutic response may take 2-4 wk

• That decreased fats, increased cholesterol, increased exercise, decreased smoking are necessary to correct condition

• To observe feet for arterial insufficiency

• To use cotton socks, well-fitted shoes; not to go barefoot

• To watch for bleeding, bruises, petechiae, epistaxis

---

permethrin

(per-meth'ren)

Elimite, Nix

Func. class.: Pediculicide

Chem. class.: Synthetic pyrethroid

Action: Acts by disrupting sodium channel current in parasite's nerve cell; delayed repolarization, paralysis of lice

Uses: Lice, nits, ticks, flea nits

Dosage and routes:

• *Adult and child:* Wash hair, towel dry; apply liberally to hair, leave on 10 min, rinse with water

Available forms: Liq 1%, cream 5%

Side effects/adverse reactions:

INTEG: Pruritus, burning, stinging, rash, tingling, numbness, edema

Contraindications: Hypersensitivity

Precautions: Head rash, children, lactation

Pharmacokinetics:

Metabolized in liver to inactive metabolites, excreted in urine

NURSING CONSIDERATIONS

Administer:

• To body area, scalp only; do not apply to face, lips, mouth, eyes, any mucous membranes, anus, or meatus

• Topical corticosteroids as ordered to decrease contact dermatitis

• Lotions of menthol or phenol to control itching

• Topical antibiotics for infection

Perform/provide:

• Isolation until areas on skin, scalp have cleared and treatment is complete

• Removal of nits by using a fine-tooth comb rinsed in vinegar after treatment

Evaluate:

• Therapeutic response: decreased crusts, nits, itching, papules in skin folds

Teach patient/family:

• To wash all inhabitants' clothing, bed linen using insecticide; preventive treatment may be required of all persons living in same house, using lotion or shampoo to decrease spread of infection

• That itching may continue for 4-6 wk

• That drug must be reapplied if accidentally washed off, or treatment will be ineffective

• Not to apply to face; apply from neck down for body lice

---

*Available in Canada only

• To treat sexual partners simultaneously

Treatment of ingestion: Gastric lavage, saline laxatives, IV diazepam for convulsions

---

perphenazine
(per-fen′a-zeen)
Trilafon, Perphenazine, Phenazine
Func. class.: Antipsychotic/neuroleptic
Chem. class.: Phenothiazine piperidine

Action: Depresses cerebral cortex, hypothalamus, limbic system, which control activity, aggression; blocks neurotransmission produced by dopamine at synapse; exhibits strong α-adrenergic, anticholinergic blocking action; as antiemetic inhibits medullary chemoreceptor trigger zone; mechanism for antipsychotic effects is unclear

Uses: Psychotic disorders, schizophrenia, alcoholism, nausea, vomiting

Dosage and routes:
Nausea/vomiting/alcoholism
• *Adult and child >12 yr:* IM 5-10 mg prn, max 15 mg in ambulatory patients, 30 mg in hospitalized patients; PO 8-16 mg/day in divided doses, up to 24 mg; IV not to exceed 5 mg, give diluted or slow IV drip

Psychiatric use in hospitalized patients
• *Adults:* PO 8-16 mg bid-qid, gradually increased to desired dose, not to exceed 64 mg/day; IM 5 mg q6h, not to exceed 30 mg/day
• *Child >12 yr:* PO 6-12 mg in divided doses

Nonhospitalized patients
• *Adult:* PO 4-8 mg tid or 8-32 mg repeat-action bid; IM 5 mg q6h

Available forms: Tabs 2, 4, 8, 16 mg; sol 16 mg/5ml; inj IM/IV 5 mg/ml; sus rel tabs 8 mg

Side effects/adverse reactions:
RESP: **Laryngospasm,** dyspnea, *respiratory depression*

CNS: Extrapyramidal symptoms: *pseudoparkinsonism, akathisia, dystonia, tardive dyskinesia, **seizures,** headache*

HEMA: Anemia, **leukopenia, leukocytosis, agranulocytosis**

INTEG: *Rash,* photosensitivity, dermatitis

EENT: Blurred vision, glaucoma

GI: Dry mouth, nausea, vomiting, anorexia, constipation, diarrhea, jaundice, weight gain

GU: Urinary retention, urinary frequency, enuresis, impotence, amenorrhea, gynecomastia

*CV: Orthostatic hypotension, **cardiac arrest,** ECG changes, **tachycardia***

Contraindications: Hypersensitivity, blood dyscrasias, coma, child <12 yr, brain damage, bone marrow depression

Precautions: Pregnancy (C), lactation, seizure disorders, hypertension, hepatic disease, cardiac disease

Pharmacokinetics:
PO: Onset erratic, peak 2-4 hr
IM: Onset 10 min, peak 1-2 hr, duration 6 hr, occasionally 12-24 hr; metabolized by liver, excreted in urine, crosses placenta, enters breast milk

Interactions/incompatibilities:
• Oversedation: other CNS depressants, alcohol, barbiturate anesthetics
• Toxicity: epinephrine
• Decreased absorption: aluminum hydroxide or magnesium hydroxide antacids

P

---

italics = common side effects   **bold italic** = life threatening reactions

- Decreased effects of: lithium, levodopa
- Increased effects of both drugs: β-adrenergic blockers, alcohol
- Increased anticholinergic effects: anticholinergics
- Incompatible with aminophylline, cefoperazone, midazolam, opium, oxytocin, pentobarbital, secobarbital, thiopental, Vit B complex

Lab test interferences:

Increase: Liver function tests, cardiac enzymes, cholesterol, blood glucose, prolactin, bilirubin, PBI, cholinesterase, ^{131}I

Decrease: Hormones (blood, urine)

False positive: Pregnancy tests, PKU

False negative: Urinary steroids, 17-OHCS

NURSING CONSIDERATIONS
Assess:

- Mental status before initial administration
- Swallowing of PO medication; check for hoarding or giving of medication to other patients
- I&O ratio; palpate bladder if low urinary output occurs
- Bilirubin, CBC, liver function studies monthly
- Urinalysis is recommended before and during prolonged therapy
- Affect, orientation, LOC, reflexes, gait, coordination, sleep pattern disturbances
- B/P standing and lying; also include pulse, respirations q4h during initial treatment; establish baseline before starting treatment; report drops of 30 mm Hg
- Dizziness, faintness, palpitations, tachycardia on rising
- Extrapyramidal symptoms including akathisia (inability to sit still, no pattern to movements), tardive dyskinesia (bizarre movements of jaw, mouth, tongue, extremities), pseudoparkinsonism (rigidity, tremors, pill rolling, shuffling gait)
- Skin turgor daily
- For neuroleptic malignant syndrome: hyperthermia, altered mental status, increased CPK, muscle rigidity
- Constipation, urinary retention daily; if these occur, increase bulk, water in diet

Administer:

- IV after diluting each 5 mg/9 ml of NaCl, shake, (1ml = 0.5 mg), give 0.5 mg or less over 1 min; may be further diluted and given as an inf
- Antiparkinsonian agent after securing order from physician; to be used if extrapyramidal symptoms occur
- Concentrate mixed in water, orange, pineapple, apricot, prune, tomato, grapefruit juice; do not mix with caffeine beverages (coffee, cola), tannics (tea), or pectinates (apple juice), since incompatibility may result; use 60 ml diluent for each 5 ml of concentrate
- Repeat-action tablets whole; do not crush or chew
- IM injection into a large muscle mass

Perform/provide:

- Decreased noise input by dimming lights, avoiding loud noises
- Supervised ambulation until stabilized on medication; do not involve in strenuous exercise program because fainting is possible; patient should not stand still for long periods
- Increased fluids to prevent constipation
- Sips of water, candy, gum for dry mouth

*Available in Canada only

- Storage in tight, light-resistant container

Evaluate:

- Therapeutic response: decrease in emotional excitement, hallucinations, delusions, paranoia, reorganization of patterns of thought, speech

Teach patient/family:

- That orthostatic hypotension occurs frequently and to rise from sitting or lying position gradually; to avoid hazardous activities until stabilized on medication
- To remain lying down after IM injection for at least 30 min
- To avoid hot tubs, hot showers, tub baths, since hypotension may occur
- To avoid abrupt withdrawal of this drug, or extrapyramidal symptoms may result; drug should be withdrawn slowly
- To avoid OTC preparations (cough, hay fever, cold) unless approved by physician, since serious drug interactions may occur; avoid use with alcohol or CNS depressants; increased drowsiness may occur
- To use a sunscreen during sun exposure to prevent burns
- Regarding compliance with drug regimen
- About necessity for meticulous oral hygiene, since oral candidiasis may occur
- To report sore throat, malaise, fever, bleeding, mouth sores; if these occur, CBC should be drawn and drug discontinued
- In hot weather, that heat stroke may occur; take extra precautions to stay cool

Treatment of overdose: Lavage if orally ingested; provide an airway; *do not induce vomiting*

phenacemide
(fe-nass'e-mide)
Phenurone
Func. class.: Anticonvulsant
Chem. class.: Hydantoin

Action: Increases seizure threshold in cortex

Uses: Refractory, generalized tonic-clonic (grand mal), complex-partial (psychomotor), absence (petit mal), atypical seizures

Dosage and routes:

- *Adult:* PO 500 mg tid, may increase by 500 mg/wk, not to exceed 5 g/day
- *Child 5-10 yr:* PO 250 mg tid, may increase by 250 mg/wk, not to exceed 1.5 g/day prn

Available forms: Tabs 500 mg

Side effects/adverse reactions:

*HEMA: **Agranulocytosis, leukopenia, aplastic anemia***

CNS: Drowsiness, dizziness, insomnia, paresthesias, depression, suicidal tendencies, aggression, headache

GI: Anorexia, weight loss, ***hepatitis,*** jaundice, nausea

GU: Nephritis, ***albuminuria***

INTEG: Rash

Contraindications: Hypersensitivity, psychiatric condition, pregnancy (D)

Precautions: Allergies, hepatic disease, renal disease

Pharmacokinetics:

PO: Duration 5 hr, metabolized by liver, excreted by kidneys

Interactions/incompatibilities:

- Paranoid signs and symptoms: ethotoin

NURSING CONSIDERATIONS
Assess:

- Blood, liver function, renal function studies

P

---

italics = common side effects   ***bold italic*** = life threatening reactions

- Drug level: drug is extremely toxic
- Mental status: mood, sensorium, affect, memory (long, short); psychosis is common
- Respiratory depression: respirations <10/min, shallow
- Blood dyscrasias: fever, sore throat, bruising, rash, jaundice

Administer:
- With food to decrease GI symptoms

Evaluate:
- Therapeutic response: decreased seizures

Teach patient/family:
- To notify physician if sore throat, fever, rash, fatigue, bleeding, bruising occur (blood dyscrasia)
- To notify physician if dark urine, jaundice, yellow sclerae, itching occur (liver dysfunction)
- To avoid hazardous activities until stabilized on drug
- Never to withdraw abruptly
- To report personality changes

---

phenazopyridine HCl
(fen-az-eh-peer'i-deen)
Azo-Standard, Baridium, Eridium, Geridium, Phenazo,* Phenazodine, Phenazopyridine HCl, Pyridiate, Pyridium, Urodine
Func. class.: Nonnarcotic analgesic
Chem. class.: Azodye

Action: Exerts analgesic, anesthetic action on the urinary tract mucosa; exact mechanism of action unknown

Uses: Urinary tract irritation, infection

Dosage and routes:
- *Adult:* PO 100-200 mg tid

- *Child 6-12 yr:* PO 12 mg/kg/24 hr in divided doses

Available forms: Tabs 100, 200 mg

Side effects/adverse reactions:
HEMA: **Thrombocytopenia, agranulocytosis, leukopenia, neutropenia, hemolytic anemia, methemoglobinemia**
CNS: Headache, vertigo
GI: Nausea, vomiting, GI bleeding, diarrhea, heartburn, anorexia, **hepatic toxicity**
INTEG: Rash, urticaria, skin pigmentation
GU: **Renal toxicity**, orange-red urine

Contraindications: Hypersensitivity, hepatic disease

Precautions: Pregnancy (B), renal disease

Pharmacokinetics: Metabolized by liver, excreted by kidneys, crosses placenta, duration 6-8 hr

Lab test interferences:
Interference: Bilirubin, urinary glucose tests, urinalysis, PSP excretion, urinary ketones, steroids, proteins
False positive: Clinitest

NURSING CONSIDERATIONS
Assess:
- Liver function studies: AST, ALT, bilirubin if patient is on long-term therapy
- Hepatotoxicity: dark urine, clay-colored stools, yellowing of skin and sclera, itching, abdominal pain, fever, diarrhea if patient is on long-term therapy
- Allergic reactions: rash, urticaria; if these occur, drug may have to be discontinued

Administer:
- To patient crushed or whole; chewable tablets may be chewed
- With food or milk to decrease gastric symptoms

Evaluate:
• Therapeutic response: decrease in pain

Teach patient/family:
• To report any symptoms of hepatotoxicity
• Not to exceed recommended dosage and to take with meals
• To read label on other OTC drugs; many contain aspirin
• Discontinue after pain is relieved but continue to take concurrent prescribed antibiotic until finished
• Urine may turn red-orange, may stain clothing

Treatment of overdose: Methylene blue 1-2 mg/kg IV or 100-200 mg Vit C PO

---

phendimetrazine tartrate

(fen-dye-me′tra-zeen)
Adipost, Anorex, Bacarate, Bontril PDM, Bontril Slow-Release, Ditall, Dyrexan-OD, Melfiat-105 Unicelles, Metra, Phenazine-35, Phenzine, Obalan, Obeval, Plegine, Phendimetrazine Tartrate, Prelu-2, Sprx-105, Slyn-LL, Trimstat, TrimTabs, Weh-Less, Wehless Timecelles, X-Trozine, X-Trozine LA, Weightrol

Func. class.: Anorexiant
Chem. class.: Morpholine derivative

Controlled Substance Schedule IV

Action: Increases release of norepinephrine, dopamine in cerebral cortex to reticular activating system

Uses: Exogenous obesity

Dosage and routes:
Adult: PO 35 mg bid-tid 1 hr ac, not to exceed 70 mg tid, sus rel 105 mg qd ac AM

Available forms: Tabs 35 mg, caps 35 mg, sus rel cap 105 mg

Side effects/adverse reactions:
HEMA: **Bone marrow depression, leukopenia, agranulocytosis**
CNS: Hyperactivity, insomnia, restlessness, dizziness, tremor headache, fatigue, malaise, euphoria, depression, confusion
INTEG: Urticaria, rash, erythema
GI: Nausea, anorexia, dry mouth, diarrhea, constipation, cramps, vomiting
GU: Dysuria, impotence, menstrual irregularities, change in libido, urinary frequency
CV: Palpitations, tachycardia, hypertension
EENT: Blurred vision, mydriasis, eye irritation

Contraindications: Hypersensitivity, hyperthyroidism, hypertension, glaucoma, severe arteriosclerosis, severe cardiovascular disease, children <12 yr, agitated states, drug abuse

Precautions: Drug abuse, anxiety, pregnancy (C), lactation, convulsive disorders

Pharmacokinetics:
PO: Onset 30 min, peak 1-3 hr, duration 4-20 hr, metabolized by liver, excreted by kidneys, crosses placenta, excreted in breast milk, half-life 2-10 hr

Interactions/incompatibilities:
• Hypertensive crisis: MAOIs or within 14 days of MAOIs, furazolidone
• Decreased effect of phendimetrazine: tricyclics, phenothiazides, haloperidol
• Decreased effect of: guanethidine

NURSING CONSIDERATIONS

Assess:
• VS, B/P, since this drug may reverse antihypertensives; check pa-

P

---

italics = common side effects   ***bold italic*** = life threatening reactions

tients with cardiac disease more often
• CBC, urinalysis; in diabetes: blood sugar, urine sugar; insulin changes may have to be made, since eating will decrease
• Height, growth rate in children; growth rate may decrease

Administer:
• At least 6 hr before hs to avoid sleeplessness
• For obesity only if patient is on weight reduction program, including dietary changes, exercise; patient will develop tolerance; loss of weight won't occur without additional methods; give 1 hr before meals
• Gum, hard candy, frequent sips of water for dry mouth

Teach patient/family:
• Not to crush or chew sus rel preps or to take more than prescribed amount
• To decrease caffeine consumption (coffee, tea, cola, chocolate), which may increase irritability, stimulation
• To avoid OTC preparations unless approved by physician
• To taper off drug over several weeks, or depression, increased sleeping, lethargy will ensue
• To avoid alcohol ingestion
• To avoid hazardous activities until patient is stabilized on medication
• To get needed rest; patients will feel more tired at end of day

Treatment of overdose: Administer fluids, hemodialysis or peritoneal dialysis; antihypertensive for increased B/P; ammonium Cl for increase excretion

phenelzine sulfate
(fen'el-zeen)
Nardil
Func. class.: Antidepressant MAOI
Chem. class.: Hydrazine

Action: Increases concentrations of endogenous epinephrine, norepinephrine, serotonin, dopamine in storage sites in CNS by inhibition of MAO; increased concentration reduces depression

Uses: Depression, when uncontrolled by other means

Dosage and routes:
• *Adult:* PO 45 mg/day in divided doses; may increase to 60 mg/day; dose should be reduced to 15 mg/day, not to exceed 90 mg/day

Available forms: Tabs 15 mg

Side effects/adverse reactions:
HEMA: Anemia
CNS: Dizziness, drowsiness, confusion, headache, anxiety, tremors, stimulation, weakness, hyperreflexia, mania, insomnia, fatigue, weight gain
GI: Constipation, dry mouth, nausea, vomiting, *anorexia,* diarrhea, weight gain
GU: Change in libido, frequency
INTEG: Rash, flushing, increased perspiration
CV: Orthostatic hypotension, hypertension, dysrhythmias, hypertensive crisis
EENT: Blurred vision
ENDO: SIADH-like syndrome
Contraindications: Hypersensitivity to MAOIs, elderly, hypertension, CHF, severe hepatic disease, pheochromocytoma, severe renal disease, severe cardiac disease
Precautions: Suicidal patients, convulsive disorders, severe de-

pression, schizophrenia, hyperactivity, diabetes mellitus, pregnancy (C)

Pharmacokinetics:
Metabolized by liver, excreted by kidneys

Interactions/incompatibilities:
• Increased pressor effects: guanethidine, clonidine, indirect acting sympathomimetics (ephedrine)
• Increased effects of: direct-acting sympathomimetics (epinephrine), alcohol, barbiturates, benzodiazepines, CNS depressants, levodopa
• Hyperpyretic crisis, convulsions, hypertensive episode: tricyclic antidepressants, meperidine
• Increased hypoglycemic effect: insulin

NURSING CONSIDERATIONS
Assess:
• B/P (lying, standing), pulse; if systolic B/P drops 20 mm Hg, hold drug, notify physician
• Blood studies: CBC, leukocytes, cardiac enzymes if patient is receiving long-term therapy
• Hepatic studies: ALT, AST, bilirubin; hepatotoxicity may occur
• Toxicity: increased headache, palpitation; discontinue drug immediately; prodromal signs of hypertensive crisis
• Mental status changes: mood, sensorium, affect, memory (long, short); increase in psychiatric symptoms
• Urinary retention, constipation, edema; take weight weekly
• Withdrawal symptoms: headache, nausea, vomiting, muscle pain, weakness

Administer:
• Increased fluids, bulk in diet if constipation occurs
• With food or milk for GI symptoms

• Crushed if patient is unable swallow medication whole
• Dosage hs if oversedation occurs during day
• Gum, hard candy, or frequent sips of water for dry mouth
• Phentolamine for severe hypertension

Perform/provide:
• Storage in tight container in cool environment
• Assistance with ambulation during beginning therapy, since drowsiness/dizziness occurs, especially elderly
• Safety measures including side rails
• Checking to see PO medication swallowed

Evaluate:
• Therapeutic response: decreased depression

Teach patient/family:
• That therapeutic effects may take 1-4 wk
• To avoid driving, other activities requiring alertness
• To avoid alcohol ingestion, CNS depressants, OTC medications: cold, weight loss, hay fever, cough syrup
• Not to discontinue medication quickly after long-term use
• To avoid high-tyramine foods: cheese (aged), sour cream, beer, wine, pickled products, liver, raisins, bananas, figs, avocados, meat tenderizers, chocolate, yogurt; increased caffeine
• To report headache, palpitation, neck stiffness

Treatment of overdose: Lavage, activated charcoal, monitor electrolytes, vital signs, diazepam IV, NaHCO$_3$

P

---

italics = common side effects   ***bold italic*** = life threatening reactions

…bital, …rbital sodium

(fee … bar'bi-tal)

Barbita, Phenobarbital, Phenobarbital Sodium, Solfoton

Func. class.: Anticonvulsant
Chem. class.: Barbiturate

Controlled Substance Schedule IV

Action: Decreases impulse transmission; increases seizure threshold at cerebral cortex level

Uses: All forms of epilepsy, status epilepticus, febrile seizures in children, sedation, insomnia, hyperbilirubinemia, chronic cholestasis

Dosage and routes:

Seizures

• *Adult:* PO 100-200 mg/day in divided doses tid or total dose hs
• *Child:* PO 4-6 mg/kg/day in divided doses q12h; may be given as single dose

Status epilepticus

• *Adult:* IV INF 10 mg/kg; run no faster than 50/mg/min; may give up to 20 mg/kg
• *Child:* IV INF 5-10 mg/kg; may repeat q10-15min up to 20 mg/kg; run no faster than 50 mg/min

Insomnia

• *Adult:* PO/IM 100-320 mg
• *Child:* PO/IM 3-6 mg/kg

Sedation

• *Adult:* PO 30-120 mg/day in 2-3 divided doses
• *Child:* PO 6 mg/kg/day in 3 divided doses

Preoperative sedation

• *Adult:* IM 100-200 mg 1-1½ hr before surgery
• *Child:* PO 6 mg/kg/day in 3 divided doses

Hyperbilirubinemia

• *Neonate:* PO 7 mg/kg/day on days 1-5 after birth; IM 5 mg/kg/day on day 1, then PO on days 2-7 after birth

Chronic cholestasis

• *Adult:* PO 90-180 mg/day in 2-3 divided doses
• *Child <12 yr:* PO 3-12 mg/kg/day in 2-3 divided doses

Available forms: Caps 16 mg; elix 15, 20 mg/5 ml; tabs 8, 15, 16, 30, 32, 60, 65, 100 mg; inj 30, 60, 65, 130 mg/ml

Side effects/adverse reactions:

CNS: Paradoxical excitement (elderly), drowsiness, lethargy, hangover headache, flushing, hallucinations, coma
GI: Nausea, vomiting
INTEG: Rash, urticaria, Stevens-Johnson syndrome, angioedema, local pain, swelling, necrosis, thrombophlebitis

Contraindications: Hypersensitivity to barbiturates, porphyria, hepatic disease, respiratory disease, nephritis, hyperthyroidism, diabetes mellitus, elderly, lactation, pregnancy (D)

Precautions: Anemia

Pharmacokinetics:

IV: Onset 5 min, peak 30 min, duration 4-6 hr
IM/SC: Onset 10-30 min, duration 4-6 hr
PO: Onset 20-60 min, peak 8-12 hr, duration 6-10 hr; metabolized by liver, excreted by kidneys, crosses placenta, excreted in breast milk, half-life 53-118 hr

Interactions/incompatibilities:

• Increased effects: CNS depression, alcohol, chloramphenicol, valproic acid, disulfiram, nondepolarizing skeletal muscle relaxants, sulfonamides
• Decreased effects: Theophylline, oral anticoagulants, corticoste-

roids, OCs, metronidazole, doxycycline, quinidine
• Increased orthostatic hypotension: furosemide
• Incompatible with atropine,
benzquinamide, brompheniramine,
butorphanol, cefazolin, cephalothin, chlordiazepoxide, chlorpheniramine, chlorpromazine, cimetidine, clindamycin, codeine,
dimenhydrate, droperidol, erythromycin, glycopyrrolate, hydrocortisone, insulin, kanamycin, levarterenol, levorphanol, meperidine, methadone, midazolam,
morphine, nalbuphine, opium,
penicillins, pentazocine, phenytoin, prochlorperazine, promazine,
promethazine, ranitidine, streptomycin, succinylcholine, tetracycline, triflupromazine, vancomycin, NaCO₃, fructose sol

NURSING CONSIDERATIONS
Assess:
• Mental status: mood, sensorium,
affect, memory (long, short)
• Respiratory depression
• Blood dyscrasias: fever, sore
throat, bruising, rash, jaundice
• Convulsion activity: type, dura-
tion, precipitating factors
• Blood studies, liver function tests
during long-term treatment
• Therapeutic blood level periodi-
cally: 15-40 mg/ml
• Respiratory status: rate, rhythm,
depth

Administer:
• IV after slow dilution with at least
10 ml sterile H_2O for inj regardless
of dose; give 65 mg or less/min;
titrate to patient response
• Give IM inj deeply into large
muscle mass to prevent tissue
sloughing; use <5 ml in each site

Perform/provide:
• Supervision of ambulation for
dizziness, drowsiness

Evaluate:
• Therapeutic response: ᴄ
seizures, increased sedation

Teach patient/family:
• To use medication exactly as ordered
• To avoid other CNS depressants,
including alcohol
• To avoid hazardous activities until stabilized on drug; drowsiness
may occur
• Never to withdraw drug abruptly;
withdrawal symptoms may occur
• That therapeutic effects (PO) may
not be seen for 2-3 wk

Treatment of overdose: Calcium
gluconate IV

phenolphthalein
(fee-nol-thay'leen)
Alophen, Correctol, Espotabs,
Evac-U-Gen, Evac-U-Lax, Ex-
Lax, Feen-A-Mint, Lax-Pills,
Modane, Phenolax, Prulet

Func. class.: Laxative, stimu-
lant/irritant
Chem. class.: Diphenylmethane

Action: Directly acts on intestinal
smooth muscle by increasing motor
activity; thought to irritate colonic
intramural plexus
Uses: Constipation, preparation for
bowel surgery or examination
Dosage and routes:
• *Adult:* PO 60-270 mg hs
• *Child >6 yr:* 30-60 mg/day
• *Child 2-5 yr:* 15-20 mg/day
Available forms: Tabs 60 mg; chew
tab 60, 64.8, 80, 90, 97.2 mg;
chew gum 97.2 mg; susp 22 mg/5
ml
Side effects/adverse reactions:
INTEG: Rash, urticaria, **Stevens-
Johnson syndrome**

---

italics = common side effects   **bold italic** = life threatening reactions

*halein

*decreased

ıorexia,

ctrolyte,

ersensitiv-

abdominal

pain, ᵧ, fecal im-

paction

Pharmacokinetics:

PO: Onset 6-8 hr; excreted in feces

Lab test interferences:

BSP test

NURSING CONSIDERATIONS

Assess:

• Blood, urine electrolytes if drug is used often by patient

• I&O ratio to identify fluid loss

• Cause of constipation; identify whether fluids, bulk, or exercise is missing from life-style

• Cramping, rectal bleeding, nausea, vomiting; if these symptoms occur, drug should be discontinued

Administer:

• Alone for better absorption

• In morning or evening (oral dose)

Evaluate:

• Therapeutic response: decrease in constipation

Teach patient/family:

• To keep out of children's reach; some is fruit or chocolate flavored

• To swallow tabs whole; do not chew

• Not to use laxatives for long-term therapy; bowel tone will be lost

• That normal bowel movements do not always occur daily

• Not to use in presence of abdominal pain, nausea, vomiting

• To notify physician if constipation unrelieved or if symptoms of electrolyte imbalance occur: muscle cramps, pain, weakness, dizziness

• That urine, feces may turn pink to yellow-brown

---

phenoxybenzamine HCl

(fen-ox-ee-ben'za-meen)

Dibenzyline

Func. class.: Antihypertensive

Chem. class.: α-Adrenergic blocker

Action: α-Adrenergic blocker that binds to α-adrenergic receptors, dilating peripheral blood vessels, lowers peripheral resistance, lowers blood pressure

Uses: Pheochromocytoma

Dosage and routes:

• *Adult:* PO 10 mg bid, increase by 10 mg qod, usual range: 20-40 mg bid-tid

Available forms: Caps 10 mg

Side effects/adverse reactions:

GI: Dry mouth, nausea, vomiting, diarrhea

CV: Postural hypotension, tachycardia, palpitations

CNS: Dizziness, flushing, drowsiness, sedation, weakness, confusion, headache, malaise

GU: Inhibition of ejaculation

EENT: Nasal congestion, dry mouth, miosis

INTEG: Allergic contact dermatitis

Contraindications: Hypersensitivity, CHF, angina, cerebral vascular insufficiency, coronary arteriosclerosis

Precautions: Severe renal disease, severe pulmonary disease, pregnancy (C)

Pharmacokinetics:

PO: Onset 2 hr, peak 4-6 hr, duration 3-4 days; half-life 24 hr, metabolized in liver, excreted in urine, bile

Interactions/incompatibilities:

• Hypotensive response: epinephrine, antihypertensives

---

*Available in Canada only

NURSING CONSIDERATIONS
Assess:
- Electrolytes: K, Na, Cl, CO_2
- Weight daily, I&O
- B/P lying, standing before starting treatment, q4h after
- Nausea, vomiting, diarrhea
- Skin turgor, dryness of mucous membranes for hydration status

Administer:
- Starting with low dose, gradually increasing to prevent side effects
- Gum, frequent rinsing of mouth or hard candy for dry mouth
- With food or milk for GI symptoms

Evaluate:
- Therapeutic response: decreased B/P, increased peripheral pulses

Teach patient/family:
- To avoid alcoholic beverages
- To report dizziness, palpitations, fainting
- To change position slowly, or fainting may occur
- To take drug exactly as prescribed
- To avoid all OTC products: cough, cold, allergy, unless directed by physician

Treatment of overdose: Administer IV saline, norepinephrine, elevate legs, discontinue drug

---

phensuximide
(fen-sux'i-mide)
Kapseals, Milontin
Func. class.: Anticonvulsant
Chem. class.: Succinimide

Action: Inhibits spike, wave formation in absence seizures (petit mal), decreases amplitude, frequency, duration

Uses: Absence (petit mal) seizures

Dosage and routes:
- *Adult and child:* PO 500 mg-1 g bid or tid
Available forms: Caps 500 mg
Side effects/adverse reactions:
*HEMA: **Agranulocytosis, aplastic anemia, thrombocytopenia, leukocytosis, eosinophilia, pancytopenia***
CNS: Drowsiness, dizziness, fatigue, euphoria, lethargy, anxiety, depression, irritability, insomnia, aggressiveness, weakness, headache
GI: Nausea, vomiting, heartburn, anorexia, diarrhea, abdominal pain, cramps, constipation
GU: Vaginal bleeding, ***hematuria, renal damage,*** urinary frequency
INTEG: Urticaria, pruritic erythema, hirsutism, ***Stevens-Johnson syndrome***
EENT: Myopia, gum hypertrophy, tongue swelling, blurred vision
Contraindications: Hypersensitivity to succinimide derivatives
Precautions: Lactation, hepatic disease, pregnancy (D), renal disease
Pharmacokinetics:
PO: Peak 1-4 hr, metabolized by liver, excreted by kidneys, half-life 5-12 hr
Interactions/incompatibilities:
- Antagonist effect: tricyclic antidepressants (imipramine, doxepin)
- Decreased effects of: estrogens, oral contraceptives
Lab test interferences:
Increase: Coombs' test

NURSING CONSIDERATIONS
Assess:
- Renal studies: urinalysis, BUN, urine creatinine q6mo
- Blood studies: CBC, Hct, Hgb, reticulocyte counts q3mo
- Hepatic studies: AST, ALT, bilirubin, creatinine q6mo

---

italics = common side effects   ***bold italic*** = life threatening reactions

• Drug levels during initial treatment, therapeutic range (40-80 μg/ml)
• Mental status: mood, sensorium, affect, behavioral changes; if mental status changes, notify physician
• Eye problems; need for ophthalmic exam before, during, after treatment (slit lamp, fundoscopy, tonometry)
• Allergic reaction: red raised rash; if this occurs, drug should be discontinued
• Blood dyscrasias: fever, sore throat, bruising, rash, jaundice
• Toxicity: bone marrow depression, nausea, vomiting, ataxia, diplopia

Administer:
• With food, milk to decrease GI symptoms

Perform/provide:
• Hard candy, frequent rinsing of mouth, gum for dry mouth
• Assistance with ambulation during early part of treatment; dizziness occurs

Evaluate:
• Therapeutic response: decreased seizures

Teach patient/family:
• To carry ID card or Medic Alert bracelet stating drugs taken, condition, physician's name, phone number
• To avoid driving, other activities that require alertness
• To avoid alcohol ingestion, CNS depressants; increased sedation may occur
• Not to discontinue medication quickly after long-term use
• To call physician if sore throat, fever, malaise, bruises, epistaxis occur
• That drug may color urine pink or red

Treatment of overdose: Lavage, activated charcoal, monitor electrolytes, VS; do not induce vomiting

phentermine HCl
(fen'ter-meen)
Adipex-P, Fastin, Ionamin, Obephen, Obe-Nix, Phentermine Resin, Phentermine HCl, Phentrol
Func. class.: Cerebral stimulant
Chem. class.: Sympathomimetic amine

Controlled Substance Schedule IV

Action: Stimulates satiety center by action on adrenergic pathways

Uses: Exogenous obesity

Dosage and routes:
• *Adult:* PO 8 mg tid 30 min before meals or 15-37.5 mg qd before breakfast

Available forms: Tabs 8, 15, 30, 37.5 mg; caps 15, 18.75, 30, 37.5 mg; caps time rel 15, 30 mg

Side effects/adverse reactions:
CNS: Hyperactivity, insomnia, restlessness, dizziness, tremor, headache
GI: Nausea, anorexia, dry mouth, constipation, unpleasant taste
GU: Impotence, change in libido
CV: Palpitations, tachycardia, hypertension
INTEG: Urticaria
EENT: Blurred vision

Contraindications: Hypersensitivity, hyperthyroidism, hypertension, glaucoma, severe arteriosclerosis, angina pectoris, cardiovascular disease, pregnancy (C), child <12 yr

Precautions: Pregnancy (C), lactation, drug abuse, anxiety

Pharmacokinetics:
CON REL: Duration 10-14 hr; me-

tabolized by liver, excreted by kidneys

Interactions/incompatibilities:
• Hypertensive crisis: MAOIs or within 14 days of MAOIs
• Increased effect of phentermine: acetazolamide, antacids, sodium bicarbonate
• Decreased effect of phentermine: tricyclics, ascorbic acid, ammonium chloride
• Decreased effect of: guanethidine, other antihypertensives
• Decreased insulin requirements: diabetes mellitus

NURSING CONSIDERATIONS
Assess:
• VS, B/P, since this drug may reverse antihypertensives; check patients with cardiac disease more often
• CBC, urinalysis, in diabetes: blood sugar, urine sugar; insulin changes may have to be made, since eating will decrease
• Height and growth rate in children; growth rate may be decreased
• Mental status: mood, sensorium, affect, stimulation, insomnia, aggressiveness
• Physical dependency: should not be used for extended periods; dose should be discontinued gradually; tolerance occurs with long-term use
• Withdrawal symptoms: headache, nausea, vomiting, muscle pain, weakness

Administer:
• At least 6 hr before hs to avoid sleeplessness
• For obesity only if patient is on weight reduction program including dietary changes, exercise; patient will develop tolerance, and loss of weight won't occur without additional methods; give 30 min before meals

• Gum, hard candy, frequent sips of water for dry mouth

Perform/provide:
• Check to see PO medication has been swallowed

Evaluate:
• Therapeutic response: decreased weight

Teach patient/family:
• To decrease caffeine consumption (coffee, tea, cola, chocolate), which may increase irritability, stimulation
• To avoid OTC preparations unless approved by physician
• To taper off drug over several weeks, or depression, increased sleeping, lethargy may ensue
• To avoid alcohol ingestion
• To avoid hazardous activities until patient is stabilized on medication
• To get needed rest; patients will feel more tired at end of day

Treatment of overdose: Administer fluids; hemodialysis or peritoneal dialysis; antihypertensive for increased B/P; ammonium Cl for increased excretion

phentolamine mesylate

(fen-tole'a-meen)
Regitine, Rogitine*
Func. class.: Antihypertensive
Chem. class.: α-Adrenergic blocker

Action: α-Adrenergic blocker, binds to α-adrenergic receptors, dilating peripheral blood vessels, lowering peripheral resistances, lowering blood pressure
Uses: Hypertension, pheochromocytoma, prevention, treatment of dermal necrosis following extrav-

asation of norepinephrine or dopamine

Dosage and routes:

***Treatment of hypertensive epi-
sodes in pheochromocytoma***

• *Adult:* 5 mg IV/IM, repeat if
necessary

• *Child:* 1 mg IV/IM, repeat if
necessary

• *Adult:* 2.5 mg IV, if negative repeat with 5 mg IV

• *Child:* 0.5 mg IV, if negative repeat with 1 mg IV

Prevention, treatment of necrosis

• *Adult:* 5-10 mg/10 ml NS injected into area of norepinephrine
extravasation within 12 hr

Available forms: Inj IM, IV 5 mg/
ml; tabs 25, 50 mg (only injectable
form available in US)

Side effects/adverse reactions:

*GI: Dry mouth, nausea, vomiting,
diarrhea, abdominal pain*

*CV: Hypotension, tachycardia, an-
gina, dysrhythmias, **myocardial infarction***

CNS: Dizziness, flushing, weakness

EENT: Nasal congestion

Contraindications: Hypersensitivity, myocardial infarction, coronary insufficiency, angina

Precautions: Pregnancy (C), lactation

Pharmacokinetics:

IV: Peak 2 min, duration 10-15 min

IM: Peak 15-20 min, duration 3-4
hr; metabolized in liver, excreted in
urine

Interactions/incompatibilities:

• Increased effects of: epinephrine,
antihypertensives

• Incompatible with iron salts

NURSING CONSIDERATIONS

Assess:

• Electrolytes: K, Na, Cl, CO_2

• Weight daily, I&O

• B/P lying, standing before starting treatment, q4h after

• Nausea, vomiting, diarrhea,
edema in feet, legs daily; skin turgor, dryness of mucous membranes
for hydration status, postural hypotension, cardiac system: pulse,
ECG

Administer:

• IV after diluting 5 mg/1 ml sterile H_2O for inj; may be further diluted with 5-10 ml sterile H_2O for
inj; give 5 mg or less/min

• Gum, frequent rinsing of mouth
or hard candy for dry mouth

• With vasopressor nearby

• After discontinuing all medication for 24 hr

Evaluate:

• Therapeutic response: decreased
B/P

Teach patient/family:

• That bed rest is required during
treatment, 1 hr after

Treatment of overdose: Administer norepinephrine; discontinue
drug

---

phenylbutazone

(fen-ill-byoo'-ta-zone)

Butazolidin, Phenylbutazone

Func. class.: Nonsteroidal antiinflammatory

Chem. class.: Pyrazolone derivative

Action: Inhibits prostaglandin synthesis by decreasing an enzyme
needed for biosynthesis; analgesic,
antiinflammatory, antipyretic

Uses: Mild to moderate pain, osteoarthritis, rheumatoid arthritis,
acute gouty arthritis

Dosage and routes:

Pain

• *Adult:* PO 100-200 mg tid-qid,
then after desired response 100 mg
tid-qid, not to exceed 600 mg/day

Acute Arthritis

• *Adult:* PO 400 mg, then 100 mg q4h × 4 days or until desired response

Available forms: Tabs 100 mg; caps 100 mg

Side effects/adverse reactions:

GI: Nausea, anorexia, vomiting, diarrhea, jaundice, *cholestatic hepatitis,* constipation, flatulence, cramps, dry mouth, peptic ulcer

CNS: Dizziness, drowsiness, fatigue, tremors, confusion, insomnia, anxiety, depression

CV: Tachycardia, peripheral edema, palpitations, dysrhythmias, pericarditis, myocarditis, cardiac decompensation

INTEG: Purpura, rash, pruritus, sweating

GU: Nephrotoxicity: dysuria, hematuria, oliguria, azotemia

HEMA: Bone marrow suppression

EENT: Tinnitus, hearing loss, blurred vision

Contraindications: Hypersensitivity, asthma, severe renal disease, severe hepatic disease, pregnancy (D), children <14 yr, ulcer disease

Precautions: Lactation, children, bleeding disorders, GI disorders, cardiac disorders, hypersensitivity to other antiinflammatory agents

Pharmacokinetics:

PO: Peak 2 hr, half-life 3-3½ hr; metabolized in liver, excreted in urine (metabolites), excreted in breast milk, 98% protein binding

Interactions/incompatibilities:

• Increased action of: coumarin, phenytoin, sulfonamides when used with this drug

NURSING CONSIDERATIONS

Assess:

• Renal, liver, blood studies: BUN, creatinine, AST, ALT, Hgb, before treatment, periodically thereafter

• Record patient's weight and I&O daily

• Audiometric, ophthalmic exam before, during, after treatment

• For history of peptic ulcer disease

• For eye, ear problems: blurred vision, tinnitus (may indicate toxicity)

Administer:

• With food to decrease GI symptoms; best to take on empty stomach to facilitate absorption

Perform/provide:

• Storage at room temperature

Evaluate:

• Therapeutic response: decreased pain, stiffness, swelling in joints, ability to move more easily

Teach patient/family:

• To report blurred vision or ringing, roaring in ears (may indicate toxicity)

• To avoid driving or other hazardous activities if dizziness or drowsiness occurs

• To report change in urine pattern, weight increase, edema, pain increase in joints, fever, blood in urine (indicates nephrotoxicity)

• That therapeutic effects may take up to 1 mo

• To report black, tarry stools or unusual bleeding, bruising

• To take with full glass of water

---

phenylephrine HCl

(fen-ill-ef'rin)

Neo-Synephrine

Func. class.: Adrenergic, direct acting

Chem. class.: Substituted phenylethylamine

Action: Powerful and selective (α_1) receptor agonist causing contraction of blood vessels

Uses: Hypotension, paroxysmal

---

supraventricular tachycardia, shock, maintain B/P during spinal anesthesia

Dosage and routes:

Hypotension

• *Adult:* SC/IM 2-5 mg, may repeat q10-15min if needed IV 0.1-0.5 mg, may repeat q10-15min if needed

PVCs

• *Adult:* IV BOL 0.5 mg given rapidly, not to exceed prior dose by >0.1 mg; total dose >1 mg

Shock

• *Adult:* IV INF 10 mg/500 ml D₅W given 100-180 gtts/min, then 40-60 gtts/min titrated to B/P

Available forms: Inj IV, SC, IM, 1% (10 mg/ml)

Side effects/adverse reactions:

CNS: Headache, anxiety, tremor, insomnia, dizziness

CV: Palpitations, tachycardia, hypertension, ectopic beats, angina, reflex bradycardia

GI: Nausea, vomiting

INTEG: Necrosis, tissue sloughing with extravasation, ***gangrene***

Contraindications: Hypersensitivity, ventricular fibrillation, tachydysrhythmias, pheochromocytoma, narrow-angle glaucoma

Precautions: Pregnancy (C), lactation, arterial embolism, peripheral vascular disease, elderly, hyperthyroidism, bradycardia, myocardial disease, severe arteriosclerosis

Pharmacokinetics:

IV: Duration 20-30 min

IM/SC: Duration 45-60 min

Interactions/incompatibilities:

• Do not use within 2 wk of MAOIs, or hypertensive crisis may result

• Dysrhythmias: general anesthetics, bretylium

• Decreased action of phenylephrine: α-blockers

• Increase in B/P: oxytocics

• Increased pressor effect: tricyclic antidepressant, MAOIs, guanethidine

• Incompatible with alkaline solutions: NaHCO₃, iron salts, phenytoin

NURSING CONSIDERATIONS

Assess:

• I&O ratio, notify MD if output <30 ml/hr

• ECG during administration continuously; if B/P increases, drug is decreased

• B/P and pulse q5min after parenteral route

• CVP or PWP during infusion if possible

• For paresthesias and coldness of extremities; peripheral blood flow may decrease

Administer:

• Plasma expanders for hypovolemia

• IV after diluting 1 mg/9 ml sterile H₂O for inj; give dose over ½-1 min; may be diluted 10 mg/500 ml of D₅W or NS; titrate to patient response; low (normal B/P) check for extravasation, check site for infiltration, use infusion pump

Perform/provide:

• Storage of reconstituted sol if refrigerated for no longer than 24 hr

• Elimination of discolored sol

Evaluate:

• Therapeutic response: increase B/P with stabilization

Teach patient/family:

• The reason for drug administration

• To report pain at infusion site immediately

Treatment of overdose: Administer an α-blocker

---

*Available in Canada only

phenylephrine HCl (nasal)

(fen-ill-ef'rin)

Alconefrin, Alconefrin-25, Alconefrin-50, Duration, Neo-Synephrine, Nōstril, Rhinall-10, Sinex, St. Joseph Measured Dose

Func. class.: Nasal decongestant

Chem. class.: Sympathomimetic amine

Action: Produces vasoconstriction (rapid, long-acting) of arterioles, thereby decreasing fluid exudation, mucosal engorgement

Uses: Nasal congestion

Dosage and routes:
• *Adult:* INSTILL 2-3 gtts or sprays to nasal mucosa bid (0.25%-1%); TOP apply to nasal mucosa q3-4h prn
• *Child 6-12 yr:* INSTILL 1-2 gtts or sprays (0.25%) q3-4h prn
• *Child <6 yr:* INSTILL 2-3 gtts or sprays (0.125%) q3-4h prn

Available forms: Sol 0.125%, 0.16%, 0.2%, 0.25%, 0.5%, 1%; jelly 0.5%

Side effects/adverse reactions:
GI: Nausea, vomiting, anorexia
EENT: Irritation, burning, sneezing, stinging, dryness, rebound congestion
INTEG: Contact dermatitis
CNS: Anxiety, restlessness, tremors, weakness, insomnia, dizziness, fever, headache

Contraindications: Hypersensitivity to sympathomimetic amines

Precautions: Child <6 yr, elderly, diabetes, cardiovascular disease, hypertension, hyperthyroidism, increased ICP, prostatic hypertrophy, pregnancy (C), glaucoma

Interactions/incompatibilities:
• Hypertension: MAOIs, β-adrenergic blockers
• Hypotension: methyldopa, mecamylamine, reserpine

NURSING CONSIDERATIONS
Assess:
• Redness, swelling, pain in nasal passages

Administer:
• No more than q4h
• For <4 consecutive days

Perform/provide:
• Environmental humidification to decrease nasal congestion, dryness
• Storage in light-resistant containers; do not expose to high temperatures

Evaluate:
• Therapeutic response: decreased nasal congestion

Teach patient/family:
• That stinging may occur for a few applications; drying of mucosa may be decreased by environmental humidification
• To notify physician if irregular pulse, insomnia, dizziness, or tremors occur
• Proper administration to avoid systemic absorption

phenylephrine HCl (optic)

(fen-ill-ef'rin)

AK-Dilate Ophthalmic, AK-Nefrin Ophthalmic, Isopto Frin, Neo-Synephrine 2.5%, Neo-Synephrine 10% Plain, Neo-Synephrine Viscous, Phenylephrine HCl, 2.5% Mydfrin Ophthalmic, Phenoptic, Relief, Prefrin

Func. class.: Ophthalmic vasoconstrictor

Chem. class.: Direct sympathomimetic amine (α-agonist)

Action: Vasoconstriction of eye arterioles; decreases eye engorgement by stimulation of α-adrenergic receptors

Uses: Topical ocular vasoconstrictor in uveitis, open-angle glaucoma, prior to surgery, diagnostic procedures, refraction without cycloplegia

Dosage and routes:
Eye irritation
• *Adult:* INSTILL 2 gtts of a 0.12% sol; may repeat q3-4h
Refraction/ophthalmoscopic exam
• *Adult:* Sol 1 gtt of 2.5%
Uveitis/glaucoma/surgery
• *Adult and child:* INSTILL 1 gtt of a 2.5% or 10% sol in upper surface of cornea
Available forms: Sol 10%, 2.5%, 0.12%

Side effects/adverse reactions:
CNS: Headache, dizziness, weakness
CV: Bradycardia, hypertension, dysrhythmias, *tachycardia, CV collapse,* palpitation
EENT: Stinging, lacrimation, blurred vision, conjunctival allergy
Contraindications: Hypersensitivity, narrow-angle glaucoma
Precautions: Severe hypertension, diabetes, hyperthyroidism, elderly, severe arteriosclerosis, cardiac disease, infants, pregnancy (C)
Pharmacokinetics:
INSTILL: Peak 1 hr, duration 0.5-7 hr depending on strength
Interactions/incompatibilities:
• Increased pressor effects: MAOIs, tricyclic antidepressants, H_1 antihistamines, guanethedine
NURSING CONSIDERATIONS
Assess:
• B/P, pulse; systemic absorption does occur
Perform/provide:
• Storage in tight, light-resistant container; do not use discolored solutions

Evaluate:
• Therapeutic response: decreased eye irritation

Teach patient/family:
• To report change in vision, blurring, loss of sight; breathing trouble, sweating, flushing
• Method of instillation: tilt head backward, hold dropper over eye, drop medication inside lower lid, using pressure on inside corner of eye hold 1 min, do not touch dropper to eye
• That blurred vision will decrease with repeated use of drug
• To notify physician of headache, spots, redness, pain; discontinue use
• To use sunglasses if photophobia occurs
• To use exactly as prescribed

phenytoin sodium/ phenytoin sodium extended/phenytoin sodium prompt
(fen'i-toy-in)
Dilantin, Dilantin Capsules, Di-Phen, Diphenylan, Phenytoin Oral Suspension
Func. class.: Anticonvulsant
Chem. class.: Hydantoin

Action: Inhibits spread of seizure activity in motor cortex
Uses: Generalized tonic-clonic seizures; status epilepticus; nonepileptic seizures associated with Reye's syndrome or after head trauma; migraines, trigeminal neuralgia, Bell's palsy, ventricular dysrhythmias uncontrolled by antidysrhythmics
Dosage and routes:
Seizures
• *Adult:* IV loading dose 900 mg-

1.5 g run at 50 mg/min; if patient has received phenytoin, 100-300 mg run at 50 mg/min; PO loading dose 900 mg-1.5 g divided tid, then 300 mg/day (extended) or divided tid (extended/prompt)
• *Child:* IV loading dose 15 mg/kg run at 50 mg/min; if patient has received phenytoin, 5-7 mg/kg run at 50 mg/min; may repeat in 30 min; PO loading dose of 15 mg/kg divided q8-12h, then 5-7 mg/kg in divided doses q12h
Neuritic pain
• *Adult:* PO 200-400 mg/day
Ventricular dysrhythmias
• *Adult:* PO loading dose 1 g divided over 24 hr, then 500 mg/day × 2 days; IV 250 mg given over 5 min until dysrhythmias subside or 1 g is given or 100 mg q15min until dysrhythmias subside or 1 g is given
• *Child:* PO 3-8 mg/kg or 250 mg/m²/day as single dose or divided in 2 doses; IV 3-8 mg/kg given over several min, or 250 mg/m²/day as single dose or divided in 2 doses
Available forms: Susp 30, 125 mg/5 ml; tabs, chewable 50 mg; inj 50 mg/ml; caps ext 30, 100 mg; caps prompt 30, 100 mg

Side effects/adverse reactions:
CNS: Drowsiness, dizziness, insomnia, paresthesias, depression, suicidal tendencies, aggression, headache, confusion, slurred speech
CV: Hypotension, *ventricular fibrillation*
EENT: Nystagmus, diplopia, blurred vision
GI: Nausea, vomiting, constipation, anorexia, weight loss, *hepatitis,* jaundice, gingival hyperplasia
GU: Nephritis

*HEMA: **Agranulocytosis, leukopenia, aplastic anemia, thrombocytopenia, megaloblastic anemia***
INTEG: Rash, *lupus erythematosus, Stevens-Johnson syndrome,* hirsutism

Contraindications: Hypersensitivity, psychiatric condition, pregnancy (D), bradycardia, SA and AV block, Stokes-Adams syndrome
Precautions: Allergies, hepatic disease, renal disease

Pharmacokinetics:
PO-ER: Onset 2-24 hr, peak 4-12 hr, duration 12-36 hr
PO: Onset 2-24 hr, peak 1½-2½ hr, duration 6-12 hr, metabolized by liver, excreted by kidneys
IV: Onset 1-2 hr, duration 12-24 hr

Interactions/incompatibilities:
• Decreased effects of phenytoin: alcohol (chronic use), antihistamines, antacids, antineoplastics, CNS depressants, rifampin, folic acid
• Incompatible with any drug in sol or syringe

Lab test interferences:
Decrease: Dexamethasone, metyrapone test serum, PBI, urinary steroids
Increase: Glucose, alk phosphatase, BSP

NURSING CONSIDERATIONS
Assess:
• Drug level: toxic level 30-50 μg/ml
• Blood studies: CBC, platelets q2wk until stabilized, then qmo × 12, then q3mo; discontinue drug if neutrophils are <1600/mm³
• Mental status: mood, sensorium, affect, memory (long, short)
• Respiratory depression; rate, depth, character
• Blood dyscrasias: fever, sore throat, bruising, rash, jaundice

P

---

italics = common side effects   ***bold italic*** = life threatening reactions

Administer:
• IV after diluting with special diluent provided (2.2 ml/100 mg, 5.2 ml/250 mg) (1 ml/50 mg); place vial in warm water to dissolve powder; give through Y-tube or 3-way stopcock; inject slowly <50 mg/min; clear IV tubing first with NS sol; use in-line filter; discard 4 hr after preparation; inject into large veins to prevent purple glove syndrome

Evaluate:
• Therapeutic response; decrease in severity of seizures, ventricular dysrhythmias

Teach patient/family:
• To take PO doses divided with or after meals to decrease adverse effects
• That if diabetic, urine glucose should be monitored
• That urine may turn pink
• Not to discontinue drug abruptly; seizures may occur
• Proper brushing of teeth using a soft toothbrush, flossing to prevent gingival hyperplasia; need to see dentist frequently
• To avoid hazardous activities until stabilized on drug
• To carry Medic Alert ID stating drug use
• That heavy use of alcohol may diminish effect of drug; to avoid OTC medications
• Not to change brands or forms once stabilized on therapy; brands may vary

physostigmine salicylate/physostigmine sulfate

(fi-zoe-stig′meen)
Isopto Eserine Solution/Eserine Sulfate Ointment, Fisostin
Func. class.: Miotic
Chem. class.: Cholinesterase inhibitor

Action: Increases concentration of acetylcholine at cholinergic transmission sites, causing prolonged, exaggerated action; produces constriction of ciliary muscles, iris sphincter, causing iris to be pulled away from anterior chamber angle, aiding in aqueous humor drainage

Uses: Wide-angle glaucoma

Dosage and routes:
• *Adult and child:* INSTILL OINT ¼ inch strip of 0.25% oint in conjunctival sac; INSTILL SOL 1-2 gtts of a 0.25%-0.5% sol in conjunctival sac qd-qid

Available forms: Oint 0.25% (sulfate); sol 0.25% (salicylate)

Side effects/adverse reactions:
*CNS: **Convulsions,*** headache
CV: Hypertension, hypotension, bradycardia, irregular pulse
GI: Nausea, vomiting, abdominal cramps
*RESP: **Bronchospasm,*** dyspnea, ***pulmonary edema***
EENT: Blurred vision, conjunctivitis, allergic reactions, rhinorrhea, salivation, eye, brow pain, lacrimation, twitching of eyelids

Contraindications: Hypersensitivity, inflammatory disease of iris or ciliary body

Precautions: Epilepsy, parkinsonism, bradycardia, pregnancy (C), asthma, bronchitis, diabetes mellitus, CV disease

Interactions/incompatibilities:
• Benzalkonium chloride in solution or syringe

Pharmacokinetics:

Miosis: Onset 20-30 min, duration 12-36 hr

Intraocular pressure: Peak 2-6 hrs, duration 12-36 hrs

NURSING CONSIDERATIONS

Administer:
• Topically to conjunctival sac
• Immediately after reconstituting; discard unused portion

Perform/provide:
• Only clear sol, never pink or brown

Evaluate
• Therapeutic response: decreased intraocular pressure

Teach patient/family:
• To report change in vision, blurring or loss of sight, trouble breathing, sweating, flushing
• Method of instillation, including pressure on lacrimal sac for 1 min, not to touch dropper to eye
• That long-term therapy may be required
• That blurred vision will decrease with repeated use of drug
• That drug is often irritating to eye, rarely tolerated for prolonged periods
• That drug may be prescribed for bedtime use to prevent nocturnal rise in ocular tension
• That maximal effect of topical application is reached in 30 min, may last 12-36 hr
• To observe eyes for irritation, development of cataracts

---

physostigmine salicylate

(fi-zoe-stig′meen)
Antilirium
Func. class.: Antidote, reversible anticholinesterase
Chem. class.: Tertiary amine

Action: Increases acetylcholine at cholinergic nerve terminals; reverses central, peripheral anticholinergic effects

Uses: To reverse CNS effects of diazepam; anticholinergic, tricyclic antidepressant, Alzheimer's disease, hereditary ataxia

Dosage and routes:

Overdose of anticholinergics
• *Adult:* IM/IV 2 mg; give no more than 1 mg/min; may repeat
• *Pediatric:* IM/IV inj 0.02 mg/kg, not more than 0.5 mg/min; may repeat at 5-10 min intervals until max dose of 2 mg

Postanesthesia
• *Adult:* IM/IV 0.5-1 mg; give no more than 1 mg/min (IV); can repeat at 10 to 30 min intervals

Available forms: Inj IM, IV 1 mg/ml

Side effects/adverse reactions:

INTEG: Rash, urticaria

CNS: Dizziness, headache, sweating, weakness, *convulsions,* incoordination, *paralysis,* hallucination, delirium, drowsiness

GI: Nausea, diarrhea, vomiting, cramps, increased salivary and gastric secretions

CV: Bradycardia, hypotension, syncope

GU: Frequency, incontinence, urgency

RESP: Respiratory depression, bronchospasm, constriction, dyspnea

P

---

italics = common side effects   ***bold italic*** = life threatening reactions

EENT: Miosis, blurred vision, lacrimation

Contraindications: Hypotension, obstruction of intestine or renal system, asthma, gangrene, CV disease, choline esters, depolarizing neuromuscular blocking agents, diabetes

Precautions: Seizure disorders, bronchial asthma, coronary occlusion, hyperthyroidism, dysrhythmias, peptic ulcer, megacolon, poor GI motility, pregnancy (C), Parkinson's disease, bradycardia, lactation

Pharmacokinetics:
IM/IV: Peak 5 min, duration 45-60 min; crosses blood-brain barrier, excreted in urine

Interactions/incompatibilities:
• Decreased action of: gallamine, metocurine, pancuronium, tubocurarine, atropine
• Increased action of: decamethonium, succinylcholine
• Decreased action of physostigmine: aminoglycosides, anesthetics, procainamide, quinidine
• Considered incompatible with any drug in sol or syringe

NURSING CONSIDERATIONS
Assess:
• VS; respiration q8h
• I&O ratio; check for urinary retention or incontinence
• Drug should be discontinued if toxicity occurs

Administer:
• IV undiluted, give through Y-tube or 3-way stopcock; give 1 mg or less/1-3 min or 0.5 mg or less over 1 min or more (child)
• Only with atropine sulfate available for cholinergic crisis
• Only after all other cholinergics have been discontinued
• Increased doses if tolerance occurs

Perform/provide:
• Storage at room temperature
Evaluate:
• Therapeutic response: LOC—alert
Treatment of overdose: Can cause cholinergic crisis; atropine is an antagonist

---

phytonadione (vitamin K₁)
(fye-toe-na-dye'one)
AquaMEPHYTON, Konakion, Mephyton
Func. class.: Vitamin K₁, fat-soluble vitamin

Action: Needed for adequate blood clotting (factors II, VII, IX, X)
Uses: Vit K malabsorption, hypoprothrombinemia, prevention of hypoprothrombinemia caused by oral anticoagulants

Dosage and routes:
Hypoprothrombinemia caused by Vit K malabsorption
• *Adult:* PO/IM 2-25 mg may repeat or increase to 50 mg
• *Child:* PO/IM 5-10 mg
• *Infants:* PO/IM 2 mg
Prevention of hemorrhagic disease of the newborn
• *Neonate:* SC/IM 0.5-1 mg after birth, repeat in 6-8 hr if required
Hypoprothrombinemia caused by oral anticoagulants
• *Adult:* PO/SC/IM 2.5-10 mg, may repeat 12-48 hr after PO dose or 6-8 hr after SC/IM dose, based on PT
Available forms: Tabs 5 mg; inj aqueous colloidal IM, IV; inj aqueous dispersion 2, 10 mg/ml, IM only

Side effects/adverse reactions:
CNS: Headache, *brain damage* (large doses)

GI: Nausea, decrease liver function tests

HEMA: **Hemolytic anemia, hemoglobinuria, hyperbilirubinemia**

INTEG: Rash, urticaria

Contraindications: Hypersensitivity, severe hepatic disease, last few weeks of pregnancy

Precautions: Pregnancy (C), neonates

Pharmacokinetics:

PO/INJ: Metabolized, crosses placenta

Interactions/incompatibilities:

• Decreased action of phytonadione: cholestyramine, mineral oil

• Decreased action of: oral anticoagulants

• Incompatible with Vits C and B$_{12}$, dextran, pentobarbital, phenobarbital, phenytoin, vancomycin, warfarin

NURSING CONSIDERATIONS

Assess:

• Pro-time during treatment (2-sec deviation from control time, bleeding time, and clotting time); monitor for bleeding, pulse, and BP

• Nutritional status: liver (beef), spinach, tomatoes, coffee, asparagus, broccoli, cabbage, lettuce, greens

Administer:

• IV after diluting with D$_5$ NS 10 ml or more; give 1 mg/min or more

• IV only when other routes not possible (deaths have occurred)

Perform/provide

• Storage in tight, light-resistant container

Evaluate:

• Therapeutic response: decreased bleeding tendencies, decreased pro-time, decreased clotting time

Teach patient/family

• Not to take other supplements, unless directed by physician

• Necessary foods to be included in diet

• To avoid IM injections, use soft toothbrush, don't floss, use electric razor until coagulation defect corrected

• To report symptoms of bleeding

• Not to use OTC medications unless approved by physician

• Emphasize importance of frequent lab tests to monitor coagulation factors

---

pilocarpine HCl/pilocarpine nitrate

(pye-loe-kar'peen)

Adsorbocarpine, Akarpine, Isopto Carpine, Miocarpine,* Pilagan, Pilocar, Pilocarpine HCl, Pilopine HS, Piloptic-1, Piloptic-2, Pilostat

Func. class.: Direct-acting miotic

Chem. class.: Cholinergic agonist

Action: Acts directly on cholinergic receptor sites; induces miosis, spasm of accommodation, fall in intraocular pressure, caused by stimulation of ciliary, pupillary sphincter muscles, which leads to pulling away of iris from filtration angle, resulting in increased outflow of aqueous humor

Uses: Primary glaucoma, early stages of wide-angle glaucoma (less useful in advanced stages), chronic open-angle glaucoma, acute narrow-angle glaucoma before emergency surgery; also neutralizes mydriatics used during eye exam; may be used alternately with mydriatics to break adhesions between iris and lens

Dosage and routes:

• *Adult and child:* INSTILL SOL

---

italics = common side effects   ***bold italic*** = life threatening reactions

1-2 gtts of 1% or 2% solution in eye q6-8h; INSTILL 20-40 µg/hr (Ocusert) in cul-de-sac of eye

Available forms: 0.25% to 10% sol; Ocusert Pilo 20, 40; 4% gel

Side effects/adverse reactions:

CV: Hypotension, tachycardia

RESP: **Bronchospasm**

GI: Nausea, vomiting, abdominal cramps, diarrhea

GU: Bladder tightness

EENT: Blurred vision, browache, twitching of eyelids, eye pain with change in focus

Contraindications: Hypersensitivity

Precautions: Bronchial asthma, hypertension, pregnancy (C), bradycardia, hyperthyroidism, coronary artery disease, obstruction of GI/urinary tracts (or if strength of walls of these structures in question, peptic ulcers), epilepsy, parkinsonism, asthma

NURSING CONSIDERATIONS

Assess:
• Heart rate, respiratory status, B/P
• Replacement of ocular systems qwk; check system each hs, AM

Administer:
• After shaking vial to mix drug to clear solution; push stopper to mix sterile water with powder
• After cleaning stopper with alcohol
• Wipe away excess solution promptly to prevent its flow into lacrimal system, producing systemic symptoms
• With atropine readily available as antidote
• Immediately after reconstituting; discard unused portion

Perform/provide:
• Protect solution from light
• Store Ocusert systems and sol at 36°-46° F (2°-8° C), 46°-86° F 8°-

30° C; refrigerate gel until dispensed to patient; discard unused sol after 8wk

Evaluate:
• Therapeutic response: decreased intraocular pressure

Teach patient/family:
• To report change in vision, blurring or loss of sight, trouble breathing, sweating, flushing
• Method of instillation, including pressure on lacrimal sac for 1 min, not to touch dropper to eye
• That long-term therapy may be required
• That blurred vision will decrease with repeated use of drug
• To discontinue use if local hypersensitivity reaction occurs
• That acuity in dim light will be reduced
• Not to drive while using drug

---

pinacidil

(pye-na'si-dil)
Pindac

Func. class.: Antihypertensive
Chem. class.: Vasodilator—peripheral

Action: Directly relaxes arteriolar smooth muscle, causing vasodilation

Uses: Severe hypertension not responsive to other therapy; topically to treat alopecia

Dosage and routes:
• *Adult:* PO 12.5-25 mg bid

Available forms: Tabs 12.5, 25 mg

Side effects/adverse reactions:

CV: Severe rebound hypertension, tachycardia, angina, increased T wave, *CHF,* pulmonary edema, edema, Na and water retention

CNS: Drowsiness, dizziness, sedation, headache, depression

GI: Nausea, vomiting, diarrhea, constipation, dry mouth
GU: Gynecomastia, breast tenderness
INTEG: Pruritus, **Stevens-Johnson syndrome**, rash, hirsutism
Contraindications: Acute myocardial infarction, dissecting aortic aneurysm, hypersensitivity, pheochromocytoma
Precautions: Pregnancy (C), lactation, children, renal disease, CAD, post MI
Pharmacokinetics:
Peak 1 hr, 60% protein bound; metabolized in the liver; excreted in urine, feces (active metabolites); half-life 1½-3 hr
Interactions/incompatibilities:
• Orthostatic hypotension: guanethidine
• Reduced effect of pinacidil: nonsteroidal antiinflammatory drugs
Lab test interferences:
Increase: Renal function studies
Decrease: Hgb/Hct/RBC
NURSING CONSIDERATIONS
Assess:
• Electrolytes: K, Na, Cl; CO_2
• Renal function studies: AST, ALT, alk phosphatase
• B/P, pulse
• Weight daily, I&O, nausea
• Edema in feet, legs daily
• Skin turgor, dryness of mucous membranes for hydration status
• Rales, dyspnea, orthopnea
Administer:
• With meals for better absorption, to decrease GI symptoms
• With β-blocker and/or diuretic
Evaluate:
• Therapeutic response: decreased B/P or increased hair growth
Teach patient/family:
• That body hair will increase but is reversible after treatment is discontinued

• Not to discontinue drug abruptly
• To report pitting edema, dizziness, weight gain >5 lb, shortness of breath, bruising or bleeding, heart rate >20 beats/min over normal, severe indigestion, dizziness, light-headedness, panting, new or aggravated symptoms of angina
• To take drug exactly as prescribed or serious side effects may occur
Treatment of overdose: Administer normal saline IV, phenylephrine, angiotensin II, vasopressor; dopamine may reverse hypotension

---

pindolol
(pin'doe-lole)
Visken
Func. class.: Antihypertensive
Chem. class.: Nonselective β-blocker

Action: Competitively blocks stimulation of β-adrenergic receptor within vascular smooth muscle; produces chronotropic, inotropic activity (decreases rate of SA node discharge, increases recovery time), slows conduction of AV node, decreases heart rate, which decreases O_2 consumption in myocardium; also decreases renin-aldosterone-angiotensin system, at high doses inhibits β-2 receptors in bronchial system
Uses: Mild to moderate hypertension
Dosage and routes:
• *Adult:* PO 5 mg bid, usual dose 15 mg/day (5 mg tid), may increase by 10 mg/day q3-4wk to a max of 60 mg/day
Available forms: Tabs 5, 10 mg
Side effects/adverse reactions:
CV: Hypotension, bradycardia, **CHF,** edema, chest pain, palpita-

---

tion, claudication, tachycardia, *AV block*

CNS: Insomnia, dizziness, hallucinations, anxiety, fatigue

GI: Nausea, vomiting, *ischemic colitis,* diarrhea, *abdominal pain, mesenteric arterial thrombosis*

INTEG: Rash, alopecia, pruritus, fever

HEMA: Agranulocytosis, thrombocytopenia, purpura

EENT: Visual changes, sore throat, *double vision,* dry burning eyes

GU: Impotence, frequency

RESP: Bronchospasm, dyspnea, cough, rales

MISC: Joint pain, muscle pain

Contraindications: Hypersensitivity to β-blockers, cardiogenic shock, 2nd, 3rd degree heart block, sinus bradycardia, CHF, cardiac failure, bronchial asthma

Precautions: Major surgery, pregnancy (B), lactation, diabetes mellitus, renal disease, thyroid disease, COPD, well-compensated heart failure, CAD, nonallergic bronchospasm

Pharmacokinetics:

PO: Peak 2-4 hr; half-life 3-4 hr, excreted 30%-45% unchanged; 60%-65% metabolized by liver; excreted in breast milk

Interactions/incompatibilities:

• Increased hypotension, bradycardia: reserpine, hydralazine, methyldopa, prazosin, anticholinergics

• Decreased antihypertensive effects: indomethacin, sympathomimetics

• Increased hypoglycemic effect: insulin

• Decreased bronchodilation: theophyllines, β2 agonists

Lab test interferences:

Increase: Liver function tests, renal function tests

NURSING CONSIDERATIONS
Assess:

• I&O, weight daily

• B/P during initial treatment, periodically thereafter; pulse q4h, note rate, rhythm, quality

• Apical, radial pulse before administration; notify physician of any significant changes

• Baselines in renal, liver function tests before therapy begins

• Edema in feet, legs daily

• Skin turgor, dryness of mucous membranes for hydration status

Administer:

• PO ac, hs; tablet may be crushed or swallowed whole

• Reduced dosage in renal dysfunction

Perform/provide:

• Storage in dry area at room temperature; do not freeze

Evaluate:

• Therapeutic response: decreased B/P after 1-2 wk

Teach patient/family:

• To take with or immediately after meals

• Not to discontinue drug abruptly; taper over 2 wk; may cause precipitate angina

• Not to use OTC products containing α-adrenergic stimulants (nasal decongestants, OTC cold preparations) unless directed by physician

• To report bradycardia, dizziness, confusion, depression, fever, sore throat, shortness of breath to physician

• To take pulse at home; advise when to notify physician

• To avoid alcohol, smoking, Na intake

• To comply with weight control, dietary adjustments, modified exercise program

- To carry Medic Alert ID to identify drug, allergies
- To avoid hazardous activities if dizziness is present
- To report symptoms of CHF: difficult breathing, especially on exertion or when lying down, night cough, swelling of extremities
- To take medication at bedtime to prevent orthostatic hypotension
- To wear support hose to minimize effects of orthostatic hypotension

Treatment of overdose: Lavage, IV atropine for bradycardia, IV theophylline for bronchospasm, digitalis, O_2, diuretic for cardiac failure, hemodialysis, hypotension; give vasopressor (norepinephrine)

pipecuronium bromide

Arduran

Func. class.: Neuromuscular blocker (nondepolarizing)
Chem. class.: Synthetic curariform

Action: Inhibits transmission of nerve impulses by binding with cholinergic receptor sites, antagonizing action of acetylcholine

Uses: Facilitation of endotracheal intubation, skeletal muscle relaxation during mechanical ventilation, surgery, or general anesthesia

Dosage and routes: Dosage is individualized; in patients with normal renal function who are not obese, initial dose is 70-85 μg/kg; maintenance dose ranges from 10-15 μg/kg

Available forms: Inj IV 10-mg vials

Side effects/adverse reactions:

CV: Bradycardia, tachycardia, increased or decreased B/P, ventricular extrasystole, ***myocardial isch-emia, cardiovascular accident, thrombosis, atrial fibrillation***

RESP: ***Prolonged apnea, broncho-spasm, cyanosis, respiratory depression***

GU: ***Anuria***

EENT: Increased secretions

CNS: Hypesthesia, CNS depression

MS: Weakness to prolonged skeletal muscle relaxation

INTEG: Rash, urticaria

METABOLIC: Hypoglycemia, hyperkalemia, increased creatinine

Contraindications: Hypersensitivity to bromide ion

Precautions: Pregnancy (C), renal disease, cardiac disease, lactation, children <3 mo, fluid and electrolyte imbalances, neuromuscular diseases, respiratory disease, obesity

Pharmacokinetics:

IV: Onset 30-45 sec, peak 3-5 min: metabolized (small amounts), excreted in urine (unchanged), crosses placenta

Interactions/incompatibilities:

- Increased neuromuscular blockade: aminoglycosides, quinidine, local anesthetics, polymyxin antibiotics, enflurane, isoflurane, tetracyclines, halothane, magnesium, colistin

NURSING CONSIDERATIONS

Assess:

- For electrolyte imbalances (K, Mg); may lead to increased action of this drug
- Vital signs (B/P, pulse, respirations, airway) until fully recovered: rate, depth, pattern of respirations, strength of hand grip
- I&O ratio; check for urinary retention, frequency, hesitancy
- Recovery: decreased paralysis of face, diaphragm, leg, arm, rest of body
- Allergic reactions: rash, fever,

P

---

italics = common side effects   ***bold italic*** = life threatening reactions

respiratory distress, pruritus; drug should be discontinued

Administer:
• Using nerve stimulator by anesthesiologist to determine neuromuscular blockade
• Atropine to counteract muscarinic effects
• After succinylcholine effects subside
• Anticholinesterase to reverse neuromuscular blockade
• By slow IV over 1-2 min (only by qualified persons, usually an anesthesiologist)
• Only fresh solution

Perform/provide:
• Storage in refrigerator; do not store in plastic container or syringe
• Reassurance if communication is difficult during recovery from neuromuscular blockade
• Use of reconstituted solution within 24 hr, or discard
• Frequent (q2h) instillation of artificial tears and covering eyes to prevent drying of cornea

Evaluate:
• Therapeutic response: paralysis of jaw, eyelid, head, neck, rest of body

Treatment of overdose: Neostigmine, atropine; monitor VS; may require mechanical ventilation

---

piperacillin sodium
(pi-per'a-sill-in)
Pipracil

Func. class.: Broad-spectrum antibiotic
Chem. class.: Extended-spectrum penicillin

Action: Interferes with cell wall replication of susceptible organisms; osmotically unstable cell wall

swells and bursts from osmotic pressure

Uses: Respiratory, skin, urinary tract, bone infections; gonorrhea; pneumonia; effective for gram-positive cocci *(S. aureus, S. pyogenes, S. viridans, S. faecalis, S. bovis, S. pneumoniae)*, gram-negative cocci *(N. gonorrhoeae, N. meningitidis)*, gram-positive bacilli, *C. perfringens, C. tetani*, gram-negative bacilli *(Bacteroides, F. nucleatum, E. coli, Klebsiella, P. mirabilis, M. morganii, P. vulgaris, P. rehgesii, Enterobacter, Citrobacter, P. aeruginosa, Serratia, Acinetobacter, Peptococcus, Peptostreptococcus, Eubacterium)*

Dosage and routes:
Systemic infections
• *Adult and child >12 yr:* IM/IV 100-300 mg/kg/day in divided doses q4-6h
Prophylaxis of surgical infections
• *Adult:* IV 2g ½-1 hr before procedure; may be repeated during surgery or after surgery
Available forms: Inj IM, IV 2, 3, 4, 40 g; IV INF 2, 3, 4 g

Side effects/adverse reactions:
HEMA: Anemia, increased bleeding time, ***bone marrow depression***
GI: Nausea, vomiting, diarrhea, increased AST, ALT, abdominal pain, glossitis, colitis
GU: ***Oliguria, proteinuria, hematuria***, *vaginitis, moniliasis,* ***glomerulonephritis***
CNS: Lethargy, hallucinations, anxiety, depression, twitching, ***coma, convulsions***
META: Hypokalemia, hypernatremia

Contraindications: Hypersensitivity to penicillins; neonates
Precautions: Pregnancy (B); hypersensitivity to cephalosporins; CHF

Pharmacokinetics:
IM: Peak 30-50 min
IV: Peak 20-30 min
Half-life 0.7-1.33 hr; excreted in urine, bile, breast milk; crosses placenta

Interactions/incompatibilities:
• Decreased antimicrobial effect of piperacillin: tetracyclines, erythromycins, aminoglycosides IV
• Increased piperacillin concentrations: aspirin, probenecid
• Incompatible in sol with aminoglycosides, amphotericin B, chloramphenicol, lincomycin, polymyxin B, promethazine, tetracycline, Vit B with C

Lab test interferences:
False positive: Urine glucose, urine protein, Coombs' test

NURSING CONSIDERATIONS
Assess:
• I&O ratio; report hematuria, oliguria, since penicillin in high doses is nephrotoxic
• Any patient with compromised renal system, since drug is excreted slowly in poor renal system function; toxicity may occur rapidly
• Liver studies: AST, ALT
• Blood studies: WBC, RBC, H&H, bleeding time
• Renal studies: urinalysis, protein, blood
• C&S before drug therapy; drug may be taken as soon as culture is taken
• Bowel pattern before and during treatment
• Skin eruptions after administration of penicillin to 1 wk after discontinuing drug
• Respiratory status: rate, character, wheezing, tightness in chest
• Allergies before initiation of treatment, reaction of each medi-

cation; highlight allergies on chart, Kardex

Administer:
• IV after diluting 1 g or less/5 ml or more sterile H_2O or 0.9% NaCl; shake; give dose over 3-5 min; may further dilute to 50-100 ml with D_5W, 0.9% NS, and give over ½ hr; discontinue primary IV
• Drug after C&S has been completed

Perform/provide:
• Adrenalin, suction, tracheostomy set, endotracheal intubation equipment on unit
• Adequate intake of fluids (2 L) during diarrhea episodes
• Scratch test to assess allergy after securing order from physician; usually done when penicillin is only drug of choice
• Storage at room temperature, reconstituted solution for 24 hr or 7 days refrigerated

Evaluate:
• Therapeutic response: absence of fever, purulent drainage, redness, inflammation

Teach patient/family:
• That culture may be taken after completed course of medication
• To report sore throat, fever, fatigue; (may indicate superimposed infection)
• To wear or carry Medic Alert ID if allergic to penicillins
• To notify nurse of diarrhea
Treatment of overdose: Withdraw drug, maintain airway, administer epinephrine, aminophylline, O_2, IV corticosteroids for anaphylaxis

---

italics = common side effects   ***bold italic*** = life threatening reactions

piperacillin sodium and tazobactam sodium

(pi-per'a-sill-in)
Zosyn

Func. class.: Broad-spectrum antibiotic

Chem. class.: Extended-spectrum penicillin/β-lactamase inhibitor

Action: Interferes with cell wall replication of susceptible organisms; osmotically unstable cell wall swells and bursts from osmotic pressure

Uses: Moderate to severe infections: piperacillin-resistant, β-lactamase producing strains causing infections in respiratory, skin, urinary tract, bone infections, gonorrhea, pneumonia; effective for resistant *S. aureus*, resistant *E. coli*, *B. fragilis*, *B. ovatus*, *B. thetaiotaomicron*, *B. vulgatus*

Dosage and routes:
• *Adult:* IV INF 12-15 gm day given 3.375 g q6hr over 30 min × 7-10 days

Available forms: Powder for inj IV 2 gm piperacillin/0.25 gm tazobactam, 3 gm piperacillin/0.375 gm tazobactam, 4 gm piperacillin/0.5 gm tazobactam

Side effects/adverse reactions:
CNS: Lethargy, hallucinations, anxiety, depression, twitching, *coma, convulsions*

GI: Nausea, vomiting, diarrhea, increased AST, ALT, abdominal pain, glossitis, colitis

GU: Oliguria, proteinuria, hematuria, vaginitis, moniliasis, glomerulonephritis

HEMA: Anemia, increased bleeding time, *bone marrow depression*

META: Hypokalemia, hypernatremia

Contraindications: Hypersensitivity to penicillins, neonates

Precautions: Pregnancy (B), hypersensitivity to cephalosporins, CHF

Pharmacokinetics:
IV: Peak completion of IV, duration 6 hr
Half-life 0.7-1.2 hr; excreted in urine, bile, breast milk; crosses placenta; 33% bound to plasma proteins

Interactions/incompatibilities:
• Decreased antimicrobial effect of piperacillin: tetracyclines, erythromycins, aminoglycosides IV
• Increased piperacillin concentrations: aspirin, probenecid
• Incompatible with aminoglycosides, amphotericin B, chloramphenicol, lincomycin, polymyxin B, promethazine, tetracycline, Vit B with C, lactated ringers sol

Lab test interferences:
False positive: Urine glucose, urine protein, Coombs' test
Decreased: Hct, Hgb, electrolytes
Increased: platelet count, eosinophilia, neutropenia, leukopenia, serum creative, PTT, AST, ALT, alk phosphatase, bilirubin, BUN, electrolytes

NURSING CONSIDERATIONS
Assess:
• I&O ratio; report hematuria, oliguria, since penicillin in high doses is nephrotoxic
• Any patient with compromised renal system, since drug is excreted slowly in poor renal system function; toxicity may occur rapidly
• Liver studies: AST, ALT
• Blood studies: WBC, RBC, H & H, bleeding time
• Renal studies: urinalysis, protein, blood

---

* Available in Canada only

- C&S before drug therapy; drug may be given as soon as culture is taken
- Bowel pattern before and during treatment
- Skin eruptions after administration of penicillin to 1 wk after discontinuing drug
- Respiratory status: rate, character, wheezing, tightness in chest
- Allergies before initiation of treatment, reaction of each medication; highlight allergies on chart

Administer:
- IV after diluting 5 ml 0.9% NaCl for injection or sterile H_2O for injection, dextran 6% in saline, dextrose 5%, KCl 40 mEq, bacteriostatic saline/parabens, bacteriostatic saline/benzyl alcohol, bacteriostatic H_2O/benzyl alcohol per 1 g piperacillin; shake well; further dilute in at least 50 ml compatible IV sol and run as INT INF over at least 30 min
- Drug after C&S is complete

Perform/provide:
- Adrenalin, suction, tracheostomy set, endotracheal intubation equipment on unit
- Adequate intake of fluids (2 L) during diarrhea episodes
- Scratch test to assess allergy after securing order from physician; usually done when penicillin is only drug of choice
- Discard any portion after 24 hr if stored at room temperature or after 48 hr if refrigerated; use single-dose vials immediately after reconstitution; stable in ambulatory IV pump for 12 hr

Evaluate:
- Therapeutic response: absence of fever, purulent drainage, redness, inflammation; culture shows decreased organisms

Teach patient/family:
- That culture may be taken after completed course of medication
- To report sore throat, fever, fatigue (may indicate superimposed infection)
- To wear or carry Medic Alert ID if allergic to penicillins
- To notify nurse of diarrhea

Treatment of overdose:
Withdraw drug, maintain airway, administer epinephrine, aminophylline, O_2, IV corticosteroids for anaphylaxis

---

piperazine citrate
(pi'per-a-zeen)
Piperazine
Func. class.: Anthelmintic

Action: Causes paralysis in worm, leading to expulsion by normal peristalsis

Uses: Pinworm, roundworm

Dosage and routes:
Pinworm
- *Adult and child:* PO 65 mg/kg × 7-8 days, not to exceed 2.5 g/day

Roundworm
- *Adult:* PO 3.5 g in single dose × 2 days
- *Child:* PO 75 mg/kg/day in a single dose × 2 days

Available forms: Tabs 250, syr 500 mg/5 ml

Side effects/adverse reactions:
HEMA: Hemolytic anemia
INTEG: Rash, urticaria, photosensitivity
RESP: Bronchospasm
CNS: Dizziness, headache, paresthesia, convulsions, fever, headache, ataxia
EENT: Blurred vision, nystagmus, strabismus, cataracts, rhinorrhea
GI: Nausea, vomiting, anorexia, diarrhea, abdominal cramps

---

italics = common side effects **bold italic** = life threatening reactions

Contraindications: Hypersensitivity, renal disease, hepatic disease, seizures

Precautions: Severe malnutrition, seizure disorders, anemia, pregnancy (B)

Pharmacokinetics:

PO: Excreted in urine (unchanged)

Interactions/incompatibilities:

• Increased extrapyramidal symptoms: phenothiazines

Lab test interferences:

Decrease: Serum uric acid

NURSING CONSIDERATIONS

Assess:

• Stools during entire treatment, 1, 3 mo after treatment; specimens must be sent to lab while still warm

• For allergic reaction: rash, itching, urticaria

• For infection in other family members, since infection from person to person is common

Administer:

• Powder for oral suspension in 57 ml H$_2$O, milk, or fruit juice

• May be crushed or chewed if unable to swallow whole

• Laxatives if constipated; not needed for drug to work

• Second course after 1 wk off drug, if infection is severe

Perform/provide:

• Storage in tight container at room temperature

Evaluate:

• Therapeutic response: expulsion of worms, 3 negative stool cultures after completion of treatment

Teach patient/family:

• Proper hygiene after BM, including hand-washing technique, tell patient to avoid putting fingers in mouth

• That infected person should sleep alone; do not shake bed linen; change bed linen daily, wash in hot water; change and wash undergarments daily

• To clean toilet qd with disinfectant (green soap solution)

• Need for compliance with dosage schedule and duration of treatment

• That urine may turn orange or red

• To avoid hazardous activities, since drowsiness occurs

• That seizures may recur in patient who is controlled on medication

---

pirbuterol acetate
(purr-byoo′-ter-ole)
Maxair

Func. class.: Bronchodilator
Chem. class.: β-Adrenergic agonist

Action: Causes bronchodilation with little effect on heart rate by action on β-receptors, causing increased cAMP and relaxation of smooth muscle

Uses: Reversible bronchospasm (prevention, treatment) including asthma; may be given with theophylline or steroids

Dosage and routes:

• *Adult and child >12 yr:* Aerosol 1-2 inh (0.4 mg) q4-6h; do not exceed 12 inh/day

Available forms: Aerosol delivers 0.2 mg pirbuterol/actuation

Side effects/adverse reactions:

CNS: Tremors, anxiety, insomnia, headache, dizziness, stimulation, restlessness, hallucinations, drowsiness, irritability

EENT: Dry nose and mouth, irritation of nose, throat

CV: Palpitations, tachycardia, hypertension, angina, hypotension, dysrhythmias

GI: Gastritis, nausea, vomiting, anorexia

MS: Muscle cramps

---

*Available in Canada only

RESP: **Bronchospasm,** dyspnea, coughing

Contraindications: Hypersensitivity to sympathomimetics, tachycardia

Precautions: Lactation, pregnancy (C), cardiac disorders, hyperthyroidism, diabetes mellitus, prostatic hypertrophy

Pharmacokinetics:

INH: Onset 3 min, peak ½-1 hr, duration 5 hr

Interactions/incompatibilities:

• Increased action of: other aerosol bronchodilators

• Increased action of pirbuterol: tricyclic antidepressants, antihistamines, sodium levothyroxine

• Decreased action of pirbuterol: β-blockers

• Increased dysrhythmias: halogenated hydrocarbon anesthetics

NURSING CONSIDERATIONS

Assess:

• Respiratory function: vital capacity, forced expiratory volume, ABGs, B/P

Administer:

• After shaking; exhale, place mouthpiece in mouth, inhale slowly, hold breath, remove, exhale slowly

• Gum, sips of water for dry mouth

Perform/provide:

• Storage in light-resistant container, do not expose to temperatures over 86° F (30° C)

Evaluate:

• Therapeutic response: absence of dyspnea, wheezing over 1 hr

Teach patient/family:

• Not to use OTC medications; extra stimulation may occur

• Use of inhaler; review package insert with patient

• To avoid getting aerosol in eyes

• To wash inhaler in warm water and dry qd, rinse mouth after use; if used with inhalers containing glucocorticosteroids, wait 5 min before using steroid inhaler

• About all aspects of drug; avoid smoking, smoke-filled rooms, persons with respiratory infections

• To keep fluid intake >2 L/day to liquefy thick secretions

Treatment of overdose: Administer a β-adrenergic blocker

piroxicam

(peer-ox'i-kam)

Feldene

Func. class.: Nonsteroidal antiinflammatory

Chem. class.: Oxicam derivative

Action: Inhibits prostaglandin synthesis by decreasing an enzyme needed for biosynthesis; possesses analgesic, antiinflammatory, antipyretic properties

Uses: Mild to moderate pain, osteoarthritis, rheumatoid arthritis

Dosage and routes:

• *Adult:* PO 20 qd or 10 mg bid

Available forms: Caps 10, 20 mg

Side effects/adverse reactions:

GI: Nausea, anorexia, vomiting, diarrhea, jaundice, **cholestatic hepatitis,** constipation, flatulence, cramps, dry mouth, peptic ulcer, **bleeding, ulceration, perforation**

CNS: Dizziness, drowsiness, fatigue, tremors, confusion, insomnia, anxiety, depression, headache

CV: Tachycardia, peripheral edema, palpitations, dysrhythmias

INTEG: Purpura, rash, pruritus, sweating, photosensitivity

GU: **Nephrotoxicity: dysuria, hematuria, oliguria, azotemia**

HEMA: **Blood dyscrasias**

EENT: Tinnitus, hearing loss, blurred vision

---

italics = common side effects   **bold italic** = life threatening reactions

P

Contraindications: Hypersensitivity, asthma, severe renal disease, severe hepatic disease, ulcer disease, cardiac disease

Precautions: Pregnancy (C), lactation, children, bleeding disorders, GI disorders, cardiac disorders, hypersensitivity to other antiinflammatory agents

Pharmacokinetics:

PO: Peak 2 hr, half-life 3-3½ hr; metabolized in liver; excreted in urine (metabolites); excreted in breast milk; 99% protein binding

Interactions/incompatibilities:

• Increased action of: coumarin, phenytoin, sulfonamides

NURSING CONSIDERATIONS

Assess:

• Renal, liver, blood studies: BUN, creatinine, AST, ALT, Hgb, before treatment, periodically thereafter

• Audiometric, ophthalmic exam before, during, after treatment

• For eye, ear problems: blurred vision, tinnitus (may indicate toxicity)

Administer:

• With food to decrease GI symptoms; best to take on empty stomach to facilitate absorption; take drug same time qd

Perform/provide:

• Storage at room temperature

Evaluate:

• Therapeutic response: decreased pain, stiffness, swelling in joints; ability to move more easily

Teach patient/family:

• To report blurred vision or ringing, roaring in ears (may indicate toxicity)

• To avoid driving, other hazardous activities if dizziness or drowsiness occurs

• Patient should drink at least 6-8 glasses of water/day

• To report change in urine pattern, weight increase, edema, pain increase in joints, fever, blood in urine (indicates nephrotoxicity)

• That therapeutic effects may take up to 1 mo

• To avoid ASA, other OTC meds, alcohol; advise patient to use sunscreen

plasma protein fraction

Plasmanate, Plasma Plex, Plasmatein, PPF Protenate

Func. class.: Blood derivative
Chem. class.: Human plasma in NaCl

Action: Exerts similar oncotic pressure as human plasma, expands blood volume

Uses: Hypovolemic shock, hypoproteinemia, ARDS, preoperative cardiopulmonary bypass, acute liver failure

Dosage and routes:

Shock

• *Adult:* IV INF 250-500 ml (12.5-25 g protein), not to exceed 10 ml/min

• *Child:* IV INF 22-33 ml/kg at 5-10 ml/min

Hypoproteinemia

• *Adult:* IV INF 1000-1500 ml qd, not to exceed 8 ml/min

Available forms: Inj IV 50 mg/ml

Side effects/adverse reactions:

GI: Nausea, vomiting, increased salivation

INTEG: Rash, urticaria, cyanosis

CNS: Fever, chills, headache, paresthesias, flushing

RESP: Altered respirations, dyspnea, pulmonary edema

CV: Fluid overload, hypotension, erratic pulse

Contraindications: Hypersensitiv-

ity, CHF, severe anemia, renal insufficiency

Precautions: Decreased salt intake, decreased cardiac reserve, lack of albumin deficiency, hepatic disease, renal disease, pregnancy (C)

Pharmacokinetics:
Metabolized as a protein/energy source

Interactions/incompatibilities:
• Incompatible with sol containing alcohol or norepinephrine

Lab test interferences:
False increase: Alk phosphatase

NURSING CONSIDERATIONS
Assess:
• Blood studies: Hct, Hgb; if serum protein declines, dyspnea, hypoxemia can result
• B/P (decreased), pulse (erratic), respiration during infusion
• I&O ratio; urinary output may decrease
• CVP, pulmonary wedge pressure (increases if overload occurs)
• Allergy: fever, rash, itching, chills, flushing, urticaria, nausea, vomiting, or hypotension requires discontinuation of infusion; use new lot if therapy reinstituted
• Increased CVP reading: distended neck veins indicate circulatory overload; SOB, anxiety, insomnia, expiratory rales, frothy blood-tinged cough, cyanosis indicate pulmonary overload

Administer:
• No dilution required; use infusion pump, use large-gauge needle (≥20G), discard unused portion, infuse slowly
• Within 4 hr of opening

Perform/provide:
• Adequate hydration before administration
• Storage—check type of albumin, date; may have to refrigerate

Evaluate:
• Therapeutic repsonse: increased B/P, decrease edema, increased serum albumin

---

plicamycin (mithramycin)
(plik-a-mi'cin)
Mithracin
Func. class.: Antineoplastic, antibiotic
Chem. class.: Crystalline aglycone

Action: Inhibits DNA, RNA, protein synthesis; derived from *Streptomyces plicatus;* replication is decreased by binding to DNA; demonstrates Ca-lowering effect not related to its tumoricidal activity; also acts on osteoclasts and blocks action of parathyroid hormone; a vesicant

Uses: Testicular cancer, hypercalcemia, hypercalciuria, symptomatic treatment of advanced neoplasms

Dosage and routes:
Testicular tumors
• *Adult:* IV 25-30 μg/kg/day × 8-10 days, not to exceed 30 μg/kg/day

Hypercalcemia/hypercalciuria
• *Adult:* IV 25 μg/kg/day × 3-4 days, repeat at intervals of 1 wk

Available forms: Inj IV 2.5 mg/vial powder

Side effects/adverse reactions:
META: Decreased serum Ca, P, K
HEMA: **Hemorrhage, thrombocytopenia,** decreased pro-time, WBC count
GI: Nausea, vomiting, anorexia, diarrhea, stomatitis, increased liver enzymes
GU: Increased BUN, creatinine, ***proteinuria***

---

italics = common side effects   ***bold italic*** = life threatening reactions

INTEG: Rash, cellulitis, *extravasation,* facial flushing

CNS: Drowsiness, weakness, lethargy, headache, flushing, fever, depression

Contraindications: Hypersensitivity, thrombocytopenia, bone marrow depression, bleeding disorders, pregnancy (X)

Precautions: Renal disease, hepatic disease, electrolyte imbalances

Pharmacokinetics: Crosses blood-brain barrier, excreted in urine; little known about pharmacokinetics

Interactions/incompatibilities:

• Increased toxicity: other antineoplastics or radiation

• Considered incompatible with any drugs in sol or syringe

NURSING CONSIDERATIONS

Assess:

• CBC, differential, platelet count qwk; withhold drug if WBC is <4000/mm³ or platelet count is <50,000/mm³; notify physician of results

• Renal function studies: BUN, serum uric acid, urine CrCl, electrolytes before, during therapy

• I&O ratio; report urine output <30 ml/hr

• Monitor temperature q4h; fever may indicate beginning infection

• Liver function tests before, during therapy: bilirubin, AST, ALT, alk phosphatase prn or monthly

• Alkalosis if severe vomiting is present

• Toxicity: facial flushing, epistaxis, increased pro-time, thrombocytopenia; drug should be discontinued

• Bleeding: hematuria, guaiac stools, bruising or petechiae, mucosa or orifices q8h

• Food preferences; list likes, dislikes

• Inflammation of mucosa, breaks in skin

• Yellowing of skin and sclera, dark urine, clay-colored stools, itchy skin, abdominal pain, fever, diarrhea

• Buccal cavity q8h for dryness, sores, ulceration, white patches, oral pain, bleeding, dysphagia

• Local irritation, pain, burning at injection site

• Frequency of stools, characteristics, cramping

• Acidosis, signs of dehydration: rapid respirations, poor skin turgor, decreased urine output, dry skin, restlessness, weakness

Administer:

• IV dilute 2.5 mg/4.9 ml of sterile H_2O; (1 ml = 500 µg) dilute single dose in 1000 ml of D_5W run over 4-6 hr

• EDTA for extravasation, apply ice compress

• Antiemetic 30-60 min before giving drug and 4-10 hr after treatment to prevent vomiting

• Slow IV infusion using 20G, 21G needle

• Transfusion for anemia

• Antispasmodic for diarrhea, phenothiazine for nausea and vomiting

Perform/provide:

• Liquid diet: carbonated beverages; gelatin may be added if patient is not nauseated or vomiting

• Rinsing of mouth tid-qid with water; brushing of teeth with baking soda bid-tid with soft brush or cotton-tipped applicators for stomatitis; unwaxed dental floss

• Usage immediately after mixing

Evaluate:

• Therapeutic response: decreased tumor size, spread of malignancy

Teach patient/family:

• To report any complaints or side effects to nurse or physician

• To avoid foods with citric acid, hot or rough texture

• To report to physician any bleeding, white spots, ulcerations in the mouth; tell patient to examine mouth qd

• To avoid driving, activities requiring alertness; drowsiness may occur

• To report leg cramps, tingling of fingertips, weakness; may indicate hypocalcemia

• To avoid crowds, persons with infections when granulocyte count is low

---

podophyllum resin
(poe-doe-fil' um)
Pod-Ben-25, Podocon-25, Podofilm,* Podofin
Func. class.: Keratolytic
Chem. class.: Podophyllum derivative

Action: Arrests mitosis by binding to tubulin, protein subunit of spindle microtubules; also interferes with movements of chromosomes

Uses: Venereal warts, keratoses, multiple superficial epitheliomatoses

Dosage and routes:
Warts
• *Adult:* TOP cover wart, cover with wax paper, bandage for 1-4 hr, wash, may repeat qwk if needed
Keratoses/epitheliomatoses
• *Adult:* TOP apply qd with applicator, let dry, remove tissue, may reapply if needed
Available forms: Sol 11.5%, 25%

Side effects/adverse reactions:
*HEMA: **Thrombocytopenia, leukopenia***
INTEG: Irritation of unaffected areas
CNS: Peripheral neuropathy

MISC: Paresthesia, nausea, vomiting, diarrhea, abdominal pain, confusion, dizziness, ***stupor, convulsions coma, death***

Contraindications: Hypersensitivity, pregnancy (X), bleeding, warts, lactation, poor blood circulation, diabetes

Interactions/incompatibilities:
• Necrosis of skin: when used with other keratolytic

NURSING CONSIDERATIONS
Assess:
• Platelets, WBC if systemic absorption occurs
• Allergic reactions: irritation, redness, itching, stinging, burning; drug should be discontinued
• Blood dyscrasias if systemic absorption is suspected: decrease platelets
• CNS toxicity: peripheral neuropathy; drug should be discontinued

Administer:
• Only to affected area; cover normal skin with petrolatum for protection; do not apply to broken or inflamed skin; applied only by physician, not to be dispensed to patient
• Only to small areas or for short periods, or absorption (systemic) may occur

Evaluate:
• Therapeutic response: decrease in size and number of lesions

Teach patient/family:
• That discomfort will begin after 24 hr, subside in 2-4 days
• To use soap and water to clean area and remove drug

Poliovirus vaccine, live, oral, trivalent
Orimune
Func. class.: Vaccine

Action: Produces specific antibodies for poliomyelitis
Uses: Prevention of polio

---

italics = common side effects   ***bold italic*** = life threatening reactions

Dosage and routes:
• *Adult and child >2 yr:* PO 0.5 ml, given q8wk × 2 doses, then 0.5 ml ½-1 yr after dose 2
• *Infant:* PO 0.5 ml at 2, 4, 18 mo
Available forms: Oral vaccine
Side effects/adverse reactions:
SYST: Paralysis

Contraindications: Hypersensitivity, active infection, allergy to neomycin/streptomycin, immunosuppression, vomiting or diarrhea
Precautions: Pregnancy
Interactions/incompatibilities:
• Do not use TB skin test or other live virus vaccines within 6 wk of vaccine
• Do not use within 3 mo of transfusion of whole blood, plasma, or use with immune serum globulin
NURSING CONSIDERATIONS
Assess:
• For anaphylaxis: inability to breathe, bronchospasm
Administer:
• Only PO
• Do not administer within 1 mo of other live virus vaccines
Perform/Provide:
• Storage at 7° F (−13° C)
• Written record of immunization
Evaluate:
• For history of allergies, skin conditions (eczema, psoriasis, dermatitis), reactions to vaccinations

---

polymyxin B sulfate
(pol-i-mix'in)
Aerosporin, Polymyxin B Sulfate
Func. class.: Antibacterial
Chem. class.: Polymyxin

Action: Interferes with phospholipids, penetrates cell wall; immediately changes bacterial membrane, causing leakage of essential metabolites

Uses: Serious *P. aeruginosa, E. aerogenes, K. pneumoniae, E. coli, H. influenzae* infections or when other antibiotics cannot be used
Dosage and routes:
• *Adult and child:* IV INF 15,000-25,000 U/kg/day in divided doses q12h, or 25,000 U/kg/day in divided doses q4-8h
P. aeruginosa/H. influenzae
• *Adult and child >2 yr:* INTRATHECAL 50,000 U/day × 3-4 days, then 50,000 U/qod × 2 wk after CSF negative, glucose normal
• *Child <2 yr:* INTRATHECAL 20,000 U/day × 3-4 days, then 25,000 U qod × 2 wk after CSF negative
Available forms: Inj IV, intrathecal, 500,000 U
Side effects/adverse reactions:
INTEG: Urticaria
CNS: Dizziness, confusion, weakness, drowsiness, paresthesia, slurred speech, *coma, seizures,* headache, stiff neck
RESP: Paralysis
GU: Proteinuria, hematuria, azotemia, leukocyturia
Contraindications: Hypersensitivity, severe renal disease
Precautions: Pregnancy (B)
Pharmacokinetics:
IM: Peak 2 hr, half-life 4½-6 hr, excreted in urine unchanged (60%)
IV: Data not available
Interactions/incompatibilities:
• Increased skeletal muscle relaxation: anesthetics, neuromuscular blockers (tubocurarine decamethonium, succinylcholine, gallamine)
• Increased nephrotoxicity, neurotoxicity: aminoglycosides
• Incompatible with amphotericin B, cephalosporins, penicillins,

chloramphenicol, strong acidic/alkalinic agents, chlorothiazide, heparin, magnesium sulfate, prednisolone, tetracycline

NURSING CONSIDERATIONS

Assess:

• I&O ratio; report hematuria, oliguria

• Any patient with compromised renal system; drug is excreted slowly in poor renal system function; toxicity may occur rapidly; monitor BUN, creatinine

• Renal studies: urinalysis, protein, blood

• C&S before drug therapy; drug may be given as soon as culture is taken; C&S may be done after completion of therapy

• Skin eruptions, itching; drug should be discontinued

• Respiratory status: rate, character, dyspnea, symptoms of neuromuscular blockade, tightness in chest; discontinue drug if these occur

• Allergies before initiation of treatment, reaction of each medication; place allergies on chart, Kardex in bright red letters; notify all people giving drugs

• For flushing of face, dizziness, disorientation, weakness, paresthesia, blurred vision, slurred speech, restlessness, irritability; indicate neurotoxicity

• For headache, fever, stiff neck; after intrathecal administration, indicate meningeal irritation

Administer:

• IV after diluting 500,000 U/5 ml sterile H_2O or NS for inj (100,000 U/ml), then dilute each dose with 300-500 ml D_5W given as a cont inf over 60-90 min

• Intrathecal after reconstituting with 10 ml NS to yield 50,000 U/ml

Perform/provide:

• Storage in dark area at room temperature

• Do not use procaine HCl in intrathecal injection

• Adrenalin, suction, tracheostomy set, endotracheal intubation equipment on unit

Evaluate:

• Therapeutic response: absence of fever, purulent drainage, C&S negative

Teach patient/family:

• To report sore throat, fever, fatigue; may indicate superimposed infection

Treatment of overdose: Withdraw drug, maintain airway, administer epinephrine, aminophylline, O_2, IV corticosteroids

---

polymyxin B sulfate (ophthalmic)

(pol-ee-mix'in)

Func. class.: Antiinfective (ophthalmic)

Action: Inhibits cell wall permeability in susceptible organisms

Uses: Superficial external ocular infections

Dosage and routes:

• *Adult and child:* INSTILL 1-2 gtts bid-qid × 7-10 days

Available forms: Powder for sol; 500,000 U

Side effects/adverse reactions:

EENT: Poor corneal wound healing, temporary visual haze, overgrowth of nonsusceptible organisms

Contraindications: Hypersensitivity

Precautions: Antibiotic hypersensitivity, pregnancy (B), varicella, vaccinia, mycobacterial or fungal infections

---

italics = common side effects   ***bold italic*** = life threatening reactions

NURSING CONSIDERATIONS
Assess:
• Allergy: itching, lacrimation, redness, swelling
Administer:
• After washing hands; cleanse crusts or discharge from eye before application
• After reconstituting powder to 20-50 ml
Perform/provide:
• Storage in refrigerator
Evaluate:
• Therapeutic response: absence of redness, inflammation, tearing
Teach patient/family:
• To use drug exactly as prescribed
• Not to use eye makeup, towels, washcloths, eye medication of others; reinfection may occur
• That drug container tip should not be touched to eye
• To report itching, increased redness, burning, stinging, swelling; drug should be discontinued

potassium bicarbonate/potassium acetate/ potassium chloride/ potassium gluconate/ potassium phosphate

Effer-K, K-Lyte, K-Lyte DS, Klorvess, Tri-K, Twin-K, Cena-K, Gen-K, K⁺10, K-Tab, K-Norm, K-Dur 10, K-Dur 20, K-Lyte/Cl, K-Lease, K⁺ Care, Kaon-Cl, Kaon-Cl-10, Kaochlor, Kaochlor S-F, Kato, Kay Ciel, Klor, Klor-Con, Klor-Con 8, Klor-Con 10, Klor-Con/25, Klortrix, Klorvess, Micro-K, Micro KLS, Potachlor, Potage, Potasalan, Potassium Chloride, Rum-K, Slow-K, Ten-K, Urocit-K, Kao-Nor, Kaylixir, K-G Elixir, My-K Elixir, Potassium Gluconate

Func. class.: Electrolyte
Chem. class.: Potassium

Action: Needed for adequate transmission of nerve impulses and cardiac contraction, renal function, intracellular ion maintenance
Uses: Prevention and treatment of hypokalemia
Dosage and routes:
Potassium bicarbonate
• *Adult:* PO dissolve 25-50 mEq in water qd-qid
Potassium acetate—hypokalemia
• *Adult and child:* PO 40-100 mEq/day in divided doses 2-4 days
Hypokalemia (prevention)
• *Adult and child:* PO 20 mEq/day in 2-4 divided doses
Potassium chloride
• *Adult:* PO 40-100 mEq in divided doses tid-qid; IV 20 mEq/hr when diluted as 40 mEq/1000 ml, not to exceed 150 mEq/day

Potassium gluconate
• *Adult:* PO 40-100 mEq in divided doses tid-qid
Potassium phosphate
• *Adult:* IV 1 mEq/hr in sol of 60 mEq/L, not to exceed 150 mEq/day; PO 40-100 mEq/day in divided doses
Available forms: Tabs for sol 6.5, 25 mEq/inj for prep of IV 2, 4 mEq/caps ext rel 8, 10 mEq; powder for sol 3.3, 5, 6.7, 10, 13.3 mEq/5 ml; tabs 4, 13.4 mEq; tabs ext rel 6.7, 8, 10 mEq; inj for prep of IV 1.5, 2, 2.4, 3, 3.2 mEq/ml; elix 6.7 mEq/5 ml; tabs 2, 5 mEq; oral sol 2.375 mEq/5 ml; inj for prep of IV 4.4, 4.7 mEq/ml
Side effects/adverse reactions:
CNS: Confusion
CV: Bradycardia, *cardiac depression, dysrhythmias, arrest, peaking T waves, lowered R and depressed RST, prolonged P-R interval, widened QRS complex*
GI: Nausea, vomiting, cramps, pain, *diarrhea,* ulceration of small bowel
GU: Oliguria
INTEG: Cold extremities, rash
Contraindications: Renal disease (severe), severe hemolytic disease, Addison's disease, hyperkalemia, acute dehydration, extensive tissue breakdown
Precautions: Cardiac disease, K-sparing diuretic therapy, systemic acidosis, pregnancy (A)
Interactions/incompatibilities:
• Hyperkalemia: potassium phosphate IV and products containing Ca or Mg; K-sparing, diuretic, or other K products
• Incompatible with amikacin, amphotericin B, dobutamine, fat emulsion, penicillin G sodium
Pharmacokinetics:
PO: Excreted by kidneys and in

feces; onset of action ≈ 30 min
IV: Immediate onset of action
NURSING CONSIDERATIONS
Assess:
• ECG for peaking T waves, lowered R, depressed RST, prolonged P-R interval, widening QRS complex, hyperkalemia; drug should be reduced or discontinued
• K level during treatment (3.5-5.0 mg/dl is normal level)
• I&O ratio; watch for decreased urinary output; notify physician immediately
• Cardiac status: rate, rhythm, CVP, PWP, PAWP, if being monitored directly
Administer:
• Through large-bore needle, to decrease vein inflammation, check for extravasation
• In large vein, avoiding scalp vein in child (IV)
• IV after diluting in large volume of IV sol and give as an inf, slowly by IV; INF to prevent toxicity; never give IV bolus or IM
• PO, with or pc meal; dissolve effervescent tabs, powder in 8 oz cold water or juice; do not give IM, SC
Perform/provide:
• Storage at room temperature
Evaluate:
• Therapeutic response: absence of fatigue, muscle weakness, and decreased thirst and urinary output, cardiac changes
Teach patient/family:
• To add potassium-rich foods to diet: bananas, orange juice, avocados; whole grains, broccoli, carrots, prunes, cocoa after this medication is discontinued
• To avoid OTC products: antacids, salt substitutes, analgesics, vitamin preparations, unless specifically directed by physician

P

---

italics = common side effects   ***bold italic*** = life threatening reactions

• To report hyperkalemia symptoms (lethargy, confusion, diarrhea, nausea, vomiting, fainting, decreased output) or continued hypokalemia symptoms (fatigue, weakness, polyuria, polydipsia, cardiac changes)
• Take capsules with full glass of liquid
• To dissolve powder or tablet completely in at least 120 ml water or juice
• Not to chew time-release or extended-release preparations
• Emphasize importance of regular follow-up

---

potassium iodide
Pima, Potassium Iodide Solution, SSKI, Thyro-Block
Func. class.: Thyroid hormone antagonist
Chem. class.: Iodine product

Action: Inhibits secretion of thyroid hormone, fosters colloid accumulation in thyroid follicles, decreases vascularity of gland
Uses: Preparation for thyroidectomy, thyrotoxic crisis, neonatal thyrotoxicosis, radiation protectant, thyroid storm
Dosage and routes:
Thyrotoxic crisis
• *Adult and child:* PO 1 ml in water tid after meals (strong iodine sol)
Preparation for thyroidectomy
• *Adult and child:* PO 0.1-0.3 ml tid (strong iodine sol) or 5 gtts in water tid pc × 2-3 wk before surgery (potassium iodide sol)
Available forms: Sol 5%, 10%, 21 mg/gtt; tabs 130, 300 mg; inj IV 10%, 20%
Side effects/adverse reactions:
ENDO: Hypothyroidism, hyperthyroid adenoma

INTEG: Rash, urticaria, *angineurotic edema,* acne, mucosal hemorrhage, fever
CNS: Headache, confusion, paresthesias
GI: Nausea, diarrhea, vomiting, small-bowel lesions, upper gastric pain
MS: Myalgia, arthralgia, weakness
EENT: Metallic taste, stomatitis, salivation, periorbital edema, sore teeth and gums, cold symptoms
Contraindications: Hypersensitivity to iodine, pulmonary edema, pulmonary TB, pregnancy (D)
Precautions: Lactation, children
Pharmacokinetics:
PO: Onset 24-48 hr, peak 10-15 days after continuous therapy, uptake by thyroid gland or excreted in urine; crosses placenta
Interactions/incompatibilities:
• Hypothyroidism: lithium, other antithyroid agents
Lab test interferences:
Interferes: Urinary 17-OHCS
NURSING CONSIDERATIONS
Assess:
• Pulse, B/P, temperature
• I&O ratio; check for edema: puffy hands, feet, periorbit; indicate hypothyroidism
• Weight qd; same clothing, scale, time of day
• T_3, T_4, which is increased; serum TSH, which is decreased; free thyroxine index, which is increased if dosage is too low; discontinue drug 3-4 wk before RAIU
• Overdose: peripheral edema, heat intolerance, diaphoresis, palpitations, dysrhythmias, severe tachycardia, increased temperature delirium, CNS irritability
• Hypersensitivity: rash; enlarged cervical lymph nodes may indicate drug may have to be discontinued

---

• Hypoprothrombinemia: bleeding, petechiae, ecchymosis
• Clinical response: after 3 wk should include increased weight, pulse; decreased T_4

Administer:
• Strong iodine solution after diluting with water or juice to improve taste
• Through straw to prevent tooth discoloration
• With meals to decrease GI upset
• At same time each day, to maintain drug level
• Lowest dose that relieves symptoms, discontinue before RAI

Perform/provide:
• Fluids to 3-4 L/day, unless contraindicated

Evaluate:
• Therapeutic response: weight gain, decreased pulse, T_4, size of thyroid gland

Teach patient/family:
• To abstain from breast-feeding after delivery
• To keep graph of weight, pulse, mood
• To avoid OTC products that contain iodine
• That seafood, other iodine products may be restricted
• Not to discontinue this medication abruptly; thyroid crisis may occur; stress patient response
• That response may take several months if thyroid is large
• To discontinue drug, notify physician if fever, rash, metallic taste, swelling of throat, burning of mouth, throat, sore gums, teeth, severe GI distress, enlargement of thyroid, cold symptoms occur

potassium iodide (SSKI)
Pima, Iosat, Thyro-Block
Func. class.: Expectorant

Action: Increases respiratory tract fluid by decreasing surface tension, adhesiveness, which increases removal of mucus

Uses: Bronchial asthma, emphysema, bronchitis, nuclear radiation protection

Dosage and routes:
• *Adult:* PO 0.3-0.6 ml q4-6h
• *Child:* PO 0.25-1 ml saturated sol bid-qid

Radiation protection:
• *Adult:* PO 0.13 ml SSKI before or after initial exposure
• *Infant <1 yr:* Half adult dose

Available forms: Sol 1 g/ml

Side effects/adverse reactions:
EENT: Burning mouth, throat, eye irritation, swelling of eyelids
GI: Gastric irritation
ENDO: Iodism, goiter, myxedema
RESP: **Pulmonary edema**
INTEG: **Angioedema,** rash
CNS: Frontal headache, ***CNS depression,*** fever, parkinsonism

Contraindications: Hypersensitivity to iodides, pulmonary TB, pregnancy (D), hyperthyroidism, hyperkalemia, acute bronchitis

Precautions: Hypothyroidism, cystic fibrosis, lactation

Pharmacokinetics: Excreted in urine

Interactions/incompatibilities:
• Increased hypothyroid effects: lithium, antithyroid drugs
• Dysrhythmias, hyperkalemia: K-sparing diuretics, K-containing medication

NURSING CONSIDERATIONS
Assess:
• Cough: type, frequency, character including sputum

P

Administer:
• Decreased dose to elderly patients; excretion may be slowed
• Diluted water or fruit juice to improve taste, decrease nausea
Perform/provide:
• Storage at room temperature in tight container
• Increased fluids to liquefy secretions
Evaluate:
• Therapeutic response: absence of cough
Teach patient/family:
• Not to use if pregnant
• Symptoms of iodism: eruptions, burning of oral cavity, eye irritation
• Symptoms of hyperthyroidism: CNS depression, fever, glomerulonephritis
• To discontinue, notify physician if fever, rash, metallic taste occur

---

povidone iodine
(poe'vi-done)
Acu-Dyne, Betadine, Biodine Topical 1%, Efo-Dine, Iodex Regular, Mallisol, Operand Povidone-Iodine, Pharmadine, Polydine, Proviodine*
Func. class.: Disinfectant
Chem. class.: Iodophor

Action: Destroys a wide variety of microorganisms by local irritation, germicidal action
Uses: Cleansing wounds, disinfection, preoperative skin preparation
Dosage and routes:
• *Adult and child:* Use sol as needed, topical only
Available forms: Top sol 1.5%, 3%
Side effects/adverse reactions:
GU: Renal damage
META: Metabolic acidosis
INTEG: Irritation
Contraindications: Hypersensi-

tivity to iodine, pregnancy (vaginal antiseptic) (D)
Precautions: Extensive burns
Interactions/incompatibilities:
• Do not use with alcohol or hydrogen peroxide
NURSING CONSIDERATIONS
Assess:
• For allergies to seafood; drug should not be used
Perform/provide:
• Storage in tight, light-resistant container
• Bandaging of areas if needed
Evaluate:
• Area of the body involved: irritation, rash, breaks, dryness, scales
Teach patient/family:
• To discontinue use if rash, irritation, or redness occurs

---

pralidoxime chloride
(pra-li-dox'eem)
Protopam chloride, 2-PAM
Func. class.: Cholinesterase reactivator
Chem. class.: Quaternary ammonium oxide

Action: Reactivated enzyme metabolizes and inactivates acetylcholine at both muscarinic and nicotinic sites in the periphery
Uses: Cholinergic crisis in myasthenia gravis, organophosphate poisoning antidote, relief of paralysis of respiratory muscles; used as an adjunct to systemic atropine administration
Dosage and routes:
Anticholinesterase overdose
• *Adult:* IV 1-2 g, then 250 mg q5min until desired response
Organophosphate poisoning
• *Adult:* IV INF 1-2 g/100 ml NS over 15-30 min; may repeat in 1 hr; PO 1-3 g q5h

---

• *Child:* IV INF 20-40 mg/kg/ dose diluted in 100 ml NS over 15-30 min

Available forms: Inj IV 600 mg/2 ml; tabs 500 mg; emergency kit 1 g/20-ml vial

Side effects/adverse reactions:

CNS: Dizziness, headache, drowsiness, blurred vision, diplopia, impaired accommodation

GI: Nausea

MS: Weakness, muscle rigidity

CV: Tachycardia

RESP: Hyperventilation, ***laryngospasm***

Contraindications: Hypersensitivity, carbamate insecticide poisoning

Precautions: Myasthenia gravis, pregnancy (C), renal insufficiency, children, lactation

Pharmacokinetics:

PO: Peak 2-3 hr

IV: Peak 5-15 min

IM: Peak 10-20 min

Half-life 1½ hr, metabolized in liver, excreted in urine (unchanged)

Interactions/incompatibilities:

• Avoid use with aminophylline, morphine, phenothiazines, reserpine, succinylcholine, theophylline in organophosphate poisoning

• Incompatible with any drug in sol or syringe

NURSING CONSIDERATIONS

Assess:

• For 48-72 hr after poisoning

• B/P, VS, I&O ratio; observe for decreased urinary output for 48-72 hr after poisoning to determine atropine toxicity from poisoning effects

• Respiratory status: rate, rhythm, characteristics

Administer:

• Only with emergency equipment available

• As soon as possible after poisoning; within 4 hr

• IV after diluting 1 g/20 ml sterile H₂O for inj; further dilute/100 ml NS and give 1 g or less/5 min; may be given as an inf over 15-30 min

• Slowly (IV) after dilution with sterile water

• Concurrent atropine 2-4 mg IV or IM if cyanosis is present, to block accumulated acetylcholine in respiratory center; repeat q5-10min until toxicity occurs: dry mouth, flushing, tachycardia, delirium, hallucinations

• Only with edrophonium (Tensilon) on unit for myasthenia gravis patient

Evaluate:

• Airway, need for assistance with respiration

---

pramoxine HCl (topical)

(pra-mox′-een)

Itch-X, Phicon, Pramegel, Prax, Procto Foam, Tronolane, Tronothane HCl

Func. class.: Topical anesthetic

Action: Inhibits nerve impulses from sensory nerves, which produces anesthesia

Uses: Pruritus, sunburn, toothache, sore throat, cold sores, oral pain, rectal pain and irritation

Dosage and routes:

• *Adult and child:* TOP apply q3-4h; REC apply 1 full applicator bid-tid and after each BM

Available forms: Aero, cream, gel, lotion 1%; rec oint 1%; rec or top aero, cream 1%

Side effects/adverse reactions:

INTEG: Rash, irritation, sensitization

Contraindications: Hypersensitiv-

P

---

italics = common side effects   ***bold italic*** = life threatening reactions

ity, infants <1 yr, application to large areas

Precautions: Child <6 yr, sepsis, pregnancy (C), denuded skin

NURSING CONSIDERATIONS
Assess:
• Allergy: rash, irritation, reddening, swelling
• Infection: if affected area is infected, do not apply

Administer:
• After cleansing and drying of affected area
• Rectal aerosol using applicator or tissue
• Directly, using gauze

Evaluate:
• Therapeutic response: absence of pain, itching of affected area

Teach patient/family:
• To report rash, irritation, redness, swelling
• How to apply
• Not for long-term use, consult physician after 4 wk of use

---

pravastatin
(prav-i-sta'tin)
Pravachol
Func. class.: Antihyperlipidemic

Action: Inhibits HMG-CoA reductase enzyme, which reduces cholesterol synthesis

Uses: As an adjunct in primary hypercholesterolemia (types IIa, IIb)

Dosage and routes:
• *Adult:* PO 10-20 mg qd at hs (range 10-40 mg qd)

Available forms: Tabs 10, 20 mg

Side effects/adverse reactions:
INTEG: Rash, pruritus
GI: Nausea, constipation, diarrhea, dyspepsia, flatus, abdominal pain, heartburn, *liver dysfunction,* pancreatitis, *hepatitis*

EENT: Lens opacities, common cold, rhinitis, cough
MS: Muscle cramps, myalgia, *myositis, rhabdomyolysis*
CNS: Headache, dizziness, psychic disturbances

Contraindications: Hypersensitivity, pregnancy (X), lactation, active liver disease

Precautions: Past liver disease, alcoholism, severe acute infections, trauma, hypotension, uncontrolled seizure disorders, severe metabolic disorders, electrolyte imbalances

Pharmacokinetics: Peak 1-1½ hr, metabolized by the liver, highly protein bound, excreted in urine, feces; crosses placenta, excreted in breast milk

Interactions/incompatibilities:
• Increased effects of: coumadin
• Decreased bioavailability of pravastatin: bile acid sequestrants

Lab test interferences:
Increase: CPK, liver function tests

NURSING CONSIDERATIONS
Assess:
• Cholesterol levels periodically during treatment
• Liver function studies: baseline, q6wk during the first 3 mo, q8wk for remainder of yr, then q6mo; AST, ALT, liver function tests may increase
• Renal studies in patients with compromised renal system: BUN, I&O ratio, creatinine

Administer:
• Without regard to meals, hs

Perform/provide:
• Storage in cool environment in tight container protected from light

Evaluate:
• Therapeutic response: decrease in cholesterol to desired level after 8 wk

Teach patient/family:
• That treatment will take several years

• That blood work will be necessary during treatment
• To report blurred vision, severe GI symptoms, dizziness, headache
• That previously prescribed regimen will continue: low-cholesterol diet, exercise program

---

prazepam
(pra′ze-pam)
Centrax
Func. class.: Antianxiety
Chem. class.: Benzodiazepine

Controlled Substance Schedule IV

Action: Potentiates the actions of GABA, especially in limbic system and reticular formation

Uses: Anxiety

Dosage and routes:
• *Adult:* PO 20-60 mg in divided doses or 20 mg at hs
Available forms: Caps 5, 10, 20 mg; tabs 10 mg

Side effects/adverse reactions:
CNS: Dizziness, drowsiness, confusion, headache, anxiety, tremors, stimulation, fatigue, insomnia, weakness
GI: Constipation, dry mouth, nausea, vomiting, anorexia, diarrhea
INTEG: Rash, dermatitis, itching
CV: Orthostatic hypotension, **ECG changes, tachycardia,** hypotension, palpitations, syncope
EENT: Blurred vision, tinnitus, mydriasis

Contraindications: Hypersensitivity to benzodiazepines, narrow-angle glaucoma, psychosis, pregnancy (D), child <18 yr

Precautions: Elderly, debilitated, hepatic disease, renal disease

Pharmacokinetics:
PO: Peak 6 hr, duration up to 48 hr; metabolized by liver; excreted by kidneys; crosses placenta, breast milk; half-life 30-100 hr

Interactions/incompatibilities:
• Decreased effects of prazepam: oral contraceptives, valproic acid
• Increased effects of prazepam: CNS depressants, alcohol, disulfiram, oral contraceptives, cimetidine

Lab test interferences:
Increase: AST, ALT, serum bilirubin, LDH
Decrease: RAIU
False increase: 17-OHCS

NURSING CONSIDERATIONS
Assess:
• B/P (lying, standing), pulse; if systolic B/P drops 20 mm Hg, hold drug, notify physician
• Blood studies: CBC
• Hepatic studies: AST, ALT, bilirubin, CrCl
• Mental status: mood, sensorium, affect
• Physical dependency, withdrawal symptoms: headache, nausea, vomiting, muscle pain, weakness, tremors, **convulsions** after long-term use
• Check to see PO medication has been swallowed

Administer:
• With food or milk for GI symptoms
• Crushed if patient is unable to swallow medication whole
• Gum, hard candy, frequent sips of water for dry mouth

Perform/provide:
• Assistance with ambulation during beginning therapy, since drowsiness, dizziness occur
• Safety measures including side rails

Evaluate:
• Therapeutic response: decreased anxiety

---

italics = common side effects   ***bold italic*** = life threatening reactions

Teach patient/family:
• Not to be used for everyday stress or used longer than 4 mo; not to use more than prescribed amount; may be habit forming
• To avoid OTC preparations (cough, cold, hay fever) unless approved by physician
• To avoid driving, other activities that require alertness
• To avoid alcohol ingestion, other psychotropic medications
• Not to discontinue medication quickly after long-term use
• To rise slowly or fainting may occur, especially elderly
Treatment of overdose: Lavage, VS, supportive care, flumazenil

---

praziquantel
(pray-zi-kwon'tel)
Biltricide
Func. class.: Anthelmintic
Chem. class.: Pyrazinoisoquiolone derivative

Action: Causes contraction, paralysis, leading to dislodgement of suckers; they are carried to liver, where phagocytosis takes place
Uses: Schistosomiasis, liver flukes, lung flukes, intestinal flukes, tapeworms

Dosage and routes:
• *Adult and child >4 yr:* PO 20 mg/kg q4-6h × 1 day
Available forms: Tabs 600 mg
Side effects/adverse reactions:
INTEG: Rash, pruritus, urticaria, internal hypertension
CNS: Dizziness, headache, drowsiness, malaise, increased seizure activity, fever, sweating
GI: Nausea, vomiting, anorexia, diarrhea, abdominal pain, increased liver enzymes

Contraindications: Hypersensitivity, lactation
Precautions: Child <4 yr, seizure disorders, pregnancy (B)
Pharmacokinetics:
PO: Peak 1-3 hr, half-life 48-90 min; metabolized by liver (metabolites); excreted in urine, breast milk, CSF

NURSING CONSIDERATIONS
Assess:
• Liver function test: AST, ALT; watch for increase
• Stools during entire treatment, 1, 3 mo after treatment; specimens must be sent to lab while still warm
• For allergic reaction: rash, urticaria, pruritus
• For diarrhea during expulsion of worms
• For CSF reaction: headache, high fever; if these occur, drug should be discontinued, physician notified
Administer:
• Corticosteroids as ordered to reduce CNS effects (cerebral cysticercosis)
• Laxatives before treatment to cleanse bowel
• PO with liquids during meals to avoid GI symptoms; not to be chewed
Perform/provide:
• Storage in tight container in cool environment
Evaluate:
• Therapeutic response: expulsion of worms, 3 negative stool cultures after completion of treatment
Teach patient/family:
• To avoid driving, hazardous activities on day of treatment and day after treatment
• Proper hygiene after BM, including hand-washing technique; tell patient to avoid putting fingers in mouth
• Tablets taste very bitter; keeping

---

*Available in Canada only

in mouth too long may cause gagging/vomiting
• Need for compliance with dosage schedule, duration of treatment
• To refrain from breast-feeding on day of treatment, 72 hr after
Treatment of overdose: Fast-acting laxative

---

prazosin HCl
(pra′zoe-sin)
Minipress, Prazosin
Func. class.: Antihypertensive
Chem. class.: α₁-Adrenergic blocker

Action: Peripheral blood vessels dilate, peripheral resistance drops; reduction in blood pressure results from α-adrenergic receptors being blocked
Uses: Hypertension, refractory CHF, Raynaud's vasospasm
Dosage and routes:
• *Adult:* PO 1 mg bid or tid, increasing to 20 mg qd in divided doses if required, usual range 6-15 mg/day, not to exceed 1 mg initially
Available forms: Caps 1, 2, 5 mg
Side effects/adverse reactions:
CV: Palpitations, orthostatic hypotension, tachycardia, edema, rebound hypertension
CNS: Dizziness, headache, drowsiness, anxiety, depression, vertigo, weakness, fatigue
GI: Nausea, vomiting, diarrhea, constipation, abdominal pain
GU: Urinary frequency, incontinence, impotence, priapism, H₂O, Na retention
EENT: Blurred vision, epistaxis, tinnitus, dry mouth, red sclera
Contraindications: Hypersensitivity

Precautions: Pregnancy (C), children
Pharmacokinetics:
PO: Onset 2 hr, peak 1-3 hr, duration 6-12 hr; half-life 2-3 hr, metabolized in liver, excreted via bile, feces (>90%), in urine (<10%)
Interactions/incompatibilities:
• Increased hypotensive effects: β-blockers, nitroglycerin
• Decreased effect: indomethacin
Lab test interferences:
Increased: Urinary norepinephrine, VMA
NURSING CONSIDERATIONS
Assess:
• B/P during initial treatment, periodically thereafter
• Pulse, jugular venous distention q4h
• BUN, uric acid if on long-term therapy
• Weight daily, I&O
• Edema in feet, legs daily
• Skin turgor, dryness of mucous membranes for hydration status
• Rales, dyspnea, orthopnea q30min
Perform/provide:
• Storage in tight containers in cool environment
Evaluate:
• Therapeutic response: decreased B/P
Teach patient/family:
• Fainting occasionally occurs after 1st dose; do not drive or operate machinery for 4 hr after 1st dose, or take 1st dose at bedtime
Treatment of overdose: Administer volume expanders or vasopressors, discontinue drug, place in supine position

P

---

prednicarbate
(pred-ni-car'bate)
Dermatop
Func. class.: Topical corticosteroid

Action: Antipruritic, antiinflamatory

Uses: Psoriasis, eczema, contact dermatitis, pruritus

Dosage and routes:
• *Adult and child:* Apply to affected area bid-qid

Available forms: Cream 0.1%

Side effects/adverse reactions:
INTEG: Burning, dryness, itching, irritation, acne, folliculitis, hypertrichosis, perioral dermatitis, hypopigmentation, atrophy, striae, miliaria, allergic contact dermatitis, secondary infection

Contraindications: Hypersensitivity to corticosteroids, fungal infections

NURSING CONSIDERATIONS
Assess:
• Temperature; if fever develops, drug should be discontinued

Administer:
• Only to affected areas; do not get in eyes
• Medication, then cover with occlusive dressing (only if prescribed), seal to normal skin, change q12h; use occlusive dressing with extreme caution (group II potency); systemic absorption may occur
• Only to dermatoses; do not use on weeping, denuded, or infected areas

Perform/provide:
• Cleansing before application of drug; apply to slightly moist skin; use gloves, cotton-tipped applicator

• Treatment for a few days after area has cleared
• Storage at room temperature

Evaluate:
• Therapeutic response: absence of severe itching, patches on skin, flaking
• For systemic absorption: increased temperature, inflammation, irritation

Teach patient/family:
• To avoid sunlight on affected area; burns may occur

prednisolone/prednisolone acetate/prednisolone phosphate/prednisolone tebutate
(pred-niss'oh-lone)
Delta-Cortef, Prednisolone, Prelone, Articulose-50, Key-Pred 25, Key-Pred 50, Predaject-50, Predalone 50, Predcor-25, Predcor-50, Prednisolone Acetate, Hydeltrasol, Key-Pred-SP, Pediapred, Hydeltra-T.B.A., Predalone-T.B.A., Prednisol TBA, Prednisolone Tebutate
Func. class.: Corticosteroid
Chem. class.: Glucocorticoid, immediate acting

Action: Decreases inflammation by suppression of migration of polymorphonuclear leukocytes, fibroblasts; reversal to increase capillary permeability and lysosomal stabilization

Uses: Severe inflammation, immunosuppression, neoplasms

Dosage and routes:
• *Adult:* PO 2.5-15 mg bid-qid; IM 2-30 mg (acetate, phosphate) q12h; IV 2-30 mg (phosphate) q12h, 2-30 mg in joint or soft tissue (phos-

phate), 4-40 mg in joint of lesion (tebutate), 0.25-1 ml qwk in joints (acetate-phosphate)

Available forms: Tabs 5 mg; inj 25, 50, 100 mg/ml acetate; inj 20 mg/ml terbutate; inj 20 mg/ml phosphate; inj 80 mg/ml acetate/phosphate

Side effects/adverse reactions:

INTEG: Acne, poor wound healing, ecchymosis, petechiae

CNS: **Depression,** flushing, sweating, headache, mood changes

*CV: Hypertension, **circulatory collapse, thrombophlebitis, embolism,** tachycardia*

HEMA: **Thrombocytopenia**

MS: Fractures, osteoporosis, weakness

*GI: Diarrhea, nausea, abdominal distention, **GI hemorrhage,** increased appetite, pancreatitis*

EENT: Fungal infections, increased intraocular pressure, blurred vision

Contraindications: Psychosis, hypersensitivity, idiopathic thrombocytopenia, acute glomerulonephritis, amebiasis, fungal infections, nonasthmatic bronchial disease, child <2 yr

Precautions: Pregnancy (C), diabetes mellitus, glaucoma, osteoporosis, seizure disorders, ulcerative colitis, CHF, myasthenia gravis

Pharmacokinetics:

PO: Peak 1-2 hr, duration 2 days
IM: Peak 3-45 hr

Interactions/incompatibilities:

• Decreased action of prednisolone: cholestyramine, colestipol, barbiturates, rifampin, ephedrine, phenytoin, theophylline

• Decreased effects of: anticoagulants, anticonvulsants, antidiabetics, ambenonium, neostigmine, isoniazid, toxoids, vaccines, anti-cholinesterases, salicylates, somatrem

• Increased side effects: alcohol, salicylates, indomethacin, amphotericin B, digitalis, cyclosporine, diuretics

• Increased action of prednisolone: salicylates, estrogens, indomethacin, oral contraceptives, ketoconazole, macrolide antibiotics

• Incompatible with calcium gluconate/gluceptate, dimenhydrinate, metaraminol, methotrexate, polymyxin B, prochlorperazine, promazine, promethazine

Lab test interferences:

Increase: Cholesterol, Na, blood glucose, uric acid, Ca, urine glucose

Decrease: Ca, K, T_4, T_3, thyroid ^{131}I uptake test, urine 17-OHCS, 17-KS, PBI

False negative: Skin allergy tests

NURSING CONSIDERATIONS
Assess:

• K, blood sugar, urine glucose while on long-term therapy; hypokalemia and hyperglycemia

• Weight daily, notify physician if weekly gain of >5 lb

• B/P q4h, pulse, notify physician if chest pain occurs

• I&O ratio; be alert for decreasing urinary output and increasing edema

• Plasma cortisol levels during long-term therapy (normal level: 138-635 nmol/L SI units when drawn at 8 AM)

• Infection: increased temperature, WBC, even after withdrawal of medication; drug masks symptoms of infection

• K depletion: paresthesias, fatigue, nausea, vomiting, depression, polyuria, dysrhythmias, weakness

P

• Edema, hypertension, cardiac symptoms
• Mental status: affect, mood, behavioral changes, aggression

Administer:
• IV undiluted or added to NaCl or D₅ and given by IV INF; give 10 mg or less/1 min; decrease rate if burning occurs
• After shaking suspension (parenteral)
• Titrated dose; use lowest effective dose
• IM inj deeply in large mass, rotate sites, avoid deltoid, use 21G needle
• In one dose in AM to prevent adrenal suppression; avoid SC administration; may damage tissue
• With food or milk to decrease GI symptoms

Perform/provide:
• Assistance with ambulation in patient with bone tissue disease to prevent fractures

Evaluate:
• Therapeutic response: ease of respirations, decreased inflammation

Teach patient/family:
• That ID as steroid user should be carried
• To notify physician if therapeutic response decreases; dosage adjustment may be needed
• Not to discontinue this medication abruptly, or adrenal crisis can result
• To avoid OTC products: salicylates, alcohol in cough products, cold preparations unless directed by physician
• About cushingoid symptoms
• Symptoms of adrenal insufficiency: nausea, anorexia, fatigue, dizziness, dyspnea, weakness, joint pain

---

prednisolone acetate (suspension)/prednisolone sodium phosphate (solution)
(pred-niss'oh-lone)
Econopred, Econopred Plus, Pred-Forte, Pred-Mild, AK-Pred, Inflamase Forte, Inflamase Mild Ophthalmic, Metreton Ophthalmic
Func. class.: Ophthalmic antiinflammatory
Chem. class.: Analog of hydrocortisone

Action: Decreases inflammation, resulting in decreases in pain, photophobia, hyperemia, cellular infiltration

Uses: Inflammation of eye, lids, conjunctiva, cornea, uveitis, iridocyclitis, allergic condition, burns, foreign bodies

Dosage and routes:
• *Adult and child:* INSTILL 1-2 gtts into conjunctival sac q1h × 2 days, if needed, then bid-qid

Available forms: Susp 0.12%, 0.125%, 1%; sol 0.125%, 0.5%, 1%

Side effects/adverse reactions:
*EENT: **Increased intraocular pressure,*** poor corneal wound healing, increased possibility of corneal infections, glaucoma exacerbation, ***optic nerve damage,*** decreased acuity, visual field

Contraindications: Hypersensitivity, acute superficial herpes simplex, fungal/viral diseases of eye or conjunctiva, active diabetes mellitus, ocular TB, infections of the eye

Precautions: Corneal abrasions, glaucoma, pregnancy (C), lactation, children

---

NURSING CONSIDERATIONS
Administer:
• After shaking, suspension
Perform/provide:
• Storage in tight, light-resistant container
Evaluate:
• Therapeutic response: absence of swelling, redness, exudate
Teach patient/family:
• Instillation method: pressure on lacrimal duct for 1 min
• Not to share eye medications with others
• Not to use if purulent drainage is present
• Not to discontinue abruptly; taper over 1-2 wk

---

prednisone

(pred′ni-sone)
Deltasone, Liquid Pred, Meticorten, Orasone, Panasol-S, Prednicen-M, Prednisone, Prednisone Intensol Concentrate, Sterapred, Sterapred OS
Func. class.: Corticosteroid
Chem. class.: Intermediate-acting glucocorticoid

Action: Decreases inflammation by suppression of migration of polymorphonuclear leukocytes, fibroblasts, reversal to increase capillary permeability, and lysosomal stabilization
Uses: Severe inflammation, immunosuppression, neoplasms, multiple sclerosis, collagen disorders, dermatologic disorders
Dosage and routes:
• *Adult:* PO 1.5-2.5 mg bid-qid, then qd or qod; maintenance up to 250 mg/day
Nephrosis
• *Child 18 mo-4 yr:* 7.5-10 mg qid initially

• *Child 4-10 yr:* 15 mg qid initially
• *Child >10 yr:* 20 mg qid initially
Multiple sclerosis
• *Adult:* PO 200 mg/day × 1 wk, then 80 mg qod × 1 mo
Available forms: Tabs 1, 2.5, 5, 10, 20, 25, 50 mg; oral sol 5 mg/5 ml; syr 5 mg/5 ml
Side effects/adverse reactions:
CNS: Depression, flushing, sweating, headache, mood changes
CV: Hypertension, *circulatory collapse, thrombophlebitis, embolism,* tachycardia
EENT: Fungal infections, increased intraocular pressure, blurred vision
GI: Diarrhea, nausea, abdominal distention, *GI hemorrhage,* increased appetite, pancreatitis
HEMA: Thrombocytopenia
INTEG: Acne, poor wound healing, ecchymosis, petechiae
MS: Fractures, osteoporosis, weakness
Contraindications: Psychosis, hypersensitivity, idiopathic thrombocytopenia, acute glomerulonephritis, amebiasis, fungal infections, nonasthmatic bronchial disease, child <2 yr, AIDS, TB
Precautions: Pregnancy (C), diabetes mellitus, glaucoma, osteoporosis, seizure disorders, ulcerative colitis, CHF, myasthenia gravis, renal disease, esophagitis, peptic ulcer
Pharmacokinetics:
Well absorbed PO
PO: Peak 1-2 hr, duration 1-1½ days, half-life 3½-4 hr; crosses placenta, enters breast milk, metabolized by the liver after conversion
Interactions/incompatibilities:
• Decreased action of prednisone: cholestyramine, colestipol, barbiturates, rifampin, ephedrine, phenytoin, theophylline
• Decreased effects of: anticoagu-

P

lants, anticonvulsants, antidiabetics, ambenonium, neostigmine, isoniazid, toxoids, vaccines, anticholinesterases, salicylates, somatrem

• Increased side effects: alcohol, salicylates, indomethacin, amphotericin B, digitalis, cyclosporine, diuretics

• Increased action of prednisone: salicylates, estrogens, indomethacin, oral contraceptives, ketoconazole, macrolide antibiotics

Lab test interferences:

Increase: Cholesterol, Na, blood glucose, uric acid, Ca, urine glucose

Decrease: Ca, K, T_4, T_3, thyroid ^{131}I uptake test, urine 17-OHCS, 17-KS, PBI

False negative: Skin allergy tests

NURSING CONSIDERATIONS

Assess:

• Adrenal insufficiency: nausea, vomiting, anorexia, confusion, hypotension

• K, blood sugar, urine glucose while on long-term therapy; hypokalemia and hyperglycemia

• Weight daily; notify physician of weekly gain >5 lb

• B/P q4h, pulse; notify physician of chest pain; monitor for rales, crackles, dyspnea if edema is present

• I&O ratio; be alert for decreasing urinary output, increasing edema

• Plasma cortisol levels during long-term therapy (normal level: 138-635 nmol/L SI units when drawn at 8 AM)

• Infection: increased temperature, WBC, even after withdrawal of medication; drug masks symptoms of infection

• K depletion: paresthesias, fatigue, nausea, vomiting, depression, polyuria, dysrhythmias, weakness

• Edema, hypertension, cardiac symptoms

• Mental status: affect, mood, behavioral changes, aggression

Administer:

• Titrated dose; use lowest effective dose

• With food or milk to decrease GI symptoms

Perform/provide:

• Assistance with ambulation in patient with bone tissue disease to prevent fractures

Evaluate:

• Therapeutic response: ease of respirations, decreased inflammation

Teach patient/family:

• That ID as steroid user should be carried; information on drug being taken and condition

• To notify physician if therapeutic response decreases; dosage adjustment may be needed

• To avoid vaccinations while on this drug

• Not to discontinue this medication abruptly, or adrenal crisis can result

• To avoid OTC products: salicylates, alcohol in cough products, cold preparations unless directed by physician

• About cushingoid symptoms: moon face, weight gain

• That drug causes immunosuppression; to report any symptoms of infection (increased temperature, sore throat, cough)

• Symptoms of adrenal insufficiency; nausea, anorexia, fatigue, dizziness, dyspnea, weakness, joint pain

---

primaquine phosphate

(prim'a-kween)

Func. class.: Antimalarial
Chem. class.: Synthetic 8-aminoquinolone

Action: Unknown; thought to destroy exoerythrocytic forms by gametocidal action

Uses: Malaria caused by *P. vivax*

Dosage and routes:
• *Adult:* PO 15 mg (base) qd × 2 wk; 26.3-mg tab is 15-mg base
• *Child:* PO 0.3 mg/kg × 2 wk

Available forms: Tabs 26.3 mg

Side effects/adverse reactions:
INTEG: Pruritus, skin eruptions
CNS: Headache
EENT: Blurred vision, difficulty focusing
GI: Nausea, vomiting, anorexia, cramps
CV: Hypertension
*HEMA: **Agranulocytosis, granulocytopenia, leukopenia, hemolytic anemia, leukocytosis,** mild anemia, **methemoglobinemia***

Contraindications: Hypersensitivity, anemia, lupus erythematosus, methemoglobinemia, porphyria, rheumatoid arthritis, methemoglobin reductase deficiency, G-6-PD deficiency

Precautions: Pregnancy (C)

Pharmacokinetics:
PO: Metabolized by liver (metabolites), half-life 3.7-9.6 hr

Interactions/incompatibilities:
• Toxicity: quinacrine

NURSING CONSIDERATIONS
Assess:
• Ophthalmic test if long-term treatment or drug dosage >150 mg/day
• Liver studies qwk: AST, ALT, bilirubin, if on long-term therapy
• Blood studies: CBC, since blood dyscrasias occur
• Allergic reactions: pruritus, rash, urticaria
• Blood dyscrasias: malaise, fever, bruising, bleeding (rare)
• For renal status: dark urine, hematuria, decreased output
• For hemolytic reaction: chills, fever, chest pain, cyanosis; drug should be discontinued immediately

Administer:
• Before or after meals at same time each day to maintain drug level

Evaluate:
• Therapeutic response: decreased symptoms of malaria

Teach patient/family:
• To report visual problems, fever, fatigue, dark urine, bruising, bleeding; may indicate blood dyscrasias

primidone

(pri'mi-done)

Mysoline, Primidone, Sertan*

Func. class.: Anticonvulsant
Chem. class.: Barbiturate derivative

Action: Raises seizure threshold by conversion of drug to phenobarbital

Uses: Generalized tonic-clonic (grand mal), complex-partial psychomotor seizures

Dosage and routes:
• *Adult and child >8 yr:* PO 250 mg/day; may increase by 250 mg/wk, not to exceed 2 g/day in divided doses qid
• *Child <8 yr:* PO 125 mg/day; may increase by 125 mg/wk, not to exceed 1 g/day in divided doses qid

P

italics = common side effects   ***bold italic*** = life threatening reactions

Available forms: Tabs 50, 250 mg; susp 250 mg/5 ml

Side effects/adverse reactions:

*HEMA: **Thrombocytopenia, leukopenia, neutropenia, eosinophilia, megaloblastic anemia,** decreased serum folate level, lymphadenopathy

*CNS: **Stimulation, drowsiness,** dizziness, confusion, sedation, headache, flushing, hallucinations, coma, psychosis, ataxia, vertigo

GI: Nausea, vomiting, anorexia

INTEG: Rash, edema, alopecia, lupuslike syndrome

EENT: Diplopia, nystagmus, edema of eyelids

GU: Impotence, polyuria

Contraindications: Hypersensitivity, porphyria, pregnancy (D)

Precautions: COPD, hepatic disease, renal disease, hyperactive children

Pharmacokinetics:

PO: Peak 4 hr; excreted by kidneys, in breast milk; half-life 3-24 hr

Interactions/incompatibilities:

• Increased blood levels: alcohol, heparin, CNS depressants, isoniazid, phenytoin, phenobarbital

NURSING CONSIDERATIONS

Assess:

• Drug level: therapeutic level 5-12 μg/ml; CBC should be done q6mo

• Mental status: mood, sensorium, affect, memory (long, short)

• Respiratory depression or wheezing

• Blood dyscrasias: fever, sore throat, bruising, rash, jaundice

Administer:

• Shake liquid susp well

Evaluate:

• Therapeutic response: decreased seizures

Teach patient/family:

• Not to withdraw drug quickly; withdrawal symptoms may occur

• To avoid hazardous activities until stabilized on drug

---

probenecid
(proe-ben'e-sid)
Benemid, Benuryl,* Probalan, Probenecid
Func. class.: Uricosuric
Chem. class.: Sulfonamide derivative

Action: Inhibits tubular reabsorption of urates, with increased excretion of uric acids

Uses: Gonorrhea, hyperuricemia in gout, gouty arthritis, adjunct to cephalosporin or penicillin treatment

Dosage and routes:

Gonorrhea

• *Adult:* PO 1 g with 3.5 g ampicillin or 1 g ½ hr before 4.8 million U of aqueous penicillin G procaine injected into 2 sites IM

Gout/gouty arthritis

• *Adult:* PO 250 mg bid for 1 wk, then 500 mg bid, not to exceed 2 g/day; maintenance: 500 mg/day × 6 mo

Adjunct in penicillin/cephalosporin treatment

• *Adult and child >50 kg:* PO 500 mg qid

• *Child <50 kg:* PO 25 mg/kg, then 40 mg/kg in divided doses qid

Available forms: Tabs 0.5 g

Side effects/adverse reactions:

CNS: Drowsiness, headache

CV: Bradycardia

GU: Glycosuria, thirst, frequency, **nephrotic syndrome**

GI: Gastric irritation, nausea, vomiting, anorexia, **hepatic necrosis**

INTEG: Rash, dermatitis, pruritus, fever

META: Acidosis, hypokalemia, hyperchloremia, hyperglycemia

RESP: **Apnea,** irregular respirations

Contraindications: Hypersensitivity, severe hepatic disease, blood dyscrasias, severe renal disease, CrC <50 mg/min, history of uric acid calculus

Precautions: Pregnancy (B), severe respiratory disease, lactation, cardiac edema, child <2 yr

Pharmacokinetics:

PO: Peak 2-4 hr, duration 8 hr, half-life 8-10 hr; metabolized by liver; excreted in urine; crosses placenta

Interactions/incompatibilities:

• Increased activity of: oral anticoagulants

• Increased toxicity: sulfa drugs, dapsone, clofibrate, PAS, indomethacin, rifampin, naproxen, methotrexate, pantothenic acid, oral hypoglycemics

• Decreased action of probenecid: alcohol, salicylates, nitrofurantoin, diazoxides, diuretics

• Decreased action of: oral hypoglycemics

Lab test interferences:

False positive: Urine glucose with copper sulfate test (Clinitest)

False positive: Theophylline levels

Increase: BSP/urinary PSP

Decrease: Urinary 17-KS

NURSING CONSIDERATIONS

Assess:

• Uric acid levels (3-7 mg/dl)

• Respiratory rate, rhythm, depth; notify physician of abnormalities

• Electrolytes, CO_2 before, during treatment

• Urine pH, output, glucose during beginning treatment

• For CNS symptoms: confusion, twitching, hyperreflexia, stimulation, headache; may indicate overdose

Administer:

• After meals or with milk if GI symptoms occur

• Increase fluid intake to 2-3 L/day to prevent urinary calculi

Perform/provide:

• Low purine diet restricting organ meats, anchovies, sardines, meat gravy, dried beans, meat extracts

Evaluate:

• Therapeutic response: absence of pain, stiffness in joints

Teach patient/family

• To avoid high-purine foods; alcohol, urinary calculi may form

• To avoid OTC preparations (aspirin) unless directed by physician

---

probucol

(proe'byoo-kole)

Lorelco

Func. class.: Antilipemic

Action: Increases bile acid excretion, catabolism of LDL-cholesterol; increases HDL reverse cholesterol transport and blocks oxidation of LDL-cholesterol

Uses: Severe hypercholesterolemia when other treatment unsuccessful

Dosage and routes:

Adult: PO 500 mg bid with breakfast, supper

Available forms: Tabs 250, 500 mg

Side effects/adverse reactions:

GI: Nausea, vomiting, diarrhea, flatulence, anorexia

CV: Palpitations, dysrhythmias, **myocardial infarction,** prolonged QT interval

EENT: Visual disturbances, ptosis, tinnitus

CNS: Insomnia, dizziness, palpitations, paresthesias, syncope

Contraindications: Hypersensitivity

Precautions: Dysrhythmias, pregnancy (B), lactation, children

---

italics = common side effects   **bold italic** = life threatening reactions

Pharmacokinetics:
PO: Excreted in bile, feces
Interactions/incompatibilities:
• Do not use with clofibrate
Lab test interferences:
Increase: Liver function studies, CPK, blood glucose, uric acid, BUN

NURSING CONSIDERATIONS
Assess:
• Hepatic function if patient is on long-term therapy
• Bowel pattern daily; increase bulk, water in diet if constipation develops
Administer:
• Drug with meals if GI symptoms occur
Evaluate:
• Therapeutic response: decreased cholesterol levels, (hyperlipidemia), diarrhea, pruritus (excess bile area)
Teach patient/family:
• That compliance is necessary, since toxicity may result if doses are missed
• That risk factors should be decreased: high fat diet, smoking, alcohol consumption, absence of exercise
• Birth control should be practiced while on this drug

---

procainamide HCl
(proe-kane-a′mide)
Procan SR, Promine, Procainamide, Pronestyl, Sub-Quin, Rhythmin
Func. class.: Antidysrhythmic (Class IA)
Chem. class.: Procaine HCl amide analog

Action: Depresses excitability of cardiac muscle to electrical stimulation and slows conduction in atrium, bundle of His, and ventricle
Uses: PVCs, atrial fibrillation, PAT, ventricular tachycardia, atrial dysrhythmias, ventricular tachycardia
Dosage and routes:
Atrial fibrillation/PAT
• *Adult:* PO 1-1.25 g, may give another 750 mg if needed; if no response, 500 mg-1g q2h until desired response; maintenance 50 mg/kg in divided doses q6h
Ventricular tachycardia
• *Adult:* PO 1g; maintenance 50 mg/kg/day given in 3 hr intervals; SUS REL TABS 500 mg-1.25 g q6h
Other dysrhythmias
• *Adult:* IV BOL 100 mg q5min, given 25-50 mg/min, not to exceed 500 mg; or 17 mg/kg total then IV INF 2-6 mg/min
Available forms: Caps 250, 375, 500 mg; tabs 250, 375, 500 mg; tabs sus rel 250, 500, 750, 1000 mg; inj IV 100, 500 mg/ml
Side effects/adverse reactions:
CNS: Headache, dizziness, confusion, psychosis, restlessness, irritability, weakness
GI: Nausea, vomiting, anorexia, diarrhea, hepatomegaly
CV: Hypotension, **heart block, cardiovascular collapse, arrest**
HEMA: SLE syndrome, **agranulocytosis, thrombocytopenia, neutropenia, hemolytic anemia**
INTEG: Rash, urticaria, edema, swelling (rare), pruritus
Contraindications: Hypersensitivity, myasthenia gravis, severe heart block
Precautions: Pregnancy (C), lactation, children, renal disease, liver disease, CHF, respiratory depression
Pharmacokinetics:
PO: Peak 1-2 hr, duration 3 hr (8 hr extended)

IM: Peak 10-60 min, duration 3 hr; half-life 3 hr, metabolized in liver to active metabolites, excreted unchanged by kidneys (60%)

Interactions/incompatibilities:

• Increased effects of: neuromuscular blockers, anticholinergics, antihypertensives

• Increased procainamide effects: cimetidine

• Decreased effects of procainamide: barbiturates

• Increased toxicity: other antidysrhythmics

• Incompatible with phenytoin

NURSING CONSIDERATIONS

Assess:

• ECG continuously to determine increased PR or QRS segments; if these develop, discontinue immediately; watch for increased ventricular ectopic beats, maximum need to rebolus

• Blood levels, 3-10 μg/ml

• B/P continuously for fluctuations

• I&O ratio; electrolytes (K, Na, Cl)

• Malignant hyperthermia: tachypnea, tachycardia, changes in B/P, increased temperature

• Cardiac rate, respiration: rate, rhythm, character

• Respiratory status: rate, rhythm, lung fields; watch for respiratory depression

• CNS effects: dizziness, confusion, psychosis, paresthesias, convulsions; drug should be discontinued

• Lung fields; bilateral rales may occur in CHF patient

• Increased respiration, increased pulse; drug should be discontinued

Administer:

• IV after diluting 100 mg/ml of D₅W or sterile H₂O for inj; give 20 mg or less/1 min; may dilute 1 g/ 250-500 ml D₅W, run at 2-6 mg/ min

• IM injection in deltoid; aspirate to avoid intravascular administration; check IV site q8h for infiltration or extravasation

Evaluate:

• Therapeutic response: decreased dysrhythmias

---

procaine HCl

(proe′-kane)

Novocain, Unicaine

Func. class.: Local anesthetic

Chem. class.: Ester

Action: Competes with calcium for sites in nerve membrane that control sodium transport across cell membrane; decreases rise of depolarization phase of action potential

Uses: Spinal anesthesia, epidural, peripheral nerve block, perineum, lower extremities, infiltration

Dosage and routes:

Varies by route of anesthesia

Available forms: Inj 1%, 2%, 10%

Side effects/adverse reactions:

CNS: Anxiety, restlessness, ***convulsions, LOC,*** drowsiness, disorientation, tremors, shivering

*CV: **Myocardial depression, cardiac arrest, dysrhythmias,*** bradycardia, hypotension, hypertension, fetal bradycardia

GI: Nausea, vomiting

EENT: Blurred vision, tinnitus, pupil constriction

INTEG: Rash, urticaria, allergic reactions, edema, burning, skin discoloration at injection site, tissue necrosis

*RESP: **Status asthmaticus, respiratory arrest, anaphylaxis***

Contraindications: Hypersensitiv-

ity, child <12 yr, elderly, severe liver disease

Precautions: Elderly, severe drug allergies, pregnancy (C)

Pharmacokinetics:
Onset 2-5 min, duration 1 hr; metabolized by liver, excreted in urine (metabolites)

Interactions/incompatibilities:
• Dysrhythmias: epinephrine, halothane, enflurane
• Hypertension: MAOIs, tricyclic antidepressants, phenothiazines
• Decreased action of procaine: chloroprocaine

NURSING CONSIDERATIONS
Assess:
• B/P, pulse, respiration during treatment
• Fetal heart tones if drug is used during labor
• Allergic reactions: rash, urticaria, itching
• Cardiac status: ECG for dysrhythmias, pulse, B/P during anesthesia

Administer:
• Only drugs that are not cloudy, do not contain precipitate
• Only with crash cart, resuscitative equipment nearby
• Only drugs without preservatives for epidural or caudal anesthesia

Perform/provide:
• Use of new solution; discard unused portions

Evaluate:
• Therapeutic response: anesthesia necessary for procedure

Treatment of overdose: Airway, O₂, vasopressor, IV fluids, anticonvulsants for seizures

procarbazine HCl
(proe-kar′ba-zeen)
Matulane, Natulan*
Func. class.: Antineoplastic, miscellaneous
Chem. class.: Hydrazine derivative

Action: Inhibits DNA, RNA, protein synthesis; has multiple sites of action; a nonvesicant

Uses: Lymphoma, Hodgkin's disease, cancers resistant to other therapy

Dosage and routes:
• *Adult:* PO 2-4 mg/kg/day for first wk; maintain dosage of 4-6 mg/kg/day until platelets and WBC fall; after recovery, 1-2 mg/kg/day
• *Child:* PO 50 mg/day for 7 days, then 100 mg/m² until desired response, leukopenia, or thrombocytopenia occurs; 50 mg/day is maintenance after bone marrow recovery

Available forms: Caps 50 mg

Side effects/adverse reactions:
*HEMA: **Thrombocytopenia, anemia, leukopenia, myelosuppression, bleeding tendencies**,* purpura, petechiae, epistaxis
GI: Nausea, vomiting, anorexia, diarrhea, constipation, dry mouth, stomatitis
EENT: Retinal hemorrhage, nystagmus, photophobia, diplopia
INTEG: Rash, pruritus, dermatitis, alopecia, herpes, hyperpigmentation
CNS: Headache, dizziness, insomnia, hallucinations, confusion, coma, pain, chills, fever, sweating, paresthesias
RESP: Cough, pneumonitis
MS: Arthralgias, myalgias

GU: Azoospermia, cessation of menses

Contraindications: Hypersensitivity, thrombocytopenia, bone marrow depression

Precautions: Renal disease, hepatic disease, pregnancy (D), radiation therapy

Pharmacokinetics: Half-life 1 hr; concentrates in liver, kidney, skin; metabolized in liver, excreted in urine

Interactions/incompatibilities:
• Increased CNS depression: barbiturates, antihistamines, narcotics, hypotensive agents, phenothiazines
• Disulfiram-like reaction: ethyl alcohol, MAOIs, tricyclic antidepressants, tyramine foods, sympathomimetic drugs
• Hypertension: guanethidine, levodopa, methyldopa, reserpine
• Increased hypoglycemia: insulin, oral hypoglycemics

NURSING CONSIDERATIONS
Assess:
• CBC, differential, platelet count weekly; withhold drug if WBC is <4000/mm³ or platelet count is <100,000/mm³; notify physician of these results
• Renal function studies: BUN, serum uric acid, urine CrCl, electrolytes before, during therapy
• I&O ratio, report fall in urine output to <30 ml/hr
• Monitor temperature q4h; fever may indicate beginning infection
• Liver function tests before, during therapy: bilirubin, AST, ALT, alk phosphatase prn or monthly
• CNS changes: confusion, paresthesias, neuropathies, drug should be discontinued
• Toxicity: facial flushing, epistaxis, increased pro-time, thrombocytopenia; drug should be discontinued
• Bleeding: hematuria, guaiac stools, bruising or petechiae, mucosa or orifices q8h
• Food preferences; list likes, dislikes
• Effects of alopecia on body image; discuss feelings about body changes
• Inflammation of mucosa, breaks in skin
• Yellowing of skin and sclera, dark urine, clay-colored stools, itchy skin, abdominal pain, fever, diarrhea
• Buccal cavity q8h for dryness, sores or ulceration, white patches, oral pain, bleeding, dysphagia
• Alkalosis if vomiting is severe
• GI symptoms: frequency of stools, cramping
• Acidosis, signs of dehydration: rapid respirations, poor skin turgor, decreased urine output, dry skin, restlessness, weakness

Administer:
• In divided doses and at hs to minimize nausea and vomiting
• Nonphenothiazine antiemetic 30-60 min before giving drug and 4-10 hr after treatment to prevent vomiting
• Transfusion for anemia
• Antispasmodic for GI symptoms

Perform/provide:
• Liquid diet: carbonated beverages; gelatin may be added if patient is not nauseated or vomiting
• Storage in tight, light-resistant container in cool environment

Evaluate:
• Therapeutic response: decreased tumor size, spread of malignancy

Teach patient/family:
• To report any complaints, side effects to nurse or physician: cough, shortness of breath, fever, chills,

sore throat, bleeding, bruising, vomiting blood, black tarry stools
• That hair may be lost during treatment and wig or hairpiece may make patient feel better; tell patient that new hair may be different in color, texture
• To avoid foods with citric acid, hot or rough texture
• To report any bleeding, white spots, ulcerations in mouth to physician; tell patient to examine mouth qd
• To avoid driving or activities requiring alertness; dizziness may occur
• That contraceptive measures are recommended during therapy
• To avoid ingestion of alcohol, tyramine-containing foods; cold, hay fever, weight-reducing products may cause serious drug interactions
• To avoid crowds, persons with infections if granulocytes are low

---

prochlorperazine edisylate/prochlorperazine maleate
(proe-klor-per'a-zeen)
Compazine, Stemetil*
Func. class.: Antiemetic
Chem. class.: Phenothiazine, piperazine derivative

Action: Acts centrally by blocking chemoreceptor trigger zone, which in turn acts on vomiting center
Uses: Nausea, vomiting
Dosage and routes:
Postoperative nausea/vomiting
• *Adult:* IM 5-10 mg 1-2 hr before anesthesia; may repeat in 30 min; IV 5-10 mg 15-30 min before anesthesia; IV INF 20 mg/L D₅W or NS 15-30 min before anesthesia, not to exceed 40 mg/day

Severe nausea/vomiting
• Adult: PO 5-10 mg tid-qid; SUST REL 15 mg qd in AM or 10 mg q12h; REC 25 mg/bid; IM 5-10 mg; may repeat q4h, not to exceed 40 mg/day
• *Child 18-39 kg:* PO 2.5 mg tid or 5 mg bid; do not exceed 15 mg/day; IM 0.132 mg/kg
• *Child 14-17 kg:* PO/REC 2.5 mg bid-tid, not to exceed 10 mg/day; IM 0.132 mg/kg
• *Child 9-13 kg:* PO/REC 2.5 mg qd-bid, not to exceed 7.5 mg/day; IM 0.132 mg/kg
Available forms: Oral sol 5 mg/ml; inj 5 mg/ml; tabs 5, 10, 25 mg; caps ext rel 10, 15, 30 mg
Side effects/adverse reactions:
CNS: Euphoria, depression, extrapyramidal symptoms, restlessness, tremor, dizziness
GI: Nausea, vomiting, anorexia, dry mouth, diarrhea, constipation, weight loss, metallic taste, cramps
CV: Circulatory failure, tachycardia
RESP: Respiratory depression
Contraindications: Hypersensitivity to phenothiazines, coma, seizure, encephalopathy, bone marrow depression
Precautions: Children <2 yr, pregnancy (C), elderly
Pharmacokinetics:
PO: Onset 30-40 min, duration 3-4 hr
EX REL: Onset 30-40 min, duration 10-12 hr
REC: Onset 60 min, duration 3-4 hr
IM: Onset 10-20 min, duration 12 hr; metabolized by liver; excreted by kidneys; crosses placenta; excreted in breast milk
Interactions/incompatibilities:
• Decreased effect of prochlorperazine: barbiturates, antacids
• Increased anticholinergic action:

anticholinergics, antiparkinson drugs, antidepressants
• Incompatible with aminophylline, amobarbital, amphotericin B, ampicillin, calcium, cephalothin, chloramphenicol, chlorothiazide, dexamethasone, dimenhydrinate, epinephrine, erythromycin, heparin, hydrocortisone, hydromorphone, kanamycin, methicillin, methohexital, midazolam, penicillin G, pentobarbital, phenobarbital, phenytoin, prednisolone, secobarbital, tetracycline, thiopental, vancomycin
• Do not mix with other drug in syringe or sol

NURSING CONSIDERATIONS
Assess:
• VS, B/P; check patients with cardiac disease more often
• Respiratory status before, during, after administration of emetic; check rate, rhythm, character; respiratory depression can occur rapidly with elderly or debilitated patients

Administer:
• IM injection in large muscle mass; aspirate to avoid IV administration
• IV after diluting 5 mg/9 ml of NaCl for inj (1 ml = 0.5 mg); give 5 mg or less/min; may dilute 10-20 mg/L NaCl and give as infusion; can cause contact dermatitis

Evaluate:
• Therapeutic response: absence of nausea, vomiting

Teach patient/family:
• To avoid hazardous activities, activities requiring alertness; dizziness may occur
• To avoid alcohol while taking this drug

procyclidine HCl
(proe-sye'kli-deen)
Kemadrin, Procyclid*
Func. class.: Cholinergic blocker
Chem. class.: Tertiary amine

Action: Centrally acting anticholinergic
Uses: Parkinson symptoms, extrapyramidal disorders
Dosage and routes:
• *Adult:* PO 2.5 mg tid pc, titrated to patient response
Available forms: Tabs 5 mg
Side effects/adverse reactions:
MS: Weakness, cramping
INTEG: Rash, urticaria, dermatoses
MISC: Increased temperature, flushing, decreased sweating, hyperthermia, heat stroke, numbness of fingers
CNS: Confusion, anxiety, restlessness, irritability, delusions, hallucinations, headache, sedation, depression, incoherence, dizziness, light-headedness, memory loss
EENT: Blurred vision, photophobia, dilated pupils, difficulty swallowing, mydriasis, increased intraocular tension, angle-closure glaucoma
CV: Palpitations, tachycardia, postural hypotension, bradycardia
GI: Dryness of mouth, constipation, nausea, vomiting, abdominal distress, paralytic ileus, *epigastric distress*
GU: Hesitancy, retention, dysuria
Contraindications: Hypersensitivity, narrow-angle glaucoma, myasthenia gravis, GI/GU obstruction, child <3 yr, megacolon, stenosing peptic ulcer, prostatic hypertrophy

P

---

italics = common side effects   ***bold italic*** = life threatening reactions

Precautions: Pregnancy (C), elderly, lactation, tachycardia, children, kidney, liver disease, drug abuse, hypotension, hypertension, psychiatric patients, prostatic hypertrophy

Pharmacokinetics:
PO: Onset 30-45 min, duration 4-6 hr

Interactions/incompatibilities:
• Decreased action of: haloperidol, levodopa
• Increased anticholinergic effect: antihistamines, MAOIs, phenothiazines, amantadine

NURSING CONSIDERATIONS
Assess:
• I&O ratio; retention commonly causes decreased urinary output
• Heart rate, rhythm, B/P
• Parkinsonism: shuffling gait, muscle rigidity, involuntary movements
• Urinary hesitancy, retention; palpate bladder if retention occurs
• Constipation, especially elderly; increase fluids, bulk, exercise; if this occurs, palpate abdomen
• For tolerance over long-term therapy; dose may have to be increased or changed
• Mental status: affect, mood, CNS depression, worsening of mental symptoms during early therapy

Administer:
• With or after meals for GI upset; may give with fluids other than water
• At hs to avoid daytime drowsiness in patient with parkinsonism

Perform/provide:
• Storage at room temperature in tight container
• Hard candy, frequent drinks, sugarless gum to relieve dry mouth

Evaluate:
• Therapeutic response: decreased involuntary movements

Teach patient/family:
• Not to discontinue this drug abruptly; to taper off over 1 wk
• To avoid driving, other hazardous activities; drowsiness may occur
• To avoid OTC medication: cough, cold preparations with alcohol, antihistamines unless directed by physician
• To avoid alcohol

---

progesterone
(proe-jess'ter-one)
Progestasert, Progesterone, Gesterol 50, Progesterone in Oil
Func. class.: Progestogen
Chem. class.: Progesterone derivative

Action: Inhibits secretion of pituitary gonadotropins, which prevents follicular maturation, ovulation; stimulates growth of mammary tissue; antineoplastic action against endometrial cancer

Uses: Contraception, amenorrhea, premenstrual syndrome, abnormal uterine bleeding

Dosage and routes:
Amenorrhea/uterine bleeding
• Adult: IM 5-10 mg qd × 6-8 doses
Contraception
• Adult: INSERT 1 placed in uterine cavity, active for 1 yr
PMS
• Adult: REC SUPP/VAG SUPP 200-400 mg
Available forms: Inj IM 25, 50, 100 mg/ml; IU system 38 mg, rec supp, vag supp

Side effects/adverse reactions:
CNS: Dizziness, headache, migraines, depression, fatigue
CV: Hypotension, thrombophlebitis, edema, ***thromboembolism,***

---

stroke, pulmonary embolism, myocardial infarction

GI: Nausea, vomiting, anorexia, cramps, increased weight, *cholestatic jaundice*

EENT: Diplopia

GU: Amenorrhea, cervical erosion, breakthrough bleeding, dysmenorrhea, vaginal candidiasis, breast changes, *gynecomastia, testicular atrophy, impotence,* endometriosis, *spontaneous abortion*

INTEG: Rash, urticaria, acne, hirsutism, alopecia, oily skin, seborrhea, purpura, melasma

META: Hyperglycemia

Contraindications: Breast cancer, hypersensitivity, thromboembolic disorders, reproductive cancer, genital bleeding (abnormal, undiagnosed), cerebral hemorrhage, pregnancy (X)

Precautions: Lactation, hypertension, asthma, blood dyscrasias, gallbladder disease, CHF, diabetes mellitus, bone disease, depression, migraine headache, convulsive disorders, hepatic disease, renal disease, family history of breast or reproductive tract cancer

Pharmacokinetics:
IM: Duration 24 hr

Excreted in urine, feces; metabolized in liver

Lab test interferences:
Increase: Alk phosphatase, nitrogen (urine), pregnanediol, amino acids, factors VII, VIII, IX, X
Decrease: GTT, HDL

NURSING CONSIDERATIONS
Assess:
• Weight daily; notify physician of weekly weight gain >5 lb
• B/P at beginning of treatment and periodically
• I&O ratio; be alert for decreasing urinary output, increasing edema
• Liver function studies: ALT, AST, bilirubin periodically during long-term therapy
• Edema, hypertension, cardiac symptoms, jaundice
• Mental status: affect, mood, behavioral changes, depression
• Hypercalcemia

Administer:
• Titrated dose; use lowest effective dose
• Oil solution deeply in large muscle mass IM; rotate sites
• In one dose in AM
• With food or milk to decrease GI symptoms
• After warming to dissolve crystals

Perform/provide:
• Storage in dark area

Evaluate:
• Therapeutic response: decreased abnormal uterine bleeding, absence of amenorrhea

Teach patient/family:
• About cushingoid symptoms
• To report breast lumps, vaginal bleeding, edema, jaundice, dark urine, clay-colored stools, dyspnea, headache, blurred vision, abdominal pain, numbness or stiffness in legs, chest pain
• To report suspected pregnancy
• To monitor blood sugar if diabetic

---

promazine HCl
(proe'ma-zeen)
Promanyl,* Promazine, Prozine, Sparine

Func. class.: Antipsychotic/neuroleptic
Chem. class.: Phenothiazine, aliphatic

Action: Depresses cerebral cortex, hypothalamus, limbic system, which control activity, aggression;

---

italics = common side effects   ***bold italic*** = life threatening reactions

blocks neurotransmission produced by dopamine at synapse; exhibits a strong α-adrenergic, anticholinergic blocking action; as antiemetic, inhibits medullary chemoreceptor trigger zone; mechanism for antipsychotic effects is unclear

Uses: Psychotic disorders, schizophrenia, nausea, vomiting, alcohol withdrawal

Dosage and routes:
Psychosis
• *Adult:* PO 10-200 mg q4-6h, max dose 1000 mg/day; IM 50-150 mg, followed in 30 min with additional dose up to a total dose of 300 mg
• *Child >12 yr:* PO 10-25 mg q4-6h

Nausea/vomiting
• *Adult:* PO 25-50 mg q4-6h; IM 50 mg; IV not recommended, but may use in concentrations of <25 mg/ml

Available forms: Tabs 25, 50, 100 mg; syr 10 mg/5ml; inj IV, IM 25, 50 mg/ml

Side effects/adverse reactions:
*RESP: **Laryngospasm,** dyspnea, **respiratory depression***

*CNS: Extrapyramidal symptoms: pseudoparkinsonism, akathisia, dystonia, tardive dyskinesia, drowsiness, headache, **seizures***

*HEMA: Anemia, **leukopenia, leukocytosis, agranulocytosis***

INTEG: Rash, photosensitivity, dermatitis

EENT: Blurred vision, glaucoma, dry eyes

GI: Dry mouth, nausea, vomiting, anorexia, constipation, diarrhea, jaundice, weight gain

GU: Urinary retention, urinary frequency, enuresis, impotence, amenorrhea, gynecomastia

*CV: Orthostatic hypotension, **cardiac arrest,** ECG changes, **tachycardia***

Contraindications: Hypersensitivity, blood dyscrasias, coma, child <12 yr, brain damage, bone marrow depression, glaucoma

Precautions: Pregnancy (C), lactation, seizure disorders, hypertension, hepatic disease, cardiac disease

Pharmacokinetics:
PO: Onset erratic, peak 2-4 hr
IM: Onset 15 min, peak 1 hr, duration 4-6 hr; metabolized by liver, excreted in urine, crosses placenta, enters breast milk

Interactions/incompatibilities:
• Oversedation: other CNS depressants, alcohol, barbiturate anesthetics
• Toxicity: epinephrine
• Decreased absorption: aluminum hydroxide, magnesium hydroxide antacids
• Decreased effects of: lithium, levodopa
• Increased effects of both drugs: β-adrenergic blockers, alcohol
• Increased anticholinergic effects: anticholinergics
• Incompatible with aminophylline, amobarbital, ampicillin, atropine, chloramphenicol, chlorothiazide, dimenhydrinate, epinephrine, heparin, hydrocortisone, methicillin, methohexital, nafcillin, penicillin G, pentobarbital, phenobarbital, phenytoin, prednisolone, thiopental, warfarin, $NaCO_3$

Lab test interferences:
Increase: Liver function tests, cardiac enzymes, cholesterol, blood glucose, prolactin, bilirubin, PBI, cholinesterase, ^{131}I

Decrease: Hormones (blood and urine)

False positive: Pregnancy tests, PKU

False negative: Urinary steroids, 17-OHCS, pregnancy tests

---

* Available in Canada only

NURSING CONSIDERATIONS
Assess:
• Mental status before initial administration
• Swallowing of PO medication; check for hoarding or giving of medication to other patients
• I&O ratio; palpate bladder if urinary output is low
• Bilirubin, CBC, liver function studies monthly
• Urinalysis is recommended before and during prolonged therapy
• Affect, orientation, LOC, reflexes, gait, coordination, sleep pattern disturbances
• B/P standing and lying; also include pulse, respirations, q4h during initial treatment; establish baseline before starting treatment; report drops of 30 mm Hg
• *Dizziness, faintness, palpitations, tachycardia* on rising
• Extrapyramidal symptoms including akathisia (inability to sit still, no pattern to movements), tardive dyskinesia (bizarre movements of jaw, mouth, tongue, extremities), pseudoparkinsonism (rigidity, tremors, pill rolling, shuffling gait)
• For neuroleptic malignant syndrome: muscle rigidity, altered mental status, hyperthermia, increased CPK
• Skin turgor daily
• Constipation, urinary retention daily; if these occur increase bulk and water in diet

Administer:
• Reduced dose in elderly
• IV undiluted; give at 25 mg/min or less over 1 min; may dilute 25-60 mg/9 ml NaCl for inj
• Antiparkinsonian agent, after securing order from physician to be used if EPS occur
• Syrup mixed in citrus- or chocolate-flavored drinks
• IM injection into large muscle mass

Perform/provide:
• Decreased noise input by dimming lights, avoiding loud noises
• Supervised ambulation until stabilized on medication; do not involve in strenuous exercise program because fainting is possible; patient should not stand still for long periods
• Increased fluids to prevent constipation
• Sips of water, candy, gum for dry mouth
• Storage in tight, light-resistant container; avoid contact with hands

Evaluate:
• Therapeutic response: decrease in emotional excitement, hallucinations, delusions, paranoia; reorganization of patterns of thought, speech

Teach patient/family:
• That orthostatic hypotension occurs frequently and to rise from sitting or lying position gradually, to avoid hazardous activities until stabilized on medication
• To remain lying down for at least 30 min after IM injection
• To avoid hot tubs, hot showers, tub baths, since hypotension may occur
• To avoid abrupt withdrawal of this drug, or extrapyramidal symptoms may result; drugs should be withdrawn slowly
• To avoid OTC preparations (cough, hay fever, cold) unless approved by physician, since serious drug interactions may occur; avoid use with alcohol, CNS depressants; increased drowsiness may occur
• To use a sunscreen during sun exposure to prevent burns

P

italics = common side effects   ***bold italic*** = life threatening reactions

• Regarding compliance with drug regimen
• About extrapyramidal symptoms and necessity for meticulous oral hygiene, since oral candidiasis may occur
• To report sore throat, malaise, fever, bleeding, mouth sores; if these occur, CBC should be drawn and drug discontinued
• That in hot weather, heat stroke may occur; take extra precautions to stay cool

Treatment of overdose: Lavage if orally ingested; provide an airway; *do not induce vomiting*

---

promethazine HCl
(proe-meth'a-zeen)

Anergan 25, Anergan 50, Pentazine, Phenameth, Phenazine 25, Phenazine 50, Phenergan, Phenergan Fortis, Phenergan Plain, Phenoject-50, Pro 50, Prometh-50, Promethazine HCl, Prorex 25, Prorex 50, Prothazine, Prothazine Plain, V-Gan 25, V-Gan 50

Func. class.: Antihistamine, H_1-receptor antagonist
Chem. class.: Phenothiazine derivative

Action: Acts on blood vessels, GI, respiratory system by competing with histamine for H_1-receptor site; decreases allergic response by blocking histamine

Uses: Motion sickness, rhinitis, allergy symptoms, sedation, nausea, preoperative and postoperative sedation

Dosage and routes:
Nausea
• *Adult:* PO/IM 25 mg; may repeat 12.5-25 mg q4-6h
• *Child:* PO/IM 0.5 mg/lb q4-6h

Motion sickness
• *Adult:* PO 25 mg bid
• *Child:* PO/IM/REC 12.5-25 mg bid

Allergy/rhinitis
• *Adult:* PO 12.5 mg qid, or 25 mg hs
• *Child:* PO 6.25-12.5 mg tid or 25 mg hs

Sedation
• *Adult:* PO/IM 25-50 mg hs
• *Child:* PO/IM/REC 12.5-25 mg hs

Sedation (preoperative/postoperative)
• *Adult:* PO/IM/IV 25-50 mg
• *Child:* PO/IM/IV 12.5-25 mg

Available forms: Tabs 12.5, 25, 50 mg; syr 6.25, 25 mg/5 ml; supp 12.5, 25, 50 mg; inj 25, 50 mg/ml

Side effects/adverse reactions:
CNS: Dizziness, drowsiness, poor coordination, fatigue, anxiety, euphoria, confusion, paresthesia, neuritis
CV: Hypotension, palpitations, tachycardia
RESP: Increased thick secretions, wheezing, chest tightness
HEMA: Thrombocytopenia, agranulocytosis, hemolytic anemia
GI: Constipation, dry mouth, nausea, vomiting, anorexia, diarrhea
INTEG: Rash, urticaria, photosensitivity
GU: Retention, dysuria, frequency
EENT: Blurred vision, dilated pupils, tinnitus, nasal stuffiness, dry nose, throat, mouth, photosensitivity

Contraindications: Hypersensitivity to H_1-receptor antagonist, acute asthma attack, lower respiratory tract disease

Precautions: Increased intraocular pressure, renal disease, cardiac disease, hypertension, bronchial asthma, seizure disorder, stenosed

---

peptic ulcers, hyperthyroidism, prostatic hypertrophy, bladder neck obstruction, pregnancy (C)

Pharmacokinetics:

PO: Onset 20 min, duration 4-6 hr; metabolized in liver; excreted by kidneys, GI tract (inactive metabolites)

Interactions/incompatibilities:

• Increased CNS depression: barbiturates, narcotics, hypnotics, tricyclic antidepressants, alcohol

• Decreased effect of: oral anticoagulants, heparin

• Increased effect of promethazine: MAOIs

• Incompatible with aminophylline, calcium gluconate, carbenicillin, chloramphenicol, chlordiazepoxide, chlorothiazide, codeine, dextran, dimenhydrinate, heparin, hydrocortisone, methicillin, methohexital, methylprednisolone, morphine, penicillin G, pentobarbital, phenobarbital, phenytoin, secobarbital, thiopental, Vit B with C

Lab test interferences:

False negative: Skin allergy test

False positive: Urine pregnancy test

NURSING CONSIDERATIONS
Assess:

• I&O ratio; be alert for urinary retention, frequency, dysuria; drug should be discontinued if these occur

• CBC during long-term therapy; blood dyscrasias

• Respiratory status: rate, rhythm, increase in bronchial secretions, wheezing, chest tightness

• Cardiac status: palpitations, increased pulse, hypotension

Administer:

• IV after diluting each 25-50 mg/9 ml of NaCl for inj; give 25 mg or less/2 min

• With meals if GI symptoms occur; absorption may slightly decrease

• Deep IM in large muscle; rotate site

• When used for motion sickness, 30 min before travel

Perform/provide:

• Hard candy, gum, frequent rinsing of mouth for dryness

• Storage in tight, light-resistant container

Evaluate:

• Therapeutic response: absence of running, congested nose, rashes, absence of motion sickness, nausea; sedation

Teach patient/family:

• That drug may cause photosensitivity; to avoid prolonged sunlight

• To notify physician if confusion, sedation, hypotension occurs

• To avoid driving, other hazardous activity if drowsiness occurs

• To avoid concurrent use of alcohol, other CNS depressants

Treatment of overdose: Administer ipecac syrup or lavage, diazepam, vasopressors, barbiturates (short-acting)

P

---

propafenone
(proe-pa-fen'one)
Rythmol
Func. class.: Antidysrhythmic, (Class IC)

Action: Slows conduction velocity; reduces membrane responsiveness; inhibits automaticity; increases ratio of effective refractory period to action potential duration; β-blocking activity

Uses: Life-threatening dysrhythmias, sustained ventricular tachycardia

italics = common side effects   ***bold italic*** = life threatening reactions

Dosage and routes:
• *Adult:* PO 300-900 mg/day in divided doses, 150 mg q8h; allow a 3-4 day interval before increasing dose

Available forms: Tabs 150, 300 mg

Side effects/adverse reactions:

INTEG: Rash

CV: Dysrhythmias, palpitations, AV block, intraventricular conduction delay, AV dissociation, CHF, **sudden death,** atrial flutter

HEMA: **Leukopenia, agranulocytosis, granulocytopenia, thrombocytopenia,** anemia

CNS: Headache, dizziness, abnormal dreams, syncope, confusion, **seizures**

GI: Nausea, vomiting, constipation, dyspepsia, cholestasis, **hepatitis,** abnormal liver function studies, dry mouth

RESP: Dyspnea

EENT: Blurred vision, altered taste, tinnitus

Contraindications: 2nd or 3rd degree AV block, right bundle branch block, cardiogenic shock, hypersensitivity, bradycardia, uncontrolled CHF, sick-sinus node syndrome, marked hypotension, bronchospastic disorders

Precautions: CHF, hypokalemia, hyperkalemia, recent MI, nonallergic branchospasm, pregnancy (C), lactation, children, hepatic or renal disease

Pharmacokinetics:
Peak 3-5 hr, half-life 2-10 hr; metabolized in liver; excreted in urine (metabolite)

Interactions/incompatibilities:
• Increased effect of propafenone: cimetidine, quinidine
• Increased anticoagulation: warfarin
• Increased digoxin level: digoxin
• Increased β-blocker effect: propranolol, metoprolol

Lab test interferences:
Increase: CPK

NURSING CONSIDERATIONS
Assess:
• GI status: bowel pattern, number of stools
• Cardiac status: rate, rhythm, quality
• Chest x-ray film, pulmonary function test during treatment
• I&O ratio; check for decreasing output
• B/P for fluctuations
• Lung fields; bilateral rales may occur in CHF patient
• Increased respiration, increased pulse; drug should be discontinued
• Toxicity: fine tremors, dizziness
• Cardiac rate: respiration, rate, rhythm, character continuously

Evaluate:
• Therapeutic response: absence of dysrhythmias

Treatment of overdose: O₂, artificial ventilation, ECG; administer dopamine for circulatory depression, diazepam or thiopental for convulsions

---

propantheline bromide
(proe-pan'the-leen)
Banlin,* Pro-Banthine, Propanthel, Propantheline Bromide

Func. class.: GI anticholinergic
Chem. class.: Synthetic quaternary ammonium compound

Action: Inhibits muscarinic actions of acetylcholine at postganglionic parasympathetic neuroeffector sites

Uses: Treatment of peptic ulcer disease, irritable bowel syndrome, duodenography, urinary incontinence

Dosage and routes:
• *Adult:* PO 15 mg tid ac, 30 mg hs
• *Elderly:* PO 7.5 mg tid ac
Available forms: Tabs 7.5, 15 mg
Side effects/adverse reactions:
CNS: Confusion, stimulation in elderly, headache, insomnia, dizziness, drowsiness, anxiety, weakness, hallucinations
*GI: Dry mouth, constipation, **paralytic ileus,*** heartburn, nausea, vomiting, dysphagia, absence of taste
GU: Hesitancy, retention, impotence
CV: Palpitations, tachycardia
EENT: Blurred vision, photophobia, mydriasis, cycloplegia, increased ocular tension
INTEG: Urticaria, rash, pruritus, anhidrosis, fever, allergic reactions
Contraindications: Hypersensitivity to anticholinergics, narrow-angle glaucoma, GI obstruction, myasthenia gravis, paralytic ileus, GI atony, toxic megacolon
Precautions: Hyperthyroidism, coronary artery disease, dysrhythmias, CHF, ulcerative colitis, hypertension, hiatal hernia, hepatic disease, renal disease, pregnancy (C), urinary retention, prostatic hypertrophy
Pharmacokinetics:
PO: Onset 30-45 min, duration 6 hr; metabolized by liver, GI system, excreted in urine, bile
Interactions/incompatibilities:
• Increased anticholinergic effect: amantadine, tricyclic antidepressants, MAOIs, H₁ antihistamines
• Decreased effect of: phenothiazines, levodopa, ketoconazole
NURSING CONSIDERATIONS
Assess:
• VS, cardiac status: checking for

dysrhythmias, increased rate, palpitations
• I&O ratio; check for urinary retention or hesitancy
• GI complaints: pain, bleeding (frank or occult), nausea, vomiting, anorexia
Administer:
• ½-1 hr ac for better absorption
• Decreased dose to elderly patients; metabolism may be slowed
• Gum, hard candy, frequent rinsing of mouth for dryness of oral cavity
Perform/provide:
• Storage in tight container protected from light
• Increased fluids, bulk, exercise to patient's life-style to decrease constipation
Evaluate:
• Therapeutic response: absence of epigastric pain, bleeding, nausea, vomiting
Teach patient/family:
• To avoid driving, other hazardous activities until stabilized on medication; may cause blurred vision
• To avoid alcohol, other CNS depressants; will enhance sedating properties of this drug
• To drink plenty of fluids
• To report dysphagia

P

propofol
(proe-po'foel)
Diprivan
Func. class.: General anesthetic

Controlled Substance Schedule II
Action: Produces dose-dependent CNS depression
Uses: Induction or maintenance of anesthesia as part of balanced anesthetic technique

italics = common side effects   ***bold italic*** = life threatening reactions

Dosage and routes:
Induction
• *Adult:* IV 2-2.5 mg/kg, approximately 40 mg q10sec until induction onset
• *Elderly:* 1-1.5 mg/kg, approximately 20 mg q10sec until induction onset
Maintenance
• *Adult:* 0.1-0.2 mg/kg/min (6-12 mg/kg/hr)
• *Elderly:* 0.05-0.1 mg/kg/min (3-6 mg/kg/hr)
Intermittent bolus
• *Adult:* Increments of 25-50 mg as needed
Available forms: Inj 10 mg/ml in 20 ml amp
Side effects/adverse reactions:
CNS: Movement, headache, jerking, fever, dizziness, shivering, tremor, confusion, somnolence, paresthesia, agitation, abnormal dreams, euphoria, fatigue
GI: Nausea, vomiting, abdominal cramping, dry mouth, swallowing, hypersalivation
MS: Myalgia
GU: Urine retention, green urine
EENT: Blurred vision, tinnitus, eye pain, strange taste
CV: Bradycardia, hypotension, hypertension, PVC, PAC, tachycardia, abnormal ECG, ST segment depression, *asystole*
RESP: Apnea, cough, hiccups, dyspnea, hypoventilation, sneezing, wheezing, tachypnea, hypoxia
INTEG: Flushing, phlebitis, hives, burning/stinging at injection site
Contraindications: Hypersensitivity, hyperlipidemia
Precautions: Elderly, respiratory depression, severe respiratory disorders, cardiac dysrhythmias, pregnancy (B), labor and delivery, lactation, children

Pharmacokinetics:
Onset 40 sec, rapid distribution, half-life 1-8 min, terminal elimination half-life 5-10 hr; 70% excreted in urine; metabolized in liver by conjugation to inactivate metabolites
Interactions/incompatibilities:
• Increased CNS depression: alcohol, narcotics, sedative/hypnotics, antipsychotics, skeletal muscle relaxants, inhalational anesthetics
NURSING CONSIDERATIONS
Assess:
• Injection site: phlebitis, burning/stinging
• ECG for changes: PVC, PAC, ST segment changes
• CNS changes: movement, jerking, tremors, dizziness, LOC, pupil reaction
• Allergic reactions: hives
• Respiratory dysfunction: respiratory depression, character, rate, rhythm; notify physician if respirations are <10/min
Administer:
• After diluting with D$_5$W mixed in lipid base; use only glass containers when mixing, not stable in plastic
• By IV infusion only
• Alone; do not mix with other agents before using
• Only with resuscitative equipment available
• Only by qualified persons trained in anesthesia
Perform/provide:
• Storage in light-resistant area at room temperature
• Coughing, turning, deep breathing for postoperative patients
• Safety measures: side rails, nightlight, call bell within reach
Evaluate:
• Therapeutic response: induction of anesthesia
Treatment of overdose: Discon-

---

* Available in Canada only

tinue drug; administer vasopressor agents or anticholinergics, artificial ventilation

propoxyphene HCl/ propoxyphene napsylate

(proe-pox'i-feen)
Darvon Pulvules, Dolene, Propoxyphene HCl

Func. class.: Narcotic analgesics
Chem. class.: Synthetic opiate

Controlled Substance Schedule IV

Action: Depresses pain impulse transmission at the spinal cord level by interacting with opioid receptors

Uses: Mild to moderate pain

Dosage and routes:

• *Adult:* PO 65 mg q4h prn (HCl)
• *Adult:* PO 100 mg q4h prn (napsylate)

Available forms: HCl: tabs 32, 65 mg; napsylate: tabs 100 mg; susp 10 mg/ml

Side effects/adverse reactions:

CNS: Drowsiness, dizziness, confusion, headache, sedation, euphoria, **convulsions, hyperthermia**
GI: Nausea, vomiting, anorexia, constipation, cramps
GU: Urinary retention, dysuria
INTEG: Rash, urticaria, bruising, flushing, diaphoresis, pruritus
EENT: Tinnitus, blurred vision, miosis, diplopia
CV: Palpitations, bradycardia, change in B/P, **dysrhythmias**
*RESP: **Respiratory depression***

Contraindications: Hypersensitivity to ASA products (some preparations), addiction (narcotic)

Precautions: Addictive personality, pregnancy (C), lactation, increased intracranial pressure, MI

(acute), severe heart [...] spiratory depression, h[...] ease, renal disease, child <[...]

Pharmacokinetics:

PO: Onset 15-30 min, peak 2-3 hr, duration 4-6 hr
REC: Onset slow; duration 4-6 hr
Metabolized by liver, excreted by kidneys (as metabolites), crosses placenta, excreted in breast milk, half-life 12 hr (metabolites)

Interactions/incompatibilities:

• Increased effects with other CNS depressants: alcohol, narcotics, sedative/hypnotics, antipsychotics, skeletal muscle relaxants

Lab test interferences:

Increase: Amylase

NURSING CONSIDERATIONS
Assess:

• I&O ratio; check for decreasing output; may indicate urinary retention
• CNS changes: dizziness, drowsiness, hallucinations, euphoria, LOC, pupil reaction
• Allergic reactions: rash, urticaria
• Respiratory dysfunction: respiratory depression, character, rate, rhythm; notify physician if respirations are <10/min
• Need for pain medication; physical dependence

Administer:

• With antiemetic if nausea, vomiting occur
• When pain is beginning to return; determine dosage interval by patient response

Perform/provide:

• Storage in light-resistant area at room temperature
• Assistance with ambulation
• Safety measures: side rails, nightlight, call bell within easy reach

Evaluate:

• Therapeutic response: decrease in pain

---

italics = common side effects   ***bold italic*** = life threatening reactions

...of CNS

...icy may ...nded pe-

...toms may occur: nau... ...ng, cramps, fever, faintness, anorexia

Treatment of overdose: Naloxone (Narcan) 0.2-0.8 IV, O_2, IV fluids, vasopressors

---

propranolol HCl

(proe-pran'oh-lole)

Betachron, Inderal, Inderal LA, Inderal 10, Inderal 20, Inderal 40, Inderal 60, Inderal 80, Ipran, Propranolol HCl, Propranolol Intensol

Func. class.: Antihypertensive, antianginal

Chem. class.: β-Adrenergic blocker

Action: Nonselective β-blocker with negative inotropic, chronotropic, dromotropic properties

Uses: Chronic stable angina pectoris, hypertension, supraventricular dysrhythmias, migraine, prophylaxis, MI, pheochromocytoma, essential tremor, tetralogy of Fallot, cyanotic spells

Dosage and routes:

Dysrhythmias

• *Adult:* PO 10-30 mg tid-qid; IV BOL 0.5-3 mg over 1 mg/min; may repeat in 2 min

Hypertension

• *Adult:* PO 40 mg bid or 80 mg qd (sus rel) initially; usual dose 120-240 mg/day bid-tid or 120-160 mg qd (sus rel)

Angina

• *Adult:* PO 80-320 mg in divided doses bid-qid or 80 mg qd (sus rel); usual dose 160 mg qd (sus rel)

MI

• *Adult:* PO 180-240 mg/day tid-qid

Pheochromocytoma

• *Adult:* PO 60 mg/day × 3 days preoperatively in divided doses or 30 mg/day in divided doses (inoperable tumor)

Migraine

• *Adult:* PO 80 mg/day (sus rel) or in divided doses; may increase to 160-240 mg/day in divided doses

Essential tremor

• *Adult:* PO 40 mg bid; usual dose 120 mg/day

Available forms: Caps ext rel 80, 120, 160 mg; tabs 10, 20, 40, 60, 80, 90 mg; inj 1 mg/ml, oral sol 4 mg, 8 mg/ml, conc oral sol 80 mg/ml, ext rel cap 60 mg

Side effects/adverse reactions:

RESP: Dyspnea, respiratory dysfunction, *bronchospasm*

CV: Bradycardia, hypotension, CHF, palpitations, AV block, peripheral vascular insufficiency, vasodilation

HEMA: Agranulocytosis, thrombocytopenia

GI: Nausea, vomiting, diarrhea, colitis, constipation, cramps, dry mouth, hepatomegaly, gastric pain, acute pancreatitis

GU: Impotence, decreased libido, urinary tract infections

MS: Joint pain, arthralgia, muscle cramps, pain

MISC: Facial swelling, weight change, Raynaud's phenomenon

INTEG: Rash, pruritus, fever

CNS: Depression, hallucinations, dizziness, fatigue, lethargy, paresthesias, bizarre dreams, disorientation

EENT: Sore throat, *laryngospasm,* blurred vision, dry eyes

---

*Available in Canada only

META: Hyperglycemia, hypoglycemia

Contraindications: Hypersensitivity to this drug, cardiac failure, cardiogenic shock, 2nd or 3rd degree heart block, bronchospastic disease, sinus bradycardia, CHF

Precautions: Diabetes mellitus, pregnancy (C), renal disease, lactation, hyperthyroidism, COPD, hepatic disease, children, myasthenia gravis, peripheral vascular disease, hypotension, CHF

Pharmacokinetics:

PO: Onset 30 min, peak 1-1½ hr
IV: Onset 2 min, peak 15 min, duration 3-6 hr; immediate rel half-life 3-5 hr; sus rel half-life 8-11 hr; metabolized by liver; crosses placenta, blood-brain barrier; excreted in breast milk

Interactions/incompatibilities:

• AV block: digitalis, calcium channel blockers
• Increased negative inotropic effects: verapamil, disopyramide
• Increased effects of: reserpine, digitalis, neuromuscular blocking agents
• Decreased β-blocking effects: norepinephrine, isoproterenol, barbiturates, rifampin, dopamine, dobutamine, smoking
• Increased β-blocking effect: cimetidine
• Increased hypotension: quinidine, haloperidol, hydralazine
• Incompatible with any drug in sol or syringe

Lab test interferences:

Increase: Serum K, serum uric acid, ALT/AST, alk phosphatase, LDH

Decrease: Blood glucose

NURSING CONSIDERATIONS
Assess:

• B/P, pulse, respirations during beginning therapy
• Weight qd, report gain of 5 lb
• I&O ratio, CrCl if kidney damage is diagnosed
• ECG if using as antidysrhythmic
• Hepatic enzymes: AST, ALT, bilirubin
• Pain: duration, time started, activity being performed, character
• Tolerance if taken over long period of time
• Headache, light-headedness, decreased B/P; may indicate a need for decreased dosage

Administer:

• Do not give with aluminum-containing antacid; may decrease GI absorption
• IV undiluted or diluted 10 ml D₅W for inj; give 1 mg or less/min; may be diluted in 50 ml NaCl and run 1 mg over 10-15 min
• With 8 oz of water on empty stomach

Perform/provide:

• Protection from light (injection)

Evaluate:

• Therapeutic response: decreased B/P, dysrhythmias

Teach patient/family:

• Not to discontinue abruptly, to take drug at same time each day
• To avoid OTC drugs unless approved by physician
• To avoid hazardous activities if dizziness occurs
• Stress importance of compliance with complete medical regimen
• To make position changes slowly to prevent fainting
• To decrease dosage over 2 weeks to prevent cardiac damage

P

---

italics = common side effects   ***bold italic*** = life threatening reactions

propylthiouracil (PTU)
(proe-pill-thye-oh-yoor′a-sill)
Propylthiouracil, Propyl-Thyra-cil*

Func. class.: Thyroid hormone antagonist
Chem. class.: Thioamide

Action: Blocks synthesis peripherally of T₃, T₄ (triiodothyronine, thyroxine), inhibits organification of iodine

Uses: Preparation for thyroidectomy, thyrotoxic crisis, hyperthyroidism, thyroid storm

Dosage and routes:
Thyrotoxic crisis
• *Adult and child:* PO same as hyperthyroidism with iodine and propranolol

Preparation for thyroidectomy
• *Adult:* 600-1200 mg/day
• *Child:* 10 mg/kg/day in divided doses

Hyperthyroidism
• *Adult:* PO 100 mg tid increasing to 300 mg q8h if condition is severe; continue to euthyroid state, then 100 mg qd-tid
• *Child >10 yr:* PO 100 mg tid; continue to euthyroid state, then 25 mg tid to 100 mg bid
• *Child 6-10 yr:* PO 50-150 mg in divided doses q8h

Available forms: Tabs 50 mg

Side effects/adverse reactions:
INTEG: Rash, urticaria, pruritus, alopecia, hyperpigmentation, lupuslike syndrome
GU: Nephritis
CNS: Drowsiness, headache, vertigo, fever, paresthesias, neuritis
*HEMA: **Agranulocytosis, leukopenia, thrombocytopenia, hypothrombinemia, lymphadenopathy,*** bleeding, vasculitis, periarteritis

*GI: Nausea, diarrhea, vomiting, **jaundice, hepatitis,*** loss of taste
MS: Myalgia, arthralgia, nocturnal muscle cramps

Contraindications: Hypersensitivity, pregnancy (D), lactation

Precautions: Infection, bone marrow depression, hepatic disease

Pharmacokinetics:
PO: Onset 30-40 min, duration 2-4 hr, half-life 1-2 hr; excreted in urine, bile, breast milk; crosses placenta

Interactions/incompatibilities:
• Increased anticoagulant effect: heparin, oral anticoagulants

Lab test interferences:
Increases: Pro-time, AST/ALT, alk phosphatase

NURSING CONSIDERATIONS
Assess:
• Pulse, B/P, temperature
• I&O ratio; check for edema: puffy hands, feet, periorbits; indicates hypothyroidism
• Weight qd; same clothing, scale, time of day
• T₃, T₄, which are increased; serum TSH, which is decreased; free thyroxine index, which is increased if dosage is too low; discontinue drug 3-4 wk before RAIU
• Blood work: CBC for blood dyscrasias: leukopenia, thrombocytopenia, agranulocytosis; LFTs
• Overdose: peripheral edema, heat intolerance, diaphoresis, palpitations, dysrhythmias, severe tachycardia, increased temperature delirium, CNS irritability
• Hypersensitivity: rash, enlarged cervical lymph nodes; drug may have to be discontinued
• Hypoprothrombinemia: bleeding, petechiae, ecchymosis
• Clinical response: after 3 wk should include increased weight, pulse; decreased T₄

- Bone marrow depression: sore throat, fever, fatigue

Administer:
- With meals to decrease GI upset
- At same time each day to maintain drug level
- Lowest dose that relieves symptoms

Perform/provide:
- Storage in light-resistant container
- Fluids to 3-4 L/day, unless contraindicated

Evaluate:
- Therapeutic response: weight gain, decreased pulse, decreased T_4, decreased B/P

Teach patient/family:
- To abstain from breast-feeding after delivery
- To take pulse daily
- To report redness, swelling, sore throat, mouth lesions, which indicate blood dyscrasias
- To keep graph of weight, pulse, mood
- To avoid OTC products that contain iodine
- That seafood, other iodine products may be restricted
- Not to discontinue this medication abruptly; thyroid crisis may occur; stress patient response
- That response may take several months if thyroid is large
- Symptoms/signs of overdose: periorbital edema, cold intolerance, mental depression
- Symptoms of inadequate dose: tachycardia, diarrhea, fever, irritability

protamine sulfate
(proe'ta-meen)
Func. class.: Heparin antagonist
Chem. class.: Low-molecular-weight protein

Action: Binds heparin, making it ineffective

Uses: Heparin overdose

Dosage and routes:
- *Adult:* IV 1 mg of protamine/90-115 U heparin given; administer slowly 1-3 min; give undiluted to 1%, not to exceed 50 mg/10 min

Available forms: Inj IV 10 mg/ml

Side effects/adverse reactions:
CV: Hypotension, bradycardia, ***circulatory collapse***
GI: Nausea, vomiting, anorexia
INTEG: *Rash,* dermatitis, urticaria
CNS: Lassitude
HEMA: Bleeding, ***anaphylaxis***
RESP: Dyspnea, pulmonary edema, severe respiratory distress

Contraindications: Hypersensitivity

Precautions: Pregnancy (C), lactation, children, allergy to fish

Pharmacokinetics:
IV: Onset 5 min, duration 2 hr

Interactions/incompatibilities:
- Considered incompatible with any drug in sol or syringe

NURSING CONSIDERATIONS
Assess:
- Blood studies (Hct, platelets, occult blood in stools) q3mo
- Coagulation tests (APTT, ACT) 15 min after dose, then in several hours
- VS, B/P, pulse of 30 min; plus 3 hr after dose
- Skin rash, urticaria, dermatitis
- Allergy to fish; use with caution in these patients

---

italics = common side effects   ***bold italic*** = life threatening reactions

Administer:
• IV after diluting 50 mg/5 ml sterile bacteriostatic H_2O for inj; shake, give 20 mg or less over 1-3 min; may further dilute with equal volume of NaCl or D_5W and run over 2-3 hr; titrate to APTT, ACT; use infusion pump
Perform/provide:
• Storage at 36°-46° F (2°-8° C)
Evaluate:
• Therapeutic response: reversal of heparin overdose

---

protriptyline HCl
(proe-trip′te-leen)
Triptil*, Vivactil
Func. class.: Tricyclic antidepressant
Chem. class.: Dibenzocycloheptene—secondary amine

Action: Blocks reuptake of norepinephrine, serotonin into nerve endings, increasing action of norepinephrine, serotonin in nerve cells
Uses: Depression
Dosage and routes:
• *Adult:* PO 15-40 mg/day in divided doses; may increase to 60 mg/day
Available forms: Tabs 5, 10 mg
Side effects/adverse reactions:
HEMA: Agranulocytosis, thrombocytopenia, eosinophilia, leukopenia
CNS: Dizziness, drowsiness, confusion, headache, anxiety, tremors, stimulation, weakness, insomnia, nightmares, EPS (elderly), increased psychiatric symptoms, paresthesia, seizures
GI: Diarrhea, dry mouth, nausea, vomiting, *paralytic ileus,* increased appetite, cramps, epigas-

tric distress, jaundice, *hepatitis,* stomatitis, constipation
GU: Retention, acute renal failure
INTEG: Rash, urticaria, sweating, pruritus, photosensitivity
CV: Orthostatic hypotension, ECG changes, tachycardia, *hypertension,* palpitations
EENT: Blurred vision, tinnitus, mydriasis
Contraindications: Hypersensitivity to tricyclic antidepressants, recovery phase of myocardial infarction, convulsive disorders, prostatic hypertrophy
Precautions: Suicidal patients, severe depression, increased intraocular pressure, narrow-angle glaucoma, urinary retention, cardiac disease, hepatic disease, hyperthyroidism, electroshock therapy, elective surgery, pregnancy (C)
Pharmacokinetics:
PO: Onset 15-30 min, peak 24-30 hr, duration 4-6 hr; therapeutic effect 2-3 wk; metabolized by liver, excreted by kidneys, crosses placenta, half-life 54-98 hr
Interactions/incompatibilities:
• Decreased effects of: guanethidine, clonidine, indirect-acting sympathomimetics (ephedrine)
• Increased effects of: direct-acting sympathomimetics (epinephrine), alcohol, barbiturates, benzodiazepines, CNS depressants
• Hyperpyretic crisis, convulsions, hypertensive episode: MAOI (pargyline [Eutonyl])
Lab test interferences:
Increase: Serum bilirubin, blood glucose, alk phosphatase
False increase: Urinary catecholamines
Decrease: VMA, 5-HIAA
NURSING CONSIDERATIONS
Assess:
• B/P (lying, standing), pulse q4h;

if systolic B/P drops 20 mm Hg, hold drug, notify physician; take vital signs q4h in patients with cardiovascular disease
• Blood studies: CBC, leukocytes, differential, cardiac enzymes if patient is receiving long-term therapy
• Hepatic studies: AST, ALT, bilirubin
• Weight qwk; appetite may increase with drug
• ECG for flattening of T wave, bundle branch block, AV block, dysrhythmias in cardiac patients
• EPS primarily in elderly: rigidity, dystonia, akathisia
• Mental status changes: mood, sensorium, affect, suicidal tendencies, increase in psychiatric symptoms: depression, panic
• Urinary retention, constipation; constipation is more likely to occur in children
• Withdrawal symptoms: headache, nausea, vomiting, muscle pain, weakness; do not usually occur unless drug was discontinued abruptly
• Alcohol consumption; if alcohol is consumed, hold dose until morning

Administer:
• Increased fluids, bulk in diet if constipation occurs
• With food or milk for GI symptoms
• Dosage hs if oversedation occurs during day; may take entire dose hs; elderly may not tolerate once/day dosing
• Gum, hard candy, or frequent sips of water for dry mouth

Perform/provide:
• Storage in tight, light-resistant container at room temperature
• Assistance with ambulation during beginning therapy, since drowsiness/dizziness occurs
• Safety measures including side rails, primarily in elderly
• Checking to see PO medication swallowed

Evaluate:
• Therapeutic response: decreased depression

Teach patient/family:
• That therapeutic effects may take 2-3 wk
• To use caution in driving, other activities requiring alertness because of drowsiness, dizziness, blurred vision
• To avoid alcohol ingestion, other CNS depressants
• Not to discontinue medication quickly after long-term use; may cause nausea, headache, malaise
• To wear sunscreen or large hat, since photosensitivity occurs

Treatment of overdose: ECG monitoring; induce emesis; lavage, activated charcoal; administer anticonvulsant

---

pseudoephedrine HCl/pseudoephedrine sulfate

(soo-doe-e-fed'rin)

Afrinol Repetabs, Allerid, Cenafed, Cenafed Syrup, Children's Sudafed, Decofed Syrup, DeFed-60, Dorcol Children's Decongestant, Drixoral Non-Drowsy Formula, Eltor,* Efidac/24, Genaphed, Halofed, Myfedrine, Novafed, Pedia Care Infant's Decongestant, Pseudoephedrine HCl, Pseudogest Decongestant, Pseudo Syrup, Sinustat, Sudafed, Sudafed 12 hour, Sudrin

Func. class.: Adrenergic
Chem. class.: Substituted phenylethylamine

Action: Primary activity through

α-effects on respiratory mucosal membranes reducing congestion hyperemia, edema; minimal bronchodilation secondary to β-effects

Uses: Nasal decongestant

Dosage and routes:
• *Adult:* PO 60 mg q6h; EXT REL 60-120 mg q12h or q24h
• *Child 6-12 yr:* PO 30 mg q6h, not to exceed 120 mg/day
• *Child 2-6 yr:* PO 15 mg q6h, not to exceed 60 mg/day

Available forms: Caps ext rel 120 mg; sol 15 mg, 30 mg/5 ml, 7.5 mg/0.8 ml; tabs 30, 60, 120 mg

Side effects/adverse reactions:
CNS: Tremors, anxiety, insomnia, headache, dizziness, anxiety, hallucinations, *seizures*
EENT: Dry nose, irritation of nose and throat
CV: Palpitations, tachycardia, hypertension, chest pain, *dysrhythmias*
GI: Anorexia, nausea, vomiting, dry mouth
GU: Dysuria

Contraindications: Hypersensitivity to sympathomimetics, narrow-angle glaucoma

Precautions: Pregnancy (C), cardiac disorders, hyperthyroidism, diabetes mellitus, prostatic hypertrophy

Pharmacokinetics:
PO: Onset 15-30 min, duration 4-6 hr, 8-12 hr (extended release); metabolized in liver, excreted in feces and breast milk

Interactions/incompatibilities:
• Do not use with MAOIs or tricyclic antidepressants; hypertensive crisis may occur
• Decreased effect of this drug: methyldopa, urinary acidifiers, rauwolfia alkaloids
• Increased effect of this drug: urinary alkalizers

NURSING CONSIDERATIONS
Perform/provide:
• Storage at room temperature
Evaluate:
• Therapeutic response: Decreased nasal congestion
Teach patient/family:
• Reason for drug administration
• Not to use continuously, or more than recommended dose, or rebound congestion may occur
• To check with physician before using other drugs, as drug interactions may occur
• To avoid taking near hs; stimulation can occur
• Not to use if stimulation, restlessness, or tremors occur

---

psyllium
(sill'i-um)
Effer-Syllium, Fiberall, Fiberall Natural Flavor and Orange Flavor, Hydrocil Instant Powder, Konsyl, Konsyl-D, Metamucil, Metamucil Instant Mix Lemon Lime, Metamucil Instant Mix Orange, Metamucil Orange Flavor, Metamucil Sugar Free, Metamucil Sugar Free Orange Flavor, Modane Bulk, Natural Vegetable Reguloid, Perdiem, Pro-Lax, Prodiem Plain,* Reguloid Natural, Reguloid Orange, Reguloid Sugar Free Orange, Reguloid Sugar Free Regular, Serutan, Siblin, Syllact, V-Lax

Func. class.: Bulk laxative
Chem. class.: Psyllium colloid

Action: Bulk-forming laxative
Uses: Chronic constipation, ulcerative colitis, irritable bowel syndrome
Dosage and routes:
• *Adult:* PO 1-2 tsp in 8 oz H₂O bid

or tid, then 8 oz H$_2$O or 1 premeasured packet in 8 oz H$_2$O bid or tid, then 8 oz H$_2$O

• *Child >6 yr:* 1 tsp in 4 oz H$_2$O hs

Available forms: Chew pieces 1.7 g/piece; pdr 309, 390, 430, 450, 486, 500, 600, 630, 654, 672, 791, 919, 950 mg/g, 1 g/g

Side effects/adverse reactions:

GI: Nausea, vomiting, anorexia, diarrhea, cramps

Contraindications: Hypersensitivity, intestinal obstruction, abdominal pain, nausea/vomiting, fecal impaction

Precautions: Pregnancy (C)

Pharmacokinetics: Excreted in feces, not absorbed in GI tract

NURSING CONSIDERATIONS

Assess:

• Blood, urine electrolytes if used often by patient

• I&O ratio to identify fluid loss

• Cause of constipation; identify whether fluids, bulk, or exercise is missing from life-style

• Cramping, rectal bleeding, nausea, vomiting; if these symptoms occur, drug should be discontinued

Administer:

• Alone for better absorption

• In morning or evening (oral dose)

• After mixing with H$_2$O immediately before use

• With 8 oz H$_2$O or juice followed by another 8 oz of fluid

Evaluate:

• Therapeutic response: decrease in constipation or decreased diarrhea in colitis

Teach patient/family:

• To maintain adequate fluid consumption

• That normal bowel movements do not always occur daily

• Not to use in presence of abdominal pain, nausea, vomiting

• To notify physician if constipation unrelieved or if symptoms of electrolyte imbalance occur: muscle cramps, pain, weakness, dizziness, excessive thirst

pyrantel pamoate
(pi-ran'tel)
Antiminth, Combantrin,* Pin-X, Reese's Pinworm
Func. class.: Anthelmintic
Chem. class.: Pyrimidine derivative

Action: Causes paralysis in worm by neuroblockade, caused by stimulation of ganglionic receptors; worms are expelled by normal peristalsis

Uses: Pinworms, roundworms

Dosage and routes:

• *Adult and child >2 yr:* PO 11 mg/kg as single dose, not to exceed 1 g; repeat in 2 wk for pinworms

Available forms: Oral susp 250 mg/5 ml

Side effects/adverse reactions:

INTEG: Rash

CNS: Dizziness, headache, drowsiness, insomnia, fever, weakness

GI: Nausea, vomiting, anorexia, diarrhea, distention

Contraindications: Hypersensitivity

Precautions: Seizure disorders, hepatic disease, dehydration, anemia, child <2 yr, pregnancy (C)

Pharmacokinetics:

PO: Peak 1-3 hr; metabolized in liver; excreted in feces, urine (unchanged/metabolites)

Interactions/incompatibilities:

• Antagonizes effect of pyrantel: piperazine

NURSING CONSIDERATIONS

Assess:

• Stools during entire treatment;

P

italics = common side effects   ***bold italic*** = life threatening reactions

specimens must be sent to lab while still warm
• For allergic reaction: rash
• For diarrhea during expulsion of worms

Administer:
• PO after meals to avoid GI symptoms
• After shaking suspension

Perform/provide:
• Storage in tight, light-resistant container in cool environment

Evaluate:
• Therapeutic response: expulsion of worms, 3 negative stool cultures after completion of treatment

Teach patient/family:
• Proper hygiene after BM, including hand washing technique; tell patient to avoid putting fingers in mouth
• That infected person should sleep alone; not to shake bed linen; change bed linen qd, wash in hot water
• To clean toilet qd with disinfectant (green soap solution)
• Need for compliance with dosage schedule, duration of treatment
• To drink fruit juice to help expel worms
• To wear shoes, wash all fruits, vegetables well before eating

---

pyrazinamide

(peer-a-zin'a-mide)
Pyrazinamide, Tebrazid*

Func. class.: Antitubercular agent
Chem. class.: Pyrazinoic acid amine/nicoturimide analog

Action: Bactericidal interference with lipid, nucleic acid biosynthesis

Uses: Tuberculosis, as an adjunct when other drugs are not feasible

Dosage and routes:
• *Adult:* PO 20-35 mg/kg/day in 3-4 divided doses, not to exceed 3 g/day
Available forms: Tabs 500 mg

Side effects/adverse reactions:
INTEG: Photosensitivity, urticaria
CNS: Headache
GI: **Hepatotoxicity,** abnormal liver function tests, peptic ulcer
GU: Urinary difficulty, increased uric acid
HEMA: **Hemolytic anemia**

Contraindications: Hypersensitivity

Precautions: Pregnancy (C), child <13 yr

Pharmacokinetics:
PO: Peak 2 hr, half-life 9-10 hr; metabolized in liver, excreted in urine (metabolites/unchanged drug)

Lab test interferences:
Increase: PBI
Decrease: 17-KS

NURSING CONSIDERATIONS
Assess:
• Signs of anemia: Hct, Hgb, fatigue
• Temperature if <101° F (38° C), drug should be reduced
• Liver studies qwk: ALT, AST, bilirubin
• Renal status before, qmo: BUN, creatinine, output, sp gr, urinalysis
• Hepatic status: decreased appetite, jaundice, dark urine, fatigue

Administer:
• With meals to decrease GI symptoms
• After C&S is completed; qmo to detect resistance

Evaluate:
• Therapeutic response: decreased symptoms of TB, culture negative

Teach patient/family:
• That compliance with dosage schedule, length is necessary

• To avoid alcohol while taking this drug

pyrethrins
(peer'e-thrins)
A-200 Pyrinate, Barc, Pyrinyl, RID, TISIT, Triple X
Func. class.: Pediculocide
Chem. class.: Pyrethrin/piperonyl butoxide/petroleum distillate

Action: Causes paralysis, death of organism by acting as a contact poison

Uses: Head, body, pubic lice; nits; scabies

Dosage and routes:
• *Adult and child:* Apply undiluted to infested area; allow application to remain no longer than 10 min, wash thoroughly with warm water, soap, or shampoo; remove dead lice, eggs with fine-toothed comb; do not exceed 2 consecutive applications within 24 hr; may repeat in 7-10 days
• *Adult and child:* CREAM/LOTION wash area with soap, water; remove visible crusts, apply to skin surfaces, remove with soap, water in 8-12 hr; may reapply in 1 wk if needed; SHAMPOO using 30 ml, work into lather, rub for 5 min, rinse, dry with towel
Available forms: Gel, liq, shampoo, cream, lotion

Side effects/adverse reactions:
INTEG: Irritation, pruritus, urticaria, eczema

Contraindications: Hypersensitivity, inflammation of skin, abrasions, or breaks in skin

Precautions: Child/infant, ragweed sensitivity, pregnancy (C)

NURSING CONSIDERATIONS
Administer:
• To body areas, scalp only; do not apply to face, lips, mouth, eyes, any mucous membrane, anus, or meatus; apply from neck down for body lice
• Topical corticosteroids as ordered to decrease contact dermatitis
• Lotions of menthol or phenol to control itching
• Topical antibiotics for infection

Perform/provide:
• Storage in tight container
• Isolation until areas on skin, scalp have cleared and treatment is complete
• Removal of nits by using a fine-toothed comb rinsed in vinegar after treatment

Evaluate:
• Therapeutic response: decreased nits, crusts

Teach patient/family:
• To discontinue use and notify physician if irritation or infection occurs
• To flush with water in case of contact with eyes
• To wash all inhabitants' clothing, bed linen using insecticide; preventive treatment may be required of all persons living in same house, using lotion or shampoo to decrease spread of infection
• That itching may continue for 4-6 wk
• That drug must be reapplied if accidentally washed off, or treatment will be ineffective
• To use externally only
• To treat sexual partners simultaneously

P

---

italics = common side effects   ***bold italic*** = life threatening reactions

pyridostigmine bromide

(peer-id-oh-stig'meen)
Mestinon, Regonol

Func. class.: Cholinergic
Chem. class.: Tertiary amine carbamate

Action: Inhibits destruction of acetylcholine, which increases concentration at sites where acetylcholine is released; this facilitates transmission of impulses across myoneural junction

Uses: Nondepolarizing muscle relaxant antagonist, myasthenia gravis

Dosage and routes:
Myasthenia gravis
• *Adult:* PO 60-180 mg bid-qid, not to exceed 1.5 g/day; IM/IV ⅓₀ of PO dose, sus rel 180-540 mg qd or bid at intervals of at least 6 hr

Tubocurare antagonist
• *Adult:* 0.6-1.2 mg IV atropine, then 10-30 mg

Available forms: Tabs 60 mg; tabs sus rel 180 mg; syr 60 mg/5 ml; inj IM/IV 5 mg/ml

Side effects/adverse reactions:
INTEG: Rash, urticaria, flushing
CNS: Dizziness, headache, sweating, weakness, *convulsions,* incoordination, paralysis, drowsiness, LOC
GI: Nausea, diarrhea, vomiting, cramps, increased salivary and gastric secretions, peristalsis
CV: Tachycardia, dysrhythmias, bradycardia, AV block, hypotension, ECG changes, *cardiac arrest,* syncope
GU: Frequency, incontinence, urgency
RESP: Respiratory depression, bronchospasm, constriction, laryngospasm, respiratory arrest

EENT: Miosis, blurred vision, lacrimation, visual changes

Contraindications: Bradycardia; hypotension; obstruction of intestine, renal system; bromide sensitivity

Precautions: Seizure disorders, bronchial asthma, coronary occlusion, hyperthyroidism, dysrhythmias, peptic ulcer, megacolon, poor GI motility, pregnancy (C)

Pharmacokinetics:
PO: Onset 20-30 min, duration 3-6 hr
IM/IV/SC: Onset 2-15 min, duration 2½-4 hr; metabolized in liver, excreted in urine

Interactions/incompatibilities:
• Decreased action: gallamine, metocurine, pancuronium, tubocurarine, atropine
• Increased action: decamethonium, succinylcholine
• Decreased action of pyridostigmine: aminoglycosides, anesthetics, procainamide, quinidine, mecamylamine, polymyxin, magnesium, corticosteroids, antidysrhythmics
• Considered incompatible with any drug in sol or syringe

NURSING CONSIDERATIONS
Assess:
• VS, respiration q8h
• I&O ratio; check for urinary retention or incontinence
• Bradycardia, hypotension, bronchospasm, headache, dizziness, convulsions, respiratory depression; drug should be discontinued if toxicity occurs

Administer:
• IV undiluted, give through Y-tube or 3-way stopcock, give 0.5 mg or less/min
• Only with atropine sulfate available for cholinergic crisis

• Only after all other cholinergics have been discontinued
• Increased doses if tolerance occurs
• Larger doses after exercise or fatigue
• On empty stomach for better absorption

Perform/provide:
• Storage at room temperature

Evaluate:
• Therapeutic response: increased muscle strength, hand grasp, improved gait, absence of labored breathing (if severe)

Teach patient/family:
• Not to crush or chew sus rel prep
• That drug is not a cure, only relieves symptoms
• To wear Medic Alert ID specifying myasthenia gravis, drugs taken

Treatment of overdose:
Discontinue drug, atropine 1-4 mg IV

---

pyridoxine HCl (vitamin B$_6$)

(peer-i-dox-een)
Beesix, Nestrex, Pyridoxine HCl, Vitamin B$_6$, Rodex TD, Hexa-Betalin

Func. class.: Vitamin B$_6$, water soluble

Action: Needed for fat, protein, carbohydrate metabolism; enhances glycogen release from liver and muscle tissue; needed as coenzyme for metabolic transformations of a variety of amino acids

Uses: Vit B$_6$ deficiency associated with inborn errors of metabolism, seizures, isoniazid therapy, oral contraceptives, alcoholic polyneuritis

Dosage and routes:
Vit B$_6$ deficiency
• *Adult:* PO/IM/IV 2.5-10 mg until corrected, then 2-5 mg qd
• *Child:* PO/IM/IV 100 mg until desired response

Inborn errors of metabolism
• *Adult:* IM/IV/PO 600 mg or less qd, then 50 mg qd for life
• *Child:* IM/PO/IV 100 mg, then 2-10 mg IM or 10-100 mg PO qd

Deficiency caused by isoniazid
• *Adult:* PO 100 mg qd × 3 wk, then 50 mg qd
• *Child:* PO dose titrated to patient response

Prevention of deficiency caused by isoniazid
• *Adult:* PO 10-50 mg qd
• *Child:* PO 0.5-1.5 mg qd
• *Infant:* PO 0.1-0.5 mg qd

Available forms: Tabs 10, 25, 50, 100, 200, 250, 500 mg; tabs time rel 500 mg; inj IM-IV 100 mg/ml; oral cap 500 mg

Side effects/adverse reactions:
CNS: Paresthesia, flushing, warmth, lethargy (rare with normal renal function)
INTEG: Pain at injection site

Contraindications: Hypersensitivity

Precautions: Pregnancy (A), lactation, children, Parkinson's disease

Pharmacokinetics:
PO/INJ: Half-life 2-3 wk, metabolized in liver, excreted in urine

Interactions/incompatibilities:
• Decreased effects of: levodopa
• Decreased effects of pyridoxine: oral contraceptives, INH, cycloserine, hydralazine, penicillamine
• Incompatible with alkaline sol, iron salts

NURSING CONSIDERATIONS
Assess:
• Pyridoxine levels throughout treatment

---

italics = common side effects   ***bold italic*** = life threatening reactions

• Nutritional status: yeast, liver, legumes, bananas, green vegetables, whole grains

Administer:

• IV undiluted or added to most IV sol; give 50 mg or less / 1 min if undiluted

• IM rotate sites; burning or stinging at site may occur

• Z-track to minimize pain

Perform / provide:

• Storage in tight, light-resistant container

Evaluate:

• Therapeutic response: absence of nausea, vomiting, anorexia, skin lesions, glossitis, stomatitis, edema, convulsions, restlessness, paresthesia

Teach patient / family:

• To avoid vitamin supplements unless directed by physician

• To keep out of children's reach

• To increase meat, bananas, potatoes, lima beans, whole grain cereals

• To discuss birth control status with physician

---

pyrimethamine

(peer-i-meth'a-meen)

Daraprim, Fansidar (with sulfadoxine)

Func. class.: Antimalarial
Chem. class.: Folic acid antagonist

Action: Inhibits folic acid metabolism in parasite, prevents transmission by stopping growth of fertilized gametes

Uses: Malaria prophylaxis, *P. vivax*

Dosage and routes:

Prophylaxis of malaria

• *Adult:* PO 1 tab qwk or 2 tabs q2wk (Fansidar)

• *Child 9-14 yr:* PO ¾ tab qwk or 1½ tabs q2wk (Fansidar)

• *Child >10 yr:* PO 25 mg qwk

• *Child 4-10 yr:* PO 12.5 mg qwk

• *Child 4-8 yr:* PO ½ tab qwk or 1 tab q2wk (Fansidar)

• *Child <4 yr:* PO ¼ tab qwk or ½ tab q2wk (Fansidar)

• *Child <4 yr:* PO 6.25 mg qwk

Acute attacks of malaria

• *Adult:* PO 2-3 tabs as a single dose (Fansidar) alone or with quinine or primaquine

• *Child 9-14 yr:* 2 tabs

• *Child 4-8 yr:* 1 tab

• *Child <4 yr:* ½ tab

Toxoplasmosis

• *Adult:* PO 100 mg, then 25 mg qd × 4-5 wk, with 1 g sulfadiazine q6h

• *Child:* PO 1 mg/kg, then 0.25 mg/kg qd × 4-5 wk, with sulfadiazine 100 mg/kg/day in divided doses q6h

Available forms: Tabs 25 mg; combo tabs 500 mg sulfadoxine / 25 mg pyrimethamine

Side effects / adverse reactions:

RESP: Respiratory failure

INTEG: Skin eruptions, photosensitivity

CNS: Stimulation, irritability, *convulsions,* tremors, ataxia, fatigue

GI: Nausea, vomiting, cramps, anorexia, diarrhea, atrophic glossitis, gastritis

HEMA: Thrombocytopenia, leukopenia, pancytopenia, megaloblastic anemia, decreased folic acid, *agranulocytosis*

Contraindications: Hypersensitivity, chloroquine-resistant malaria, megaloblastic anemia caused by folate deficiency

Precautions: Blood dyscrasias, seizure disorder, pregnancy (C), lactation, G-6-PD disease, renal, hepatic disease

---

Pharmacokinetics:
PO: Peak 2 hr, half-life 111 hr; metabolized in liver, highly protein bound, excreted in urine (metabolites)

Interactions/incompatibilities:
• Synergestic action: paraaminobenzoic acid or folic acid
• Increased bone marrow suppression: antibiotics

NURSING CONSIDERATIONS
Assess:
• Folic acid level; megaloblastic anemia occurs
• Blood studies, CBC, platelets, since blood dyscrasias occur; twice weekly if dosage is increased
• For toxicity: vomiting, anorexia, seizure, blood dyscrasia, glossitis; drug should be discontinued immediately

Administer:
• Leucovorin IM 3-9 mg/day × 3 days if folic acid deficiency occurs
• Before or after meals at same time each day to maintain drug level, to decrease GI symptoms

Perform/provide:
• Storage in tight, light-resistant containers

Evaluate:
• Therapeutic response: decreased symptoms of malaria

Teach patient/family:
• To report visual problems, fever, fatigue, bruising, bleeding; may indicate blood dyscrasias

Treatment of overdose: Gastric lavage, short-acting barbiturate, leucovorin, respiratory support if needed

quazepam
Doral
Func. class.: Sedative-hypnotic
Chem. class.: Benzodiazepine derivative

Controlled Substance Schedule IV (USA)

Action: Produces CNS depression at the limbic, thalamic, hypothalamic levels of CNS; may be mediated by neurotransmitter γ-aminobutyric acid (GABA); results are sedation, hypnosis, skeletal muscle relaxation, anticonvulsant activity, anxiolytic action

Uses: Insomnia

Dosage and routes:
Adult: PO 7.5 mg hs; may increase if needed

Available forms: Tabs 7.5, 15 mg

Side effects/adverse reactions:
*HEMA: **Leukopenia, granulocytopenia** (rare)*
CNS: Lethargy, drowsiness, daytime sedation, dizziness, confusion, light-headedness, headache, anxiety, irritability, weakness, tremor, depression
GI: Nausea, vomiting, diarrhea, heartburn, abdominal pain, constipation, anorexia, taste alteration
CV: Chest pain, pulse changes, palpitations, tachycardia
MISC: Joint pain, congestion, dermatitis, sweating

Contraindications: Hypersensitivity to benzodiazepines, pregnancy, lactation

Precautions: Hepatic disease, renal disease, suicidal individuals, drug abuse, elderly, psychosis, child <18 yr, lactation, depression, pulmonary insufficiency

Pharmacokinetics:
PO: Onset 15-45 min, duration 7-8 hr; metabolized by liver, excreted

italics = common side effects   ***bold italic*** = life threatening reactions

by kidneys (inactive/active metabolites), crosses placenta, excreted in breast milk

Interactions/incompatibilities:
• Increased effects of quazepam: cimetidine, disulfiram, OC
• Decreased effects: smoking, rifampin, theophylline with increased levels of phenytoin and digoxin
• Increased CNS depression: alcohol, CNS depressants
• Decreased effect of quazepam: antacids

Lab test interferences:
Increase: AST/ALT, serum bilirubin
Decrease: RAI uptake

NURSING CONSIDERATIONS
Assess:
• Blood studies: Hct, Hgb, RBCs (if on long-term therapy)
• Hepatic studies: AST, ALT, bilirubin
• Mental status: mood, sensorium, affect, memory (long, short)
• Blood dyscrasias: fever, sore throat, bruising, rash, jaundice, epistaxis (rare)
• Type of sleep problem: falling asleep, staying asleep

Administer:
• After removal of cigarettes to prevent fires
• After trying conservative measures for insomnia
• ½-1 hr before hs for sleeplessness
• On empty stomach for fast onset, but may be taken with food if GI symptoms occur

Perform/provide:
• Assistance with ambulation after receiving dose
• Safety measure: side rails, nightlight, call bell within easy reach
• Checking to see PO medication has been swallowed

• Storage in tight container in cool environment

Evaluate:
• Therapeutic response: ability to sleep at night, decreased amount of early morning awakening

Teach patient/family:
• To avoid driving or other activities requiring alertness until drug is stabilized
• To avoid alcohol ingestion, CNS depressants; serious CNS depression may result
• That effects may take two nights for benefits to be noticed
• Alternative measures to improve sleep: reading, exercise several hours before hs, warm bath, warm milk, TV, self-hypnosis, deep breathing
• That hangover is common in elderly but less common than with barbiturates

Treatment of overdose: Lavage, activated charcoal; monitor electrolytes, vital signs

---

quinacrine HCl
(kwin'a-kreen)
Atabrine HCl
Func. class.: Anthelmintic
Chem. class.: Acridine dye derivative

Action: Causes worm scolex to detach from GI tract; inhibits DNA synthesis in susceptible parasites
Uses: Giardiasis, tapeworms (cestodiasis), malaria
Dosage and routes:
• *Adult:* PO 100 mg tid × 5-7 days
• *Child:* PO 7 mg/kg/day in 3 divided doses pc × 5 days, not to exceed 300 mg/day; may repeat in 2 wk if needed; administer 1-3 mo for malaria

Tapeworm

• *Adults and children >14yr:* 4 doses of 200 mg PO given 10 min apart (800 mg total)

• *Children 11-14 yr:* 200 mg PO given 10 min apart 3 times (600 mg total)

Available forms: Tabs 100 mg

Side effects/adverse reactions:

INTEG: Rash, dermatitis, yellow pigmentation of skin, urticaria

CNS: Dizziness, headache, insomnia, restlessness, confusion, behavioral changes, psychosis, ***convulsions,*** nightmares

EENT: Bad taste, oral irritation, corneal deposits, retinopathy

GI: Nausea, vomiting, anorexia, diarrhea, cramps, hepatitis

GU: Yellow discoloration of urine

*HEMA: **Aplastic anemia, agranulocytosis***

Contraindications: Hypersensitivity, porphyria, psoriasis

Precautions: Seizure disorders, elderly, psychosis, alcoholism, hepatic disease, depression, child <12 yr, G-6-PD deficiency, pregnancy (C), hepatic disease

Pharmacokinetics:

PO: Peak 8 hr, metabolized by the liver (slowly), excreted primarily in urine, crosses placenta, high protein bindings

Interactions/incompatibilities:

• Increased toxicity: primaquine, hepatotoxic drugs

• Disulfiram-like reaction: alcohol

Lab test interferences:

False positive: Adrenal function tests

Increase: 17-OHCS (Mattingly method)

NURSING CONSIDERATIONS

Assess:

• Stools during entire treatment, collect entire stools × 48 hr, pass through sieve, check for scolex (yellow tapeworms)

• CBC, ophthalmic exam if used for long-term treatment

• Stools 2 wk after last dose for giardiasis

• For allergic reaction (rash), visual problems (halos, blurring, inability to focus)

• For infection in other family members, since infection from person to person is common

• Mental status: affect, mood, behavioral changes

Administer:

• By duodenal tube for pork tapeworm; prevents vomiting, transportation of parasites into stomach

• Bland liquid diet, no fat, no residue 24-48 hr before beginning therapy; patient should be fasting night before, given saline enemas, cleansing enema before beginning therapy (tapeworms only)

• Laxatives before treatment to cleanse bowel; $NaCO_3$ with each dose for nausea and vomiting

• After meals with fluids for giardiasis, malaria

• In jam or honey to disguise bitter taste of pulverized tablets (children)

Perform/provide:

• Storage in tight containers

Evaluate:

• Therapeutic response: expulsion of worms, 3 negative stool cultures after completion of treatment

Teach patient/family:

• Proper hygiene after BM, including hand-washing technique; tell patient to avoid putting fingers in mouth

• To clean toilet qd with disinfectant (green soap solution)

• Need for compliance with dosage schedule, duration of treatment

---

italics = common side effects   ***bold italic*** = life threatening reactions

• That skin, urine may turn deep yellow
• To report any visual changes
• Not to drink alcohol
Treatment of overdose: Induce vomiting

---

quinapril
(kwye'na-preel)
Accupril
Func. class.: Antihypertensive
Chem. class.: Angiotensin-converting enzyme (ACE) inhibitor

Action: Selectively suppresses renin-angiotensin-aldosterone system; inhibits ACE, prevents conversion of angiotensin I to angiotensin II; results in dilation of arterial, venous vessels
Uses: Hypertension, alone or in combination with thiazide diuretics
Dosage and routes:
• *Adult:* PO 10 mg qd initially, then 20-80 mg/day divided bid or qd
Available forms: Tabs 5, 10, 20, 40 mg
Side effects/adverse reactions:
CV: Hypotension, postural hypotension, syncope, palpitations, angina pectoris, MI, tachycardia, vasodilation
GU: Increased BUN, creatinine, decreased libido, impotence, urinary tract infection
*HEMA: **Thrombocytopenia, agranulocytosis***
*INTEG: **Angioedema,** rash, sweating, photosensitivity, pruritus
RESP: Cough, bronchitis
META: Hyperkalemia
GI: Nausea, constipation, vomiting, gastritis, GI hemorrhage, dry mouth
CNS: Headache, dizziness, fatigue, somnolence, depression, malaise, nervousness, vertigo

MISC: Back pain, amblyopia, pharyngitis
MS: Arthralgia, arthritis, myalgia
Contraindications: Hypersensitivity to ACE inhibitors, pregnancy (D), children
Precautions: Impaired renal, liver function, dialysis patients, hypovolemia, blood dyscrasias, COPD, asthma, elderly, lactation
Pharmacokinetics:
PO: Peak ½-1 hr, serum protein binding, 97%, half-life 2 hr, metabolized by liver (metabolites), metabolites excreted in urine
Interactions/incompatibilities:
• Increased hypotension: diuretics, other antihypertensives, ganglionic blockers, adrenergic blockers, phenothiazines
• Use caution with vasodilators, hydralazine, prazosin, potassium-sparing diuretics, sympathomimetics, K supplements
• Decreased absorption of: tetracycline
• Reduced hypotensive effect of quinipril: indomethacin
• Increased toxicity: lithium, digoxin
Lab test interferences:
False positive: Urine acetone
NURSING CONSIDERATIONS
Assess:
• Blood studies: neutrophils, decreased platelets
• B/P, orthostatic hypotension, syncope
• Renal studies: protein, BUN, creatinine; watch for increased levels; may indicate nephrotic syndrome
• Baselines in renal, liver function tests before therapy begins
• K levels, although hyperkalemia rarely occurs
• Dip-stick of urine for protein qd in first morning specimen; if pro-

tein is increased, a 24-hr urinary protein should be collected
• Edema in feet, legs daily
• Allergic reactions: rash, fever, pruritus, urticaria; drugs should be discontinued if antihistamines fail to help
• Renal symptoms: polyuria, oliguria, frequency, dysuria

Administer:
• IV infusion of 0.9% NaCl (as ordered) to expand fluid volume if severe hypotension occurs

Perform/provide:
• Supine or Trendelenburg position for severe hypotension

Evaluate:
• Therapeutic response: decrease in B/P

Teach patient/family:
• To take 1 hr before meals; not to take antacids within 1-2 hr of quinapril
• Not to discontinue drug abruptly
• Not to use OTC products (cough, cold, allergy); not to use salt substitutes containing potassium unless directed by physician
• To comply with dosage schedule, even if feeling better
• To rise slowly to sitting or standing position to minimize orthostatic hypotension
• To notify physician of mouth sores, sore throat, fever, swelling of hands or feet, irregular heartbeat, chest pain, persistent dry cough
• To report excessive perspiration, dehydration, vomiting, diarrhea; may lead to fall in B/P
• That drug may cause dizziness, fainting, light-headedness; may occur during 1st few days of therapy
• That drug may cause skin rash or impaired taste perception
• How to take B/P, and normal readings for age group

Treatment of overdose: 0.9% NaCl IV INF, hemodialysis

---

quinestrol
(kwin-ess'trole)
Estrovis
Func. class.: Estrogen
Chem. class.: Nonsteroidal synthetic estrogen

Action: Needed for adequate functioning of female reproductive system; affects release of pituitary gonadotropins, inhibits ovulation, promotes adequate calcium use in bone structures

Uses: Menopause, atrophic vaginitis, kraurosis vulvae, female castration, female hypogonadism, primary ovarian failure

Dosage and routes:
• *Adult:* PO 100 μg qd × 1 wk, then 100 μg qwk starting 2 wk after beginning treatment; may increase to 200 μg/wk

Available forms: Tabs 100 μg

Side effects/adverse reactions:
CNS: Dizziness, headache, migraine, depression
CV: Hypotension, thrombophlebitis, edema, *thromboembolism, stroke, pulmonary embolism, myocardial infarction*
GI: Nausea, vomiting, diarrhea, anorexia, pancreatitis, cramps, constipation, increased appetite, increased weight, *cholestatic jaundice*
EENT: Contact lens intolerance, increased myopia, astigmatism
GU: Amenorrhea, cervical erosion, breakthrough bleeding, dysmenorrhea, vaginal candidiasis, breast changes, *gynecomastia, testicular atrophy, impotence*
INTEG: Rash, urticaria, acne, hir-

italics = common side effects   ***bold italic*** = life threatening reactions

sutism, alopecia, oily skin, seborrhea, purpura, melasma
META: Folic acid deficiency, hypercalcemia, hyperglycemia
Contraindications: Breast cancer, thromboembolic disorders, reproductive cancer, genital bleeding (abnormal, undiagnosed), pregnancy (X)
Precautions: Hypertension, asthma, blood dyscrasias, gallbladder disease, CHF, diabetes mellitus, bone disease, depression, migraine headache, convulsive disorders, hepatic disease, renal disease, family history of cancer of breast or reproductive tract
Pharmacokinetics:
PO: Degraded in liver, excreted in urine, crosses placenta, excreted in breast milk
Interactions/incompatibilities:
• Decreased action of: anticoagulants, oral hypoglycemics
• Toxicity: tricyclic antidepressants
• Decreased action of quinestrol: anticonvulsants, barbiturates, phenylbutazone, rifampin
• Increased action of: corticosteroids

NURSING CONSIDERATIONS
Assess:
• Urine glucose in patient with diabetes; increased urine glucose may occur
• Weight daily; notify physician of weekly weight gain >5 lb; if increase, diuretic may be ordered
• B/P q4h; watch for increase caused by H_2O, Na retention
• I&O ratio; be alert for decreasing urinary output and increasing edema
• Liver function studies, including AST, ALT, bilirubin, alk phosphatase

• Edema, hypertension, cardiac symptoms, jaundice, calcemia
• Mental status: affect mood, behavioral changes, aggression
Administer:
• Titrated dose; use lowest effective dose
• With food or milk to decrease GI symptoms
Evaluate:
• Therapeutic response: reversal of menopause or decrease in tumor size in prostatic cancer
Teach patient/family:
• To weigh weekly, report gain >5 lb
• To report breast lumps, vaginal bleeding, edema, jaundice, dark urine, clay-colored stools, dyspnea, headache, blurred vision, abdominal pain, numbness or stiffness in legs, chest pain; male to report impotence or gynecomastia

---

quinidine gluconate/ quinidine polygalacturonate/quinidine sulfate
(kwin'i-deen)
Quinaglute Dura-Tabs, Quinalan, Quinidine Gluconate, Cardioquin, Quinidex Extentabs, Quinidine Sulfate, Quinora
Func. class.: Antidysrhythmic (Class IA)
Chem. class.: Quinine dextro isomer

Action: Prolongs action, potential duration, and effective refractory period, thus decreasing myocardial excitability; anticholinergic properties
Uses: PVCs, atrial fibrillation, PAT, ventricular tachycardia, atrial dysrhythmias

Dosage and routes:
Atrial fibrillation/flutter
• *Adult:* PO 200 mg q2-3h × 5-8 doses; may increase qd until sinus rhythm is restored; max 4 g/day given only after digitalization
Paroxysmal supraventricular tachycardia
• *Adult:* PO 400-600 mg q2-3h
All other dysrhythmias
• *Adult:* PO 50-200 mg as a test dose, then 200-400 mg q4-6h; IM 600 mg, then 400 mg q2h, after test dose (gluconate); IV INF 800 mg in 40 ml D$_5$W run at 16 mg/min
Available forms: (Gluconate) tabs sus rel 324, 330 mg; inj IM gluconate 80 mg/ml (sulfate) tabs 100, 200, 300 mg; caps 200, 300 mg; tabs sus rel 300 mg; inj IV (polygalacturonate) tabs 275 mg, sulfate 200 mg/ml
Side effects/adverse reactions:
CNS: Headache, dizziness, involuntary movement, confusion, psychosis, restlessness, irritability, syncope, excitement
EENT: Cinchonism: tinnitus, blurred vision, hearing loss, mydriasis, disturbed color vision
GI: Nausea, vomiting, anorexia, *diarrhea,* **hepatotoxicity**
CV: Hypotension, bradycardia, PVCs, **heart block, cardiovascular collapse, arrest**
HEMA: **Thrombocytopenia,** hemolytic anemia, agranulocytosis, hypoprothrombinemia
RESP: Dyspnea, *respiratory depression*
INTEG: Rash, urticaria, angioedema, swelling, photosensitivity
Contraindications: Hypersensitivity, blood dyscrasias, severe heart block, myasthenia gravis
Precautions: Pregnancy (C), lactation, children, renal disease, K

imbalance, liver disease, CHF, respiratory depression
Pharmacokinetics:
PO: Peak 0.5-6 hr, duration 6-8 hr; half-life 6-7 hr, metabolized in liver, excreted unchanged by kidneys
Interactions/incompatibilities:
• Increased effects of: neuromuscular blockers, digoxin, coumadin
• Increased effects of quinidine: cimetidine, propranolol, thiazides, sodium bicarbonate, carbonic anhydrase inhibitors, antacids, hydroxide suspensions
• May decrease effects of quinidine: barbiturates, phenytoin, rifampin, nifedipine
• Additive vagolytic effect: anticholinergic blockers
• Additive cardiac depression: other antidysrhythmics, phenothiazines, reserpine
• Considered incompatible with any drug in sol or syringe
Lab test interferences:
Increase: CPK
NURSING CONSIDERATIONS
Assess:
• ECG continuously to determine increased PR or QRS segments; if these develop, discontinue or reduce dose
• Blood levels (therapeutic level 2-6 μg/ml)
• B/P continuously for fluctuations
• Cinchonism: tinnitus, headache, nausea, dizziness, fever, vertigo, tremor; may lead to hearing loss
• Cardiac rate, respiration: rate, rhythm, character, continuously
• Respiratory status: rate, rhythm, lung fields for rales
• CNS effects: dizziness, confusion, psychosis, paresthesias, convulsions; drug should be discontinued

---

italics = common side effects   ***bold italic*** = life threatening reactions

• Lung fields; bilateral rales may occur in CHF patient
• Increased respiration, increased pulse; drug should be discontinued

Administer:
• IV after diluting 800 mg/40 ml or more D_5; give 16 mg or less over 1 min as infusion; use infusion pump
• IM injection in deltoid; aspirate to avoid intravascular administration
• An AV node blocker (digoxin, verapamil) before starting quinidine to avoid increased ventricular rate

Evaluate:
• Therapeutic response: decreased dysrhythmias

Treatment of overdose: O_2, artificial ventilation, ECG, administer dopamine for circulatory depression, administer diazepam or thiopental for convulsions

---

quinine sulfate
(kwye′nine)
Formula Q, Legatrin, M-Kya, Novoquine,* Quinamm, Quinine Sulfate, Quiphile, Q-Vel
Func. class.: Antimalarial
Chem. class.: Cinchona tree alkaloid

Action: Inhibits parasite replications, transcription of DNA to RNA by forming complexes with DNA of parasite
Uses: *Plasmodium falciparum* malaria, nocturnal leg cramps
Dosage and routes:
• *Adult:* PO 650 mg q8h × 10 days, given with pyrimethamine 25 mg q12h × 3 days, with sulfadiazine 500 mg qid × 5 days
Available forms: Caps 130, 195, 200, 300, 325 mg; tabs 260, 325 mg

Side effects/adverse reactions:
RESP: Dyspnea
INTEG: Pruritus, pigmentary changes, skin eruptions, lichen planuslike eruptions, flushing, facial edema, sweating
*HEMA: **Thrombocytopenia, purpura, hypothrombinemia, hemolysis***
CNS: Headache, stimulation, fatigue, irritability, **convulsion,** bad dreams, dizziness, fever, confusion, anxiety
EENT: Blurred vision, corneal changes, retinal changes, difficulty focusing, tinnitus, vertigo, deafness, photophobia, diplopia, night blindness
GU: Renal tubular damage, anuria
GI: Nausea, vomiting, anorexia, diarrhea, epigastric pain
CV: Angina, dysrhythmias, tachycardia, hypotension, **acute circulatory failure**
ENDO: Hypoglycemia
Contraindications: Hypersensitivity, G-6-PD deficiency, retinal field changes, pregnancy (X)
Precautions: Blood dyscrasias, severe GI disease, neurologic disease, severe hepatic disease, psoriasis, cardiac dysrhythmias, tinnitus
Pharmacokinetics:
PO: Peak 1-3 hr, metabolized in liver, excreted in urine, half-life 4-5 hr
Interactions/incompatibilities:
• Toxicity: $NaHCO_3$, acetazolamide
• Decreased absorption: magnesium or aluminum salts
• Increase levels of: digoxin, digitoxin, neuromuscular blockers, other anticoagulants

Lab test interferences:
Increase: 17-KS
Interference: 17-OHCS

NURSING CONSIDERATIONS
Assess:
• B/P, pulse, watch for hypotension, tachycardia
• Liver studies weekly: ALT, AST, bilirubin
• Blood studies, CBC, since blood dyscrasias occur
• For cinchonism: nausea, blurred vision, tinnitus, headache, difficulty focusing

Administer:
• Before or after meals at same time each day to maintain drug level

Perform/provide:
• Storage in tight, light-resistant container

Evaluate:
• Therapeutic response: decreased symptoms of malaria

Teach patient/family:
• To avoid OTC preparations: cold preparations, tonic water

---

rabies immune globulin, human
Hyperab, Imogam
Func. class.: Immune serum
Chem. class.: IgG

Action: Provides passive immunity; given with HDCV; may be used regardless of time of bite, treatment

Uses: Exposure to rabies

Dosage and routes:
• *Adult and child:* IM 20 IU/kg given at same time as 1st rabies vaccine; infiltrate wound with ½ dose, then administer rest IM, 1 ml dose on each of days 3, 7, 14, 28 after 1st dose

Available forms: Inj IM 125 IU/ml

Side effects/adverse reactions:
INTEG: Pain at injection site, rash, pruritus
MS: Arthralgia
SYST: Lymphadenopathy, **anaphylaxis**, fever
CNS: Headache, fatigue, malaise
GI: Abdominal pain

Contraindications: Hypersensitivity to equine products and thimerosal

Interactions/incompatibilities:
• Decreased action of rabies immune globulin: corticosteroids, immunosuppressants

NURSING CONSIDERATIONS
Administer:
• Test dose: dilute drug either with 1:100 or 1:1000 0.9% NaCl for injection, inject 0.1 ml 0.9% NaCl in other arm intradermally, check for wheal ≥10 mm after 10 min; if present, drug should not be used
• Only after epinephrine 1:1000, resuscitative equipment are available
• Only if human immune serum is not available
• As soon as possible after exposure

Perform/provide:
• Storage at 36°-46°F (2°-8°C)

Evaluate:
• Allergic reactions: dyspnea, rash, pruritus, eruptions

Teach patient/family:
• That pain, swelling, itching may occur at injection site
• To take acetaminophen to alleviate headache, fever, and pain

---

radioactive iodine (sodium iodide) ¹³¹I
Func. class.: Antithyroid
Chem. class.: Radiopharmaceutical

Action: Converted to protein-

R

bound iodine by thyroid gland for use when needed

Uses:

High dose: Thyroid cancer, hyperthyroidism

Low dose: Visualization to determine thyroid cancer, diagnostic aid in thyroid function studies

Dosage and routes:

Thyroid cancer

• *Adult:* PO 50-150 mCi, may repeat depending on clinical status

Hyperthyroidism

• *Adult:* PO 4-10 mCi, depending on serum thyroxine level

Available forms: Caps 1-50, 0.8-100 mCi; oral sol 7.05 mCi/ml, 3.5-150 mCi/vial

Side effects/adverse reactions:

ENDO: Hypothyroidism, *hyperthyroid adenoma,* transient thyroiditis

INTEG: Alopecia

HEMA: Eosinophilia, lymphedema, leukemia, bone marrow depression, leukopenia, anemia

GI: Nausea, diarrhea, vomiting

EENT: Sore throat, cough

Contraindications: Recent MI, lactation, large nodular goiter, pregnancy (X), age <30 yr, vomiting/diarrhea, acute hyperthyroidism, use of thyroid drugs

Pharmacokinetics:

PO: Onset 3-6 days; excreted in urine, sweat, feces; crosses placenta; excreted in breast milk; excreted in 56 days

Interactions/incompatibilities:

• Hypothyroidism: lithium

• Decreased uptake if recent intake of stable iodine, thyroid, antithyroid drugs

NURSING CONSIDERATIONS

Assess:

• Weight qd in same clothing, scale, time of day

• Blood work, including CBC for blood dyscrasias (leukopenia,

thrombocytopenia, agranulocytosis)

• Overdose: peripheral edema, heat intolerance, diaphoresis, palpitations, dysrhythmias, severe tachycardia, increased temperature delirium, CNS irritability

• Hypersensitivity: rash, enlarged cervical lymph nodes; drug may have to be discontinued

• Hypoprothrombinemia: bleeding, petechiae, ecchymosis

• Clinical response: after 3 wk should include increased weight, pulse; decreased T_4

• Bone marrow depression: sore throat, fever, fatigue

Administer:

• Only after discontinuing all other antithyroid agents × 5-7 days

• After NPO overnight, food delays action

• During or within 10 days after menstruation

Perform/provide:

• Limited contact with patient ½ hr/day for each person

• Adequate rest after treatment

• Fluids to 3-4 L/day for 48 hr after agent is administered to remove agent from body

Evaluate:

• Therapeutic response: weight gain, decreased pulse, decreased T_4, B/P

Teach patient/family:

• To empty bladder often during treatment; avoids irradiation of gonads

• To report redness, swelling, sore throat, mouth lesions; indicate blood dyscrasias

• To avoid extended contact with children, spouse for 1 week

• That bathroom may be used by entire family

• Not to take antithyroid agents but propranolol, which decreases hy-

perthyroid symptoms, until total effects of ^{131}I has taken effect (about 6 wk)
• To avoid coughing, expectorating for 24 hr (saliva and vomiting are highly radioactive for 6-8 hr)

---

ramipril
(ra-mi'pril)
Altace

Func. class.: Antihypertensive
Chem. class.: Angiotensin-converting enzyme (ACE) inhibitor

Action: Selectively suppresses renin-angiotensin-aldosterone system; inhibits ACE, prevents conversion of angiotensin I to angiotensin II; results in dilation of arterial, venous vessels

Uses: Hypertension, alone or in combination with thiazide diuretics

Dosage and routes:
• *Adult:* PO 2.5 mg qd initially, then 2.5-20 mg/day divided bid or qd; renal impairment: 1.25 mg qd with CrCl <40 ml/min/1.73 m², increase as needed to maximum or 5 mg/day

Available forms: Caps 1.25, 2.5, 5, 10 mg

Side effects/adverse reactions:
CV: Hypotension, chest pain, palpitations, angina, syncope, dysrhythmia
GU: Proteinuria, increased BUN, creatinine, impotence
HEMA: Decreased Hct, Hgb, *eosinophilia, leukopenia*
INTEG: Angioedema, rash, sweating, photosensitivity, pruritus
RESP: Cough, dyspnea
META: Hyperkalemia
GI: Nausea, constipation, vomiting, dyspepsia, dysphagia, anorexia, diarrhea, abdominal pain
CNS: Headache, dizziness, anxiety,

insomnia, paresthesia, fatigue, depression, malaise, vertigo, *convulsions,* hearing loss
MS: Arthralgia, arthritis, myalgia

Contraindications: Hypersensitivity to ACE inhibitors, pregnancy (D), lactation, children

Precautions: Impaired renal, liver function, dialysis patients, hypovolemia, blood dyscrasias, CHF, COPD, asthma, elderly

Pharmacokinetics:
PO: Peak ½-1 hr, serum protein binding 97%, half-life 1-2 hr, metabolized by liver (metabolites excreted in urine, feces)

Interactions/incompatibilities:
• Increased hypotension: diuretics, other antihypertensives, ganglionic blockers, adrenergic blockers
• Increased toxicity: vasodilators, hydralazine, prazosin, K-sparing diuretics, sympathomimetics, K supplements
• Decreased absorption: antacids
• Decreased antihypertensive effect: indomethacin
• Increased serum levels of: digoxin, lithium
• Increased hypersensitivity: allopurinol

Lab test interferences:
False positive: Urine acetone

NURSING CONSIDERATIONS 🇷
Assess:
• Blood studies: neutrophils, decreased platelets
• B/P, orthostatic hypotension, syncope
• Renal studies: protein, BUN, creatinine; watch for increased levels that may indicate nephrotic syndrome
• Baselines in renal, liver function tests before therapy begins
• K levels, although hyperkalemia rarely occurs
• Dipstick of urine for protein qd

---

italics = common side effects   ***bold italic*** = life threatening reactions

in first morning specimen; if protein is increased, a 24-hr urinary protein should be collected
• Edema in feet, legs daily
• Allergic reactions: rash, fever, pruritus, urticaria; drugs should be discontinued if antihistamines fail to help
• Renal symptoms: polyuria, oliguria, frequency, dysuria

Administer:
• IV infusion of 0.9% NaCl (as ordered) to expand fluid volume if severe hypotension occurs

Perform/provide:
• Storage in tight container at 48° F (30° C) or less
• Supine or Trendelenburg position for severe hypotension

Evaluate:
• Therapeutic response: decrease in B/P

Teach patient/family:
• Not to discontinue drug abruptly
• Not to use OTC products (cough, cold, allergy) unless directed by physician; not to use salt substitutes containing potassium without consulting physician
• To comply with dosage schedule, even if feeling better
• To rise slowly to sitting or standing position to minimize orthostatic hypotension
• To notify physician of: mouth sores, sore throat, fever, swelling of hands or feet, irregular heartbeat, chest pain
• To report excessive perspiration, dehydration, vomiting, diarrhea; may lead to fall in B/P
• That drug may cause dizziness, fainting, light-headedness; may occur during 1st few days of therapy
• That drug may cause skin rash or impaired perspiration
• How to take B/P, and normal readings for age group

Treatment of overdose: 0.9% NaCl IV INF, hemodialysis

---

ranitidine
(ra-nye′ te-deen)
Zantac
Func. class.: H$_2$ histamine receptor antagonist

Action: Inhibits histamine at H$_2$ receptor site in parietal cells, which inhibits gastric acid secretion

Uses: Duodenal ulcer, Zollinger-Ellison syndrome, gastric ulcers, hypersecretory conditions, gastroesophageal reflux disease, stress ulcers

Dosage and routes:
• *Adult:* PO 150 mg bid, 300 mg hs; IM 50 mg q6-8h; IV BOL 50 mg diluted to 20 ml over 5 min q6-8h; IV INT INF 50 mg/100 ml D$_5$ over 15-20 min, q6-8h

Available forms: Tabs 150, 300 mg; inj 25 mg/ml IM, IV

Side effects/adverse reactions:
CNS: Headache, sleeplessness, dizziness, confusion, agitation, depression, hallucination
GI: Constipation, abdominal pain, diarrhea, nausea, vomiting, *hepatotoxicity*
GU: Impotence, gynecomastia
CV: Tachycardia, bradycardia, PVCs
EENT: Blurred vision, increased ocular pressure
INTEG: Urticaria, rash, fever

Contraindications: Hypersensitivity

Precautions: Pregnancy (B), lactation, child <12 yr, hepatic disease, renal disease

Pharmacokinetics:
PO: Peak 2-3 hr, duration 8-12 hr; metabolized by liver; excreted in urine, breast milk; half-life 2-3 hr

Interactions/incompatibilities:
• Increased toxicity: anticoagulants, metoprolol
• Decreased absorption of: ketoconazole
• Decreased absorption of ranitidine: antacids, diazepam
• Incompatible with amphotericin B, chlorpromazine, clindamycin, diazepam, hydroxyzine, midazolam, opium, pentobarbital, phenobarbital; do not add any other drugs to premixed ranitidine

Lab test interferences:
Increase: AST/ALT, alk phosphatase, creatinine, LDH, bilirubin
False positive: Urine protein

NURSING CONSIDERATIONS
Assess:
• Gastric pH (>5 should be maintained)
• I&O ratio, BUN, creatinine
• Mental status: confusion, dizziness, depression, anxiety, weakness, tremors, psychosis, diarrhea, abdominal discomfort, jaundice; report immediately
• GI complaints: nausea, vomiting, diarrhea, cramps

Administer:
• With meals for prolonged effect
• Antacids 1 hr before or 1 hr after ranitidine
• IV after diluting 50 mg/20 ml of NS, D_5W, $D_{10}W$, LR, $NaCO_3$ 5% and give 50 mg or less/5 min or more; may dilute 50 mg/50-100 ml of NS, D_5W, $D_{10}W$, LR, $NaCO_3$ 5% and give over 15-20 min

Perform/provide:
• Storage at room temperature

Evaluate:
• Therapeutic response: decreased abdominal pain

Teach patient/family:
• That gynecomastia, impotence may occur but are reversible
• To avoid driving, other hazardous

activities until patient is stabilized on this medication
• To avoid black pepper, caffeine, alcohol, harsh spices, extremes in temperature of food
• That drug must be continued for prescribed time to be effective

---

reserpine
(re-ser'peen)
Novoreserpine,* Serpalan
Func. class.: Antihypertensive
Chem. class.: Antiadrenergic agent

Action: Inhibits norepinephrine release, depleting norepinephrine stores in adrenergic nerve endings
Uses: Hypertension; relief in agitated psychotic states unable to tolerate phenothiazines or requiring antihypertensive medication

Dosage and routes:
Hypertension
• *Adult:* PO 0.25-0.5 mg qd × 1-2 wk, then 0.1-0.25 mg qd maintenance
• *Child:* PO 0.07 mg/kg or 2 mg/m^2 given with hydralzine IM q12-24h

Pyschiatric disorders
• *Adult:* 0.5 mg/day (range 0.1-1 mg)

Available forms: Tabs 0.2, 0.1, 0.25, 1 mg; time rel caps 0.5 mg; inj 2.5 mg/ml

Side effects/adverse reactions:
CV: Bradycardia, chest pain, dysrhythmias, prolonged bleeding time, *thrombocytopenia,* purpura
CNS: Drowsiness, fatigue, lethargy, dizziness, depression, anxiety, headache, increased dreaming, nightmares, convulsions, parkinsonism, EPS (high doses)
GI: Nausea, vomiting, cramps,

italics = common side effects   ***bold italic*** = life threatening reactions

peptic ulcer, dry mouth, increased appetite, anorexia

INTEG: Rash, purpura, alopecia, flushing, warm feeling, pruritus, ecchymosis

EENT: Lacrimation, miosis, blurred vision, ptosis, dry mouth, epistaxis

GU: Impotence, dysuria, nocturia, Na and H_2O retention, edema, breast engorgement, galactorrhea, gynecomastia

RESP: **Bronchospasm,** dyspnea, cough, rales

Contraindications: Hypersensitivity, depression, suicidal patients, active peptic ulcer disease, ulcerative colitis, pregnancy (D), Parkinson's disease

Precautions: Lactation, seizure disorders, renal disease

Pharmacokinetics:

PO: Peak 4 hr, duration 2-6 wk; half-life 50-100 hr; metabolized by liver; excreted in urine, feces; crosses placenta, blood-brain barrier; excreted in breast milk

Interactions/incompatibilities:

• Increased hypotension: diuretics, hypotension, β-blockers, methotrimeprazine

• Dysrhythmias: cardiac glycosides

• Increased cardiac depression: quinidine, procainamide

• Excitation, hypertension: MAOIs

• Increased CNS depression: barbiturates, alcohol, narcotics

• Increased pressor effects: epinephrine, isoproterenol, norepinephrine

• Decreased pressor effects: ephedrine, amphetamine

Lab test interferences:

Increase: VMA excretion, 5-HIAA excretion

Interferences: 17-OHCS, 17-KS

NURSING CONSIDERATIONS

Assess:

• Renal function studies in renal impairment (BUN, creatinine)

• Bleeding time; check for ecchymosis, thrombocytopenia, purpura

• I&O in renal disease patient

• Cardiac status: B/P, pulse; watch for hypotension, bradycardia

• Edema in feet, legs daily; take weight daily

• Skin turgor, dryness of mucous membranes for hydration status

• Symptoms of CHF: edema, dyspnea, wet rales

Evaluate:

• Therapeutic response: decreased hypertension

Teach patient/family:

• To avoid driving, hazardous activities if drowsiness occurs

• Not to discontinue drug abruptly

• Not to use OTC products (cough, cold preparations) unless directed by physician

• To report bradycardia, dizziness, confusion, depression, fever, sore throat

• That impotence, gynecomastia may occur but are reversible

• To rise slowly to sitting or standing position to minimize orthostatic hypotension

• That therapeutic effect may take 2-4 wk

Treatment of overdose: Lavage, IV atropine for bradycardia, supportive therapy

---

Rh₀ (D) immune globulin, human

HypoRho-D, MICRhoGAM, Mini-Gamulin RH

Func. class.: Immunizing agent
Chem. class.: IgG

Action: Supresses immune response of nonsensitized Rh₀ (D or Dᵘ)-negative patients who are exposed to Rh₀ (D or Dᵘ)-positive blood

Uses: Prevention of isoimmunization in Rh-negative women exposed to Rh-positive blood given after abortions, miscarriages, amniocentesis

Dosage and routes:

Obstetrical use

• *Adult:* IM 1 vial if fetal packed RBCs <15 ml, or 2 vials if fetal packed RBCs >15 ml; given within 72 hr of delivery or miscarriage

Transfusion error

• *Adult:* IM Give within 72 hr

Available forms: Inj IM single-dose vial

Side effects/adverse reactions:

INTEG: Irritation at injection site, fever

CNS: Lethargy

MS: Myalgia

Contraindications: Previous immunization with this drug, Rh₀ (O)-positive/Dᵘ-positive patient

NURSING CONSIDERATIONS
Assess:

• Allergies, reactions to immunizations; previous immunization with this drug

Administer:

• After sending newborn's cord blood to lab after delivery for crossmatch, type; infant must be Rh-positive, with Rh-negative mother

• IM in deltoid; aspirate

• Only equal lot numbers of drug, cross-match

• Only MICRhoGAM for abortions or miscarriages < 12 wk unless fetus or father is Rh⁻; unless patient is Rh₀ (D)-positive, Dᵘ-positive, Rh antibodies are present

Evaluate:

• Allergic reaction: rash, urticaria, nausea, fever, wheezing

Perform/provide:

• Storage in refrigerator

Teach patient/family:

• How drug works; that drug must be given after subsequent deliveries if subsequent babies are Rh positive

---

riboflavin (vitamin B₂)

(rye′boo-flay-vin)

Riobin-50 and others

Func. class.: Vitamin B₂, water soluble

Action: Needed for respiratory reactions by catalyzing proteins and for normal vision

Uses: Vit B₂ deficiency or polyneuritis; cheilosis adjunct with thiamine

Dosage and routes:

• *Adult and child >12 yr:* PO 5-50 mg qd

• *Child <12 yr:* PO 2-10 mg qd

Available forms: Tabs 5, 10, 25, 50, 100 mg

Side effects/adverse reactions:

GU: Yellow discoloration of urine (large doses)

Contraindications: Child <12 yr

Precautions: Pregnancy (A)

Pharmacokinetics:

PO: Half-life 65-85 min, 60% protein-bound, unused amounts excreted in urine (unchanged)

Interactions/incompatibilities:

• Decreased action of: tetracyclines

Lab test interferences:

• May cause false elevations of urinary catecholamines

NURSING CONSIDERATIONS
Assess:

• Nutritional status: liver, eggs, dairy products, yeast, whole grain, green vegetables

Administer:

• With food for better absorption

R

---

italics = common side effects   ***bold italic*** = life threatening reactions

Perform/provide:
• Storage in tight, light-resistant container

Evaluate:
• Therapeutic response: absence of headache, GI problems, cheilosis, skin lesions, depression, burning, itchy eyes, anemia

Teach patient/family:
• That urine may turn bright yellow
• About addition of needed foods that are rich in riboflavin
• To avoid alcohol

---

rifabutin
(rif'-a-byoo-ten)
Mycobutin
Func. class.: Antimycobacterial agent
Chem. class.: Rifamycin S derivative

Action: Inhibits DNA-dependent RNA polymerase in susceptible strains of *E. coli* and *B. subtilis;* mechanism of action against *M. avium* unknown

Uses: Prevention of *M. avium* complex in patients with advanced HIV infection

Dosage and routes:
• *Adult:* 300 mg qd (may take as 150 mg bid)
Available forms: Caps 150 mg

Side effects/adverse reactions:
INTEG: Rash
MS: Asthenia, arthralgia, myalgia
MISC: Flulike syndrome, shortness of breath, chest pressure
GI: Nausea, vomiting, anorexia, diarrhea, heartburn, hepatitis
GU: Hematuria
CNS: Headache, fatigue, anxiety, confusion, insomnia
HEMA: Hemolytic anemia, eosinophilia, thrombocytopenia, leukopenia

Contraindications: Hypersensitivity, active TB

Precautions: Pregnancy (B), lactation, hepatic disease, blood dyscrasias, children

Pharmacokinetics:
PO: Peak 2-3 hr, duration >24 hr, half-life 3 hr; metabolized in liver (active/inactive metabolites), excreted in urine primarily as metabolites

Interactions/incompatibilities:
• Decreased action: barbiturates, clofibrate, corticosteroids, dapsone, anticoagulants, sulfonylureas, estrogens, digitoxin and digoxin, oral contraceptives, theophylline, β-blockers
• Rifabutin does not appear to alter the acetylation of INH

Lab test interferences:
Interference: Folate level, Vit B_{12}, BSP, gallbladder studies

NURSING CONSIDERATIONS
Assess:
• Signs of anemia: Hct, Hgb, fatigue
• Liver studies qwk: ALT, AST, bilirubin
• Renal status before, qmo: BUN, creatinine, output, sp gr, urinalysis
• Hepatic studies: decreased appetite, jaundice, dark urine, fatigue

Administer:
• With food if GI upset occurs
• Antiemetic if vomiting occurs
• After C&S is completed; qmo to detect resistance

Evaluate:
• Therapeutic response: not used for active TB because of risk of development of resistance to rifampin; culture negative

Teach patient/family:
• That patients using oral contraceptives should consider using nonhormonal methods of birth control,

since rifabutin may decrease their efficacy
• That compliance with dosage schedule, duration is necessary
• That scheduled appointments must be kept; relapse may occur
• That urine, feces, saliva, sputum, sweat, tears may be colored red-orange; soft contact lenses may be permanently stained
• To report flulike symptoms: excessive fatigue, anorexia, vomiting, sore throat; unusual bleeding, yellowish discoloration of skin, eyes

---

rifampin
(rif'am-pin)
Rifadin, Rimactane, Rofact*
Func. class.: Antitubercular
Chem. class.: Rifamycin B derivative

Action: Inhibits DNA-dependent polymerase, decreases tubercle bacilli replication
Uses: Pulmonary tuberculosis, meningococcal carriers (prevention)
Dosage and routes:
• *Adult:* PO/IV 600 mg/day as single dose 1 hr ac or 2 hr pc
• *Child >5 yr:* PO/IV 10-20 mg/kg/day as single dose 1 hr ac or 2 hr pc, not to exceed 600 mg/day, with other antituberculars
Meningococcal carriers
• *Adult:* PO/IV 600 mg bid × 2 days
• *Child >5 yr:* PO/IV 10 mg/kg bid × 2 days, not to exceed 600 mg/dose
• *Infant 3 mo-1 yr:* 5 mg/kg PO bid for 2 days
Available forms: Caps 150, 300 mg
Side effects/adverse reactions:
INTEG: Rash, pruritus, urticaria

EENT: Vis...
MS: Atoxia,
MISC: Fluliko
disturbances,
breath
GI: Nausia, vo
diarrhea, *pseudo..   ...us colitis,* heartburn, sore mouth and tongue, pancreatitis
GU: Hematuria, acute renal failure, hemoglobinuria
CNS: Headache, fatigue, anxiety, drowsiness, confusion
HEMA: Hemolytic anemia, eosinophilia, thrombocytopenia, leukopenia
Contraindications: Hypersensitivity
Precautions: Pregnancy (C), lactation, hepatic disease, blood dyscrasias
Pharmacokinetics:
PO: Peak 2-3 hr, duration >24 hr, half-life 3 hr; metabolized in liver (active/inactive metabolites), excreted in urine as free drug (30% crosses placenta), excreted in breast milk
Interactions/incompatibilities:
• Decreased action: barbiturates, clofibrate, corticosteroids, dapsone, anticoagulants, antidiabetics, hormones, digoxin, PAS, alcohol, oral contraceptives
• Hepatotoxicity: INH
• Incompatible with sodium lactate
Lab test interferences:
Interference: Folate level, vit B_{12}, BSP, gallbladder studies
NURSING CONSIDERATIONS
Assess:
• Signs of anemia: Hct, Hgb, fatigue
• Liver studies qwk: ALT, AST, bilirubin
• Renal status before, qmo: BUN, creatinine, output, sp gr, urinalysis

---

italics = common side effects   ***bold italic*** = life threatening reactions

status: decreased appetite, jaundice, dark urine, fatigue

Administer:
• IV after diluting each 600 mg/10 ml of sterile water for inj (60 mg/ml), agitate, withdraw dose and dilute in 100 ml or 500 ml of D_5W or NS given as an inf over 3 hr, or if diluted in 100 ml, give over ½ hr
• On empty stomach, 1 hr ac or 2 hr pc
• Antiemetic if vomiting occurs
• After C&S is completed; qmo to detect resistance

Evaluate:
• Therapeutic response: decreased symptoms of TB, culture negative

Teach patient/family:
• That compliance with dosage schedule, duration is necessary
• That scheduled appointments must be kept; relapse may occur
• To avoid alcohol while taking drug
• That urine, feces, saliva, sputum, sweat, tears may be colored red-orange; soft contact lenses may be permanently stained
• To report flulike symptoms: excessive fatigue, anorexia, vomiting, sore throat; unusual bleeding, yellowish discoloration of skin, eyes

---

rimantadine
(rye-man'ta-deen)
Flumadine
Func. class.: Synthetic antiviral
Chem. class.: Tricyclic amine

Action: Prevents uncoating of nucleic acid in viral cell, preventing penetration of virus to host; causes release of dopamine from neurons

Uses: Prophylaxis or treatment of influenza type A

Dosage and routes:
Influenza type A prophylaxis
• *Adult:* PO 100 mg bid; in renal hepatic disease, lower dose to 100 mg/day
• *Child <10 yr:* PO 5 mg/kg/day, not to exceed 150 mg
Treatment
• *Adult:* PO 100 mg bid; in renal or hepatic disease, lower dose to 100 mg/day; start treatment at onset of symptoms, continue for at least 1 wk
Available forms: Tabs 100 mg; syringe 50 mg/5 ml

Side effects/adverse reactions:
CNS: Headache, dizziness, fatigue, depression, hallucinations, tremors, **convulsions,** insomnia, poor concentration, asthenia, gait abnormalities
CV: Pallor, palpitations, hypertension
EENT: Tinnitus, taste abnormality, eye pain
GI: Nausea, vomiting, constipation, dry mouth, anorexia, abdominal pain, diarrhea, dyspepsia
INTEG: Rash

Contraindications: Hypersensitivity, lactation, child <1 yr, pregnancy (C)

Precautions: Epilepsy, hepatic disease, renal disease

Pharmacokinetics:
PO: Peak 6 hr, elimination half-life 25½ hr, plasma protein binding (40%)

Interactions/incompatibilities:
• Decreased peak concentration of rimantadine: acetaminophen, aspirin

NURSING CONSIDERATIONS
Assess:
• I&O ratio; report frequency, hesitancy in renal disease

---

* Available in Canada only

- Bowel pattern before, during treatment
- Skin eruptions, photosensitivity after administration of drug
- Respiratory status: rate, character, wheezing, tightness in chest
- Allergies before initiation of treatment, reaction of each medication; list allergies on chart in bright red letters
- Signs of infection

Administer:
- Before exposure to influenza; continue for 10 days after contact
- At least 4 hr before hs to prevent insomnia
- After meals for better absorption, to decrease GI symptoms
- In divided doses to prevent CNS disturbances: headache, dizziness, fatigue, drowsiness

Perform/provide:
- Storage in tight, dry container

Evaluate:
- Therapeutic response: absence of fever, malaise, cough, dyspnea in infection

Teach patient/family:
- About aspects of drug therapy: need to report dyspnea, dizziness, poor concentration, behavioral changes
- To avoid hazardous activities if dizziness occurs

Treatment of overdose:
Withdraw drug, maintain airway, administer epinephrine, aminophylline, O_2, IV corticosteroids, physostigmine

---

ritodrine HCl
(ri'toe-dreen)
Yutopar
Func. class.: Tocolytic, uterine relaxant
Chem. class.: β_2-adrenergic agonist

Action: Reduces frequency, intensity of uterine contractions by stimulation of the β_2 receptors in uterine smooth muscle

Uses: Management of preterm labor

Dosage and routes:
- Adult: IV INF 150 mg/500 ml (0.3 mg/ml) given 0.1 mg/min, increased gradually by 0.05 mg/min q10min until desired response; PO 10 mg given ½ hr before termination of IV, then 10 mg q2h × 24 hr, then 10-20 mg q4-6h, not to exceed 120 mg/day

Available forms: Tabs 10 mg; inj 10 mg/ml, 15 mg/ml

Side effects/adverse reactions:
MISC: Erythema, rash, dyspnea, hyperventilation, glycosuria, lactic acidosis
META: Hyperglycemia, hypokalemia
CNS: Headache, restlessness, anxiety, nervousness, sweating, chills, drowsiness, tremor
GI: Nausea, vomiting, anorexia, malaise, bloating, constipation, diarrhea
CV: Altered maternal, fetal heart rate, B/P, dysrhythmias, palpitation, chest pain

Contraindications: Hypersensitivity, eclampsia, hypertension, dysrhythmias, thyrotoxicosis, before 20th wk of pregnancy, antepartum hemorrhage, intrauterine fetal death, maternal cardiac disease, pulmonary hypertension, uncontrolled diabetes, pheochromocytoma, bronchial asthma

Precautions: Migraine, sulfite sensitivity, pregnancy-induced hypertension, hypertension, diabetes

Pharmacokinetics:
PO: Peak ½-1 hr
IV: Immediate, distribution half-life 6 min, 2nd phase 1½-2½ hr, elimination phase >10 hr; metabolized

---

italics = common side effects   ***bold italic*** = life threatening reactions

in liver; 90% excreted in urine, crosses placenta

Interactions/incompatibilities:

• Pulmonary edema: corticosteroids

• Increased CV effects of ritodrine: magnesium sulfate, diazoxide, meperidine, potent general anesthetics

• Increased effects of: sympathomimetic amines

• Systemic hypertension: atropine

• Decreased action of ritodrine: β-blockers

• Considered incompatible with any drug in sol or syringe

Lab test interferences:

Increase: Blood glucose, free fatty acids, insulin, GTT

Decrease: K

NURSING CONSIDERATIONS
Assess:

• Maternal, fetal heart tones during infusion

• Intensity, length of uterine contractions

• Fluid intake to prevent fluid overload; discontinue if this occurs

• Blood glucose in diabetics

Administer:

• Only clear sol

• After dilution: 150 mg/500 ml D_5W or NS, give at 0.3 mg/ml

• Using infusion pump, or monitor carefully

Perform/provide:

• Positioning of patient in left lateral recumbent position to decrease hypotension, increase renal blood flow

Evaluate:

• Therapeutic response: decreased intensity, length of contraction, absence of preterm labor, decreased B/P

Teach patient/family:

• To remain in bed during infusion

---

salicylic acid

Calicylic Creme, Clear Away, Clear Away Plantar, Compound W, Duofilm, Freezone, Gordofilm, Hydrisalic, Keralyt, Lactisol, Lactisol Forte, Mediplast, Mosco, Occlusal, Occlusal HP, Off-Ezy Wart Remover, Panscol, Paplex Ultra, Pediapatch, Sal-Acid, Salacid 25%, Salacid 60%, Salactic Film, Salicylic Acid Creme 60%, Sal Plant, Trans-Ver-Sal, Trans-Plantar, Vergogel Duoplant for Feet, Verukan HP Paplex, Viranol Gel Ultra, Viranol, Wart-Off, Wart Remover

Func. class.: Keratolytic

Action: Corrects abnormal keratinization and causes peeling of skin

Uses: Dandruff, seborrheic dermatitis, psoriasis, multiple superficial epitheliomatoses

Dosage and routes:

• *Adult:* TOP apply as needed, cover at night

Available forms: Powder, cream 2%, 2.5%, 10%; gel 6%, 17%; oint 3%, 25%, 60%; plaster 40%; pledgets 0.5%; shampoo 2%, 4%; solution 13.6%, 17%; stick 2%; susp 2%, liquid 12%, 16.7%, 17%, 20%, 26%

Side effects/adverse reactions:

INTEG: Irritation, drying

CNS: Salicylism: hearing loss, tinnitus, dizziness, confusion, headache, hyperventilation

Contraindications: Hypersensitivity, diabetes, impaired circulation, use on moles, genital or facial warts

Precautions: Pregnancy (C), diabetes

NURSING CONSIDERATIONS
Assess:

• Platelets, WBC if systemic absorption occurs

---

* Available in Canada only

- Salicylism: tinnitus, hearing loss, dizziness, confusion, headache, hyperventilation
- Allergic reactions: irritation, redness

Administer:
- Only to intact skin; do not use on inflamed, denuded skin
- After wetting skin; wash thoroughly each AM after treatment
- Using an occlusive dressing to increase absorption, apply more often to areas where occlusion is impossible

Evaluate:
- Therapeutic response: decrease in dandruff, size of lesions

Teach patient/family:
- To avoid contact with eyes, mucous membranes
- To apply lotion if drying occurs
- To avoid applying to large areas; salicylate toxicity may occur

---

salsalate
(sal-sa'late)
Amigesic, Argesic-SA, Arthra-G, Disalcid, Mono-gesic, Salflex, Salsalate, Salsitab
Func. class.: Nonnarcotic analgesic
Chem. class.: Salicylate

Action: Blocks formation of peripheral prostaglandins, which cause pain and inflammation; antipyretic action results from inhibition of hypothalamic heat-regulating center; does not inhibit platelet aggregation
Uses: Mild to moderate pain or fever, including arthritis, juvenile rheumatoid arthritis
Dosage and routes:
- *Adult:* PO 3 g/day in divided doses

Available forms: Caps 500 mg; tabs 500, 750 mg
Side effects/adverse reactions:
*HEMA: **Thrombocytopenia, agranulocytosis, leukopenia, neutropenia, hemolytic anemia,*** increased pro-time
CNS: Stimulation, drowsiness, dizziness, confusion, ***convulsions,*** headache, flushing, hallucinations, coma
GI: Nausea, vomiting, GI bleeding, diarrhea, heartburn, anorexia, **hepatotoxicity**
INTEG: Rash, urticaria, bruising
EENT: Tinnitus, hearing loss
CV: Rapid pulse, ***pulmonary edema***
RESP: Wheezing, hyperpnea
ENDO: Hypoglycemia, hyponatremia, hypokalemia, alteration in acid-base balance
Contraindications: Hypersensitivity to salicylates, NSAIDs, GI bleeding, bleeding disorders, children < 3 yr, Vit K deficiency
Precautions: Anemia, hepatic disease, renal disease, Hodgkin's disease, pregnancy (C), lactation
Pharmacokinetics: Metabolized by liver; excreted by kidneys; half-life 1 hr; highly protein bound; crosses blood-brain barrier and placenta slowly
Interactions/incompatibilities:
- Decreased effects of salsalate: antacids, steroids, urinary alkalizers
- Increased blood loss: alcohol, heparin, ibuprofen, warfarin
- Increased effects of: anticoagulants, insulin, methotrexate, probenecid
- Decreased effects of: spironolactone, sulfinpyrazone, sulfonylmides, loop diuretics
- Toxic effects: PABA

S

---

italics = common side effects   ***bold italic*** = life threatening reactions

• Decreased blood sugar levels: salicylates

Lab test interferences:

Increase: Coagulation studies, liver function studies, serum uric acid, amylase, CO_2, urinary protein

Decrease: Serum K, PBI, cholesterol, blood glucose

Interfere: Urine catecholamines, pregnancy test

NURSING CONSIDERATIONS
Assess:

• Liver function studies: AST, ALT, bilirubin if patient is on long-term therapy

• Renal function studies: BUN, urine creatinine if patient is on long-term therapy

• Blood studies: CBC, Hct, Hgb, pro-time if patient is on long-term therapy

• I&O ratio; decreasing output may indicate renal failure (long-term therapy)

• Hepatotoxicity: dark urine, clay-colored stools, yellowing of skin and sclera, itching, abdominal pain, fever, diarrhea if patient is on long-term therapy

• Allergic reactions: rash, urticaria; if these occur, drug may have to be discontinued

• Renal dysfunction: decreased urine output

• Ototoxicity: tinnitus, ringing, roaring in ears; audiometric testing is needed before, after long-term therapy

• Visual changes: blurring, halos, corneal and retinal damage

• Edema in feet, ankles, legs

• Drug history; there are many drug interactions

Administer:

• To patient crushed or whole; chewable tablets may be chewed

• With food or milk to decrease gastric symptoms; give 30 min before or 2 hr after meals

• With full glass of water

Evaluate:

• Therapeutic response: decreased pain, fever

Teach patient/family:

• To report any symptoms of hepatotoxicity, renal toxicity, visual changes, ototoxicity, allergic reactions (long-term therapy)

• Not to exceed recommended dosage; acute poisoning may result

• To read label on other OTC drugs; many contain aspirin

• That therapeutic response takes 2 wk (arthritis)

• To avoid alcohol ingestion; GI bleeding may occur

Treatment of overdose: Lavage, activated charcoal, monitor electrolytes, VS

---

sargramostim (GM-CSF)
(sare-gram′o-stim)
Leukine, Prokine
Func. class.: Biologic modifier

Action: Stimulates proliferation and differentiation of hematopoietic progenitor cells

Uses: Acceleration of myeloid recovery in patients with non-Hodgkin's lymphoma, acute lymphoblastic leukemia, autologous bone marrow transplantation in Hodgkin's disease; bone marrow transplantation failure or engraftment delay

Dosage and routes:

Myeloid reconstitution after autologous bone marrow transplantation

• *Adult:* IV 250 μg/m²/day × 3 wks; give over 2 hr, 2-4 hr after autologous bone marrow infusion, and not less than 24 hr after last dose of antineoplastics and 12 hr after last dose of radiotherapy, bone marrow transplantation failure, or engraftment delay

• *Adult:* IV 250 μg/m²/day × 14 days; give over 2 hr; may repeat in 7 days, may repeat 500 μg/m²/day × 14 days after another 7 days if no improvement

Available forms: Powder for inj lyophilized 250, 500 μg

Side effects/adverse reactions:

CNS: Fever, malaise, CNS disorder

GI: Nausea, vomiting, diarrhea, anorexia, *GI hemorrhage,* stomatitis, *liver damage*

HEMA: **Blood dyscrasias, hemorrhage**

INTEG: Alopecia, rash, peripheral edema

GU: Urinary tract disorder, abnormal kidney function

Contraindications: Hypersensitivity to GM-CSF, yeast products; excessive leukemic myeloid blast in the bone marrow or peripheral blood

Precautions: Pregnancy (C), lactation, children; renal, hepatic, lung disease; cardiac disease; pleural, pericardial effusions

Pharmacokinetics: Half-life 2 hr, detected within 5 min after administration, peak 2 hr

Interactions/incompatibilities:

• Do not use this drug concomitantly with antineoplastics

• Increased myeloproliferation: lithium, corticosteroids

• Do not add other medications to inf sol

NURSING CONSIDERATIONS
Assess:

• Blood studies: CBC, differential count before treatment and twice weekly; leukocytosis may occur (WBC >50,000 cells/mm³, ANC >20,000 cells/mm³)

• Renal and hepatic studies before

treatment: BUN, creatinine, urinalysis; AST, ALT, alk phosphatase; twice weekly monitoring is needed in renal, hepatic disease

• For hypersensitive reactions, rashes, and local injection site reactions; usually transient

• For increased fluid retention in cardiac disease

Administer:

• After reconstituting with 1 ml sterile water for inj without preservative; do not reenter vial; discard unused portion; direct reconstitution sol at side of vial; rotate contents; do not shake

• Dilute in 0.9% NaCl inj to prepare IV infusion; if final concentration is <10 μg/ml, add human albumin to make a final concentration of 0.1% to the NaCl before adding sargramostim to prevent adsorption; for a final concentration of 0.1% albumin, add 1 mg human albumin/1 ml 0.9% NaCl inj; give within 6 hr after reconstitution

Perform/provide:

• Storage in refrigerator; do not freeze

Evaluate:

• Therapeutic response: WBC and differential recovery

---

scopolamine (transdermal)

(skoe-pol'-a-meen)

Transderm-Scōp

Func. class.: Antiemetic, anticholinergic

Chem. class.: Belladonna alkaloid

Action: Competitive antagonism of acetylcholine at receptor site in eye, smooth muscle, cardiac muscle, glandular cells; inhibition of vestibular input to the CNS, re-

---

sulting in inhibition of vomiting reflex

Uses: Prevention of motion sickness

Dosage and routes:

• *Adult:* PATCH 1 placed behind ear 4-5 hr before travel

• Not recommended for children

Available forms: Patch, 0.5 mg delivered in 72 hr

Side effects/adverse reactions:

INTEG: Rash, erythema

GU: Difficult urination

CNS: Dizziness, drowsiness, confusion, disorientation, memory disturbances, hallucinations

EENT: Blurred vision, altered depth perception, *dilated pupils,* photophobia, *dry mouth;* dry, itchy, red eyes; acute narrow-angle glaucoma

Contraindications: Hypersensitivity, glaucoma

Precautions: Children, elderly, pregnancy (C); pyloric, urinary, bladder neck, intestinal obstruction; liver, kidney disease

Pharmacokinetics:

PATCH: Onset 4-5 hr, duration 72 hr

Interactions/incompatibilities:

• Increased anticholinergic effects: antihistamines, antidepressants

NURSING CONSIDERATIONS

Teach patient/family:

• To avoid hazardous activities, activities requiring alertness; dizziness may occur

• To wash, dry hands before and after applying to surface behind ear

• To change patch q72h

• To apply at least 4 hr before traveling

• If blurred vision, severe dizziness, drowsiness occurs, to discontinue use, use another type of antiemetic

• To read label of all OTC medications; if any scopolamine is found in product, avoid use

• To keep out of children's reach

---

scopolamine hydrobromide

(skoe-pol′a-meen)

Func. class.: Cholinergic blocker

Chem. class.: Belladonna alkaloid

Action: Inhibits acetylcholine at receptor sites in autonomic nervous system, which controls secretions, free acids in stomach; blocks central muscarinic receptors, which decreases involuntary movements

Uses: Reduction of secretions before surgery, calm delirium, motion sickness

Dosage and routes:

Parkinson symptoms

• *Adult:* IM/SC/IV 0.3-0.6 mg tid-qid diluted using dilution provided

• *Child:* SC 0.006 mg/kg tid-qid or 0.2 mg/m^2

Preoperatively

• *Adult:* SC 0.4-0.6 mg

Available forms: Inj 0.3, 0.4, 0.86, 1 mg/ml

Side effects/adverse reactions:

CNS: Confusion, anxiety, restlessness, irritability, delusions, hallucinations, headache, sedation, depression, incoherence, dizziness, excitement, delirium, flushing, weakness

INTEG: Urticaria

MISC: Suppression of lactation, nasal congestion, decreased sweating

EENT: Blurred vision, photophobia, dilated pupils, difficulty swallowing, mydriasis, cycloplegia

CV: Palpitations, tachycardia, postural hypotension, paradoxical bradycardia

GI: Dryness of mouth, constipation, nausea, vomiting, abdominal distress, *paralytic ileus*

GU: Hesitancy, retention

Contraindications: Hypersensitivity, narrow-angle glaucoma, myasthenia gravis, GI/GU obstruction, hypersensitivity to belladonna, barbiturates

Precautions: Pregnancy (C), elderly, lactation, prostatic hypertrophy, CHF, hypertension, dysrhythmia, children, gastric ulcer

Pharmacokinetics:

SC/IM: Peak 30-45 min, duration 7 hr

IV: Peak 10-15 min, duration 4 hr Excreted in urine, bile, feces (unchanged)

Interactions/incompatibilities:

• Increased anticholinergic effect: alcohol, narcotics, antihistamines, phenothiazines, tricyclics

• Do not mix with diazepam, chloramphenicol, pentobarbital, sodium bicarbonate in syringe or sol

NURSING CONSIDERATIONS

Assess:

• I&O ratio; retention commonly causes decreased urinary output

• Parkinsonism, extrapyramidal symptoms: shuffling gait, muscle rigidity, involuntary movements

• Urinary hesitancy, retention; palpate bladder if retention occurs

• Constipation; increase fluids, bulk, exercise if this occurs

• For tolerance over long-term therapy; dose may have to be increased or changed

• Mental status: affect, mood, CNS depression, worsening of mental symptoms during early therapy

Administer:

• Parenteral dose with patient re-

cumbent to prevent postural hypotension

• With or after meals for GI upset; may give with fluids other than H_2O

• At hs to avoid daytime drowsiness in patient with parkinsonism

• Parenteral dose slowly; keep in bed for at least 1 hr after dose

• With analgesic to avoid behavioral changes when given as a preop

Perform/provide:

• Storage at room temperature in light-resistant container

• Hard candy, frequent drinks, sugarless gum to relieve dry mouth

Evaluate:

• Therapeutic response: decreased secretions

Teach patient/family:

• Not to discontinue this drug abruptly; to taper off over 1 wk

• To avoid driving, other hazardous activities; drowsiness may occur

• To avoid OTC medication: cough, cold preparations with alcohol, antihistamines unless directed by physician

scopolamine hydrobromide (optic)

(skoe-pol'a-meen)

Isopto-Hyoscine

Func. class.: Mydriatic

Chem. class.: Synthetic alkaloid

Action: Blocks response of iris sphincter muscle, muscle of accommodation of ciliary body to cholinergic stimulation, resulting in dilation, paralysis of accommodation

Uses: Uveitis, iritis, cycloplegia, mydriasis

Dosage and routes:

• *Adult:* INSTILL 1-2 gtts before

S

refraction or 1-2 gtts qd-tid for iritis or uveitis
• *Child:* INSTILL 1 gtt bid × 2 days before refraction
Available forms include: Sol 0.25%
Side effects/adverse reactions:
CV: Tachycardia
CNS: Confusion, somnolence, flushing, fever
EENT: Blurred vision, photophobia, increased intraocular pressure, irritation, edema
Contraindications: Hypersensitivity, children <6 yr, narrow-angle glaucoma, increased intraocular pressure, infants
Precautions: Children, elderly, hypertension, hyperthyroidism, diabetes, pregnancy (C), lactation, Down syndrome
Pharmacokinetics:
INSTILL: Peak 20-30 min, duration 3-7 days
NURSING CONSIDERATIONS
Assess:
• Eye pain; discontinue use
Evaluate:
• Therapeutic response: decrease in inflammation, cycloplegic refraction
Teach patient/family:
• To report change in vision; blurring or loss of sight; trouble breathing; inhibition of sweating; flushing
• Method of instillation: pressure on lacrimal sac for 1 min; do not touch dropper to eye
• That blurred vision will decrease with repeated use of drug
• Not to engage in hazardous activities until able to see
• Wait 5 min to use other drops
• Do not blink more than usual

secobarbital/secobarbital sodium

(see-koe-bar′bi-tal)
Secobarbital Sodium, Secogen Sodium,* Seconal Sodium, Seconal Sodium Pulvules, Seral,* Secretin-Ferring
Func. class.: Sedative/hypnotic-barbiturate
Chem. class.: Barbitone (short acting)

Controlled Substance Schedule II (USA), Schedule G (Canada)
Action: Depresses activity in brain cells primarily in reticular activating system in brain stem; selectively depresses neurons in posterior hypothalamus, limbic structures; decreases seizure activity by inhibition of epileptic activity in CNS
Uses: Insomnia, sedation, preoperative medication, status epilepticus, acute tetanus convulsions
Dosage and routes:
Insomnia
• *Adult:* PO/IM 100-200 mg hs
• *Child:* IM 3-5 mg/kg, not to exceed 100 mg, not to inject >5 ml in one site; REC 4-5 mg/kg
Sedation/preoperatively
• *Adult:* PO 200-300 mg 1-2 hr preoperatively
• *Child:* PO 50-100 mg 1-2 hr preoperatively; REC 4-5 mg/kg 1-2 hr preoperatively
Status epilepticus
• *Adult and child:* IM/IV 250-350 mg
Acute psychotic agitation
• *Adult and child:* IM/IV 5.5 mg/kg q3-4h
Available forms: Caps 50, 100 mg; tabs 100 mg, inj IM, IV 50 mg/ml; powder, rec supp 200 mg

Side effects/adverse reactions:

CNS: Lethargy, drowsiness, hangover, dizziness, paradoxical stimulation in the elderly and children, light-headedness, dependency, CNS depression, mental depression, slurred speech

GI: Nausea, vomiting, diarrhea, constipation

INTEG: Rash, urticaria, pain, abscesses at injection site, angioedema, thrombophlebitis, ***Stevens-Johnson syndrome***

CV: Hypotension, bradycardia

RESP: Depression, ***apnea, laryngospasm, bronchospasm***

*HEMA: **Agranulocytosis, thrombocytopenia, megaloblastic anemia*** (long-term treatment)

Contraindications: Hypersensitivity to barbiturates, respiratory depression, addiction to barbiturates, severe liver impairment, porphyria, uncontrolled severe pain

Precautions: Anemia, pregnancy (D), lactation, hepatic disease, renal disease, hypertension, elderly, acute/chronic pain

Pharmacokinetics:

IM: Onset 10-15 min, duration 4-6 hr

REC: Onset slow, duration 3-6 hr; metabolized by liver, excreted by kidneys (metabolites); half-life 15-40 hr

Interactions/incompatibilities:

• Do not mix with other drugs in sol or syringe

• Increased CNS depression: alcohol, MAOIs, sedative, narcotics

• Decreased effect of: oral anticoagulants, corticosteroids, griseofulvin, quinidine

• Decreased half-life of doxycycline

• Incompatible with atracurium, benzquinamide, chlordiazepoxide, chlorpromazine, cimetidine, clindamycin, codeine, diphenhydramine, droperidol, ephedrine, erythromycin, glycopyrrolate, hydrocortisone, insulin, isoproterenol, levarterenol, levorphanol, meperidine, methadone, methyldopate, penicillin G, pentazocine, phenytoin, prochlorperazine, promethazine, streptomycin, succinycholine, tetracycline, vancomycin

Lab test interferences:

False increase: Sulfobromophthalein

NURSING CONSIDERATIONS

Assess:

• VS q30min after parenteral route for 2 hr

• Blood studies: Hct, Hgb, RBCs, serum folate, Vit D (if on long-term therapy); pro-time in patients receiving anticoagulants

• Hepatic studies: AST, ALT, bilirubin; if increased, the drug is usually discontinued

• Unresolved pain, as drug may cause severe stimulation if pain is present

• Mental status: mood, sensorium, affect, memory (long, short)

• Physical dependency: more frequent requests for medication, shakes, anxiety

• Barbiturate toxicity: hypotension; pulmonary constriction; cold, clammy skin; cyanosis of lips; insomnia; nausea; vomiting; hallucinations; delirium; weakness; mild symptoms may occur in 8-12 hr without drug

• Respiratory dysfunction: depression, character, rate, rhythm; hold drug if respirations <10/min or if pupils dilated

• Blood dyscrasias: fever, sore throat, bruising, rash, jaundice, epistaxis

• Perianal irritation if rectal forms used

S

---

italics = common side effects   ***bold italic*** = life threatening reactions

Administer:
• IV after diluting with sterile H_2O for inj; rotate; give 50 mg or less over 1 min; titrate to patient response
• After removal of cigarettes to prevent fires
• IM injection in deep large muscle mass to prevent tissue sloughing and abscesses
• After conservative measures for insomnia have been tried
• Within 30 min of mixing with sterile water for injection; reconstitute after rotating ampule; do not shake; do not use cloudy solution; may be given directly or indirectly
• IV only with resuscitative equipment available; administer at <100 mg/min (only by qualified personnel)
• ½-1 hr before hs for sleeplessness
• On empty stomach for best absorption
• For <14 days, since drug is not effective after that; tolerance develops
• Crushed or whole
• Alone; do not mix with other drugs or inject if there is precipitate
• After cleansing enema if given rectally preoperatively in children

Perform/provide:
• Assistance with ambulation after receiving dose
• Safety measure: side rails, nightlight, call bell within easy reach
• Checking to see PO medication has been swallowed
• Storage of suppositories in refrigerator; do not use aqueous solutions containing precipitate

Evaluate:
• Therapeutic response: ability to sleep at night, decreased amount of early morning awakening if taking drug for insomnia, or decrease in number, severity of seizures if taking drug for seizure disorder

Teach patient/family:
• That morning hangover is common
• That drug is indicated only for short-term treatment of insomnia and is probably ineffective after 2 wk
• That physical dependency may result when used for extended periods (45-90 days depending on dose)
• To avoid driving other activities requiring alertness
• To avoid alcohol ingestion, CNS depressants; serious CNS depression may result
• Not to discontinue medication quickly after long-term use; drug should be tapered over 1-2 wk
• To tell all prescribers that barbiturate is being taken
• That withdrawal insomnia may occur after short-term use; do not start using drug again; insomnia will improve in 1-3 nights; may experience increased dreaming
• That effects may take 2 nights for benefits to be noticed
• Alternative measures to improve sleep (reading, exercise several hours before hs, warm bath, warm milk, TV, self-hypnosis, deep breathing)

Treatment of overdose: Lavage, activated charcoal, warming blanket, vital signs, hemodialysis, I&O ratio

selegiline HCl
(L-Deprenyl)
(sel-ee-gill'ene)
Eldepryl

Func. class.: Antiparkinson agent
Chem. class.: Levorotatory acetylenic derivative of phenethylamine

Action: Increased dopaminergic activity by inhibition of MAO type B activity; not fully understood

Uses: Adjunct management of Parkinson's disease in patients being treated with levodopa/carbidopa who have had a poor response to therapy

Dosage and routes:
• *Adult:* PO 10 mg/day in divided doses 5 mg at breakfast and lunch, after 2-3 days begin to reduce the dose of levodopa/carbidopa 10%-30%

Available forms: Tabs 5 mg

Side effects/adverse reactions:
CNS: Increased tremors, chorea, restlessness, blepharospasm, increased bradykinesia, grimacing, tardive dyskinesia, dystonic symptoms, involuntary movements, increased apraxia, hallucinations, dizziness, mood changes, nightmares, delusions, lethargy, apathy, overstimulation, sleep disturbances, headache, migraine, numbness, muscle cramps, confusion, anxiety, tiredness, vertigo, personality change, back/leg pain
CV: Orthostatic hypotension, hypertension, dysrhythmia, palpitations, angina pectoris, hypotension, tachycardia, edema, sinus bradycardia, syncope
GI: Nausea, vomiting, constipation, weight loss, anorexia, diarrhea, heartburn, rectal bleeding, poor appetite, dysphagia
GU: Slow urination, nocturia, prostatic hypertrophy, hesitation, retention, frequency, sexual dysfunction
INTEG: Increased sweating, alopecia, hematoma, rash, photosensitivity, facial hair
RESP: Asthma, shortness of breath
EENT: Diplopia, dry mouth, blurred vision, tinnitus

Contraindications: Hypersensitivity

Precautions: Pregnancy (C), lactation, children

Pharmacokinetics:
Rapidly absorbed, peak ½-2 hr; rapidly metabolized (active metabolites: N-desmethyldeprenyl, amphetamine, methamphetamine), metabolites excreted in urine

Interactions/incompatibilities:
• **Fatal interaction:** opioids (especially meperidine); do not administer together

Lab test interferences:
False positive: urine ketones, urine glucose
False negative: urine glucose (glucose oxidase)
False increase: uric acid, urine protein
Decrease: VMA

NURSING CONSIDERATIONS
Assess:
• B/P, respiration
• Mental status: affect, mood behavioral changes, depression; perform suicide assessment

Administer:
• Drug until NPO before surgery
• Adjusting dosage to patient response
• With meals; limit protein taken with drug
• At doses <10 mg/day because of risks associated with nonselective inhibition of MAO

S

Perform/provide:
• Assistance with ambulation, during beginning therapy

Evaluate:
• Therapeutic response: decrease in akathisia, increased mood

Teach patient/family:
• To change positions slowly to prevent orthostatic hypotension
• To report side effects: twitching, eye spasms; indicate overdose
• To use drug exactly as prescribed; if drug is discontinued abruptly, parkinsonian crisis may occur
• To avoid foods high in tyramine: cheese, pickled products, wine, beer, large amounts of caffeine
• Not to exceed recommended dose of 10 ml because might precipitate a hypertensive crisis; report severe headache or other unusual symptoms

Treatment of overdose: IV fluids for hypertension, IV dilute pressure agent for B/P titration

---

selenium sulfide
(see-leen'ee-um)
Exsel, Head and Shoulders Intensive Treatment, Selenium Sulfide, Selsun, Selsun Blue
Func. class.: Local antiseborrheic, antifungal

Action: Appears to have cytostatic effect on epidural cells and reduces corneocyte production

Uses: Dandruff, seborrhea; dermatitis of the scalp, versicolor

Dosage and routes:
• *Adult and child:* TOP wash hair with 1-2 tsp, leave on 2-3 min; rinse, repeat; use 2 applications/wk × 2 wk, then q3-4 wk or as needed

Available forms: Shampoo lotion 1%, 2.5%

Side effects/adverse reactions:
INTEG: Oiliness of hair/scalp, alopecia, discoloration of hair, skin irritation

Contraindications: Hypersensitivity to sulfur preparations, inflamed skin

Precautions: Infants, pregnancy (C)

NURSING CONSIDERATIONS

Assess:
• Area of body involved, including time involved, what helps or aggravates condition

Perform/provide:
• Thorough hair rinsing after use
• Storage at room temperature in tight container

Evaluate:
• Toxicity: tremors, perspiration, pain in abdomen, weakness, anorexia

Teach patient/family:
• To avoid contact with eyes, genital area
• To discontinue use if rash or irritation occurs
• That drug may damage jewelry; remove before application
• That drug is not be taken internally

---

senna
(sin'na)
Black Draught, Dr. Caldwell Senna Laxative, Fletcher's Castoria, Gentlax, Senexon, Senna-Gen, Senokot, Senokotxtra, Senolax
Func. class.: Laxative-stimulant
Chem. class.: Anthraquinone

Action: Stimulates peristalsis by action on Auerbach's plexus

Uses: Constipation; bowel preparation for surgery or examination

---

Dosage and routes:
• *Adult:* PO 1-8 tabs (Senokot)/day
½ to 4 tsp of granules added to
water or juice; REC SUPP 1-2 hs;
SYR 1-4 tsp hs, 7.5-15 ml; (Black
Draught) ¾ oz dissolved in 2.5 oz
liquid given between 2-4 PM the day
before procedure (X-Prep)
• *Child >27 kg:* ½ adult dose; do
not use Black Draught for children
• *Child 1 mo-1 yr:* SYR 1.25-2.5
ml (Senokot) hs
Available forms: Supp 625 mg, 30
mg sennosides; powder 662 mg/g,
6, 15 mg sennosides/3g; tabs 8.6
sennosides, 180 mg
Side effects/adverse reactions:
*GI: Nausea, vomiting, anorexia,
cramps,* diarrhea
META: Hypocalcemia, enteropathy,
alkalosis, hypokalemia, ***tetany***
Contraindications: Hypersensitivity, GI bleeding, obstruction, CHF,
lactation, abdominal pain, nausea/
vomiting, appendicitis, acute surgical abdomen
Precautions: Pregnancy (C)
Pharmacokinetics:
PO: Onset 6-24 hr; metabolized by
liver, excreted in feces
Interactions/incompatibilities:
• Do not use with disulfiram (An-
tabuse)
NURSING CONSIDERATIONS
Assess:
• Blood, urine electrolytes if drug
is used often by patient
• I&O ratio to identify fluid loss
• Cause of constipation; identify
whether fluids, bulk, or exercise is
missing from life-style
• Cramping, rectal bleeding, nau-
sea, vomiting; if these symptoms
occur, drug should be discontinued
Administer:
• In morning or evening (oral dose)
Evaluate:
• Therapeutic response: decrease in
constipation

Teach patient/family:
• That urine, feces may turn yellow-brown to red
• Not to use laxatives for long-term
therapy; bowel tone will be lost
• That normal bowel movements
do not always occur daily
• Not to use in presence of abdominal pain, nausea, vomiting
• To notify physician if constipation unrelieved or of symptoms of
electrolyte imbalance: muscle
cramps, pain, weakness, dizziness,
excessive thirst

---

sertraline
(sir′trall-en)
Zoloft
Func. class.: Antidepressant

Action: Inhibits serotonin reuptake
Uses: Major depression
Dosage and routes:
• *Adult:* PO 50 mg qd; may increase to a maximum of 200 mg/
day; do not change dose at intervals
of <1 wk; administer qd in AM, PM
Available forms: Tabs 50, 100 mg
Side effects/adverse reactions:
CNS: Insomnia, agitation, somnolence, dizziness, headache, tremor,
fatigue, paresthesia, twitching,
confusion, ataxia
GU: Male sexual dysfunction, micturition disorder
GI: Diarrhea, nausea, constipation,
anorexia, dry mouth, dyspepsia,
vomiting, flatulence
CV: Palpitations, chest pain, hypotension
EENT: Vision abnormalities
Contraindications: Hypersensitivity
Precautions: Pregnancy (B), lactation, elderly, hepatic, renal disease, epilepsy

S

---

italics = common side effects   ***bold italic*** = life threatening reactions

Pharmacokinetics:
PO: Peak 6-10 hr, plasma protein binding 99%, elimination half-life 25 hr, extensively metabolized, metabolite excreted in urine

Interactions/incompatibilities:
• Increased effects of: alcohol, diazepam, tolbutamide, warfarin
• Fatal reactions: MAOIs
• Altered lithium levels: lithium

Lab test interferences:
Increase: Serum bilirubin, blood glucose, alk phosphatase
Decreased: VMA, 5-HIAA
False increase: Urinary catecholamines

NURSING CONSIDERATIONS
Assess:
• Mental status: mood sensorium, affect, suicidal tendencies, increase in psychiatric symptoms, depression, panic
• B/P (lying/standing), pulse q4h; if systolic B/P drops 20 mm Hg, hold drug, notify physician; take vital signs q4h in patients with cardiovascular disease
• Weight weekly; appetite may decrease with drug
• Urinary retention, constipation, especially in elderly
• Withdrawal symptoms: headache, nausea, vomiting, muscle pain, weakness; do not usually occur unless drug is discontinued abruptly
• Alcohol consumption; if alcohol is consumed, hold dose until morning

Administer:
• Increased fluids, bulk in diet if constipation, urinary retention occur
• With food or milk for GI symptoms
• Crushed if patient is unable to swallow medication whole

• Gum, hard candy, frequent sips of water for dry mouth

Perform/provide:
• Storage at room temperature; do not freeze
• Assistance with ambulation during therapy, since drowsiness, dizziness occur
• Safety measures, including side rails, primarily for elderly
• Checking to see that PO medication is swallowed

Evaluate:
• Therapeutic response: significant improvement in depression

Teach patient/family:
• That therapeutic effect may take 2-3 wk
• To use caution in driving, other activities requiring alertness, because drowsiness, dizziness, blurred vision may occur
• Not to discontinue medication quickly after long-term use; may cause nausea, headache, malaise
• To avoid alcohol, other CNS depressants
• To notify physician if pregnant or plan to become pregnant or breastfeed

---

silver nitrate
Func. class.: Keratolytic

Action: Antiinfective, astringent, caustic
Uses: Cauterization of lesions, warts, burns (low concentrations)
Dosage and routes:
• *Adult and child:* TOP apply to area to be treated
Available forms: Sticks, sol 10%, 25%, 50%
Side effects/adverse reactions:
INTEG: Skin discoloration
Contraindications: Hypersensitivity

---

silver sulfadiazine (topical)

Interactions/incompatibilities:
• Not to be used with alkalies, phosphates, thimerosal, benzalkonium chloride, halogenated acids
NURSING CONSIDERATIONS
Administer:
• After moistening stick with water
• To burns using a wet dressing (low concentrations 0.125%)
Evaluate:
• Therapeutic response: absence of lesions, healing of burned areas
Perform/provide:
• Storage in cool area
Teach patient/family:
• To avoid contact with clothing or unaffected areas; discoloration may occur

---

silver nitrate 1% (ophthalmic)
Func. class.: Antiinfective

Action: Inhibits metabolic actions in susceptible organisms
Uses: Prevention, treatment of gonorrheal ophthalmia neonatorum
Dosage and routes:
• *Neonate:* INSTILL 2 gtts of 1% solution into each eye
Available forms: Sol
Side effects/adverse reactions:
EENT: Redness, discharge, edema, swelling
Contraindications: Hypersensitivity
Precautions: Antibiotic hypersensitivity, pregnancy (C)
NURSING CONSIDERATIONS
Administer:
• After washing hands
Perform/provide:
• Storage at room temperature in tight, light-resistant container
Evaluate:
• Allergy: itching, lacrimation, redness, swelling

---

silver protein, mild
Argyrol S.S. 10%, Argyrol S.S. 20%

Func. class.: Disinfectant
Chem. class.: Silver colloidal compound

Action: Destroys gram-positive, gram-negative organisms
Uses: Eye, nose, throat, swelling, infection
Dosage and routes:
• *Adult and child:* TOP sol use as needed
Available forms: Top sol 5%, 10%, 25%; eyedrops 20%
Side effects/adverse reactions:
INTEG: Irritation, discoloration of tissue
Contraindications: Hypersensitivity
Precautions: Pregnancy (C)
NURSING CONSIDERATIONS
Administer:
• To area to be treated only; do not apply to healthy skin
Perform/provide:
• Storage in tight container
Evaluate:
• Area of body involved: irritation, rash, breaks, dryness, scales

---

silver sulfadiazine (topical)
(sul-fa-dye′a-zeen)
Silvadene, SSD, SSD AF
Func. class.: Local antiinfective
Chem. class.: Sulfonamide

Action: Interferes with bacterial cell wall synthesis, broad-spectrum
Uses: Burns (2nd, 3rd degree); prevention of wound sepsis

italics = common side effects   ***bold italic*** = life threatening reactions

Dosage and routes:
• *Adult and child:* TOP apply ¹⁄₁₆ in to affected area qd-bid
Available forms: Cream 10 mg/g
Side effects/adverse reactions:
INTEG: Rash, urticaria, stinging, burning, itching, pain, skin necrosis, erythema
HEMA: Reversible leukopenia
Contraindications: Hypersensitivity, child <2 mo
Precautions: Impaired renal function, pregnancy (C), impaired hepatic function, lactation
NURSING CONSIDERATIONS
Assess:
• Allergic reaction: burning, stinging, swelling, redness
• Renal function studies; check for crystalluria
Administer:
• Using aseptic technique, use sterile gloves
• Enough medication to cover burns completely; keep covered with medication at all times
• After cleansing debris before each application; bathe daily
• Analgesic before application if needed
Perform/provide:
• Storage at room temperature in dry place
Evaluate:
• Therapeutic response: relief of infection
Teach patient/family:
• That drug may be continued until graft can be done

---

simethicone
(si-meth′-i-kone)
Extra Strength Gas-X, Gas-X, Mylicon, Mylicon 80, Ovol,* Phazyme, Phazyme 95, Phazyme 125
Func. class.: Antiflatulent

Action: Disperses, prevents gas pockets in GI system
Uses: Flatulence
Dosage and routes:
• *Adult and child >12 yr:* PO 40-100 mg pc, hs
Available forms: Chew tabs 40, 80 mg; tabs 50, 60, 95, 125 mg; drops 40 mg/0.6 ml
Side effects/adverse reactions:
GI: Belching, rectal flatus
Contraindications: Hypersensitivity
Precautions: Pregnancy (C)
NURSING CONSIDERATIONS
Evaluate:
• Therapeutic response: absence of flatulence
Teach patient/family:
• That tablets must be chewed
• To shake suspension well before pouring

---

simvastatin
(sem-va-sta′-tin)
Zocor
Func. class.: Antihyperlipidemic
Chem. class.: Synthetically derived fermentation product

Action: Inhibits HMG-CoA reductase enzyme, which reduces cholesterol synthesis
Uses: As an adjunct in primary hypercholesterolemia (types IIa, IIb)
Dosage and routes:
• *Adult:* PO 5-10 mg qd in PM ini-

tially; usual range 5-40 mg/day qd in PM, not to exceed 40 mg/day; dosage adjustments may be made in 4-wk intervals or more

Available forms: Tabs 5, 10, 20, 40 mg

Side effects/adverse reactions:

INTEG: Rash, pruritus, alopecia

GI: Nausea, constipation, diarrhea, dyspepsia, flatus, abdominal pain, heartburn, *liver dysfunction,* pancreatitis

EENT: Lens opacities

MS: Muscle cramps, myalgia, *myositis, rhabdomyolysis*

CNS: Headache, tremor, vertigo, peripheral neuropathy

Contraindications: Hypersensitivity, pregnancy (X), lactation, active liver disease

Precautions: Past liver disease, alcoholism, severe acute infections, trauma, hypotension, uncontrolled seizure disorders, severe metabolic disorders, electrolyte imbalances

Pharmacokinetics: Peak 1-2 ½ hr, metabolized in liver (active metabolites), highly protein bound, excreted primarily in bile, feces

Interactions/incompatibilities:

• Increased effects of: coumadin

• Increased myalgia, myositis: cyclosporine, gemfibrozil, niacin, erthyromycin

• Increased serum level of: digoxin

Lab test interferences:

Increase: CPK, liver function tests

NURSING CONSIDERATIONS

Assess:

• Cholesterol levels periodically during treatment

• Liver function studies q1-2mo during the first 1½ yr of treatment; AST, ALT, liver function tests may increase

• Renal studies in patients with compromised renal system: BUN, I&O ratio, creatinine

• Eyes [...] after t[...] lens op[...]

Admin[...]

• Total [...]

Perfor[...]

• Storag[...] tight contai[...]

Evaluate:

• Therapeutic response: decrease in cholesterol to desired level after 8 wk

Teach patient/family:

• That treatment will take several years

• That blood work and eye exam will be necessary during treatment

• To report blurred vision, severe GI symptoms, dizziness, headache

• That previously prescribed regimen will continue: low-cholesterol diet, exercise program

sodium bicarbonate

Func. class.: Alkalinizer

Chem. class.: NaHCO₃

Action: Orally neutralizes gastric acid, which forms water, NaCl, CO_2; increases plasma bicarbonate, which buffers H^+ ion concentration; reverses acidosis

Uses: Acidosis (metabolic), cardiac arrest, alkalinization (systemic/urinary) antacid

Dosage and routes:

Acidosis

• *Adult and child:* IV INF 2-5 mEq/kg over 4-8 hr depending on CO_2, pH

Cardiac arrest

• *Adult and child:* IV BOL 1 mEq/kg, then 0.5 mEq/kg q10 min, then doses based an ABGs

• *Infant:* IV INF not to exceed 8 mEq/kg/day based on ABGs (4.2% sol)

S

---

italics = common side effects   ***bold italic*** = life threatening reactions

325 mg-2 g qid
PO 12-120 mg/kg/day

ult: PO 300 mg-2 g chewed, taken with H_2O qd-qid
Available forms: Tabs 325, 520, 650 mg; powder; inj 4%, 4.2%, 5%, 7.5%, 8.4%

Side effects/adverse reactions:
CNS: Irritability, headache, confusion, stimulation, tremors, *twitching, hyperreflexia,* **tetany,** weakness, **convulsions** caused by alkalosis
CV: Irregular pulse, **cardiac arrest,** water retention, edema, weight gain
GI: Flatulence, *belching, distention,* **paralytic ileus,** acid rebound
META: Alkalosis
GU: Calculi
RESP: Shallow, slow respirations, cyanosis, **apnea**
Contraindications: Hypertension, peptic ulcer, renal disease, hypocalcemia
Precautions: CHF, cirrhosis, toxemia, renal disease, pregnancy (C)
Pharmacokinetics:
PO: Onset 2 min, duration 10 min
IV: Onset 15 min, duration 1-2 hr, excreted in urine
Interactions/incompatibilities:
• Increases effects: amphetamines, mecamylamine, quinine, quinidine, pseudoephedrine, flecainide, anorexants
• Decreases effects: lithium, chlorpropamide, barbiturates, salicylates, benzodiazepines
• Increased Na and decreased K: corticosteroids
• Incompatible with atropine, Ca, carmustine, cefotaxime, chlorpromazine, cisplatin, codeine, corticotropin, dobutamine, dopamine, epinephrine, glycopyrrolate, hydromorphone, insulin, isoproterenol, labetalol, levarterenol, levorphanol, lincomycin, magnesium sulfate, meperidine, methadone, methicillin, morphine, penicillin G, pentobarbital, pentazocine, phenobarbital, procaine, promazine, secobarbital, streptomycin, succinylcholine, tetracycline, thiopental, vancomycin

Lab test interferences:
Increase: Urinary urobilinogen
False positive: Urinary protein, blood lactate

NURSING CONSIDERATIONS
Assess:
• Respiratory and pulse rate, rhythm, depth, lung sounds; notify physician of abnormalities
• Fluid balance (I&O, weight qd, edema); notify physician of fluid overload
• Electrolytes, blood pH, PO_2, HCO_3, during treatment; ABGs frequently during emergencies
• Urine pH, urinary output, during beginning treatment
• Extravasation with IV administration (tissue sloughing, ulceration, and necrosis)
• Weight daily with initial therapy
• Alkalosis: irritability, confusion, twitching, hyperreflexia stimulation, slow respirations, cyanosis, irregular pulse
• Milk-alkali syndrome: confusion, headache, nausea, vomiting, anorexia, urinary stones, hypercalcemia
Administer:
• IV in prepared sol or diluted in an equal amount of compatible sol given 2-5mEq/kg over 4-8 hr, not to exceed 50mEq/hr; slower rate in children
Evaluate:
• Therapeutic response: ABGs,

electrolytes, blood pH, HCO₃ WNL
Teach patient/family:
• To chew antacid tablets and drink 8 oz water
• Not to take antacid with milk, or milk-alkali syndrome may result
• Not to use antacid for more than 2 weeks
• To notify physician if indigestion is accompanied by chest pain, dyspnea, diarrhea, dark, tarry stools
• About sodium-restricted diet; to avoid use of baking soda for indigestion

---

sodium biphosphate/ sodium phosphate

Enemeez, Fleet Enema, Phospho-Soda, Saf-tip Phosphate Enema/Sal-Hepatica
Func. class.: Laxative, saline

Action: Increases water absorption in the small intestine by osmotic action
Uses: Constipation, bowel or rectal preparation for surgery, examination
Dosage and routes:
• *Adult:* PO 5-20 ml with H₂O; powder 4 g dissolved in H₂O; sol 20-46 ml mixed with 4 oz cold H₂O; enema 2-4.5 oz
Available forms: Powder, sol
Side effects/adverse reactions:
GI: Nausea, cramps, diarrhea
META: Electrolyte, fluid imbalances
Contraindications: Hypersensitivity, rectal fissures, abdominal pain, nausea/vomiting, appendicitis, acute surgical abdomen, ulcerated hemorrhoids, Na-restricted diets (Sal-Hepatica, PhosphoSoda)
Precautions: Pregnancy (C)

Pharmacokinetics: Excreted in feces
NURSING CONSIDERATIONS
Assess:
• Blood, urine electrolytes if drug is used often by patient
• I&O ratio to identify fluid loss
• Cause of constipation; identify whether fluids, bulk, or exercise is missing from life-style
• Cramping, rectal bleeding, nausea, vomiting; if these symptoms occur, drug should be discontinued
Administer:
• Alone for better absorption; do not take within 1 hr of other drugs
Evaluate:
• Therapeutic response: decrease in constipation
Teach patient/family:
• Not to use laxatives for long-term therapy; bowel tone will be lost
• That normal bowel movements do not always occur daily
• Not to use in presence of abdominal pain, nausea, vomiting
• To notify physician if constipation unrelieved or if symptoms of electrolyte imbalance occur: muscle cramps, pain, weakness, dizziness, excessive thirst
• To maintain adequate fluid consumption

---

sodium chloride, hypertonic

Adsorbonac Ophthalmic Solution, AK-NaCl, Dey-Pak Sodium Chloride 3% and 10%, Muro-128 Ophthalmic, Muroptic-S
Func. class.: Miscellaneous ophthalmic agent
Chem. class.: Hyperosmolar ophthalmic

Action: Reduces corneal edema by

S

---

osmosis of water through corneal epithelium, which is semipermeable

Uses: Reduces corneal edema

Dosage and routes:
• *Adult:* INSTILL 1-2 gtts q3-4h or ointment hs

Available forms: Sol 2%, 5%; oint 5%

Side effects/adverse reactions:
EENT: Stinging

Contraindications: Hypersensitivity

NURSING CONSIDERATIONS
Perform/provide:
• Storage in tight container

Evaluate:
• Therapeutic response: decreased corneal edema

Teach patient/family:
• Method of instillation, including pressure on lacrimal sac for 1 min, and not to touch dropper to eye
• That blurred vision is common with oint
• To report double vision, rapid change in vision, appearance of floating spots, acute redness of eyes

---

sodium fluoride

ACT, Checkmate, Fluor-A-Day,* Fluorigard, Fluorinse, Fluoritab, Fluotic,* Flura, Flura-Drops, Flura-Loz, Gel II, Gel-Kam, Gel-Tin, Karidium, Karigel, Karigel-N, Listermint with Fluoride, Loz-Tabs, Luride, Luride-SF, Luride Lozi-Tabs, Luride 0.25 Lozi-Tabs, Luride 0.5 Lozi-Tabs, Minute-Gel, Pediaflor, Pharmaflur, Pharmaflur 1.1, Pharmaflur df, Phos-Flur, Point-Two, Prevident, Sodium Fluoride, Stop, Thera-Flur, Thera-Flur-N

Func. class.: Trace elements
Chem. class.: Fluorideion

Action: Needed for hard tooth enamel and for resistance to periodontal disease; reduces acid production by dental bacteria

Uses: Prevention of dental caries

Dosage and routes:
• *Adult and child >12 yr:* TOP 10 ml 0.2% sol qd after brushing teeth, rinse mouth for >1 min with sol
• *Child 6-12 yr:* TOP 5 ml 0.2% sol
• *Child >3 yr:* PO 1 mg qd
• *Child <3 yr:* PO 0.5 mg

Available forms: Tabs chewable 0.25 mg; tabs 0.5, 1 mg, tabs effervescent 10 mg; drops 0.125, 0.25, 0.5 mg/ml; rinse supplements 0.2 mg/ml, rinse 0.01%, 0.02%, 0.09%; gel 0.1%, 0.5%, 1.23%

Side effects/adverse reactions:
ACUTE OVERDOSE: Black tarry stools, bloody vomit, diarrhea, decreased respiration, increased salivation, watery eyes
CHRONIC OVERDOSE: Hypocalcemia and tetany, respiratory arrest, sores in mouth, constipation, loss of appetite, nausea, vomiting, weight loss, discoloration of teeth (white, black, brown)

Contraindications: Hypersensitivity, pregnancy (D)

Precautions: Child < 6 yr

Pharmacokinetics:
PO: Excreted in urine and feces; crosses placenta, breast milk

Interactions/incompatibilities:
• Avoid use with dairy products

NURSING CONSIDERATIONS
Assess:
• Use in children
• Nutritional status: increase fluoride content of water, decrease carbohydrate snacks, increase fish, tea, mineral water

Administer:
• Drops after meals with fluids or undiluted tablets; may be chewed;

---

do not swallow whole; may be given with water or juice; avoid milk

Evaluate:
• Therapeutic response: absence of dental caries

Teach patient/family:
• To monitor children using gel or rinse; not to be swallowed
• Not to drink, eat, or rinse mouth for at least ½ hr
• Not to use during pregnancy
• To apply after brushing and flossing hs
• To store out of children's reach

sodium polystyrene sulfonate

(pol-ee-stye′-reen)
Kayexalate, SPS Suspension
Func. class.: Potassium-removing resin
Chem. class.: Cation exchange resin

Action: Removes potassium by exchanging sodium for potassium in body; occurs primarily in large intestine

Uses: Hyperkalemia in conjunction with other measures

Dosage and routes:
• *Adult:* PO 15 g qd-qid; rectal enema 30-50 g/100 ml of sorbitol warmer to body temperature q6h
• *Child:* 1 mEq of K exchanged/g of resin, approximate dose 1g/kg q6h

Available forms: Susp, 15 g polystyrene sulfonate, 21.5 ml sorbitol, 15 g (65 mEq) Na/60 ml; powder

Side effects/adverse reactions:
GI: Constipation, anorexia, nausea, vomiting, diarrhea (sorbitol), fecal impaction, gastric irritation
META: Hypocalcemia, hypokalemia, hypomagnesemia, Na retention

Precautions: Pregnancy (C), renal failure, CHF, severe edema, severe hypertension

Interactions/incompatibilities:
• Decreased effect of sodium polystyrene: antacids, laxatives

NURSING CONSIDERATIONS
Assess:
• Bowel function daily
• Hypotension: confusion, irritability, muscular pain, weakness
• Serum K, Ca, Mg, Na, acid-base balance

Administer:
• Oral dose as susp mixed with H_2O or syrup (20-100 ml)
• Mild laxative as ordered to prevent constipation and fecal impaction
• Sorbitol as ordered to prevent constipation
• Retention enema after mixing with warm water; introduce by gravity, continue stirring, flush with 100 ml of fluid, clamp, and leave in place

Perform/provide:
• Retention of enema for at least ½-1 hr
• Irrigation of colon after enema with 1-2 qt of nonsodium solution, drain
• Storage of freshly prepared solution for 24 hr at room temperature

Evaluate:
• Therapeutic response: K level WNL

sodium thiosalicylate

Rexolate, Tusal
Func. class.: Nonnarcotic analgesic
Chem. class.: Salicylate

Action: Blocks pain impulses in

CNS that occur in response to inhibition of prostaglandin synthesis; antipyretic action results from inhibition of hypothalamic heat-regulating center

Uses: Mild to moderate pain (rheumatic fever, acute gout)

Dosage and routes:

Pain
• *Adult:* IM 50-100 mg qd or qod

Rheumatic fever
• *Adult:* IM 100-150 mg q4-6h × 3 days, then 100 mg bid

Arthritis
• *Adult:* IM 100 mg/day

Available forms: Inj IM 50 mg/ml

Side effects/adverse reactions:

HEMA: *Thrombocytopenia, agranulocytosis, leukopenia, neutropenia, hemolytic anemia,* increased pro-time

CNS: stimulation, drowsiness, dizziness, confusion, *convulsions,* headache, flushing, hallucinations, *coma*

GI: *Nausea, vomiting, GI bleeding, diarrhea, heartburn,* anorexia, *hepatitis*

INTEG: Rash, urticaria, bruising

EENT: tinnitus, hearing loss

CV: Rapid pulse, *pulmonary edema*

RESP: Wheezing, hyperpnea

ENDO: Hypoglycemia, hyponatremia, hypokalemia

Contraindications: Hypersensitivity to salicylates, GI bleeding, bleeding disorders, children < 3 yr, Vit K deficiency, peptic ulcer

Precautions: Anemia, hepatic disease, renal disease, Hodgkin's disease, pregnancy (C), lactation

Pharmacokinetics:

PO: Onset 15-30 min, peak 1-2 hr, duration 4-6 hr

REC: Onset slow, duration 4-6 hr, Metabolized by liver, excreted by kidneys, crosses placenta, excreted in breast milk, half-life 1-3½ hr

Interactions/incompatibilities:
• Decreased effects of sodium thiosalicylate: antacids, steroids, urinary alkalizers
• Increased blood loss: alcohol, heparin
• Increased effects of: anticoagulants, insulin, methotrexate
• Decreased effects of: probenecid, spironolactone, sulfinpyrazone, sulfonylmides
• Toxic effects: PABA

Lab test interferences:

Increase: Coagulation studies, liver function studies, serum uric acid, amylase, CO_2, urinary protein

Decrease: Serum K, PBI, cholesterol, blood glucose

Interfere: Urine catecholamines, pregnancy test

NURSING CONSIDERATIONS
Assess:
• Liver function studies: ALT, AST, bilirubin if patient is on long-term therapy
• Renal function studies: BUN, urine creatinine if patient is on long-term therapy
• Blood studies: CBC, Hct, Hgb, pro-time if patient is on long-term therapy
• I&O ratio; decreasing output may indicate renal failure (long-term therapy)
• Hepatotoxicity: dark urine, clay-colored stools, yellowing of skin and sclera, itching, abdominal pain, fever, diarrhea if patient is on long-term therapy
• Allergic reactions: rash, urticaria; if these occur, drug may have to be discontinued
• Renal dysfunction: decreased urine output
• Ototoxicity: tinnitus, ringing, roaring in ears; audiometric testing

is needed before, after long-term therapy
• Visual changes: blurring, halos, corneal, retinal damage
• Edema in feet, ankles, legs
• Prior drug history; many drug interactions

Evaluate:
• Therapeutic response: decreased pain

Teach patient/family:
• To report any symptoms of hepatotoxicity, renal toxicity, visual changes, ototoxicity, allergic reactions (long-term therapy)
• Not to exceed recommended dosage; acute poisoning may result
• To read label on other OTC drugs; many contain aspirin
• That therapeutic response takes 2 wk (arthritis)
• To avoid alcohol ingestion; GI bleeding may occur

Treatment of overdose: Lavage, activated charcoal, monitor electrolytes, VS

---

somatotropin (human growth hormone)
(soe-ma-toe-troe′pin)
Humatrope*

Func. class.: Pituitary hormone
Chem. class.: Growth hormone

Action: Stimulates growth
Uses: Pituitary growth hormone deficiency (hypopituitary dwarfism)
Dosage and routes:
• *Child:* IM 2 IU 3 × /wk, less than 48 hr between doses, may give 4 IU if growth is <1 inch/6 mo
Available forms: Inj IM, IV 2, 4, 10 IU

Side effects/adverse reactions:
GU: Hypercalciuria
INTEG: Rash, urticaria, pain, inflammation at injection site

CNS: Headache, growth of intracranial tumor
*ENDO: **Hyperglycemia, ketosis, hypothyroidism***
*SYST: **Antibodies to growth hormone***

Contraindications: Hypersensitivity to benzyl alcohol, closed epiphyses, intracranial lesions
Precautions: Diabetes mellitus, hypothyroidism, pregnancy (C)
Pharmacokinetics:
Half-life 15-60 min, duration 7 days; metabolized in liver
Interactions/incompatibilities:
• Decreased growth: glucocorticosteroids
• Epiphyseal closure: androgens, thyroid hormones

NURSING CONSIDERATIONS
Assess:
• Growth hormone antibodies if patient fails to respond to therapy
• Thyroid function tests: T_3, T_4, T_7, TSH to identify hypothyroidism
• Allergic reaction: rash, itching, fever, nausea, wheezing
• Hypercalciuria: urinary stones; groin, flank pain; nausea, vomiting, frequency, hematuria, chills
• Growth rate of child at intervals during treatment

Administer:
• IM; rotate injection site
• After reconstituting 10 IU/5 ml bacteriostatic H_2O for injection, do not shake

Perform/provide:
• Storage in refrigerator for <1 mo if reconstituted <1 wk; do not use discolored or cloudy sol

Evaluate:
• Therapeutic response: growth in children

S

---

italics = common side effects   ***bold italic*** = life threatening reactions

sotalol hydrochloride

(soe-ta′-lole)
Betapace
Func. class.: Antidysrhythmic
Chem. class.: Nonselective
β-blocker

Action: Blockade of B_1 and B_2 receptors leads to antidysrhythmic effect

Uses: Life-threatening ventricular dysrhythmias

Dosage and routes:
• *Adult:* PO initial 80 mg bid, may increase to a total of 240-320 mg/day

Available forms: Tabs 80, 160, 240 mg

Side effects/adverse reactions:

CV: Orthostatic hypotension, bradycardia, CHF, chest pain, ventricular dysrhythmias, AV block, peripheral vascular insufficiency, palpitations

CNS: Dizziness, mental changes, drowsiness, fatigue, headache, catatonia, depression, anxiety, nightmares, paresthesia, lethargy, insomnia, decreased concentration

GI: Nausea, vomiting, diarrhea, dry mouth, flatulence, constipation, anorexia

INTEG: Rash, alopecia, urticaria, pruritus, fever

HEMA: Agranulocytosis, thrombocytopenic purpura (rare), thrombocytopenia, leukopenia

EENT: Tinnitus, visual changes, sore throat, double vision, dry burning eyes

GU: Impotence, dysuria, ejaculatory failure, urinary retention

RESP: Bronchospasm, dyspnea, wheezing, nasal stuffiness, pharyngitis

MS: Joint pain, arthralgia, muscle cramps, pain

OTHER: Facial swelling, decreased exercise tolerance, weight change, Raynaud's disease

Contraindications: Hypersensitivity to β-blockers, cardiogenic shock, heart block (2nd or 3rd degree), sinus bradycardia, CHF, bronchial asthma, congenital or acquired long QT syndrome

Precautions: Major surgery, pregnancy (B), lactation, diabetes mellitus, renal disease, thyroid disease, COPD, well-compensated heart failure, CAD, nonallergic bronchospasm, electrolyte disturbances, bradycardia, cardiac dysrhythmias, peripheral vascular disease

Pharmacokinetics:
PO: Onset 1-2 hr, peak 2-4 hr, duration 8-12 hr, half-life 12 hr; metabolized by liver (metabolites inactive), excreted unchanged in urine, crosses placenta, excreted in breast milk

Interactions/incompatibilities:
• Increased hypotension: diuretics, other antihypertensives, nitroglycerin, prazosin
• Decreased β-blocker effects: sympathomimetics, nonsteroidal antiinflammatory agents, salicylates
• Increased hypoglycemia effect: insulin
• Increased effects of: lidocaine
• Decreased bronchodilating effects of: theophylline
• Decreased hypoglycemic effects of: sulfonylureas

Lab test interferences:
• *False increase:* Urinary catecholamines
• *Interference:* Glucose, insulin tolerance tests

NURSING CONSIDERATIONS
Assess:
• I&O, weight daily

---

* Available in Canada only

• B/P pulse q4h; note rate, rhythm, quality
• Apical/radial pulse before administration: notify physician of any significant changes
• Baselines in renal, liver function tests before therapy begins
• Edema in feet, legs daily
• Skin turgor, dryness of mucous membranes for hydration status

Administer:
• PO: ac, hs; tablet may be crushed or swallowed whole
• Reduced dosage in renal dysfunction

Perform/provide:
• Storage in dry area at room temperature; do not freeze

Evaluate:
• Therapeutic response: decreased B/P after 1-2 wk

Teach patient/family:
• Not to discontinue drug abruptly; taper over 2 wk or may precipitate angina
• Not to use OTC products containing α-adrenergic stimulants (nasal decongestants, OTC cold preparations) unless directed by physician
• To report bradycardia, dizziness, confusion, depression, fever
• To take pulse at home; advise when to notify physician
• To avoid alcohol, smoking, sodium intake
• To comply with weight control, dietary adjustments, modified exercise program
• To carry Medic Alert ID to identify drug being taken, allergies
• To avoid hazardous activities if dizziness is present
• To report symptoms of CHF: difficult breathing, especially on exertion or when lying down; night cough, swelling of extremities
• To take medication to minimize orthostatic hypotension

• To wear support hose to minimize effects of orthostatic hypotension
Treatment of overdose: Lavage, IV atropine for bradycardia, IV theophylline for bronchospasm, digitalis, O_2, diuretic for cardiac failure; hemodialysis is useful for removal; administer vasopressor (norepinephrine) for hypotension, isoproterenol for heart block

---

spectinomycin hydrochloride

(spek-ti-noe-mye′sin)
Trobicin
Func. class.: Antibiotic
Chem. class.: Aminocyclitol

Action: Inhibits bacterial synthesis by binding to 30S subunit on ribosomes
Uses: Gonorrhea
Dosage and routes:
• *Adult:* IM 2-4 g as single dose
Available forms: Inj IM 2, 4 g
Side effects/adverse reactions:
CNS: Dizziness, chills, fever, insomnia, headache, anxiety
HEMA: Anemia
GI: Nausea, vomiting, increased BUN
GU: Decreased urine output
INTEG: Pain at injection site, urticaria, rash, pruritus, fever
Contraindications: Hypersensitivity, syphilis
Precautions: Pregnancy (B), infants, children
Pharmacokinetics:
IM: Peak 1-2 hr, duration >8 hr, half-life 1-3 hr, excreted in urine (active form)
NURSING CONSIDERATIONS
Assess:
• Gonorrhea culture after treatment
• I&O ratio; report decreased output

S

• Liver studies: AST, ALT, serum alk phosphatase following multiple doses
• Blood studies: Hct, Hgb, BUN if multiple diagnoses given
• Serologic test for gonorrhea 3 mo after treatment
• Allergies before treatment, reaction of each medication

Administer:
• After shaking vial
• IM in deep muscle mass
• With 20G needle; no more than 5 ml per site

Perform/provide:
• Storage at room temperature; reconstituted sol should be discarded after 24 hr
• Treatment of partner; report infection

Evaluate:
• Therapeutic response: negative gonorrhea culture after treatment

---

spironolactone
(speer'on-oh-lak'tone)
Alatone, Aldactone, Novospiroton, Sincomen
Func. class.: Potassium-sparing diuretic
Chem. class.: Aldosterone antagonist

Action: Competes with aldosterone at receptor sites in distal tubule, resulting in excretion of sodium chloride, water, retention of potassium, phosphate
Uses: Edema, hypertension, diuretic-induced hypokalemia, primary hyperaldosteronism (diagnosis, short-term treatment, long-term treatment), nephrotic syndrome, cirrhosis of the liver with ascites

Dosage and routes:
Edema/hypertension
• *Adult:* PO 25-200 mg/qd in single or divided doses
• *Child:* PO 3.3 mg/kg/day in single or divided doses
Hypokalemia
• *Adult:* PO 25-100 mg/day; if PO, K supplements are unable to be used
Primary hyperaldosteronism diagnosis
• *Adult:* PO 400 mg/day × 4 days or 4 wk depending on test, then 100-400 mg/day maintenance
Available forms: Tab 25, 50, 100 mg
Side effects/adverse reactions:
CNS: Headache, confusion, drowsiness, lethargy, ataxia
GI: Diarrhea, cramps, **bleeding,** gastritis, *vomiting,* anorexia, nausea
CV: dysrythmias
INTEG: Rash, pruritus, urticaria
ENDO: Impotence, gynecomastia, irregular menses, amenorrhea, postmenopausal bleeding, hirsutism, deepening voice
HEMA: Decreased WBCs, platelets
ELECT: Hyperchloremic metabolic acidosis, **hyperkalemia,** hyponatremia
Contraindications: Hypersensitivity, anuria, severe renal disease, hyperkalemia, pregnancy (D)
Precautions: Dehydration, hepatic disease, lactation
Pharmacokinetics:
PO: Onset 24-48 hr, peak 48-72 hr; metabolized in liver, excreted in urine, crosses placenta
Interactions/incompatibilities:
• Increased action of: antihypertensives, digitalis, lithium
• Increased hyperkalemia: K-sparing diuretics, K products, ACE inhibitors, salt substitutes

---

* Available in Canada only

• Decreased effect of spironolactone: ASA

Lab test interferences:

Interference: 17-OHCS, 17-KS, radioimmunoassay, digoxin assay

NURSING CONSIDERATIONS
Assess:

• Electrolytes: Na, Cl, K, BUN, serum creatinine, ABGs, CBC

• Weight, I&O daily to determine fluid loss; effect of drug may be decreased if used qd; ECG periodically for patients with long-term therapy

• Signs of metabolic acidosis: drowsiness, restlessness

• Rashes, temperature elevation qd

• Confusion, especially in elderly; take safety precautions if needed

• Hydration: skin turgor, thirst, dry mucous membranes

Administer:

• In AM to avoid interference with sleep

• With food; if nausea occurs, absorption may be decreased slightly

Evaluate:

• Therapeutic response: improvement in edema of feet, legs, sacral area daily if medication is being used in CHF

Teach patient/family:

• To avoid foods with high K^+ content: oranges, bananas, salt substitutes, dried apricots, dates

• That drowsiness, ataxia, mental confusion may occur; observe caution in driving

• To notify physician of cramps, diarrhea, lethargy, thirst, headache, skin rash, menstrual abnormalities, deepening voice, breast enlargement

Treatment of overdose: Lavage if taken orally; monitor electrolytes, administer IV fluids, monitor hydration, renal, CV status

---

stanozolol
(stan-oh'zoe'lole)
Winstrol

Func. class.: Androgenic anabolic steroid

Chem. class.: Halogenated testosterone derivative

Action: Increases weight by building body tissue; increases potassium, phosphorus, chloride, and nitrogen levels; increases bone development

Uses: Prevention of hereditary angioedema, aplastic anemia to increase hemoglobin

Dosage and routes:

Aplastic anemia (possibly effective)

• *Adult:* PO 2 mg tid

• *Child 6-12 yr:* PO up to 2 mg tid

• *Child <6 yr:* PO 1 mg bid

Angioedema

• *Adult:* PO 2 mg tid, then decrease q1-3 mo, down to 2 mg qd or q2d

Available forms: Tabs 2 mg

Side effects/adverse reactions:

INTEG: Rash, acneiform lesions, oily hair, skin, flushing, sweating, acne vulgaris, alopecia, hirsutism

CNS: Dizziness, headache, fatigue, tremors, paresthesias, flushing, sweating, anxiety, lability, insomnia, carpal tunnel syndrome

MS: Cramps, spasms

CV: Increased B/P

GU: **Hematuria,** amenorrhea, vaginitis, decreased libido, decreased breast size, clitoral hypertrophy, testicular atrophy

GI: Nausea, vomiting, constipation, weight gain, ***cholestatic jaundice***

EENT: Conjunctional edema, nasal congestion

ENDO: Abnormal GTT

S

---

italics = common side effects   ***bold italic*** = life threatening reactions

Contraindications: Severe renal disease, severe cardiac disease, severe hepatic disease, hypersensitivity, pregnancy (X), lactation, genital bleeding (abnormal)

Precautions: Diabetes mellitus, CV disease, MI

Pharmacokinetics:

PO: Metabolized in liver, excreted in urine, crosses placenta, excreted in breast milk

Interactions/incompatibilities:

• Increased effects of: oral antidiabetics, oxyphenbutazone
• Increased PT: anticoagulants
• Edema: ACTH, adrenal steroids
• Decreased effects of: insulin

Lab test interferences:

Increase: Serum cholesterol, blood glucose, urine glucose

Decrease: Serum Ca, serum K, T_4, T_3, thyroid ^{131}I uptake test, urine 17-OHCS

NURSING CONSIDERATIONS
Assess:

• Weight daily, notify physician if weekly weight gain is >5 lb
• B/P q4h
• I&O ratio; be alert for decreasing urinary output, increasing edema
• Growth rate in children, since growth rate may be uneven (linear/bone growth) when used for extended period
• Electrolytes: K, Na, Cl, Ca; cholesterol
• Liver function studies: ALT, AST, bilirubin
• Edema, hypertension, cardiac symptoms, jaundice
• Mental status: affect, mood, behavioral changes, aggression
• Signs of masculinization in female: increased libido, deepening of voice, breast tissue, enlarged clitoris, menstrual irregularities; male: gynecomastia, impotence, testicular atrophy

• Hypercalcemia: lethargy, polyuria, polydipsia, nausea, vomiting, constipation; dosage may have to be decreased
• Hypoglycemia in diabetics, since oral antidiabetic action is increased

Administer:

• Titrated dose; use lowest effective dose

Perform/provide:

• Diet with increased calories and protein; decrease Na if edema occurs
• Supportive drug of anemia

Evaluate:

• Therapeutic response: occurs in 4-6 wk in osteoporosis

Teach patient/family:

• That drug must be combined with complete health plan: diet, rest, exercise
• To notify physician if therapeutic response decreases
• Not to discontinue this medication abruptly
• About change in sex characteristics
• Women to report menstrual irregularies
• That 1-3-mo course is necessary for response in breast cancer
• Procedure for use of buccal tablets (requires 30-60 min to dissolve; change absorption site with each dose; do not eat, drink, chew, or smoke while tablet is in place)

---

streptokinase
(strep-toe-kye′nase)
Kabikinase, Streptase
Func. class.: Thrombolytic enzyme
Chem. class.: β-Hemolytic streptococcus filtrate (purified)

Action: Activates conversion of plasminogen to plasmin (fibrinolysin): plasmin breaks down clots (fibrin), fibrinogen, factors V, VII; occlusion of venous access lines

Uses: Deep vein thrombosis, pulmonary embolism, arterial thrombosis, arterial embolism, arteriovenous cannula occlusion, lysis of coronary artery thrombi after MI, acute evolving transmural MI

Dosage and routes:

Lysis of coronary artery thrombi
• *Adult:* CC 20,000 IU, then 2000 IU/min over 1 hr as IV INF

Arteriovenous cannula occlusion
• *Adult:* IV INF 250,000 IU/2 ml sol into occluded limb of cannula run over ½ hr; clamp for 2 hr; aspirate contents; flush with NaCl sol and reconnect

Thrombosis/embolism
• *Adult:* IV INF 250,000 IU over ½ hr, then 100,000 IU/hr for 72 hr for deep thrombosis; 100,000 IU/hr over 24-72 hr for pulmonary embolism

Acute evolving transmural MI
• *Adult:* IV INF 1,500,000 IU diluted to a volume of 45 ml; give within 1 hr

Available forms: Inj IV 250,000, 600,000, 750,000 IU

Side effects/adverse reactions:
CNS: Headache, fever
EENT: Periorbital edema
GI: Nausea
HEMA: Decreased Hct, **bleeding**
INTEG: Rash, urticaria, phlebitis at IV inf site, itching, flushing
MS: Low back pain
RESP: Altered respirations, SOB, ***bronchospasm***
SYST: ***GI, GU, intracranial retroperitoneal bleeding, surface bleeding, anaphylaxis***

Contraindications: Hypersensitivity, active bleeding, intraspinal surgery, neoplasms of the CNS, ulcerative colitis, enteritis, severe hypertension, severe renal disease, hepatic disease, hypocoagulation, COPD, subacute bacterial endocarditis, rheumatic valvular disease, cerebral embolism/thrombosis/hemorrhage, intraarterial diagnostic procedure or surgery (10 days), recent major surgery

Precautions: Arterial emboli from left side of heart, pregnancy (C)

Pharmacokinetics:
IV: Onset immediate, duration <12 hr; excreted in bile, urine, half-life <20 min

Interactions/incompatibilities:
• Bleeding potential: aspirin, indomethacin, phenylbutazone, anticoagulants
• Considered incompatible with any drug in sol or syringe

Lab test interferences:
Increase: PT, APTT, TT

NURSING CONSIDERATIONS
Assess:
• Allergy: fever, rash, itching, chills; mild reaction may be treated with antihistamines
• For bleeding during 1st hr of treatment; hematuria, hematemesis, bleeding from mucous membranes, epistaxis, ecchymosis
• Blood studies (Hct, platelets, PTT, PT, TT, APTT) before starting therapy; PT or APTT must be less than ×2 control before starting therapy TT ot PT q3-4h during treatment
• For hypersensitive reactions: fever, rash, dyspnea; drug should be discontinued
• VS, B/P, pulse, respirations, neuro signs, temp at least q4h; temp >104° F (40° C) indicate internal bleeding, cardiac rhythm following intracoronary administration; systolic pressure increase of >25 mm Hg, should be reported to physician

---

italics = common side effects   ***bold italic*** = life threatening reactions

• For neurologic changes that may indicate intracranial bleeding
• Retroperitoneal bleeding: back pain, leg weakness, diminished pulses
• For streptokinase reactions previously

Administer:

• As soon as thrombi identified; not useful for thrombi over 1 wk old
• Cryoprecipitate or fresh frozen plasma if bleeding occurs
• Loading dose at beginning of therapy; may require increase loading doses
• Heparin after fibrinogen level >100 mg/dl; heparin infusion to increase PTT to 1.5-2 × baseline for 3-7 days
• After reconstituting with 5 ml NS or D₅W; do not shake; further dilute to total volume of 45 ml; may be diluted to 500 ml in 45 ml increments; may dilute vial in 15 ml NS, further dilute 750,000 IU/50 ml NS or D₅W; further dilute 1,500,000 IU dose/100 ml or more
• About 10% patients have high streptococcal antibody titers requiring increased loading doses
• IV therapy using 0.8 μm filter

Perform/provide:

• Storage of reconstituted sol in refrigerator; discard after 24 hr
• Bed rest during entire course of treatment
• Avoidance of venous or arterial puncture, inj, rectal temp; any invasive treatment
• Treatment of fever with acetaminophen or aspirin
• Pressure for 30 sec to minor bleeding sites; inform physician if this does not attain hemostasis; apply pressure dressing

Evaluate:

• Therapeutic response: resolution of thrombosis, embolism

---

streptomycin sulfate
(strep-toe-mye′sin)

Func. class.: Antibiotic
Chem. class.: Aminoglycoside

Action: Interferes with protein synthesis in bacterial cell by binding to ribosomal subunit, causing inaccurate peptide sequence to form in protein chain, causing bacterial death

Uses: Sensitive strains of *M. tuberculosis,* nontuberculous infections caused by sensitive strains of *Y. pestus, Brucella, H. influenzae, K. pneumoniae, E. coli, E. aerogenes, S. viridans, F. tularensis, Proteus*

Dosage and routes:
Tuberculosis

• *Adult:* IM 1g qd × 2-3 mo, then 1 g 2-3 ×/week given with other antitubercular drugs
• *Child:* IM 20-40 mg/kg/day in divided doses given with other antitubercular drugs; max 15 mg/kg/day

Streptococcal endocarditis

• *Adult:* IM 1 g q12h × 1 wk with penicillin, then 500 mg bid × 1 wk

Enterococcal endocarditis

• *Adult:* IM 1 g q12h × 2 wk, then 500 mg q12h × 4 wk with penicillin max 15 mg/kg/day

Available forms: Inj IM 1, 5 g: 400 mg/ml

Side effects/adverse reactions:

GU: **Oliguria, hematuria, renal damage, azotemia, renal failure, nephrotoxicity**

CNS: Confusion, depression, numbness, tremors, **convulsions,** muscle twitching, **neurotoxicity**

EENT: **Ototoxicity,** deafness, visual disturbances

HEMA: **Agranulocytosis, throm-**

---

bocytopenia, leukopenia, eosino-philia, anemia

GI: Nausea, vomiting, anorexia, increased ALT, AST, bilirubin, hepatomegaly, ***hepatic necrosis,*** splenomegaly

CV: Hypotension, myocarditis, palpitations

INTEG: Rash, burning urticaria, dermatitis, alopecia

Contraindications: Severe renal disease, hypersensitivity

Precautions: Neonates, mild renal disease, pregnancy (B), myasthenia gravis, lactation, hearing deficits, elderly, Parkinson's disease

Pharmacokinetics:

IM: Onset rapid, peak 1-2 hr; plasma half-life 2-2½ hr; not metabolized, excreted unchanged in urine, crosses placental barrier

Interactions/incompatibilities:

• Increased ototoxicity, neurotoxicity, nephrotoxicity: other aminoglycosides, amphotericin B, polymyxin, vancomycin, ethacrynic acid, furosemide, mannitol, methoxyflurane, cisplatin, cephalosporins, bacitracin

• Do not mix in sol or syringe: carbenicillin, ticarcillin, amphotericin B, cephalothin, erythromycin, heparin

• Increased effects: nondepolarizing muscle relaxants, succinylcholine, warfarin

NURSING CONSIDERATIONS
Assess:

• Weight before treatment; calculation of dosage is usually done based on ideal body weight, but may be calculated on actual body weight

• I&O ratio, urinalysis daily for proteinuria, cells, casts; report sudden change in urine output

• Serum peak 20-30 min after IM injection, trough level drawn 8 hr

• Urine pH if drug is used for UTI; urine should be kept alkaline

• Renal impairment by securing urine for CrCl testing, BUN, serum creatinine; lower dosage should be given in renal impairment (CrCl <80 ml/min)

• Deafness by audiometric testing, ringing, roaring in ears, vertigo; assess hearing before, during, after treatment

• Dehydration: high sp gr, decrease in skin turgor, dry mucous membranes, dark urine

• Overgrowth of infection: increased temperature, malaise, redness, pain, swelling, perineal itching, diarrhea, stomatitis, change in cough, sputum

• C&S before starting treatment to identify infecting organism

• Vestibular dysfunction: nausea, vomiting, dizziness, headache; drug should be discontinued if severe

• Injection sites for redness, swelling, abscesses; use warm compresses at site

Administer:

• IM injection in large muscle mass; rotate injection sites

• Drug in evenly spaced doses to maintain blood level

Perform/provide:

• Adequate fluids of 2-3 L/day unless contraindicated to prevent irritation of tubules

• Supervised ambulation, other safety measures with vestibular dysfunction

Evaluate:

• Therapeutic effect: absence of fever, draining wounds, negative C&S after treatment

Teach patient/family:

• To report headache, dizziness, symptoms of overgrowth of infection, renal impairment

italics = common side effects   ***bold italic*** = life threatening reactions

• To report loss of hearing, ringing, roaring in ears, fullness in head
Treatment of overdose: Hemodialysis; monitor serum levels of drug

---

streptozocin
(strep-toe-zoe′sin)
Zanosar
Func. class.: Antineoplastic alkylating agent
Chem. class.: Nitrosourea

Action: Alkylates DNA, RNA; inhibits enzymes that allow synthesis of amino acids in proteins; is also responsible for cross-linking DNA strands; activity is not cell cycle phase specific
Uses: Metastatic islet cell carcinoma of pancreas
Dosage and routes:
• *Adult:* IV 500 mg/m² × 5 days q6wk until desired response; alternate with 1 g/m² qwk × 2 wk, not to exceed 1.5 g/m² in 1 dose
Available forms: Inj IV 1 g
Side effects/adverse reactions:
*HEMA: **Thrombocytopenia, leukopenia, pancytopenia***
CNS: Confusion, depression, lethargy
GI: Nausea, vomiting, diarrhea, weight loss, **hepatotoxicity**
*GU: **Azotemia, anuria,** hypophosphatemia, glycosuria, renal tubular acidosis, **renal toxicity***
Contraindications: Hypersensitivity
Precautions: Radiation therapy, children, lactation, pregnancy (C), hepatic disease, renal disease
Pharmacokinetics:
IV: Metabolized by liver, excreted in urine, half-life 5 min, terminal 35-40 min
Interactions/incompatibilities:
• Increased toxicity: neurotoxic agents, other antineoplastics

• Increased action of: doxorubicin
• Decreased effect of streptozocin: phenytoin
• Considered incompatible in sol or syringe with any other drug
NURSING CONSIDERATIONS
Assess:
• CBC, differential, platelet count weekly; withhold drug if WBC is <4000 or platelet count is <75,000; notify physician of results
• Renal function studies: BUN, serum uric acid, phosphate urine CrCl before, during therapy
• I&O ratio; report fall in urine output of 30 ml/hr
• Monitor temperature q4h (may indicate beginning infection)
• Liver function tests before, during therapy (bilirubin, AST, ALT, LDH) as needed or monthly, blood sugar levels qd and observe for hypoglycemia
• Bleeding: hematuria, guaiac, bruising or petechiae, mucosa or orifices q8h
• Food preferences; list likes, dislikes
• Inflammation of mucosa, breaks in skin
• Yellowing of skin and sclera, dark urine, clay-colored stools, itchy skin, abdominal pain, fever, diarrhea
• Local irritation, pain, burning, discoloration at injection site
• Symptoms indicating severe allergic reaction: rash, urticaria, itching, flushing
Administer:
• Antiemetic 30-60 min before giving drug to prevent vomiting
• Antibiotics for prophylaxis of infection
• IV after diluting 1 g/9.5 ml 0.9% NaCl or D₅; may be further diluted

---

in 50-250 mg; may be given directly over 5-15 min
• Using 21G, 23G, 25G needle
• Topical or systemic analgesics for pain
• Local or systemic drugs for infection

Perform/provide:
• Storage protected from light; refrigerate reconstituted sol; stable for 48 hr at room temperature
• Strict medical asepsis, protective isolation if WBC levels are low
• Special skin care
• Warm compresses at injection site for inflammation
• Adequate hydration that may reduce renal toxicity

Evaluate:
• Therapeutic response: decreased tumor size, spread of malignancy

Teach patient/family:
• Of protective isolation precautions
• To report signs of infection: increased temperature, sore throat, flu symptoms
• To report signs of anemia: fatigue, headache, faintness, shortness of breath, irritability
• To avoid use of razors, commercial mouthwash
• To avoid use of aspirin products, ibuprofen

---

succimer
(suk-si′mer)
Chemet
Func. class.: Heavy metal antagonist
Chem. class.: Chelating agent

Action: Binds with ions of lead to form a water-soluble complex excreted by kidneys

Uses: Lead poisoning in children with lead levels above 45 µg/dl; may be beneficial in mercury, arsenic poisoning

Dosage and routes:
• *Child:* PO 10 mg/kg or 350 mg/m^2 q8h × 5 days, then 10 mg/kg or 350 mg/m^2 q12h × 2 wk; another course may be required depending on lead levels; allow 2 wk between courses

Available forms: Caps 100 mg

Side effects/adverse reactions:
SYST: Back, stomach, head, rib flank pain, abdominal cramps, chills, fever, flulike symptoms, head cold, headache
HEMA: Increased platelets, intermittent eosinophilia
GU: Proteinuria, decreased urination, voiding difficulties
INTEG: Rash, urticaria, pruritus
META: Increased AST, ALT, alk phosphatase, cholesterol
GI: Nausea, vomiting, diarrhea, metallic taste, anorexia
CNS: Drowsiness, dizziness, paresthesia, sensorimotor neuropathy
EENT: Otitis media, watery eyes, film in eyes, plugged ears
RESP: Sore throat, rhinorrhea, nasal congestion, cough

Contraindications: Hypersensitivity

Precautions: Pregnancy (C), lactation, children <1 yr

Pharmacokinetics:
PO: Peak 1-2 hr, 49% excreted as 39% in feces, 9% urine, 1% as CO_2 from the lungs

Interactions/incompatibilities:
• Not recommended to be used concurrently with other chelating agents

NURSING CONSIDERATIONS
Assess:
• Hepatic, renal studies: ALT, AST, alk phosphatase, BUN, creatinine, serum lead level
• I&O

S

---

italics = common side effects   **bold italic** = life threatening reactions

- For lead sources in home, school environment
- Allergic reactions: rash, pruritus, urticaria; drug should be discontinued if antihistamines fail to help

Administer:
- To children who cannot swallow capsule by separating the capsule and sprinkling content on food or in a spoon followed by a drink

Perform/provide:
- Adequate fluids; check hydration status daily

Evaluate:
- Therapeutic response: decrease in serum lead level

Teach patient/family:
- That therapeutic effect may take 1-3 mo
- To report urticaria, rash

---

succinylcholine chloride

(suk-sin-ill-koe'leen)
Anectine, Anectine Flo-Pack, Brevidil M* (Bromide Salt), Min-I-Mix, Quelicin, Scaline,* Succinylcholine Chloride Min-I-Mix, Sucostrin, Sux-Cert*

Func. class.: Neuromuscular blocker (depolarizing-ultra short)

Action: Inhibits transmission of nerve impulses by binding with cholinergic receptor sites, antagonizing action of acetylcholine

Uses: Facilitation of endotracheal intubation, skeletal muscle relaxation during orthopedic manipulations

Dosage and routes:
- *Adult:* IV 25-75 mg, then 2.5 mg/min as needed; IM 2.5 mg/kg, not to exceed 150 mg
- *Child:* IV/IM 1-2 mg/kg, not to exceed 150 mg IM

Available forms: Inj IM, IV 20, 50, 100 mg/ml; powder for inj 100, 500 mg/vial, 1 g/vial

Side effects/adverse reactions:
CV: Bradycardia, tachycardia; increased, decreased B/P, *sinus arrest, dysrhythmias*
RESP: Prolonged apnea, bronchospasm, cyanosis, respiratory depression
EENT: Increased secretions, increased intraocular pressure
MS: Weakness, muscle pain, fasciculations, prolonged relaxation
HEMA: Myoglobulinemia
INTEG: Rash, flushing, pruritus, urticaria

Contraindications: Hypersensitivity, malignant hyperthermia, decreased plasma pseudocholinesterase, penetrating eye injuries, acute narrow angle glaucoma

Precautions: Pregnancy (C), cardiac disease, severe burns, fractures—fasciculations may increase damage—lactation, children <2 yr, electrolyte imbalances, dehydration, neuromuscular disease, respiratory disease, collagen diseases, glaucoma, eye surgery, penetrating eye wounds, elderly or debilitated patients

Pharmacokinetics:
IV: Onset 1 min, peak 2-3 min, duration 6-10 min
IM: Onset 2-3 min
Hydrolyzed in urine (active/inactive metabolites)

Interactions/incompatibilities:
- Increased neuromuscular blockade: aminoglycosides, clindamycin, lincomycin, quinidine, local anesthetics, polymyxin antibiotics, lithium, narcotic analgesics, thiazides, enflurane, isoflurane, Mg salts, oxytocin
- Dysrhythmias: theophylline
- Incompatible with barbiturates,

chlorpromazine, nafcillin, alkaline sol

NURSING CONSIDERATIONS
Assess:
• For electrolyte imbalances (K, Mg); may lead to increased action of this drug
• Vital signs (B/P, pulse, respirations, airway) until fully recovered; rate, depth, pattern of respirations, strength of hand grip
• I&O ratio; check for urinary retention, frequency, hesitancy
• Recovery: decreased paralysis of face, diaphragm, leg, arm, rest of body
• Allergic reactions: rash, fever, respiratory distress, pruritus; drug should be discontinued

Administer:
• Using nerve stimulator by anesthesiologist to determine neuromuscular blockade
• Anticholinesterase to reverse neuromuscular blockade
• IV INF; dilute 1-2 mg/ml in D$_5$, isotonic saline sol, give 0.5-10 mg/min, titrate to patient response; may be given directly over 1 min
• Deep IM, preferably high in deltoid muscle

Perform/provide:
• Storage in refrigerator, powder at room temp; close tightly
• Reassurance if communication is difficult during recovery from neuromuscular blockade; postoperative stiffness is normal, soon subsides

Evaluate:
• Therapeutic response: paralysis of jaw, eyelid, head, neck, rest of body

Treatment of overdose: Edrophonium or neostigmine, atropine, monitor VS; may require mechanical ventilation

---

sucral___

(soo-kral'fa___
Carafate, Su___

Func. class.: ___
Chem. class.: A___ ___y-droxide/sulfated sucrose

Action: Forms a complex that adheres to ulcer site, adsorbs pepsin
Uses: Duodenal ulcer
Dosage and routes:
• *Adult:* PO 1 g qid 1 hr ac, hs
Available forms: Tabs 1 g
Side effects/adverse reactions:
CNS: Drowsiness, dizziness
GI: Dry mouth, constipation, nausea, gastric pain, vomiting
INTEG: Urticaria, rash, pruritus
Contraindications: Hypersensitivity
Precautions: Pregnancy (B), lactation, children
Pharmacokinetics:
PO: Duration up to 5 hr
Interactions/incompatibilities:
• Decreased action of: tetracyclines, phenytoin, fat-soluble vitamins

NURSING CONSIDERATIONS
Assess:
• Gastric pH (>5 should be maintained)
Perform/provide:
• Storage at room temperature
Evaluate:
• Therapeutic response: absence of pain, or GI complaints
Teach patient/family:
• To avoid black pepper, caffeine, alcohol, harsh spices, extremes in temperature of food
• To take on empty stomach
• To take full course of therapy
• To avoid antacids within ½ hr of drug

---

italics = common side effects   ***bold italic*** = life threatening reactions

...entanil citrate

(soo-fen'ta-nil)
Sufenta
Func. class.: Narcotic analgesic
Chem. class.: Opiate, synthetic

Controlled Substance Schedule II
Action: Inhibits ascending pain pathways in CNS, increases pain threshold, alters pain perception
Uses: Primary anesthetic, adjunct to general anesthetic
Dosage and routes:
Primary anesthetic
• *Adult:* IV 8-30 μg/kg given with 100% O_2, a muscle relaxant
Adjunct
• *Adult:* IV 1-8 μg/kg given with nitrous oxide/O_2
Available forms: Inj IV 50 μg/ml
Side effects/adverse reactions:
CNS: Drowsiness, dizziness, confusion, headache, sedation, euphoria
GI: Nausea, vomiting, anorexia, constipation, cramps
GU: Increased urinary output, dysuria, urinary retention
INTEG: Rash, urticaria, bruising, flushing, diaphoresis, pruritus
EENT: Tinnitus, blurred vision, miosis, diplopia
CV: Palpitations, bradycardia, change in B/P
RESP: Respiratory depression
Contraindications: Hypersensitivity, addiction (narcotic)
Precautions: Addictive personality, pregnancy (C), lactation, increased intracranial pressure, MI (acute), severe heart disease, respiratory depression, hepatic disease, renal disease, child <18 yr
Pharmacokinetics:
Half-life 1-2 hr

Interactions/incompatibilities:
• Increased effects with other CNS depressants: alcohol, narcotics, sedative/hypnotics, antipsychotics, skeletal muscle relaxants
Lab test interferences:
Increase: Amylase
NURSING CONSIDERATIONS
Assess:
• I&O ratio; check for decreasing output (may indicate urinary retention)
• CNS changes: dizziness, drowsiness, hallucinations, euphoria, LOC, pupil reaction
• Allergic reactions: rash, urticaria
• Respiratory dysfunction: respiratory depression, character, rate, rhythm; notify physician if respirations are <10/min
• Need for pain medication, physical dependence
Administer:
• IV undiluted over 1-2 min or give as INF
• With antiemetic if nausea, vomiting occur
Perform/provide:
• Storage in light-resistant area at room temperature
• Safety measures: side rails, nightlight, call bell within easy reach
Evaluate:
• Therapeutic response: maintenance of anesthesia
Teach patient/family:
• To report any symptoms of CNS changes, allergic reactions
Treatment of overdose: Naloxone (Narcan) 0.2-0.8 IV, O_2, IV fluids, vasopressors

---

* Available in Canada only

sulfacetamide sodium (ophthalmic)

(sul-fa-see′ta-mide)

AK-Sulf, Bleph-10 Liquifilm, Bleph-10 S.O.P., Cetamide, Isopto Cetamide, Ophthacet, Sodium Sulamyd, Sodium Sulfacetamide 10%, Sodium Sulfacetamide 15%, Sodium Sulfacetamide 30%, Soss-10, Sulf-10, Sulfair 15

Func. class.: Antibacterial
Chem. class.: Sulfonamide

Action: Inhibits folic acid synthesis by preventing PABA use, which is necessary for bacterial growth

Uses: Conjunctivitis, superficial eye infections, corneal ulcers, adjunct to systemic sulfonamide therapy in treatment of trachoma

Dosage and routes:

• *Adult and child:* INSTILL 1-2 gtts q2-3h; TOP apply ½-1 inch oint into conjunctival sac qid-tid and at bedtime

Available forms: Sterile ophth sol 10%, 15%, 30%; sterile ophth oint 10%

Side effects/adverse reactions:

EENT: Burning, stinging, swelling

Contraindications: Hypersensitivity, infants <2 mo, varicella, vaccinia, viral disease, mycobacterial/fungal infection of the eye, epithelial herpes simplex, keratitis

Precautions: Antibiotic hypersensitivity, pregnancy (C), lactation, children, dry eye

Interactions/incompatabilities:

• Incompatable with silver preparations

NURSING CONSIDERATIONS

Assess:

• Allergy: itching, lacrimation, redness, swelling

Administer:

• After washing hands; cleanse crusts or discharge from eye before application

Perform/provide:

• Storage at room temperature

Evaluate:

• Therapeutic response: absence of redness, inflammation, tearing

Teach patient/family:

• To use drug exactly as prescribed

• Not to use eye makeup, towels, washcloths, eye medication of others; reinfection may occur

• That drug container tip should not be touched to eye

• To report itching, increased redness, burning, stinging; drug should be discontinued

• That drug may cause blurred vision when ointment is applied; may cause sensitivity to bright light

sulfadiazine

(sul-fa-dye′a-zeen)

Func. class.: Antibiotic
Chem. class.: Sulfonamide, intermediate acting

Action: Interferes with bacterial biosynthesis of proteins by competitive antagonism of PABA

Uses: Urinary tract infections, rheumatic fever prophylaxis, adjunctive in toxoplasmosis

Dosage and routes:

Urinary tract infections

• *Adult:* PO 2-4 g, then 1-2 g q6h × 10 days

• *Child:* PO 75 mg/kg or 2 g/m², then 150 mg/kg/day or 4 g/m² in 4-6 divided doses, max. 6 g/day

Rheumatic fever prophylaxis

• *Child >30 kg:* PO 1 g qd

• *Child <30 kg:* PO 500 mg qd

Available forms: Tabs 500 mg

S

Side effects/adverse reactions:

SYST: Anaphylaxis

GI: Nausea, vomiting, abdominal pain, stomatitis, *hepatitis,* glossitis, pancreatitis, diarrhea, *enterocolitis,* anorexia

CNS: Headache, insomnia, hallucinations, depression, vertigo, fatigue, anxiety, *convulsions,* drug fever, chills, drowsiness

HEMA: Leukopenia, thrombocytopenia, agranulocytosis, hemolytic anemia, aplastic anemia

INTEG: Rash, dermatitis, urticaria, *Stevens-Johnson syndrome,* erythema, photosensitivity, alopecia

GU: Renal failure, toxic nephrosis, increased BUN, creatinine, crystalluria, hematuria, proteinuria

CV: Allergic myocarditis

Contraindications: Hypersensitivity to sulfonamides, sulfonylureas, thiazide and loop diuretics, salicylates, pregnancy at term

Precautions: Pregnancy (C), lactation, impaired hepatic function, severe allergy, bronchial asthma, renal dysfunction

Pharmacokinetics:

PO: Rapidly absorbed, onset ½ hr; peak 3-6 hr, 30%-50% bound to plasma proteins, half-life 8-10 hr; excreted in urine, breast milk; crosses placenta, metabolized in liver

Interactions/incompatibilities:

• Decreased effectiveness: oral contraceptives

• Increased hypoglycemic response: sulfonylurea agents

• Increased anticoagulant effects: oral anticoagulants

• Decreased renal excretion of: methotrexate

• Decreased hepatic clearance of: phenytoin

Lab test interferences:

False positive: Urinary glucose test (Benedict's method)

NURSING CONSIDERATIONS

Assess:

• I&O ratio; note color, character, pH of urine if drug administered for urinary tract infections; output should be 800 ml less than intake; if urine is highly acidic, alkalization may be needed

• Kidney function studies: BUN, creatinine, urinalysis if on long-term therapy

• Blood dyscrasias: skin rash, fever, sore throat, bruising, bleeding, fatigue, joint pain

• Allergic reaction: rash, dermatitis, urticaria, pruritus, dyspnea, bronchospasm

Administer:

• With full glass of H_2O to maintain adequate hydration; increase fluids to 2 L/day to decrease crystallization in kidneys

• Medication after C&S; repeat C&S after full course of medication completed

• With resuscitative equipment available; severe allergic reaction may occur

Perform/provide:

• Storage in tight, light-resistant container at room temperature

Evaluate:

• Therapeutic response: absence of pain, fever, C&S negative

Teach patient/family:

• To take each oral dose with full glass of water to prevent crystalluria

• To complete full course of treatment to prevent superimposed infection

• To avoid sunlight or use sunscreen to prevent burns

• To avoid OTC medication (aspirin, Vit C) unless directed by physician

• To use alternative contraceptive measures; decreased effectiveness

of oral contraceptives may result
• To notify physician if skin rash, sore throat, fever, mouth scores, unusual bruising, bleeding occur

---

sulfamethizole
(sul-fa-meth'i-zole)
Sulfasol, Thiosulfil
Func. class.: Antibiotic
Chem. class.: Sulfonamide, short acting

Action: Interferes with bacterial biosynthesis of proteins by competitive antagonism of PABA
Uses: UTIs
Dosage and routes:
• *Adult:* PO 0.5-1 g tid-qid
• Child >2 mo: PO 30-45 mg/kg/day in divided doses q6h
Available forms: Tabs 250, 500 mg
Side effects/adverse reactions:
SYST: Anaphylaxis
GI: Nausea, vomiting, abdominal pain, stomatitis, *hepatitis,* glossitis, pancreatitis, diarrhea, *enterocolitis*
CNS: Headache, confusion, insomnia, hallucinations, depression, vertigo, fatigue, anxiety, *convulsions,* drug fever, chills
HEMA: Leukopenia, neutropenia, thrombocytopenia, agranulocytosis, hemolytic anemia
INTEG: Rash, dermatitis, urticaria, *Stevens-Johnson syndrome,* erythema, photosensitivity
GU: Renal failure, toxic nephrosis, increased BUN, creatinine, crystalluria
CV: Allergic myocarditis
Contraindications: Hypersensitivity to sulfonamides, pregnancy at term
Precautions: Pregnancy (C), lactation, impaired hepatic function, severe allergy, bronchial asthma

Pharmacokinetics:
PO: Rapidly absorbed, peak 2 hr, 90% bound to plasma proteins, excreted in urine, breast milk, crosses placenta
Interactions/incompatibilities:
• Decreased absorption of: digoxin
• Decreased effectiveness: oral contraceptives
• Increased hypoglycemic response: sulfonylurea agents
• Increased anticoagulant effects: oral anticoagulants
• Decreased renal excretion of: methotrexate
• Decreased hepatic clearance of: phenytoin
Lab test interferences:
False positive: Urinary glucose test (Benedict's method)
NURSING CONSIDERATIONS
Assess:
• I&O ratio; note color, character, pH of urine if drug administered for UTIs; output should be 800 ml less than intake; if urine is highly acidic, alkalization may be needed
• Kidney function studies: BUN, creatinine, urinalysis if on long-term therapy
• Blood dyscrasias: skin rash, fever, sore throat, bruising, bleeding, fatigue, joint pain
• Allergic reaction: rash, dermatitis, urticaria, pruritus, dyspnea, bronchospasm
Administer:
• With full glass of H_2O to maintain adequate hydration; increase fluids to 2 L/day to decrease crystallization in kidneys
• Medication after C&S; repeat C&S after full course of medication completed
• With resuscitative equipment available; severe allergic reactions may occur

S

---

italics = common side effects   ***bold italic*** = life threatening reactions

Perform/provide:
• Storage in tight, light-resistant container at room temperature
Evaluate:
• Therapeutic response: absence of pain, fever, C&S negative
Teach patient/family:
• To take each oral dose with full glass of H_2O to prevent crystalluria
• To complete full course of treatment to prevent superimposed infection
• To avoid sunlight or use sunscreen to prevent burns
• To avoid OTC medication (aspirin, Vit C) unless directed by physician
• To use alternative contraceptive measures; decreased effectiveness of oral contraceptives may result
• To notify physician of skin rash, sore throat, fever, mouth sores, unusual bruising, bleeding

---

sulfamethoxazole
(sul-fa-meth-ox′a-zole)
Gantanol, Urobak
Func. class.: Antibiotic
Chem. class.: Sulfonamide, intermediate acting

Action: Interferes with bacterial biosynthesis of proteins by competitive antagonism of PABA
Uses: UTIs, lymphogranuloma venereum, systemic infections
Dosage and routes:
• *Adult:* PO 2 g, then 1 g bid or tid for 7-10 days
• Child >2 mo: PO 50-60 mg/kg then 25-30 mg/kg bid, not to exceed 75 mg/kg/day
Lymphogranuloma venereum
• Adult: PO 1 g bid × 14 days
Available forms: Tabs 500 mg; oral susp 500 mg/5ml

Side effects/adverse reactions:
*SYST: **Anaphylaxis***
GI: Nausea, vomiting, abdominal pain, stomatitis, ***hepatitis,*** glossitis, pancreatitis, diarrhea, ***enterocolitis,*** anorexia
CNS: Headache, insomnia, hallucinations, depression, vertigo, fatigue, anxiety, convulsions, drug fever, chills, drowsiness
*HEMA: **Leukopenia, thrombocytopenia, agranulocytosis, hemolytic anemia, aplastic anemia***
INTEG: Rash, dermatitis, urticaria, ***Stevens-Johnson syndrome,*** erythema, photosensitivity, alopecia
*GU: **Renal failure, toxic nephrosis,*** increased BUN, creatinine, crystalluria, hematuria, proteinuria
*CV: **Allergic myocarditis***
Contraindications: Hypersensitivity to sulfonamides, sulfonylureas, thiazide and loop diuretics, salicylates, pregnancy at term
Precautions: Pregnancy (C), lactation, impaired hepatic function, severe allergy, bronchial asthma
Pharmacokinetics:
PO: Poorly absorbed, peak 3-4 hr, 50%-70% bound to plasma proteins, half-life 7-12 hr; excreted in urine (unchanged 90%), breast milk; crosses placenta
Interactions/incompatibilities:
• Decreased effectiveness: oral contraceptives
• Increased hypoglycemic response: sulfonylurea agents
• Increased anticoagulant effects: oral anticoagulants
• Decreased renal excretion of: methotrexate
• Decreased hepatic clearance of: phenytoin
Lab test interferences:
False positive: Urinary glucose test (Benedict's method)

NURSING CONSIDERATIONS
Assess:
• I&O ratio; note color, character, pH of urine if drug administered for urinary tract infections; output should be 800 ml less than intake; if urine is highly acidic, alkalization may be needed
• Kidney function studies: BUN, creatinine, urinalysis if on long-term therapy
• Blood dyscrasias: skin rash, fever, sore throat, bruising, bleeding, fatigue, joint pain
• Allergic reaction: rash, dermatitis, urticaria, pruritus, dyspnea, bronchospasm

Administer:
• With full glass of H_2O to maintain adequate hydration; increase fluids to 2 L/day to decrease crystallization in kidneys
• Medication after C&S; repeat C&S after full course of medication completed
• With resuscitative equipment available; severe allergic reaction may occur

Perform/provide:
• Storage in tight, light-resistant container at room temperature

Evaluate:
• Therapeutic response: absence of pain, fever, C&S negative

Teach patient/family:
• To take each oral dose with full glass of H_2O to prevent crystalluria
• To complete full course of treatment to prevent superimposed infection
• To avoid sunlight or use sunscreen to prevent burns
• To avoid OTC medication (aspirin, Vit C) unless directed by physician
• To use alternative contraceptive measures; decreased effectiveness of oral contraceptives may result

• To notify physician if skin rash, sore throat, fever, mouth sores, unusual bruising, bleeding occur

---

sulfasalazine
(sul-fa-sal′a-zeen)
Azulfidine, Azulfidine EN-Tabs, Salazopyrin,* Sulfasalazine
Func. class.: Antiinflammatory
Chem. class.: Sulfonamide

Action: Prodrug to deliver sulfapyridine and 5-aminosalicylic acid to colon

Uses: Ulcerative colitis

Dosage and routes:
• *Adult:* PO 3-4 g/day in divided doses; maintenance 1.5-2 g/day in divided doses q6h
• *Child >2 yrs.:* PO 40-60 mg/kg/day in 4-6 divided doses, then 20-30 mg/kg/day in 4 doses, max 2 g/day

Available forms: Tabs 500 mg; oral susp 250 mg/5ml; enteric-coated tabs 500 mg

Side effects/adverse reactions:
*SYST: **Anaphylaxis***

GI: Nausea, vomiting, abdominal pain, stomatitis, **hepatitis**, glossitis, pancreatitis, diarrhea

CNS: Headache, confusion, insomnia, hallucinations, depression, vertigo, fatigue, anxiety, **convulsions,** drug fever, chills

*HEMA: **Leukopenia, neutropenia, thrombocytopenia, agranulocytosis, hemolytic anemia***

INTEG: Rash, dermatitis, urticaria, **Stevens-Johnson syndrome,** erythema, photosensitivity

*GU: **Renal failure, toxic nephrosis,*** increased BUN, creatinine, crystalluria

*CV: **Allergic myocarditis***

Contraindications: Hypersensitivity to sulfonamides or salicylates,

---

italics = common side effects   ***bold italic*** = life threatening reactions

S

pregnancy at term, child <2 yr intestinal, urinary obstruction

Precautions: Pregnancy (C), lactation, impaired hepatic function, severe allergy, bronchial asthma, impaired renal function

Pharmacokinetics:

PO: Partially absorbed, peak 1½-6 hr, half-life 5-10 hr, excreted in urine as sulfasalazine (15%), sulfapyridine (60%), 5-aminosalicylic acid and metabolites (20%-33%), in breast milk; crosses placenta

Interactions/incompatibilities:
• Decreased absorption of: digoxin, folic acid
• Decreased effectiveness: oral contraceptives
• Increased hypoglycemic response: sulfonylurea agents
• Increased anticoagulant effects: oral anticoagulants
• Decreased renal excretion of: methotrexate
• Decreased hepatic clearance of: phenytoin

Lab test intereferences:

False positive: Urinary glucose test

NURSING CONSIDERATIONS

Assess:
• I&O ratio; note color, amount, character, pH of urine if drug administered for urinary tract infections; output should be 800 ml less than intake; if urine is highly acidic, alkalization may be needed
• Kidney function studies: BUN, creatinine, urinalysis if on long-term therapy
• Blood dyscrasias: skin rash, fever, sore throat, bruising, bleeding, fatigue, joint pain
• Allergic reaction: rash, dermatitis, urticaria, pruritus, dyspnea, bronchospasm

Administer:
• With full glass of H_2O to maintain adequate hydration; increase fluids to 2 L/day to decrease crystallization in kidneys
• Medication after C&S; repeat C&S after full course of medication completed
• With resuscitative equipment available; severe allergic reaction may occur
• Total daily dose in evenly spaced doses and after meals to help minimize GI intolerance

Perform/provide:
• Storage in tight, light-resistant container at room temperature

Evaluate:
• Therapeutic response: absence of fever, mucus in stools

Teach patient family:
• To take each oral dose with full glass of H_2O to prevent crystalluria
• To complete full course of treatment to prevent superimposed infection
• To avoid sunlight or use sunscreen to prevent burns
• To avoid OTC medication (aspirin, Vit C) unless directed by physician
• To use alternative contraceptive measures; decreased effectiveness of oral contraceptives may result
• To notify physician if skin rash, sore throat, fever, mouth sores, unusual bruising, bleeding occur

---

sulfinpyrazone
(sul-fin-peer′a-zone)
Anturan,* Anturane
Func. class.: Uricosuric
Chem. class.: Pyrazolone

Action: Inhibits tubular reabsorption of urates, with increased excretion of uric acid; inhibits prostaglandin synthesis, which decreases platelet aggregation

Uses: Inhibition of platelet aggregation, gout
Dosage and routes:
Inhibition of platelet aggregation
• *Adult:* PO 200 mg qid
Gout/gouty arthritis
• *Adult:* PO 100-200 mg bid × 1 wk, then 200-400 mg bid, not to exceed 800 mg/day
Available forms: Tabs 100 mg; caps 200 mg
Side effects/adverse reactions:
CNS: Dizziness, *convulsions, coma*
EENT: Tinnitus
GU: Renal calculi, hypoglycemia
GI: Gastric irritation, nausea, vomiting, anorexia, hepatic necrosis, GI bleeding
INTEG: Rash, dermatitis, pruritus, fever, photosensitivity
HEMA: Agranulocytosis (rare)
RESP: Apnea, irregular respirations
Contraindications: Hypersensitivity to pyrazolone derivatives, severe hepatic disease, blood dyscrasias, severe renal disease, CrCl <50 mg/min, active peptic ulcer, GI inflammation, renal calculi
Precautions: Pregnancy (C), lactation
Pharmacokinetics:
PO: Peak 1-2 hr, duration 4-6 hr, half-life 3 hr; metabolized by liver, excreted in urine
Interactions/incompatibilities:
• Increased toxicity: sulfa drugs, dapsone, clofibrate, PAS, indomethacin, rifampin, naproxen, methotrexate, pantothenic acid, tolbutamide, warfarin
• Decreased effects of sulfinpyrazone: salicylates, xanthines
NURSING CONSIDERATIONS
Assess:
• Uric acid levels (3-7 mg/dl)
• Respiratory rate, rhythm, depth; notify physician of abnormalities
• Renal function

• Bleeding tendencies, RBC and Hct
• I & O
• Electrolytes, CO_2 before, during treatment
• Urine pH, output, glucose during beginning treatment
Lab test interferences:
Increase: PSP, aminohippuric acid
False positive: Clinitest
Administer:
• With glass of milk
• With food for GI symptoms
• Increased fluids to prevent calculi; alkalinization of urine may be required
Evaluate:
• Therapeutic response: absence of pain, stiffness in joints
Teach patient/family:
• To avoid aspirin, alcohol, high purine diet

---

sulfisoxazole
(sul-fi-sox'a-zole)
Gantrisin, Novosoxazole,* Sulfisoxazole
Func. class.: Antibiotic
Chem. class.: Sulfonamide, short acting

Action: Interferes with bacterial biosynthesis of proteins by competitive antagonism of PABA
Uses: Urinary tract, systemic infections; chancroid; trachoma; toxoplasmosis; acute otitis media; lymphogranuloma venereum, eye infections
Dosage and routes:
• *Adult:* PO 2-4 g loading dose, then 1-2 g qid × 7-10 days
• *Child >2 mo:* PO 75 mg/kg or 2 g/m² loading dose, then 120-150 mg/kg/day or 4 g/m²/day in divided doses q6h, not to exceed 6 g/day

Available forms: Tabs 500 mg; syr, pediatric susp 500 mg/5 ml

Side effects/adverse reactions:
SYST: Anaphylaxis
GI: Nausea, vomiting, abdominal pain, stomatitis, *hepatitis,* glossitis, pancreatitis, diarrhea, *enterocolitis,* anorexia
CNS: Headache, insomnia, hallucinations, depression, vertigo, fatigue, anxiety, *convulsions,* drug fever, chills, drowsiness
HEMA: Leukopenia, thrombocytopenia, agranulocytosis, hemolytic anemia, aplastic anemia
INTEG: Rash, dermatitis, urticaria, *Stevens-Johnson syndrome,* erythema, photosensitivity, alopecia
GU: Renal failure, toxic nephrosis, increased BUN, creatinine, crystalluria, hematuria, proteinuria
CV: Allergic myocarditis

Contraindications: Hypersensitivity to sulfonamides and sulfonylureas, thiazide and loop diuretics, salicylates; pregnancy at term

Precautions: Pregnancy (C), lactation, impaired hepatic function, severe allergy, bronchial asthma

Pharmacokinetics:
PO: Rapidly absorbed, peak 2-4 hr, 85% protein bound; half-life 4-7 hr, excreted in urine, crosses placenta

Interactions/incompatibilities:
• Decreased effectiveness of: oral contraceptives
• Increased hypoglycemic response: sulfonylurea agents
• Increased anticoagulant effect: oral anticoagulants
• Decreased renal excretion of: methotrexate
• Decreased hepatic clearance of: phenytoin

Lab test interferences:
False positive: Urinary glucose test

NURSING CONSIDERATIONS
Assess:
• I&O ratio; note color, character, pH of urine if drug administered for urinary tract infections; output should be 800 ml less than intake; if urine is highly acidic, alkalization may be needed
• Kidney function studies: BUN, creatinine, urinalysis if on long-term therapy
• Blood dyscrasias: skin rash, fever, sore throat, bruising, bleeding, fatigue, joint pain
• Allergic reaction: rash, dermatitis, urticaria, pruritus, dyspnea, bronchospasm

Administer:
• With full glass of H_2O to maintain adequate hydration; increase fluids to 2 L/day to decrease crystallization in kidneys
• Medication after C&S; repeat C&S after full course of medication completed
• With resuscitative equipment available; severe allergic reaction may occur

Perform/provide:
• Storage in tight, light-resistant container at room temperature

Evaluate:
• Therapeutic response: absence of pain, fever, C&S negative

Teach patient/family:
• Take each oral dose with full glass of H_2O to prevent crystalluria
• To complete full course of treatment to prevent superimposed infection
• To avoid sunlight or use sunscreen to prevent burns; avoid hazardous activities if dizziness occurs
• To avoid OTC medication (aspirin, Vit C) unless directed by physician
• To use alternative contraceptive measures; decreased effectiveness of oral contraceptives may result
• To notify physician if skin rash,

sore throat, fever, mouth sores, unusual bruising, bleeding occur

sulindac
(sul-in'dak)
Clinoril, Novosudac,* Sulindac
Func. class.: Nonsteroidal antiinflammatory
Chem. class.: Indeneacetic acid derivative

Action: Inhibits prostaglandin synthesis by decreasing an enzyme needed for biosynthesis; analgesic, antiinflammatory, antipyretic

Uses: Mild to moderate pain, osteoarthritis, rheumatoid, gouty arthritis, ankylosing spondylitis

Dosage and routes:
Arthritis
• *Adult:* PO 150 mg bid, may increase to 200 mg bid
Bursitis/acute arthritis
• *Adult:* PO 200 mg bid × 1-2 wk, then reduce dose
Available forms: Tabs 100, 150, 200 mg

Side effects/adverse reactions:
GI: Nausea, anorexia, vomiting, diarrhea, jaundice, ***cholestatic hepatitis,*** constipation, flatulence, cramps, dry mouth, peptic ulcer, ***bleeding, ulceration, perforation***
CNS: Dizziness, drowsiness, fatigue, tremors, confusion, insomnia, anxiety, depression
CV: Tachycardia, peripheral edema, palpitations, dysrhythmias
INTEG: Purpura, rash, pruritus, sweating, photosensitivity
GU: ***Nephrotoxicity: dysuria, hematuria, oliguria, azotemia***
HEMA: ***Blood dyscrasias***
EENT: Tinnitus, hearing loss, blurred vision

Contraindications: Hypersensitivity, asthma, severe renal disease, severe hepatic disease, active ulcers

Precautions: Pregnancy (C), lactation, children, bleeding disorders, GI disorders, cardiac disorders, hypersensitivity to other antiinflammatory agents

Pharmacokinetics:
PO: Peak 2 hr, half-life 3-3½ hr; metabolized in liver, excreted in urine (metabolites); excreted in breast milk, 93% protein binding

Interactions/incompatibilities:
• Increased action of: coumarin, phenytoin, sulfonamides

NURSING CONSIDERATIONS
Assess:
• Renal, liver, blood studies: BUN, creatinine, AST, ALT, Hgb, before treatment, periodically thereafter
• Have BP checked monthly; drug causes Na retention
• Audiometric, ophthalmic exam before, during, after treatment
• For eye, ear problems: blurred vision, tinnitus (may indicate toxicity)

Administer:
• With food to decrease GI symptoms; best to take on empty stomach to facilitate absorption; tablet may be crushed

Perform/provide:
• Storage at room temperature

Evaluate:
• Therapeutic response: decreased pain, stiffness, swelling in joints, ability to move more easily

Teach patient/family:
• To report blurred vision or ringing, roaring in ears (may indicate toxicity)
• To avoid driving or other hazardous activities if dizziness or drowsiness occurs
• To report change in urine pattern, weight increase, edema, pain increase in joints, fever, blood in urine (indicates nephrotoxicity)

S

---

italics = common side effects   ***bold italic*** = life threatening reactions

- That therapeutic effects may take up to 1 mo
- To avoid alcohol and aspirin
- To take with full glass of water
- To use sunscreen

---

sumatriptan succinate
(summa-trip′-tan)
Imitrex
Func. class.: Migraine agent
Chem. class.: 5HT-1-like receptor agonist

Action: Binds selectively to the vascular 5-HT-1 receptor subtype and exerts antimigraine effect; causes vasoconstriction

Uses: Acute treatment of migraine with or without aura and cluster headache

Dosage and routes:
• *Adult:* SC 6 mg or less; may repeat in 1 hr; not to exceed 12 mg/24 hr
Available forms: SC inj 6 mg (12 mg/ml); unit-of-use syringes (0.5 in/ml); self-dosing system, 6-mg single-dose vial (0.5 ml in 2 ml)

Side effects/adverse reactions:
NEURO: Tingling, hot sensation, burning, feeling of pressure, tightness, numbness, dizziness, sedation, headache, anxiety, fatigue, cold sensation
CV: Flushing
RESP: Chest tightness, pressure
EENT: Throat, mouth, nasal discomfort, vision changes
GI: Abdominal discomfort
MS: Weakness, neck stiffness, myalgia
INTEG: Injection site reaction, sweating

Contraindications: Angina pectoris, history of MI, documented silent ischemia, Prinzmetal's angina, ischemic heart disease, IV use, concurrent ergotamine-containing preparations, uncontrolled hypertension, hypersensitivity, basilar or hemiplegic migraine

Precautions: Postmenopausal women, men >40 yr, risk factors for CAD, hypercholesterolemia, obesity, diabetes, impaired hepatic or renal function, pregnancy (C), lactation, children, elderly

Pharmacokinetics: Onset of pain relief 10 min–2 hr, peak 10-20 min, 10%-20% plasma protein binding, metabolized in the liver (metabolite), excreted in urine, feces

NURSING CONSIDERATIONS
Assess:
- Tingling, hot sensation, burning, feeling of pressure, numbness, flushing, infection site reaction
- For stress level, activity, recreation, coping mechanisms of patient
- Neurologic status: LOC, blurring vision, nausea, vomiting, tingling in extremities preceding headache
- Ingestion of tyramine foods (pickled products, beer, wine, aged cheese), food additives, preservatives, colorings, artificial sweeteners, chocolate, caffeine, which may precipitate these types of headaches

Perform/provide:
- Quiet, calm environment with decreased stimulation for noise, bright light, excessive talking

Evaluate:
- Therapeutic response: decrease in frequency, severity of headache

Teach patient/family:
- Use of self-dosing system; not to exceed 12 mg/24 hr
- To report any side effects to physician

• To use contraception when taking drug

---

tacrine HCl (tetrahydroaminoacridine, THA)
(tack'rin)
Cognex
Func. class.: Reversible cholinesterase

Action: Elevates acetylcholine concentrations (cerebral cortex) by slowing degradation of acetylcholine released in cholinergic neurons; does not alter underlying dementia

Uses: Treatment of mild to moderate dementia in Alzheimer's disease

Dosage and routes:
• *Adult:* PO 10 mg qid × 6 wk, then 20 mg qid × 6 wk, increase at 6-wk intervals if patient tolerating drug well and if transaminase is WNL

Available forms: Tabs 10, 20, 30, 40 mg

Side effects/adverse reactions:
*CNS: **Dizziness, confusion, insomnia,** tremor, **ataxia, somnolence, anxiety, agitation, depression, hallucinations, hostility, abnormal thinking,** chills, fever*
CV: Hypotension or hypertension
*GI: **Nausea, vomiting, anorexia, abdominal pain, constipation,** dyspepsia, flatulence*
*GU: **Frequency, UTI, incontinence***
*INTEG: **Rash,** flushing*
*RESP: **Rhinitis, URI, cough,** pharyngitis*

Contraindications: Hypersensitivity to this drug or acridine derivatives, patients treated with this drug who developed jaundice with a total bilirubin of >3 mg/dl

Precautions: Sick sinus syndrome, history of ulcers, GI bleeding, hepatic disease, bladder obstruction, asthma, pregnancy (C), lactation, children

Pharmacokinetics: Rapidly absorbed PO, 55% bound to plasma proteins, metabolized to metabolites, elimination half-life 2-4 hr

Interactions/incompatibilities:
• Decreased activity of: anticholinergics
• Increased elimination half-life of: theophylline
• Synergistic effect: succinylcholine, cholinesterase inhibitors, cholinergic agonists

NURSING CONSIDERATIONS
Assess:
• B/P, hypotension or hypertension
• Mental status: affect, mood, behavioral changes, depression; complete suicide assessment; hallucinations, confusion
• GI status: nausea, vomiting, anorexia, constipation, abdominal pain; add bulk and increase fluids for constipation
• GU status: urinary frequency, incontinence

Administer:
• Dosage adjusted to patient's response no more than q6wk

Perform/provide:
• Assistance with ambulation during beginning therapy; dizziness, ataxia may occur

Evaluate:
• Therapeutic response: decrease in confusion, improved mood

Teach patient/family:
• To report side effects: twitching, eye spasms; indicate overdose
• To use drug exactly as prescribed:

---

italics = common side effects   ***bold italic*** = life threatening reactions

at regular intervals, preferably between meals; may be taken with meals for GI upset
• To notify physician of nausea, vomiting, diarrhea (dose increase or beginning treatment) or rash, very dark or very light stools, jaundice (delayed onset)
• Not to increase or abruptly decrease dose; serious consequences may result

Treatment of overdose:
Withdraw drug, administer tertiary anticholinergics, provide supportive care

---

talbutal
(tal′byoo-tal)
Lotusate
Func. class.: Sedative/hypnotic barbiturate (intermediate acting)
Chem. class.: Barbitone

Controlled Substance Schedule II (USA), Schedule G (Canada)
Action: Depresses activity in brain cells, primarily in reticular activating system in brain stem; selectively depresses neurons in posterior hypothalamus, limbic structures
Uses: Insomnia, short-term only
Dosage and routes:
• *Adult:* PO 120 mg hs
Available forms: Tabs 120 mg
Side effects/adverse reactions:
CNS: Lethargy, drowsiness, hangover, dizziness, paradoxical stimulation in elderly and children, light-headedness, dependency, CNS depression, mental depression, slurred speech
GI: Nausea, vomiting, diarrhea, constipation
INTEG: Rash, urticaria, pain, abscesses at injection site, angio-

edema, thrombophlebitis, *Stevens-Johnson syndrome*
CV: Hypotension, bradycardia
RESP: Depression, apnea, *laryngospasm, bronchospasm*
HEMA: Agranulocytosis, thrombocytopenia, megaloblastic anemia (long-term treatment)
Contraindications: Hypersensitivity to barbiturates, respiratory depression, addiction to barbiturates, severe liver impairment, porphyria, pregnancy (D), uncontrolled severe pain
Precautions: Anemia, lactation, hepatic disease, renal disease, hypertension, elderly, acute/chronic pain
Pharmacokinetics:
Onset 30-45 min, duration 4-6 hr; metabolized by liver, excreted by kidneys (metabolites)
Interactions/incompatibilities:
• Increased CNS depression: alcohol, MAOIs, sedative, narcotics
• Decreased effect of: oral anticoagulants, corticosteroids, griseofulvin, quinidine
• Decreased half-life of: doxycycline
Lab test interferences:
False increase: Sulfobromophthalein
NURSING CONSIDERATIONS
Assess:
• Blood studies: Hct, Hgb, RBCs, if blood dyscrasias are suspected
• Hepatic studies: AST, ALT, bilirubin, if hepatic damage has occurred
• Mental status: mood, sensorium, affect, memory (long, short)
• Physical dependency: more frequent requests for medication, shakes, anxiety
• Barbiturate toxicity: hypotension; pupillary constriction; cold, clammy skin; cyanosis of lips; in-

---

somnia; nausea; vomiting; hallucinations; delirium; weakness; mild symptoms may occur in 8-12 hr without drug
• Respiratory dysfunction: respiratory depression, character, rate, rhythm; hold drug if respirations are < 10/min or if pupils are dilated (rare)
• Blood dyscrasias: fever, sore throat, bruising, rash, jaundice, epistaxis (rare)

Administer:
• After removal of cigarettes to prevent fires
• After trying conservative measures for insomnia
• ½-1 hr before hs for sleeplessness
• On empty stomach for best absorption
• For < 14 days, since drug is not effective after that; tolerance develops
• Crushed or whole

Perform/provide:
• Assistance with ambulation after receiving dose
• Safety measure: side rails, nightlight, call bell within easy reach
• Checking to see PO medication has been swallowed
• Storage in tight container in cool environment

Evaluate:
• Therapeutic response: ability to sleep at night, decreased amount of early morning awakening

Teach patient/family:
• That morning hangover is common
• That drug is indicated only for short-term treatment of insomnia and is probably ineffective after 2 wk
• That physical dependency may result when used for extended periods of time (45-90 days depending on dose)

tamox

• To avoid
ties requirin
curs within
• To avoid
depressants;
sion may resu.
• To tell all prescribers that barbiturate is being taken
• That withdrawal insomnia may occur after short-term use; do not start using drug again; insomnia will improve in 1-3 nights; may experience increased dreaming
• That effects may take 2 nights for benefits to be noticed
• Alternative measures to improve sleep (reading, exercise several hours before hs, warm bath, warm milk, TV, self-hypnosis, deep breathing)

Treatment of overdose: Lavage, activated charcoal, warming blanket, vital signs, hemodialysis, I&O ratio

---

tamoxifen citrate
(ta-mox′i-fen)
Nolvadex, Tamofen,* Tamone*

Func. class.: Antineoplastic
Chem. class.: Antiestrogen hormone

Action: Inhibits cell division by binding to cytoplasmic estrogen receptors; resembles normal cell complex but inhibits DNA synthesis and estrogen response of target tissue

Uses: Advanced breast carcinoma that has not responded to other therapy in estrogen-receptor-positive patients (usually postmenopausal)

Dosage and routes:
• *Adult:* PO 10-20 mg bid
Available forms: Tabs 10 mg

---

italics = common side effects   **bold italic** = life threatening reactions

oxifen citrate

...cts/adverse reactions:
... Thrombocytopenia, leuko-
...a
...: Nausea, vomiting, altered taste
(anorexia)
GU: Vaginal bleeding, pruritus
vulvae
INTEG: Rash, alopecia
CV: Chest pain
*CNS: Hot flashes, headache, light-
headedness,* depression
META: Hypercalcemia
EENT: Ocular lesions, retinopathy,
corneal opacity, blurred vision
(high doses)
Contraindications: Hypersensitiv-
ity, pregnancy (D)
Precautions: Leukopenia, throm-
bocytopenia, lactation, cataracts
Pharmacokinetics:
PO: Peak 4-7 hr, half-life 7 days (1
wk terminal), excreted primarily in
feces
Lab test interferences:
Increase: Serum Ca
NURSING CONSIDERATIONS
Assess:
• CBC, differential, platelet count
weekly; withhold drug if WBC
is <3500 or platelet count is
<100,000; notify physician of re-
sults
• Bleeding: hematuria, guaiac,
bruising, petechiae, mucosa or orifices q8h
• Food preferences; list likes, dislikes
• Effects of alopecia on body image; discuss feelings about body
changes
• Symptoms indicating severe allergic reactions: rash, pruritus, urticaria, purpuric skin lesions, itching, flushing
Administer:
• Antacid before oral agent; give
drug after evening meal, before
bedtime

• Antiemetic 30-60 min before giv-
ing drug to prevent vomiting
Perform/provide:
• Liquid diet, if needed including
cola, Jell-O; dry toast or crackers
may be added if patient is not nauseated or vomiting
• Increase fluid intake to 2-3 L/day
to prevent dehydration
• Nutritious diet with iron, vitamin
supplements as ordered
• Storage in light-resistant container at room temperature
Evaluate:
• Therapeutic response: decreased
tumor size, spread of malignancy
Teach patient/family:
• To report any complaints, side effects to nurse or physician
• That vaginal bleeding, pruritus, hot flashes, can occur, are
reversible after discontinuing treatment
• To report immediately decreased
visual acuity, which may be irreversible; stress need for routine eye
exams, who should be told about
tamoxifen therapy
• To report vaginal bleeding immediately
• That tumor flare—increase in
size of tumor, increased bone
pain—may occur: and will subside
rapidly; may take analgesics for
pain
• That premenopausal women must
use mechanical birth control because ovulation may be induced
• That hair may be lost during treatment; a wig or hairpiece may make
patient feel better; new hair may be
different in color, texture

* Available in Canada only

temazepam

(te-maz'e-pam)

Restoril, Temazepam

Func. class.: Sedative-hypnotic

Chem. class.: Benzodiazepine

Controlled Substance Schedule IV (USA), Schedule F (Canada)

Action: Produces CNS depression at limbic, thalamic, hypothalamic levels of the CNS; may be mediated by neurotransmitter γ-aminobutyric acid (GABA); results are sedation, hypnosis, skeletal muscle relaxation, anticonvulsant activity, anxiolytic action

Uses: Insomnia

Dosage and routes:

• *Adult:* PO 15-30 mg hs

Available forms: Caps 15, 30 mg

Side effects/adverse reactions:

*HEMA: **Leukopenia, granulocytopenia** (rare)*

CNS: Lethargy, drowsiness, daytime sedation, dizziness, confusion, light-headedness, headache, anxiety, irritability

GI: Nausea, vomiting, diarrhea, heartburn, abdominal pain, constipation, anorexia

CV: Chest pain, pulse changes

Contraindications: Hypersensitivity to benzodiazepines, pregnancy (X), lactation, intermittent porphyria

Precautions: Anemia, hepatic disease, renal disease, suicidal individuals, drug abuse, elderly, psychosis, child < 15 yr, acute narrow-angle glaucoma, seizure disorders

Pharmacokinetics:

PO: Onset 30-45 min, duration 6-8 hr, half-life 10-20 hr; metabolized by liver, excreted by kidneys, crosses placenta, excreted in breast milk

Interactions/incompatibilities:

• Increased effects of: cimetidine, disulfiram, oral contraceptives

• Increased action of both drugs: alcohol, CNS depressants

• Decreased effect of: antacids, theophylline, smoking, rifampin

Lab test interferences:

Increase: ALT/AST, serum bilirubin

Decrease: RAI uptake

False increase: Urinary 17-OHCS

NURSING CONSIDERATIONS

Assess:

• Blood studies: Hct, Hgb, RBCs (if on long-term therapy)

• Hepatic studies: AST, ALT, bilirubin (if on long-term therapy)

• Mental status: mood, sensorium, affect, memory (long, short)

• Blood dyscrasias: fever, sore throat, bruising, rash, jaundice, epistaxis (rare)

• Type of sleep problem: falling asleep, staying asleep

Administer:

• After removal of cigarettes to prevent fires

• After trying conservative measures for insomnia

• ½-1 hr before hs for sleeplessness

• On empty stomach for fast onset, but may be taken with food if GI symptoms occur

Perform/provide:

• Assistance with ambulation after receiving dose

• Safety measure: side rails, nightlight, call bell within easy reach

• Checking to see PO medication has been swallowed

• Storage in tight container in cool environment

Evaluate:

• Therapeutic response: ability to sleep at night, decreased amount of early morning awakening if taking drug for insomnia

---

italics = common side effects   ***bold italic*** = life threatening reactions

Teach patient/family:
• To avoid driving, other activities requiring alertness until drug is stabilized
• To avoid alcohol ingestion, CNS depressants; serious CNS depression may result
• That effects may take 2 nights for benefits to be noticed
• Alternative measures to improve sleep: reading, exercise several hours before hs, warm bath, warm milk, TV, self-hypnosis, deep breathing
• That hangover, memory impairment are common in elderly but less common than with barbiturates
Treatment of overdose: Lavage, activated charcoal; monitor electrolytes, VS

---

teniposide (VM 26)
(ten-i-poe-side)
Vumon
Func. class.: Antineoplastic
Chem. class.: Semisynthetic podophyllotoxin

Action: Inhibits mitotic activity through metaphase to mitosis; also inhibits cells from entering mitosis, depresses DNA, RNA synthesis
Uses: Childhood acute lymphoblastic leukemia (ALL)
Dosage and routes:
• *Child IV inf:* Combo teniposide 165 mg/m² and cytarabine 300 mg/m² 2×/wk × 8-9 doses or combo teniposide 250 mg/m² and vincristine 1.5 mg/m² qwk × 4-8 wk and prednisone 40 mg/m² PO × 28 days
Available forms: Inj IV 10 mg/ml
Side effects/adverse reactions:
HEMA: Thrombocytopenia, leukopenia, neutropenia, myelosuppression, anemia

GI: Nausea, vomiting, anorexia, *hepatotoxicity,* diarrhea, stomatitis
INTEG: Rash, alopecia, phlebitis
RESP: Bronchospasm
CV: Hypotension
CNS: Headache, fever
GU: Nephrotoxicity
SYST: Anaphylaxis
Contraindications: Hypersensitivity, bone marrow depression, severe hepatic disease, severe renal disease, bacterial infection, pregnancy (D)
Precautions: Renal disease, hepatic disease, lactation, children, gout, depression
Pharmacokinetics:
Half-life terminal 5 hr, metabolized in liver, excreted in urine, crosses placental barrier
Interactions/incompatibilities:
• Plasma clearance of methotrexate may be increased: methotrexate
• Increased toxicity: sodium salicylate, sulfamethizole, tolbutamide
NURSING CONSIDERATIONS
Assess:
• CBC, differential, platelet count weekly; withhold drug if WBC is <4000 or platelet count is <75,000; notify physician of results
• Renal function studies: BUN, serum uric acid, urine CrCl, electrolytes before, during therapy
• I&O ration; report fall in urine output of 30 ml/hr
• Monitor temperature q4h; may indicate beginning infection
• Liver function tests before, during therapy (bilirubin, AST, ALT, LDH) as needed or monthly
• RBC, Hct, Hgb since these may be decreased
• Bleeding: hematuria, guaiac stools, bruising or petechiae, mucosa or orifices q8h

---

*Available in Canada only

• Food preferences; list likes, dislikes
• Effects of alopecia on body image; discuss feelings about body changes
• Yellowing of skin and sclera, dark urine, clay-colored stools, itchy skin, abdominal pain, fever, diarrhea
• Buccal cavity q8h for dryness, sores or ulceration, white patches, oral pain, bleeding, dysphagia
• Local irritation, pain, burning, discoloration at injection site
• Symptoms indicating severe allergic reaction: rash, pruritus, urticaria, purpuric skin lesions, itching, flushing
• Symptoms of anaphylaxis: flushing, restlessness, coughing, difficulty breathing
• Frequency of stools, characteristics: cramping, acidosis; signs of dehydration: rapid respirations, poor skin turgor, decreased urine output, dry skin, restlessness, weakness

Administer:
• After diluting in D$_5$ or 0.9% NaCl to a concentration of 0.1, 0.2, 0.4, or 1 mg/ml; infuse over 30-60 min or longer; prepare and use glass or polyolefin plastic bags or containers
• Antiemetic 30-60 min before giving drug and prn to prevent vomiting
• Allopurinol or sodium bicarbonate to maintain uric acid levels, alkalinization of urine
• Hyaluronidase 150 U/ml to 1 ml NaCl to infiltration area, ice compress
• Transfusion for anemia
• Antispasmodic

Perform/provide:
• Storage in refrigerator of unopened amps; do not freeze

• Liquid diet: cola, Jell-O; dry toast or crackers may be added if patient is not nauseated or vomiting
• Increase fluid intake to 2-3 L/day to prevent urate deposits, calculi formation
• Diet low in purines: organ meats (kidney, liver), dried beans, peas, to maintain alkaline urine
• Nutritious diet with iron, vitamin supplements
• HOB raised to facilitate breathing

Evaluate:
• Therapeutic response: remission of ALL

Teach patient/family:
• To report any complaints or side effects to nurse or physician
• To report any changes in breathing, coughing, fever, chills, rapid heartbeat
• That hair may be lost during treatment, a wig or hairpiece may make patient feel better; tell patient that new hair may be different in color, texture
• To make position changes slowly to prevent fainting

---

terazosin HCl
(ter-ay′zoe-sin)
Hytrin
Func. class.: Antihypertensive
Chem. class.: α$_1$-Adrenergic blocker

Action: Decreases total vascular resistance, which is responsible for a decrease in B/P; this occurs by blockade of α$_1$-adrenoreceptors
Uses: Hypertension, as a single agent or in combination with diuretics or β-blockers, BPH

Dosage and routes:
• *Adult:* PO 1 mg hs, may increase dose slowly to desired response; not to exceed 20 mg/day

---

Available forms: Tabs 1, 2, 5 mg
Side effects/adverse reactions:
CV: Palpitations, orthostatic hypotension, tachycardia, edema, rebound hypertension
CNS: Dizziness, headache, drowsiness, anxiety, depression, vertigo, weakness, fatigue
GI: Nausea, vomiting, diarrhea, constipation, abdominal pain
GU: Urinary frequency, incontinence, impotence, priapism
EENT: Blurred vision, epistaxis, tinnitus, dry mouth, red sclera, nasal congestion, sinusitis
RESP: Dyspnea
Contraindications: Hypersensitivity
Precautions: Pregnancy (C), children, lactation
Pharmacokinetics:
Peak 1 hr, half-life 9-12 hr, highly bound to plasma proteins; metabolized in liver, excreted in urine, feces
Interactions/incompatibilities:
• Increased hypotensive effects: β-blockers, nitroglycerin, verapamil, nifedipine

NURSING CONSIDERATIONS
Assess:
• B/P, pulse, jugular venous distention q4h
• BUN, uric acid if on long-term therapy
• Weight daily, I&O
• Skin turgor, dryness of mucous membranes for hydration status
• Rales, dyspnea, orthopnea q30min
Perform/provide:
• Storage in tight container in cool environment
Evaluate:
• Therapeutic response: decreased B/P, edema in feet, legs
Teach patient/family:
• That fainting occasionally occurs after first dose; not to drive or operate machinery for 4 hr after first dose or after an increase in dose; or take first dose hs
• To rise slowly from sitting/lying position

---

terbinafine cream
(ter-been'-a-feen)
Lamisil
Func. class.: Topical antifungal
Chem. class.: Synthetic allylamine derivative

Action: Interferes with cell membrane permeability in fungi such as *T. rubrum, T. mentagrophytes, T. tonsurans, E. floccosum, M. canis, M. audouinii, M. gypseum, Candida,* broad-spectrum antifungal
Uses: Tinea cruris, tinea corporis, tinea pedis
Dosage and routes: Massage into affected area, surrounding area qd or bid, continue for 7-14 days, not to exceed 4 wk
Available forms: Cream 1%
Side effects/adverse reactions:
INTEG: Burning, stinging, dryness, itching, local irritation
Contraindications: Hypersensitivity
Precautions: Pregnancy (B), lactation, children
NURSING CONSIDERATIONS
Assess:
• For continuing infection: increased size, number of lesions
Administer:
• To affected area, surrounding area; do not cover with occlusive dressings
Perform/provide:
• Storage below 30° C (86° F)
Evaluate:
• Therapeutic response: decrease in size, number of lesions

Teach patient/family:
• To wear cotton clothing
• To use clean towel, dry well
• To avoid contact with mucous membranes
• Not to cover areas unless directed to by physician
• To report excessive itching, burning
• How to apply; massage cream into affected area and surrounding skin in AM, PM; effects observed within 1 wk, continue 1-2 wk after symptoms decrease

---

terbutaline sulfate
(ter-byoo′te-leen)
Brethaire, Brethine, Bricanyl
Func. class.: Selective β₂-agonist

Func. class.: Selective β_2-agonist
Chem. class.: Catecholamine

Action: Relaxes bronchial smooth muscle by direct action on β_2-adrenergic receptors through accumulation of cAMP at β-adrenergic receptor sites

Uses: Bronchospasm, premature labor

Dosage and routes:
Bronchospasm
• *Adult and child >12 yr:* INH 2 puffs q1min, then q4-6h; PO 2.5-5 mg q8h; SC 0.25 mg q8h
Premature labor
• *Adult:* IV INF: 0.01 mg/min, increased by 0.005 mg q10min, not to exceed 0.025 mg/min; SC 0.25 mg q1h; PO 5 mg q4h × 48 hr, then 5 mg q6h as maintenance for above doses

Available forms: Tabs 2.5, 5 mg; aerosol 0.2 mg/actuation

Side effects/adverse reactions:
CNS: Tremors, anxiety, insomnia, headache, dizziness, stimulation
CV: Palpitations, tachycardia, hypertension, dysrhythmias, ***cardiac arrest***
GI: Nausea, vomiting

Contraindications: Hypersensitivity to sympathomimetics, narrow-angle glaucoma, tachydysrhythmias

Precautions: Pregnancy (B), cardiac disorders, hyperthyroidism, diabetes mellitus, prostatic hypertension, lactation, elderly, hypertensive, glaucoma

Pharmacokinetics:
PO: Onset ½ hr, Peak 1-2 hr, duration 4-8 hr
SC: Onset 6-15 min, Peak ½-1 hr, duration 1½-4 hr
INH: Onset 5-30 min, Peak 1-2 hr, duration 3-6 hr

Interactions/incompatibilities:
• Increased effects of both drugs: other sympathomimetics
• Decreased action: β-blockers
• Hypertensive crisis: MAOIs
• Incompatible with bleomycin
• Considered incompatible in sol or syringe with any other drug

NURSING CONSIDERATIONS
Assess:
• Respiratory function: vital capacity, forced expiratory volume, ABGs, B/P, pulse, respiratory pattern, lung sounds, sputum before and after treatment
• Tolerance over long-term therapy; dose may have to be changed; monitor for rebound bronchospasm

Administer:
• With food; may be crushed
• IV after diluting each 5 mg/1 L D₅W for inf
• IV, run 10 μg/min; may increase 5 μg q10 min, titrate to response; after ½-1 hr taper dose by 5 μg; switch to PO as soon as possible
• 2 hr before hs to avoid sleeplessness

T

Perform/provide:

• Storage at room temperature; do not use discolored sol

Evaluate:

• Therapeutic response: absence of dyspnea, wheezing

Teach patient/family:

• Not to use OTC medications; extra stimulation may occur

• Use of inhaler; review package insert with patient

• To avoid getting aerosol in eyes; burning, stinging, will occur

• To wash inhaler in warm water and dry qd, rinse mouth after use

• On all aspects of drug; avoid smoking, smoke-filled rooms, persons with respiratory infections

• To increase fluids >2 L/day; allow 15 min between inhalation of this drug and inhaler containing steroid

• Take on time; if missed, do not make up after one hour; wait till next dose

Treatment of overdose: Administer an α-blocker, then norepinephrine for severe hypotension

---

terconazole

(ter-kon'-a-zole)
Terazol 3, Terazol 7
Func. class.: Local antiinfective
Chem. class.: Antifungal

Action: Interferes with fungal DNA replication; binds sterols in fungal cell membranes, which increases permeability, leaking of nutrients

Uses: Vaginal, vulval, vulvovaginal candidiasis (moniliasis)

Dosage and routes:

• *Adult:* Vag 5 g (1 applicator) hs × 7 days

Available forms: Vag cream 0.4%

Side effects/adverse reactions:

GU: Vulvovaginal burning, itching, pelvic cramps

INTEG: Rash, urticaria, stinging, burning

MISC: Headache, body pain

Contraindications: Hypersensitivity

Precautions: Children <2 yr, pregnancy, lactation

NURSING CONSIDERATIONS
Assess:

• Allergic reaction: burning, stinging, swelling, redness

Administer:

• Enough medication to cover lesions completely

• After cleansing with soap, water before each application; dry well

Perform/provide:

• Storage at room temperature in dry place

Evaluate:

• Therapeutic response: decrease in size, number of lesions

Teach patient/family:

• To use medical asepsis (hand washing) before, after each application

• To avoid use of OTC creams, ointments, lotions unless directed by physician

• To avoid contact with eyes

• To continue during menses, even if symptoms subside; to refrain from sexual intercourse during treatment

• To complete full treatment regimen

---

terfenadine

(ter-fen'-a-deen)
Seldane
Func. class.: Antihistamine
Chem. class.: Butyrophenone derivative

Action: Acts on blood vessels, GI,

respiratory systems by competing with histamine for H$_1$-receptor site; decreases allergic response by blocking histamine

Uses: Rhinitis, allergy symptoms

Dosage and routes:
• *Adult and child >12 yr:* PO 60 mg bid
• *Child <12 yr:* PO 15-30 mg bid

Available forms: Tabs 60 mg

Side effects/adverse reactions:
CV: **Life-threatening dysrhythmias** (rare)
CNS: Dizziness, poor coordination
RESP: Increased thick secretions
GI: Anorexia, increased liver function tests, dry mouth
GU: Retention

Contraindications: Hypersensitivity, severe hepatic disease

Precautions: Pregnancy (C)

Pharmacokinetics:
PO: Peak 1-2 hr, 97% bound to plasma proteins; half-life is biphasic 3½ hr, 16-23 hr

Interactions/incompatibilities:
• Not to be taken with ketoconazole, erythromycin

Lab test interferences:
False negative: Skin allergy tests

NURSING CONSIDERATIONS
Assess:
• I&O ratio; be alert for urinary retention, frequency, dysuria; drug should be discontinued if these occur
• CBC during long-term therapy
• Respiratory status: rate, rhythm, increase in bronchial secretions, wheezing, chest tightness

Administer:
• With meals if GI symptoms occur; absorption may slightly decrease

Perform/provide:
• Hard candy, gum, frequent rinsing of mouth for dryness

• Storage in tight, light-resistant container

Evaluate:
• Therapeutic response: absence of running or congested nose, rash

Teach patient/family:
• To notify physician of confusion, sedation, hypotension
• Not to exceed recommended dose; dysrhythmias may occur

Treatment of overdose: Administer ipecac syrup or lavage, diazepam, vasopressors, barbiturates (short-acting)

---

terpin hydrate
(ter′pin)
Func. class.: Expectorant

Action: Direct action on respiratory tract, which increases fluids, allows for expectoration

Uses: Bronchial secretions

Dosage and routes:
• *Adult:* ELIX 5-10 ml q4-6h

Available forms: Elix terpin hydrate codeine 10 mg codeine/85 mg terpin hydrate; elix, plain 85 mg/5 ml

Side effects/adverse reactions:
GI: Nausea, vomiting, anorexia

Contraindications: Hypersensitivity, child <12 yr

Precautions: Pregnancy (C)

NURSING CONSIDERATIONS
Assess:
• Cough: type, frequency, character, including sputum

Administer:
• With glass of water or food to decrease GI irritation

Perform/provide:
• Storage at room temperature

Evaluate:
• Therapeutic response: absence of thick secretions

T

---

italics = common side effects   ***bold italic*** = life threatening reactions

Teach patient/family:
• To avoid driving, other hazardous activities until patient is stabilized on this medication (if combined with codeine, drowsiness occurs)
• Not to exceed recommended dosage

---

testolactone
(tess-toe-lak′tone)
Teslac
Func. class.: Antineoplastic
Chem. class.: Androgen hormone

Action: Acts on adrenal cortex to suppress activity; reduces estrone synthesis
Uses: Advanced breast carcinoma in postmenopausal women; prostatic cancer
Dosage and routes:
• *Adult:* PO 250 mg qid
Available forms: Tabs 50 mg
Side effects/adverse reactions:
GI: Nausea, vomiting, anorexia, glossitis
GU: Urinary retention, ***renal failure***
INTEG: Rash, nail changes, facial hair growth
CV: Orthostatic hypertension, edema
CNS: Paresthesias, dizziness
EENT: Deepening voice
META: Hypercalcemia
Contraindications: Hypersensitivity, premenopausal women, carcinoma of male breast
Precautions: Renal disease, hypercalcemia, cardiac disease, pregnancy (C)
Pharmacokinetics: None known
Interactions/incompatibilities:
• Enhanced effects of: oral anticoagulants

Lab test interferences:
Increase: Urinary 17-OHCS
Decrease: Estradiol
NURSING CONSIDERATIONS
Assess:
• CA⁺ levels
• B/P q4h; tell patient to rise slowly from sitting or lying down
• Food preferences; list likes, dislikes
• Edema in feet; joint, stomach pain; shaking
• Symptoms indicating severe allergic reaction: rash, pruritus, urticaria, purpuric skin lesions, itching, flushing
• Anorexia, nausea, vomiting, constipation, weakness, loss of muscle tone (indicating hypercalcemia)
Administer:
• For mo or longer for desired response
Evaluate:
• Therapeutic response: decreased tumor size, spread of malignancy
Teach patient/family:
• To recognize and report signs of hepatotoxicity, hypercalcemia, virilization (in females), bleeding if on anticoagulants

---

testosterone
(tess-toss′ter-one)
Andro 100, Histerone-50, Histerone 100, Tesamone, Testosterone Aqueous
Func. class.: Androgenic anabolic steroid
Chem. class.: Halogenated testosterone derivative

Action: Increases weight by building body tissue, increases potassium, phosphorus, chloride, nitrogen levels, bone development
Uses: Breast engorgement, breast

---

* Available in Canada only

cancer in postmenopausal women, eunuchoidism, eunuchism, male climacteric

Dosage and routes:

Breast engorgement

- *Adult:* IM 25-50 mg/day × 3-4 days

Breast cancer

- *Adult:* IM 100 mg 3 ×/wk

Male climacteric/eunuchoidism/eunuchism

- *Adult:* IM 10-25 mg 2-5 ×/wk

Available forms: Inj IM 25, 50, 100 mg/ml

Side effects/adverse reactions:

INTEG: Rash, acneiform lesions, oily hair, skin, flushing, sweating, acne vulgaris, alopecia, hirsutism

CNS: Dizziness, headache, fatigue, tremors, paresthesias, flushing, sweating, anxiety, lability, insomnia

MS: Cramps, spasms

CV: Increased B/P

GU: Hematuria, amenorrhea, vaginitis, decreased libido, decreased breast size, clitoral hypertrophy, testicular atrophy

GI: Nausea, vomiting, constipation, weight gain, ***cholestatic jaundice***

EENT: Carpal tunnel syndrome, conjunctival edema, nasal congestion

ENDO: Abnormal GTT

Contraindications: Severe renal disease, severe cardiac disease, severe hepatic disease, hypersensitivity, pregnancy (X), lactation, genital bleeding (abnormal)

Precautions: Diabetes mellitus, CV disease, MI

Pharmacokinetics:

PO: Metabolized in liver, excreted in urine, crosses placenta, excreted in breast milk

Interactions/incompatibilities:

- Increased effects of: oral antidiabetics, oxyphenbutazone

- Increased PT: anticoagulants
- Edema: ACTH, adrenal steroids
- Decreased effects of: insulin

Lab test interferences:

Increase: Serum cholesterol, blood glucose, urine glucose

Decrease: Serum Ca, serum K, T_4, T_3, thyroid ^{131}I uptake test, urine 17-OHCS, 17-KS

NURSING CONSIDERATIONS

Assess:

- Weight daily; notify physician if weekly weight gain is >5 lb
- B/P q4h
- I&O ratio; be alert for decreasing urinary output, increasing edema
- Growth rate in children, since growth rate may be uneven (linear/bone growth) when used for extended period
- Electrolytes: K, Na, Cl, Ca; cholesterol
- Liver function studies: ALT, AST, bilirubin
- Edema, hypertension, cardiac symptoms, jaundice
- Mental status: affect, mood, behavioral changes, aggression
- Signs of masculinization in female: increased libido, deepening of voice, decreased breast tissue, enlarged clitoris, menstrual irregularities; male: gynecomastia, impotence, testicular atrophy
- Hypercalcemia: lethargy, polyuria, polydipsia, nausea, vomiting, constipation; drug may need to be decreased
- Hypoglycemia in diabetics, since oral anticoagulant action is decreased

Administer:

- Titrated dose; use lowest effective dose
- IM deep into upper outer quadrant of gluteal muscle

Perform/provide:

- Diet with increased calories and

---

italics = common side effects   ***bold italic*** = life threatening reactions

protein; decrease Na if edema occurs

• Supportive drug of anemia

Evaluate:

• Therapeutic response: occurs in 4-6 wk in osteoporosis

Teach patient/family:

• Drug must be combined with complete health plan: diet, rest, exercise

• To notify physician if therapeutic response decreases

• Not to discontinue this medication abruptly

• About changes in sex characteristics

• Women to report menstrual irregularities

• That 1-3-mo course is necessary for response in breast cancer

---

testosterone cypionate/testosterone enanthate/testosterone propionate

Andro L.A. 200, Delatest, Delatestryl, Durathate-200, Everone 100, Everone 200, Testone LA 100, Testone LA 200, Testosterone Enanthate, Testrin PA, Andro-Cyp 100, Andro-Cyp 200, Andronate 100, Andronate 200, depAndro 100, depAndro 200, Depotest 100, Depotest 200, Depo-Testosterone, Duratest-100, Duratest-200, Testosterone Cypionate, Testred Cypionate, Testex, Testosterone Propionate

Func. class.: Androgenic anabolic steroid

Chem. class.: Halogenated testosterone derivative

Action: Increases weight by building body tissue, increases potassium, phosphorus, chloride, nitrogen levels, increases bone development

Uses: Female breast cancer, eunuchoidism, male climacteric, oligospermia, impotence, osteoporosis

Dosage and routes:

Oligospermia

• *Adult:* IM 100-200 mg q4-6wk (cypionate or enanthate)

Breast cancer

• *Adult:* IM 50-100 mg 3 ×/wk (propionate) or 200-400 mg q2-4wk (cypionate or enanthate)

Male climacteric/eunuchoidism/eunuchism

• *Adult:* IM 10-25 mg 2-4 ×/wk (propionate)

Available forms: Propionate inj IM 25, 50, 100 mg/ml; enanthate inj IM 100, 200 mg/ml; cypionate inj IM 50, 100, 200 mg/ml

Side effects/adverse reactions:

INTEG: Rash, acneiform lesions, oily hair and skin, flushing, sweating, acne vulgaris, alopecia, hirsutism

CNS: Dizziness, headache, fatigue, tremors, paresthesias, flushing, sweating, anxiety, lability, insomnia, carpal tunnel syndrome

MS: Cramps, spasms

CV: Increased B/P

GU: Hematuria, amenorrhea, vaginitis, decreased libido, decreased breast size, clitoral hypertrophy, testicular atrophy

GI: Nausea, vomiting, constipation, weight gain, *cholestatic jaundice*

EENT: Conjunctival edema, nasal congestion

ENDO: Abnormal GTT

Contraindications: Severe renal disease, severe cardiac disease, severe hepatic disease, hypersensitivity, pregnancy (X), lactation, genital bleeding (abnormal)

Precautions: Diabetes mellitus, CV disease, MI

Pharmacokinetics:

PO: Metabolized in liver, excreted in urine, breast milk; crosses placenta

Interactions/incompatibilities:

• Increased effects of: oral antidiabetics, oxyphenbutazone

• Increased PT: anticoagulants

• Edema: ACTH, adrenal steroids

• Decreased effects of: insulin

Lab test interferences:

Increase: Serum cholesterol, blood glucose, urine glucose

Decrease: Serum Ca, serum K, T$_4$, T$_3$, thyroid ^{131}I uptake test, urine 17-OHCS, 17-KS, PBI

NURSING CONSIDERATIONS

Assess:

• Weight daily; notify physician if weekly weight gain is >5 lb

• B/P q4h

• I&O ratio; be alert for decreasing urinary output, increasing edema

• Growth rate in children, since growth rate may be uneven (linear/bone growth) if used for extended periods

• Electrolytes: K, Na, Cl, Ca; cholesterol

• Liver function studies: ALT, AST, bilirubin

• Edema, hypertension, cardiac symptoms, jaundice

• Mental status: affect, mood, behavioral changes, aggression

• Signs of masculinization in female: increased libido, deepening of voice, decreased breast tissue, enlarged clitoris, menstrual irregularities; male: gynecomastia, impotence, testicular atrophy

• Hypercalcemia: lethargy, polyuria, polydipsia, nausea, vomiting, constipation; drug may have to be decreased

• Hypoglycemia in diabetics, since oral antidiabetic action is increased

Administer:

• Titrated dose; use lowest effective dose

• IM deep into upper outer quadrant of gluteal muscle

Perform/provide:

• Diet with increased calories, protein; decrease Na if edema occurs

• Supportive drug of anemia

Evaluate:

• Therapeutic response: occurs in 4-6 wk in osteoporosis

Teach patient/family:

• That drug needs to be combined with complete health plan: diet, rest, exercise

• To notify physician if therapeutic response decreases

• Not to discontinue this medication abruptly

• About changes in sex characteristics

• Women to report menstrual irregularities

• That 1-3-mo course is necessary for response in breast cancer

• Procedure for use of buccal tablets (requires 30-60 min to dissolve, change absorption site with each dose; do not eat, drink, chew, or smoke while tablet is in place)

tetanus toxoid, adsorbed; tetanus toxoid

Func. class.: Toxoid

Action: Produces specific antibodies to tetanus

Uses: Tetanus toxoid: used for prophylactic treatment of wounds

Dosage and routes:

• *Adult and child:* IM 0.5 ml q4-6

wk × 2 doses, then 0.5 ml 1 yr after dose 2 (adsorbed); SC/IM 0.5 ml q4-8wk × 3 doses, then 0.5 ml ½-1 yr after dose 3, booster dose 0.5 ml q10 yr

Available forms: Inj adsorbed IM 5, 10 LfU/0.5 ml; inj IM, SC 4, 5 LfU/0.5 ml

Side effects/adverse reactions:
GI: Nausea, vomiting, anorexia
INTEG: Skin abscess, urticaria, itching, swelling, erythema, induration at injection site
CV: Tachycardia, hypotension
SYST: Lymphadenitis, *anaphylaxis*
CNS: Crying, fretfulness, fever, drowsiness

Contraindications: Hypersensitivity, active infection, poliomyelitis outbreak, immunosuppression

Precautions: Pregnancy (C), elderly

NURSING CONSIDERATIONS
Assess:
• For skin reactions: swelling, rash, urticaria
• For history of allergies, skin conditions (eczema, psoriasis, dermatitis), reactions to vaccinations
• For anaphylaxis: inability to breathe, bronchospasm

Administer:
• At least 4 wk apart × 3 doses for children >6 wk old
• Only with epinephrine 1:1000 on unit to treat laryngospasm

Perform/provide
• Written record of immunization

Teach patient/family:
• That doses are given at least 4 wk apart × 3 doses; booster needed at 10-yr intervals

---

tetracaine/tetracaine HCl (topical)
(tet′-ra-cane)
Pontocaine
Func. class.: Topical anesthetic

Action: Inhibits nerve impulses from sensory nerves, which produces anesthesia

Uses: Pruritus, sunburn, toothache, sore throat, cold sores, oral pain, rectal pain and irritation, control of gagging

Dosage and routes:
• *Adult and child:* TOP apply to affected area 1 oz for adult ¼ oz for child

Available forms: Sol 2%; aero spray, liq, 0.5% oint, gel, 1% cream

Side effects/adverse reactions:
INTEG: Rash, irritation, sensitization burning, stinging, tenderness

Contraindications: Hypersensitivity, infants <1 yr, application to large areas, PABA allergies

Precautions: Child <6 yr, sepsis, pregnancy (C), denuded skin

NURSING CONSIDERATIONS
Assess:
• Allergy: rash, irritation, reddening, swelling
• Infection: if affected area is infected, do not apply

Administer:
• After cleansing and drying of affected area

Evaluate:
• Therapeutic response: absence of pain, itching of affected area

Teach patient/family:
• To report rash, irritation, redness, swelling
• How to apply solution

---

tetracaine HCl
(tet'-ra-caine)
Pontocaine Eye, Pontocaine
HCl, Tetracaine
Func. class.: Ophthalmic anesthetic
Chem. class.: Ester

Action: Decreases ion permeability by stabilizing neuronal membrane
Uses: Cataract extraction, tonometry, gonioscopy, removal of foreign objects, corneal suture removal, glaucoma surgery
Dosage and routes:
• *Adult and child:* INSTILL 1-2 gtts before procedure; oint ½-1 in to lower conjunctival fornix
Available forms include: Sol 0.5%; oint 0.5%
Side effects/adverse reactions:
EENT: Blurred vision, stinging, burning, lacrimation, photophobia, conjunctival redness
INTEG: Contact dermatitis
SYST: CNS stimulation, CNS and CV depression
Contraindications: Hypersensitivity to PABA
Precautions: Abnormal levels of plasma esterases, allergies, hyperthyroidism, hypertension, cardiac disease, pregnancy (C)
Pharmacokinetics:
Instill: Onset 13-30 sec, duration 15-20 min
Interactions/incompatibilities:
• Decreases antibacterial action of: sulfonamides
NURSING CONSIDERATIONS
Assess:
• Previous hypersensitivity to anesthetics
Perform/provide:
• Protective covering for eye
• Storage at room temperature in

tight, light-resistant container; refrigerate
Teach patient/family:
• To report change in vision, with blurring or loss of sight, trouble breathing, sweating, flushing
• Not to touch or rub eye, which may further damage eye
• That someone must drive the patient home after the appointment

tetracaine HCl
(tet-ra'-kane)
Pontocaine
Func. class.: Local anesthetic
Chem. class.: Ester

Action: Competes with calcium for sites in nerve membrane that control sodium transport across cell membrane; decreases rise of depolarization phase of action potential
Uses: Spinal anesthesia, epidural and peripheral nerve block, perineum, lower extremities
Dosage and routes:
Varies with route of anesthesia
Available forms: Inj 0.2%, 0.3%, 1%; powder
Side effects/adverse reactions:
CNS: Anxiety, restlessness, ***convulsions, LOC,*** drowsiness, disorientation, tremors, shivering
*CV: **Myocardial depression, cardiac arrest, dysrhythmias,*** bradycardia, hypotension, hypertension, fetal bradycardia
GI: Nausea, vomiting
EENT: Blurred vision, tinnitus, pupil constriction
INTEG: Rash, urticaria, allergic reactions, edema, burning, skin discoloration at injection site, tissue necrosis
*RESP: **Status asthmaticus, respiratory arrest, anaphylaxis***

italics = common side effects   ***bold italic*** = life threatening reactions

Contraindications: Hypersensitivity, severe liver disease, heart block
Precautions: Elderly, severe drug allergies, pregnancy (C), lacation, children
Pharmacokinetics:
Onset 15 min, duration 3 hr; metabolized by liver, excreted in urine (metabolites)
Interactions/incompatibilities:
• Dysrhythmias: epinephrine, halothane, enflurane
• Hypertension: MAOIs, tricyclic antidepressants, phenothiazines
• Decreased action of tetracaine: chloroprocaine
• Decreased action of: sulfonamides

NURSING CONSIDERATIONS
Assess:
• B/P, pulse, respiration during treatment
• Fetal heart tones if drug is used during labor
• Allergic reactions: rash, urticaria, itching
• Cardiac status: ECG for dysrhythmias, pulse, B/P, during anesthesia
Administer:
• Only drugs that are not cloudy, do not contain precipitate
• Only with crash cart, resuscitative equipment nearby
• Only drugs without preservatives for epidural or caudal anesthesia
Perform/provide:
• Use of new solution, discard unused portions, store in refrigerator
Evaluate:
• Therapeutic response: anesthesia necessary for procedure
Treatment of overdose: Airway, O₂, vasopressor, IV fluids, anticonvulsants for seizures

tetracycline HCl
(tet-ra-sye′kleen)
Achromycin, Achromycin V, Cefracycline,* Medicycline,* Neo-Tetrine,* Nor-Tet, Novotetra,* Panmycin, Robitet, Sumycin 250, Sumycin 500, Sumycin Syrup, Teline, Teline 500, Tetracap, Tetracycline HCl, Tetracycline HCl Syrup, Tetracyn, Tetralan 250, Tetralan 500, Tetralan Syrup, Tetralean,* Tetram
Func. class.: Broad-spectrum antibiotic/antiinfective
Chem. class.: Tetracycline

Action: Inhibits protein synthesis and phosphorylation in microorganisms; bacteriostatic
Uses: Syphilis, chlamydia trachomatis, gonorrhea, lymphogranuloma venereum, uncommon gram-positive, gram-negative organisms, rickettsial infections
Dosage and routes:
• *Adult:* PO 250-500 mg q6h; IM 250 mg/day or 150 mg q12h; IV 250-500 mg q8-12h
• *Child >8 yr:* PO 25-50 mg/kg/day in divided doses q6h; IM 15-25 mg/kg/day in divided doses q8-12h; IV 10-20 mg/kg/day in divided doses q12h
Gonorrhea
• *Adult:* PO 1.5 g, then 500 mg qid for a total of 9 g × 7 days
Chlamydia trachomatis
• *Adult:* PO 500 mg qid × 7 days
Syphilis
• *Adult:* PO 2-3 g in divided doses × 10-15 days; if syphilis duration > 1 yr, must treat 30 days
Brucellosis
• *Adult:* PO 500 mg qid × 3 wk with 1 g streptomycin IM 2 ×/day

× 1 wk, and 1 × /day the second wk
Urethral syndrome in women
• *Adult:* PO 500 mg qid × 7 days
Rape Victims
• *Adult:* PO 500 mg qid × 7 days
Acne
• *Adult:* 1 g/day in divided doses; maintenance 125-500 mg/day
Available forms: Oral susp 125 mg/5 ml, caps 100, 200, 500 mg; tabs 100, 250, 500 mg; powder for inj
Side effects/adverse reactions:
CNS: Fever, headache, paresthesia
HEMA: ***Eosinophilia, neutropenia, thrombocytopenia, leukocytosis, hemolytic anemia***
EENT: Dysphagia, glossitis, decreased calcification of deciduous teeth, oral candidiasis, oral ulcers
GI: Nausea, abdominal pain, *vomiting, diarrhea,* anorexia, enterocolitis, *hepatotoxicity,* flatulence, abdominal cramps, epigastric burning, stomatitis
CV: Pericarditis
GU: Increased BUN
INTEG: Rash, urticaria, *photosensitivity, increased pigmentation,* ***exfoliative dermatitis,*** pruritus, ***angioedema***
Contraindications: Hypersensitivity to tetracyclines, children <8 yr, pregnancy (D), lactation
Precautions: Renal disease, hepatic disease
Pharmacokinetics:
PO: Peak 2-3 hr, duration 6 hr, half-life 6-10 hr; excreted in urine, crosses placenta, excreted in breast milk, 20%-60% protein bound
Interactions/incompatibilities:
• Decreased effect of tetracycline: antacids, $NaHCO_3$, dairy products, alkali products, iron, kaolin/pectin
• Increased effect: anticoagulants

• Decreased effect of: penicillins, oral contraceptives
• Nephrotoxicity: methoxyflurane
• Incompatible in sol with amikacin, aminophylline, amobarbital, amphotericin B, Ca, carbenicillin, cefazolin, cephalothin, cephapirin, chloramphenicol, chlorothiazide, dimenhydrinate, erythromycin, heparin, hydrocortisone, methicillin, methohexital, methyldopate, methylprednisolone, metoclopramide, oxacillin, penicillins, pentobarbital, phenobarbital, phenytoin, polymyxin B, prochlorperazine, secobarbital, thiopental, warfarin, fat emulsion 10%
Lab test interferences:
False negative: Urine glucose with Clinistix or Tes-Tape
False increase: Urinary catecholamines
NURSING CONSIDERATIONS
Assess:
• Signs of anemia: Hct, Hgb, fatigue
• I&O ratio
• Blood studies: PT, CBC, AST, ALT, BUN, creatinine
• Allergic reactions: rash, itching, pruritus, angioedema
• Nausea, vomiting, diarrhea; administer antiemetic, antacids as ordered
• Overgrowth of infection: increased temperature, malaise, redness, pain, swelling, drainage, perineal itching, diarrhea, changes in cough or sputum
Administer:
• IM: deep; no more than 2 ml/injection site
• IV after diluting 250 mg or less/5 ml of sterile H_2O; may be further diluted with 100 ml or more D_5W or NS; give 100 mg or less over 5 min or more; use sol within 12 hr
• After C&S obtained

italics = common side effects   ***bold italic*** = life threatening reactions

• 2 hr before or after ferrous products; 3 hr after antacid or kaolin/pectin products

Perform/provide:

• Storage in tight, light-resistant container at room temperature

Evaluate:

• Therapeutic response: decreased temperature, absence of lesions, negative C&S

Teach patient/family:

• To avoid sun exposure, since burns may occur; sunscreen does not seem to decrease photosensitivity

• Diabetic should avoid use of Clinistix, Diastix, or Tes-Tape for urine glucose testing

• That all prescribed medication must be taken to prevent superimposed infection

• To avoid milk products, antacids, or separate by 2 hrs; take with a full glass of water

---

tetracycline HCl (ophthalmic)

(tet-ra-sye'kleen)

Achromycin Ophthalmic

Func. class.: Antiinfective

Action: Inhibits bacterial protein synthesis

Uses: Infection of eye, ophthalmia neonatorum

Dosage and routes:

• *Adult and child:* Instill 1-2 gtts bid-qid as needed

Ophthalmia neonatorum

• *Neonate:* TOP 1-2 gtts into each eye immediately after delivery; SOL, 1 gtt q6-12h more frequently

Available forms: Oint 1%, Susp 1%

Side effects/adverse reactions:

EENT: Poor corneal wound healing,

overgrowth of nonsusceptible organisms

Contraindications: Hypersensitivity, pregnancy (D), varicella, vaccinia, mycobacterial, fungal infections of the eye, epithelial herpes simplex keratitis

Precautions: Antibiotic hypersensitivity

NURSING CONSIDERATIONS

Assess:

• Allergy: itching, lacrimation, redness, swelling

Administer:

• After washing hands; cleanse crusts or discharge from eye before application

Perform/provide:

• Storage at room temperature in light-resistant container

Evaluate:

• Therapeutic response: absence of redness, inflammation, tearing

Teach patient/family:

• To use drug exactly as prescribed, shake well before using

• Not to use eye make-up, towels, washcloths, or eye medication of others, or reinfection may occur

• That drug container tip should not be touched to eye

• To report itching, increased redness, burning, stinging, swelling; drug should be discontinued

• That drug may cause blurred vision when ointment is applied

---

tetracycline HCl (topical)

(tet-ra-sye'kleen)

Achromycin, Topicycline

Func. class.: Local antiinfective

Chem. class.: Tetracycline

Action: Interferes with microorganism protein synthesis

Uses: Acne vulgaris, skin abrasions

Dosage and routes:
• *Adult and child >12 yr:* TOP apply to affected area bid
Available forms: Oint 3%; sol 0.22%

Side effects/adverse reactions:
INTEG: Rash, urticaria, stinging, burning, redness, swelling, photosensitivity

Contraindications: Hypersensitivity, pregnancy (D)

Precautions: Lactation, children, hepatic, renal disease

NURSING CONSIDERATIONS
Assess:
• Allergic reaction: burning, stinging, swelling, redness

Administer:
• Enough medication to cover lesions completely
• After cleansing with soap, water before each application; dry well

Perform/provide:
• Storage at room temperature in dry place; use within 2 mo or discard

Evaluate:
• Therapeutic response: decrease in size, number of lesions

Teach patient/family:
• To apply with glove to prevent further infection
• To avoid use of OTC creams, ointments, lotions unless directed by physician
• To use medical asepsis (hand washing) before, after each application, avoid eyes, nose, mouth
• To notify physician if condition worsens
• That some stinging may occur
• To avoid sunlight, ultraviolet light, or burning may occur
• That staining of clothing and skin may occur

tetrahydrozoline HCl
(tet-ra-hi-droz′-o-leen)
Collyrium Fresh Eye Drops, Eyesine, Murine Plus Eye Drops, Optigene 3 Eye Drops, Soothe Eye Drops, Tetrahydrozoline HCl, Visine Eye Drops

Func. class.: Ophthalmic vasoconstrictor
Chem. class.: Direct sympathomimetic amine

Action: Vasoconstriction of eye arterioles; decreases eye engorgement by stimulation of α-adrenergic receptors

Uses: Ocular congestion, irritation, itching, redness

Dosage and routes:
• *Adult and child >2 yr:* INSTILL 1-2 gtts bid or tid
Available forms: Sol 0.05%

Side effects/adverse reactions:
CNS: Headache, dizziness, weakness
CV: Reflex bradycardia, hypertension, dysrhythmias, tachycardia, *CV collapse,* palpitation
EENT: Stinging, lacrimation, blurred vision, conjunctival allergy

Contraindications: Hypersensitivity, narrow-angle glaucoma

Precautions: Severe hypertension, diabetes, hyperthyroidism, elderly, severe arteriosclerosis, cardiac disease, infants, pregnancy (C), lactation, diabetes, asthma, coronary artery disease

Pharmacokinetics:
INSTILL: Duration 2-3 hr

Interactions/incompatibilities:
• Increased pressor effects: MAOIs, tricyclic antidepressants
• Increased side effects: β blockers
• Sensitized myocardium: anesthetics

italics = common side effects   ***bold italic*** = life threatening reactions

NURSING CONSIDERATIONS
Assess:

• B/P, pulse; systemic absorption does occur

Perform/provide:

• Storage in tight, light-resistant container; do not use discolored sol

Evaluate:

• Therapeutic response: decreased eye irritation, itching

Teach patient/family:

• To report change in vision, blurring, loss of sight; breathing trouble, sweating, flushing

• Method of instillation: tilt head backward, hold dropper over eye, drop medication inside lower lid, using pressure on inside corner of eye; hold 1 min; do not touch dropper to eye

• That blurred vision will decrease with repeated use of drug

• To notify physician of headache, spots, redness, pain; discontinue use

• To use sunglasses if photophobia occurs

• To use exactly as prescribed

• Do not use for longer than 72 hr without physician approval

---

tetrahydrozoline HCl
(tet-ra-hi-drozz'o-leen)
Tyzine HCl, Tyzine Pediatric
Func. class.: Nasal decongestant
Chem. class.: Sympathomimetic amine

Action: Produces vasoconstriction (rapid, long-acting) of arterioles, thereby decreasing fluid exudation, mucosal engorgement

Uses: Nasal congestion

Dosage and routes:

• *Adult and child >6 yr:* INSTILL 2-4 gtts or sprays q4-6h prn (0.1%)

• *Child 2-6 yr:* INSTILL 2-3 gtts q4-6h prn (0.05%)

Available forms: Sol 0.05%, 0.1%

Side effects/adverse reactions:

GI: Nausea, vomiting, anorexia

EENT: Irritation, burning, sneezing, stinging, dryness, rebound congestion

INTEG: Contact dermatitis

CNS: Anxiety, restlessness, tremors, weakness, insomnia, dizziness, fever, headache

Contraindications: Hypersensitivity to sympathomimetic amines

Precautions: Child <6 yr, elderly, diabetes, cardiovascular disease, hypertension, hyperthyroidism, increased ICP, prostatic hypertrophy, pregnancy (C), glaucoma

Interactions/incompatibilities:

• Hypertension: MAOIs, β-adrenergic blockers

• Hypotension: methyldopa, mecamylamine, reserpine

NURSING CONSIDERATIONS
Assess:

• Redness, swelling, pain in nasal passages

Administer:

• No more than q4h

• For <4 consecutive days

Perform/provide:

• Environmental humidification to decrease nasal congestion, dryness

• Storage in light-resistant containers; do not expose to high temperatures

Evaluate:

• Therapeutic response: decreased nasal congestion

Teach patient/family:

• That stinging may occur for several applications; drying of mucosa may be decreased by environmental humidification

• To notify physician of irregular pulse, insomnia, dizziness, or tremors

• Proper administration to avoid systemic absorption

---

theophylline, theophylline sodium glycinate

(thee-off'i-lin)

Accurbron, Aerolate III, Aerolate Jr., Aerolate Slo-Phyllin, Aerolate Sr., Aquaphyllin, Asmalix, Bronkodyl, Constant-T, Elixomin, Elixophyllin, Elixophyllin SR, Lanophyllin, Quibron-T Dividose, Quibron-T/SR Dividose, Respbid, Slo-Bid Gyrocaps, Slo-Phyllin Gyrocaps, Sustaire, Theolair-SR, Theo-24, Theobid Duracaps, Theobid Jr. Duracaps, Theochron, Theoclear-80, Theoclear L.A., Theo-Dur, Theo-Dur Sprinkle, Theolair, Theolair-SR, Theophylline, Theophylline and 5% Dextrose, Theophylline Extended Release, Theophylline Oral, Theophylline S.R., Theo-Sav, Theospan-SR, Theostat 80, Theovent, Theox, T-Phyl, Uniphyl

Func. class.: Spasmolytic
Chem. class.: Xanthine, ethylenediamide

Action: Relaxes smooth muscle of respiratory system by blocking phosphodiesterase, which increases cAMP

Uses: Bronchial asthma, bronchospasm of COPD, chronic bronchitis

Dosage and routes:

Bronchospasm, bronchial asthma
• *Adult:* PO 100-200 mg q6h; dosage must be individualized; REC 250-500 mg q8-12h
• *Child:* PO 50-100 mg q6h, not to exceed 12 mg/kg/24 hr

COPD, chr...
• *Adult:* PO ...
(sodium glyc...
• *Child >12* ...
q6-8h pc (sod...
• *Child 6-12 y...*
pc (sodium glycina...
• *Child 3-6 yr:* PO 110-165 mg q6-8h pc (sodium glycinate)
• *Child 1-3 yr:* PO 55-110 mg q6-8h pc (sodium glycinate)

Available forms: Caps 50, 100, 200, 250 mg; tabs 100, 125, 200, 225, 250, 300 mg; tabs time-release 100, 200, 250, 300, 400, 500 mg; caps time-release 50, 65, 100, 125, 130, 200, 250, 260, 300, 400, 500 mg; elix 80, 11.25 mg/15 ml; sol 80 mg/15 ml; liq 80, 150, 160 mg/15 ml; susp 300 mg/15 ml

Side effects/adverse reactions:

CNS: Anxiety, restlessness, insomnia, dizziness, convulsions, headache, light-headedness, muscle twitching
CV: Palpitations, sinus tachycardia, hypotension, other dysrhythmias, fluid retention with tachycardia
GI: Nausea, vomiting, anorexia, diarrhea, bitter taste, dyspepsia, gastric distress
RESP: Increased rate
INTEG: Flushing, urticaria

Contraindications: Hypersensitivity to xanthines, tachydysrhythmias

Precautions: Elderly, CHF, cor pulmonale, hepatic disease, active peptic ulcer disease, diabetes mellitus, hyperthyroidism, hypertension, children, pregnancy (C)

Pharmacokinetics:

SOL: Peak 1 hr, metabolized in liver, excreted in urine and breast milk, crosses placenta

Interactions/incompatibilities:
• Increased action of theophylline:

T

---

italics = common side effects   ***bold italic*** = life threatening reactions

e, propranolol, erythro-
, troleandomycin
May increase effects of: antico-
agulants
• Cardiotoxicity: β-blockers
• Decreased effect of: lithium

NURSING CONSIDERATIONS
Assess:
• Theophylline blood levels (therapeutic level is 10-20 μg/ml); toxicity may occur with small increase
above 20 μg/ml
• Monitor I&O; diuresis occurs;
dehydration may result in elderly
or children
• Signs of toxicity: irritability, insomnia, restlessness, tremors, nausea, vomiting
• Respiratory rate, rhythm, depth;
auscultate lung fields bilaterally;
notify physician of abnormalities
• Allergic reactions: rash, urticaria;
if these occur, drug should be discontinued
Administer:
• PO after meals to decrease GI
symptoms; absorption may be affected
Evaluate:
• Therapeutic response: ability to
breathe more easily
Teach patient/family
• To check OTC medications, current prescription medications for
ephedrine, which will increase
stimulation, to avoid alcohol, caffeine chocolate
• To avoid hazardous activities;
dizziness may occur
• That if GI upset occurs, to take
drug with 8 oz H$_2$O; avoid food;
absorption may be decreased
• Not to crush, dissolve, or chew
slow-release products
• That contents of bead-filled capsule may be sprinkled over food for
children's use
• To notify physician of toxicity:

nausea, vomiting, anxiety, insomnia, convulsions
• To notify physician of change in
smoking habit; dosage may have to
be changed

---

thiabendazole
(thye-a-ben′da-zole)
Mintezol
Func. class.: Antihelmintic
Chem. class.: Benzimadazole
derivative

Action: Inhibits anaerobic metab-
olism, disrupts microtubules
Uses: Pinworm, roundworm,
threadworm, whipworm, trichino-
sis, hookworm, cutaneous larva
migrans (creeping eruption)
Dosage and routes:
• *Adult and child:* PO 25 mg/kg in
2 doses qd × 2-5 days, not to exceed 3 g/day
Available forms: Tabs, chew 500
mg; oral susp 500 mg/5 ml
Side effects/adverse reactions:
*SYST: **Anaphylaxis***
*GU: **Hematuria, nephrotoxicity,***
enuresis, abnormal smell of urine
INTEG: Rash, pruritus, erythema,
Stevens-Johnson syndrome
CNS: Dizziness, headache, drowsiness, fever, flushing, ***convulsions,***
behavioral changes
EENT: Tinnitus, blurred vision,
xanthopsia
GI: Nausea, vomiting, anorexia,
diarrhea, jaundice, liver damage,
epigastric distress
CV: Hypotension, bradycardia
Contraindications: Hypersensi-
tivity
Precautions: Severe malnutrition,
hepatic disease, renal disease,
anemia, severe dehydration,
child <14 kg, pregnancy (C)

Pharmacokinetics:

PO: Peak 1-2 hr, metabolized completely by liver, excreted in feces and urine

NURSING CONSIDERATIONS

Assess:

• Stools periodically during entire treatment

Administer:

• Susp after shaking

• PO after meals to avoid GI symptoms

Perform/provide:

• Storage in tight container

Evaluate:

• Therapeutic response: stools negative for helminthics

Teach patient/family:

• Proper hygiene after BM, including hand-washing technique; tell patient to avoid putting fingers in mouth

• That infected person should sleep alone; not to shake bed linen; to change bed linen qd

• To clean toilet qd with disinfectant (green soap solution)

• Need for compliance with dosage schedule, duration of treatment

• To drink fruit juice to remove mucus that intestinal tapeworms burrow in; aids in expulsion of worms

• To avoid hazardous activities if drowsiness occurs

Treatment of overdose: Induce emesis or gastric lavage

---

thiamine HCl (vitamin B₁)

Betaxin,* Betalin S, Biamine, Revitonus, Thiamilate, Thiamine HCl

Func. class.: Vitamin B₁

Chem. class.: Water soluble

Action: Needed for pyruvate metabolism

Uses: Vitamin B₁ deficiency or polyneuritis, cheilosis adjunct with thiamine beriberi, Wernicke-Korsakoff syndrome, pellagra, metabolic disorders

Dosage and routes:

Beriberi

• *Adult:* IM 10-500 mg tid × 2 wk, then 5-10 mg qd × 1 mo

• *Child:* IM 10-50 mg qd × 4-6 wk

Anemia/alcoholism/pregnancy/pellagra

• *Adult:* PO 100 mg qd

• *Child:* PO 10-50 mg qd in divided doses

Beriberi with cardiac failure

• *Adult and child:* IV 100-500 mg

Wernicke's encephalopathy

• *Adult:* IV 500 mg or less, then 100 mg bid

Available forms: Tabs 5, 10, 25, 50, 100, 250, 500 mg; inj IM, IV 100, 200 mg/ml

Side effects/adverse reactions:

CNS: Weakness, restlessness

GI: Hemorrhage, *nausea, diarrhea*

CV: **Collapse, pulmonary edema,** hypotension

INTEG: **Angioneurotic edema,** cyanosis, sweating, warmth

SYST: **Anaphylaxis**

EENT: Tightness of throat

Contraindications: Hypersensitivity

Precautions: Pregnancy (A)

Pharmacokinetics:

PO/INJ: Unused amounts excreted in urine (unchanged)

Interactions/incompatibilities:

• Incompatible with amobarbital, phenobarbital, sulfites, carbonates, citrates

NURSING CONSIDERATIONS

Assess:

• Thiamine levels throughout treatment

• Nutritional status: yeast, beef,

T

liver, whole or enriched grains, legumes

Administer:

• IV undiluted or diluted with IV sol and given as an INF at a rate of 100 mg or less/5 min or more

• By IM injection; rotate sites if pain and inflammation occur; do not mix with alkaline solutions; Z-track to minimize pain

• Application of cold may decrease pain

Perform/provide:

• Storage in tight, light-resistant container

Evaluate:

• Therapeutic response: absence of nausea, vomiting, anorexia, insomnia, tachycardia, paresthesias, depression, muscle weakness

Teach patient/family:

• Necessary foods to be included in diet: yeast, beef, liver, legumes, whole grain

---

thiethylperazine maleate

(thye-eth-il-per'-a-zeen)

Torecan

Func. class.: Antiemetic

Chem. class.: Phenothiazine, piperazine derivative

Action: Acts centrally by blocking chemoreceptor trigger zone, which in turn acts on vomiting center

Uses: Nausea, vomiting

Dosage and routes:

• *Adult:* PO/IM/REC 10 mg/qd-tid

Available forms: Tabs 10 mg; supp 10 mg; inj 5 mg/ml

Side effects/adverse reactions:

GU: Urinary retention, dark urine

CNS: Euphoria, depression, restlessness, tremor, extrapyramidal

symptoms, *convulsions,* drowsiness

GI: Nausea, vomiting, anorexia, dry mouth, diarrhea, constipation, weight loss, metallic taste, cramps

CV: Circulatory failure, tachycardia, postural hypotension, ECG changes

RESP: Respiratory depression

Contraindications: Hypersensitivity to phenothiazines, coma, seizure, encephalopathy, bone marrow depression

Precautions: Children <2 yr, pregnancy (C), elderly

Pharmacokinetics:

PO: Onset 45-60 min

REC: Onset 45-60 min, metabolized by liver, excreted by kidneys, crosses placenta, excreted in breast milk

Interactions/incompatibilities:

• Decreased effect of thiethylperazine: barbiturates, antacids

• Increased anticholinergic action: anticholinergics, antiparkinson drugs, antidepressants

• Do not mix with other drug in syringe or sol

NURSING CONSIDERATIONS

Assess:

• VS, B/P; check patients with cardiac disease more often

• Respiratory status before, during, after administration of emetic; check rate, rhythm, character; respiratory depression can occur rapidly with elderly or debilitated patients

Administer:

• IM injection in large muscle mass; aspirate to avoid IV administration

Evaluate:

• Therapeutic response: absence of nausea, vomiting

Teach patient/family:

• To avoid hazardous activities, activities requiring alertness; dizziness may occur

thioguanine (6-TG)
(thye-oh-gwah'neen)
Thioguanine, Lanvis*

Func. class.: Antineoplastic-antimetabolite
Chem. class.: Purine analog

Action: Interferes with synthesis, utilization of purine nucleotides; S phase of cell cycle specific

Uses: Acute leukemias, chronic granulocytic leukemia, lymphomas, multiple myeloma, solid tumors

Dosage and routes:
• *Adult and child:* PO 2 mg/kg/day, then increase slowly to 3 mg/kg/day after 4 wk

Available forms: Tabs 40 mg

Side effects/adverse reactions:
*HEMA: **Thrombocytopenia, leukopenia, myelosuppression, anemia***
*GI: Nausea, vomiting, anorexia, diarrhea, stomatitis, **hepatotoxicity**, gastritis, jaundice*
*GU: **Renal failure**, hyperuricemia, oliguria*
INTEG: Rash, dermatitis, dry skin

Contraindications: Prior drug resistance, leukopenia (<2500/mm³), thrombocytopenia (<100,000/mm³), anemia, pregnancy (D)

Precautions: Liver disease

Pharmacokinetics: Oral form absorbed only 30%, metabolized in liver, only small amounts excreted in urine (unchanged)

Interactions/incompatibilities:
• Increased toxicity: radiation, other antineoplastics

Lab test interferences:
Increase: Uric acid (blood, urine)

NURSING CONSIDERATIONS
Assess:
• CBC, differential, platelet count weekly; withhold drug if WBC is <3500/mm³ or platelet count is <100,000/mm³; notify physician of these results; drug should be discontinued
• Renal function studies: BUN, serum uric acid, urine CrCl, electrolytes before, during therapy
• I&O ratio; report fall in urine output to <30 ml/hr
• Monitor temperature q4h; fever may indicate beginning infection
• Liver function tests before, during therapy: bilirubin, alk phosphatase, AST, ALT
• Bleeding time, coagulation time during treatment
• Bleeding: hematuria, guaiac, bruising, petechiae, mucosa or orifices q8h
• Food preferences; list likes, dislikes
• Hepatotoxicity: yellowing of skin and sclera, dark urine, clay-colored stools, pruritus, abdominal pain, fever, diarrhea
• Buccal cavity q8h for dryness, sores, ulceration, white patches, oral pain, bleeding, dysphagia
• Symptoms indicating severe allergic reaction: rash, urticaria, itching, flushing

Administer:
• Antacid before oral agent; give drug after evening meal before bedtime
• Antiemetic 30-60 min before giving drug to prevent vomiting
• Allopurinol or sodium bicarbonate to maintain uric acid levels, alkalinization of urine
• Antibiotics for prophylaxis of infection
• Topical or systemic analgesics for pain
• Transfusion for anemia

T

Perform/provide:
• Strict medical asepsis, protective isolation if WBC levels are low
• Liquid diet: carbonated beverage, Jell-O; dry toast, crackers may be added when patient is not nauseated or vomiting
• Increase fluid intake to 2-3 L/day to prevent urate deposits, calculi formation, unless contraindicated
• Diet low in purines: absence of organ meats (kidney, liver), dried beans, peas to maintain alkaline urine
• Rinsing of mouth tid-qid with water, club soda, brushing of teeth bid-tid with soft brush or cotton-tipped applicators for stomatitis; use unwaxed dental floss
• Nutritious diet with iron, vitamin supplements as ordered
• Storage in tightly closed container in cool environment

Evaluate:
• Therapeutic response: decreased tumor size, spread of malignancy

Teach patient/family:
• Why protective isolation precautions are needed
• To report any complaints, side effects to nurse or physician: black tarry stools, chills, fever, sore throat, bleeding, bruising, cough, shortness of breath, dark, bloody urine
• To avoid foods with citric acid, hot or rough texture if stomatitis is present
• To report stomatitis: any bleeding, white spots, ulcerations in mouth; tell patient to examine mouth qd, report symptoms
• That contraceptive measures are recommended during therapy
• To drink 10-12 (8 oz) glasses of fluid/day

---

thiopental sodium
(thye-oh-pen'tal)
Pentothal, Thiopental Sodium
Func. class.: General anesthetic
Chem. class.: Barbiturate

Controlled Substance Schedule III

Action: Acts in reticular-activating system to produce anesthesia

Uses: Short general anesthesia, narcoanalysis, induction anesthesia before other anesthetics

Dosage and routes:
Induction
• *Adult:* IV 210-280 mg or 3-5 ml/kg
General anesthetic
• *Adult:* IV 50-75 mg given at 20-40 sec intervals
Narcoanalysis
• *Adult:* IV 200 mg/min, not to exceed 50 ml/min
Sedation or narcosis
• *Adult:* Rec 12-20 mg/lb

Available forms: Inj IV, rectal sus

Side effects/adverse reactions:
*RESP: **Respiratory depression, bronchospasm***
CNS: Retrograde amnesia, prolonged somnolence
CV: Tachycardia, hypotension, ***myocardial depression, dysrhythmias***
EENT: Sneezing, coughing
INTEG: Chills, *shivering,* necrosis, pain at injection site
MS: Muscle irritability

Contraindications: Hypersensitivity, status asthmaticus, hepatic/intermittent porphyrias

Precautions: Severe cardiovascular disease, renal disease, hypotension, liver disease, myxedema, myasthenia gravis, asthma, increased

---

intracranial pressure, pregnancy (C)

Pharmacokinetics:

IV: Onset 30-40 sec; half-life 11½ hr; crosses placenta

Interactions/incompatibilities:

• Increased action: CNS depressants

• Incompatible with amikacin, aminophylline, atracurium, benzquinamide, Ca, cephalothin, cephapirin, cimetidine, clindamycin, chlorpromazine, codeine, dimenhydrinate, diphenhydramine, doxapram, droperidol, ephedrine, glycopyrrolate, hydromorphone, insulin, levarterenol, levorphanol, magnesium sulfate, meperidine, methadone, methylprednisolone, morphine, penicillins, procaine, prochlorperazine, promazine, promethazine, succinylcholine, tetracycline, tubocurarine, Ringer's sol, NaCO$_3$

NURSING CONSIDERATIONS

Assess:

• VS q3-5min during IV administration, after dose, q4h postoperatively

• Extravasation; if it occurs, use nitroprusside or chloroprocaine to decrease pain, increase circulation

• Dysrhythmias or myocardial depression

Administer:

• IV after diluting 500 mg/20 ml sterile H$_2$O for inj; give each 25 mg or less/min, titrate to response

• Only with crash cart, resuscitative equipment nearby

Evaluate:

• Therapeutic response: maintenance of anesthesia

---

thioridazine HCl

(thye-or-rid' a-zeen)

Mellaril, Mellaril Concentrate, Mellaril-5, Novoridazine,* Thioridazine HCl

Func. class.: Antipsychotic/neuroleptic

Chem. class.: Phenothiazine, piperidine

Action: Depresses cerebral cortex, hypothalamus, limbic system, which control activity, aggression; blocks neurotransmission produced by dopamine at synapse; exhibits strong α-adrenergic, anticholinergic blocking action; mechanism for antipsychotic effects is unclear

Uses: Psychotic disorders, schizophrenia, behavioral problems in children, alcohol withdrawal as adjunct, anxiety, major depressive disorders, organic brain syndrome

Dosage and routes:

Psychosis

• *Adult:* PO 25-100 mg tid, max dose 800 mg/day; dose is gradually increased to desired response, then reduced to minimum maintenance

Depression/behavioral problems/organic brain syndrome

• *Adult:* PO 25 tid, range from 10 mg bid-qid to 50 mg tid-qid

• *Child 2-12 yr:* PO 0.5-3 mg/kg/day in divided doses

Available forms: Tabs 10, 15, 25, 50, 100, 150, 200, 300 mg; conc 30, 100 mg/ml; susp 25, 100 mg/5 ml, syrup 10 mg/15 ml

Side effects/adverse reactions:

RESP: **Laryngospasm,** dyspnea, **respiratory depression**

CNS: Extrapyramidal symptoms (rare): pseudoparkinsonism, akathisia, dystonia, tardive dyskinesia, **seizures,** headache, confusion

---

italics = common side effects   **bold italic** = life threatening reactions

HEMA: Anemia, **leukopenia, leukocytosis, agranulocytosis**
INTEG: Rash, photosensitivity, dermatitis
EENT: Blurred vision, glaucoma, dry eyes
GI: Dry mouth, nausea, vomiting, anorexia, constipation, diarrhea, jaundice, weight gain
GU: Urinary retention, urinary frequency, enuresis, impotence, amenorrhea, gynecomastia
CV: Orthostatic hypotension, **cardiac arrest,** ECG changes, **tachycardia**
Contraindications: Hypersensitivity, blood dyscrasias, coma, child <2 yr, brain damage, bone marrow depression
Precautions: Pregnancy (C), lactation, seizure disorders, hypertension, hepatic disease, cardiac disease
Pharmacokinetics:
PO: Onset erratic, peak 2-4 hr; metabolized by liver, excreted in urine, crosses placenta, enters breast milk, half-life 26-36 hr
Interactions/incompatibilities:
• Oversedation: other CNS depressants, alcohol, barbiturate anesthetics
• Toxicity: epinephrine
• Decreased absorption: aluminum hydroxide, magnesium hydroxide antacids
• Decreased effects of: lithium, levodopa
• Increased effects of both drugs: β-adrenergic blockers, alcohol
• Increased anticholinergic effects: anticholinergics
Lab test interferences:
Increase: Liver function tests, cardiac enzymes, cholesterol, blood glucose, prolactin, bilirubin, PBI, cholinesterase, ^{131}I

Decrease: Hormones (blood, urine)
False positive: Pregnancy tests, PKU
False negative: Urinary steroids, pregnancy tests
NURSING CONSIDERATIONS
Assess:
• Mental status before initial administration
• Swallowing of PO medication; check for hoarding or giving of medication to other patients
• I&O ratio; palpate bladder if low urinary output occurs
• Bilirubin, CBC, liver function studies monthly
• Urinalysis is recommended before and during prolonged therapy
• Affect, orientation, LOC, reflexes, gait, coordination, sleep pattern disturbances
• B/P standing and lying; also include pulse and respirations q4h during initial treatment; establish baseline before starting treatment; report drops of 30 mm Hg
• Dizziness, faintness, palpitations, tachycardia on rising
• Extrapyramidal symptoms including akathisia (inability to sit still, no pattern to movements), tardive dyskinesia (bizarre movements of jaw, mouth, tongue, extremities), pseudoparkinsonism (rigidity, tremors, pill rolling, shuffling gait)
• For neuroleptic malignant syndrome: altered mental status, muscle rigidity, increased CPK, hyperthermia
• Skin turgor daily
• Constipation, urinary retention daily; if these occur, increase bulk, water in diet
Administer:
• Antiparkinsonian agent, after securing order from physician to be

used if extrapyramidal symptoms occur

• Concentrate mixed in citrus juices or distilled or acidified tap water

Perform/provide:

• Decreased noise input by dimming lights, avoiding loud noises

• Supervised ambulation until stabilized on medication; do not involve in strenuous exercise program because fainting is possible; patient should not stand still for long periods

• Increased fluids to prevent constipation

• Sips of water, candy, gum for dry mouth

• Storage in tight, light-resistant container; avoid contact with skin

Evaluate:

• Therapeutic response: decrease in emotional excitement, hallucinations, delusions, paranoia, reorganization of patterns of thought, speech

Teach patient/family:

• That orthostatic hypotension occurs frequently, to rise from sitting or lying position gradually; to avoid hazardous activities until stabilized on medication

• To remain lying down after IM injection for at least 30 min

• To avoid hot tubs, hot showers, tub baths, since hypotension may occur

• To avoid abrupt withdrawal of thioridazine, or extrapyramidal symptoms may result; drug should be withdrawn slowly

• To avoid OTC preparations (cough, hay fever, cold) unless approved by physician, since serious drug interactions may occur; avoid use with alcohol, CNS depressants; increased drowsiness may occur

• To use a sunscreen during sun e. posure to prevent burns

• Regarding compliance with drug regimen

• About necessity for meticulous oral hygiene, since oral candidiasis may occur

• To report sore throat, malaise, fever, bleeding, mouth sores; if these occur, CBC should be drawn and drug discontinued

• In hot weather, heat stroke may occur; take extra precautions to stay cool

Treatment of overdose: Lavage if orally ingested, provide an airway; do not induce vomiting

---

thiotepa

(thye-oh-tep′a)

Thiotepa

Func. class.: Antineoplastic
Chem. class.: Alkylating agent

Action: Responsible for cross-linking DNA strands leading to cell death; activity is not cell cycle specific

Uses: Hodgkin's disease, lymphomas; breast, ovarian, lung, bladder, cancer; neoplastic effusions

Dosage and routes:

• *Adult:* IV 50.2 mg/kg × 5 days, then 0.2 mg/kg q1-3 wk

Neoplastic effusions

• *Adult:* Intracavity 10-15 mg

Bladder cancer

• *Adult:* INSTILL 60 mg/60 ml water for inj instilled in bladder for 2 hr once weekly × 4 wk

Available forms: Inj 15 mg, powder for inj

Side effects/adverse reactions:

CNS: Dizziness, headache

HEMA: ***Thrombocytopenia, leukopenia, pancytopenia***

T

---

italics = common side effects   ***bold italic*** = life threatening reactions

GI: Nausea, vomiting, anorexia, stomatitis
GU:Hyperuricemia, hematuria, amenorrhea, azoospermia
INTEG: Rash, pruritus
Contraindications: Hypersensitivity, pregnancy (D)
Precautions: Radiation therapy, bone marrow suppression, impaired renal or hepatic function
Pharmacokinetics:
Onset slow, metabolized in liver, excreted in urine
Interactions/incompatibilities:
• Increased apnea: succinylcholine
NURSING CONSIDERATIONS
Assess:
• CBC, differential, platelet count weekly; withhold drug if WBC is <4000 or platelet count is <75,000; notify physician of results
• Renal function studies: BUN, serum uric acid, urine CrCl before, during therapy
• I&O ratio, report fall in urine output of 30 ml/hr
• Monitor temperature q4h (may indicate beginning infection)
• Liver function tests before, during therapy (bilirubin, AST, ALT, LDH) as needed or monthly
• Bleeding: hematuria, guaiac, bruising or petechiae, mucosa or orifices q8h
• Food preferences; list likes, dislikes
• Inflammation of mucosa, breaks in skin
• Yellowing of skin and sclera, dark urine, clay-colored stools, itchy skin, abdominal pain, fever, diarrhea
• Buccal cavity q8h for dryness, sores, ulceration, white patches, oral pain, bleeding, dysphagia
• Symptoms indicating severe allergic reaction: rash, pruritus, urticaria, itching, flushing
Administer:
• IV after diluting 15 mg/1.5 ml of sterile H_2O for inj; give over 1-3 min; may be further diluted in 50-100 ml compatible sol
• Antiemetic 30-60 min before giving drug to prevent vomiting
• Allopurinol or sodium bicarbonate to maintain uric acid levels, alkalinization of urine
• Antibiotics for prophylaxis of infection
• Local or systemic drugs for infection
Perform/provide:
• Storage in light-resistant container; refrigerate
• Strict medical asepsis, protective isolation if WBC levels are low
• Special skin care
• Increase fluid intake to 2-3 L/day to prevent urate deposits, calculi formation
• Diet low in purines: organ meats (kidney, liver), dried beans, peas, to maintain alkaline urine
• Rinsing of mouth tid-qid with water; brushing of teeth bid-tid with soft brush or cotton-tipped applicators for stomatitis; use unwaxed dental floss
• Warm compresses at injection site for inflammation
Evaluate:
• Therapeutic response: decreased tumor size, spread of malignancy
Teach patient/family:
• Of protective isolation precautions
• That azoospermia or amenorrhea can occur; reversible after discontinuing treatment
• To avoid foods with citric acid, hot or rough texture
• To report any bleeding, white spots or ulcerations in mouth to

physician; tell patient to examine mouth qd

• To report signs of infection: increased temperature, sore throat, flu symptoms

• To report signs of anemia: fatigue, headache, faintness, shortness of breath, irritability

• To avoid use of razors, commercial mouthwash

• To avoid use of aspirin products, ibuprofen

---

thiothixene

(thye-oh-thix′een)

Navane, Thiothixene

Func. class.: Antipsychotic/neuroleptic

Chem. class.: Thioxanthene

Action: Depresses cerebral cortex, hypothalamus, limbic system, which control activity, aggression; blocks neurotransmission produced by dopamine at synapse; exhibits strong α-adrenergic blocking action; mechanism for antipsychotic effects is unclear

Uses: Psychotic disorders, schizophrenia, acute agitation

Dosage and routes:

• *Adult:* PO 2-5 mg bid-qid depending on severity of condition; dose gradually increased to 15-30 mg if needed; IM 4 mg bid-qid; max dose 30 mg qd; administer PO dose as soon as possible

Available forms: Caps 1, 2, 5, 10, 20 mg; conc 5 mg/ml; inj IM 2 mg/ml; powder for inj 5 mg/ml

Side effects/adverse reactions:

*RESP: **Laryngospasm,** dyspnea, respiratory depression*

CNS: Extrapyramidal symptoms: pseudoparkinsonism, akathisia, dystonia, tardive dyskinesia, seizures, *headache*

HEMA: Anemia, *leukopenia, leukocytosis, agranulocytosis*

INTEG: Rash, photosensitivity, dermatitis

EENT: Blurred vision, glaucoma

GI: Dry mouth, nausea, vomiting, anorexia, constipation, diarrhea, jaundice, weight gain

GU: Urinary retention, urinary frequency, enuresis, impotence, amenorrhea, gynecomastia

CV: Orthostatic hypotension, hypertension, *cardiac arrest,* ECG changes, *tachycardia*

Contraindications: Hypersensitivity, blood dyscrasias, child <12 yr, bone marrow depression, circulatory collapse, CNS depression, coma, alcoholism, CV disease, hepatic disease, Reye's syndrome, narrow-angle glaucoma

Precautions: Pregnancy (C), lactation, seizure disorders, hypertension, hepatic disease

Pharmacokinetics:

PO: Onset slow, peak 2-8 hr, duration up to 12 hr

IM: Onset 15-30 min, peak 1-6 hr, duration up to 12 hr; metabolized by liver, excreted in urine, crosses placenta, enters breast milk, half-life 34 hr

Interactions/incompatibilities:

• Oversedation: other CNS depressants, alcohol, barbiturate anesthetics

• Toxicity: epinephrine

• Decreased absorption: aluminum hydroxide, magnesium hydroxide antacids

• Decreased effects of thiothixene: lithium, levodopa

• Increased effects of both drugs: β-adrenergic blockers, alcohol

• Increased anticholinergic effects: anticholinergics

Lab test interferences:

Increase: Liver function tests, car-

---

italics = common side effects   **bold italic** = life threatening reactions

diac enzymes, cholesterol, blood glucose, prolactin, bilirubin, PBI, cholinesterase, ^{131}I

Decrease: Uric acid

NURSING CONSIDERATIONS
Assess:
• Mental status before initial administration
• Swallowing of PO medication; check for hoarding or giving of medication to other patients
• I&O ratio, palpate bladder if low urinary output occurs
• Bilirubin, CBC, liver function studies monthly
• Urinalysis is recommended before and during prolonged therapy
• Affect, orientation, LOC, reflexes, gait, coordination, sleep pattern disturbances
• B/P standing and lying; pulse and respirations q4h during initial treatment; establish baseline before starting treatment; report drops of 30 mm Hg
• Dizziness, faintness, palpitations, tachycardia on rising
• EPS including akathisia (inability to sit still, no pattern to movements), tardive dyskinesia (bizarre movements of jaw, mouth, tongue, extremities), pseudoparkinsonism (rigidity, tremors, pill rolling, shuffling gait)
• For neuroleptic malignant syndrome: muscle rigidity, altered mental status, increased CPK, hyperthermia
• Constipation, urinary retention daily; if these occur, increase bulk, water in diet

Administer:
• Antiparkinsonian agent after securing order from physician; to be used if EPS occur
• Concentrate mixed in citrus juices or distilled or acidified tap water
• IM injection into large muscle mass

Perform/provide:
• Decreased noise input by dimming lights, avoiding loud noises
• Supervised ambulation until stabilized on medication; do not involve in strenuous exercise program because fainting is possible; patient should not stand still for long periods
• Increased fluids to prevent constipation
• Sips of water, candy, gum for dry mouth
• Storage in tight, light-resistant container; keep reconstituted solutions at room temperature for up to 48 hr; avoid contact with skin

Evaluate:
• Therapeutic response: decrease in emotional excitement, hallucinations, delusions, paranoia, reorganization of patterns of thought, speech

Teach patient/family:
• That orthostatic hypotension occurs frequently, and to rise from sitting or lying position gradually; to avoid hazardous activities until stabilized on medication
• To remain lying down after IM inj for at least 30 min
• To avoid hot tubs, hot showers, tub baths, since hypotension may occur
• To avoid abrupt withdrawal of this drug, or EPS may result; drugs should be withdrawn slowly
• To avoid OTC preparations (cough, hay fever, cold) unless approved by physician, since serious drug interactions may occur; avoid use with alcohol, CNS depressants; increased drowsiness may occur
• To use a sunscreen during sun exposure to prevent burns

---

*Available in Canada only

• Regarding compliance with drug regimen
• About EPS and necessity for meticulous oral hygiene, since oral candidiasis may occur
• To report sore throat, malaise, fever, bleeding, mouth sores; if these occur, CBC should be drawn and drug discontinued
• In hot weather, heat stroke may occur; take extra precautions to stay cool

Treatment of overdose: Lavage if orally ingested; provide an airway; *do not induce vomiting*

---

thrombin
Thrombinar, Thrombogen, Thrombostat

Func. class.: Hemostatic
Chem. class.: Bovine thrombin

Action: Converts fibrinogen to fibrin, promotes clotting

Uses: GI hemorrhage, bleeding in dental, plastic, nasal, laryngeal surgery, skin grafting

Dosage and routes:
• *Adult:* TOP apply 100 U/1 ml sterile isotonic NaCl or distilled H₂O in light to moderate bleeding, or 1000-2000 U/ml sterile isotonic NaCl in severe bleeding; dry area before applying

Available forms: Powder 1000, 5000, 10,000, 20,000, 50,000 U

Side effects/adverse reactions:
INTEG: Rash, allergic reactions
*HEMA: **Intravascular clotting when entering large blood vessels***

Contraindications: Hypersensitivity to bovine products

Precautions: Pregnancy (C), children

NURSING CONSIDERATIONS
Assess:
• For allergic reactions: fever, rash,

itching, changes in VS; thrombosis formation

Administer:
• Only to area sponged free of blood
• After preparing with NS, isotonic saline
• With blood available for transfusion

Perform/provide:
• Storage in refrigerator; use reconstituted solution within 3 hr; some can be administered up to 48 hr after reconstitution if refrigerated or preferably frozen shortly after reconstituted; discard unused portion

Evaluate:
• Therapeutic response: control of bleeding

---

thyroglobulin
(thye-roe-glob'yoo-lin)
Proloid

Func. class.: Thyroid hormone
Chem. class.: Combination of natural T₄/T₃; ratio 2.5 to 1

Action: Increases metabolic rates, cardiac output, O₂ consumption, body temperature, blood volume, growth, development at cellular level

Uses: Hypothyroidism

Dosage and routes:
Hypothyroidism
Adult: 32 mg/day increasing q2-3wk to desired response; maintenance 65-200 mg/day

Available forms: Tabs 32, 65, 100, 130, 200 mg

Side effects/adverse reactions:
INTEG: Sweating, alopecia
CNS: Anxiety, insomnia, tremors, headache, heat intolerance, fever, coma, thyroid storm
CV: Tachycardia, palpitations, an-

gina, dysrhythmias, hypertension, CHF

GI: Nausea, diarrhea, increased or decreased appetite, cramps

GU: Menstrual irregularities

Contraindications: Adrenal insufficiency, myocardial infarction, thyrotoxicosis

Precautions: Elderly, angina pectoris, hypertension, ischemia, cardiac disease, pregnancy (A), lactation

Pharmacokinetics:

PO: Peak 12-48 hr, half-life 6-7 days

Interactions/incompatibilities:

• Decreased absorption of thyroglobulin: cholestyramine

• Increased effects of: anticoagulants, sympathomimetics, tricyclic antidepressants, catecholamines

• Decreased effects of: digitalis drugs, insulin, hypoglycemics

• Decreased effects of liothyronine: estrogens

Lab test interferences:

Increase: CPK, LDH, AST, PBI, blood glucose

Decrease: TSH, ^{131}I uptake test, uric acid, triglycerides

NURSING CONSIDERATIONS
Assess:

• B/P, pulse before each dose

• I&O ratio

• Weight qd in same clothing, using same scale, at same time of day

• Height, growth rate if given to a child

• T_3, T_4, which are decreased, radioimmunoassay of TSH, which is increased, radio uptake, which is decreased if patient is on too low a dose of medication

• Pro-time may require decreased anticoagulant; check for bleeding, bruising

• Increased nervousness, excitability, irritability, which may indicate too high dose of medication, usually after 1-3 wk of treatment

• Cardiac status: angina, palpitation, chest pain, change in VS

Administer:

• In AM if possible as a single dose to decrease sleeplessness

• At same time each day to maintain drug level

• Only for hormone imbalances; not to be used for obesity, male infertility, menstrual conditions, lethargy

• Lowest dose that relieves symptoms

Perform/provide:

• Removal of medication 4 wk before RAIU test

Evaluate:

• Therapeutic response: absence of depression; increased weight loss, diuresis, pulse, appetite; absence of constipation, peripheral edema, cold intolerance, pale, cool dry skin, brittle nails, alopecia, coarse hair, menorrhagia, night blindness, paresthesias, syncope, stupor, coma; rosy cheeks

Teach patient/family:

• To report excitability, irritability, anxiety, which indicate overdose

• Not to switch brands unless approved by physician

• That hypothyroid child will show almost immediate behavior/personality change

• That drug is not to be taken to reduce weight

• To avoid OTC preparations with iodine, to read labels

• To avoid iodine food, iodized salt, soybeans, tofu, turnips, some seafood, some bread

---

*Available in Canada only

thyroid USP (desiccated)

(thye-roid)

Armour Thyroid, Cholaxin,* S-P-T, Thyrar, Thyroid Strong, Thyroid USP

Func. class.: Thyroid hormone
Chem. class.: Active thyroid hormone in natural state and ratio

Action: Increases metabolic rates, increases cardiac output, O_2 consumption, body temperature, blood volume, growth, development at cellular level

Uses: Hypothyroidism, cretinism, myxedema

Dosage and routes:
Hypothyroidism
• *Adult:* PO 65 mg qd, increased by 65 mg q30d until desired response; maintenance dose 65-195 mg qd
• *Geriatric:* PO 7.5-15 mg qd, double dose q6-8wk until desired response
Cretinism/juvenile hypothyroidism
• *Child over 1 yr:* PO up to 180 mg qd titrated to response
• *Child 4-12 mo:* PO 30-60 mg qd
• *Child 1-4 mo:* PO 15-30 mg qd; may increase q2wk; titrated to response; maintenance dose 30-45 mg qd
Myxedema
• *Adult:* PO 16 mg qd, double dose q2wk, maintenance 65-195 mg/day

Available forms: Tabs 16, 32, 65, 98, 130, 195, 260, 325 mg; tabs enteric coated 32, 65, 130 mg; sugar-coated tabs 32, 65, 130, 195 mg; caps 65, 130, 195, 325 mg

Side effects/adverse reactions:
CNS: Insomnia, tremors, headache, thyroid storm

CV: Tachycardia, palpitations, angina, dysrhythmias, hypertension, **cardiac arrest**

GI: Nausea, diarrhea, increased or decreased appetite, cramps

MISC: Menstrual irregularities, weight loss, sweating, heat intolerance, fever

Contraindications: Adrenal insufficiency, myocardial infarction, thyrotoxicosis

Precautions: Elderly, angina pectoris, hypertension, ischemia, cardiac disease, pregnancy (A), lactation

Pharmacokinetics:
PO: Peak 12-48 hr, half-life 6-7 days

Interactions/incompatibilities:
• Decreased absorption of thyroid: cholestyramine
• Increased effects of: anticoagulants, sympathomimetics, tricyclic antidepressants, catecholamines
• Decreased effects of: digitalis drugs, insulin, hypoglycemics
• Decreased effects of thyroid: estrogens

Lab test interferences:
Increase: CPK, LDH, AST, PBI, blood glucose
Decrease: TSH, ^{131}I uptake test, uric acid, triglycerides

NURSING CONSIDERATIONS
Assess:
• B/P, pulse before each dose
• I&O ratio
• Weight qd in same clothing, using same scale, at same time of day
• Height, growth rate if given to a child
• T_3, T_4, which are decreased; radioimmunoassay of TSH, which is increased; radio uptake, which is decreased if patient is on too low a dose of medication
• Pro-time may require decreased

---

italics = common side effects   ***bold italic*** = life threatening reactions

anticoagulant, check for bleeding, bruising
• Increased nervousness, excitability, irritability; may indicate too high dose of medication, usually after 1-3 wk of treatment
• Cardiac status: angina, palpitation, chest pain, change in VS

Administer:
• In AM if possible as a single dose to decrease sleeplessness
• At same time each day to maintain drug level
• Only for hormone imbalances; not to be used for obesity, male infertility, menstrual conditions, lethargy
• Lowest dose that relieves symptoms

Perform/provide:
• Removal of medication 4 wk before RAIU test

Evaluate:
• Therapeutic response: absence of depression; increased weight loss, diuresis, pulse, appetite; absence of constipation, peripheral edema, cold intolerance, pale, cool dry skin, brittle nails, alopecia, coarse hair, menorrhagia, night blindness, paresthesias, syncope, stupor, coma, rosy cheeks

Teach patient/family:
• That hair loss will occur in child, is temporary
• To report excitability, irritability, anxiety; indicates overdose
• Not to switch brands unless directed by physician
• That hypothyroid child will show almost immediate behavior/personality change
• That treatment drug is not to be taken to reduce weight
• To avoid OTC preparations with iodine; read labels
• To avoid iodine food, iodized

salt, soybeans, tofu, turnips, some seafood, some bread

---

thyrotropin (thyroid-stimulating hormone, or TSH)

(thye-roe-troe′pin)
Thytropar
Func. class.: Thyroid hormone
Chem. class.: TSH

Action: Increases uptake of iodine by thyroid gland, production of thyroid hormone, release of thyroid hormone

Uses: Diagnosis and treatment of thyroid cancer, diagnosis of primary/secondary hypothyroidism

Dosage and routes:
Diagnosis of hypothyroidism
• *Adult:* IM/SC 10 Units qd × 1-3 days
Diagnosis of thyroid cancer
• *Adult:* IM/SC 10 IU qd × 3-7 days
Treatment of thyroid cancer
• *Adult:* IM/SC 10 Units qd × 3-8 days
Available forms: Powder for inj 10 IU/vial

Side effects/adverse reactions:
INTEG: Urticaria
CNS: Headache, fever
CV: Tachycardia, angina, *atrial fibrillation, CHF,* hypotension
GI: Nausea, vomiting
SYST: **Anaphylactic reactions**

Contraindications: Hypersensitivity, coronary thrombosis, untreated Addison's disease

Precautions: Angina pectoris, adrenal insufficiency, pregnancy (C), lactation, children

Pharmacokinetics:
IM/SC: Onset 8 hr, peak 24-48 hr

NURSING CONSIDERATIONS
Administer:

• After dilution with 2 ml sterile saline solution

• Three-day dose schedule for myxedema (pituitary)

• In combination with ^{131}I to treat thyroid cancer

Treatment of overdose: Discontinue drug, administer supportive care

---

ticarcillin disodium
(tye-kar-sill'in)
Ticaripen,* Ticar
Func. class.: Broad-spectrum antibiotic
Chem. class.: Extended-spectrum penicillin

Action: Interferes with cell wall replication of susceptible organisms; osmotically unstable cell wall swells, bursts from osmotic pressure.

Uses: Respiratory, soft tissue, urinary tract infections, bacterial septicemia; effective for gram-positive cocci *(S. aureus, S. faecalis, S. pneumoniae)*, gram-negative cocci *(N. gonorrhoeae)*, gram-positive bacilli *(C. perfringens, C. tetani)*, gram-negative bacilli *(Bacteroides, F. nucleatum, E. coli, P. mirabilis, Salmonella, M. morganii, P. rettgeri, Enterobacter, P. aeruginosa, Serratia, Peptococcus, Peptostreptococcus, Eubacterium)*

Dosage and routes:

• *Adult:* IV/IM 12-24 g/day in divided doses q3-6h; infuse over ½-2 hr

• *Child:* IV/IM 50-300 mg/kg/day in divided doses q4-8h

• *Neonates:* IV INF 75-100 mg/kg/8-12 hr

Available forms: Inj IM, IV 1, 3, 6, 20, 30 g, IV INF 3 g

Side effects/adverse reactions:

HEMA: Anemia, increased bleeding time, ***bone marrow depression, granulocytopenia***

GI: *Nausea, vomiting, diarrhea,* increased AST, ALT, abdominal pain, glossitis, colitis

GU: Oliguria, proteinuria, hematuria, *vaginitis, moniliasis,* ***glomerulonephritis***

CNS: Lethargy, hallucinations, anxiety, depression, twitching, ***coma, convulsions***

META: Hypokalemia

Contraindications: Hypersensitivity to penicillins

Precautions: Hypersensitivity to cephalosporins, pregnancy (B)

Pharmacokinetics:

IM: Peak 1 hr, duration 4-6 hr

IV: Peak 30-45 min, duration 4 hr, half-life 70 min; small amount metabolized in liver; excreted in urine, breast milk

Interactions/incompatibilities:

• Decreased antimicrobial effect of ticarcillin: tetracyclines, erythromycins, aminoglycosides IV

• Increased ticarcillin concentrations: aspirin, probenecid

• Incompatible in sol with aminoglycosides, tetracyclines, amphotericin B, gentamycin, amikacin, tobramycin

Lab test interferences:

False positive: Urine glucose, urine protein

NURSING CONSIDERATIONS
Assess:

• I&O ratio; report hematuria, oliguria, since penicillin in high doses is nephrotoxic

• Any patient with compromised renal system, since drug is excreted slowly in poor renal system func-

T

---

tion; toxicity may occur rapidly
• Liver studies: AST, ALT
• Blood studies: WBC, RBC, H&H, bleeding time
• Renal studies: urinalysis, protein, blood
• C&S before drug therapy; drug may be given as soon as culture is taken
• Bowel pattern before, during treatment
• Skin eruptions after administration of penicillin to 1 wk after discontinuing drug
• Respiratory status: rate, character, wheezing, tightness in chest
• Allergies before initiation of treatment, reaction of each medication; highlight allergies on chart, Kardex

Administer:
• IV after diluting 1 g or less/4 ml sterile H_2O for inj; dilute further with 10-20 ml or more D_5W, NS, or sterile H_2O for inj sol; give 1 g or less/5 min or more or by intermittent INF over ½-2 hr or by continuous INF at prescribed rate
• Drug after C&S has been completed

Perform/provide:
• Adrenalin, suction, tracheostomy set, endotracheal intubation equipment
• Adequate fluid intake (2 L) during diarrhea episodes
• Scratch test to assess allergy after securing order from physician; usually done when penicillin is only drug of choice
• Storage at room temperature, reconstituted sol for 72 hr at room temperature

Evaluate:
• Therapeutic response: absence of fever, purulent drainage, redness, inflammation

Teach patient/family:
• That culture may be taken after completed course of medication
• To report sore throat, fever, fatigue (may indicate superimposed infection)
• To wear or carry Medic Alert ID if allergic to penicillins
• To notify nurse of diarrhea

Treatment of overdose: Withdraw drug, maintain airway, administer epinephrine, aminophylline, O_2, IV corticosteroids for anaphylaxis

---

ticarcillin disodium/ clavulanate potassium
Timentin

Func. class.: Broad-spectrum antibiotic

Chem. class.: Extended-spectrum penicillin

Action: Interferes with cell wall replication of susceptible organisms; osmotically unstable cell wall swells, bursts from osmotic pressure

Uses: Respiratory, soft tissue, and urinary tract infections, bacterial septicemia; effective for gram-positive cocci *(S. aureus, S. faecalis, S. pneumoniae),* gram-negative cocci *(N. gonorrhoeae),* gram-positive bacilli *(C. perfringens, C. tetani),* gram-negative bacilli *(Bacteroides, F. nucleatum, E. coli, P. mirabilis, Salmonella, M. morganii, P. rettgeri, Enterobacter, P. aeruginosa, Serratia, Peptococcus, Peptostreptococcus, Eubacterium)*

Dosage and routes:
• *Adult:* IV INF 1 vial containing ticarcillin 3 g, clavulanate K 0.1 g q4-6h, infuse over 30 min
• *Child <60 kg:* 200-300 mg ti-

carcillin/kg/day in divided doses q4-6h

Available forms: Inj IM, IV 3 g ticarcillin and 0.1g clavulanate; IV INF 3 g ticarcillin and 0.1 g clavulanate

Side effects/adverse reactions:

HEMA: Anemia, increased bleeding time, ***bone marrow depression, granulocytopenia***

GI: Nausea, vomiting, diarrhea, increased AST, ALT, abdominal pain, glossitis, colitis

GU: Oliguria, proteinuria, hematuria, *vaginitis, moniliasis, **glomerulonephritis***

CNS: Lethargy, hallucinations, anxiety, depression, twitching, ***coma, convulsions***

META: Hyperkalemia, hypokalemia, alkalosis, hypernatremia

Contraindications: Hypersensitivity to penicillins; neonates

Precautions: Hypersensitivity to cephalosporins, pregnancy (B)

Pharmacokinetics:

IV: Peak 30-45 min, duration 4 hr, half-life 64-68 min; excreted in urine

Interactions/incompatibilities:

• Decreased antimicrobial effect of ticarcillin: tetracyclines, erythromycins, aminoglycosides IV

• Increased ticarcillin concentrations: aspirin, probenecid

• Incompatible in sol with aminoglycosides, amikacin, $NaCO_3$

Lab test interferences:

False positive: Urine glucose, urine protein Coombs' test

NURSING CONSIDERATIONS

Assess:

• I&O ratio; report hematuria, oliguria, since penicillin in high doses is nephrotoxic

• Any patient with compromised renal system, since drug is excreted slowly in poor renal system func-

tion; toxicity may occur rapidly

• Liver studies: AST, ALT

• Blood studies: WBC, RBC, H&H, bleeding time

• Renal studies: urinalysis, protein, blood

• C&S before drug therapy; drug may be given as soon as culture is taken

• Bowel pattern before, during treatment

• Skin eruptions after administration of penicillin to 1 wk after discontinuing drug

• Respiratory status: rate, character, wheezing, and tightness in chest

• Allergies before initiation of treatment, reaction of each medication; highlight allergies on chart, Kardex

Administer:

• IV after diluting 3.1 g or less/13 ml of sterile H_2O or NaCl (200 mg/ ml), shake; may further dilute in 50-100 ml or more normal saline, D_5W, or LR sol and run over ½ hr

• Drug after C&S has been completed

Perform/provide:

• Adrenalin, suction, tracheostomy set, endotracheal intubation equipment

• Adequate fluid intake (2 L) during diarrhea episodes

• Scratch test to assess allergy after securing order from physician; usually done when penicillin is only drug of choice

• Storage at room temperature, reconstituted sol for 12-24 hr or 3-7 days refrigerated

Evaluate:

• Therapeutic response: absence of fever, purulent drainage, redness, inflammation

Teach patient/family:

• That culture may be taken after

completed course of medication
• To report sore throat, fever, fatigue (may indicate superimposed infection)
• To wear or carry Medic Alert ID if allergic to penicillins
Treatment of overdose: Withdraw drug, maintain airway, administer epinephrine, aminophylline, O_2, IV corticosteroids for anaphylaxis

---

ticlopidine
(tye-klo′-pa-deen)
Ticlid
Func. class.: Platelet aggregation inhibitor

Action: Inhibits first and second phases of ADP-induced effects in platelet aggregation
Uses: Reducing the risk of stroke in high-risk patients
Dosage and routes:
• *Adult:* PO 250 mg bid with food
Available forms: Tabs 250 mg
Side effects/adverse reactions:
INTEG: Rash, pruritus
GI: Nausea, vomiting, diarrhea, GI discomfort, *cholestatic jaundice, hepatitis,* increased cholesterol, LDL, VLDL
HEMA: Bleeding (epistaxis, hematuria, conjunctival hemorrhage, GI bleeding), agranulocytosis, neutropenia, thrombocytopenia
Contraindications: Hypersensitivity, active liver disease, blood dyscrasias
Precautions: Past liver disease, renal disease, elderly, pregnancy (B), lactation, children, increased bleeding risk
Pharmacokinetics: Peak 1-3 hr, metabolized by the liver, excreted in urine, feces; half-life increases with repeated dosing
Interactions/incompatibilities:
• Increased bleeding tendencies: anticoagulants, aspirin
• Decreased plasma levels of ticlopidine: antacids
• Decreased plasma levels of: digoxin
• Increased effects of ticlopidine: cimetidine
• Increased effects of: theophylline
NURSING CONSIDERATIONS
Assess:
• Liver function studies: AST, ALT, bilirubin, creatinine if patient is on long-term therapy
• Blood studies: CBC, Hct, Hgb, pro-time if patient is on long-term therapy
Administer:
• With food to decrease gastric symptoms
Evaluate:
• Therapeutic response: absence of stroke
Teach patient/family:
• That blood work will be necessary during treatment
• To report any unusual bleeding to physician
• To take with food or just after eating to minimize GI discomfort
• To report side effects such as diarrhea, skin rashes, subcutaneous bleeding, signs of cholestasis (yellow skin and sclera, dark urine, light-colored stools)

---

timolol maleate
(tye′moe-lole)
Blocadren, Timolol maleate
Func. class.: Antihypertensive
Chem. class.: Nonselective β-blocker

Action: Competitively blocks stimulation of β-adrenergic receptor within vascular smooth muscle; produces chronotropic, inotropic activity (decreases rate of SA node discharge, increases recovery time), slows conduction of AV node, decreases heart rate, which decreases O_2 consumption in myocardium; also decreases renin-aldosterone-angiotensin system, at high doses inhibits β-2 receptors in bronchial system

Uses: Mild to moderate hypertension, sinus tachycardia, persistent atrial extrasystoles, tachydysrhythmias, prophylaxis of angina pectoris, reduction of mortality after MI

Dosage and routes:
Hypertension
• *Adult:* PO 10 mg bid, or 20 mg qd, may increase by 10 mg q2-3d, not to exceed 60 mg/day
Myocardial infarction
• *Adult:* 10 mg bid
Available forms: Tabs 5, 10, 20 mg
Side effects/adverse reactions:
CV: Hypotension, bradycardia, **CHF,** edema, chest pain, bradycardia, claudication
CNS: Insomnia, dizziness, hallucinations, anxiety
GI: Nausea, vomiting, ***ischemic colitis,*** diarrhea, *abdominal pain,* ***mesenteric arterial thrombosis***
INTEG: Rash, alopecia, pruritus, fever
HEMA: ***Agranulocytosis, thrombocytopenia, purpura***
EENT: Visual changes, sore throat, *double vision,* dry burning eyes
GU: Impotence, frequency
RESP: ***Bronchospasm,*** *dyspnea,* cough, rales
META: Hypoglycemia
MUSC: Joint pain, muscle pain
Contraindications: Hypersensitiv-

ity to β-blockers, cardiogenic shock, heart block (2nd, 3rd degree), sinus bradycardia, CHF, cardiac failure
Precautions: Major surgery, pregnancy (C), lactation, diabetes mellitus, renal disease, thyroid disease, COPD, well-compensated heart failure, CAD, nonallergic bronchospasm
Pharmacokinetics:
PO: Peak 2-4 hr; half-life 3-4 hr; excreted 30%-45% unchanged; 60%-65% metabolized by liver; excreted in breast milk
Interactions/incompatibilities:
• Increased hypotension, bradycardia: reserpine, hydralazine, methyldopa, prazosin, anticholinergics
• Decreased antihypertensive effects: idomethacin
• Increased hypoglycemic effects: insulin
• Decreased bronchodilation: theophyllines
Lab test interferences:
Increase: Liver function tests, renal function tests, K, uric acid
Decrease: Hct, Hgb, HDL
NURSING CONSIDERATIONS
Assess:
• I&O, weight daily
• B/P during initial treatment, periodically thereafter, pulse q4h; note rate, rhythm, quality
• Apical/radial pulse before administration; notify physician of any significant changes
• Baselines in renal, liver function tests before therapy begins
• Edema in feet, legs daily
• Skin turgor, dryness of mucous membranes for hydration status
Administer:
• PO ac, hs, tablet may be crushed or swallowed whole

---

italics = common side effects   ***bold italic*** = life threatening reactions

• Reduced dosage in renal dysfunction
Perform/provide:
• Storage in dry area at room temperature; do not freeze
Evaluate:
• Therapeutic response: decreased B/P after 1-2 wk
Teach patient/family:
• To take with or immediately after meals
• Not to discontinue drug abruptly; taper over 2 wk; may cause precipitate angina
• Not to use OTC products containing α-adrenergic stimulants (nasal decongestants, cold preparations) unless directed by physician
• To report bradycardia, dizziness, confusion, depression, fever, sore throat, shortness of breath to physician
• To take pulse at home; advise when to notify physician
• To avoid alcohol, smoking, sodium intake
• To comply with weight control, dietary adjustments, modified exercise program
• To carry Medic Alert ID to identify drug, allergies
• To avoid hazardous activities if dizziness is present
• To report symptoms of CHF: difficult breathing, especially on exertion or when lying down; night cough; swelling of extremities
• To take medication hs to maintain effect of orthostatic hypotension
• To wear support hose to minimize effects of orthostatic hypotension
Treatment of overdose: Lavage, IV atropine for bradycardia, IV theophylline for bronchospasm, digitalis, O_2, diuretic for cardiac failure, hemodialysis; administer vasopressor (norepinephrine)

timolol maleate (optic)
(tye'moe-lole)
Timoptic, Timoptic in Ocudose
Func. class.: β-Adrenergic blocker
Chem. class.: I-isomer

Action: Reduces production of aqueous humor by unknown mechanism
Uses: Ocular hypertension, chronic open-angle glaucoma, secondary glaucoma, aphakic glaucoma
Dosage and routes:
• *Adult:* INSTILL 1 gtt 0.25% sol in affected eye(s) bid, then 1 gtt for maintenance; may increase to 1 gtt 0.5% sol bid if needed
Available forms: Sol 0.25%, 0.5%
Side effects/adverse reactions:
CNS: Weakness, fatigue, depression, anxiety, headache, confusion
GI: Nausea, anorexia, dyspepsia
EENT: Eye irritation, conjunctivitis, keratitis
INTEG: Rash, urticaria
CV: Bradycardia, hypotension, dysrhythmias, syncope, heart block, CHF, CVA
*RESP: **Bronchospasm,** dyspnea*
Contraindications: Hypersensitivity, asthma, 2nd or 3rd degree heart block, right ventricular failure, congenital glaucoma (infants), COPD
Precautions: Nonallergic bronchospasm, diabetes, pregnancy, children, lactation, myasthenia gravis
Pharmacokinetics:
INSTILL: Onset 15-30 min, peak 1-2 hr, duration 24 hr
Interactions/incompatibilities:
• Toxicity: β-adrenergic blockers
• Increased effect: propranolol, metoprolol
• Bradycardia, asystole: verapamil

NURSING CONSIDERATIONS
Evaluate:
• Therapeutic response: decreased intraocular pressure
Teach patient/family:
• To report change in vision with blurring or loss of sight, trouble breathing, sweating, flushing, since systemic absorption may occur
• Method of instillation, including pressure on lacrimal sac for 1 min, and not to touch dropper to eye
• That long-term therapy may be required
• That blurred vision will decrease with continued use of drug

---

tiopronin
(tye-o-pro′-nen)
Thiola
Func. class.: Orphan drug
Chem. class.: Active reducing, complexing thiol compound

Action: Prevents cystine (kidney) stone formation by increasing amount of water-soluble cystine
Uses: Prevention of kidney stone formation in patients with severe homozygous cystinuria with urinary cystine greater than 500 mg/day, who are resistant to conservative treatment
Dosage and routes:
• *Adult:* PO 800-1000 mg/day, given in divided doses tid at least 1 hr before or 2 hr after meals
• *Child:* PO 15 mg/kg/day, given in divided doses tid at least 1 hr before or 2 hr after meals
Available forms: Tabs 100 mg
Side effects/adverse reactions:
MISC: Blunting of taste
INTEG: Erythema, maculopapular rash, wrinkling skin, lupuslike syndrome (fever, arthralgia, lymphadenopathy), pruritus
CNS: Drug fever
META: Vit B_6 deficiency
Contraindications: History of agranulocytosis, thrombocytopenia, aplastic anemia
Precautions: Pregnancy (C), lactation, myasthenia gravis, Goodpasture's syndrome, children <9 yr
Pharmacokinetics:
Reduction of urinary cystine of 250-500 mg on 1-2 g/day may be expected; excreted in urine 78% in 3 days

NURSING CONSIDERATIONS
Assess:
• I&O during treatment; check urine for stones; strain all urine, keep output at 2 L/day
• Diet for alkaline foods: dairy products; prevent overindulgence of Na, alkali foods, since hypercalcinuria results
• Urine pH; notify physician of pH over 7
• Urinary cystine 1 mo after treatment, q3mo thereafter
Administer:
• After adequate hydration, conservative treatment: 3 L/day fluid, 16 oz fluid at meals and hs
Perform/provide:
• Storage at room temperature
Evaluate:
• Therapeutic response: decrease in urinary cystine to <250 mg/L, absence of pain, hematuria
Teach patient/family:
• To watch for lupuslike syndrome: fever, joint pain, swollen lymph glands; drug may have to be discontinued

T

---

italics = common side effects   ***bold italic*** = life threatening reactions

tobramycin (ophthalmic)

(toe-bra-mye'sin)
Tobrex
Func. class.: Antiinfective
Chem. class.: Aminoglycoside

Action: Inhibits bacterial protein synthesis
Uses: Infection of eye
Dosage and routes:
• *Adult and child:* INSTILL 1-2 gtts q1-4h depending on infection; OINT: 1 cm bid-tid
Available forms: Oint 0.3%; sol 0.3%
Side effects/adverse reactions:
EENT: Poor corneal wound healing, visual haze, (temporary), overgrowth of nonsusceptible organisms
Contraindications: Hypersensitivity, varicella, vaccinia, mycobacterial/fungal infection, epithelial herpes, simplex keratitis
Precautions: Antibiotic hypersensitivity, pregnancy (D)
NURSING CONSIDERATIONS
Assess:
• Allergy: itching, lacrimation, redness, swelling
Administer:
• After washing hands; cleanse crusts or discharge from eye before application
• Apply pressure on lacrimal sac for 1 min
Perform/provide:
• Storage at room temperature
Evaluate:
• Therapeutic response: absence of redness, inflammation, tearing
Teach patient/family:
• To use drug exactly as prescribed
• Not to use eye make-up, towels, washcloths, or eye medication of others, or reinfection may occur
• That drug container tip should not be touched to eye
• To report itching, increased redness, burning, stinging; drug should be discontinued
• That drug may cause blurred vision when ointment is applied

tobramycin sulfate

(toe-bra-mye'sin)
Nebcin, Tobramycin Sulfate
Func. class.: Antibiotic
Chem. class.: Aminoglycoside

Action: Interferes with protein synthesis in bacterial cell by binding to ribosomal subunit, causing inaccurate peptide sequence to form in protein chain, causing bacterial death
Uses: Severe systemic infections of CNS, respiratory, GI, urinary tract, bone, skin, soft tissues caused by *P. aeruginosa, E. coli, Enterobacter, Providencia, Citrobacter, Staphylococcus, Proteus, Klebsiella, Serratia*
Dosage and routes:
• *Adult:* IM/IV 3 mg/kg/day in divided doses q8h; may give up to 5 mg/kg/day in divided doses q6-8h
• *Child:* IM/IV 6-7.5 mg/kg/day in 3-4 equal divided doses
• *Neonates <1 wk:* IM up to 4 mg/kg/day in divided doses q12h; IV up to 4 mg/kg/day in divided doses q12h diluted in 50-100 mg NS or D$_5$W; give over 30-60 min
Available forms: Inj IM, IV 10, 40 mg/ml; powder for inj 1.2 g; inj 20 mg/2 ml
Side effects/adverse reactions:
GU: Oliguria, hematuria, renal damage, azotemia, renal failure, nephrotoxicity
CNS: Confusion, depression,

numbness, tremors, *convulsions,* muscle twitching, *neurotoxicity,* dizziness, vertigo

*EENT: **Ototoxicity,** deafness, visual disturbances, tinnitus*

*HEMA: **Agranulocytosis, thrombocytopenia, leukopenia, eosinophilia,** anemia*

GI: Nausea, vomiting, anorexia, increased ALT, AST, bilirubin, hepatomegaly, ***hepatic necrosis,*** splenomegaly

CV: Hypotension, hypertension, palpitation

INTEG: Rash, burning, urticaria, dermatitis, alopecia

Contraindications: Severe renal disease, hypersensitivity to aminoglycosides

Precautions: Neonates, mild renal disease, pregnancy (D), myasthenia gravis, lactation, hearing deficits, Parkinson's disease

Pharmacokinetics:

IM: Onset rapid, peak 1 hr

IV: Onset immediate, peak 1 hr Plasma half-life 2-3 hr; not metabolized, excreted unchanged in urine, crosses placental barrier

Interactions/incompatibilities:

• Increased ototoxicity, neurotoxicity, nephrotoxicity: other aminoglycosides, amphotericin B, polymyxin, vancomycin, ethacrynic acid, furosemide, mannitol, methoxyflurane, cisplatin, cephalosporins, bacitracin, acyclovir

• Incompatible with cefamandole, clindamycin, heparin; do not mix in syringe or sol with other drugs

• Increased effects: nondepolarizing muscle relaxants, succinylcholine

NURSING CONSIDERATIONS
Assess:

• Weight before treatment; calculation of dosage is usually based on ideal body weight, but may be calculated on actual body weight

• I&O ratio, urinalysis daily for proteinuria, cells, casts; report sudden change in urine output

• VS during infusion, watch for hypotension, change in pulse

• IV site for thrombophlebitis, including pain, redness, swelling q30min; change site if needed; apply warm compresses to discontinued site

• Serum peak, drawn at 30-60 min after IV infusion or 60 min after IM injection, trough level <2 μg/ml; serum levels <12 mEq/ml

• Urine pH if drug is used for UTI; urine should be kept alkaline

• Renal impairment by securing urine for CrCl testing, BUN, serum creatinine; lower dosage should be given in renal impairment (CrCl <80 ml/min)

• Deafness by audiometric testing, ringing, roaring in ears, vertigo; assess hearing before, during, after treatment

• Dehydration: high sp gr, decrease in skin turgor, dry mucous membranes, dark urine

• Overgrowth of infection: increased temperature, malaise, redness, pain, swelling, perineal itching, diarrhea, stomatitis, change in cough, sputum

• C&S before starting treatment to identify infecting organism

• Vestibular dysfunction: nausea, vomiting, dizziness, headache; drug should be discontinued if severe

• Injection sites for redness, swelling, abscesses; use warm compresses at site

Administer:

• IV diluted in 50-100 ml NS or D₅W (adult), infuse over 20-60 min

T

---

italics = common side effects   ***bold italic*** = life threatening reactions

• IM injection in large muscle mass; rotate injection sites
• Drug in evenly spaced doses to maintain blood level
• Bicarbonate to alkalinize urine if ordered in treating UTI, as drug is most active in an alkaline environment

Perform/provide:
• Adequate fluids of 2-3 L/day unless contraindicated to prevent irritation of tubules
• Flush of IV line with NS or D_5W after infusion
• Supervised ambulation, other safety measures with vestibular dysfunction

Evaluate:
• Therapeutic response: absence of fever, draining wounds, negative C&S after treatment

Teach patient/family:
• To report headache, dizziness, symptoms of overgrowth of infection, renal impairment
• To report loss of hearing, ringing, roaring in ears, feeling of fullness in head

Treatment of overdose: Hemodialysis; monitor serum levels of drug

---

tocainide HCl
(toe-kay′nide)
Tonocard
Func. class.: Antidysrhythmic (Class IB)
Chem. class.: Lidocaine analog

Action: Decreases sodium and potassium, resulting in decreased excitability of myocardial cells
Uses: PVCs, ventricular tachycardia

Dosage and routes:
• *Adult:* PO 600 mg loading dose, then 400 mg q8h
Available forms: Tabs 400, 600 mg

Side effects/adverse reactions:
CNS: Headache, dizziness, involuntary movement, confusion, psychosis, restlessness, irritability, paresthesias, tremors, *seizures*
EENT: Tinnitus, blurred vision, hearing loss
GI: Nausea, vomiting, anorexia, diarrhea, hepatitis
CV: Hypotension, bradycardia, angina, PVCs, *heart block, cardiovascular collapse, arrest, CHF,* chest pain, tachycardia
RESP: Dyspnea, *respiratory depression, pulmonary fibrosis*
INTEG: Rash, urticaria, edema, swelling
HEMA: Blood dyscrasias: leukopenia, agranulocytosis, hypoplastic anemia, thrombocytopenia
Contraindications: Hypersensitivity to amides, severe heart block
Precautions: Pregnancy (C), lactation, children, renal disease, liver disease, CHF, respiratory depression, myasthenia gravis, blood dyscrasias

Pharmacokinetics:
PO: Peak 0.5-3 hr; half-life 10-17 hr; metabolized by liver, excreted in urine

Interactions/incompatibilities:
• Increased effects: propranolol, quinidine and all other antidysrhythmics

Lab test interferences:
Increase: CPK
Positive: ANA titer

NURSING CONSIDERATIONS
Assess:
• Chest x-ray film, pulmonary function tests, liver enzymes during treatments
• CBC during beginning treatment
• I&O ratio; check for decreasing output
• Blood levels (therapeutic level 4-10 μg/ml)

---

*Available in Canada only

- B/P continuously for fluctuations
- Lung fields; bilateral rales may occur in CHF patient
- Increased respiration, increased pulse; drug should be discontinued
- Toxicity: fine tremors, dizziness
- Blood dyscrasias: fatigue, sore throat, fever, bruising, increased temperature
- Cardiac rate, respiration: rate, rhythm, character

Evaluate:
- Therapeutic response: decreased dysrhythmia

Treatment of overdose: O_2, artificial ventilation, ECG; administer dopamine for circulatory depression, diazepam or thiopental for convulsions

---

tolazamide
(tole-az'a-mide)
Tolamide, Tolazimide, Tolinase
Func. class.: Antidiabetic
Chem. class.: Sulfonylurea (1st generation)

Action: Causes functioning β-cells in pancreas to release insulin, leading to drop in blood glucose levels; may improve binding to insulin receptors or increase the number of insulin receptors with prolonged administration; may also reduce basal hepatic glucose secretion; this drug not effective if patient lacks functioning β-cells

Uses: Type II (NIDDM) diabetes mellitus

Dosage and routes:
- *Adult:* PO 100 mg/day for FBS <200 mg/dl or 250 mg/day for FBS >200 mg/dl; dose should be titrated to patient response (1 g or less/day)

Available forms: Tabs 100, 250, 500 mg scored

Side effects/adverse reactions:
CNS: Headache, weakness, fatigue, lethargy, dizziness, vertigo, tinnitus

GI: Nausea, vomiting, diarrhea, constipation, gas, *hepatotoxicity, jaundice,* heartburn

HEMA: Leukopenia, thrombocytopenia, agranulocytosis, aplastic anemia, pancytopenia, hemolytic anemia

INTEG: Rash, (rare) allergic reactions, pruritus, urticaria, eczema, photosensitivity, erythema

ENDO: Hypoglycemia

Contraindications: Hypersensitivity to sulfonylureas, juvenile or brittle diabetes

Precautions: Pregnancy (C), elderly, cardiac disease, thyroid disease, severe hypoglycemic reactions, renal disease, hepatic disease

Pharmacokinetics:
PO: Completely absorbed by GI route; onset 4-6 hr, peak 4-8 hr, duration 12-24 hr; half-life 7 hr; metabolized in liver, excreted in urine (metabolites), breast milk, highly protein bound

Interactions/incompatibilities:
- Increased hypoglycemic reaction: oral anticoagulants, chloramphenicol, cimetidine, MAOIs, insulin, guanethidine, methyldopa, nonsteroidal antiinflammatories, salicylates, probenecid, sulfonamides, ranitidine
- Mask symptoms of hypoglycemia: β-blockers
- Decreased effects of both drugs: diazoxide
- Decreased action of tolazamide: calcium channel blockers, corticosteroids, oral contraceptives, thiazide diuretics, thyroid preparations, estrogens, phenothiazines, phenytoin, rifampin, isoniazide, phenobarbital, sympathomimetics

T

---

italics = common side effects   ***bold italic*** = life threatening reactions

• Disulfiram-like reaction: alcohol

NURSING CONSIDERATIONS
Assess:
• Hypoglycemic, hyperglycemic reaction; can occur soon after meals
Administer:
• Drug 30 min before meal
Perform/provide:
• Storage in tight container in cool environment
Evaluate:
• Therapeutic response: decrease in polyuria, polydipsia, polyphagia, clear sensorium, absence of dizziness, stable gait
Teach patient/family:
• To check for symptoms of cholestatic jaundice (dark urine, pruritus, yellow sclera); if these occur a physician should be notified
• To use a capillary blood glucose test while on this drug
• The symptoms of hypoglycemia, hyperglycemia, what to do about each; have glucagon emergency kit available
• That this drug must be taken daily; explain consequence of discontinuing drug abruptly
• To take drug in morning to prevent hypoglycemic reactions at night
• To avoid OTC medications and alcohol unless prescribed by a physician; explain disulfiram reaction
• That diabetes is a lifelong illness; drug will not cure disease
• That all food included in diet plan must be eaten to prevent hypoglycemia
• To carry a Medic Alert ID for emergency purposes
Treatment of overdose: Glucose 25g IV, via dextrose 50% sol, 50 ml or 1 mg glucagon

tolazoline HCl
(toe-laz′a-leen)
Priscoline
Func. class.: Peripheral vasodilator
Chem. class.: Imidazoline derivative

Action: Peripheral vasodilation occurs by direct relaxation on vascular smooth muscle; also has weak α- and β-adrenergic properties
Uses: Persistent pulmonary hypertension of newborn; also hypoxic pulmonary hypertension
Dosage and routes:
• *Newborn:* IV 1-2 mg/kg via scalp vein; IV INF 1-2 mg/kg/hr
Available forms: Inj SC, IM, IV 25 mg/ml
Side effects/adverse reactions:
CV: Orthostatic hypotension, tachycardia, dysrhythmias, hypertension, *cardiovascular collapse*
RESP: Pulmonary hemorrhage
GU: Edema, oliguria, hematuria
GI: Nausea, vomiting, diarrhea, peptic ulcer, *GI hemorrhage, hepatitis*
INTEG: Flushing, tingling, rash, chills, sweating, increased pilomotor activity
HEMA: Thrombocytopenia, leukopenia
Contraindications: Hypersensitivity, CVA, CAD
Precautions: Pregnancy (C), active peptic ulcer, lactation, mitral stenosis
Pharmacokinetics:
IM/SC: Peak 30-60 min, duration 3-4 hr, excreted in urine, half-life 3-10 hr
Interactions/incompatibilities:
• Increased effects with alcohol, β-blockers, antihypertensive

• Decrease B/P, rebound hypertension: epinephrine
• Incompatible with ethacrynic acid, hydrocortisone, methylprednisolone

NURSING CONSIDERATIONS
Assess:
• ABGs, electrolytes, VS in newborn
• B/P, pulse during treatment until stable; take B/P lying, standing; orthostatic hypotension is common
• Hepatic tests: AST, ALT, bilirubin; liver enzymes may increase
• Blood studies: CBC, platelets; watch for thrombocytopenia, agranulocytosis
• Hepatic involvement: nausea, vomiting, jaundice; drug should be discontinued if this occurs
• For bleeding from GI tract: coffee grounds vomitus, increased pulse, pain in upper gastric area
• Affected areas for changes in temperature, color

Administer:
• IV undiluted; give 10 mg or less over 1 min; in scalp vein may be diluted in D₅, D₅NS, LR, NS, ½NS, Ringer's sol; run over 1 hr
• Ordered analgesic if headache develops
• Intraarterially to patient in supine position
• To patient who is sitting or lying down during treatment

Perform/provide:
• Storage at room temperature, protect from light

Evaluate:
• Therapeutic response: decrease in pulmonary hypertension or pulse volume, increased temperature in extremities, ability to walk without pain

Teach patient/family:
• To report jaundice, dark urine, joint pain, fatigue, malaise, bruising, easy bleeding, which may indicate blood dyscrasias
• That it is necessary to quit smoking to prevent excessive vasoconstriction if prescribed for PVD
• To avoid hazardous activities until stabilized on medication; dizziness may occur

Treatment of overdose: Administer IV fluids, head-low position

---

tolbutamide
(tole-byoo′ta-mide)
Mobenol,* Novobutamide,* Orinase, Tolbutamide, Tolbutone*

Func. class.: Antidiabetic
Chem. class.: Sulfonylurea (1st generation)

Action: Causes functioning β-cells in pancreas to release insulin, leading to drop in blood glucose levels; may improve binding to insulin receptors or increase the number of insulin receptors with prolonged administration; may also reduce basal hepatic secretion; not effective if patient lacks functioning β-cells
Uses: Type II (NIDDM) diabetes mellitus

Dosage and routes:
• *Adult:* PO 1-2 g/day in divided doses, titrated to patient response
Available forms: Tabs 250, 500 mg scored

Side effects/adverse reactions:
CNS: Headache, weakness, paresthesia, tinnitus, dizziness, vertigo
GI: Nausea, fullness, heartburn, *hepatotoxicity, cholestatic jaundice,* taste alteration, diarrhea
HEMA: Leukopenia, thrombocytopenia, agranulocytosis, aplastic anemia, increased AST, ALT, alk phosphatase
INTEG: Rash, allergic reactions,

---

pruritus, urticaria, eczema, photosensitivity, erythema
ENDO: Hypoglycemia
MS: Joint pains
Contraindications: Hypersensitivity to sulfonylureas, juvenile or brittle diabetes
Precautions: Pregnancy (C), elderly, cardiac disease, thyroid disease, severe hypoglycemic reactions, renal disease, hepatic disease
Pharmacokinetics:
PO: Completely absorbed by GI route; onset 30-60 min, peak 3-5 hr, duration 6-12 hr; half-life 4-5 hr; metabolized in liver; excreted in urine (metabolites), breast milk; 90%-95% plasma protein bound
Interactions/incompatibilities:
• Increased hypoglycemic reaction: oral anticoagulants, chloramphenicol, cimetidine, MAOIs, insulin, guanethidine, methyldopa, nonsteroidal antiinflammatories, salicylates, probenecid, sulfonamides, ranitidine
• Mask symptoms of hypoglycemia: β-blockers
• Decreased effects of both drugs: diazoxide
• Increased effects of tolbutamide: insulin, MAOIs
• Possible disulfiram (Antabuse) reaction
• Decreased action of tolbutamide: calcium channel blockers, corticosteroids, oral contraceptives, thiazide diuretics, thyroid preparations, estrogens, phenobarbital, phenytoin, rifampin, phenothiazines, sympathomimetics
Lab test interferences:
Decrease: RAIU test
Interfere: Urinary albumin
NURSING CONSIDERATIONS
Assess:
• Hypoglycemic, hyperglycemic reaction; can occur soon after meals

Administer:
• Drug 30 min before meals
Perform/provide:
• Storage in tight container in cool environment
Evaluate:
• Therapeutic response: decrease in polyuria, polydipsia, polyphagia, clear sensorium, absence of dizziness, stable gait
Teach patient/family:
• To check for symptoms of cholestatic jaundice (dark urine, pruritus, yellow sclera); if these occur, a physician should be notified
• To use a capillary blood glucose test while on this drug
• To test urine glucose levels with Chemstrip 3× /day
• The symptoms of hypoglycemia, hyperglycemia, what to do about each; have glucagon emergency kit available
• That this drug must be taken daily; explain consequence of discontinuing drug abruptly
• To take drug in morning to prevent hypoglycemic reaction at night
• To avoid OTC medications and alcohol unless prescribed by a physician; explain disulfiram reaction
• That diabetes is a lifelong illness; drug will not cure disease
• That all food in diet plan must be eaten to prevent hypoglycemia
• To carry a Medic Alert ID for emergency purposes
Treatment of overdose: 10%-50% glucose sol IV or 1 mg glucagon

tolmetin sodium

(tole′met-in)
Tolectin DS, Tolectin 200, Tolectin 600, Tolmetin Sodium
Func. class.: Nonsteroidal antiinflammatory
Chem. class.: Pyrrole acetic acid derivative

Action: Inhibits prostaglandin synthesis by decreasing an enzyme needed for biosynthesis; analgesic, antiinflammatory, antipyretic

Uses: Mild to moderate pain, osteoarthritis, rheumatoid arthritis

Dosage and routes:
• *Adult:* PO 400 mg tid-qid, not to exceed 2 g/day
• *Child >2 yr:* PO 15-30 mg/kg/day in 3 or 4 divided doses
Available forms: Caps 400 mg; tabs 200 mg

Side effects/adverse reactions:
GI: Nausea, anorexia, vomiting, diarrhea, jaundice, ***cholestatic hepatitis,*** constipation, flatulence, cramps, dry mouth, peptic ulcer, ulceration, bleeding, perforation
CNS: Dizziness, drowsiness, fatigue, tremors, confusion, insomnia, anxiety, depression
CV: Tachycardia, peripheral edema, palpitations, dysrhythmias, hypertension
INTEG: Purpura, rash, pruritus, sweating
GU: ***Nephrotoxicity: dysuria, hematuria, oliguria, azotemia, pseudoproteinuria***
HEMA: ***Blood dyscrasias***
EENT: Tinnitus, hearing loss, blurred vision

Contraindications: Hypersensitivity, asthma, severe renal disease, severe hepatic disease, ulcer disease

Precautions: Pregnancy (B), lactation, children, bleeding disorders, GI disorders, cardiac disorders, hypersensitivity to other antiinflammatory agents, peptic ulcer disease

Pharmacokinetics:
PO: Peak 2 hr, half-life 3-3½ hr; metabolized in liver, excreted in urine (metabolites), excreted in breast milk, 99% protein binding

Interactions/incompatibilities:
• Increased action of: coumarin, phenytoin, sulfonamides when used with this drug

NURSING CONSIDERATIONS
Assess:
• Renal, liver, blood studies: BUN, creatinine, AST, ALT, Hgb before treatment, periodically thereafter
• I&O ratio
• Audiometric, ophthalmic exam before, during, after treatment
• For eye, ear problems: blurred vision, tinnitus (may indicate toxicity)

Administer:
• With food to decrease GI symptoms; best to take on empty stomach to facilitate absorption; tab may be crushed

Perform/provide:
• Storage at room temperature

Evaluate:
• Therapeutic response: decreased pain, stiffness, swelling in joints, ability to move more easily

Teach patient/family:
• To report blurred vision, ringing, roaring in ears (may indicate toxicity)
• To avoid driving, other hazardous activities if dizziness or drowsiness occurs
• To report change in urine pattern, weight increase, edema, pain increase in joints, fever, blood in urine (indicates nephrotoxicity)

---

italics = common side effects   ***bold italic*** = life threatening reactions

• That therapeutic effects may take up to 1 mo
• To drink 8 glasses water daily

---

tolnaftate (topical)
(tole-naf'tate)
Absorbine Antifungal, Absorbine Jock Itch, Absorbine Jr. Antifungal, Aftate For Athlete's Foot, Aftate For Jock Itch, Genaspor, NP-27, Quinsana Plus, Tinactin, Ting, Tolnaftate, Zeasorb-AF

Func. class.: Local antiinfective
Chem. class.: Antifungal

Action: Interferes with fungal cell membrane, which increases permeability, leaking of cell nutrients
Uses: Tinea pedis, tinea cruris, tinea corporis, tinea capitis, tinea unguium, versicolor
Dosage and routes:
• *Adult and child:* TOP apply to affected area bid for 2-6 wk, rub in
Available forms: Cream, powder, aerosol powder, aerosol liq, gel, pump spray liquid 1%
Side effects/adverse reactions:
INTEG: Rash, urticaria, stinging
Contraindications: Hypersensitivity, nail infections
Precautions: Pregnancy (C), lactation

NURSING CONSIDERATIONS
Assess:
• Allergic reaction: burning, stinging, swelling, redness
Administer:
• Aerosol powder after shaking
• Enough medication to cover lesions completely
• After cleansing with soap, water before each application; dry well
Perform/provide:
• Storage at room temperature in dry place; do not puncture or incinerate aerosol container
Evaluate:
• Therapeutic response: decrease in size, number of lesions
Teach patient/family:
• To use medical asepsis (hand washing) before, after each application
• To apply with glove to prevent further infection
• To avoid use of OTC creams, ointments, lotions unless directed by physician
• To avoid contact with eyes
• To notify physician if condition worsens or does not improve in 10 days; continue even if symptoms improve
• To complete treatment regimen

---

torsemide
(tore-sa'mide)
Demadox
Func. class.: Loop diuretic
Chem. class.: Sulfonamide derivative

Action: Acts on loop of Henle by increasing excretion of chloride, sodium, water
Uses: Treatment of hypertension and edema in CHF, hepatic disease, renal disease
Dosage and routes:
• *Adult:* PO 2.5-5 mg qd; may gradually increase dose as needed
Available forms: Tabs 5, 10, 20, 100 mg; 10 mg/ml vials of 2,5 ml
Side effects/adverse reactions:
CNS: Headache, fatigue, weakness, vertigo, paresthesias
CV: Orthostatic hypotension, chest pain, ECG changes, *circulatory collapse*
EENT: Loss of hearing, ear pain, tinnitus, blurred vision

ENDO: Hyperglycemia

ELECT: Hypokalemia, hypochloremic alkalosis, hypomagnesemia, hyperuricemia, hypocalcemia, hyponatremia, metabolic alkalosis

GI: Nausea, diarrhea, dry mouth, vomiting, anorexia, cramps, oral and gastric irritations, pancreatitis

*GU: Polyuria, **renal failure,*** glycosuria

*HEMA: **Thrombocytopenia, agranulocytosis, leukopenia, neutropenia,** anemia*

INTEG: Rash, pruritus, purpura, ***Stevens-Johnson syndrome,*** sweating, photosensitivity, urticaria

MS: Cramps, stiffness

Contraindications: Hypersensitivity to sulfonamides, anuria, hypovolemia, infants, lactation, electrolyte depletion

Precautions: Diabetes mellitus, dehydration, severe renal disease, pregnancy (C)

Pharmacokinetics:

PO: Rapidly absorbed

Duration 6 hr

Excreted in urine, feces; crosses placenta; excreted in breast milk; half-life 2-4 hr, plasma protein binding 97%-99%

Interactions/incompatibilities:

• Increased toxicity: lithium, non-depolarizing skeletal muscle relaxants, digitalis

• Increased action of: antihypertensives, oral anticoagulants, nitrates

• Increased ototoxicity: aminoglycosides, cisplatin, vancomycin

• Decreased antihypertensive effect of torsemide: indomethacin, metolazone

• Incompatible with acidic sol, Vit C, corticosteroids, diphenhydramine, dobutamine, esmolol, epinephrine, gentamicin, levarterenol, meperidine, milrione, netilmicin,

reserpine, spironolactone, tetracyclines in sol

Lab test interferences:

Interference: GTT

Incompatible with any drug in syringe

NURSING CONSIDERATIONS

Assess:

• Hearing when giving high doses

• Weight, I&O daily to determine fluid loss; effect of drug may be decreased if used qd

• Rate, depth, rhythm of respiration, effect of exertion

• B/P lying, standing; postural hypotension may occur

• Electrolytes: K, Na, Cl; include BUN, blood sugar, CBC, serum creatinine, blood pH, ABGs, uric acid, Ca, Mg

• Glucose in urine if patient is diabetic

• Signs and symptoms of metabolic alkalosis: drowsiness, restlessness

• Signs and symptoms of hypokalemia: postural hypotension, malaise, fatigue, tachycardia, leg cramps, weakness

• Rashes, temperature elevation qd

• Confusion, especially in elderly; take safety precautions if needed

Perform/provide:

• In AM to avoid interference with sleep if using drug as a diuretic

• K replacement if less than 3.0

• With food if nausea occurs; absorption may be decreased slightly

Evaluate:

• Therapeutic response: improvement in edema of feet, legs, sacral area daily if medication is being used in CHF

Teach patient/family:

• To rise slowly from lying, sitting position

• Adverse reactions: muscle cramps, weakness, nausea, dizziness

---

italics = common side effects   ***bold italic*** = life threatening reactions

• To take food or milk for GI symptoms
• To take early in day to prevent nocturia

Treatment of overdose:
Lavage if taken orally; monitor electrolytes, administer dextrose in saline; monitor hydration, CV, renal status

---

trace elements (chromium, copper, iodide, manganese, selenium, zinc)

Func. class.: Minerals

Action: Needed for adequate absorption and synthesis of amino acids
Uses: Prevention of trace element deficiency
Dosage and routes:
Chromium
• *Adult:* IV 10-15 µg qd
• *Child:* IV 0.14-0.20 µg/kg/day
Copper
• *Adult:* IV 0.5-1.5 mg/day
• *Child:* IV .05-0.2 mg/kg/day
Iodine
• *Adult:* IV 1 µg/kg/day
Manganese
• *Adult:* IV 1-3 mg/day
Selenium
• *Adult:* 40-120 µg/day
• *Child:* 3 µg/kg/day
Zinc
• *Adult:* IV 2-4 mg/day
• *Child:* IV 0.05 mg/kg/day
Available forms: Many forms available—see particular elements
Side effects/adverse reactions:
None known
Precautions: Liver, biliary disease

NURSING CONSIDERATIONS
Assess:
• Trace element levels; notify phy-

sician if low copper 0.07-0.15 mg/ml, zinc 0.05-0.15 mg/100 ml, manganese 4-20 µg/100 ml, selenium 0.1-0.19 µg/ml
• Trace element deficiency if patient is receiving TPN for extended period
Administer:
• By IV infusion, often mixed with TPN solution
Evaluate:
• Therapeutic response: absence of element deficiency

---

tranylcypromine sulfate

(tran-ill-sip'roe-meen)
Parnate
Func. class.: Antidepressant-MAOI
Chem. class.: Nonhydrazine

Action: Increases concentrations of endogenous epinephrine, norepinephrine, serotonin, dopamine in storage sites in CNS by inhibition of MAO; increased concentration reduces depression
Uses: Depression, when uncontrolled by other means
Dosage and routes:
• *Adult:* PO 10 mg bid; may increase to 30 mg/day after 2 wk
Available forms: Tabs 10 mg
Side effects/adverse reactions:
HEMA: Anemia
CNS: Dizziness, drowsiness, confusion, headache, anxiety, tremors, stimulation, weakness, hyperreflexia, mania, insomnia, fatigue, weight gain
GI: Constipation, dry mouth, nausea, vomiting, *anorexia,* diarrhea, weight gain
GU: Change in libido, frequency
INTEG: Rash, flushing, increased perspiration

CV: Orthostatic hypotension, hypertension, dysrhythmias, hypertensive crisis
EENT: Blurred vision
ENDO: **SIADH-like syndrome**
Contraindications: Hypersensitivity to MAOIs, elderly, hypertension, CHF, severe hepatic disease, pheochromocytoma, severe renal disease, severe cardiac disease
Precautions: Suicidal patients, convulsive disorders, severe depression, schizophrenia, hyperactivity, diabetes mellitus, pregnancy (C)
Pharmacokinetics:
Metabolized by liver, excreted by kidneys, crosses placenta, excreted in breast milk
Interactions/incompatibilities:
• Increased pressor effects: guanethidine, clonidine, indirect acting sympathomimetics (ephedrine)
• Increased effects of: direct-acting sympathomimetics (epinephrine), alcohol, barbiturates, benzodiazepines, CNS depressants, levodopa
• Hyperpyretic crisis, convulsions, hypertensive episode: tricyclic antidepressants, meperidine
• Hypoglycemic effect increased: insulin

NURSING CONSIDERATIONS
Assess:
• B/P (lying, standing), pulse; if systolic B/P drops 20 mm Hg, stop drug, notify physician
• Blood studies: CBC, leukocytes, cardiac enzymes if patient is receiving long-term therapy
• Hepatic studies: ALT, AST, bilirubin; hepatotoxicity may occur
• Toxicity: increased headache, palpitation; discontinue drug immediately; prodromal signs of hypertensive crisis
• Mental status changes: mood, sensorium, affect, memory (long,

short), increase in psychiatric symptoms
• Urinary retention, constipation, edema: take weight weekly
• Withdrawal symptoms: headache, nausea, vomiting, muscle pain, weakness
Administer:
• Increased fluids, bulk in diet if constipation occurs
• With food or milk for GI symptoms
• Crushed if patient is unable to swallow medication whole
• Dosage hs if oversedation occurs during day
• Gum, hard candy, frequent sips of water for dry mouth
• Phentolamine for severe hypertension
Perform/provide:
• Storage in tight container in cool environment
• Assistance with ambulation during beginning therapy for drowsiness/dizziness
• Safety measures including side rails
• Checking to see PO medication swallowed
Evaluate:
• Therapeutic response: decreased depression
Teach patient/family:
• That therapeutic effects may take 1-4 wk
• To avoid driving, other activities requiring alertness
• To avoid alcohol ingestion, CNS depressants, OTC medications: cold, weight loss, hay fever, cough syrup
• Not to discontinue medication quickly after long-term use
• To avoid high-tyramine foods: cheese (aged), sour cream, beer, wine, pickled products, liver, raisins, bananas, figs, avocados, meat

T

---

italics = common side effects   ***bold italic*** = life threatening reactions

tenderizers, chocolate, yogurt; increased caffeine
• To report headache, palpitation, neck stiffness
Treatment of overdose: Lavage, activated charcoal; monitor electrolytes, vital signs; diazepam IV, $NaHCO_3$

---

trazodone HCl

(tray'zoe-done)
Desyrel, Desyrel Dividose, Trazodone HCl
Func. class.: Antidepressant, miscellaneous
Chem. class.: Triazolopyridine

Action: Selectively inhibits serotonin uptake by brain, potentiates behavorial changes
Uses: Depression
Dosage and routes:
• *Adult:* PO 150 mg/day in divided doses; may increase by 50 mg/day q3-4d, not to exceed 600 mg/day
Available forms: Tabs 50, 100, 150, 300 mg
Side effects/adverse reactions:
HEMA: Agranulocytosis, thrombocytopenia, eosinophilia, leukopenia
CNS: Dizziness, drowsiness, confusion, headache, anxiety, tremors, stimulation, weakness, insomnia, nightmares, EPS (elderly), increase in psychiatric symptoms
GI: Diarrhea, dry mouth, nausea, vomiting, *paralytic ileus,* increased appetite, cramps, epigastric distress, jaundice, *hepatitis,* stomatitis
GU: Retention, acute renal failure, priapism
INTEG: Rash, urticaria, sweating, pruritus, photosensitivity
CV: Orthostatic hypotension, ECG

changes, tachycardia, **hypertension,** palpitations
EENT: Blurred vision, tinnitus, mydriasis
Contraindications: Hypersensitivity to tricyclic antidepressants, recovery phase of myocardial infarction, convulsive disorders, prostatic hypertrophy
Precautions: Suicidal patients, severe depression, increased intraocular pressure, narrow-angle glaucoma, urinary retention, cardiac disease, hepatic disease, hyperthyroidism, electroshock therapy, elective surgery, pregnancy (C)
Pharmacokinetics:
Metabolized by liver, excreted by kidneys, feces; half-life 4.4-7.5 hr
Interactions/incompatibilities:
• Decreased effects of: guanethidine, clonidine, indirect-acting sympathomimetics (ephedrine)
• Increased effects of: direct-acting sympathomimetics (epinephrine), alcohol, barbiturates, benzodiazepines, CNS depressants
• Hyperpyretic crisis, convulsions, hypertensive episode: MAOI (pargyline [Eutonyl])
Lab test interferences:
Increase: Serum bilirubin, blood glucose, alk phosphatase
False increase: Urinary catecholamines
Decrease: VMA, 5-HIAA
NURSING CONSIDERATIONS
Assess:
• B/P (lying, standing), pulse q4h; if systolic B/P drops 20 mm Hg, hold drug, notify physician; take vital signs q4h in patients with cardiovascular disease
• Blood studies: CBC, leukocytes, differential, cardiac enzymes if patient is receiving long-term therapy
• Hepatic studies: AST, ALT, bilirubin

• Weight qwk; appetite may increase with drug
• ECG for flattening of T wave, bundle branch block, AV block, dysrhythmias in cardiac patients
• EPS, primarily in elderly: rigidity, dystonia, akathisia
• Mental status changes: mood, sensorium, affect, suicidal tendencies, increase in psychiatric symptoms, depression, panic
• Urinary retention, constipation; constipation is more likely to occur in children
• Withdrawal symptoms: headache, nausea, vomiting, muscle pain, weakness; do not usually occur unless drug discontinued abruptly
• Alcohol consumption; if alcohol is consumed, hold dose until morning

Administer:
• Increased fluids, bulk in diet if constipation occurs, especially in elderly
• With food or milk for GI symptoms
• Dosage hs if oversedation occurs during day; may take entire dose hs; elderly may not tolerate qd dosing
• Gum, hard candy, or frequent sips of water for dry mouth

Perform/provide:
• Storage in tight, light-resistant container at room temperature
• Assistance with ambulation during beginning therapy for drowsiness/dizziness
• Safety measures, including side rails, primarily for elderly
• Checking to see PO medication swallowed

Evaluate:
• Therapeutic response: decreased depression

Teach patient/family:
• That therapeutic effects may take 2-3 wk
• To use caution in driving, other activities requiring alertness because of drowsiness, dizziness, blurred vision
• To avoid alcohol ingestion, other CNS depressants
• Not to discontinue medication quickly after long-term use; may cause nausea, headache, malaise
• To wear sunscreen or large hat, since photosensitivity occurs

Treatment of overdose: ECG monitoring; induce emesis; lavage, activated charcoal; administer anticonvulsant

---

tretinoin (vitamin A acid, retinoic acid)
(tret'i-noyn)
Retin-A, Stievaa*

Func. class.: Vitamin A acid/acne product
Chem. class.: Tretinoin derivative

Action: Decreases cohesiveness of follicular epithelium, decreases microcomedone formation

Uses: Acne vulgaris (grades 1-3); unlabeled use: skin cancer

Dosage and routes:
• *Adult and child:* TOP cleanse area, apply hs; cover lightly
Available forms: Top cream 0.1%, 0.05%, 0.025%; top gel 0.025%, 0.01%; top liq 0.05%

Side effects/adverse reactions:
INTEG: Rash, stinging, warmth, redness, erythema, blistering, crusting, peeling, contact dermatitis, hypopigmentation, hyperpigmentation

Contraindications: Hypersensitivity

Precautions: Pregnancy (B), lactation, eczema, sunburn

Pharmacokinetics:

TOP: Poor systemic absorption

Interactions/incompatibilities:

• Increase peeling: medication containing agents such as sulfur, benzoyl peroxide, resorcinol, salicylic acid

• Use with caution medicated, abrasive soaps, cleansers that have drying effect, products with high concentrations of alcohol astringents

NURSING CONSIDERATIONS
Assess:

• Area of body involved, including time involved, what helps or aggravates condition

Administer:

• Once daily before hs; cover area lightly using gauze

Perform/provide:

• Storage at room temperature

• Washing of hands after application

Evaluate:

• Therapeutic response: decrease in size and number of lesions

Teach patient/family:

• To avoid application on normal skin, getting cream in eyes, nose, other mucous membranes

• To avoid sunlight, sunlamps

• That treatment may cause warmth, stinging; dryness; peeling will occur

• That cosmetics may be used over drug; not to use shaving lotions

• That rash may occur during first 1-3 wk of therapy

• That drug does not cure condition; only relieves symptoms

• Therapeutic results may be seen in 2-3 wk but may not be optimal until after 6 wk

---

triamcinolone/triamcinolone acetonide/triamcinolone diacetate/triamcinolone hexacetonide

(trye-am-sin'oh-lone)

Aristocort, Atolone, Kenacort, Aristocort, Azmacort, Cenocort A-40, Kenaject-40, Kenalog, Kenalog-10, Kenalog-40, Tac-3, Tac-40, Triam-A, Triamcinolone Acetonide, Triamonide 40,

Amcort, Aristocort Forte, Aristocort Intralesional, Articulose L.A., Cenocort Forte, Triamcinolone, Triam Forte, Triamolone 40, Trilone, Trisoject, Aristospan Intra-Articular, Aristospan Intralesional, Tri-Kort, Trilog

Func. class.: Corticosteroid

Chem. class.: Glucocorticoid, intermediate-acting

Action: Decreases inflammation by suppression of migration of polymorphonuclear leukocytes, fibroblasts, reversal to increase capillary permeability and lysosomal stabilization

Uses: Severe inflammation, immunosuppression, neoplasms, asthma (steroid dependent), collagen, respiratory, dermatologic disorders

Dosage and routes:

• *Adult:* PO 4-48 mg/day in divided doses qd-qid; IM 40 mg qwk (acetonide, or diacetate), 5-48 mg into neoplasms (diacetate, acetonide), 2-40 mg into joint or soft tissue (diacetate, acetonide), 0.5 mg/sq in of affected intralesional skin (hexacetonide), 2-20 mg into joint or soft tissue (hexacetonide)

Asthma
• *Adult:* INH 2 tid-qid, not to exceed 16 INH/day
• *Child 6-12 yr:* INH 1-2 tid-qid, not to exceed 12 INH/day
Available forms: Tabs 1, 2, 4, 8, 16 mg; syr 2 mg/5 ml, 4.85 mg/5 ml; inj 25, 40 mg/ml diacetate; inj 3, 10, 40 mg/ml acetonide; inj 20, 5 mg/ml hexacetonide
Side effects/adverse reactions:
INTEG: Acne, poor wound healing, ecchymosis, petechiae
CNS: Depression, flushing, sweating, headache, mood changes
*CV: Hypertension, **circulatory collapse, thrombophlebitis, embolism,** tachycardia, edema*
*HEMA: **Thrombocytopenia***
MS: Fractures, osteoporosis, weakness
*GI: Diarrhea, nausea, abdominal distention, **GI hemorrhage,** increased appetite, **pancreatitis***
EENT: Fungal infections, increased intraocular pressure, blurred vision
Contraindications: Psychosis, hypersensitivity, idiopathic thrombocytopenia, acute glomerulonephritis, amebiasis, fungal infections, nonasthmatic bronchial disease, child <2 yr, AIDS, TB
Precautions: Pregnancy (C), diabetes mellitus, glaucoma, osteoporosis, seizure disorders, ulcerative colitis, CHF, myasthenia gravis, renal disease, esophagitis, peptic ulcer
Pharmacokinetics:
PO/IM: Peak 1-2 hr, 2 days, 1-6 wk (IM), half-life 2-5 hr
Interactions/incompatibilities:
• Decreased action of triamcinolone: cholestyramine, colestipol, barbiturates, rifampin, ephedrine, phenytoin, theophylline
• Decreased effects of: anticoagulants, anticonvulsants, antidiabet-

ics, ambenonium, neostigmine, isoniazid, toxoids, vaccines, anticholinesterases, salicylates, somatrem
• Increased side effects: alcohol, salicylates, indomethacin, amphotericin B, digitalis, cyclosporine, diuretics
• Increased action of triamcinolone: salicylates, estrogens, indomethacin, oral contraceptives, ketoconazole, macrolide antibiotics
Lab test interferences:
Increase: Cholesterol, Na, blood glucose, uric acid, Ca, urine glucose
Decrease: Ca, K, T_4, T_3, thyroid ^{131}I uptake test, urine 17-OHCS, 17-KS, PBI
False negative: Skin allergy tests
NURSING CONSIDERATIONS
Assess:
• K, blood sugar, urine glucose while on long-term therapy; hypokalemia and hyperglycemia
• Weight daily; notify physician if weekly gain >5 lb
• B/P q4h, pulse; notify physician if chest pain occurs
• I&O ratio; be alert for decreasing urinary output and increasing edema
• Plasma cortisol levels during long-term therapy (normal level: 138-635 nmol/L SI units when drawn at 8 AM)
• Infection: increased temperature, WBC, even after withdrawal of medication; drug masks infection symptoms
• K depletion: paresthesias, fatigue, nausea, vomiting, depression, polyuria, dysrhythmias, weakness
• Edema, hypertension, cardiac symptoms
• Mental status: affect, mood, behavioral changes, aggression

italics = common side effects   ***bold italic*** = life threatening reactions

Administer:
• After shaking suspension (parenteral)
• Titrated dose; use lowest effective dose
• IM injection deeply in large mass; rotate sites; avoid deltoid; use 21G needle
• In one dose in AM to prevent adrenal suppression; avoid SC administration; may damage tissue
• With food or milk to decrease GI symptoms

Perform/provide:
• Assistance with ambulation in patient with bone tissue disease to prevent fractures

Evaluate:
• Therapeutic response: ease of respirations, decreased inflammation

Teach patient/family:
• That ID as steroid user should be carried
• To notify physician if therapeutic response decreases; dosage adjustment may be needed
• Not to discontinue this medication abruptly; adrenal crisis can result
• To avoid OTC products: salicylates, alcohol in cough products, cold preparations unless directed by physician
• About cushingoid symptoms
• Symptoms of adrenal insufficiency: nausea, anorexia, fatigue, dizziness, dyspnea, weakness, joint pain

---

triamcinolone acetonide

(trye-am-sin'oh-lone)
Aristocort, Aristocort A, Flutex, Kenalog, Kenalog-H, Triacet, Triamcinolone Acetonide, Triderm

Func. class.: Topical corticosteroid
Chem. class.: Synthetic fluorinated agent, group II potency (0.5%), group III potency (0.1%), group IV potency (0.025%)

Action: Antipruritic, antiinflammatory

Uses: Psoriasis, eczema, contact dermatitis, pruritus

Dosage and routes:
• *Adult and child:* Apply to affected area bid-qid

Available forms: Oint 0.025%, 0.1%, 0.5%; cream 0.025%, 0.1%, 0.5%; lotion 0.025%, 0.1%; aerosol 0.2 mg/2 sec; paste 0.1%

Side effects/adverse reactions:
INTEG: Burning, dryness, itching, irritation, acne, folliculitis, hypertrichosis, perioral dermatitis, hypopigmentation, atrophy, striae, miliaria, allergic contact dermatitis, secondary infection

Contraindications: Hypersensitivity to corticosteroids, fungal infections

Precautions: Pregnancy (C), lactation, viral infections, bacterial infections

NURSING CONSIDERATIONS
Assess:
• Temperature; if fever develops, drug should be discontinued
• For systemic absorption: increased temperature, inflammation, irritation

---

Administer:

• Only to affected areas; do not get in eyes

• Medication, then cover with occlusive dressing (only if prescribed), seal to normal skin, change q12h; use occlusive dressing with extreme caution (group II potency); systemic absorption may occur

• Only to dermatoses; do not use on weeping, denuded, or infected area

Perform/provide:

• Cleansing before application of drug; apply to slightly moist skin; use gloves and a cotton-tipped applicator

• Treatment for a few days after area has cleared

• Storage at room temperature

Evaluate:

• Therapeutic response: absence of severe itching, patches on skin, flaking

Teach patient/family:

• To avoid sunlight on affected area; burns may occur

---

triamcinolone acetonide (topical-oral)

(trye-am-sin'oh-lone)
Kenalog in Orabase, Oralone Dental

Func. class.: Topical anesthetic
Chem. class.: Synthetic fluorinated adrenal corticosteroid

Action: Inhibits nerve impulses from sensory nerves
Uses: Oral pain
Dosage and routes:
• *Adult and child:* TOP press ¼ inch into affected area until film appears, repeat bid-tid
Available forms: Paste 0.1%

Side effects/adverse reactions:
INTEG: Rash, irritation, sensitization
Contraindications: Hypersensitivity, infants <1 yr, application to large areas, presence of fungal, viral, or bacterial infections of mouth or throat
Precautions: Child <6 yr, sepsis, pregnancy (C), denuded skin
NURSING CONSIDERATIONS
Assess:
• Allergy: rash, irritation, reddening, swelling
• Infection: if affected area is infected, do not apply
Administer:
• After cleansing oral cavity
Evaluate:
• Therapeutic response: absence of pain in affected area
Teach patient/family:
• To report rash, irritation, redness, swelling
• How to apply paste

---

triamterene

(trye-am'ter-een)
Dyrenium

Func. class.: Potassium-sparing diuretic
Chem. class.: Pteridine derivative

Action: Acts on distal tubule to inhibit reabsorption of sodium, chloride; increase potassium retention
Uses: Edema; may be used with other diuretics, hypertension
Dosage and routes:
• *Adults:* PO 100 mg bid pc, not to exceed 300 mg
Available forms: Cap 50, 100 mg
Side effects/adverse reactions:
GI: Nausea, diarrhea, vomiting, dry mouth, *jaundice, liver disease*

T

---

italics = common side effects   ***bold italic*** = life threatening reactions

ELECT: Hyperkalemia, hyponatremia, hypochloremia
CNS: Weakness, headache, dizziness
INTEG: Photosensitivity, rash
HEMA: ***Thrombocytopenia, megaloblastic anemia,*** low folic acid levels
GU: ***Azotemia, interstitial nephritis,*** increased BUN, creatinine, renal stones, bluish discoloration of urine
Contraindications: Hypersensitivity, anuria, severe renal disease, severe hepatic disease, hyperkalemia, pregnancy (D), lactation
Precautions: Dehydration, hepatic disease, lactation, CHF, renal disease, cirrhosis
Pharmacokinetics:
PO: Onset 2 hr, peak 6-8 hr, duration 12-16 hr; half-life 3 hr; metabolized in liver, excreted in bile and urine
Interactions/incompatibilities:
• Nephrotoxicity: indomethacin
• Enhanced action of: antihypertensives, lithium, amantadine
• Increased hyperkalemia: other K-sparing diuretics, K products, ACE inhibitors, salt substitutes
Lab test interferences:
Interference: quinidine serum levels, LDH
NURSING CONSIDERATIONS
Assess:
• Weight, I&O daily to determine fluid loss; effect of drug may be decreased if used qd
• Electrolytes: K, Na, Cl; include BUN, blood sugar, CBC, serum creatinine, blood pH, ABGs, liver function tests
• Improvement in CVP q8h
• Signs of metabolic acidosis: drowsiness, restlessness
• Rashes, temperature elevation qd
• Confusion, especially in elderly;

take safety precautions if needed
• Hydration: skin turgor, thirst, dry mucous membranes
Administer:
• In AM to avoid interference with sleep
• With food if nausea occurs; absorption may be decreased slightly
Evaluate:
• Therapeutic response: improvement in edema of feet, legs, sacral area daily if medication is being used in CHF
Teach patient/family:
• To take medication after meals for GI upset
• To avoid prolonged exposure to sunlight since photosensitivity may occur
• To avoid foods high in K: oranges, bananas, salt substitutes, dried apricots, dates
• To notify physician of weakness, headache, nausea, vomiting, dry mouth, fever, sore throat, mouth sores, unusual bleeding or bruising
Treatment of overdose: Lavage if taken orally; monitor electrolytes; administer IV fluids, dialysis; monitor hydration, CV, renal status

triazolam
(trye-ay'zoe-lam)
Halcion
Func. class.: Sedative-hypnotic
Chem. class.: Benzodiazepine

Controlled Substance Schedule IV (USA), Schedule F (Canada)
Action: Produces CNS depression at limbic, thalamic, hypothalamic levels of CNS; may be mediated by neurotransmitter γ-aminobutyric acid (GABA); results are sedation, hypnosis, skeletal muscle relaxation, anticonvulsant activity, anxiolytic action
Uses: Insomnia

Dosage and routes:
• *Adult:* PO 0.125-0.5 mg hs
• *Elderly:* PO 0.125-0.25 mg hs
Available forms: Tabs 0.125, 0.25, 0.5 mg
Side effects/adverse reactions:
*HEMA: **Leukopenia, granulocytopenia*** (rare)
CNS: Headache, lethargy, drowsiness, daytime sedation, dizziness, confusion, light-headedness, anxiety, irritability, amnesia, poor coordination
GI: Nausea, vomiting, diarrhea, heartburn, abdominal pain, constipation
CV: Chest pain, pulse changes
Contraindications: Hypersensitivity to benzodiazepines, pregnancy (X), lactation, intermittent porphyria
Precautions: Anemia, hepatic disease, renal disease, suicidal individuals, drug abuse, elderly, psychosis, child < 15 yr, acute narrow-angle glaucoma, seizure disorders
Pharmacokinetics:
PO: Onset 30-45 min, duration 6-8 hr; metabolized by liver, excreted by kidneys (inactive metabolites), crosses placenta, excreted in breast milk; half-life 2-3 hr
Interactions/incompatibilities:
• Increased effects of: cimetidine, disulfiram, erythromycin, macrolides, probenecid, isoniazid, oral contraceptives
• Increased action of both drugs: alcohol, CNS depressants
• Decreased effect of: antacids, theophylline, rifampin, smoking
Lab test interferences:
Increase: ALT, AST, serum bilirubin
Decrease: RAI uptake
False increase: Urinary 17-OHCS

NURSING CONSIDERATIONS
Assess:
• Blood studies: Hct, Hgb, RBCs, if blood dyscrasias are suspected (rare)
• Hepatic studies: AST, ALT, bilirubin if liver damage has occurred
• Mental status: mood, sensorium, affect, memory (long, short)
• Blood dyscrasias: fever, sore throat, bruising, rash, jaundice, epistaxis (rare)
• Type of sleep problem: falling asleep, staying asleep
Administer:
• After removal of cigarettes to prevent fires
• After trying conservative measures for insomnia
• ½-1 hr before hs for sleeplessness
• On empty stomach for fast onset, but may be taken with food if GI symptoms occur
Perform/provide:
• Assistance with ambulation after receiving dose
• Safety measures: side rails, nightlight, call bell within easy reach
• Checking to see PO medication has been swallowed
• Storage in tight container in cool environment
Evaluate:
• Therapeutic response: ability to sleep at night, decreased amount of early morning awakening if taking drug for insomnia
Teach patient/family:
• That dependence is possible after long-term use
• To avoid driving, other activities requiring alertness until drug is stabilized
• To avoid alcohol ingestion, CNS depressants; serious CNS depression may result
• That effects may take 2 nights for benefits to be noticed

italics = common side effects   ***bold italic*** = life threatening reactions

• Alternative measures to improve sleep: reading, exercise several hours before hs, warm bath, warm milk, TV, self-hypnosis, deep breathing

• That hangover is common in elderly but less common than with barbiturates; rebound insomnia may occur for 1-2 nights after discontinuing drug

Treatment of overdose: Lavage, activated charcoal; monitor electrolytes, VS

---

trientine HCl

(trye-en′-teen)

Syprine

Func. class.: Heavy metal antagonist

Chem. class.: Chelating agent (thiol compound)

Action: Binds with ions of lead, mercury, copper, iron, zinc to form a water-soluble complex excreted by kidneys

Uses: Wilson's disease

Dosage and routes:

• *Adult:* PO 750-2000 mg in divided doses bid-qid

• *Child:* PO 500-1500 mg in divided doses bid-qid

Available forms: Caps 125, 250 mg; tabs 250 mg

Side effects/adverse reactions:

HEMA: Anemia, *iron deficiency*

INTEG: Urticaria, fever

SYST: Hypersensitivity

GI: Epigastric distress, anorexia, heartburn

Contraindications: Hypersensitivity, cystinuria, rheumatoid arthritis, biliary cirrhosis

Precautions: Pregnancy (C), lactation, children, iron deficiency anemia

Pharmacokinetics:

PO: Peak 1 hr, metabolized in liver, excreted in urine

Interactions/incompatibilities:

• Decreased action of trientine: mineral supplements

NURSING CONSIDERATIONS

Assess:

• Monitor hepatic, renal studies: ALT/AST, alk phosphatase, BUN, creatinine, serum copper level

• Monitor I&O

• For anemia: fatigue, Hct, Hgb

• Allergic reactions (rash, urticaria); if these occur, drug should be discontinued

Administer:

• On an empty stomach, ½-1 hr before meals or 2 hr after meals

• Vit B_6 daily; depleted when this drug is used

Evaluate:

• Therapeutic response: improvement in neurologic, psychiatric symptoms

Teach patient/family:

• That therapeutic effect may take 1-3 mo or longer

• To report urticaria, fever, fatigue

---

trifluoperazine HCl

(trye-floo-oh-per′a-zeen)

Novoflurazine,* Solazine,* Stelazine, Suprazine, Terfluzine, Trifluoperazine HCl, Triflurin

Func. class.: Antipsychotic/neuroleptic

Chem. class.: Phenothiazine, piperazine

Action: Depresses cerebral cortex, hypothalamus, limbic system, which control activity, aggression; blocks neurotransmission produced by dopamine at synapse; exhibits strong α-adrenergic, anticholiner-

---

gic blocking action; mechanism for antipsychotic effects is unclear

Uses: Psychotic disorders, non-psychotic anxiety, schizophrenia

Dosage and routes:

Psychotic disorders

• *Adult:* PO 2-5 mg bid, usual range 15-20 mg/day, may require 40 mg/day or more; IM 1-2 mg q4-6h

• *Child >6 yr:* PO 1 mg qd or bid; IM *not recommended for children,* but 1 mg may be given qd or bid

Nonpsychotic anxiety

• *Adult:* PO 1-2 mg bid, not to exceed 5 mg/day; do not give longer than 12 wk

Available forms: Tabs 1, 2, 5, 10, 20 mg; conc 10 mg/ml; inj IM 2 mg/ml

Side effects/adverse reactions:

RESP: ***Laryngospasm,*** dyspnea, ***respiratory depression***

*CNS: Extrapyramidal symptoms: pseudoparkinsonism, akathisia, dystonia, tardive dyskinesia, **seizures,** headache*

HEMA: Anemia, ***leukopenia, leukocytosis, agranulocytosis***

INTEG: Rash, photosensitivity, dermatitis

EENT: Blurred vision, glaucoma, dry eyes

GI: Dry mouth, nausea, vomiting, anorexia, constipation, diarrhea, jaundice, weight gain

GU: Urinary retention, urinary frequency, enuresis, impotence, amenorrhea, gynecomastia

CV: Orthostatic hypotension, hypertension, ***cardiac arrest,*** ECG changes, ***tachycardia***

Contraindications: Hypersensitivity, cardiovascular disease, coma, blood dyscrasias, severe hepatic disease, child <6 yr, glaucoma

Precautions: Breast cancer, seizure disorders, pregnancy (C), lactation, diabetes mellitus, respiratory conditions, prostatic hypertrophy

Pharmacokinetics:

PO: Onset rapid, peak 2-3 hr, duration 12 hr

IM: Onset immediate, peak 1 hr, duration 12 hr

Metabolized by liver, excreted in urine, crosses placenta, enters breast milk

Interactions/incompatibilities:

• Oversedation: other CNS depressants, alcohol, barbiturate anesthetics

• Toxicity: epinephrine

• Decreased absorption: aluminum hydroxide, magnesium hydroxide antacids

• Decreased effects of: lithium, levodopa

• Increased effects of both drugs: β-adrenergic blockers, alcohol

• Increased anticholinergic effects: anticholinergics

Lab test interferences:

Increase: Liver function tests, cardiac enzymes, cholesterol, blood glucose, prolactin, bilirubin, PBI, cholinesterase, ^{131}I

Decrease: Hormones (blood and urine)

False positive: Pregnancy tests, PKU

False negative: Urinary steroids, 17-OHCS, pregnancy tests

NURSING CONSIDERATIONS

Assess:

• Mental status before initial administration

• Swallowing of PO medication; check for hoarding or giving of medication to other patients

• I&O ratio; palpate bladder if low urinary output occurs

• Bilirubin, CBC, liver function studies monthly

• Urinalysis is recommended be-

---

italics = common side effects   ***bold italic*** = life threatening reactions

fore and during prolonged therapy
• Affect, orientation, LOC, reflexes, gait, coordination, sleep pattern disturbances
• B/P standing and lying; also include pulse, respirations q4h during initial treatment; establish baseline before starting treatment; report drops of 30 mm Hg
• Dizziness, faintness, palpitations, tachycardia on rising
• EPS including akathisia (inability to sit still, no pattern to movements), tardive dyskinesia (bizarre movements of jaw, mouth, tongue, extremities), pseudoparkinsonism (rigidity, tremors, pill rolling, shuffling gait)
• Skin turgor daily
• Constipation, urinary retention daily; if these occur increase bulk, water in diet

Administer:
• Antiparkinsonian agent after securing order from physician, to be used if EPS occur
• Conc in 120 ml of tomato or fruit juice, milk, orange, carbonated beverage, coffee, tea, water, or semisolid foods (soup, pudding)

Perform/provide:
• Decreased stimulus by dimming lights, avoiding loud noises
• Supervised ambulation until stabilized on medication; do not involve in strenuous exercise program because fainting is possible; patient should not stand still for long periods
• Increased fluids to prevent constipation
• Sips of water, candy, gum for dry mouth
• Storage in tight, light-resistant container, oral solutions in amber bottles; slight yellowing of inj or conc is common, does not affect potency.

Evaluate:
• Therapeutic response: decrease in emotional excitement, hallucinations, delusions, paranoia, reorganization of patterns of thought, speech

Teach patient/family:
• That orthostatic hypotension occurs frequently, and to rise from sitting or lying position gradually; avoid hazardous activities until stabilized on medication
• To remain lying down after IM injection for at least 30 min
• To avoid hot tubs, hot showers, tub baths, since hypotension may occur
• To avoid abrupt withdrawal of this drug, or EPS may result; drug should be withdrawn slowly
• To avoid OTC preparations (cough, hay fever, cold) unless approved by physician, since serious drug interactions may occur; avoid use with alcohol, CNS depressants; increased drowsiness may occur
• To use a sunscreen during sun exposure to prevent burns
• Regarding compliance with drug regimen
• About necessity for meticulous oral hygiene since oral candidiasis may occur
• To report sore throat, malaise, fever, bleeding, mouth sores; if these occur, CBC should be drawn and drug discontinued
• In hot weather, that heat stroke may occur; take extra precautions to stay cool

Treatment of overdose: Lavage if orally ingested; provide an airway; *do not induce vomiting*

---

triflupromazine HCl
(trye-floo-proe′ma-zeen)
Vesprin
Func. class.: Antipsychotic/
neuroleptic
Chem. class.: Phenothiazine,
aliphatic

Action: Depresses cerebral cortex, hypothalamus, limbic system,
which control activity, aggression;
blocks neurotransmission produced
by dopamine at synapse; exhibits
strong α-adrenergic, anticholinergic blocking action; mechanism for
antipsychotic effects is unclear

Uses: Psychotic disorders, schizophrenia, acute agitation, nausea,
vomiting

Dosage and routes:
Psychosis
• *Adult:* PO 10-50 mg bid-tid depending on severity of condition;
dose is gradually increased to desired dose; IM 60 mg; not to exceed
150 mg/day
• *Child >2 yr:* PO 0.5-2 mg/kg/
day in 3 divided doses; may increase to 10 mg if needed; IM 0.2
to 0.25 mg/kg to a maximum total
dose of 10 mg/day
Nausea/vomiting
• *Adult:* PO 20-30 mg qd; IV 1-3
mg; IM 5-15 mg, q4h, max 60
mg qd
• *Child >2 yr:* PO/IM 0.2 mg/kg,
max 10 mg qd
Acute agitation
• *Adult:* IM 60-150 mg/qd in 3 divided doses
• *Child >2 yr:* IM 0.2-0.25 mg/
kg/day in divided doses, max 10
mg/qd
Available forms: Tabs 10, 25, 50
mg (Canada only); inj IM, IV 10,
20 mg/ml

Side effects/adverse reactions:
RESP: **Laryngospasm,** dyspnea, *re-*
spiratory depression
CNS: Extrapyramidal symptoms:
pseudoparkinsonism, akathisia,
dystonia, tardive dyskinesia,
drowsiness, headache, **seizures**
HEMA: Anemia, **leukopenia, leu-**
kocytosis, agranulocytosis
INTEG: Rash, photosensitivity, dermatitis
EENT: Blurred vision, glaucoma
GI: Dry mouth, nausea, vomiting,
anorexia, constipation, diarrhea,
jaundice, weight gain
GU: Urinary retention, urinary
frequency, enuresis, impotence,
amenorrhea, gynecomastia
CV: Orthostatic hypotension, hypertension, **cardiac arrest,** ECG
changes, **tachycardia**

Contraindications: Hypersensitivity, blood dyscrasias, coma, child
<2½ yr, brain damage, bone mar-
row depression

Precautions: Pregnancy (C), lactation, seizure disorders, hepatic
disease, cardiac disease

Pharmacokinetics:
PO: Onset erratic, peak 2-4 hr, duration 4-6 hr
IM: Onset 15-30 min, peak 1 hr,
duration 4-6 hr; metabolized by
liver, excreted in urine and feces,
crosses placenta, enters breast milk

Interactions/incompatibilities:
• Oversedation: other CNS depressants, alcohol, barbiturate anesthetics
• Toxicity: epinephrine
• Decreased absorption: aluminum
hydroxide, magnesium hydroxide
antacids
• Decreased effects of: lithium, levodopa
• Increased effects of both drugs:
β-adrenergic blockers, alcohol

T

---

italics = common side effects   ***bold italic*** = life threatening reactions

• Increased anticholinergic effects: anticholinergics

Lab test interferences:

Increase: Liver function tests, cardiac enzymes, cholesterol, blood glucose, prolactin, bilirubin, PBI, cholinesterase, ^{131}I

Decrease: Hormones (blood and urine)

False positive: Pregnancy tests, PKU

False negative: Urinary steroids, pregnancy tests

NURSING CONSIDERATIONS

Assess:

• Swallowing of PO medication; check for hoarding or giving of medication to other patients

• I&O ratio; palpate bladder if low urinary output occurs

• Bilirubin, CBC, liver function studies monthly

• Urinalysis is recommended before and during prolonged therapy

• Affect, orientation, LOC, reflexes, gait, coordination, sleep pattern disturbances

• B/P standing and lying; pulse, respirations q4h during initial treatment; establish baseline before starting treatment; report drops of 30 mm Hg

• For neuroleptic malignant syndrome: altered mental status, muscle rigidity, increased CPK, hyperthermia

• Dizziness, faintness, palpitations, tachycardia on rising

• Extrapyramidal symptoms, including akathisia (inability to sit still, no pattern to movements), tardive dyskinesia (bizarre movements of jaw, mouth, tongue, extremities), pseudoparkinsonism (rigidity, tremors, pill rolling, shuffling gait)

• Constipation, urinary retention daily; if these occur, increase bulk, water in the diet

Administer:

• Reduced dose to elderly

• IV after diluting 10 mg/9 ml of NS; give 1 mg or less/2 min

• Antiparkinsonian agent after securing order from physician; to be used if extrapyramidal symptoms occur

• IM injection into large muscle mass; avoid contact with skin

Perform/provide:

• Decreased stimulus by dimming lights, avoiding loud noises

• Supervised ambulation until stabilized on medication; do not involve in strenuous exercise program because fainting is possible; patient should not stand still for long periods

• Increased fluids to prevent constipation

• Sips of water, candy, gum for dry mouth

• Storage in tight, light-resistant container

Evaluate:

• Therapeutic response: decrease in emotional excitement, hallucinations, delusions, paranoia, reorganization of patterns of thought, speech

Teach patient/family:

• That orthostatic hypotension occurs frequently, and to rise from sitting or lying position gradually; to avoid hazardous activities until stabilized on medication

• To remain lying down for at least 30 min after IM injection

• To avoid hot tubs, hot showers, tub baths, since hypotension may occur

• To avoid abrupt withdrawal of this drug, or extrapyramidal symptoms may result; drug should be withdrawn slowly

• To avoid OTC preparations (cough, hay fever, cold) unless approved by physician, since serious drug interactions may occur; avoid use with alcohol, CNS depressants; increased drowsiness may occur
• To use sunscreen during sun exposure to prevent burns
• Regarding compliance with drug regimen
• About necessity for meticulous oral hygiene, since oral candidiasis may occur
• To report sore throat, malaise, fever, bleeding, mouth sores; if these occur, CBC should be drawn and drug discontinued
• That in hot weather, heat stroke may occur; take extra precautions to stay cool
Treatment of overdose: Lavage if orally ingested; provide an airway; *do not induce vomiting*

---

trifluridine (ophthalmic)

(trye-flure'i-deen)
Viroptic
Func. class.: Antiviral
Chem. class.: Pyrimidine nucleoside

Action: Inhibits viral DNA synthesis and replication
Uses: Primary keratoconjunctivitis, recurring epithelial keratitis
Dosage and routes:
• *Adult and child:* INSTILL 1 gtt q2h, not to exceed 9 gtts/day, until corneal epithelium is regrown, then 1 gtt q4h × 1 wk
Available forms: Sol 1%
Side effects/adverse reactions:
EENT: Burning, stinging, swelling, photophobia, irritation, pain
Contraindications: Hypersensitivity

Precautions: Antibiotic hypersensitivity, pregnancy (C), lactation
NURSING CONSIDERATIONS
Assess:
• Allergy: itching, lacrimation, redness, swelling
Administer:
• After washing hands; cleanse crusts or discharge from eye before application
Perform/provide:
• Storage in refrigerator
Evaluate:
• Therapeutic response: absence of redness, inflammation, tearing
Teach patient/family:
• To use drug exactly as prescribed
• Not to use eye make-up, towels, washcloths, or eye medication of others, or reinfection may occur
• That drug container tip should not be touched to eye
• To report itching, increased redness, burning, stinging; drug should be discontinued

---

trihexyphenidyl HCl

(trye-hex-ee-fen'i-dill)
Aparkane,* Aphen, Artane, Artane Sequels, Novohexidyl,* Trihexy-2, Trihexy-5, Trihexyphenidyl HCl
Func. class.: Cholinergic blocker
Chem. class.: Synthetic tertiary amine

Action: Blocks central muscarinic receptors, which decreases involuntary movements
Uses: Parkinson symptoms, drug-induced extrapyramidal symptoms
Dosage and routes:
Parkinson symptoms
• *Adult:* PO 1 mg, increased by 2 mg q3-5d to a total of 6-10 mg/day

---

italics = common side effects   ***bold italic*** = life threatening reactions

Drug-induced extrapyramidal symptoms

• *Adult:* PO 1 mg/day; usual dose 5-15 mg/day

Available forms: Tabs 2, 5 mg; caps sus-rel 5 mg; elix 2 mg/5 ml

Side effects/adverse reactions:

CNS: Confusion, anxiety, restlessness, irritability, delusions, hallucinations, headache, sedation, depression, incoherence, dizziness, flushing, weakness

EENT: Blurred vision, photophobia, dilated pupils, difficulty swallowing, dry eyes, increased intraocular tension, angle-closure glaucoma

CV: Palpitations, tachycardia, postural hypotension

INTEG: Urticaria, rash

MISC: Suppression of lactation, nasal congestion, decreased sweating, increased temperature, hyperthermia, heat stroke, numbness of fingers

MS: Weakness, cramping

GI: Dryness of mouth, constipation, nausea, vomiting, abdominal distress, *paralytic ileus*

GU: Hesitancy, retention, dysuria

Contraindications: Hypersensitivity, narrow-angle glaucoma, myasthenia gravis, GI/GU obstruction, tachycardia, myocardial ischemia, unstable CV disease, prostatic hypertrophy

Precautions: Pregnancy (C), elderly, lactation, tachycardia, abdominal obstruction, infection, children, gastric ulcer

Pharmacokinetics:

PO: Onset 1 hr, peak 2-3 hr, duration 6-12 hr, excreted in urine

Interactions/incompatibilities:

• Increased anticholinergic effects: antihistamines, phenothiazines, amantadine

• Decreased action of haloperidol

NURSING CONSIDERATIONS

Assess:

• I&O ratio; retention commonly causes decreased urinary output

• B/P, pulse frequently while dose is being determined

• Urinary hesitancy, retention; palpate bladder if retention occurs

• Constipation; increase fluids, bulk, exercise if this occurs

• For tolerance over long-term therapy; dosage may have to be increased or medication changed

• Mental status: affect, mood, CNS depression, worsening of mental symptoms during early therapy

Administer:

• With or after meals for GI upset; may give with fluids other than water

• At hs to avoid daytime drowsiness in patient with parkinsonism

Perform/provide:

• Storage at room temperature in light resistant container

• Hard candy, frequent drinks, sugarless gum to relieve dry mouth

Evaluate:

• Therapeutic response: parkinsonism: shuffling gait, muscle rigidity, involuntary movements

Teach patient/family:

• Not to discontinue this drug abruptly; to taper off over 1 wk

• To avoid driving, other hazardous activities; drowsiness may occur

• To avoid OTC medications: cough, cold preparations with alcohol, antihistamines unless directed by physician

• To avoid sudden position changes

• To avoid hot climates; overheating may occur

---

* Available in Canada only

trilostane
(trye'loe-stane)
Modrastane

Func. class.: Antineoplastic
Chem. class.: Hormone, adrenal steroid inhibitor

Action: Inhibits DNA, RNA, protein synthesis; derived from *Streptomyces verticillus;* replication is decreased by binding to DNA, which causes strand splitting; drug is phase specific in G_2, M phases

Uses: Metastatic breast cancer, adrenal cancer, suppression of adrenal function in Cushing's syndrome

Dosage and routes:
• *Adult:* PO 30 mg qid; may increase q3-4d up to 480 mg/day

Available forms: Caps 30, 60 mg

Side effects/adverse reactions:
*HEMA: **Thrombocytopenia, leukopenia, myelosuppression, anemia***
*GI: Nausea, vomiting, anorexia, **hepatotoxicity***
GU: Hirsutism
INTEG: Rash, pruritus
CV: Hypotension, tachycardia
CNS: Dizziness, headache

Contraindications: Hypersensitivity, hypothyroidism, pregnancy (X)

Precautions: Renal disease, hepatic disease, respiratory disease

Pharmacokinetics: Half-life 13 hr; metabolized in liver, excreted in urine, crosses placenta

NURSING CONSIDERATIONS
Assess:
• CBC, differential, platelet count weekly; withhold drug if WBC is <4000 or platelet count is <75,000; notify physician of results
• Renal function studies: BUN, serum uric acid, urine CrCl, electrolytes before, during therapy
• I&O ratio; report fall in urine output of 30 ml/hr
• Monitor temperature q4h (may indicate beginning infection)
• Liver function tests before, during therapy (bilirubin, AST, ALT, LDH) as needed or monthly
• RBC, Hct, Hgb, since these may be decreased
• Bleeding: hematuria, guaiac, bruising, petechiae, mucosa or orifices q8h
• Food preferences; list likes, dislikes
• Inflammation of mucosa, breaks in skin
• Yellowing of skin and sclera, dark urine, clay-colored stools, itchy skin, abdominal pain, fever, diarrhea
• Symptoms indicating severe allergic reactions: rash, pruritus, urticaria, purpuric skin lesions, itching, flushing

Administer:
• Medications by oral route; if possible avoid IM, SC, IV routes to prevent infections
• Antacid before oral agent; give last dose of drug after evening meal, before bedtime
• Antiemetic 30-60 min before giving drug to prevent vomiting
• Local or systemic drugs for infection

Perform/provide:
• Nutritious diet with iron, vitamin supplements as ordered

Evaluate:
• Therapeutic response: decreased tumor size, spread of malignancy

Teach patient/family:
• To report any complaints, side effects to nurse or physician
• That masculinization can occur, is reversible after discontinuing treatment

T

italics = common side effects   ***bold italic*** = life threatening reactions

---

trimeprazine tartrate
(trye-mep′ra-zeen)
Panectyl,* Temaril
Func. class.: Antihistamine
Chem. class.: Phenothiazine
analog, H_1-receptor antagonist

Action: Acts on blood vessels, GI,
respiratory system by competing
with histamine for H_1-receptor site;
decreases allergic response by
blocking histamine

Uses: Pruritus

Dosage and routes:
• *Adult:* PO 2.5 mg qid; TIME-
REL 5 mg bid
• *Child 3-12 yr:* PO 2.5 mg tid
or hs
• *Child 6 mo-1 yr:* PO 1.25 mg tid
or hs

Available forms: Tabs 2.5 mg;
spans 5 mg; syr 2.5 mg/5 ml

Side effects/adverse reactions:
CNS: Dizziness, drowsiness, poor
condition, fatigue, anxiety, euphoria, confusion, paresthesia,
neuritis
CV: Hypotension, palpitations,
tachycardia
RESP: Increased thick secretions,
wheezing, chest tightness
*HEMA: **Thrombocytopenia, agranulocytosis, hemolytic anemia***
GI: Dry mouth, nausea, vomiting,
anorexia, constipation, diarrhea
INTEG: Rash, urticaria, photosensitivity
GU: Retention, dysuria, frequency
EENT: Blurred vision, dilated pupils, tinnitus, nasal stuffiness, dry
nose, throat, mouth

Contraindications: Hypersensitivity to H_1-receptor antagonist, acute
asthma attack, lower respiratory
tract disease

Precautions: Increased intraocular

pressure, renal disease, cardiac
disease, hypertension, bronchial
asthma, seizure disorder, stenosed
peptic ulcers, hyperthyroidism,
prostatic hypertrophy, bladder neck
obstruction, pregnancy (C)

Interactions/incompatibilities:
• Increased CNS depression: bar-
biturates, narcotics, hypnotics, tri-
cyclic antidepressants, alcohol
• Decreased effect of: oral antico-
agulants, heparin
• Increased effect of trimeprazine:
MAOIs

Lab test interferences:
False negative: Skin allergy tests

NURSING CONSIDERATIONS
Assess:
• I&O ratio; be alert for urinary retention, frequency, dysuria; drug
should be discontinued if these
occur
• CBC during long-term therapy;
blood dyscrasias
• Respiratory status: rate, rhythm,
increase in bronchial secretions,
wheezing, chest tightness
• Cardiac status: palpitations, increased pulse, hypotension

Administer:
• Coffee, tea, cola (caffeine) to decrease drowsiness
• With meals if GI symptoms occur; absorption may slightly decrease
• Sustained-release formulation
only to adults

Perform/provide:
• Hard candy, gum, frequent rinsing of mouth for dryness
• Storage in tight container at room
temperature

Evaluate:
• Therapeutic response: decreased
itching associated with pruritus

Teach patient/family:
• To notify physician if confusion,
sedation, hypotension occurs

---

*Available in Canada only

• To avoid driving or other hazardous activity if drowsiness occurs
• To avoid concurrent use of alcohol, other CNS depressants
Treatment of overdose: Administer ipecac syrup or lavage, diazepam, vasopressors, barbiturates (short-acting)

---

trimethadione
(trye-meth-a-dye′one)
Tridione
Func. class.: Anticonvulsant
Chem. class.: Oxazolidinedione

Action: Decreases seizures in cortex, basal ganglia; decreases synaptic stimulation to low-frequency impulses
Uses: Refractory absence (petit mal) seizures
Dosage and routes:
• *Adult:* PO 300 mg tid, may increase by 300 mg/wk, not to exceed 600 mg qid
• *Child:* PO 20-50 mg/kg/day, may increase by 150-300 mg/wk
Available forms: Caps 300 mg; chew tabs 150 mg; sol 200 mg/5 ml; oral sol 40 mg/ml
Side effects/adverse reactions:
*HEMA: **Thrombocytopenia, agranulocytosis, leukopenia, neutropenia, hemolytic anemia,** in-*creased pro-time, *eosinophilia, aplastic anemia*
CNS: Drowsiness, dizziness, fatigue, paresthesia, irritability, headache, insomnia
GU: Vaginal bleeding, albuminuria, nephrosis, abdominal pain, weight loss
GI: Nausea, vomiting, bleeding gums, abnormal liver function tests
*INTEG: **Exfoliative dermatitis,*** rash, alopecia, petechiae, erythema

EENT: Photophobia, diplopia, epistaxis, retinal hemorrhage
CV: Hypertension, hypotension
Contraindications: Hypersensitivity, blood dyscrasias, pregnancy (D)
Precautions: Hepatic disease, renal disease
Pharmacokinetics:
PO: Peak 30 min-2 hr, excreted by kidneys, half-life 6-13 days
NURSING CONSIDERATIONS
Assess:
• Blood studies: Hct, Hgb, RBCs, serum folate, Vit D; hepatic studies: AST, ALT, bilirubin, creatinine; drug should be stopped if neutrophil count falls below 2500/mm³ on long-term therapy
• Mental status: mood, sensorium, affect, memory (long, short)
• Rash, alopecia, convulsions; discontinue drug if these occur
Administer:
• After diluting oral solution with H_2O, give slowly through lavage needle
• Oral with juice or milk to cover taste/smell; decreases GI symptoms
Perform/provide:
• Ventilation of room
Evaluate:
• Therapeutic response: decreased seizures
Teach patient/family:
• To notify physician of skin rash, alopecia, sore throat, fever, bruising, epistaxis or visual disturbances, particularly day blindness
• That physical dependency may result when used for extended periods
• To avoid driving, other activities that require alertness
• Not to discontinue medication quickly after long-term use; convulsions may result

italics = common side effects   ***bold italic*** = life threatening reactions

• Drug may take 1-4 wk to work; patient may still have seizures
• Report symptoms of renal damage: edema, urinary frequency, burning, cloudy urine

---

trimethaphan camsylate

(trye-meth'a-fan)
Arfonad
Func. class.: Antihypertensive
Chem. class.: Ganglionic blocker

Action: Occupies receptor site, prevents acetylcholine from attaching to postsynaptic nerve endings in sympathetic, parasympathetic ganglia

Uses: Hypertensive emergencies, production of controlled hypotension during surgery

Dosage and routes:
• *Adult:* IV INF dilute 500 mg in 500 ml of 5% dextrose injection, run at 3-4 mg/min, adjust to maintain B/P at desired rate; range 0.3-6.0 mg/min
• *Child:* 50-150 μg/kg/min
Available forms: Inj IV 50 mg/ml

Side effects/adverse reactions:
CV: Orthostatic hypotension, angina, tachycardia, edema
GI: Nausea, vomiting, anorexia, dry mouth, diarrhea, constipation, ileus
CNS: Headache, agitation, weakness, restlessness
INTEG: Rash, urticaria, pruritus
RESP: Respiratory arrest
EENT: Blurred vision, diplopia, pupillary dilation
GU: Urinary retention

Contraindications: Uncorrected respiratory insufficiency, hypersensitivity, pregnancy (C), hypovo-lemic shock, glaucoma, uncorrected anemia

Precautions: Elderly, debilitated, allergic individuals, cardiac disease, degenerative CNS disease, hepatic disease, renal disease, diabetes mellitus, Addison's disease, children

Pharmacokinetics:
IV: Onset 1-2 min, duration up to 30 min; excreted in urine, crosses placenta

Interactions/incompatibilities:
• Increased effects of diuretics, antihypertensives, anesthetics
• Do not mix with any drug in syringe or solution

NURSING CONSIDERATIONS
Assess:
• Electrolytes: K, Na, Cl, CO_2
• Renal function studies: BUN, creatinine
• B/P during initial treatment, periodically thereafter
• Weight daily, I&O
• ECG throughout treatment if there is a history of cardiac problems
• Nausea, vomiting, diarrhea
• Edema in feet, legs daily
• Skin turgor, dryness of mucous membranes for hydration status
• Constipation: number of stools, consistency; give stool softener as ordered or increase bulk in diet if constipation occurs, or antidiarrheal for diarrhea
• Respiratory dysfunction: bronchospasm, wheezing, tachypnea, respiratory arrest
• Signs of peripheral vascular collapse

Administer:
• IV infusion by microdrip regulator rate to maintain B/P
• Diluted solution only (500 mg of drug/500 ml or more of D_5W)

Perform/provide:
• Artificial ventilation equipment nearby
• Use of only freshly prepared solution
• Elevate patient's head to control B/P

Evaluate:
• Therapeutic response: decreased B/P, primarily systolic B/P

Teach patient/family:
• That lying in bed is needed during infusion

Treatment of overdose: Administer vasopressors, phenylephrine, mephentermine

---

trimethobenzamide

(trye-meth-oh-ben′za-mide)
Arrestin, T-Gen, Tebamide, Ti-con, Tigan, Trimazide, Trimethobenzamide, Trimethobenzamide HCl

Func. class.: Antiemetic, anticholinergic
Chem. class.: Ethanolamine derivative

Action: Acts centrally by blocking chemoreceptor trigger zone, which in turn acts on vomiting center

Uses: Nausea, vomiting, prevention of postoperative vomiting

Dosage and routes:
Postoperative vomiting
• *Adult:* IM/REC 200 mg before or during surgery; may repeat 3 hr after

Discontinuing anesthesia
• *Child 13-40 kg:* PO/REC 100-200 mg tid-qid
• *Child <13 kg:* PO/REC 100 mg tid-qid

Nausea/vomiting
• *Adult:* PO 250 mg tid-qid; IM/REC 200 mg tid-qid

Available forms: Caps 100, 250 mg; supp 100, 200 mg; inj IM 100 mg/ml

Side effects/adverse reactions:
CNS: Drowsiness, restlessness, headache, dizziness, insomnia, confusion, nervousness, tingling, *vertigo,* extrapyramidal symptoms
GI: Nausea, anorexia, diarrhea, vomiting, constipation
CV: Hypertension, hypotension, palpitation
INTEG: Rash, urticaria, fever, chills, flushing
EENT: Dry mouth, blurred vision, diplopia, nasal congestion, photosensitivity

Contraindications: Hypersensitivity to narcotics, shock, children (parenterally)

Precautions: Children, cardiac dysrhythmias, elderly, asthma, pregnancy (C), prostatic hypertrophy, bladder-neck obstruction, narrow-angle glaucoma, stenosing peptic ulcer, pyloroduodenal obstruction

Pharmacokinetics:
PO: Onset 20-40 min, duration 3-4 hr
IM: Onset 15 min, duration 2-3 hr; metabolized by liver, excreted by kidneys

Interactions/incompatibilities:
• Increased effect: CNS depressants
• May mask ototoxic symptoms associated with antibiotics

NURSING CONSIDERATIONS T

Assess:
• VS, B/P; check patients with cardiac disease more often
• Signs of toxicity of other drugs or masking of symptoms of disease: brain tumor, intestinal obstruction
• Observe for drowsiness, dizziness

Administer:
• IM injection in large muscle

---

mass; aspirate to avoid IV administration
• Tablets may be swallowed whole, chewed, allowed to dissolve

Evaluate:
• Therapeutic response: decreased nausea, vomiting

Teach patient/family:
• To avoid hazardous activities, activities requiring alertness; dizziness may occur; instruct patient to request assistance with ambulation
• To avoid alcohol, other depressants
• To keep out of children's reach

---

trimethoprim
(trye-meth′oh-prim)
Proloprim, Trimethoprim, Trimpex
Func. class.: Urinary antiinfective
Chem. class.: Folate antagonist

Action: Prevents bacterial synthesis by blocking enzyme reduction of dihyodrofolic acid

Uses: *E.coli, P. mirabilis, Klebsiella, Enterobacter* urinary tract infections

Dosage and routes:
• *Adult:* PO 100 mg q12h
Available forms: Tabs 100, 200 mg

Side effects/adverse reactions:
INTEG: **Exfoliative dermatitis,** pruritus, rash
HEMA: **Thrombocytopenia, leukopenia, neutropenia, megaloblastic anemia** (rare)
GI: Nausea, vomiting, abdominal pain, abnormal taste, increased AST, ALT, bilirubin, creatinine
CNS: Fever

Contraindications: Hypersensitivity, CrCl <15 ml/min, renal disease, hepatic disease, megaloblastic anemia

Precautions: Folate deficiency, pregnancy (C), lactation, fragile X chromosome, children <12 yr old

Pharmacokinetics:
PO: Peak 1-4 hr, half-life 8-11 hr; metabolized in liver, excreted in urine (unchanged 60%), breast milk; crosses placenta

Interactions/incompatabilities:
• Increased action of: phenytoin

NURSING CONSIDERATIONS
Assess:
• Nocturia; may indicate drug resistance
• Signs of infection, anemia
• AST/ALT, BUN, bilirubin, creatinine, urine cultures
• C&S before drug therapy; drug may be given as soon as culture is obtained
• Skin eruptions

Administer:
• With full glass of water

Perform/provide:
• Storage in tight, light-resistant container
• Adequate intake of fluids (2 L) to decrease bacteria in bladder

Evaluate:
• Therapeutic response: absence of pain in bladder area, negative C&S

Teach patient/family:
• Aspects of drug therapy: need to complete entire course of medication to ensure organism death (10-14 days); culture may be taken after completed course of medication
• That drug must be taken in equal intervals around clock to maintain blood levels
• To notify nurse of nausea, vomiting

---

trimetrexate glucuronate
Neutrexin

Func. class.: Antineoplastic antimetabolite
Chem. class.: Nonclassical folic acid antagonist

Action: Inhibits an enzyme that reduces folic acid, which is needed for purine biosynthesis in all cells; result is disruption of RNA, DNA, cell death; leucovorin usually transported into cells by active, carrier-mediated process; however, *Pneumocystis carinii* organisms lack carrier system; trimetrexate must be given with leucovorin to protect normal cells

Uses: Moderate to severe *P. carinii* pneumonia as an alternative to TMP/SMZ; may be useful in treating non–small cell lung, prostate, colorectal cancer

Dosage and routes:
Leucovorin must be given concurrently and for 72 hr past last trimetrexate dose
• *Adult:* IV 45 mg/m² qd over 60-90 min; with leucovorin IV 20 mg/m² over 5-10 min q 6 hr for a daily dose of 80 mg/m² or PO qid 20 mg/m² evenly spaced during the day; PO dose should be rounded to the next higher 25 mg; course is trimetrexate 21 days, leucovorin 24 days; modifications in dose must be based on hematologic toxicity
Available forms: Powder for inj lyophilized 25 mg

Side effects/adverse reactions:
CNS: confusion, fatigue, fever
*GI: Nausea, vomiting, **hepatotoxicity**,* ulcer, stomatitis
GU: Increased serum creatinine
*HEMA: **Thrombocytopenia, anemia***

INTEG: Rash, pruritus
META: Hyponatremia, hypocalcemia

Contraindications: Hypersensitivity to trimetrexate, leucovorin, methotrexate; thrombocytopenia (<25,000/mm³), severe anemia, neutropenia (<500 mm³) pregnancy (D)

Precautions: Renal disease, hepatic disease, lactation, children, seizures

Pharmacokinetics:
Terminal half-life 7-15 hr; may be 95%-98% protein bound

Interactions/incompatibilities:
Specific interactions not known; these interactions may occur:
• Increased toxicity: aspirin, sulfa drugs, other antineoplastics, radiation
• Decreased effect of trimetrexate; erythromycin, ketoconazole, fluconazole, rifampin, rifabutin, cimetidine

NURSING CONSIDERATIONS
Assess:
• CBC, differential, platelet count weekly; withhold drug if neutrophils <500/mm³ or platelet count <25,000/mm³; notify physician; drug should be discontinued; hematologic toxicity should be graded 1-4, 4 most severe
• Renal function studies: BUN, serum uric acid, urine CrCl, electrolytes before, during therapy; treatment should be interrupted when creatinine >2.5 mg/dl
• I&O ratio; report urine output <30 ml/hr
• Monitor temperature q4h; fever may indicate beginning infection; no rectal temperatures
• Liver function tests before, during therapy: bilirubin, alk phosphatase, AST, ALT; treatment should be interrupted when alk phospha-

tase or transaminase >5 × upper normal limit

• Bleeding time, coagulation time during treatment

Administer:

• Reconstitute with 2 ml D₅ or sterile H₂O (12.5 mg/ml) filter 0.22 micro prior to dilution; dilute reconstituted sol with D₅ for concentration of 0.25-2 mg/ml; give over 60 min; flush IV line thoroughly with 10 ml D₅ before, after dose

• Trimetrexate and leucovorin sol separately; leucovorin may be given before or after trimetrexate; IV line must be flushed between infusions

• If trimetrexate comes in contact with skin, wash with soap, water immediately

• Antiemetic 30-60 min before giving drug to prevent vomiting

• Topical or systemic analgesics for pain

• Transfusion for anemia

Perform/provide:

• Strict medical asepsis and protective isolation if WBC levels low

• Liquid diet: carbonated beverage, Jell-O; dry toast, crackers may be added when patient is not nauseated or vomiting

• Rinsing of mouth tid-qid with water, club soda; brushing of teeth bid-tid with soft brush or cotton-tipped applicators for stomatitis; use unwaxed dental floss

• Nutritious diet with iron, vitamin supplements

• Storage after reconstitution up to 24 hr refrigerated; do not freeze reconstituted sol; discard after 24 hr

Evaluate:

• Therapeutic response: decreased symptoms of pneumocystis

• Bleeding: hematuria, guaiac, bruising or petechiae, mucosa or orifices q8h

• Food preferences; list likes, dislikes

• Hepatotoxicity: yellowing of skin and sclera, dark urine, clay-colored stools, pruritus, abdominal pain, fever, diarrhea

• Buccal cavity q8h for dryness, sores, ulceration, white patches, oral pain, bleeding, dysphagia

• Symptoms indicating severe allergic reaction: rash, urticaria, itching, flushing

Teach patient/family:

• Why protective isolation is needed

• To report any complaints, side effects to nurse or physician: black tarry stools, chills, fever, sore throat, bleeding, bruising, cough, shortness of breath, dark or bloody urine

• To avoid foods with citric acid, hot or rough texture if stomatitis is present

• To report to physician stomatitis: any bleeding, white spots, ulcerations in mouth; tell patient to examine mouth qd, report symptoms to nurse

• To drink 10-12 glasses of fluid/day

• To avoid alcohol, salicylates

• To avoid use of razors, commercial mouthwash

---

trimipramine maleate
(tri-mip′ra-meen)
Surmontil, Trimipramine Maleate, Trisoralen
Func. class.: Antidepressant—tricyclic
Chem. class.: Tertiary amine

Action: Selectively inhibits serotonin uptake by brain; potentiates behavioral changes

Uses: Depression, enuresis in children

Dosage and routes:
• *Adult:* PO 75 mg/day in divided doses, may be increased to 200 mg/day
• *Child >6 yr:* 25 mg hs, may increase to 50 mg in children <12 yr or 75 mg in children >12 yr

Available forms: Caps 25, 50, 100 mg

Side effects/adverse reactions:
*HEMA: **Agranulocytosis, thrombocytopenia, eosinophilia, leukopenia***
CNS: Dizziness, drowsiness, confusion, headache, anxiety, tremors, stimulation, weakness, insomnia, nightmares, EPS (elderly), increase in psychiatric symptoms
GI: Diarrhea, dry mouth, nausea, vomiting, ***paralytic ileus,*** increased appetite, cramps, epigastric distress, jaundice, ***hepatitis,*** stomatitis, constipation
*GU: Retention, **acute renal failure***
INTEG: Rash, urticaria, sweating, pruritus, photosensitivity
*CV: Orthostatic hypotension, ECG changes, tachycardia, **hypertension,*** palpitations
EENT: Blurred vision, tinnitus, mydriasis

Contraindications: Hypersensitivity to tricyclic antidepressants, recovery phase of myocardial infarction, convulsive disorders, prostatic hypertrophy

Precautions: Suicidal patients, severe depression, increased intraocular pressure, narrow-angle glaucoma, urinary retention, cardiac disease, hepatic disease, hyperthyroidism, electroshock therapy, elective surgery, pregnancy (C)

Pharmacokinetics:
Metabolized by liver, excreted by kidneys, steady state 2-6 days; half-life 7-30 hr

Interactions/incompatibilities:
• Decreased effects of: guanethidine, clonidine, indirect-acting sympathomimetics (ephedrine)
• Increased effects of: direct-acting sympathomimetics (epinephrine), alcohol, barbiturates, benzodiazepines, CNS depressants
• Hyperpyretic crisis, convulsions, hypertensive episode: MAOI (pargyline [Eutonyl])

Lab test interferences:
Increase: Serum bilirubin, blood glucose, alk phosphatase
False increase: Urinary catecholamines

NURSING CONSIDERATIONS
Assess:
• B/P (lying, standing), pulse q4h; if systolic B/P drops 20 mm Hg, hold drug, notify physician; take vital signs q4h in patients with cardiovascular disease
• Blood studies: CBC, leukocytes, differential, cardiac enzymes if patient is receiving long-term therapy
• Hepatic studies: AST, ALT, bilirubin, creatinine
• Weight qwk; appetite may increase with drug
• ECG for flattening of T wave, bundle branch block, AV block, dysrhythmias in cardiac patients
• EPS primarily in elderly: rigidity, dystonia, akathisia
• Mental status changes: mood, sensorium, affect, suicidal tendencies, increase in psychiatric symptoms, depression, panic
• Urinary retention, constipation; constipation is more likely to occur in children, elderly
• Withdrawal symptoms: headache, nausea, vomiting, muscle pain, weakness; do not usually oc-

---

italics = common side effects   ***bold italic*** = life threatening reactions

cur unless drug is discontinued abruptly

• Alcohol consumption; if alcohol is consumed, hold dose until morning

Administer:

• Increased fluids, bulk in diet for constipation, urinary retention

• With food or milk for GI symptoms

• Dosage hs if oversedation occurs during day; may take entire dose hs; elderly may not tolerate once/day dosing

• Gum, hard candy, or frequent sips of water for dry mouth

Perform/provide:

• Storage in tight, light-resistant container at room temperature

• Assistance with ambulation during beginning therapy for drowsiness/dizziness

• Safety measures, including side rails, primarily for elderly

• Checking to see PO medication swallowed

Evaluate:

• Therapeutic response: decreased depression or enuresis

Teach patient/family:

• That therapeutic effects may take 2-3 wk

• To use caution in driving, other activities requiring alertness because of drowsiness, dizziness, blurred vision

• To avoid alcohol ingestion, other CNS depressants

• Not to discontinue medication quickly after long-term use; may cause nausea, headache, malaise

• To wear sunscreen or large hat, since photosensitivity occurs

Decrease: VMA, 5-HIAA

Treatment of overdose: ECG monitoring; induce emesis; lavage, activated charcoal; administer anticonvulsant

---

tripelennamine HCl

(tri-pel-enn′a-meen)
PBZ, PBZ-SR, Pelamine, Tripelennamine HCl

Func. class.: Antihistamine
Chem. class.: Ethylenediamine derivative

Action: Acts on blood vessels, GI, respiratory system by competing with histamine for H$_1$-receptor site; decreases allergic response by blocking histamine

Uses: Rhinitis, allergy symptoms

Dosage and routes:

• *Adult:* PO 25-50 mg q4-6h, not to exceed 600 mg/day; TIME-REL 100 mg bid-tid, not to exceed 600 mg/day

• *Child >5 yr:* TIME-REL 50 mg q8-12hr, not to exceed 300 mg/day

• *Child <5 yr:* PO 5 mg/kg/day in 4-6 divided doses, not to exceed 300 mg/day

Available forms: Tabs 25, 50 mg; time-rel tabs 100 mg; elix 37.5 mg/5 ml

Side effects/adverse reactions:

CNS: Dizziness, drowsiness, poor coordination, fatigue, anxiety, euphoria, confusion, paresthesia, neuritis

CV: Hypotension, palpitations, tachycardia

RESP: Increased thick secretions, wheezing, chest tightness

*HEMA: **Thrombocytopenia, agranulocytosis, hemolytic anemia***

GI: Constipation, dry mouth, nausea, vomiting, anorexia, diarrhea

INTEG: Rash, urticaria, photosensitivity

GU: Retention, dysuria, frequency

EENT: Blurred vision, dilated pupils, tinnitus, nasal stuffiness, dry nose, throat, mouth

---

** Available in Canada only

Contraindications: Hypersensitivity to H₁-receptor antagonist, acute asthma attack, lower respiratory tract disease

Precautions: Increased intraocular pressure, renal disease, cardiac disease, hypertension, bronchial asthma, seizure disorder, stenosed peptic ulcers, hyperthyroidism, prostatic hypertrophy, bladder neck obstruction, pregnancy (C)

Pharmacokinetics:

PO: Onset 15-30 min, duration 4-6 hr; detoxified in liver, excreted by kidneys

Interactions/incompatibilities:

• Increased CNS depressants: barbiturates, narcotics, hypnotics, tricyclic antidepressants, alcohol

• Decreased effect of: oral anticoagulants, heparin

• Increased effect of tripelennamine: MAOIs

Lab test interferences:

False negative: Skin allergy test

False positive: Urine pregnancy tests

NURSING CONSIDERATIONS
Assess:

• I&O ratio; be alert for urinary retention, frequency, dysuria; drug should be discontinued if these occur

• CBC during long-term therapy; blood dyscrasias

• Respiratory status: rate, rhythm, increase in bronchial secretions, wheezing, chest tightness

• Cardiac status: palpitations, increased pulse, hypotension

Administer:

• With meals if GI symptoms occur; absorption may slightly decrease

• Time-release tab to adults only

Perform/provide:

• Hard candy, gum, frequent rinsing of mouth for dryness

• Storage in tight container at room temperature

Evaluate:

• Therapeutic response: decrease itching associated with pruritus

Teach patient/family:

• All aspects of drug use; to notify physician of confusion, sedation, hypotension

• To avoid driving, other hazardous activity if drowsiness occurs

• To avoid concurrent use of alcohol, other CNS depressants

Treatment of overdose: Administer ipecac syrup or lavage, diazepam, vasopressors, barbiturates (short-acting)

---

triprolidine HCl

(trye-proe'li-deen)

Actidil, Myidil, Triprolidine HCl

Func. class.: Antihistamine

Chem. class.: Alkylamine, H₁-receptor antagonist

Action: Acts on blood vessels, GI, respiratory system by competing with histamine for H₁-receptor site; decreases allergic response by blocking histamine

Uses: Rhinitis, allergy symptoms

Dosage and routes:

• *Adult:* PO 2.5 mg tid-qid

• *Child >6 yr:* PO 1.25 mg tid-qid

• *Child 4-6 yr:* PO 0.9 mg tid-qid

• *Child 2-4 yr:* PO 0.6 mg tid-qid

• *Child 4 mo-2 yr:* 0.3 mg tid-qid

Available forms: Tab 2.5 mg; syr 1.25 mg/5 ml

Side effects/adverse reactions:

CNS: Dizziness, drowsiness, poor coordination, fatigue, anxiety, euphoria, confusion, paresthesia, neuritis

CV: Hypotension, palpitations, tachycardia

---

italics = common side effects   ***bold italic*** = life threatening reactions

RESP: Increased thick secretions, wheezing, chest tightness
*HEMA: **Thrombocytopenia, agranulocytosis, hemolytic anemia***
GI: Constipation, dry mouth, nausea, vomiting, anorexia, diarrhea
INTEG: Rash, urticaria, photosensitivity
GU: Retention, dysuria, frequency
EENT: Blurred vision, dilated pupils, tinnitus, nasal stuffiness, dry nose, throat, mouth

Contraindications: Hypersensitivity to H$_1$-receptor antagonist, acute asthma attack, lower respiratory tract disease

Precautions: Increased intraocular pressure, renal disease, cardiac disease, hypertension, bronchial asthma, seizure disorder, stenosed peptic ulcers, hyperthyroidism, prostatic hypertrophy, bladder neck obstruction, pregnancy (C)

Pharmacokinetics:
PO: Onset 20-60 min, duration 8-12 hr; detoxified in liver, excreted by kidneys (metabolites/free drug), half-life 20-24 hr

Interactions/incompatibilities:
• Increased CNS depressants: barbiturates, narcotics, hypnotics, tricyclic antidepressants, alcohol
• Decreased effect of: oral anticoagulants, heparin
• Increased effect of triprolidine: MAOIs

Lab test interferences:
False negative: Skin allergy tests

NURSING CONSIDERATIONS
Assess:
• I&O ratio; be alert for urinary retention, frequency, dysuria; drug should be discontinued if these occur
• CBC during long-term therapy; blood dyscrasias
• Respiratory status: rate, rhythm,

increase in bronchial secretions, wheezing, chest tightness
• Cardiac status: palpitations, increased pulse, hypotension
Administer:
• With meals if GI symptoms occur; absorption may slightly decrease
• Time-release formulation to adults only
Perform/provide:
• Hard candy, gum, frequent rinsing of mouth for dryness
• Storage in tight container at room temperature
Evaluate:
• Therapeutic response: decreased itching associated with pruritus
Teach patient/family:
• All aspects of drug use; to notify physician of confusion, sedation, hypotension
• To avoid driving, other hazardous activity if drowsiness occurs
• To avoid concurrent use of alcohol, other CNS depressants while taking this drug
Treatment of overdose: Administer ipecac syrup or lavage, diazepam, vasopressors, barbiturates (short-acting)

tromethamine
(troe-meth'a-meen)
Tham, Tham-E
Func. class.: Alkalinizer
Chem. class.: Amine

Action: Proton acceptor that corrects acidosis by combining with hydrogen ions to form bicarbonate and buffer; acts as diuretic (osmotic)
Uses: Acidosis (metabolic) associated with cardiac disease, COPD
Dosage and routes:
• *Adult:* 0.3 M required = kg of

weight × HCO_3 deficit (mEq/L)
• *Child:* Same as above given over 3-6 hr, not to exceed 40 ml/kg
Available forms: Inj IV 36 mg/ml, powd for inj IV 36 g
Side effects/adverse reactions:
CV: Irregular pulse, ***cardiac arrest***
META: Alkalosis, hypoglycemia
RESP: Shallow, slow respirations, cyanosis, ***apnea***
*GI: **Hepatic necrosis***
INTEG: Infection at injection site, extravasation, phlebitis
Contraindications: Hypersensitivity, anuria, uremia
Precautions: Severe respiratory disease/respiratory depression, pregnancy (C), cardiac edema, renal disease, infants
Pharmacokinetics:
IV: Excreted in urine
NURSING CONSIDERATIONS
Assess:
• Respiratory rate, rhythm, depth; notify physician of abnormalities that may indicate acidosis
• Electrolytes, blood glucose, chloride; CO_2, before, during treatment
• Urine pH, urinary output, urine glucose during beginning treatment
• I&O ratio, report large increase or decrease
• IV site for extravasation, phlebitis, thrombosis
• For signs of K^+ depletion
Administer:
• IV slowly to avoid pain at infusion site and toxicity
• IV undiluted as INF or added to priming fluid or ACD blood; give 5 ml or less/min
Evaluate:
• Therapeutic response: decreased metabolic acidosis
Teach patient/family:
• To increase K^+ in diet: bananas, oranges, cantaloupe, honeydew, spinach, potatoes, dried fruit

---

tropicamide (optic)
(troe-pik'a-mide)
Mydriacyl Ophthalmic, Tropicacyl, Tropicamide, Opticyl
Func. class.: Mydriatic, cycloplegia, anticholingeric
Chem. class.: Belladonna alkaloid

Action: Blocks response of sphincter muscle of iris and ciliary body, producing dilation and paralysis of accommodation
Uses: Fundus exam, cycloplegic refraction, dilation of pupil in inflammatory conditions of the iris and uveal tract
Dosage and routes:
• *Adult and child:* INSTILL 1-2 gtts of 1% sol, repeat in 5 min (refraction) or 1-2 gtts of 0.5% sol 15-20 min before fundus examination
Available forms: Sol 0.5%, 1%
Side effects/adverse reactions:
EENT: Blurred vision, photophobia, increased intraocular pressure, irritation, edema
SYST: Tachycardia, confusion, hallucinations, emotional changes in children, fever, flushing, dry skin, dry mouth, abdominal discomfort (infants: bladder distention, irregular pulse, drowsiness, blurred vision, ***respiratory depression***)
Contraindications: Hypersensitivity, infants <3 mo, glaucoma, conjunctivitis, elderly
Precautions: Pregnancy (C), lactation, children, Down syndrome
Pharmacokinetics:
INSTILL: Peak 20-40 min, (mydriasis), 20-35 min, (cycloplegia), duration 6 hr

---

italics = common side effects   ***bold italic*** = life threatening reactions

NURSING CONSIDERATIONS
Evaluate:
• Eye pain; discontinue use
Teach patient/family:
• To report change in vision, with blurring or loss of sight, trouble breathing, flushing
• Method of instillation, including pressure on lacrimal sac for 1 min, and not to touch dropper to eye
• That blurred vision will decrease with repeated use of drug
• Not to engage in hazardous activities until able to see
• To wait 5 min to use other drops
• Not to blink more than usual
• That dark glasses may be worn if photophobia occurs

---

tubocurarine chloride
(too-boe-kyoo-ar′een)
Tubarine,* Tubocuraine
Func. class.: Neuromuscular blocker
Chem. class.: Curare alkaloid

Action: Inhibits transmission of nerve impulses by binding with cholinergic receptor sites, antagonizing action of acetylcholine
Uses: Facilitation of endotracheal intubation, skeletal muscle relaxation during mechanical ventilation, surgery, or general anesthesia
Dosage and routes:
• *Adult:* IV BOL 0.4-0.5 mg/kg, then 0.08-0.10 mg/kg 20-45 min after 1st dose if needed for prolonged procedures
Available forms: Inj IV 3 mg/ml, 20 U/ml
Side effects/adverse reactions:
CV: Bradycardia, tachycardia, increased, decreased B/P
*RESP: **Prolonged apnea, bronchospasm, cyanosis, respiratory depression***

EENT: Increased secretions
INTEG: Rash, flushing, pruritus, urticaria
Contraindications: Hypersensitivity
Precautions: Pregnancy (C), cardiac disease, lactation, children <2 yr, electrolyte imbalances, dehydration, neuromuscular disease, respiratory disease
Pharmacokinetics:
IV: Onset 15 sec, peak 2-3 min, duration ½-1½ hr; half-life 1-3 hr, degraded in liver, kidney (minimally), excreted in urine (unchanged) crosses placenta
Interactions/incompatibilities:
• Increased neuromuscular blockade: aminoglycosides, clindamycin, lincomycin, quinidine, local anesthetics, polymyxin antibiotics, lithium, narcotic analgesics, thiazides, enflurane, isoflurane, trimethophan, Mg salts
• Dysrhythmias: theophylline
• Incompatible with barbiturates in solution or syringe; do not mix with any other drug in syringe
NURSING CONSIDERATIONS
Assess:
• For electrolyte imbalances (K, Mg); may lead to increased action of this drug
• Vital signs (B/P, pulse, respirations, airway) q15min until fully recovered; rate, depth, pattern of respirations, strength of hand grip
• I&O ratio; check for urinary retention, frequency, hesitancy
• Recovery: decreased paralysis of face, diaphragm, leg, arm, rest of body; allow to recover fully before completing neurologic assessment
• Allergic reactions: rash, fever, respiratory distress, pruritus; drug should be discontinued
Administer:
• With diazepam or morphine

---

when used for therapeutic paralysis; this drug provides no sedation alone
• Using nerve stimulator by anesthesiologist to determine neuromuscular blockade
• Anticholinesterase to reverse neuromuscular blockade
• IV undiluted 3 mg/ml; give single dose over 1-1½ sec by qualified person; diluted to 4 ml in NS given 0.5 ml/2 min myasthenia testing

Perform/provide:
• Storage in light-resistant area; use only fresh solution
• Reassurance if communication is difficult during recovery from neuromuscular blockade

Evaluate:
• Therapeutic response: paralysis of jaw, eyelid, head, neck, rest of body

Treatment of overdose: Edrophonium or neostigmine, atropine, monitor VS; may require mechanical ventilation

---

undecylenic acid (topical)
(un-de′sye-len-ik)
Caldesene, Cruex, Decylenes, Desenex, Desenex Maximum Strength, Protectol
Func. class.: Local antiinfective
Chem. class.: Antifungal, antibacterial

Action: Interferes with fungal cell membrane permeability
Uses: Tinea cruris, tinea pedis, diaper rash, minor skin irritations
Dosage and routes:
• *Adult and child:* TOP apply to affected areas bid
Available forms: Powder, oint, cream, liq, foam, soap

Side effects/adverse reactions:
INTEG: Rash, urticaria, stinging, burning
Contraindications: Hypersensitivity
Precautions: Pregnancy (C), lactation; impaired circulation; diabetes mellitus; broken, pustular skin; puncture wounds

NURSING CONSIDERATIONS
Assess:
• Allergic reaction: burning, stinging, swelling, redness
Administer:
• Enough medication to cover lesions completely
• After cleansing with soap, water before each application; dry well
Perform/provide:
• Storage at room temperature in dry place
Evaluate:
• Therapeutic response: decrease in size, number of lesions
Teach patient/family:
• To use medical asepsis (hand washing) before, after each application
• To apply with glove to prevent further infection
• To avoid use of OTC creams, ointments, lotions unless directed by physician
• To avoid inhaling and contact with eyes or other mucous membranes; to seek medical attention if symptoms persist
• To complete treatment regimen

---

uracil mustard
(yoor′a-sill)
Func. class.: Antineoplastic alkylating agent
Chem. class.: Nitrogen mustard

Action: Responsible for cross-linking DNA strands leading to cell

U

death; activity is not cell cycle specific

Uses: Hodgkin's disease, lymphomas; cervix, ovarian, lung cancer; chronic lymphocytic, myelocytic leukemia; reticulum cell sarcoma, mycosis fungoides; polycythemia vera

Dosage and routes:

• *Adult:* PO 1-2 mg/day × 3 mo or desired response, then 1 mg/day for 3 out of 4 wk until desired response or 3-5 mg × 7 days, not to exceed total dose of 0.5 mg/kg then 1 mg/day until desired response, then 1 mg/day 3 out of 4 wk

Available forms: Caps 1 mg

Side effects/adverse reactions:

*HEMA: **Thrombocytopenia, leukopenia,** anemia*

*GI: Nausea, vomiting, diarrhea, **hepatotoxicity***

GU: Amenorrhea, azoospermia

INTEG: Alopecia, dermatitis, pruritus, rash

Contraindications: Severe thrombocytopenia/leukopenia, hypersensitivity, pregnancy (X)

Precautions: Radiation therapy

Pharmacokinetics:

Excreted unchanged in urine

Interactions/incompatibilities:

• Increased toxicity: antineoplastics, radiation

NURSING CONSIDERATIONS

Assess:

• CBC, differential, platelet count weekly; withhold drug if WBC is <4000 or platelet count is <75,000; notify physician of results

• Renal function studies: BUN, serum uric acid, urine CrCl before, during therapy

• I&O ratio; report fall in urine output of 30 ml/hr

• Monitor temperature q4h (may indicate beginning infection)

• Liver function tests before, during therapy (bilirubin, AST, ALT, LDH) as needed or monthly

• Bleeding: hematuria, guaiac, bruising or petechiae, mucosa or orifices q8h

• Food preferences; list likes, dislikes

• Yellowing of skin and sclera, dark urine, clay-colored stools, itchy skin, abdominal pain, fever, diarrhea

• Effects of alopecia on body image; discuss feelings about body changes

• Inflammation of mucosa, breaks in skin

• Symptoms indicating severe allergic reaction: rash, pruritus, urticaria, itching

• Check for tartrazine dye allergy

Administer:

• Medications by oral route if possible; avoid IM, SC, IV routes to prevent infections

• Antacid before oral agent; give drug after evening meal, before bedtime

• Antiemetic 30-60 min before giving drug to prevent vomiting

• Antibiotics for prophylaxis of infection

• Topical or systemic analgesics for pain

• Local or systemic drugs for infection

Perform/provide:

• Storage in tight container at room temperature

• Strict medical asepsis, protective isolation if WBC levels are low

• Special skin care

• Liquid diet, including cola, Jell-O; dry toast or crackers may be added if patient is not nauseated or vomiting

• Increase fluid intake to 2-3 L/day to prevent urate deposits, calculi formation

Evaluate:

• Therapeutic response: decreased tumor size, spread of malignancy

Teach patient/family:

• Of protective isolation precautions

• That effect may take as long as 3 mo

• To report signs of infection: increased temperature, sore throat, flu symptoms

• To report signs of anemia: fatigue, headache, faintness, shortness of breath, irritability

• To avoid use of razors, commercial mouthwash

• To avoid use of aspirin products, ibuprofen

• That azoospermia, amenorrhea can occur, are reversible after discontinuing treatment

• That hair may be lost during treatment; a wig or hairpiece may make patient feel better; new hair may be different in color, texture

• To avoid foods with citric acid, hot or rough texture

---

urea

(yoor-ee′a)

Ureaphil, Carbamex*

Func. class.: Diuretic, osmotic
Chem. class.: Carbonic acid diamide salt

Action: Elevates plasma osmolality, increasing flow of water into the extracellular compartment

Uses: To decrease intracranial pressure, intraocular pressure

Dosage and routes:

• *Adult:* IV 1-1.5 g/kg of a 30% sol over 1-3 hr; do not exceed 120 g/day

• *Child >2 yr:* IV 0.5-1.5 g/kg, not to exceed 4 ml/min

• *Child <2 yr:* IV 0.1 g/kg, not to exceed 4 ml/min

Available forms: Inj IV 40 g/150 ml

Side effects/adverse reactions:

CNS: Dizziness, headache, disorientation, fever, syncope, *headache*

GI: Nausea, vomiting

INTEG: Venous thrombosis, phlebitis, extravasation

CV: Postural hypotension, tachycardia

Contraindications: Severe renal disease, active intracranial bleeding, marked dehydration, liver failure

Precautions: Hepatic disease, renal disease, pregnancy (C), electrolyte imbalances, lactation

Pharmacokinetics:

IV: Onset ½-1 hr, peak 1 hr, duration 3-10 hr (diuresis), 5-6 hr (intraocular pressure); half-life 1 hr; excreted in urine, crosses placenta, excreted in breast milk

Interactions/incompatibilities:

• Incompatible with whole blood, alkalines in sol or syringe

• Increased renal excretion of: lithium

NURSING CONSIDERATIONS

Assess:

• Weight, I&O daily to determine fluid loss; effect of drug may be decreased if used qd; for hourly urinary output

• Rate, depth, rhythm of respiration, effect of exertion

• B/P lying, standing, postural hypotension may occur

• Electrolytes: K, Na, Cl; include BUN, blood sugar, CBC, serum creatinine, blood pH, ABGs, liver function tests

• Signs of metabolic acidosis: drowsiness, restlessness

U

---

italics = common side effects   ***bold italic*** = life threatening reactions

• Signs of hypokalemia: postural hypotension, malaise, fatigue, tachycardia, leg cramps, weakness
• Temperature elevation, signs of extravasation
• Confusion, especially in elderly; take safety precautions if needed
• Hydration: skin turgor, thirst, dry mucous membranes

Administer:
• IV after diluting 30 g/100 ml diluent with D_5, D_{10}; run 30% sol over 1-2 hr; check for extravasation; do not exceed 4 ml/min; may cause bleeding; use IV filter
• Within minutes of reconstitution; sol becomes ammonia on standing

Evaluate:
• Therapeutic response: improvement in edema of feet, legs, sacral area daily if medication is being used in CHF

Teach patient/family:
• That drug will cause diuresis in ½ hr

Treatment of overdose: Lavage if taken orally; monitor electrolytes, administer IV fluids, monitor BUN, hydration, CV status

---

urofollitropin

(yoor-oo-foll′i-tropin)
Metrodin
Func. class.: Ovulation stimulant
Chem. class.: Gonadotropin

Action: Stimulates ovarian follicular growth in primary ovarian failure

Uses: Induction of ovulation in polycystic ovarian disease in those who have elevated LH/FSH ratios and have failed to respond to other treatment

Dosage and routes:
• *Adult:* IM 75 IU/day × 7-12 days, then 5000-10,000 U HCG 1 day after last urofollitropin if pregnancy does not occur; may repeat for 2 courses before increasing dose to 150 IU/day 7-12 days then 5000-10,000 U HCG 1 day after last urofollitropin; may repeat for 2 more courses

Available forms: Powder for injection 0.83 mg (76 IU FSH)/amp

Side effects/adverse reactions:
CNS: Malaise
GI: Nausea, vomiting, constipation, increased appetite, abdominal pain
INTEG: Rash, dermatitis, urticaria, alopecia
GU: Polyuria, frequency, birth defects, spontaneous abortions, multiple ovulation, breast pain

Contraindications: Hypersensitivity, pregnancy, undiagnosed vaginal bleeding, intracranial lesion, ovarian cyst not caused by polycystic ovarian disease

Precautions: Lactation, arterial thromboembolism

Pharmacokinetics:
Detoxified in liver, excreted in feces, stored in fat

NURSING CONSIDERATIONS
Assess:
• At same time qd to maintain drug level

Evaluate:
• Therapeutic response: ovulation, pregnancy

Teach patient/family:
• That multiple births are common after taking this drug
• To notify physician if low abdominal pain occurs; may indicate ovarian cyst, cyst rupture
• Method of taking, recording basal body temperature to determine whether ovulation has occurred
• That if ovulation can be determined (there is a slight decrease,

then a sharp increase for ovulation), to attempt coitus 3 days before and qod until after ovulation
• If pregnancy is suspected, physician must be notified immediately

---

urokinase
(yoor-oh-kin′ase)
Abbokinase, Abbokinase Open-Cath
Func. class.: Thrombolytic enzyme
Chem. class.: β-Hemolytic streptococcus filtrate (purified)

Action: Promotes thrombolysis by directly converting plasminogen to plasmin

Uses: Venous thrombosis, pulmonary embolism, arterial thrombosis, arterial embolism, arteriovenous cannula occlusion, lysis of coronary artery thrombi after myocardial infarction

Dosage and routes:
Lysis of pulmonary emboli
• *Adult:* IV 4400 IU/kg/hr × 12-24 hr, not to exceed 200 ml; then IV heparin, then anticoagulants
Coronary artery thrombosis
• *Adult:* INSTILL 6000 IU/min into occluded artery for 1-2 hr after giving IV bol of heparin 2500-10,000 U
• May also give as IV infusion of 2-3 million U over 45-90 min
Venous catheter occlusion
• *Adult:* INSTILL 5000 IU into line, wait 5 min, then aspirate, repeat aspiration attempts q5min × ½ hr; if occlusion has not been removed, then cap line and wait ½-1 hr then aspirate; may need 2nd dose if still occluded
Available forms: Inj
Side effects/adverse reactions:
*HEMA: Decreased Hct, **bleeding***

INTEG: Rash, urticaria, phlebitis at IV infusion site, itching, flushing
CNS: Headache, fever,
GI: Nausea
RESP: Altered respirations, SOB, **bronchospasm**
MS: Low back pain
CV: Hypertension, dysrhythmias
EENT: Periorbital edema
*SYST: **GI, GU, intracranial, retroperitoneal bleeding,*** surface bleeding, **anaphylaxis**
Contraindications: Hypersensitivity, active bleeding, intraspinal surgery, neoplasms of CNS, ulcerative colitis/enteritis, severe hypertension, renal disease, hepatic disease, hypocoagulation, COPD, subacute bacterial endocarditis, rheumatic valvular disease, cerebral embolism/thrombosis/hemorrhage, intraarterial diagnostic procedure or surgery (10 days), recent major surgery
Precautions: Arterial emboli from left side of heart, pregnancy (B)
Pharmacokinetics:
IV: Half-life 10-20 min; small amounts excreted in urine
Interactions/incompatibilities:
• Bleeding potential: aspirin, indomethacin, phenylbutazone, anticoagulants
• Considered incompatible with any drug in sol or syringe
NURSING CONSIDERATIONS
Assess:
• VS, B/P, pulse, resp, neurologic signs, temp at least q4h; temp >104° F (40° C) is an indicator of internal bleeding, cardiac rhythm following intracoronary administration
• For neurologic changes that may indicate intracranial bleeding
• Retroperitoneal bleeding: back pain, leg weakness, diminished pulses

---

italics = common side effects   ***bold italic*** = life threatening reactions

U

• Peripheral pulses, lung sounds, respiratory function
• Allergy: fever, rash, itching, chills; mild reaction may be treated with antihistamines
• Bleeding during 1st hr of treatment (hematuria, hematemesis, bleeding from mucous membranes, epistaxis, ecchymosis)
• Blood studies (Hct, platelets, PTT, PT, TT, APTT) before starting therapy; PT or APTT must be less than 2 × control before starting therapy TT or PT q3-4h during treatment

Administer:
• Using infusion pump, terminal filter (0.45 μm or smaller)
• IV; reconstitute only with 5.2 ml sterile water for inj (not bacteriostatic water), and roll (not shake) to enhance reconstitution; further dilute with 190 ml; give as intermittent inf or give to clear cannula by using 1 ml of diluted drug; inject into cannula slowly, clamp 5 min, aspirate clot
• As soon as thrombi identified; not useful for thrombi over 1 wk old
• Cryoprecipitate or fresh frozen plasma if bleeding occurs
• Loading dose at beginning of therapy; may require increased loading doses
• Heparin therapy after thrombolytic therapy is discontinued, TT or APTT less than 2 × control (about 3-4 hr)

Perform/provide:
• Storage in refrigerator; use immediately after reconstitution
• Bed rest during entire course of treatment; use caution in handling patients
• Avoidance of venous or arterial puncture procedures: inj, rectal temp
• Treatment of fever with acetaminophen or aspirin
• Placement of sign above patient's bed stating urokinase therapy
• Pressure for 30 sec to minor bleeding sites; 30 min to sites of arterial puncture followed by pressure dressing; inform physician if hemostasis not attained, apply pressure dressing

Evaluate:
• Therapeutic response: decreased clotting, thrombosis, embolism

Lab test interferences:
Increase: PT, APTT, TT

---

ursodiol
(your-soo'-dee-ol)
Actigall
Func. class.: Gallstone solubilizing agent
Chem. class.: Ursodeoxycholic acid

Action: Suppresses hepatic synthesis, secretion of cholesterol; inhibits intestinal absorption of cholesterol

Uses: Dissolution of radiolucent, noncalcified gallbladder stones (less than 20 mm in diameter) in which surgery is not indicated

Dosage and routes:
• *Adult:* PO 8-10 mg/kg/day in 2-3 divided doses using gallbladder ultrasound q6mo; determine if stones have dissolved; if so, continue therapy, repeat ultrasound within 1-3 mo

Available forms: Caps 300 mg

Side effects/adverse reactions:
GI: Diarrhea, nausea, vomiting, abdominal pain, constipation, stomatitis, flatulence, dyspepsia, biliary pain
INTEG: Pruritus, rash, urticaria, dry skin, sweating, alopecia

---

CNS: Headache, anxiety, depression, insomnia, fatigue
MS: Arthralgia, myalgia, back pain
OTHER: Cough, rhinitis
Contraindications: Calcified cholesterol stones, radiopaque stones, radiolucent bile pigment stones, chronic liver disease, hypersensitivity
Precautions: Pregnancy (B), lactation, children
Pharmacokinetics: 80% excreted in feces, 20% metabolized, excreted into bile, lost in feces
Interactions/incompatibilities:
• Reduced action of ursodiol: cholestyramine, colestipol, aluminum-based antacids

NURSING CONSIDERATIONS
Assess:
• GI status: diarrhea, abdominal pain, nausea, vomiting; drug may have to be discontinued if side effects are severe
• Skin for pruritus, rash, urticaria, dry skin; provide soothing lotion to lesions
• Musculoskeletal status: aches or stiffness in joints
Administer:
• For up to 9-12 mo; if no improvement is seen, discontinue drug
Evaluate:
• Therapeutic response: decreasing size of stones on ultrasound
Teach patient/family:
• That anxiety, depression, insomnia are side effects and are reversible after discontinuing drug

**valproate sodium/
valproate sodium—
valproic acid/valproic
acid**
(val-proe′ate)
Depakene Syrup, Depakote/
Depakene
Func. class.: Anticonvulsant
Chem. class.: Carboxylic acid derivative

Action: Increases levels of γ-aminobutyric acid (GABA) in brain
Uses: Simple, complex (petit mal) absence, mixed, tonic-clonic (grand mal) seizures
Dosage and routes:
• *Adult and child:* PO 15 mg/kg/day divided in 2-3 doses, may increase by 5-10 mg/kg/day qwk, not to exceed 30 mg/kg/day in 2-3 divided doses
Available forms: Caps 250 mg; tabs 125, 250, 500 mg; syr 250 mg/5 ml
Side effects/adverse reactions:
*HEMA: **Thrombocytopenia, leukopenia, lymphocytosis,** increased pro-time*
CNS: Sedation, drowsiness, dizziness, headache, incoordination, paresthesia, depression, hallucinations, behavioral changes, tremors, aggression, weakness
GI: Nausea, vomiting, constipation, diarrhea, heartburn, anorexia, cramps, **hepatic failure, pancreatitis, toxic hepatitis,** stomatitis
INTEG: Rash, alopecia, bruising
GU: Enuresis, irregular menses
Contraindications: Hypersensitivity
Precautions: MI (recovery phase), hepatic disease, renal disease, Addison's disease, pregnancy (D), lactation

V

Pharmacokinetics:
PO: Onset 15-30 min, peak 1-4 hr, duration 4-6 hr
REC: Onset slow, duration 4-6 hr
Metabolized by liver, excreted by kidneys, in feces, crosses placenta, excreted in breast milk, half-life 6-16 hr

Interactions/incompatibilities:
• Increased effects: CNS depressants
• Increased toxicity: salicylates, warfarin, sulfinpyrazone, carbamazepine, phenytoin

Lab test interferences:
False-positive: Ketones

NURSING CONSIDERATIONS
Assess:
• Blood studies: Hct, Hgb, RBCs, serum folate, pro-time, Vit D if on long-term therapy
• Hepatic studies: AST, ALT, bilirubin, creatinine, failure
• Blood levels: therapeutic level 50-100 µg/ml
• Mental status: mood, sensorium, affect, memory (long, short)
• Respiratory dysfunction: respiratory depression, character, rate, rhythm; hold drug if respirations are <12/min or if pupils are dilated

Administer:
• Tablets or capsules whole
• Elixir alone; do not dilute with carbonated beverage; do not give syrup to patients on sodium restriction
• Give with food or milk to decrease GI symptoms

Evaluate:
• Therapeutic response: decreased seizures

Teach patient/family:
• That physical dependency may result when used for extended periods
• To avoid driving, other activities that require alertness

• Not to discontinue medication quickly after long-term use; convulsions may result
• To report visual disturbances, rash, diarrhea, light-colored stools, jaundice, protracted vomiting to physician

vancomycin HCl
(van-koe-mye′sin)
Lyphocin, Vancocin, Vancoled, Vancomycin HCl
Func. class.: Antibacterial
Chem. class.: Tricyclic glycopeptide

Action: Inhibits bacterial cell wall synthesis

Uses: Resistant staphylococcal infections, pseudomembranous colitis, staphylococcal enterocolitis, endocarditis prophylaxis for dental procedures

Dosage and routes:
Serious staphylococcal infections
• *Adult:* IV 500 mg q6h or 1 g q12h
• *Child:* IV 40 mg/kg/day divided q6h
• *Neonates:* IV 15 mg/kg initially followed by 10 mg/kg q8-12h

Pseudomembranous/staphylococcal enterocolitis
• *Adult:* PO 500 mg -2 g/day in 3-4 divided doses for 7-10 days
• *Child:* PO 40 mg/kg/day divided q6h, not to exceed 2 g/day

Endocarditis prophylaxis
• *Adult:* IV 1 g over 1 hr, 1 hr before dental procedure

Available forms: Pulvules 125, 250 mg; powder for oral sol 1, 10 g; powder for inj IV 500 mg, 1 g

Side effects/adverse reactions:
CV: Cardiac arrest, vascular collapse
EENT: Ototoxicity, permanent deafness, tinnitus

*HEMA: **Leukopenia, eosinophilia, neutropenia***
*GI: **Nausea***
RESP: Wheezing, dyspnea
*SYST: **Anaphylaxis***
*GU: **Nephrotoxicity,** increased BUN, creatinine, albumin, **fatal uremia***
INTEG: Chills, fever, rash, thrombophlebitis at injection site, urticaria, pruritus, necrosis (Redman's syndrome)
Contradindications: Hypersensitivity, decreased hearing
Precautions: Renal disease, pregnancy (C), lactation, elderly, neonates
Pharmacokinetics:
Peak 5 min IV; half-life 4-8 hr; excreted in urine (active form); crosses placenta
Interactions/incompatibilities:
• Ototoxicity or nephrotoxicity: aminoglycosides, cephalosporins, colistin, polymyxin, bacitracin, cisplatin, amphotericin B
• Incompatible with aminophylline, amobarbital, chloramphenicol, chlorothiazide, dexamethasone, heparin, hydrocortisone, methicillin, penicillins, pentobarbital, phenobarbital, phenytoin, prochlorperazine, secobarbital, warfarin
NURSING CONSIDERATIONS
Assess:
• I&O ratio; report hematuria, oliguria, since nephrotoxicity may occur
• Any patient with compromised renal system; drug is excreted slowly in poor renal system function; toxicity may occur rapidly
• Blood studies: WBC
• C&S before drug therapy; drug may be given as soon as culture is taken

• Auditory function during, after treatment
• B/P during administration; sudden drop may indicate Redman's syndrome
• Signs of infection
• Hearing loss, ringing, roaring in ears; drug should be discontinued
• Skin eruptions
• Respiratory status: rate, character, wheezing, tightness in chest
• Allergies before treatment, reaction of each medication; place allergies on chart, Kardex in bright red letters; notify all people giving drugs
Administer:
• After reconstitution with 10 ml sterile water for injection (500 mg/10 ml) further dilution is needed for IV, 500 mg/100 ml NS, D₅W given as INT INF over 1 hr
• Antihistamine if Redman's syndrome occurs: decreased B/P, flushing of neck, face
• Dose based on serum concentration
Perform/provide:
• Storage at room temperature for up to 2 wk after reconstitution
• Adrenalin, suction, tracheostomy set, endotracheal intubation equipment on unit; anaphylaxis may occur
• Adequate intake of fluids (2 L) to prevent nephrotoxicity
Evaluate:
• Therapeutic response: absence of fever, sore throat
Teach patient/family:
• Aspects of drug therapy: need to complete entire course of medication to ensure organism death (7-10 days); culture may be taken after completed course of medication
• To report sore throat, fever, fatigue; could indicate superimposed infection

italics = common side effects   ***bold italic*** = life threatening reactions

• That drug must be taken in equal intervals around clock to maintain blood levels

---

vasopressin (antidiuretic hormone)

(vay-soe-press'in)
Pitressin Synthetic
Func. class.: Pituitary hormone
Chem. class.: Lysine vasopressin

Action: Promotes reabsorption of water by action on renal tubular epithelium; causes vasoconstriction
Uses: Diabetes insipidus (nonnephrogenic/nonpsychogenic), abdominal distention postoperatively, bleeding esophageal varices
Dosage and routes:
Diabetes insipidus
• *Adult:* IM/SC 5-10 units bid-qid as needed; IM/SC 2.5-5 units q2-3 days (Pitressin Tannate) for chronic therapy
• *Child:* IM/SC 2.5-10 units bid-qid as needed; IM/SC 1.25-2.5 units q2-3 days (Pitressin Tannate) for chronic therapy
Abdominal distention
• *Adult:* IM 5 units, then q3-4h, increasing to 10 units if needed (aqueous)
Available forms: Inj IM, SC 20, 5 U/ml (tannate), spray, cotton pledgets
Side effects/adverse reactions:
EENT: Nasal irritation, congestion, rhinitis
CNS: Drowsiness, headache, lethargy, flushing
GU: Vulval pain, uterine cramping
GI: Nausea, heartburn, cramps
CV: Increased B/P
MISC: Tremor, sweating, vertigo, urticaria, bronchial constriction

Contraindications: Hypersensitivity, chronic nephritis
Precautions: CAD, pregnancy (C)
Pharmacokinetics:
NASAL: Onset 1 hr, duration 3-8 hr, half-life 15 min; metabolized in liver, kidneys, excreted in urine
NURSING CONSIDERATIONS
Assess:
• Nasal mucosa if given by intranasal spray; for irritation
• Pulse, B/P, when giving drug IV or IM
• I&O ratio, weight daily; check for edema in extremities; if water retention is severe, diuretic may be prescribed
• H_2O intoxication: lethargy, behavioral changes, disorientation, neuromuscular excitability
Evaluate:
• Therapeutic response: absence of severe thirst, decreased urine output, osmolality

---

vecuronium bromide

(vek-yoo-roe'nee-um)
Norcuron
Func. class.: Neuromuscular blocker
Chem. class.: Monoquaternary analog of pancuronium

Action: Inhibits transmission of nerve impulses by binding with cholinergic receptor sites, antagonizing action of acetylcholine
Uses: Facilitation of endotracheal intubation, skeletal muscle relaxation during mechanical ventilation, surgery, general anesthesia
Dosage and routes:
• *Adult and child >9 yr:* IV BOL 0.08-0.10 mg/kg, then 0.010-0.015 mg/kg for prolonged procedures
Available forms: IV 10 mg/5 ml

Side effects/adverse reactions:

CNS: Skeletal muscle weakness or paralysis, rarely

RESP: **Prolonged apnea, possible respiratory paralysis**

Contraindications: Hypersensitivity

Precautions: Pregnancy (C), cardiac disease, lactation, children <2 yr, electrolyte imbalances, dehydration, neuromuscular disease, respiratory disease

Pharmacokinetics:

IV: Onset 15 min, peak 3-5 min, duration 45-60 min; half-life 65-75 min; not metabolized; excreted in feces; crosses placenta

Interactions/incompatibilities:

• Increased neuromuscular blockade: aminoglycosides, clindamycin, lincomycin, quinidine, local anesthetics, polymyxin antibiotics, lithium, narcotic analgesics, thiazides, enflurane, isoflurane, succinylcholine

• Dysrhythmias: theophylline

• Incompatibility unknown

NURSING CONSIDERATIONS

Assess:

• For electrolyte imbalances (K, Mg); may lead to increased action of this drug

• Vital signs (B/P, pulse, respirations, airway) q15min until fully recovered; rate, depth, pattern of respirations, strength of hand grip

• I&O ratio; check for urinary retention, frequency, hesitancy

• Recovery: decreased paralysis of face, diaphragm, leg, arm, rest of body; allow to recover fully before completing neurologic assessment

• Allergic reactions: rash, fever, respiratory distress, pruritus; drug should be discontinued

Administer:

• With diazepam or morphine when used for therapeutic paralysis; this drug provides no sedation alone

• Using nerve stimulator by anesthesiologist to determine neuromuscular blockade

• Anticholinesterase to reverse neuromuscular blockade

• IV after diluting with diluent provided; give by direct IV over 1 min; may give as continuous inf 10-20 mg/100 ml; titrate to patient response (only by qualified person)

Perform/provide:

• Storage in refrigerator; discard in 24 hr

• Reassurance if communication is difficult during recovery from neuromuscular blockade

Evaluate:

• Therapeutic response: paralysis of jaw, eyelid, head, neck, rest of body

Treatment of overdose: Edrophonium or neostigmine, atropine, monitor VS; may require mechanical ventilation

---

verapamil HCl

(ver-ap'-a-mill)

Calan, Calan SR, Isoptin, Isoptin SR, Verapamil HCl, Verelan

Func. class.: Calcium channel blocker

Chem. class.: Phenylalkylamine

Action: Inhibits calcium ion influx across cell membrane during cardiac depolarization; produces relaxation of coronary vascular smooth muscle; dilates coronary arteries; decreases SA/AV node conduction; dilates peripheral arteries

Uses: Chronic stable angina pectoris, vasospastic angina, dysrhythmias, hypertension

V

---

italics = common side effects   ***bold italic*** = life threatening reactions

Dosage and routes:
• *Adult:* PO 80 mg tid or qid, increase qwk; IV BOL 5-10 mg > 2 min, repeat if necessary in 30 min
• *Child 0-1 yr:* IV BOL 0.1-0.2 mg/kg > 2 min with ECG monitoring, repeat if necessary in 30 min
• *Child 1-15 yr:* IV BOL 0.1-0.3 mg/kg over > 2 min, repeat in 30 min, not to exceed 10 mg in a single dose

Available forms: Tabs 40, 80, 120 mg; sus rel tabs, 240 mg; inj 2.5 mg/ml

Side effects/adverse reactions:
*CV: Edema, **CHF**, bradycardia, hypotension, palpitations, AV block*
GI: Nausea, diarrhea, gastric upset, constipation, increased liver function studies
GU: Nocturia, polyuria
CNS: Headache, drowsiness, dizziness, anxiety, depression, weakness, insomnia, confusion, lightheadedness

Contraindications: Sick sinus syndrome, 2nd or 3rd degree heart block, hypotension less than 90 mm Hg systolic, cardiogenic shock, severe CHF

Precautions: CHF, hypotension, hepatic injury, pregnancy (C), lactation, children, renal disease, concomitant β-blocker therapy

Pharmacokinetics:
IV: Onset 3 min, peak 3-5 min, duration 10-20 min
PO: Onset variable, peak 3-4 hr, duration 17-24 hr, half-life (biphasic) 4 min, 3-7 hr (terminal); metabolized by liver, excreted in urine (96% as metabolites)

Interactions/incompatibilities:
• Increased hypotension: prazosin, quinidine
• Increased effects: β-blockers, antihypertensives, cimetidine
• Decreased effects of: lithium

• Increased levels of: digoxin, theophylline, cyclosporine, carbamazepine, nondepolarizing muscle relaxants
• Incompatible with albumin, amphotericin B, ampicillin, dobutamine, hydralazine, mezlocillin, nafcillin, oxacillin, NaCO₃

Lab test interferences:
Increase: Liver function tests

NURSING CONSIDERATIONS
Assess:
• Cardiac status: B/P, pulse, respiration, ECG intervals (PR, QRS, QT)

Administer:
• IV undiluted through Y-tube or 3-way stopcock of compatible sol; give over 2 min, or 3 min elderly
• Before meals, hs; sus rel give with food

Evaluate:
• Therapeutic response: decreased anginal pain, decreased B/P, dysrhythmias

Teach patient/family:
• How to take pulse before taking drug; record or graph should be kept
• To avoid hazardous activities until stabilized on drug, dizziness no longer a problem
• To limit caffeine consumption; no alcohol products
• To avoid OTC drugs unless directed by a physician
• To comply with all areas of medical regimen: diet, exercise, stress reduction, drug therapy
• To change positions slowly to prevent syncope

Treatment of overdose: Defibrillation, atropine for AV block, vasopressor for hypotension

---

vidarabine (ophthalmic)

(vye-dare′a-been)

Vira-A Ophthalmic

Func. class.: Antiviral

Chem. class.: Purine nucleoside

Action: Inhibits viral DNA synthesis by blocking DNA polymerase

Uses: Recurrent epithelial keratitis, superficial keratitis due to herpes simplex, cytomegalovirus, varicella zoster

Dosage and routes:

• *Adult and child:* TOP ½ inch oint into conjunctival sac q3h, 5 times daily

Available forms include: Oint 3%

Side effects/adverse reactions:

EENT: Burning, stinging, photophobia, pain, temporary visual haze, edema

Contraindications: Hypersensitivity

Precautions: Antibiotic hypersensitivity, pregnancy (C)

NURSING CONSIDERATIONS

Assess:

• Allergy: itching, lacrimation, redness, swelling

Administer:

• After washing hands; cleanse crusts or discharge from eye before application

Perform/provide:

• Storage at room temperature

Evaluate:

• Therapeutic response: absence of redness, inflammation, tearing

Teach patient/family:

• To use drug exactly as prescribed

• Not to use eye makeup, towels, washcloths, or eye medication of others, or reinfection may occur

• That drug container tip should not be touched to eye

• To report itching, increased redness, burning, stinging, photophobia; drug should be discontinued

• That drug may cause blurred vision when ointment is applied

• To use sunglasses to prevent photophobia

vidarabine

(vye-dare′a-been)

Vira-A

Func. class.: Antibacterial, antiviral

Chem. class.: Purine nucleoside

Action: Inhibits bacterial/viral replication by preventing DNA synthesis

Uses: Herpes simplex virus encephalitis, varicella-zoster encephalomyelitis, herpes zoster in immunosuppressed

Dosage and routes:

• *Adult and child:* IV INF 15 mg/kg/day × 10 days; infuse over 12-24 hr

Available forms: Inj IV 200 mg/ml

Side effects/adverse reactions:

CNS: Psychosis, hallucinations, dizziness, weakness, tremors, *fatal metabolic encephalopathy,* confusion, malaise, headache

GU: SIADH

HEMA: Anemia, thrombocytopenia, neutropenia

GI: Nausea, vomiting, anorexia, diarrhea, weight loss

INTEG: Pain, thrombophlebitis at injection site

Contraindications: Hypersensitivity

Precautions: Renal disease, liver disease, lactation, pregnancy (C)

Pharmacokinetics: Crosses blood-brain barrier, excreted by kidneys (metabolites), crosses placenta, half-life 1½-3 hr

Interactions/incompatibilities:

• Increased neurologic side effects: allopurinol

• Incompatible with blood, protein products

NURSING CONSIDERATIONS
Assess:

• Liver studies: AST, ALT

• Blood studies: WBC, diff, RBC, Hct, Hgb, platelets

• Renal studies: urinalysis, protein, blood

• C&S before drug therapy; drug may be taken as soon as culture is taken; C&S may be taken after therapy

• Bowel pattern before, during treatment

• Fluid overload; drug requires large volume to stay in sol

• Weakness, tremors, confusion, dizziness, psychosis; if these occur, drug may have to be decreased or discontinued

Administer:

• Shake solution; dilute to 450 mg/L IV; give fluid at constant rate over 12-24 hr, using in-line filter with mean pore diameter of 0.45 mm or less

Evaluate:

• Therapeutic response: decreased amount of lesion, itching

---

vinblastine sulfate (VLB)

(vin-blast'een)

Velban, Velbe,* Vinblastine Sulfate

Func. class.: Antineoplastic
Chem. class.: Vinca rosea alkaloid

Action: Inhibits mitotic activity, arrests cell cycle at metaphase; inhibits RNA synthesis, blocks cellular use of glutamic acid needed for purine synthesis; a vesicant

Uses: Breast, testicular cancer, lymphomas, neuroblastoma; Hodgkin's, non-Hodgkin's lymphomas; mycosis fungoides, histiocytosis, Kaposi's sarcoma

Dosage and routes:

• *Adult:* IV 0.1 mg/kg or 3.7 mg/m² qwk or q2wk, not to exceed 0.5 mg/kg or 18.5 mg/m² qwk

• Child: 2.5 mg/m² then dose of 3.75, 5.0, 6.25 and 7.5 at 7-day intervals

Available forms: Inj IV, powder 10 mg for 10 ml IV inj

Side effects/adverse reactions:

*HEMA: **Thrombocytopenia, leukopenia, myelosuppression***

*GI: Nausea, vomiting, ileus, anorexia, stomatitis, constipation, abdominal pain, GI, rectal bleeding, **hepatotoxicity,** pharyngitis*

*GU: Urinary retention, **renal failure***

INTEG: Rash, alopecia, photosensitivity

*RESP: **Fibrosis, pulmonary infiltrate***

CV: Tachycardia, orthostatic hypotension

*CNS: Paresthesias, peripheral neuropathy, depression, headache, **convulsions***

META: SIADH

Contraindications: Hypersensitivity, infants, pregnancy (D)

Precautions: Renal disease, hepatic disease

Pharmacokinetics: Half-life (triphasic) 35 min, 53 min, 19 hr, metabolized in liver, excreted in urine, feces, crosses blood-brain barrier

Interactions/incompatibilities:

• Increased action of: methotrexate

• Do not use with radiation

• Synergism: bleomycin

• Decreased phenytoin level: phenytoin
• Bronchospasm: mitomycin
• Considered incompatible with any drug in sol or syringe

NURSING CONSIDERATIONS
Assess:
• CBC, differential, platelet count weekly; withhold drug if WBC is <4000 or platelet count is <75,000; notify physician of results
• Pulmonary function tests, chest x-ray studies before, during therapy; chest x-ray film should be obtained q2wk during treatment
• Neurologic status: sensory-vibratory evaluation if side effects occur
• Renal function studies: BUN, serum uric acid, urine CrCl, electrolytes before, during therapy
• I&O ratio; report fall in urine output of 30 ml/hr
• Monitor temperature q4h; may indicate beginning infection
• Liver function tests before, during therapy (bilirubin, AST, ALT, LDH) as needed or monthly
• RBC, Hct, Hgb, since these may be decreased
• Bleeding: hematuria, guaiac, bruising or petechiae, mucosa of orifices q8h
• Dyspnea, rales, unproductive cough, chest pain, tachypnea, fatigue, increased pulse, pallor, lethargy
• Food preferences; list likes, dislikes
• Effects of alopecia on body image; discuss feelings about body changes
• Sensitivity of feet/hands, which precedes neuropathy
• Inflammation of mucosa, breaks in skin
• Yellowing of skin and sclera, dark urine, clay-colored stools, itchy skin, abdominal pain, fever, diarrhea
• Buccal cavity q8h for dryness, sores, or ulceration, white patches, oral pain, bleeding, dysphagia
• Local irritation, pain, burning, discoloration at injection site
• Symptoms indicating severe allergic reaction: rash, pruritus, urticaria, purpuric skin lesions, itching, flushing
• Frequency of stools and characteristics: cramping, acidosis; signs of dehydration: rapid respirations, poor skin turgor, decreased urine output, dry skin, restlessness, weakness

Administer:
• IV after diluting 10 mg/10 ml NaCl; give through Y-tube or 3-way stopcock or directly over 1 min
• Hyaluronidase 150 U/ml in 1 ml NaCl, warm compress for extravasation for vesicant activity treatment
• Antacid before oral agent; give drug after evening meal, before bedtime
• Antiemetic 30-60 min before giving drug and prn to prevent vomiting
• Local or systemic drugs for infection
• Transfusion for anemia
• Antispasmodic for GI symptoms

Perform/provide:
• Deep-breathing exercises with patient 3-4 × day; place in semi-Fowler's position
• Liquid diet: cola, Jell-O; dry toast or crackers may be added if patient is not nauseated or vomiting
• Increase fluid intake to 2-3 L/day to prevent urate deposits, calculi formation
• Rinsing of mouth 3-4 × day with water
• Brushing of teeth 2-3 × day

V

---

italics = common side effects   ***bold italic*** = life threatening reactions

with soft brush or cotton-tipped applicators for stomatitis; use unwaxed dental floss
• Nutritious diet with iron, vitamin supplements
• HOB raised to facilitate breathing
Evaluate:
• Therapeutic response: decreased tumor size, spread of malignancy
Teach patient/family:
• To report any complaints or side effects to the nurse or physician
• To report any changes in breathing or coughing
• That hair may be lost during treatment, a wig or hairpiece may make patient feel better; tell patient that new hair may be different in color, texture
• To report change in gait or numbness in extremities; may indicate neuropathy
• To avoid foods with citric acid, hot or rough texture
• To report any bleeding, white spots or ulcerations in mouth to physician; tell patient to examine mouth qd

---

vincristine sulfate (VCR)

(vin-kris´teen)

Oncovin, Vincasar PFS, Vincristine Sulfate

Func. class.: Antineoplastic
Chem. class.: Vinca alkaloid

Action: Inhibits mitotic activity, arrests cell cycle at metaphase; inhibits RNA synthesis, blocks cellular use of glutamic acid needed for purine synthesis; a vesicant
Uses: Breast, lung cancer, lymphomas, neuroblastoma, Hodgkin's disease, acute lymphoblastic and other leukemias, rhabdomyosarcoma, Wilms' tumor, osteogenic and other sarcomas
Dosage and routes:
• *Adult:* IV 1-2 mg/m²/wk, not to exceed 2 mg
• *Child:* IV 1.5-2 mg/m²/wk, not to exceed 2 mg
Available forms: Inj IV 1 mg/ml
Side effects/adverse reactions:
INTEG: Alopecia
HEMA: **Thrombocytopenia, leukopenia, myelosuppression, anemia**
GI: Nausea, vomiting, anorexia, stomatitis, constipation, **paralytic ileus,** abdominal pain, **hepatotoxicity**
CV: Orthostatic hypotension
CNS: Decreased reflexes, numbness, weakness, motor difficulties, CNS depression, cranial nerve paralysis, **seizures**
Contraindications: Hypersensitivity, infants, pregnancy (D)
Precautions: Renal disease, hepatic disease, hypertension, neuromuscular disease
Pharmacokinetics: Half-life (triphasic) 0.85 min, 7.4 min, 164 min; metabolized in liver; excreted in bile, feces; crosses placental barrier, blood-brain barrier
Interactions/incompatibilities:
• Increased action of: methotrexate, anticoagulants
• Do not use with radiation
• Neurotoxicity: peripheral nervous system drugs
• Decreased digoxin level: digoxin
• Decreased action of vincristine: L-asparaginase
• Acute pulmonary reactions: mitomycin-c
• Incompatible with all drugs or sol except NS, D₅
NURSING CONSIDERATIONS
Assess:
• CBC, differential, platelet count weekly; withhold drug if WBC is

<4000 or platelet count is <75,000; notify physician of results

• Renal function studies: BUN, serum uric acid, urine CrCl, electrolytes before, during therapy

• I&O ratio, report fall in urine output of 30 ml/hr

• Monitor temperature q4h; may indicate beginning infection

• Liver function tests before, during therapy (bilirubin, AST, ALT, LDH) as needed or monthly

• RBC, Hct, Hgb, since these may be decreased

• Deep tendon reflexes; drug is neurotoxic

• Sensitivity of feet/hands, which precedes neuropathy

• Bleeding: hematuria, guaiac, bruising or petechiae, mucosa of orifices q8h

• Food preferences; list likes, dislikes

• Effects of alopecia on body image, discuss feelings about body changes

• Inflammation of mucosa, breaks in skin

• Yellowing of skin and sclera, dark urine, clay-colored stools, itchy skin, abdominal pain, fever, diarrhea

• Buccal cavity q8h for dryness, sores or ulceration, white patches, oral pain, bleeding, dysphagia

• Symptoms indicating severe allergic reaction: rash, pruritus, urticaria, purpuric skin lesions, itching, flushing

• Frequency of stools, characteristics: cramping, acidosis; signs of dehydration: rapid respirations, poor skin turgor, decreased urine output, dry skin, restlessness, weakness

Administer:

• Agents to prevent constipation

• Antiemetic 30-60 min before giving drug and prn to prevent vomiting

• IV after diluting with diluent provided or 1 mg/10 ml of sterile H_2O or NaCl; give through Y-tube or 3-way stopcock or directly over 1 min

• Hyaluronidase 150 U/ml in 1 ml NaCl; apply warm compress for extravasation

• Transfusion for anemia

• Antispasmodic for GI symptoms

Perform/provide:

• Liquid diet: cola, Jell-O; dry toast or crackers may be added if patient is not nauseated or vomiting

• Rinsing of mouth 3-4 × day with water

• Brushing of teeth 2-3 × day with soft brush or cotton-tipped applicators for stomatitis; use unwaxed dental floss

• Nutritious diet with iron, vitamin supplements

Evaluate:

• Therapeutic response: decreased tumor size, spread of malignancy

Teach patient/family:

• To report change in gait or numbness in extremities; may indicate neuropathy

• To report any complaints or side effects to nurse or physician

• To report any bleeding, white spots or ulcerations in mouth to physician; tell patient to examine mouth qd

---

vitamin A
Aquasol A, Del-Vi-A, Vitamin A
Func. class.: Vitamin, fat soluble
Chem. class.: Retinol

Action: Needed for normal bone and tooth development, visual dark adaptation, skin disease, mucosa

---

italics = common side effects   ***bold italic*** = life threatening reactions

tissue repair, assists in production of adrenal steroids, cholesterol, RNA

Uses: Vitamin A deficiency

Dosage and routes:
• *Adult and child >8 yr:* PO 100,000-500,000 IU qd 3 days, then 50,000 qd × 2 wk; dose based on severity of deficiency; maintenance 10,000-20,000 IU for 2 mo
• *Child 1-8 yr:* IM 5,000-15,000 IU qd × 10 days
• *Infants <1 yr:* IM 5,000-15,000 IU × 10 days

Maintenance
• Child 4-8 yr: IM 15,000 IU qd × 2 mo
• Child <4 yr: IM 10,000 IU qd × 2 mo

Available forms: Caps 10,000, 25,000, 50,000 IU; drops 5,000 IU; inj 50,000 IU/ml

Side effects/adverse reactions:
GI: Nausea, vomiting, anorexia, abdominal pain, *jaundice*
CNS: Headache, increased intracranial pressure, intracranial hypertension, lethargy, malaise
EENT: Gingivitis, papilledema, exophthalmos, inflammation of tongue and lips
INTEG: Drying of skin, pruritus, increased pigmentation, night sweats, alopecia
MS: Arthraglia, retarded growth, hard areas on bone
META: Hypomenorrhea, hypercalcemia

Contraindications: Hypersensitivity to Vit A, malabsorption syndrome (PO)

Precautions: Lactation, impaired renal function, pregnancy (A)

Pharmacokinetics:
PO/INJ: Stored in liver, kidneys, fat; excreted (metabolites) in urine, feces

Interactions/incompatibilities:
• Decreased absorption of Vit A: mineral oil, cholestyramine, colestipol
• Increased levels of Vit A: corticosteroids, oral contraceptives
• Do not administer IV because of risk of anaphylactic shock

Lab test interferences:
False increase: Bilirubin, serum cholesterol

NURSING CONSIDERATIONS
Assess:
• Nutritional status: yellow and dark green vegetables, yellow/orange fruits, A–fortified foods, liver, egg yolks
• Vit A deficiency: decreased growth, night blindness, dry, brittle nails, hair loss, urinary stones, increased infection, hyperkeratosis of skin, drying of cornea

Administer:
• With food (PO) for better absorption

Perform/provide:
• Storage in tight, light-resistant container

Evaluate:
• Therapeutic response: increased growth rate, weight; absence of dry skin and mucous membranes, night blindness

Teach patient/family:
• Instruct patient that if dose is missed, it should be omitted
• Ophthalmic exams may be required periodically throughout therapy
• Not to use mineral oil while taking this drug
• To notify a physician of nausea, vomiting, lip cracking, loss of hair, headache
• Not to take more than the prescribed amount

Treatment of overdose: Discontinue drug

---

* Available in Canada only

vitamin D (cholecalciferol, vitamin D₃ or ergocalciferol, vitamin D₂)

Calciferol, Deltalin, Drisdol, Hytakerol, Radiostol,* Radiostol Forte*

Func. class.: Vitamin D
Chem. class.: Fat soluble

Action: Needed for regulation of calcium, phosphate levels, normal bone development, parathyroid activity, neuromuscular functioning

Uses: Vit D deficiency, rickets, renal osteodystrophy, hypoparathyroidism, hypophosphatemia, psoriasis, rheumatoid arthritis

Dosage and routes:
• *Adult:* PO/IM 12,000 IU qd, then increased to 500,000 IU/day
• *Child:* PO/IM 1500/5000 IU qd × 2-4 wk, may repeat after 2 wk or 600,000 IU as single dose
Hypoparathyroidism
• *Adult and child:* PO/IM 200,000 IU given with 4 g Ca tab

Available forms: Tabs 400, 1000, 50,000 IU; caps 25,000, 50,000; liq 8000 IU/ml; inj 500,000 IU/ml, 500,000 IU/5 ml IM

Side effects/adverse reactions:
GI: Nausea, vomiting, anorexia, cramps, diarrhea, constipation, metallic taste, dry mouth, decreased libido
CNS: Fatigue, weakness, drowsiness, **convulsions,** headache, psychosis
GU: Polyuria, nocturia, **hematuria, albuminuria, renal failure**
CV: Hypertension, dysrhythmias
MS: Decreased bone growth, early joint pain, early muscle pain
INTEG: Pruritus, photophobia

Contraindications: Hypersensitivity, hypercalcemia, renal dysfunction, hyperphosphatemia

Precautions: Cardiovascular disease, renal calculi, pregnancy (A)

Pharmacokinetics:
PO/INJ: Half-life 7-12 hr; stored in liver, duration 2 mo; excreted in bile (metabolites) and urine

Interactions/incompatibilities:
• Decreased effects of Vit D: cholestyramine, colestipol, phenobarbital, phenytoin
• Increased toxicity: diuretics (thiazides), antacids, verapamil

NURSING CONSIDERATIONS
Assess:
• Vit D levels q2 wk during treatment
• Ca, PO₄, Mg, BUN, alk phosphatase, urine Ca, creatinine
• In children, monitor height and weight
• Nutritional status: egg yolk, fortified dairy products, cod, halibut, salmon, sardines

Administer:
• IM injection in deep muscle mass; administer slowly; aspirate carefully; rotate injection sites; avoid IV administration

Evaluate:
• Therapeutic response: absence of rickets/osteomalacia, adequate Ca/phosphate levels, decrease in bone pain

Teach patient/family:
• If dose is missed, omit
• Necessary foods to be included in diet
• To avoid vitamin supplements unless directed by physician
• To keep doctor's appointments since line between therapeutic and toxic doses is narrow
• To report weakness, lethargy, headache, anorexia, loss of weight
• To report nausea, vomiting, abdominal cramps, diarrhea, consti-

pation, excessive thirst, polyuria, muscle and bone pain
• To decrease intake of antacids and laxatives containing Mg

vitamin E
Amino-Opti-E, Aquasol E, Daltose,* E-Complex-600, E-Ferol, E-Vitamin Succinate, E-200 I.U. Softgels, Gordo-Vite E, Tocopherol, Vitamin E, Vita-Plus E Softgells, Vitec

Func. class.: Vitamin E
Chem. class.: Fat soluble

Action: Needed for digestion and metabolism of polyunsaturated fats, decreases platelet aggregation, decreases blood clot formation, promotes normal growth and development of muscle tissue, prostaglandin synthesis

Uses: Vit E deficiency, impaired fat absorption, hemolytic anemia in premature neonates, prevention of retrolental fibroplasia, sickle cell anemia, supplement in malabsorption syndrome

Dosage and routes:
• *Adult:* PO/IM 60-75 IU qd, not to exceed 300 IU/day
• *Child:* PO/IM 1 mg/0.6 g of dietary fat
Available forms: Caps 50, 100, 200, 400, 500, 600, 1000 IU; 74, 165, 294, 331 mg; tabs 200, 400 IU; 331 mg; drops 50 mg/ml

Side effects/adverse reactions:
META: Altered metabolism of hormones, thyroid, pituitary, adrenal, altered immunity
MS: Weakness
CNS: Headache, fatigue
GI: Nausea, cramps, diarrhea
GU: Gonadal dysfunction
CV: Increased risk thrombophlebitis
EENT: Blurred vision

INTEG: Sterile abscess, contact dermatitis

Contraindications: None significant
Precautions: Pregnancy (A)
Pharmacokinetics:
PO: Metabolized in liver, excreted in bile

Interactions/incompatibilities:
• Increased action of: oral anticoagulants
• Decreased absorption: cholestyramine, colestipol, mineral oil, and sucralfate

NURSING CONSIDERATIONS
Assess:
• BUN, creatinine
• Vit E levels during treatment
• CBC; hemolytic anemia may occur
• Nutritional status: wheat germ, dark green leafy vegetables, nuts, eggs, liver, vegetable oils, dairy products, cereals

Administer:
• *PO:* Administer with or after meals
• *Chewable tabs:* Chew well
• *Sol:* may be dropped in mouth or mixed with food
• Topically to moisturize dry skin

Perform/provide:
• Storage in tight, light-resistant container

Evaluate:
• Therapeutic response: absence of hemolytic anemia, adequate Vit E levels, improvement in skin lesions, decreased edema

Teach patient/family:
• Necessary foods to be included in diet
• To omit if dose missed
• To avoid vitamin supplements unless directed by physician

---

* Available in Canada only

warfarin sodium

(war'far-in)

Carfin, Coumadin, Panwarfin, Sofarin, Warfarin Sodium, Warfilone Sodium,* Warnerin*

Func. class.: Anticoagulant

Action: Interferes with blood clotting by indirect means; depresses hepatic synthesis of Vit K–dependent coagulation factors (II, VII, IX, X)

Uses: Pulmonary emboli, deep vein thrombosis, myocardial infarction, atrial dysrhythmias, postcardiac valve replacement

Dosage and routes:

• *Adult:* PO/IV 10-15 mg × 3 days, then titrated to INR qd

Available forms: Tabs 1 mg, 2, 2.5, 5, 7.5, 10 mg; inj 50 mg/2 ml

Side effects/adverse reactions:

GI: Diarrhea, nausea, vomiting, anorexia, stomatitis, cramps, *hepatitis*

GU: Hematuria

INTEG: Rash, dermatitis, urticaria, alopecia, pruritus

CNS: Fever

HEMA: Hemorrhage, agranulocytosis, leukopenia, eosinophilia

Contraindications: Hypersensitivity, hemophilia, leukemia with bleeding, peptic ulcer disease, thrombocytopenic purpura, hepatic disease (severe), severe hypertension, subacute bacterial endocarditis, acute nephritis, blood dyscrasias, pregnancy (D), eclampsia, preeclampsia, lactation

Precautions: Alcoholism, elderly

Pharmacokinetics:

PO: Onset 12-24 hr, peak 1½-3 days, duration 3-5 days, half-life 1½-2½ days; metabolized in liver, excreted in urine/feces (active/in-

active metab[...] centa 99% b[...] teins

Interactions/i[...]

• Increased acti[...] lopurinol, chloramp[...], amiodarone, diflunisal, heparin, steroids, cimetidine, disulfiram, thyroid, glucagon, metronidazole, quinidine, sulindac, sulfinpyrazone, sulfonamides, clofibrate, salicylates, ethacrynic acids, indomethacin, mefenamic acid, oxyphenbutazones, phenylbutazone, cefamondole, chloral hydrate, cotrimoxazole, erythromycin, quinolone antibiotics, isoniazid, thrombolytic agents, tricyclic antidepressants

• Decreased action of warfarin: barbiturates, griseofulvin, ethchlorvynol, carbamazepine, rifampin, oral contraceptives, phenytoin, estrogens, Vit K, cholestyramine, corticosteroids, mercaptopurine, sucralfate, Vit K foods, vit supplement

• Increased toxicity: oral sulfonylureas, phenytoin

• Incompatible with amikacin, dextrose, epinephrine, metaraminol, oxytocin, promazine, tetracycline, vancomycin

Lab test interferences:

Increase: T_3 uptake

Decrease: Uric acid

NURSING CONSIDERATIONS

Assess:

• Blood studies (Hct, platelets, occult blood in stools) q3mo

• Prothrombin time, which should be 1½-2 × control, PT; often done qd initially or INR (international normalized ratio)

• Bleeding gums, petecchiae, ecchymosis, black tarry stools, hematuria

• Fever, skin rash, urticaria

---

italics = common side effects   ***bold italic*** = life threatening reactions

d dosage change q1-2wk; stable, PT q3wk

dminister:
• IV after diluting with diluent provided (50 mg/2 ml); rotate vial, give through Y-tube or 3-way stopcock at 25 mg or less/min
• At same time each day to maintain steady blood levels
• Tabs whole or crushed
• Avoiding all IM injections that may cause bleeding

Perform/provide:
• Storage in tight container

Evaluate:
• Therapeutic response: decrease of deep vein thrombosis

Teach patient/family:
• To avoid OTC preparations that may cause serious drug interactions unless directed by physician
• To use soft-bristle toothbrush to avoid bleeding gums, electric razor
• To carry a Medic Alert ID identifying drug taken
• Importance of compliance
• To report any signs of bleeding: gums, under skin, urine, stools
• To avoid hazardous activities (football, hockey, skiing), dangerous work
• Importance of avoiding unusual changes in vitamin intake, diet or life-style
• To inform dentists and other physicians of anticoagulant intake
• That smoking increases dose requirements

Treatment of overdose: Administer Vit K

xylometazoline HCl (nasal)

(xye-loe-met-az'oh-leen)
Otrivin, Otrivin Pediatric Nasal Drops, Xylometazoline HCl
Func. class.: Nasal decongestant
Chem. class.: Sympathomimetic amine

Action: Dilates arterioles of nasal membrane, which decreases congestion

Uses: Nasal congestion

Dosage and routes:
• *Adult and child >12 yr:* INSTILL 2-3 gtts or 2 sprays q8-10h (0.1%)
• *Child <12 yr:* INSTILL 2-3 gtts or 1% spray q8-10h (0.05%)

Available forms: Sol 0.05%, 0.1%

Side effects/adverse reactions:
EENT: Irritation, burning, sneezing, stinging, dryness, rebound congestion
INTEG: Contact dermatitis

Contraindications: Hypersensitivity to sympathomimetic amines

Precautions: Pregnancy (C), glaucoma

Pharmacokinetics:
INSTILL: Onset 5-10 min, duration 5-6 hr

NURSING CONSIDERATIONS
Assess:
• Redness, swelling, pain in nasal passages

Administer:
• No more than q4h
• For <4 consecutive days

Perform/provide:
• Environmental humidification to decrease nasal congestion, dryness
• Storage in light-resistant containers; do not expose to high temperatures

---

Evaluate:
• Therapeutic response: decreased nasal congestion
Teach patient/family:
• To avoid contamination of container
• That stinging may occur for a few applications; drying of mucosa may be decreased by environmental humidification
• To notify physician of irregular pulse, insomnia, dizziness, tremors
• Proper administration to avoid systemic absorption

---

zalcitabine (ddC)

(zal-sit'-a-bin)
Hivid
Func. class.: Antiviral
Chem. class.: Synthetic pyrimidine nucleoside analog of 2'-deoxycytidine

Action: Inhibits HIV replication by the conversion of this drug by cellular enzymes to an active antiviral metabolite

Uses: Advanced HIV infections in adults and children >13 yr who have been uanble to use zidovudine or who have not responded to treatment

Dosage and routes:
• *Adult:* Combined with zidovudine in advanced HIV infection: 0.75 mg administered concomitantly with 200 mg zidovudine q8h; dosage reduction not necessary for patients weighing >30 kg; in presence of peripheral neuropathy initiate dose at 0.375 mg q8h of zalcitabine

Available forms: Tabs 0.375 and 0.75 mg

Side effects/adverse reactions:
GI: Pancreatitis, diarrhea, nausea, vomiting, abdominal pa., pation, stomatitis, dysplas, abnormalities, oral ulcers, . lence, taste perversion, dry mou. oral thrush, melena, increased ALT, AST, alk phosphatase, amylase, increased bilirubin
GU: Uric acid, *toxic nephropathy,* polyuria
CNS: Headache, peripheral neuropathy, seizures, confusion, anxiety, hypertonia, abnormal thinking, asthenia, insomnia, CNS depression, pain, dizziness, chills, fever
RESP: Cough, pneumonia, dyspnea, asthma, hypoventilation
INTEG: Rash, pruritus, alopecia, sweating, acne
MS: Myalgia, arthritis, myopathy, muscular atrophy
CV: Hypertension, vasodilation, dysrhythmia, syncope, palpitation, tachycardia
EENT: Ear pain, otitis, photophobia, visual impairment
*HEMA: **Leukopenia, granulocytopenia, thrombocytopenia,** anemia
Contraindications: Hypersensitivity

Precautions: Renal, hepatic disease, pregnancy (C), lactation, children (<13 yr), patients with peripheral neuropathy

Pharmacokinetics:
PO: Elimination half-life 1.62 hr; extensive metabolism is thought to occur; administration within 5 min of food will decrease absorption

Interactions/incompatibilities:
• Increased risk of pancreatitis with agents having potential to cause pancreatitis
• Increased risk of peripheral neuropathy with other agents that can cause peripheral neuropathy: chloramphenicol, cisplatin, dapsone, disulfiram, ethionamide, glutethimide, gold, hydralazine, iodo-

---

italics = common side effects   ***bold italic*** = life threatening reactions

Z

(ddC)

...tronidazole,
...in, ribavi-
...didenosine

...: ketocona-

• Do not administer with tetracyclines
• Decreased concentrations of: fluoroquinolone antibiotics

NURSING CONSIDERATIONS
Assess:
• Neuropathy: tingling or pain in hands and feet, distal numbness
• Pancreatitis: abdominal pain, nausea, vomiting, elevated liver enzymes; drug should be discontinued, since condition can be fatal
• Children by dilated retinal examination q6mo to rule out retinal depigmentation
• CBC, differential, platelet count weekly; withhold drug if WBC is <4000 or platelet count is <75,000; notify physician of results
• Renal function studies: BUN, serum uric acid, urine CrCl before, during therapy
• Temperature: q4h; may indicate beginning infection
• Liver function tests before, during therapy (bilirubin, AST, ALT) as needed or monthly

Administer:
• Antibiotics: for prophylaxis of infection

Perform/provide:
• Strict medical asepsis, protective isolation if WBC levels are low
• Clean-up of powdered products; use wet mop or damp sponge

Evaluate:
• Therapeutic response: absence of infection; symptoms of HIV

Teach patient/family:
• To report signs of infection: increased temperature, sore throat, flu symptoms
• To report signs of anemia: fatigue, headache, faintness, shortness of breath, irritability
• To report bleeding; avoid use of razors, commercial mouthwash
• That hair may be lost during therapy; a wig or hairpiece may make patient feel better

---

zidovudine (formerly azidothymidine, or AZT)
(zid-o'-vue-dine)
Retrovir
Func. class.: Antiviral
Chem. class.: Thymidine analog

Action: Inhibits replication of HIV virus by incorporating into cellular DNA by viral reverse transcriptase, thereby terminating the cellular DNA chain

Uses: Symptomatic HIV infections (AIDS, ARC), confirmed *P. carinii* pneumonia, or absolute CD4 lymphocytes of <200/mm³

Dosage and routes:
• *Adult:* PO 200 mg q4h; may have to stop treatment if severe bone marrow depression occurs, and restart after bone marrow recovery; IV 1-2 mg/kg q4h initiate PO as soon as possible

Available forms: Caps 100 mg; Inj (IV)

Side effects/adverse reactions:
HEMA: Granulocytopenia, anemia
CNS: Fever, headache, malaise, diaphoresis, dizziness, *insomnia,* paresthesia, somnolence, chills, tremor, twitching, anxiety, confusion, depression, lability, vertigo, loss of mental acuity

GI: Nausea, vomiting, diarrhea, anorexia, cramps, *dyspepsia,* constipation, dysphagia, *flatulence,* rectal bleeding, mouth ulcer

RESP: Dyspnea

EENT: Taste change, hearing loss, photophobia

INTEG: Rash, acne, pruritus, urticaria

MS: Myalgia, arthralgia, muscle spasm

GU: Dysuria, polyuria, frequency, hesitancy

Contraindications: Hypersensitivity

Precautions: Granulocyte count <1000/mm³ or Hgb <9.5 g/dl, pregnancy (C), lactation, children, severe renal disease, severe hepatic function

Pharmacokinetics:

PO: Rapidly absorbed from GI tract, peak ½-1½ hr, metabolized in liver (inactive metabolites), excreted by kidneys

Interactions/incompatibilities:

• Toxicity: amphotericin B, dapsone, flucytosine, adriamycin, interferon vincristine, vinblastine, pentamidine, probenecid, experimental nucleoside analogs, benzodiazepines, cimetidine, morphine, sulfonamides

• Granulocytopenia: acetaminophen, aspirin, indomethacin

• Incompatible with blood, protein products

NURSING CONSIDERATIONS

Assess:

• Blood counts q2wk; watch for decreasing granulocytes, Hgb; if low, therapy may have to be discontinued and restarted after hematologic recovery; blood transfusions may be required

Administer:

• IV after diluting each 1 mg/0.25 ml or more D₅W to 4 mg/ml or less give over 1 hr

• By mouth; capsules should be swallowed whole

• Trimethoprim-sulfamethoxazole, pyrimethamine, or acyclovir as ordered to prevent opportunistic infections; if these drugs are given, watch for neurotoxicity

Perform/provide:

• Storage in cool environment; protect from light

Evaluate:

• Blood dyscrasias (anemia, granulocytopenia): bruising, fatigue, bleeding, poor healing

Teach patient/family:

• That GI complaints and insomnia resolve after 3-4 wks of treatment

• That drug is not cure for AIDS but will control symptoms

• To call physician if sore throat, swollen lymph nodes, malaise, fever occur, since other infections may occur

• That even with drug administration, patient is still infective and may pass AIDS virus on to others

• That follow-up visits must be continued since serious toxicity may occur; blood counts must be done q2wk

• That drug must be taken q4h around clock, even during night

• That serious drug interactions may occur if OTC products are ingested; check with physician before taking aspirin, acetaminophen, indomethacin

• That other drugs may be necessary to prevent other infections

• That drug may cause fainting or dizziness

---

italics = common side effects   ***bold italic*** = life threatening reactions

z

zinc sulfate
Eye-Sed Ophthalmic
Func. class.: Misc ophthalmic
Chem. class.: Zinc product

Action: Vasoconstriction occurs by action on conjunctiva
Uses: Ocular congestion, irritation, itching
Dosage and routes:
• *Adult and child >2 yr:* INSTILL 1-2 gtts bid or tid
Available forms: Sol 0.217%, 0.25%
Side effects/adverse reactions:
EENT: Eye irritation, burning
Contraindications: Hypersensitivity
Precautions: Narrow-angle glaucoma, pregnancy (C)
NURSING CONSIDERATIONS
Perform/provide:
• Storage in tight container
Evaluate:
• Therapeutic response: decreased ocular irritation, itching, congestion
Teach patient/family:
• To report change in vision, irritation
• Method of instillation; tilt head backward, hold dropper over eye, drop medication inside lower lid, using pressure on inside corner of eye hold 1 min; not to touch dropper to eye
• If pain/irritation persists discontinue use and consult physician

zinc sulfate
Orazinc, Scrip Zinc, Verazinc, Zinca-Pak, Zincate, Zinc 15, Zinc-220, Zinc Sulfate
Func. class.: Trace element

Action: Needed for adequate healing, bone and joint development (23% zinc)
Uses: Prevention of zinc deficiency, adjunct to Vit A therapy
Dosage and routes:
• *Adult:* PO 200-220 mg tid
• *Child:* PO 0.3 mg/kg/day
Available forms: Tabs 110, 200, 220 mg; caps 110, 220 mg
Side effects/adverse reactions:
GI: Nausea, vomiting, cramps, heartburn, ulcer formation
OVERDOSE: Diarrhea, rash, dehydration, restlessness
Precautions: Pregnancy (A)
Interactions/incompatibilities:
• Decreased absorption of: other covalent cations
NURSING CONSIDERATIONS
Assess:
• Zinc levels during treatment
Administer:
• With meals to decrease gastric upset; to avoid dairy products
Evaluate:
• Therapeutic response: absence of zinc deficiency
Teach patient/family:
• That element must be taken for 2 mo to be effective
• To report immediately nausea, diarrhea, rash, severe vomiting, restlessness, abdominal pain, tarry stools

zolpidem tartrate
(zole-pi'-dem)
Ambien
Func. class.: Sedative-hypnotic
Chem. class.: Nonbenzodiazepine of imidazopyridine class

Action: Produces CNS depression at limbic, thalamic, hypothalamic levels of CNS; may be mediated by neurotransmitter-amniobutyric acid (GABA); results are sedation, hypnosis, skeletal muscle relaxation, anticonvulsant activity, anxiolytic action

Uses: Insomnia, short-term treatment

Dosage and routes:
• *Adult:* PO 10 mg hs × 7-10 days only; total dose should not exceed 10 mg

Available forms: Tabs 5 mg and 10 mg (at least in U.S.)

Side effects/adverse reactions:
*HEMA: **Leukopenia, granulocytopenia (rare)***

CNS: Headache, lethargy, drowsiness, daytime sedation, dizziness, confusion, light-headedness, anxiety, irritability, amnesia, poor coordination

GI: Nausea, vomiting, diarrhea, heartburn, abdominal pain, constipation

CV: Chest pain, palpitation

Contraindications: Hypersensitivity to benzodiazepines

Precautions: Anemia, hepatic disease, renal disease, suicidal individuals, drug abuse, elderly, psychosis, child <18 yr, seizure disorders, pregnancy (B), lactation

Pharmacokinetics:
PO: Onset 1.5 hr, metabolized by liver, excreted by kidneys (inactive metabolites), crosses placenta, excreted in breast milk; half-life 2-3 hr

Interactions/incompatibilities:
• Increased action of both drugs: alcohol, CNS depressants

Lab test interferences:
• *Increase:* ALT, AST, serum bilirubin
• *Decrease:* RAI uptake
• *False increase:* Urinary 17-OHCS

NURSING CONSIDERATIONS
Assess:
• Blood studies: Hct, Hgb, RBCs, if blood dyscrasias are suspected (rare)
• Hepatic studies: AST, ALT, bilirubin if liver damage has occurred
• Mental status: mood, sensorium, affect, memory (long, short)
• Blood dyscrasias: fever, sore throat, bruising, rash, jaundice, epistaxis (rare)
• Type of sleep problem: falling asleep, staying asleep

Administer:
• After removal of cigarettes to prevent fires
• After trying conservative measures for insomnia
• ½-1 hr before hs for sleeplessness
• On empty stomach for fast onset but may be taken with food if GI symptoms occur

Perform/provide:
• Assistance with ambulation after receiving dose
• Safety measure: side rails, nightlight, call bell within easy reach
• Checking to see PO medication has been swallowed
• Storage in tight container in cool environment

Evaluate:
• Therapeutic response: ability to sleep at night, decreased amount of early morning awakening if taking drug for insomnia

Teach patient/family:
• That dependence is possible after long-term use
• To avoid driving or other activities requiring alertness until drug is stabilized
• To avoid alcohol ingestion or CNS depressants; serious CNS depression may result
• That effects may take 2 nights for benefits to be noticed
• Alternative measures to improve

---

italics = common side effects   ***bold italic*** = life threatening reactions

z

sleep: reading, exercise several hours before hs, warm bath, warm milk, TV, self-hypnosis, deep breathing

• That hangover is common in elderly but less common than with barbiturates; rebound insomnia may occur for 1-2 nights after discontinuing drug

Treatment of overdose: Lavage, activated charcoal; monitor electrolytes, vital signs

Appendix a

Weights and equivalents

METRIC SYSTEM
Weight

kilogram	= kg	=	1000 grams
gram	= g	=	1 gram
milligram	= mg	=	0.001 gram
microgram	= μg	=	0.001 milligram

Volume

liter	= L	=	1 L
milliliter	= ml	=	0.001 L

AVOIRDUPOIS WEIGHT

1 ounce (oz) = 437.5 grains
1 pound (lb) = 16 ounces = 7000 grains

METRIC AND APOTHECARY EQUIVALENTS
Exact weight equivalents

Metric	Apothecary
1 mg	1/64.8 grain
64.8 mg	1 grain
324 mg	5 grains
1 g	15.432 grains
31.103 g	1 ounce = 480 grains

Exact volume equivalents

Metric	Apothecary		
1.00 ml	16.23 minims		
3.69 ml	1 fluidram	=	60 minims
29.57 ml	1 fluidounce	=	480 minims
473.16 ml	1 pint	=	7680 minims
946.33 ml	1 quart	=	15,360 minims

Appendix b

Formulas for drug calculations

Surface area rule:

$$\text{Child dose} = \frac{\text{Surface area (m}^2)}{1.73\text{m}^2} \times \text{Adult dose}$$

Calculating strength of a solution:

Solution Strength: *Desired Solution:*

$$\frac{x}{100} = \frac{\text{Amount of drug desired}}{\text{Amount of finished solution}}$$

Calculating flow rate for IV:

$$\text{Rate of Flow} = \frac{\text{Amount of fluid} \times \text{Administration set calibration}}{\text{Running time}}$$

$$\frac{x}{1} = \frac{\text{(ml) (gtt/min)}}{\text{min}}$$

Calculation of medication dosages:

Formula method:

$$\frac{\text{Amount ordered}}{\text{Amount on hand}} \times \text{Vehicle}$$

$$= \text{Number of tablets, capsules, or amount of liquid}$$

Vehicle is the drug form or amount of liquid containing the dosage. Amounts used in calculation by formula must be in same system.

Ratio—proportion method:

1 tablet: tablet in mg on hand:: x tablet order in mg
           Know or have:: Want to know or order

Multiply means and extremes, divide both sides by known amount to get X. Amounts used in equation must be in same system.

Dimensional analysis method:

$$\text{Order in mg} \times \frac{1 \text{ tablet or capsule}}{\text{What 1 tablet or capsule is in mg}}$$

$$= \text{Tablets or capsules to be given}$$

If amounts are in different systems:

$$\text{Order in mg} \times \frac{1 \text{ tablet or capsule}}{\text{What 1 tablet or capsule is in g}} \times \frac{1}{1000 \text{ mg}}$$

$$= \text{Tablets or capsules to be given}$$

Appendix c

Commonly used antibiotics in adults and children

amoxicillin
  Adult: PO 750 mg-1.5 g qd in divided doses q8h
  Child: PO 20-40 mg/kg/day in divided doses q8h
ampicillin
  Adult: PO 1-2 g qd in divided doses q6h
      IM/IV 2-8 g qd in divided doses q4-6h
  Child: PO 50-100 mg/kg/day in divided doses q6h
      IM/IV 100-200 mg/kg/day in divided doses q6h
cefaclor
  Adult: PO 250-500 mg q8h
  Child: PO 24-40 mg/kg/day in divided doses q8h
cephalexin
  Adult: PO 250-500 mg q6h
  Child: PO 25-50 mg/kg/day in 4 equal doses
chloramphenicol
  Adult and child >3 mo: 50-100 mg/kg/day in divided doses q6h
clindamycin
  Adult: PO 150-450 mg q6h
      IM/IV 300 mg q6-12h
  Child >1 mo: PO 8-25 mg/kg/day in divided doses q6-8h
      IM/IV 15-40 mg/kg/day in divided doses q6-8h
erythromycin
  Adult: 250 mg-500 mg q6h
  Child: 30-50 mg/kg/day in divided doses q6h
gentamicin
  Adult: IV INF 3-5 mg/kg/day in divided doses q8h
  Child: IV/IM 2-2.5 mg/kg q8h
  Neonates and infants: IV/IM 2.5 mg/kg q8h
kanamycin
  Adult and child: IV INF/IM 15 mg/kg/day in divided doses
      q8-12h
methicillin
  Adult: IM/IV 4-12 g/day in divided doses q4-6h
  Child: IM/IV 50-300 mg/kg/day in divided doses q4-12h
      PO 25-50 mg/kg/day in divided doses q6h
  Neonates: IM 10 mg/kg q12h
nafcillin
  Adult: PO/IM/IV 2-6 g/day in divided doses q4-6h

Child: IM 25 mg/kg q12h
oxacillin
Adult: PO 2-6 g/day in divided doses q4-6h
IM/IV 2-12 g/day in divided doses q4-6h
Child: PO/IM/IV 50-100 mg/kg/day in divided doses q6h
penicillin G benzathine
Adult: IM 1.2 million U
penicillin G potassium
Adult: PO 400,000-500,000 U q6-8h
Child <12 yr: PO 25,000-90,000 U/kg/day in 3-6 divided doses
penicillin G procaine
Adult and child: IM 600,000-1.2 million U in 1-2 doses/day
Newborn: IM 50,000 U/kg qd
nitrofurantoin
Adult and child >12 yr: PO 50-100 mg qid pc
sulfisoxazole
Adult: PO 2-4 g loading dose, then 1-2 g qid
Child >2 mo: PO 75 mg/kg or 2 g/m^2 loading dose, then 150
mg/kg/day or 4 g/m^2 day in divided doses q6h
ticarcillin
Adult: IV/IM 12-24 g/day in divided doses q3-6h
Child: IV/IM 50-300 mg/kg/day in divided doses q4-8h
Neonates: IV INF 75-100 mg/kg q8-12h

Appendix d

Nomogram for calculation of body surface area

Place a straight edge from the patient's height in the left column to his weight in the right column. The point of intersection on the body surface area column indicates the body surface area (BSA). Reproduced from Behrman RE, and Vaughn VC (editors): Nelson's textbook of pediatrics, ed 12, Philadelphia, 1983. WB Saunders.

Appendix e

Home care medication record

Patient's Name	Age	Sex	Allergies	
Pharmacy		Caffeine		Smoking
Physician		Alcohol		Herb tea/home rem.
OTC medications: Name, dose, route, regimen		Tube feeding?	Ostomy?	Difficulty swallowing?
Antacids, antidiarrheals/laxatives, hemorrhoidal, emetic/ antiemetic, cough/cold, analgesics, vitamins/minerals/iron, sleep aids, ophthalmic/otic, topical/lotion/ointments, other		COMMENTS:		

	PRESCRIPTION MEDICATIONS MT = Medication teaching sheet requested? Yes (Y) or No (N)							
Date ordered	Medication—strength, route, frequency of administration	N/C	MT	Indication	Side effects discussed with patient	Date given	Date return

COMMENTS TO PHARMACIST

White—chart	Yellow—pharmacist	Pink—nurse	NURSE	DATE

Appendix f

Controlled substance chart

Drugs	United States	Canada
Heroin, LSD, peyote, marijuana, mescaline	Schedule I	Schedule H
Opium (morphine), meperidine, amphetamines, cocaine, short-acting barbiturates (secobarbital)	Schedule II	Schedule G
Glutethimide, paregoric, phendimetrazine	Schedule III	Schedule F
Chloral hydrate, chlordiazepoxide, diazepam, mazindol, meprobamate, phenobarbital (Canada-G)	Schedule IV	Schedule F
Antidiarrheals with opium (Canada-G), antitussives	Schedule V	Schedule F

Appendix g

FDA pregnancy categories

A No risk demonstrated to the fetus in any trimester

B No adverse effects in animals, no human studies available

C Only given after risks to the fetus are considered; animal studies have shown adverse reactions, no human studies available

D Definite fetal risks, may be given in spite of risks if needed in life-threatening conditions

X Absolute fetal abnormalities; not to be used anytime during pregnancy

APPENDIX

Appendix h

Bibliography

Clark JB, Queener SF, Karb VB: *Pharmacological basis of nursing practice,* ed 3, St Louis, 1990, Mosby–Year Book.

Drug Information 92: Bethesda, 1992, American Hospital Formulary Service.

Facts and Comparisons: Philadelphia, updated monthly, JB Lippincott.

Gahart BL: *Intravenous medications,* ed 9, St Louis, 1993, Mosby–Year Book.

Goodman A and others: *Goodman and Gilman's The pharmacological basis of therapeutics,* ed 8, *New York, 1990, Pergamon Press.*

McKenry LM and Salerno E: Mosby's pharmacology in nursing, ed 18, St Louis, 1992, Mosby–Year Book.

Mediphor Editorial Group: *Drug interaction facts,* Philadelphia, updated quarterly, JB Lippincott.

Appendix i

Combination products

Aceta with Codeine, Empracet with Codeine No. 3, Tylenol with Codeine No. 3: acetaminophen 300 mg with codeine phosphate 30 mg

Alazide, Altexide: spironolactone 25 mg with hydrochlorothiazide 25 mg

Aldactazide 25/25: spironolactone 25 mg with hydrochlorothiazide 25 mg

Aldactazide 50/50: spironolactone 50 mg with hydrochlorothiazide 50 mg

Aldoclor-15: methyldopa 250 mg with chlorothiazide 15 mg

Aldoclor-150: methyldopa 250 mg with chlorothiazide 150 mg

Aldoclor-250: methyldopa 250 mg with chlorothiazide 250 mg

Aldoril-15: methyldopa 250 mg with hydrochlorothiazide 15 mg

Aldoril-25: methyldopa 250 mg with hydrochlorothiazide 25 mg

Aldoril D30: methyldopa 500 mg with hydrochlorothiazide 30 mg

Aldoril D50: methyldopa 500 mg with hydrochlorothiazide 50 mg

Amaphen with Codeine No. 3: acetaminophen 325 mg with butalbital 50 mg, caffeine 40 mg, codeine phosphate 30 mg

Ambenyl: diphenhydramine HCl 12.5 mg/5 ml with codeine phosphate 10 mg/5 ml

Anexsia: hydrocodone bitartrate 7.5 mg with acetaminophen 325 mg

Anexsia with Codeine, Empirin with Codeine 30 mg No. 3: codeine 30 mg with acetaminophen 325 mg

Anguen No. 1: pentaerythritol tetranitrate 20 mg, phenobarbital 15 mg

Anodynos-DHC, DIA-Gesic: acetaminophen 150 mg with aspirin 230 mg, caffeine 30 mg, hydrocodone bitartrate 5 mg

Antrocol: atropine sulfate 0.195 mg with phenobarbital 16 mg

Antrocol Elixir: atropine sulfate 0.039 mg/ml with phenobarbital 3 mg/ml

Apresazide 25/25: hydralazine HCl 25 mg with hydrochlorothiazide 25 mg

Apresazide 50/50: hydralazine HCl 50 mg with hydrochlorothiazide 50 mg

Apresazide 100/50: hydralazine HCl 100 mg with hydrochlorothiazide 50 mg

Apresodex, Apresoline-Esidrix: hydralazine HCl 25 mg with hydrochlorothiazide 15 mg

Aralen Phosphate with Primaquine Phosphate: chloroquine phosphate 300 mg (of chloroquine) with primaquine phosphate 45 mg (of primaquine)

Arcotrate No. 3: pentaerythritol tetranitrate 20 mg, phenobarbital 8 mg

A.S.A. and Codeine Compound No. 3 Pulvules: codeine 30 mg with aspirin 380 mg, caffeine 30 mg

Ascriptin with Codeine No. 2: aspirin 325 mg with codeine phosphate 15 mg, buffers

Ascriptin with Codeine No. 3: aspirin 325 mg with codeine phosphate 30 mg, buffers

Atropine, Demerol Injection: meperidine HCl 50 mg/ml with atropine sulfate 0.4 mg/ml

Atropine, Demerol Injection: meperidine HCl 75 mg/ml with atropine sulfate 0.4 mg/ml

Augmentin, Clavulin: amoxicillin 250 mg with clavulanate potassium 125 mg; amoxicillin 500 mg with clavulanate potassium 125 mg; amoxicillin 125 mg with potassium clavulanate 31.5 mg/5 ml; amoxicillin 250 mg with potassium clavulanate 31.5 mg/5 ml

Axotal: aspirin 650 mg with butalbital 50 mg

Azo Gantanol, Azo Sulfamethoxazole, UroGantanol: sulfamethoxazole 500 mg with phenazopyridine HCl 100 mg

Azo-Gantrisin, Azo-Suldiazo, Azo-Sulfamethoxazole: sulfisoxazole 500 mg with phenazopyridine HCl 50 mg

B-A-C: aspirin 650 mg with butalbital 50 mg, caffeine 40 mg, buffers

B-A-C No. 3: aspirin 325 mg with butalbital 50 mg, caffeine 40 mg, codeine phosphate 30 mg, buffers

Bancap: acetaminophen 325 mg with butalbital 50 mg

Bancap HC, Dolacet, Hydrocet, Zydone: hydrocodone bitartrate 5 mg with acetaminophen 500 mg

Barbidonna: belladonna alkaloids, atropine sulfate 0.025 mg, hyoscyamine sulfate 0.1286 mg, phenobarbital 16 mg, scopolamine hydrobromide 0.0074 mg

Barbidonna Elixir: belladonna alkaloids, atropine sulfate 0.034 mg/5 ml, hyoscyamine sulfate 0.0174 mg/5 ml, phenobarbital 21.6 mg/ml, scopolamine hydrobromide 0.01 mg/5 ml

Barbidonna No. 2: belladonna alkaloids, atropine sulfate 0.025 mg, hyoscyamine sulfate 0.1286 mg, phenobarbital 32 mg, scopolamine hydrobromide 0.0074 mg

BC Powder: aspirin 650 mg with caffeine 32 mg, salicylamide 195 mg

Belap, Pheno-Bella: belladonna extract 10.8 mg (0.135 mg of alkaloids of belladonna leaf) with phenobarbital 16.2 mg

Belladenal-S: levorotatory belladonna alkaloids malates 0.25 mg (of levorotatory belladonna alkaloids) with phenobarbital 50 mg

Bellalphen, Donnatal, Hyosophen: belladonna alkaloids atropine sulfate 0.0194 mg, hyoscyamine sulfate 0.1037 mg, phenobarbital 16.2 mg, scopolamine hydrobromide 0.0065 mg

Bellergal-S: ergotamine tartrate 0.6 mg with levorotatory belladonna alkaloids malates 0.2 mg (of lavorotatory belladonna alkaloids 40 mg)

Benadryl: diphenhydramine HCl 25 mg with pseudoephedrine HCl 60 mg

Benylin: diphenhydramine HCl 12.5 mg/5 ml with pseudo-ephedrine HCl 30 mg/5 ml

Benylin DM: dextromethorphan hydrobromide 5 mg/5 ml with guaifenesin 100 mg/5 ml

Bexophene, Darvon Compound-

COMBINATION PRODUCTS

65, Dolene Compound-65, Doxaphene Compound, Propoxyphene-AC, Propoxyphene Compound-65: propoxyphene HCl 65 mg with aspirin 389 mg, caffeine 32.4 mg

Bicillin C-R: 150,000 units (of penicillin G) per ml with penicillin G benzathine 150,000 units (of penicillin G) per ml

Bicillin C-R: penicillin G procaine 300,000 units (of penicillin G) per ml with penicillin G benzathine 300,000 units (of penicillin G) per ml

Bicillin C-R 900/300: penicillin G procaine 150,000 units (of penicillin G) per ml with penicillin G benzathine 450,000 units (of penicillin G) per ml

Biphetamine 12½: dextroamphetamine 6.25 mg, amphetamine 6.25 mg

Biphetamine 20: dextroamphetamine 10 mg, amphetamine 10 mg

Bitrate: pentaerythritol tetranitrate 15 mg, phenobarbital 20 mg

Blanex: chlorzoxazone 250 mg, acetaminophen 300 mg

Bromo-seltzer: acetaminophen 325 mg/capful measure with citric acid 2.224 g/capful measure, sodium bicarbonate 2.871 g/capful measure

Butibel: belladonna extract 15 mg (0.187 mg of alkaloids of belladonna leaf) with butabarbital sodium 15 mg

Butibel Elixir: belladonna extract 15 mg (0.187 mg of alkaloids of belladonna leaf) with butabarbital sodium 15 mg

Cafergot: ergotamine tartrate 1 mg with caffeine 100 mg

Cafergot suppositories: ergotamine tartrate 2 mg, caffeine 100 mg

Caladryl: diphenhydramine HCl 1% with calamine 8%, camphor 0.1%

Calcidrine: codeine 8.4 mg/5 ml with calcium iodide anhydrous 152 mg/5 ml

CAM-AP-ES: hydrochlorothiazide 15 mg, hydralazine 25 mg, reserpine 0.1 mg

Cantri, Vagilia: sulfisoxazole 10% with allantoin 2%, aminacrine HCl 0.2%

Capital and Codeine: codeine 30 mg with acetaminophen 325 mg

Capital with Codeine: acetaminophen 120 mg/5 ml with codeine 12 mg/5 ml

Capozide 25/15: captopril 25 mg with hydrochlorothiazide 15 mg

Capozide 25/25: captopril 25 mg with hydrochlorothiazide 25 mg

Capozide 50/15: captopril 50 mg with hydrochlorothiazide 15 mg

Capozide 50/25: captopril 50 mg with hydrochlorothiazide 25 mg

Carisoprodol Compound, Soprodol Compound, Soma Compound, Soprodol Compound: risoprodol 200 mg with aspirin 325 mg

Clindex, Clinoxide, Clipoxide, Librax, Lidox, Lidoxide: clidinium bromide 2.5 mg with chlordiazepoxide HCl 5 mg

Chardonna-2: belladonna extract 15 mg (0.187 mg of alkaloids of belladonna leaf) with phenobarbital 15 mg

Cherapas, Ser-A-Gen, Ser-Ap-Es, Serathide, Serpazide, Tri-Hydroserpine, Unipres: reserpine 0.1 mg with hydralazine HCl 25 mg, hydrochlorothiazide 15 mg

Children's Hold 4 Hour: dextromethorphan hydrobromide 3.75 mg with phenylpropanolamine HCl 6.25 mg

Chlorofon-F, Chlorzone Forte, Paracet Forte, Parafon Forte, Zoxaphen: chlorzoxazone 250 mg with acetaminophen 300 mg

Chloroserp-250, Chloroserpine-250, Diupres-250: reserpine 0.125 mg with chlorothiazide 250 mg

Chloroserp-500, Chloropserpine-500, Diupres-500: reserpine 0.125 mg with chlorothiazide 500 mg

Clindex, Clinoxide, Clipoxide, Librax, Lidox: chlordiazepoxide HCl 5 mg with clidinium bromide 2.5 mg

Co-Gesic, Damacet-P, Duradyne, Hy-Phen, Norcet, Vicodin: hydrocodone bitartrate 5 mg with acetaminophen 500 mg

Codalan No. 1: acetaminophen 500 mg with caffeine 30 mg, codeine phosphate 8 mg

Codalan No. 2: acetaminophen 500 mg with caffeine 30 mg, codeine phosphate 15 mg

Codalan No. 3: acetaminophen 500 mg with caffeine 30 mg, codeine phosphate 30 mg

Codoxy, Percodan, Roxiprin: oxycodone HCl 4.5 mg, oxycodone terephthalate 0.38 mg with aspirin 325 mg

Combipres 0.1 mg: clonidine HCl 0.1 mg with chlorthalidone 15 mg

Combipres 0.2 mg: clonidine HCl 0.2 mg with chlorthalidone 15 mg

Comtrex: dextromethorphan hydrobromide 10 mg with acetaminophen 325 mg, chlorpheniramine maleate 2 mg, phenylpropanolamine hydrochloride 12.5 mg

Comtrex: dextromethorphan hydrobromide 3.3 mg/5 ml with acetaminophen 108.3 mg/5 ml, chlorpheniramine maleate 0.67 mg/5 ml, phenylpropanolamine HCl 4.2 mg/5 ml

Conar: dextromethorphan hydrobromide 15 mg with acetaminophen 300 mg, guaifenesin 100 mg, phenylephrine HCl 10 mg

Conar Expectorant: dextromethorphan hydrobromide 15 mg/5 ml with guaifenesin 100 mg/5 ml, phenylephrine HCl 10 mg/5 ml

Conar Syrup: dextromethorphan hydrobromide 15 mg/5 ml with phenylephrine HCl 10 mg/5 ml

Congespirin: phenylpropanolamine HCl 6.25 mg/5 ml with acetaminophen 130 mg/5 ml

Congespirin, Aspirin-Free: acetaminophen 81 mg with phenylephrine HCl 81 mg

Contac Jr.: dextromethorphan hydrobromide 5 mg/5 ml with acetaminophen 160 mg/5 ml, pseudoephedrine HCl 15 mg/5 ml

Contac Severe Cold Formula, Nyquil Nighttime Cold Medicine, Nytime Cold Medicine, Quiet Nite: dextromethorphan hydrobromide 5 mg/5 ml with acetaminophen 167 mg/5 ml, doxylamine succinate 1.25 mg/5 ml, pseudoephedrine HCl 10 mg/5 ml

Copavin Pulvules: codeine sulfate 15 mg with papaverine HCl 15 mg

Corzide 40/5: bendroflumethiazide 5 mg with nadolol 40 mg

Corzide 80/5: bendroflumethiazide 5 mg with nadolol 80 mg

CoTylenol: dextromethorphan hydrobromide 5 mg/5 ml with acetaminophen 108.3 mg/5 ml, chlorpheniramine maleate 0.67

COMBINATION PRODUCTS

mg/5 ml, pseudoephedrine HCl 10 mg/5 ml

CoTylenol Cold Medication Tablets: dextromethorphan hydrobromide 15 mg with acetaminophen 325 mg, chlorpheniramine maleate 2 mg, pseudoephedrine HCl 30 mg

Cremacoat 3: dextromethorphan hydrobromide 6.7 mg/5 ml with guaifenesin 66.7 mg/5 ml, phenylpropanolamine HCl 12.5 mg/5 ml

Cremacoat 4: dextromethorphan hydrobromide 6.7 mg/5 ml with doxylamine succinate 2.5 mg/5 ml, phenylpropanolamine HCl 12.5 mg/5 ml

Cyclomydril Ophthalmic: cyclopentolate HCl 0.2%, phenylephrine HCl 1%

Cystex: methenamine 165 mg, salicylamide 65 mg, sodium salicylate 97 mg, benzoic acid 32 mg

Damason-P: hydrocodone bitartrate 5 mg with aspirin 224 mg, caffeine 32 mg

Darvocet-N 50, Propoxyphene Napsylate with Acetaminophen Tablets: acetaminophen 325 mg with propoxyphene napsylate 50 mg

Darvocet-N 100, Doxapap-N, Propacet 100: propoxyphene napsylate 100 mg with acetaminophen 650 mg

Darvon Compound Pulvules: aspirin 389 mg with caffeine 32.4 mg propoxyphene HCl 32 mg

Darvon Compound-65 Pulvules, Dolene Compound-65, SK-65-Compound: aspirin 389 mg with caffeine 32.4 mg, propoxyphene HCl 65 mg

Darvon with A.S.A. Pulvules: aspirin 325 mg with propoxyphene HCl 65 mg

Darvon-N and A.S.A.: aspirin 325 mg with propoxyphene napsylate 100 mg

Decadron with Xylocaine: dexamethasone PO$_4$ 4 mg, lidocaine HCl 10 mg/ml

Deconamine: pseudoephedrine HCl 60 mg with chlorpheniramine maleate 4 mg

Demerol APAP: acetaminophen 300 mg with meperidine HCl 50 mg

Demi-Regroton: chlorthalidone 25 mg with reserpine 0.125 mg

Deprol: meprobamate 400 mg with benactyzine HCl 1 mg

Dihydrocodeine Compound Modified, Synalgos: aspirin 356.4 mg with caffeine 30 mg and dihydrocodeine bitartrate 16 mg

Dilantin with Phenobarbital: phenytoin sodium 100 mg, phenobarbital 32 mg

Dilantin with Phenobarbital: phenobarbital 16 mg, phenytoin sodium 100 mg

Dimetane-DX Cough Syrup: dextromethorphan hydrobromide 10 mg/5 ml with brompheniramine maleate 2 mg/5 ml, pseudoephedrine HCl 30 mg/5 ml

Dimycor: pentaerythritol tetranitrate 10 mg, phenobarbital 15 mg

Diupres-250: chlorothiazide 250 mg, reserpine 0.125 mg

Diupres-500: chlorothiazide 500 mg, reserpine 0.125 mg

Diurese, Matatensin No. 4, Trichlormethiazide with Reserpine Tablets, Trichlortensin: trichlormethiazide 4 mg with reserpine 0.1 mg

Diutensen: methyclothiazide 2.5 mg with cryptenamine tannates 2 mg (of cryptenamine)

Diutensen: reserpine 0.1 mg with methyclothiazide 2.5 mg

Diutensin-R: methyclothiazide 25 mg with reserpine 0.1 mg

Dolene AP-65: acetaminophen 650 mg with propoxyphene HCl 65 mg

Donnagel-PG: powdered opium 24 mg, Kaolin 6 g, pectin 142.8 mg, hyoscyamine SO₄ 0.1037 mg, atropine SO₄ 0.0194 mg, scopolamine hydrobromide 0.0065 mg, alcohol 5%/30 ml susp

Donnagel Suspension: Kaolin 6 g, pectin 142.8 mg, hyoscyamine SO₄ 0.1037 mg, atropine SO₄ 0.0194 mg, scopolamine hydrobromide 0.0065 mg, alcohol 3.8%/30 ml susp

Donnatal: belladonna alkaloids atropine sulfate 0.0194 mg, hyoscyamine sulfate 0.1037 mg, phenobarbital 32.4 mg, scopolamine hydrobromide 0.0065 mg

Donnatal Elixir, Hyosophen Elixir: belladonna alkaloids atropine sulfate 0.0194 mg/5 ml, hyoscyamine sulfate 0.1037 mg/5 ml, phenobarbital 16.2 mg/5 ml, scopolamine hydrobromide 0.0065/5 ml

Donnatal Extentabs: belladonna alkaloids atropine sulfate 0.0582 mg, hyoscyamine sulfate 0.3111 mg, phenobarbital 48.6 mg, scopolamine hydrobromide 0.0195 mg

Donnatal, Hyosophen: belladonna alkaloids atropine sulfate 0.0194 mg, hyoscyamine sulfate 0.1037 mg, phenobarbital 16.2 mg, scopolamine hydrobromide 0.0065 mg

Dorcol Children's Cough Syrup: dextromethorphan hydrobromide 5 mg/5 ml with guaifenesin 50 mg/5 ml, pseudoephedrine HCl 15 mg/5 ml

DUO-Medihaler: isoproterenol HCl 160 μg/metered spray with phenylephrine bitartrate 240 μg/metered spray

Dyazide: hydrochlorothiazide 25 mg with triamterene 50 mg

E-Pilo: epinephrine bitartrate 1%, pilocarpine HCl 1%, 2%, 3%, 4%, 6%

Empirin with Codeine 15 mg No. 2: codeine 15 mg with aspirin 325 mg

Empirin with Codeine 60 mg No. 4: aspirin 325 mg with codeine phosphate 60 mg

Empracet with Codeine Phosphate 60 mg No. 4, Tylenol with Codeine No. 4: acetaminophen 300 mg with codeine phosphate 60 mg

Endecon, Phenapap No. 2: phenylpropanolamine HCl 25 mg with acetaminophen 325 mg

Enduronyl-Forte, Eserdine Forte, Methyclothiazide and Deserpidine Tablets 5 mg/0.5 mg, Methy-Deserpidine Forte, Methy-Deserpidine Strong: methyclothiazide 5 mg with deserpidine 0.5 mg

Enduronyl, Eserdine, Methychlothiazide, Deserpidine Tablets 5 mg/0.25 mg: deserpidine 0.25 mg with methychlothiazide 5 mg

Entex: guaifenesin 200 mg with phenylephrine HCl 5 mg with phenylpropanolamine HCl 45 mg

Entex LA: guaifenesin 400 mg with phenylpropanolamine HCl 75 mg

Epromate, Equagesic, Equazine-M, Hepto-M, Mepro Compound, Meprogesic, Micranin: meprobamate 200 mg with aspirin 325 mg

COMBINATION PRODUCTS

Equagesic, Equazine-M, Mepro-Analgesic, Mepor Compound, Micrainin: aspirin 325 mg with meprobamate 200 mg

Ergocaff: ergotamine tartrate 1 mg, caffeine 100 mg

Esgic, Fioricet: acetaminophen 325 mg with butalbital 50 mg, caffeine 40 mg

Esimil: guanethidine monosulfate 10 mg (equivalent to guanethidine sulfate 8.4 mg) with hydrochlorothiazide 25 mg

Estratest: esterified estrogens 1.25 mg, methyltestosterone 2.5 mg

Estratest HS: esterified estrogens 0.625 mg, methyltestosterone 1.25 mg

Etrafon 2-10: perphenazine 2 mg, amitriptyline HCl 10 mg

Etrafon: perphenazine 2 mg, amitriptyline HCl 10 mg

Etrafon-A: perphenazine 4 mg, amitriptyline HCl 10 mg

Etrafon-Forte: perphenazine 4 mg, amitriptyline HCl 25 mg

Euthroid-½: levothyroxine sodium 30 µg, liothyronine sodium 7.5 µg

Euthroid-1: levothyroxine sodium 60 µg, liothyronine sodium 15 µg

Euthroid-2: levothyroxine sodium 120 µg, liothyronine sodium 30 µg

Euthroid-3: levothyroxine sodium 180 µg, liothyronine sodium 45 µg

Eutron Filmtab: pargyline HCl 25 mg with methyclothiazide 5 mg

Excedrin: acetaminophen 194 mg with aspirin 227 mg, caffeine 33 mg, buffers

Excedrin: aspirin 250 mg with acetaminophen 250 mg, caffeine 65 mg

Excedrin P.M.: acetaminophen 500 mg with diphenhydramine citrate 38 mg

Exna-R Tablets: benzthiazide 50 mg, reserpine 0.125 mg

Femguard, Sulfa-Gyn, Sultrin, Sulfa, Trysul: miscellaneous sulfonamide-sulfonamide sulfabenzamide 3.7%, sulfacetamide 2.85%, sulfiazole 3.42%, and urea 0.64%

Fermalox: ferrous SO_4 200 mg, magnesium hydroxide, dried aluminum hydroxide gel 200 mg

Ferocyl: iron (fumarate) 50 mg, docusate sodium 100 mg

Ferro-Sequels: iron (fumarate) 50 mg, docusate sodium 100 mg

Fiorinal: aspirin 325 mg with butalbital 50 mg, caffeine 40 mg

Fiorinal with Codeine No. 1: aspirin 325 mg with butalbital 50 mg, caffeine 40 mg, codeine phosphate 7.5 mg

Fiorinal with Codeine No. 2: aspirin 325 mg with butalbital 50 mg, caffeine 40 mg, and codeine phosphate 15 mg

Fiorinal with Codeine No. 3: aspirin 325 mg with butalbital 50 mg, caffeine 40 mg, codeine phosphate 30 mg

Gemnisyn: acetaminophen 325 mg with aspirin 325 mg

Hexalol: methenamine 40.8 mg, phenyl salicylate 18.1 mg, atropine SO_4 0.03, hyoscyamine 0.03 mg, benzoic acid 4.5 mg, methylene blue 5.4 mg

Hybephen: belladonna alkaloids atropine sulfate 0.0233 mg, hyoscyamine sulfate 0.1277 mg, phenobarbital 15 mg, scopolamine hydrobromide 0.0094 mg

Hydergine: dihydroergocorine mesylate 0.167 mg

Hydrogesic: hydrocodone bitartrate 7.5 mg with acetaminophen 650 mg

Hydromox R: quinethazone 50 mg with reserpine 0.125 mg
Hydropres-25, Hydro-Reserpine-25, Hydroserp, Hydroserpine No. 1, Hydrosine 25 mg, Mallopress: reserpine 0.125 mg with hydrochlorothiazide 25 mg
Hydropres-50, Hydro-Reserpine-50, Hydroserp, Hydroserpine No. 2, Hydrosine 50 mg, Hydrotensin, Hydroserpalan: reserpine 0.125 mg with hydrochlorothiazide 50 mg
Inderide 40/25, Propranolol HCl, Hydrochlorothiazide Tablets 40/25: propranolol HCl 40 mg with hydrochlorothiazide 25 mg
Inderide 80/25, Propranolol HCl, Hydrochlorothiazide Tablets 80/25: propranolol HCl 80 mg with hydrochlorothiazide 25 mg
Inderide LA 80/50: propranolol HCl 80 mg with hydrochlorothiazide 50 mg
INH: isoniazid 1 tablet, isoniazid 300 mg
Iophen DM, Tussi-Organidin DM: dextromethorphan hydrobromide 10 mg/5 ml with iodinated glycerol 30 mg/5 ml
Isoptop-ES: pilocarpine HCl 2%, physostigmine salicylate 0.25%
Kinesed: belladonna alkaloids atropine sulfate 0.02 mg, hyoscyamine sulfate 0.12 mg, phenobarbital 16 mg, scopolamine hydrobromide 0.007 mg
Levsin with Phenobarbital Tablets, Anaspaz: hyoscyamine sulfate 0.125 mg with phenobarbital
Levsinex with Phenobarbital Elixir: hyoscyamine sulfate 0.125 mg/5 ml with phenobarbital 15 mg/5 ml
Levsinex with Phenobarbital Time-caps: hyoscyamine sulfate

0.375 mg with phenobarbital 45 mg
Levsin-PB: hyoscyamine sulfate 0.125 mg/ml with phenobarbital 15 mg/ml
Librax: chlordiazepoxide HCl 5 mg, clidinium bromide 2.5 mg
Limbitrol 5-12.5: chlordiazepoxide 5 mg, amitriptyline HCl 12.5 mg
Limbitrol 10-25: chlordiazepoxide 10 mg, amitriptyline HCl 25 mg
Lobac: chlorzoxazone 250 mg, acetaminophen 300 mg
Lopressor HCT 50/25: metoprolol tartrate 50 mg with hydrochlorothiazide 25 mg
Lopressor HCT 100/25: metoprolol tartrate 100 mg with hydrochlorothiazide 25 mg
M-KYA, Q-VEL: quinine SO_4 64.8 mg, vit. E. 400 U, lecithin
Maxzide: hydrochlorothiazide 50 mg with triamterene 75 mg
Mediqueall: dextromethorphan hydrobromide 15 mg with pseudoephedrine HCl 30 mg
Menrium 5-2: chlordiazepoxide 5 mg with esterified estrogens 0.2 mg
Menrium 5-4: chlordiazepoxide 5 mg with esterified estrogens 0.4 mg
Menrium 10-4: chlordiazepoxide 10 mg with esterified estrogens 0.4 mg
Mepergan: meperidine HCl 25 mg/ml with promethazine HCl 25 mg/ml
Mepergan Fortis: meperidine HCl 50 mg with promethazine HCl 25 mg
Metatensin No. 2: reserpine 0.1 mg with trichlormethiazide 2 mg
Midol Caplets: aspirin 454 mg

COMBINATION PRODUCTS

with caffeine 32.4 mg, cinnamedrine HCl 14.9 mg

Midol PMS Caplets: acetaminophen 500 mg with pamabrom 25 mg, pyrilamine maleate 15 mg

Migral: ergotamine tartrate 1 mg, caffeine 50 mg, cyclizine HCl 25 mg

Milprem-200, PMB 200: meprobamate 200 mg with conjugated estrogens 0.45 mg

Milprem-400, PMB 400: meprobamate 400 mg with conjugated estrogens 0.45 mg

Minizide 1: prazosin HCl 1 mg (of prazosin) with polythiazide 0.5 mg

Minizide 2: prazosin HCl 2 mg (of prazosin) with polythiazide 0.5 mg

Minizide 5: prazosin HCl 5 mg (of prazosin) with polythiazide 0.5 mg

Mixtard injection: 100 mg/ml isophane purified pork insulin susp, purified pork insulin inj

Moduretic: amiloride HCl 5 mg, hydrochlorothiazide 50 mg

Morphine, Atropine Sulfate Injection: morphine sulfate 16 mg/ml with atropine sulfate 0.4 mg/ml

Murocoll-2: scopolamine hydrobromide 0.3%, phenylephrine hydrochloride 10%

Mus-Lax: chlorzoxazone 250 mg, acetaminophen 300 mg

Myapap with Codeine, Tylenol with Codeine: acetaminophen 120 mg/5 ml with codeine phosphate 12 mg/5 ml

Mysteclin F: amphotericin B 25 mg/5 ml with tetracycline equivalent to tetracycline HCl 25 mg/5 ml

Mysteclin-F: amphotericin B 50 mg with tetracycline equivalent to tetracycline HCl 250 mg

Mysteclin-F: tetracycline equivalent to 125 mg tetracycline HCl per 5 ml with amphotericin B 25 mg/5 ml

Mysteclin-F: tetracycline equivalent to 350 mg tetracycline HCl with amphotericin B 50 mg/5 ml

Mysteclin-F Syrup: tetracycline equivalent to 125 mg tetracycline HCl per 5 ml with amphotericin B 25 mg/5 ml

Naldecon-DX Adult: dextromethorphan hydrobromide 15 mg/5 ml with guaifenesin 200 mg/5 ml, phenylpropanolamine HCl 18 mg/5 ml

Naldecon-DX Children's Syrup: dextromethorphan hydrobromide 7.5 mg/5 ml with guaifenesin 100 mg/5 ml, phenylpropanolamine HCl 9 mg/5 ml

Naldegisic: acetaminophen 325 mg with pseudoephedrine HCl 15 mg

Naquival: trichlormethiazide 4 mg, reserpine 0.1 mg

Naturetin with K 2.5, mg: bendroflumethiazide 2.5, potassium chloride 500 mg

Naturetin with K 5 mg: bendroflumethiazide 5 mg with potassium chloride 500 mg

Neosporin G.U. Irrigant: polymyxin B sulfate 200,000 units (of polymyxin B)

Nitrotym-Plus: nitroglycerin 2.5 mg, butabarbital 48 mg

Norgesic: orphenadrine citrate 25 mg, aspirin 385 mg, caffeine 30 mg

Norgesic Forte: orphenadrine citrate 50 mg, aspirin 770 mg, caffeine 60 mg

Normozide 100/25: labetalol hydrochloride 100 mg, hydrochlorothiazide 25 mg

Normozide 200/25: labetalol hydrochloride 200 mg, hydrochlorothiazide 25 mg

Normozide 300/25: labetalol hydrochloride 300 mg, hydrochlorothiazide 25 mg

Novahistine Cough and Cold Formula: dextromethorphan hydrobromide 10 mg/5 ml with chlorpheniramine maleate 2 mg/5 ml, pseudoephedrine HCl 30 mg/5 ml

Opium and Belladonna: powdered opium 60 mg with belladonna extract 15 mg (equivalent to belladonna alkaloids 0.2 mg)

Oreticyl 25: deserpidine 0.125 mg with hydrochlorothiazide 25 mg

Oreticyl 50: deserpidine 0.125 mg with hydrochlorothiazide 50 mg

Oreticyl Forte: deserpidine 0.25 mg with hydrochlorothiazide 50 mg

Ornex: phenylpropanolamine HCl 12.5 mg with acetaminophen 325 mg

Orthoxicol Cough Syrup: dextromethorphan hydrobromide 10 mg/5 ml with methoxyphenamine HCl 17 mg/5 ml

Oxymycin, Terramycin Intramuscular Solution: oxytetracycline 50 mg/ml with lidocaine 2%

Pamprin: acetaminophen 325 mg with pamabrom 25 mg, pyrilamine maleate 12.5 mg

Pamprin Maximum Cramp Relief: acetaminophen 500 mg with pamabrom 25 mg, pyrilamine maleate 15 mg

Paracet Forte: chlorzoxazone 250 mg, acetaminophen 300 mg

Parepectolin: opium 15 mg, kaolin 5.85 g, pectin 162 mg, alcohol 0.69%/30 ml susp

Pathibamate-200: meprobamate

200 mg with tridihexethyl chloride 25 mg

Pathibamate-400: meprobamate 400 mg with tridihexethyl chloride 25 mg

Pediazole: erythromycin ethylsuccinate 200 mg (of erythromycin) per 5 ml with sulfisoxazole acetyl 600 mg (of sulfisoxazole) per 5 ml

Penntuss: codeine polistirex equivalent to codeine 10 mg/5 ml with chlorpheniramine polistirex equivalent to chlorpheniramine maleate 4 mg/5 ml

Perbuzem: pentaerythritol tetranitrate 10 mg, butabarbital 15 mg

Percodan-Demi: aspirin 325 mg with oxycodone HCl 2.25 mg, oxycodone terephthalate 0.19 mg

Percogesic: acetaminophen 325 mg with phenyltoloxamine citrate 30 mg

Peri-Colace: docusate sodium 100 mg with cusanthranol 30 mg

Persistin: salsalate 487.5 mg with aspirin 162.5 mg

Phenaphen with Codeine No. 2: acetaminophen 325 mg with codeine phosphate 15 mg

Phenaphen with Codeine No. 2, Proval No. 3: codeine 30 mg with acetaminophen 325 mg

Phenaphen with Codeine No. 3, Proval No. 2: acetaminophen 325 mg with codeine phosphate 30 mg

Phenaphen with Codeine No. 4: acetaminophen 325 mg with codeine phosphate 60 mg

Phenaphen-650 with Codeine: acetaminophen 650 mg with codeine phosphate 30 mg

Phenergan: promethazine HCl 6.25 mg/5 ml with phenylephrine HCl 5 mg/5 ml

Phenergan-D: promethazine HCl

6.25 mg with pseudoephedrine HCl 60 mg

Phenergan VC Syrup, Promethazine HCl VC: promethazine HCl 6.25 mg/5 ml with phenylephrine HCl 5 mg/5 ml

Phenergan with Dextromethorphan: dextromethorphan hydrobromide 15 mg/5 ml with promethazine HCl 6.35 mg/5 ml

Phrenilin: acetaminophen 325 mg with butalbital 50 mg

Phrenilin Forte: acetaminophen 650 mg, butalbital 50 mg

Phrenilin with Codeine No. 3: acetaminophen 325 mg, butalbital 50 mg, codeine phosphate 30 mg

Polycillin-PRB: ampicillin trihydrate 3.5 g with probenecid 1 g

Polyflex: chlorzoxazone 250 mg, acetaminophen 300 mg

Propoxyphene HCl/65, Wygesic: acetaminophen 650 mg, propoxyphene HCl 65 mg

Principen with Probenecid: ampicillin trihydrate 3.5 g with probenecid 1 g

Prunicodeine: terpin hydrate 29 mg/5 ml, codeine sulfate 10 mg/5 ml

Rautrax: rauwolfia 50 mg, flumethiazide 400 mg, potassium chloride 400 mg

Rautrax-N: bendroflumethiazide 4 mg, rauwolfia serpentina 50 mg, potassium chloride 400 mg

Rauzide: bendroflumethiazide 4 mg, rauwolfia serpentina 50 mg

Regroton: reserpine 0.25 mg, chlorthalidone 50 mg

Renese-R: reserpine 0.25 mg, polythiazide 2 mg

Rifamate: isoniazid 150 mg with rifampin 300 mg

Rimactane: isoniazid 2 capsules, rifampin 300 mg

Rimactane: rifampin 1 tablet, isoniazid 300 mg

Rimactane: rifampin 2 capsules, rifampin 300 mg

Robaxisal, Robomol/ASA: methocarbamol 400 mg, aspirin 325 mg

Robitussin-DM: dextromethorphan hydrobromide 15 mg/5 ml, guaifenesin 100 mg/5 ml

Roxicet: oxycodone HCl 5 mg/5 ml, acetaminophen 325 mg/5 ml

S-A-C: salicylamide 230 mg, acetaminophen 150 mg, caffeine 30 mg

Salimeth Forte: salicylamide 600 mg, acetaminophen 250 mg

S.B.P.: secobarbital sodium 50 mg, butabarbital sodium 30 mg, phenobarbital 15 mg

Ser-a-Gen: hydrochlorothiazide 15 mg, hydralazine hydrochloride 25 mg, resepine 0.1 mg

Serpasil-Apresoline HCl No. 1: hydralazine HCl 25 mg, reserpine 0.1 mg

Serpasil-Apresoline HCl No. 2: hydralazine HCl 25 mg, reserpine 0.2 mg

Serpasil-Esidrix No. 1: reserpine 0.1 mg, hydrochlorothiazide 25 mg

Serpasil-Esidrix No. 2: reserpine 0.1 mg, hydrochlorothiazide 50 mg

Simron: iron (gluconate) 10 mg, polysorbate 20, 400 mg

Sine-Aid: acetaminophen 325 mg, pseudoephedrine HCl 30 mg

Sine-Aid Extra Strength Caplets, Tylenol Sinus Maximum Strength Caplets: acetaminophen 500 mg, pseudoephedrine HCl 30 mg

Sine-Off Extra Strength, Sinutab: acetaminophen 500 mg, pseudoephedrine HCl 30 mg

Sinubid: acetaminophen 600 mg,

phenylpropanolamine HCl 100 mg, phenyltoloxamine citrate 66 mg

Sinutab Maximum Nighttime: acetaminophen 167 mg/5 ml, diphenhydramine HCl 8.3 mg/5 ml, pseudoephedrine HCl 10 mg/5 ml

Sinutab II Maximum, Tylenol maximum strength sinus: acetaminophen 500 mg, pseudoephedrine HCl 30 mg

SK-APAP with Codeine, Tylenol with Codeine No. 2: codeine 5 mg with acetaminophen 300 mg

Skelez: chlorzoxazone 250 mg, acetaminophen 300 mg

Soma Compound: carisoprodol 200 mg, aspirin 325 mg

Soma Compound with Codeine: codeine 16 mg, aspirin 325 mg, carisoprodol 200 mg

Spec-T: Phenylpropanolamine 10.5 mg with Benzocaine 10 mg, Phenylephrine HCl 5 mg

Spec-T Sore Throat Cough Suppressant: dextromethorphan hydrobromide 10 mg with benzocaine 10 mg

Spironazide: spironolactone 25 mg, hydrochlorothiazide 25 mg

Spirozide: spironolactone 25 mg, hydrochlorothiazide 25 mg

Sudafed Cough Syrup: dextromethorphan hydrobromide 5 mg/ 5 ml with guaifenesin 100 mg/5 ml, pseudoephedrine HCl 15 mg/ 5 ml

Sultrin: miscellaneous sulfonamide-sulfonamide sulfabenzamide 184 mg, sulfacetamide 143.75 mg, sulfathiazole 172.5 mg, urea 31.83 mg

Talacen: pentazocine HCl 25 mg (of pentazocine) with acetaminophen 650 mg

Talwin Compound Caplets: aspirin 325 mg with pentazocine HCl 12.5 mg (of pentazocine)

Tenoretic 50: atenolol 50 mg with chlorthalidone 25 mg

Tenoretic 100: atenolol 100 mg with chlorthalidone 25 mg

Terpin Hydrate and Codeine: terpin hydrate 85 mg/5 ml with dextromethorphan hydrobromide 10 mg/5 ml (with alcohol 39%-44%)

Terramycin Intramuscular Solution: oxytetracycline 125 mg/ml with lidocaine 2%

T-Gesic: hydrocodone bitartrate 5 mg with acetaminophen 325 mg, butalbital 30 mg, caffeine 40 mg

Thiacide: methenamine mandelate 500 mg, potassium acid phosphate 250 mg

Thyrolar-¼: levothyroxine sodium 12.5 mg, liothyronine sodium 3.1 μg

Thyrolar-½: levothyroxine sodium 25 μg, liothyronine sodium 6.25 μg

Thyrolar-1: levothyroxine sodium 50 μg, liothyronine sodium 12.5 μg

Thyrolar-2: levothyroxine sodium 100 μg, liothyronine sodium 25 μg

Thyrolar-3: levothyroxine sodium 150 μg, liothyronine sodium 37.5 μg

Timentin Inj: ticarcillin disodium 3 g with clavulanate potassium 100 mg

Timolide 10/25: timolol maleate 10 mg with hydrochlorothiazide 25 mg

TracTabs 2X: methenamine 120 mg, methylene blue 6 mg, phenyl salicylate 30 mg, atropine 0.06, hyoscyamine SO$_4$ 0.03 mg, benzoic acid 7.5 mg

Trendar: acetaminophen 325 mg with pamabrom 25 mg

Triaminic-DM Cough Formula: dextromethorphan hydrobromide 10 mg/5 ml with phenylpropanolamine HCl 12.5 mg/5 ml
Triaminicol: dextromethorphan hydrobromide 10 mg/5 ml with chlorpheniramine maleate 2 mg/5 ml, phenylpropanolamine HCl 12.5 mg/5 ml
Triavil 2-10, Triavil 4-10, Triavil 2-25, Triavil 4-25 (see Etrafon—same products)
Triavil 4-50: perphenazine 4 mg, amitriptyline HCl 50 mg
Tri-Barb Capsules: phenobarbital 32 mg, butabarbital sodium 32 mg, secobarbital sodium 32 mg
Trigesic: aspirin 230 mg with acetaminophen 125 mg, caffeine 30 mg
Triple Sulfa: sulfadiazine 167 mg, sulfamerazine 167 mg, sulfamethazine 167 mg
Tuinal 200 mg Pulvules: secobarbital sodium 100 mg with amobarbital sodium 100 mg
Tylenol with Codeine No. 1: acetaminophen 300 mg with codeine phosphate 7.5 mg
Tylenol with Codeine No. 2: acetaminophen 300 mg with codeine phosphate 15 mg
Tylenol with Codeine No. 3: acetaminophen 300 mg with codeine phosphate 30 mg
Tylenol with Codeine No. 4: acetaminophen 300 mg with codeine phosphate 60 mg
Tylox: acetaminophen 500 mg with oxycodone HCl 5 mg
Unasyn Inj: ampicillin sodium 1 g with sulbactam sodium 500 mg; ampicillin sodium 2 g with sulbactam sodium 1 g
Unipres: hydrochlorothiazide 15 mg, reserpine 0.1 mg, hydralazine hydrochloride 25 mg
Urisedamine: methenamine mandelate 500 mg, hyoscyamine 0.15 mg
Urobiotic-250: oxytetracycline HCl 250 mg (of oxytetracycline) with phenazopyridine HCl 50 mg, sulfamethizole 250 mg
Uroquid-Acid No. 2: methenamine mandelate 500 mg, sodium acid phosphate 500 mg
Vanquish Caplets: aspirin 227 mg with acetaminophen 194 mg, caffeine 30 mg, buffers
Vaseretic: enalapril maleate 10 mg with hydrochlorothiazide 25 mg
Vicks Childrens Cough Syrup: dextromethorphan hydrobromide 3.5 mg/5 ml with guaifenesin 25 mg/5 ml
Vicks Cough Silencers: dextromethorphan hydrobromide 2.5 mg with benzocaine 1 mg
Vicks Daycare: dextromethorphan hydrobromide 10 mg with acetaminophen 325 mg, guaifenesin 100 mg, pseudoephedrine HCl 30 mg
Vicks Daycare: dextromethorphan hydrobromide 3.3 mg/5 ml with acetaminophen 108.3 mg/5 ml, guaifenesin 33.3 mg/5 ml, pseudoephedrine HCl 10 mg/5 ml
Vicks Formula 44 Cough Control Discs: dextromethorphan hydrobromide 5 mg with benzocaine 1.25 mg
Vicks Formula 44 Cough Mixture: dextromethorphan hydrobromide 15 mg/5 ml with doxylamine succinate 3.75 mg/5 ml
Vicks Formula 44D: dextromethorphan hydrobromide 10 mg/5 ml with guaifenesin 66.7 mg/5 ml, pseudoephedrine HCl 20 mg/5 ml
Vicks Formula 44M: dextro-

methorphan hydrobromide 7.4 mg/5 ml with acetaminophen 125 mg/5 ml, guaifenesin 50 mg/5 ml, pseudoephedrine HCl 15 mg/5 ml

Wigraine: ergotamine tartrate 1 mg, caffeine 100 mg, levorotatory belladonna alkaloids 0.1 mg, phenacetin 130 mg

Wigraine Suppositories: ergotamine tartrate 2 mg, caffeine 100 mg, tartaric acid 21.5 mg

Wyanoids: belladonna extract 15 mg (0.19 mg of alkaloids of belladonna leaf) with ephedrine 3 mg

Zoxaphen: chlorzoxazone 250 mg, acetaminophen 300 mg

Ziradyl: diphenhydramine HCl 2% with zinc oxide 2%

Appendix j

Selected new drugs

fenofibrate
(fen-oh-fee'brate)
Lipidil
Func. class.: Antilipemic
Chem. class.: Aryloxisobutyric acid derivative

Action: Inhibits biosynthesis of low-density and very low-density lipoproteins, which are responsible for triglyceride development; mobilizes triglycerides from tissue; increases excretion of neutral sterols
Uses: Types IV, V hyperlipidemia
Dosage and routes:
• *Adult:* PO 100 mg/day
Available forms: Caps 100 mg
Side effects/adverse reactions:
CNS: Fatigue, weakness, drowsiness, dizziness
CV: Angina, dysrhythmias, thrombophlebitis, *pulmonary emboli*
GI: Nausea, vomiting, dyspepsia, increased liver enzymes, stomatitis, flatulence, hepatomegaly, gastritis, increased cholethiasis, weight gain
GU: Decreased libido, impotence, dysuria, proteinuria, oliguria, *hematuria*
HEMA: Leukopenia, anemia, *eosinophilia,* bleeding
INTEG: Rash, urticaria, pruritus, dry hair and skin, alopecia
MISC: Polyphagia, weight gain
MS: Myalgias, arthralgias
Contraindications: Severe hepatic disease, severe renal disease, primary biliary cirrhosis
Precautions: Peptic ulcer, pregnancy (C), lactation
Pharmacokinetics: Not known
Interactions/incompatibilities:
• Increased effects of: sulfonylureas, insulin
• Increased toxicity of fenofibrate: probenecid
• Increased anticoagulant effects of: oral anticoagulants
• Decreased effects of fenofibrate: rifampin
Lab test interferences:
Increase: Liver function studies, CPK, BSP, thymol turbidity
NURSING CONSIDERATIONS
Assess:
• Renal and hepatic levels if patient is on long-term therapy
Administer:
• Drug with meals if GI symptoms occur
Evaluate:
• Therapeutic response: decreased triglycerides, diarrhea, pruritus (excess bile acids)
• Bowel pattern daily; increase bulk, water in diet if constipation develops
Teach patient/family:
• That patient compliance is needed, since toxicity may result if doses are missed
• That risk factors should be decreased: high-fat diet, smoking, alcohol consumption, absence of exercise

• That birth control should be practiced while on this drug
• To report GU symptoms: decreased libido, impotence, dysuria, proteinuria, oliguria, hematuria

---

granisetron
(grane-iss'e-tron)
Kytril
Func. class.: Antiemetic
Chem. class.: 5-HT₃ receptor antagonist

Action: Prevents nausea, vomiting by blocking serotonin peripherally, centrally, and in the small intestine
Uses: Prevention of nausea, vomiting associated with cancer chemotherapy including high-dose cisplatin
Dosage and routes:
• *Adult:* IV 10 mcg/kg over 5 min, 30 min before the start of cancer chemotherapy
Available forms: Inj
Side effects/adverse reactions:
CNS: Headache
GI: Diarrhea, constipation, increased AST, ALT
MISC: Rash, ***bronchospasm***
Contraindications: Hypersensitivity
Precautions: Pregnancy (B), lactation, children, elderly
Pharmacokinetics: Not known
Interactions/incompatibilities: Unknown
NURSING CONSIDERATIONS
Assess:
• For absence of nausea, vomiting during chemotherapy
• Hypersensitive reaction: rash, bronchospasm
Administer:
• IV over 5 min
Perform/provide:
• Storage at room temperature for 48 hr after dilution

Evaluate:
• Therapeutic response: absence of nausea, vomiting during cancer chemotherapy
Teach patient/family:
• To report diarrhea, constipation, rash, changes in respirations

---

perindopril
(per-in-doe'pril)
Aceon
Func. class.: Diuretic; carbonic anhydrase inhibitor
Chem. class.: Sulfonamide derivative

Action: Inhibits carbonic anhydrase activity in proximal renal tubules to decrease reabsorption of water, sodium, potassium, bicarbonate; decreases carbonic anhydrase in CNS, increasing seizure threshold
Uses: Essential hypertension
Dosage and routes:
• *Adult:* PO 4 mg qd, max 16 mg/day
Available forms: Tabs 2, 4, 8 mg
Side effects/adverse reactions:
CNS: Drowsiness, paresthesia, anxiety, depression, headache, dizziness, confusion, stimulation, fatigue, ***convulsions,*** sedation, nervousness
EENT: Myopia, tinnitus
ENDO: Hyperglycemia
GI: Nausea, vomiting, anorexia, constipation, diarrhea, melena, weight loss, ***hepatic insufficiency,*** taste alterations
GU: Frequency, hypokalemia, polyuria, ***uremia,*** glucosuria, hematuria, dysuria, crystalluria, renal calculi
*HEMA: **Aplastic anemia, hemolytic anemia, leukopenia, agranulocy-***

SELECTED NEW DRUGS

tosis, thrombocytopenia, purpura, pancytopenia
INTEG: Rash, pruritus, urticaria, fever, Stevens-Johnson syndrome, photosensitivity

Contraindications: Hypersensitivity to sulfonamides, severe renal disease, severe hepatic disease, electrolyte imbalances (hyponatremia, hypokalemia), hyperchloremic acidosis, Addison's disease, COPD

Precautions: Hypercalciuria, pregnancy (C)

Pharmacokinetics: Unknown

Interactions/incompatibilities:
• Increased action of: amphetamines, procainamide, quinidine, tricyclics, flecainide, ephedrine, pseudoephedrine
• Increased excretion of: barbiturates, ASA, lithium
• Toxicity: salicylates
• Hypokalemia: with other diuretics, corticosteroids, amphotericin B
• IV compatibility: cimetidine, D_5W, $D_{10}W$, NaCl, LR, Ringer's Sol

NURSING CONSIDERATIONS
Assess:
• Weight daily, I&O daily to determine fluid loss; effect of drug may be decreased if used qd
• Rate, depth, rhythm of respiration, effect of exertion
• B/P lying, standing; postural hypotension may occur
• Electrolytes: K, Na, Cl; include BUN, blood sugar, CBC, serum creatinine, blood pH, ABGs, liver function tests

Administer:
• In AM to avoid interference with sleep if using drug as diuretic
• K replacement if K level is less than 3
• With food if nausea occurs; absorption may be decreased slightly

Perform/provide:
• Storage in dark, cool area; use reconstituted sol within 24 hr

Evaluate:
• Therapeutic response: improvement in B/P
• Signs of metabolic acidosis: drowsiness, restlessness
• Signs of hypokalemia: postural hypotension, malaise, fatigue, tachycardia, leg cramps, weakness
• Rashes, temperature elevation qd
• Confusion, especially in elderly; take safety precautions if needed

Teach patient/family:
• To notify physician of sore throat, unusual bleeding, bruising, paresthesias, tremors, flank pain, skin rash
• To avoid hazardous activities if drowsiness occurs

Treatment of overdose: Lavage if taken orally; monitor electrolytes; administer dextrose in saline; monitor hydration, CV, renal status

risperidone
(res-pare'a-done)
Risperdal
Func. class.: Antipsychotic/neuroleptic
Chem. class.: Benzisoxazole derivative

Action: Unknown; may be mediated through both dopamine type 2 (D_2) and serotonin type 2 (5-HT_2) antagonism

Uses: Psychotic disorders

Dosage and routes:
• *Adult:* PO 1 mg bid, with incremental increases of 1 mg bid on days 2 and 3 to a dose of 3 mg bid by day 3; then do not increase dose for at least 1 wk

Available forms: Tabs 1, 2, 3, 4 mg

Side effects/adverse reactions:
CNS: Extrapyramidal symptoms, pseudoparkinsonism, akathisia, dystonia, tardive dyskinesia, drowsiness, insomnia, agitation, anxiety, headache, seizures, neuroleptic malignant syndrome
CV: Orthostatic hypotension, *tachycardia*
EENT: Blurred vision
GI: Nausea, vomiting, *anorexia, constipation,* jaundice, weight gain
RESP: Rhinitis
Contraindications: Hypersensitivity, lactation, seizure disorders
Precautions: Children, renal disease, pregnancy (C), hepatic disease, elderly, breast cancer
Pharmacokinetics:
PO: Extensively metabolized by liver to a major active metabolite, plasma protein binding 90%
Interactions/incompatibilities:
• Increased sedation: other CNS depressants, alcohol
• Increased EPS: other antipsychotics, lithium
Lab test interferences:
Not known
NURSING CONSIDERATIONS
Assess:
• Mental status before initial administration
• Swallowing of PO medication; check for hoarding or giving of medication to other patients
• I&O ratio; palpate bladder if urinary output is low
• Bilirubin, CBC, liver function studies monthly
• Urinalysis before, during prolonged therapy
• Affect, orientation, LOC, reflexes, gait, coordination, sleep pattern disturbances
• B/P standing and lying; also pulse, respirations; take these q4h during initial treatment; establish

baseline before starting trea., report drops of 30 mm Hg; watch for ECG changes
• Dizziness, faintness, palpitations, tachycardia on rising
• Extrapyramidal symptoms, including akathisia (inability to sit still, no pattern to movements), tardive dyskinesia (bizarre movements of the jaw, mouth, tongue, extremities), pseudoparkinsonism (rigidity, tremors, pill rolling, shuffling gait)
• For neuroleptic malignant syndrome: hyperthermia, increased CPK, altered mental status, muscle rigidity
• Skin turgor daily
• Constipation, urinary retention daily; if these occur, increase bulk and water in diet
Administer:
• Reduced dose in elderly
• Antiparkinsonian agent, after securing order from physician, to be used if extrapyramidal symptoms occur
Perform/provide:
• Decreased stimulus by dimming lights, avoiding loud noises
• Supervised ambulation until patient is stabilized on medication; do not involve in strenuous exercise program because fainting is possible; patient should not stand still for a long time
• Increased fluids to prevent constipation
• Sips of water, candy, gum for dry mouth
• Storage in tight, light-resistant container
Evaluate:
• Therapeutic response: decrease in emotional excitement, hallucinations, delusions, paranoia; reorganization of patterns of thought, speech

Teach patient/family:
• That orthostatic hypotension may occur and to rise from sitting or lying position gradually
• To avoid hot tubs, hot showers, tub baths, since hypotension may occur
• To avoid abrupt withdrawal of this drug; EPS may result; drug should be withdrawn slowly
• To avoid OTC preparations (cough, hay fever, cold) unless approved by physician, since serious drug interactions may occur; avoid use with alcohol, CNS depressants; increased drowsiness may occur
• To avoid hazardous activities if drowsiness or dizziness occurs
• Regarding compliance with drug regimen
• To report impaired vision, tremors, muscle twitching
• In hot weather, that heat stroke may occur; take extra precautions to stay cool

Treatment of overdose: Lavage if orally ingested; provide airway; *do not induce vomiting*

---

salmeterol xinafoate

(sal-met′er-ole)
Serevent
Func. class.: Adrenergic β₂ agonist

Action: Causes bronchodilation by action on β₂ (pulmonary) receptors by increasing levels of cAMP, which relaxes smooth muscle; with very little effect on heart rate, maintains improvement in FEV from 3 to 12 hr; prevents nocturnal asthma symptoms

Uses: Prevention of exercise-induced asthma, bronchospasm

Dosage and routes:
• *Adult:* INH 2 puffs bid (AM and PM)
Available forms: Aerosol

Side effects/adverse reactions:
CNS: Tremors, anxiety, insomnia, headache, dizziness, stimulation, restlessness, hallucinations, flushing, irritability
CV: Palpitations, tachycardia, hypertension, angina, hypotension, dysrhythmias
EENT: Dry nose, irritation of nose and throat
GI: Heartburn, nausea, vomiting
MS: Muscle cramps
RESP: Bronchospasm

Contraindications: Hypersensitivity to sympathomimetics, tachydysrhythmias, severe cardiac disease

Precautions: Lactation, pregnancy (C), cardiac disorders, hyperthyroidism, diabetes mellitus, hypertension, prostatic hypertrophy, narrow-angle glaucoma, seizures

Pharmacokinetics:
INH: Onset 5-15 min, peak 4 hr, duration 12 hr, metabolized in liver, excreted in urine; crosses placenta, breast milk, blood-brain barrier

Interactions/incompatibilities:
• Increased action of: aerosol bronchodilators
• Increased action of salmeterol: tricyclic antidepressants, MAOIs
• May inhibit action of salmeterol: other β-blockers

NURSING CONSIDERATIONS
Assess:
• Respiratory function: vital capacity, forced expiratory volume, ABGs, lung sounds, heart rate and rhythm

Administer:
• After shaking; exhale, place mouthpiece in mouth, inhale

slowly, hold breath, remove, exhale slowly
• Gum, sips of water for dry mouth
Perform/provide:
• Storage in light-resistant container; do not expose to temperatures over 86° F (30° C)
Evaluate:
• Therapeutic response: absence of dyspnea, wheezing
Teach patient/family:
• Not to use OTC medications; extra stimulation may occur
• Use of inhaler; review package insert with patient
• To avoid getting aerosol in eyes
• To wash inhaler in warm water qd and dry
• To avoid smoking, smoke-filled rooms, persons with respiratory infections
Treatment of overdose: β$_2$-Adrenergic blocker

---

venlafaxine HCl
(ven-laa-fax'een)
Effexor
Func. class.: Second-generation antidepressant

Action: Potent inhibitor of neuronal serotonin and norepinephrine uptake, weak inhibitor of dopamine; no muscarinic, histaminergic, or α-adrenergic receptors in vitro
Uses: Depression
Dosage and routes:
• **Adult:** PO 75 mg/day in 2 or 3 divided doses; taken with food, may be increased to 150 mg/day; if needed, may be further increased to 225 mg/day; increments of 75 mg/day should be made at intervals of no less than 4 days; some hospitalized patients may require

up to 375 mg/day in 3 divided doses
Available forms: Tabs scored 25, 37.5, 50, 75, 100 mg
Side effects/adverse reactions:
CNS: Emotional lability, vertigo, apathy, ataxia, CNS stimulation, euphoria, hallucinations, hostility, increased libido, hypertonia, hypotonia, psychosis
CV: Migraine, angina pectoris, extrasystoles, hypotension, syncope, thrombophlebitis
EENT: Abnormal vision, ear pain, cataract, conjunctivitis, corneal lesions, dry eyes, otitis media, photophobia
GI: Dysphagia, eructation, colitis, gastritis, gingivitis, rectal hemorrhage, stomatitis, stomach and mouth ulceration
GU: Anorgasmia, dysuria, hematuria, metrorrhagia, vaginitis, impaired urination, albuminuria, amenorrhea, kidney calculus, cystitis, nocturia, breast and bladder pain, polyuria, uterine hemorrhage, vaginal hemorrhage, moniliasis
INTEG: Ecchymosis, acne, alopecia, brittle nails, dry skin, photosensitivity
META: Peripheral edema, weight gain, diabetes mellitus, edema, glycosuria, hyperlipemia, hypokalemia
MS: Arthritis, bone pain, bursitis, myasthenia tenosynovitis
RESP: Bronchitis, dyspnea, asthma, chest congestion, epistaxis, hyperventilation, laryngitis
SYST: Accidental injury, malaise, neck pain, enlarged abdomen, cyst, facial edema, hangover effect, hernia
Contraindications: Hypersensitivity
Precautions: Mania, pregnancy

SELECTED NEW DRUGS

(C), lactation, children, elderly, hypertensions, seizure disorder

Pharmacokinetics: Well absorbed, extensively metabolized in the liver to an active metabolite; 87% of drug recovered in urine; 27% protein binding; elimination half-life 5-7, 11-13 hours respectively

Interactions/incompatibilities: Hyperthermia, rigidity, rapid fluctuations of vital signs, mental status changes: MAOIs

NURSING CONSIDERATIONS
Assess:
• B/P lying, standing; pulse q/4 h; if systolic B/P drops 20 mm Hg, hold drug, notify physician; take vital signs q4h in patients with cardiovascular disease
• Blood studies: CBC, leukocytes, differential cardiac enzymes if patient is receiving long-term therapy
• Hepatic studies: AST, ALT, bilirubin
• Weight qwk; appetite may increase with drug
• With food or milk for GI symptoms
• Gum, hard candy, or frequent sips of water for dry mouth
• Mental status: mood, sensorium, affect, suicidal tendencies, increase in psychiatric symptoms; depression, panic

• Withdrawal symptoms: headache, nausea, vomiting, muscle pain, weakness; not usual unless drug is discontinued abruptly

Perform/provide:
• Storage in tight container at room temperature; do not freeze
• Assistance with ambulation during beginning therapy, since drowsiness, dizziness occur
• Checking to see if PO medication swallowed

Evaluate:
• Therapeutic response; decreased depression

Teach patient/family:
• To dispense in small amounts because of suicide potential, especially in the beginning of therapy
• To use with caution when driving or other activities requiring alertness because of drowsiness, dizziness, blurred vision
• To avoid alcohol ingestion, other CNS depressants
• Not to discontinue medication quickly after long-term use; may cause nausea, headache, malaise
• To wear sunscreen or large hat, since photosensitivity occurs

Treatment of overdose: ECG monitoring; induce emesis; lavage, activated charcoal; administer anticonvulsant

Index

Entries can be identified as follows: generic name, Trade Name, DRUG CATEGORY, *Combination Product*.

Entries can be identified as follows: generic name, Trade Name, DRUG CATEGORY, *Combination Product*.

Entries can be identified as follows: generic name, Trade Name, DRU~ *Combination Product*.

Entries can be identified as follows: generic name, Trade Name, DRUG CATEGORY, *Combination Product*.

Entries can be identified as follows: generic name, Trade Name, DRUG CATEGORY, *Combination Product*.

Entries can be identified as follows: generic name, Trade Name, DRUG CATEGORY,
Combination Product.

Entries can be identified as follows: generic name, Trade Name, DRUG CATEGORY, *Combination Product*.

Entries can be identified as follows: generic name, Trade Name, DRUG CATEGORY, *Combination Product*.

Entries can be identified as follows: generic name, Trade Name, DRUG CATEGORY, *Combination Product*.

Entries can be identified as follows: generic name, Trade Name, DRUG CATEGORY, *Combination Product*.

Entries can be identified as follows: generic name, Trade Name, DRUG CATEGORY, *Combination Product*.

Entries can be identified as follows: generic name, Trade Name, DRUG CATEGORY, *Combination Product*.

Entries can be identified as follows: generic name, Trade Name, DRUG CATEGORY, *Combination Product*.

Entries can be identified as follows: generic name, Trade Name, DRUG CATEGORY, *Combination Product*.

Entries can be identified as follows: generic name, Trade Name, DRUG CATEGORY, *Combination Product.*

Entries can be identified as follows: generic name, Trade Name, DRUG CATEGORY, *Combination Product*.

Entries can be identified as follows: generic name, Trade Name, DRUG CATEGORY, *Combination Product*.

Entries can be identified as follows: generic name, Trade Name, DRUG CATEGORY, *Combination Product.*

Entries can be identified as follows: generic name, Trade Name, DRUG CATEGORY, *Combination Product.*

Entries can be identified as follows: generic name, Trade Name, DRUG CATEGORY, *Combination Product*.

Entries can be identified as follows: generic name, Trade Name, DRUG CATEGORY,
Combination Product.

Entries can be identified as follows: generic name, Trade Name, DRUG CATEGORY, *Combination Product*.

Entries can be identified as follows: generic name, Trade Name, DRUG CATEGORY, *Combination Product.*

Entries can be identified as follows: generic name, Trade Name, DRUG CATEGORY, *Combination Product*.

Entries can be identified as follows: generic name, Trade Name, DRUG CATEGORY, *Combination Product*.

Entries can be identified as follows: generic name, Trade Name, DRUG CATEGORY, *Combination Product*.

Entries can be identified as follows: generic name, Trade Name, DRUG CATEGORY, *Combination Product*.

Entries can be identified as follows: generic name, Trade Name, DRUG CATEGORY, *Combination Product*.

Entries can be identified as follows: generic name, Trade Name, DRUG CATEGORY, *Combination Product*.

Entries can be identified as follows: generic name, Trade Name, DRUG CATEGORY,
Combination Product.

Entries can be identified as follows: generic name, Trade Name, DRUG CATEGORY,
Combination Product.

Entries can be identified as follows: generic name, Trade Name, DRUG CATEGORY, *Combination Product*.

Entries can be identified as follows: generic name, Trade Name, DRUG CATEGORY, *Combination Product*.

Entries can be identified as follows: generic name, Trade Name, DRUG CATEGORY, *Combination Product*.

Entries can be identified as follows: generic name, Trade Name, DRUG CATEGORY, *Combination Product*.

Entries can be identified as follows: generic name, Trade Name, DRUG CATEGORY, *Combination Product*.

Entries can be identified as follows: generic name, Trade Name, DRUG CATEGORY, *Combination Product*.

Entries can be identified as follows: generic name, Trade Name, DRUG CATEGORY, *Combination Product.*

Entries can be identified as follows: generic name, Trade Name, DRUG CATEGORY, *Combination Product*.

Entries can be identified as follows: generic name, Trade Name, DRUG CATEGORY, *Combination Product*.

Entries can be identified as follows: generic name, Trade Name, DRUG CATEGORY,
Combination Product.

Entries can be identified as follows: generic name, Trade Name, DRUG CATEGORY, *Combination Product*.

Entries can be identified as follows: generic name, Trade Name, DRUG CATEGORY, *Combination Product*.

Entries can be identified as follows: generic name, Trade Name, DRUG CATEGORY, *Combination Product*.

Entries can be identified as follows: generic name, Trade Name, DRUG CATEGORY, *Combination Product*.

Entries can be identified as follows: generic name, Trade Name, DRUG CATEGORY, *Combination Product*.

Entries can be identified as follows: generic name, Trade Name, DRUG CATEGORY, *Combination Product*.

Epogen is BP

Outstanding References Available Upon Request

MOSBY'S DIAGNOSTIC AND LABORATORY TEST REFERENCE
2nd Edition
Kathleen Deska Pagana, Timothy James Pagana
1995 (0-8151-6628-1)

This comprehensive and up-to-date reference features over 600 diagnostic and lab tests organized alphabetically for quick reference. Relevant information on the test, related nursing care, and patient teaching is easily accessible.

INTRAVENOUS MEDICATIONS
11th Edition
Betty L. Gahart
July 1994 (0-8016-6740-2)

The eleventh edition of this reliable handbook remains the most popular portable IV medications reference for students and professional nurses. Virtually all drugs available for IV use are presented in a clinically functional format. This edition includes new IV drugs recently approved by the FDA and highlights more than 1000 new drug facts.

To order call toll-free 800-426-4545. In Canada call 800-268-4178. We look forward to hearing from you soon!

NMA198   **M** Mosby

IV Drug/Solution Compatibility Chart

	D$_5$	D$_{10}$	D$_5$ ½S	S	NS	R	LR	OTHER
Acetazolamide	C	C	C	C	C	C	C	
Acyclovir	C							
Alpha$_1$-proteinase inhibitor								Sterile water for inj
Alprostadil	C	C			C			
Alteplase								Sterile water for inj
Amdinocillin	C	C	C	C	C	C	C	D$_5$ in R
Amikacin	C				C			
Aminocaproic acid			C	C	C	C		D in distilled water
Ammonium Cl					C			May add KCl to solution
Amphotericin B	C							
Ampicillin	C				C			
Amrinone lactate					C			0.45% saline
Antithrombin III	C				C			Sterile water for inj
Ascorbic acid	C				C	C	C	Sodium lactate
Azlocillin	C		C		C			
Atenolol	C				C			0.45% saline
Aztreonam	C	C			C	C	C	Normosol-R
Bretylium tosylate	C				C			
Cefamandole	C				C			
Cefazolin	C				C			
Cefotetan	C				C			
Cefoxitin	C	C			C	C	C	Aminosol
Ceftrazidime	C		C	C	C	C	C	M/G Sodium lactate

This chart is not inclusive and is based on manufacturers' recommendations.

Key

C	= Compatible	D$_5$S	= Dextrose 5% in saline 0.9%
C$_5$	= Dextrose 5%	NS	= Sodium chloride 0.9% (normal saline)
D$_{10}$	= Dextrose 10%	R	= Ringer's solution
D$_5$½S	= Dextrose 5% in saline 0.45%	LR	= Lactated Ringer's solution

	D5	D10	D5 ½S	D5 S	NS	R	LR	OTHER
Ceftriaxone	C				C			
Cefuroxime	C		C	C		C		M/G Sodium lactate
Cephalothin	C				C	C	C	M/G Sodium lactate
Cephapirin	C				C			
Ciprofloxacin	C				C			
Cyclosporine	C				C			Use only glass containers
Dobutamine	C				C			Sodium lactate
Dopamine	C		C	C	C		C	M/G Sodium lactate
Doxycycline	C				C			Invert sugar 10%
Edetate Na	C	C						Isotonic saline
Ganciclovir	C				C	C	C	
Gentamicin	C				C			Normosol-R
Heparin Na	C	C			C	C		
Ifosfamide	C				C		C	Sterile water for inj
Isoproterenol	C			C	C	C		Invert sugar 5% & 10%
Kanamycin	C				C			
Metaraminol	C			C	C	C	C	Normosol-R
Methicillin	C			C				
Metoclopramide	C			C		C	C	
Mezlocillin	C	C	C	C	C	C	C	Fructose 5%
Moxalactam	C	C	C	C	C	C	C	M/G Sodium lactate
Netilmicin	C	C		C	C	C	C	Normosol-R
Norepinephrine	C	C		C			C	
Nitroglycerin	C	C			C			
Piperacillin	C			C	C		C	
Ritodrine	C							
Ticarcillin	C				C		C	
Tobramycin	C				C			
Vidarabine	C	C			C			

Syringe Compatibility

	Atropine	Buprenorphine	Butorphanol	Chlorpromazine	Codeine	Diazepam	Dimenhydrinate	Diphenhydramine	Droperidol	Fentanyl	Glycopyrrolate	Heparin
Atropine			C	C		I	C	C	C	C	C	
Buprenorphine												
Butorphanol	C			C		I	I	C	C	C		
Chlorpromazine	C		C			I	I	C	C	C	C	C
Codeine						I						
Diazepam	I		I	I	I		I	I	I	I	I	
Dimenhydrinate	C		I	I		I		C	C	C	I	
Diphenhydramine	C		C	C		I	C		C	C	C	
Droperidol	C		C	C		I	C	C		C	C	I
Fentanyl	C		C	C		I	C	C	C		C	
Glycopyrrolate	C			C		I	I	C	C	C		
Heparin			I	C		I			I			
Hydroxyzine	C		C	C		I	I	C	C	C	C	
Meperidine	C		C	C		I	C	C	C	C	C	I
Metoclopramide	C		C	C		I	C	C	C	C		
Midazolam	C		C	C		I	C	C	C	C		
Morphine	C		C	C		I	C	C	C	C	C	I
Nalbuphine	C					I			C			
Pentazocine	C		C	C		I	C	C	C	C	I	I
Pentobarbital	C		I	I	I	I	I	I	I	I	I	
Perphenazine	C		C	C		I	C	C	C	C		
Prochlorperazine	C		C	C		I	I	C	C	C	C	
Promazine	C			C		I	I	C	C	C		
Promethazine	C		C	C		I	I	C	C	C	C	
Ranitidine	C			C			C	C		C	C	
Scopolamine Hbr	C		C	C		I	C	C	C	C	C	
Secobarbital	I		I	I	I	I	I	I	I	I	I	
Thiethylperazine			C			I						

Developed by Providence Memorial Hospital, El Paso, Texas.
NOTE: Give within 15 minutes of mixing. C, compatible;
I, incompatible; □, no documented information.